Contents

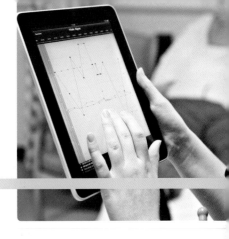

KU-272-497

Part 1   Introduction 1

Part 2   Clinical presentations at a glance 27

Cardiovascular disease

Respiratory disease

Ophthalmology

Rheumatology

Dermatology

Women's health

Other acute medical emergencies

Part 3 Diseases and treatments at a glance 172

Cardiovascular disease

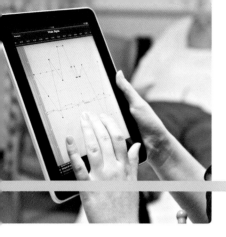

Preface to third edition

Medicine is a wonderful and exciting subject. Partly this excitement comes from the pure unadulterated intellectual joy of understanding the functioning of humans in health and disease better, an understanding based on a powerful and growing biological science, one which pushes the frontiers of our knowledge back at an accelerating rate with each passing year. The most amazing advances have been made in the treatment of many illnesses; what is true today for them may be true tomorrow for most diseases. Advances in basic sciences feed through into 'landmark' clinical trials at an ever increasing rate; indeed rarely a week goes by without another key experiment or trial being published. For this reason, now is perhaps the most exciting time ever to be involved in medicine. The medical student rapidly becomes a part of this seething intellectual community. This in itself is reason enough to study medicine.

Medicine, however, is not just about science. It is a profoundly human subject. Indeed, the opportunity to directly study human suffering and then immediately to relieve it is, in large part, what separates medicine from other subjects. Other disciplines try to understand suffering; this almost always occurs from a distance, in the abstract, by the inspection of data, or by the use of philosophical argument. Medicine, being practical, sees and feels human suffering. Most doctors experience human suffering every day of their working lives. This can lead to a far more profound understanding of humans and of the communities in which we all live. Our experience of human suffering has a profound impact on us. Doctors' experience of suffering can itself make them into better people, more humane, more understanding and more tolerant. The study of medicine is therefore an adventure, but one that requires hard work. Furthermore, what is worth studying is worth excelling in. It should be the aim of every student of medicine to be an outstanding clinician. What makes for excellence in clinical medicine? In part, it is the ability to turn symptoms rapidly into the right diagnosis, to then turn the diagnosis into a treatment plan, then to communicate all this effectively and accurately to a patient and their family. No book can teach you this entirely by itself. Books, however, can help, and the prime aim of this book is to help you reach a diagnosis, and to introduce you to some of the principles of treatment.

How is a diagnosis established? First, the patient's symptoms are fully explored, so as to completely understand what patients are actually experiencing. Second, a full examination is undertaken, to reveal diagnostic clinical signs. Third, the history and physical examination are synthesized, so that important facts are emphasized and unimportant ones rejected. This synthesis allows one to establish a differential diagnosis, ordered according to probability. This differential diagnosis is narrowed down to a diagnosis using appropriate investigations. Accurate diagnosis allows for effective treatment. *This book will help you acquire all these skills.*

There is an aphorism in medicine that in 80% of cases the history establishes the diagnosis, in 10% the examination does, and only in 10% of cases do investigations provide the answer. *History taking* is a real skill, one which you should work hard to acquire; you only have to see an experienced clinician take a history to realize the beauty and skill of a concise and accurate history taking. The acquisition of this skill will be amply rewarded over the years. Do not be deluded into thinking that just because history taking uses a skill we are all familiar with, which is speech, that it is easy. It is not, and it requires time, patience and diligence to acquire. *This book will help you acquire this vitally important skill.* The critical aspect of history taking is to make sense of it as you go along, and not just to ask questions 'by rote'. How do you do this? Well, to understand the nuances of the history, you need to know quite a lot about diseases, particularly those most prevalent in your local community. An understanding of epidemiology helps. Thus 'browsing' through the third part of the book as background reading will help. Use spare moments during the day to do this. However, though acquiring background knowledge will help, I think the very best way to learn medicine is to 'hang' your facts around individual patients, as this really 'fixes' information down in the memory. Thus, whenever you see a patient, look up their symptoms in this book, so as to understand better how symptoms are turned into a diagnosis. You will learn most if for each and every case you see you draw up a differential diagnosis, ordered according to probability. Stick your neck out! This means that you will have a personal investment in the diagnosis; you will feel proud when you are right. This is a good feeling, and will encourage you! When you are wrong, you will learn, and this is more important. Indeed, it is true to say that you will learn more from your mistakes than from your triumphs. When wrong, you should always ask 'why?' Was my reasoning defective? Did I miss a vital part of the history? Did I misinterpret a sign? The most important part of any case is to ask, 'What have I learnt from this case?' It may relate to your knowledge of the biology of the disease, to your clinical skills, to communication, to how the hospital works, etc. You can learn from each and every case. If you take the opportunity to do so you will make an outstanding doctor. Good luck.

Patrick Davey, 2010

Preface to fourth edition

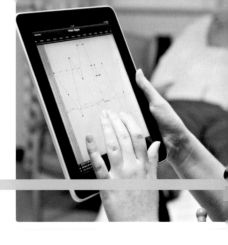

Despite appearances, modern medicine in many ways remains old-fashioned. Empathy, compassion, efficiency, tact, knowledge, motor skills, resilience, kindness, all matter as much as always, but nothing matters as much as the ability to make a diagnosis. Diagnosis is central to everything doctors do; unless we establish what the problem is correctly, we cannot give the right treatment. Furthermore, our diagnostic skills cannot rest once we have made the initial diagnosis, we need to keep re-evaluating the diagnosis in response to treatment, and be aware that as treatment progresses new diagnoses may emerge, indeed, often do. Indeed, one could say that the unique role a doctor carries out in the modern health care system is to make a diagnosis and take responsibility for it. Almost everything else doctors do can be done by others, for example, by nurses, technicians, social workers, etc. What we do that uniquely adds value, and considerable value (so justifying doctors high salaries), is being an effective diagnostician. So, the skill that you should learn during your undergraduate and training years above all others is how to make a diagnosis.

How do doctors make a diagnosis? It is not easy to explain the thought process that leads to a diagnosis and it will vary between cases from a snap decision to a very carefully considered process. To make a diagnosis you need knowledge, and skills – skills in history taking, examination, and interpretation of diagnostic tests, understanding their strengths and weaknesses. Clearly, a diagnosis should fit the key facts of the case – the demographics, the symptoms and, if present, the signs (and perhaps just as importantly, the absence of signs indicating other diagnoses). The problem is that usually there is not just one possible, or even probable diagnosis, there are a number, there is a differential diagnosis. You should establish this differential diagnosis for every case. The thoughts that you put into this process is what will make you a doctor. My advice would be to list the two most likely diagnoses, and then the most likely dangerous diagnosis. This approach will work in many cases, but not all; for these you will need to have more possible diagnoses up your sleeve! Over time, you will look forward to the less than straightforward challenges. They can be frustrating, provoke great anxiety on your part, but eventually they are what make you a doctor.

I would like to add a very short word on what diagnosis is not – too many times I see written in the notes as the diagnosis 'Chest pain? cause', or 'Exclude ACS', or 'ACS' (as if there is no other diagnoses). All of these are wrong, and indicate the sort of thinking that will damage your patient (you will miss profound and serious diagnoses unless you actually think of them), and possibly lead you to the law courts ('chest pain? cause' for example means that you are unlikely to have thought of aortic dissection, you will therefore miss the diagnosis, and your patient may die). I cannot emphasise strongly enough that you must not use these sorts of vague or syndromic diagnoses, you must carefully construct a differential diagnosis for all your patients, for their sake and yours.

I very much hope that the material in this book aids you in your search to becoming a brilliant diagnostician. I have included here the preface to the previous edition, which explains in slightly greater detail how I think you should undertake this challenge.

May I wish you great success in medicine.

Patrick Davey
Oxford, 2014

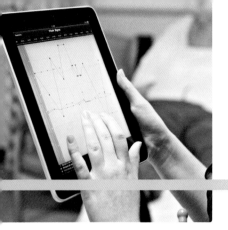

Contributors

Contributors to the fourth edition

Chris B. Bunker
Consultant Dermatologist and Professor of Dermatology
University College London
London, UK

Arani Chandrakumar
Specialist Registrar in Dermatology
University College Hospital
London, UK

Graham Collins
Consultant in Haematology
Department of Haematology
John Radcliffe Hospital
Oxford, UK

Patrick Davey
Consultant Cardiologist
Northampton General Hospital
Northampton, and
Honorary Senior Lecturer
Department of Cardiovascular Medicine
John Radcliffe Hospital
Oxford, UK

Suzanne Donnelly
Senior Lecturer and Director of Clinical Education
School of Medicine and Medical Sciences
University College Dublin
Dublin, Ireland

Daniel Glass
Specialist Registrar in Dermatology
University College Hospital
London, UK

Jonathan Gleadle
Professor of Medicine and Consultant Nephrologist
Flinders University
Flinders Medical Centre
Adelaide, South Australia

Mark Juniper
Consultant in Respiratory and Intensive Care Medicine
Great Western Hospital
Swindon, UK

David Keeling
Consultant Haematologist
Oxford University Hospitals
Oxford, UK

David Lalloo
Professor of Tropical Medicine
Liverpool School of Tropical Medicine
Liverpool, UK

Grace McGeogh
Core medical trainee Year 2
University College Hospital
London, UK

Richard Penson
Associate Professor
Harvard Medical School
Boston, MA, USA

Anna Rathmell
Oxford, UK

Jeremy Shearman
Consultant Gastroenterologist
South Warwickshire NHS Foundation Trust
Warwick, UK

Gavin Spickett
Consultant Clinical Immunologist
Regional Department of Immunology
Royal Victoria Infirmary
Newcastle-Upon-Tyne, UK

David Sprigings
Consultant Cardiologist
Northampton General Hospital
Northampton, UK

Jeremy Steele
Consultant Medical Oncologist
St Bartholomew's Hospital
London, UK

Kevin Talbot
Professor
Nuffield Department of Clinical Neurosciences
John Radcliffe Hospital
Oxford, UK

Laura Tookman
Academic Clinical Research Fellow
Barts Cancer Institute
Queen Mary, University of London
London, UK

Helen E. Turner
Consultant in Endocrinology
OCDEM, Churchill Hospital
Oxford, UK

Chin Whybrew
GP Principal
Stoke Road Surgery
Cheltenham, UK

Matt Wise
Consultant in Critical Care
Cardiff University
Cardiff, UK

Paul Wordsworth
Professor of Rheumatology
Nuffield Orthopaedic Centre
Windmill Road
Oxford, UK

Contributors to earlier editions

Keith Channon
Professor of Cardiovascular Medicine and Honorary
Consultant Cardiologist
Department of Cardiovascular Medicine
University of Oxford
John Radcliffe Hospital
Oxford, UK

Peggy Frith
Consultant Ophthalmic Physician
Oxford Eye Hospital
John Radcliffe Hospital
Oxford, UK

Tim J. Littlewood
Consultant Haematologist
Department of Haematology
John Radcliffe Hospital
Oxford, UK

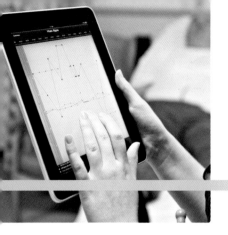

Acknowledgements

The editor, contributing authors and publishers would like to thank all those people who gave their time and expertise to advise us during the writing process of both this and previous editions. The specialist reviewers and medical students who reviewed material for the first edition were invaluable in shaping the final book and we would like to thank them unreservedly for their contribution. Thanks to Yassir Javaid for assistance with preparation of the cardiovascular MCQs.

In addition, we would like to acknowledge the following individuals and companies for their kind permission to re-use material. Although the majority of the artwork in *Medicine at a Glance* is new, some tables and figures have been redrawn from other sources. The editor and publishers have made every effort to contact all the copyright holders to obtain their permission to reproduce copyright material. However, if any have been inadvertently overlooked, the publisher will be pleased to make the necessary arrangements at the first opportunity.

Books

Abraham, S., Kulkarni, K., Madhu, R. & Provan, D. The Hands-on Guide to Data Interpretation. Blackwell Publishing, Oxford, 2010.

Baran, R. & Dawber, R. Diseases of the Nails and their Management, 2nd edn. Blackwell Science, Oxford, 2001.

Baran, R., de Berker, D. & Dawber, R. Manual of Nail Disease and Surgery. Blackwell Science, Oxford, 1997.

Bourke, S. & Brewis, R. Lecture Notes on Respiratory Medicine, 5th edn. Blackwell Science, Oxford, 1998.

Champion, R.H., Burton, J.L. Burns, T. & Breathnach, S. (eds) Rook's Textbook of Dermatology, 6th edn. Blackwell Science, Oxford, 1998.

Chapel, H., Heaney, M., Misbah, S. & Snowden, N. Essentials of Clinical Immunology, 4th edn. Blackwell Science, Oxford, 1999.

Chowdhury, R, Wilson, I, Rofe, C & Lloyd-Jones, G. Radiology at a Glance. Wiley Blackwell, Oxford, 2010

Gleadle, J. History and Examination at a Glance, 2nd edn. Wiley-Blackwell, Oxford, 2007.

Haslett, C., Boon, N., Colledge, N. et al. Davidson's Principles and Practice of Medicine, 18th edn. Churchill Livingstone, Edinburgh, 1999.

Hoffbrand, V., Moss, P. & Pettit, J. Essential Haematology, 4th edn. Blackwell Science, Oxford, 2001.

Howlett, D. & Ayers, B. The Hands-on Guide to Imaging. Blackwell Publishing, Oxford, 2004.

Hunter, J. & Savin, J. Clinical Dermatology, 2nd edn. Blackwell Science, Oxford, 1994.

Katona, C., Cooper, C. & Robertson, M. Psychiatry at a Glance, 4th edn. Wiley-Blackwell, Oxford, 2008.

Kumar, P. & Clark, M. (eds) Clinical Medicine, 4th edn. W.B. Saunders, Philadelphia, 1998.

Leach, R. Critical Care Medicine at a Glance. Blackwell Publishing, Oxford, 2004.

Mehta, A. & Hoffbrand, V. Haematology at a Glance. Blackwell Science, Oxford, 2000.

Munro, J. & Edwards, C. McLeod's Clinical Examination, 10th edn. Churchill Livingstone, Edinburgh, 2000.

Norwitz, E. & Schorge, J. Obstetrics and Gynecology at a Glance, 4th edn. Wiley Blackwell, Oxford, 2013.

Olver, J. & Cassidy, L. Ophthalmology at a Glance. Blackwell Publishing, Oxford, 2005.

Patel, P.R. Lecture Notes: Radiology, 2nd edn. Blackwell Publishing, Oxford, 2005.

Patton, K. Handbook for Anatomy and Physiology. Mosby, St Louis, 2000.

Rubenstein, E. & Federman, D.D. (eds) Scientific American Medicine, Wed MD Professional Publishing, 2003.

Sherlock, S. & Dooley, J. Diseases of the Liver and Biliary System, 11th edn. Blackwell Science, Oxford, 2002.

Warlow, C.P., Dennis, M.S., van Gijn, J. et al. (eds) Stroke: A Practical Guide, 2nd edn. Blackwell Science, Oxford, 2001.

Waye, J.D., Rex, D. & Williams, C. Colonoscopy: Principles and Practice. Blackwell Publishing, Oxford, 2003 (figures used are by Dr Michael Macari).

Weatherall, D. (ed.) Oxford Textbook of Medicine, 3rd edn. Oxford University Press, Oxford, 1995.

Journals

Hamm C.W. et al. ESC Guidelines for the management of acute coronary syndromes in patients presenting without persistent ST-segment elevation: The Task Force for the management of acute coronary syndromes (ACS) in patients presenting without persistent ST-segment elevation of the European Society of Cardiology (ESC). Eur Heart J 2011: 32(23): 2999–3054. doi:10.1093/eurheartj/ehr236. Reproduced with permission of Oxford University Press (UK) © European Society of Cardiology.

European Heart Rhythm Association et al. Guidelines for the management of atrial fibrillation: the Task Force for the Management of Atrial Fibrillation of the European Society of Cardiology (ESC). Eur Heart J 2010: 31(19): 2369–429. Reproduced with permission of Oxford University Press.

Langford, C. & Hoffman, G. Wegener's granulomatosis. Thorax 1999: 54; 629–37.

Soteriodes, E.S., Evans, J.C., Lanon, M.G. et al. Incidence and prognosis of syncope. New Engl J Med 2002: 347; 878–85.

Thadhani, R., Pascual, M. & Bonventre, J.V. Acute renal failure. N Engl J Med 1996: 334; 1448–60.

Other

Adult Advanced Life Support Guidelines. Resuscitation Council, 2010.

Special thanks to Dr Mansel Heaney for providing the cANCA figure for Chapter 147.

Nelson, M., Department of Medical Illustration and Photography, Chelsea and Westminster Hospital, London.

National Institute for Health and Care Excellence. CG 103 Delirium: diagnosis, prevention and management. London, 2010. NICE. Available from http://guidance.nice.org.uk/CG103. Reproduced with permission.

NEWS: standardising the assessment of acute illness severity in the NHS. Report of a working party. London, RCP, 2012. Reproduced with permission from the Royal College of Physicians. The chart is reproduced for reference only. For clinical use, please visit www.rcplondon.ac.uk/resources/national-early-warning-score-news where full-sized versions with instructions and guidance for use may be downloaded.

ONS: Cancer Statistics Registrations: Registrations of Cancers Diagnosed in 2001 England. ONS, Crown copyright, 2004.

World Health Organization. The World Health Report 2000: Health Systems: Improving Performance. Reproduced with permission of WHO.

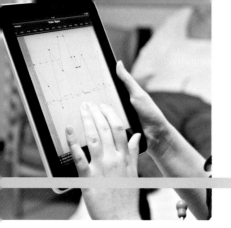

Abbreviations

AA	autoantibody		ASD	atrial septal defect
AAA	abdominal aortic aneurysm		ASO	antistreptolysin O
Ab	antibody		AST	aspartate transaminase
ABC	airway, breathing and circulation		α₁-AT	α_1-antitrypsin
ABG	arterial blood gas		ATLL	adult T-cell lymphoma/leukaemia
ABPA	allergic bronchopulmonary aspergillosis		ATN	acute tubular necrosis
AC	acromioclavicular		ATP	adenosine triphosphate
ACE	angiotensin-converting enzyme		AV	atrioventricular
ACS	acute coronary syndrome		AVNRT	atrioventricular nodal re-entrant tachycardia
ACTH	adrenocorticotrophic hormone		AVRT	atrioventricular re-entrant tachycardia
ADC	apparent diffusion coefficient		AXR	abdominal X-ray
ADH	antidiuretic hormone		BAL	bronchoalveolar lavage
ADP	adenosine diphosphate		BBB	bundle branch block
A&E	Accident and Emergency		BCC	basal cell carcinoma
AF	atrial fibrillation		BCE	basal cell epithelioma
AFB	acid-fast bacilli		BCG	bacilli Calmette–Guérin
Ag	antigen		bd	*bis die* (twice a day)
AIDS	acquired immune deficiency syndrome		BDZ	benzodiazepine
AIHA	autoimmune haemolytic anaemia		BE	base excess
AION	anterior ischaemic optic neuropathy		BLS	basic life support
AKI	acute kidney injury		BM	Boehringer Mannheim bedside testing stix
ALL	acute lymphoid leukaemia		BMD	bone mineral density
ALP	alkaline phosphatase		BMI	body mass index
ALS	advanced life support		BMZ	basement membrane zone
ALT	alanine transaminase		BNF	*British National Formulary*
AMA	antimitochondrial antibody		BOOP	bronchiolitis obliterans organizing pneumonia
AML	acute myeloid leukaemia		BP	blood pressure
ANA	antinuclear antibody		bpm	beats per minute
ANCA	antineutrophil cytoplasmic antibody		BRVO	branch retinal vein occlusion
ANF	antinuclear factor		CABG	coronary artery bypass graft
Ao	aorta		CAD	coronary artery disease
APC	activated protein C		CAH	congenital adrenal hyperplasia
APKD	adult polycystic kidney disease		CAM	Confusion Assessment Method
APS	antiphospholipid syndrome		cAMP	cyclic adenosine monophosphate
APTT	activated partial thromboplastin time		CBD	common bile duct
AR	aortic regurgitation		CBT	cognitive behavioural therapy
ARB	angiotensin receptor blockers		CCP	cyclic citrullinated peptide
ARDS	adult respiratory distress syndrome		CCU	coronary care unit
ART	anti-retroviral therapy		CF	cystic fibrosis
AS	ankylosing spondylitis		CFA	cryptogenic fibrosis alveolitis

CFS	chronic fatigue syndrome	**DHEA**	dehydoepiandrosterone
CFTR	cystic fibrosis transmembrane conductance regulator	**DHF/DSS**	dengue haemorrhagic fever/dengue shock syndrome
cGMP	cyclic guanosine monophosphate	**DIC**	disseminated intravascular coagulation
CHAD	cold haemagglutinin disease	**DIP**	distal interphalangeal
CHB	complete heart block	**DKA**	diabetic ketoacidosis
CHD	congenital heart disease	**DM**	dermatomyositis, diabetes mellitus
CHF	chronic heart failure	**DMARD**	disease-modifying antirheumatic drug
CHOP	cyclophosphamide, hydroxydaunorubicin, oncovin, prednisolone	**DMSA**	[^{99m}Tc] mercaptosuccinic acid
CIDP	chronic idiopathic demyelinating polyneuropathy	**DNA**	deoxyribonucleic acid
		DNAR	'do not attempt resuscitation'
CJD	Creutzfeldt–Jakob disease	**dsDNA**	double-stranded DNA
CK	creatine kinase	**DTPA**	diethylene triamine penta-acetic acid
CLD	chronic liver disease	**DU**	duodenal ulcer
CLL	chronic lymphoblastic leukaemia	**D&V**	diarrhoea and vomiting
CLO	*Campylobacter*-like organism test	**DVT**	deep venous thrombosis
CMC	carpometacarpal	**DWI**	diffusion-weighted imaging
CML	chronic myeloid leukaemia	**EAA**	extrinsic allergic alveolitis
CMV	cytomegalovirus	**EBV**	Epstein–Barr virus
CNS	central nervous system	**ECG**	electrocardiogram
CO	carbon monoxide	**ECT**	electroconvulsant therapy
CO$_2$	carbon dioxide	**EDH**	extradural haematoma
COPD	chronic obstructive pulmonary disease	**EEG**	electroencephalograph
COX	cyclo-oxygenase	**EGFR**	epidermal growth factor receptor
CP	chest pain	**ELISA**	enzyme-linked immunosorbent assay
CPAP	continuous positive airway pressure	**EM**	electron microscopy
CPK	creatine phosphokinase	**EMG**	electromyography
CPR	cardiopulmonary resuscitation	**EN**	erythema nodosum
CREST	calcinosis, Raynaud's, oesophagitis, sclerodactyly telangiectasia	**ENT**	ear, nose, throat
		ER	oestrogen receptor
CRF	chronic renal failure	**ERA**	enteric reactive arthritis
CRH	corticotrophin-releasing hormone	**ERCP**	endoscopic retrograde cholangiopancreatography
CRP	C-reactive protein		
CRT	cardiac resynchronization therapy	**ESR**	erythrocyte sedimentation rate
CRVO	central retinal vein occlusion	**ESRF**	end-stage renal failure
CS	Churg–Strauss; coronary sinus	**ETG**	epidermal transglutamase
CSF	cerebrospinal fluid	**EULAR**	European League Against Rheumatism
CT	computed tomography	**EUS**	endoscopic ultrasound
CVA	cerebrovascular accident	**FAB**	French–American–British
CVID	common variable immunodeficiency	**FBC**	full blood count
CVP	central venous pressure; cyclophosphamide, vincristine, prednisolone	**FDG**	flurodeoxyglucose
		FDP	fibrin degradation product
CWP	coal worker's pneumoconiosis	**FEV$_1$**	forced expiratory volume in 1 second
CXR	chest X-ray	**FFA**	free fatty acid
CYP	cytochrome P450	**FFP**	fresh frozen plasma
DAS	disease activity score	**FLAIR**	fluid-attenuated inversion recovery sequences
DC	direct current	**FNA**	fine needle aspirate
DCIS	ductal carcinoma *in situ*	**FNAC**	fine needle aspiration cytology
DCM	dilated cardiomyopathies	**FOB**	faecal occult blood
ddAVP	deamino-D-arginine vasopressin	**α-FP**	alpha fetoprotein
DEXA	dual emission X-ray absorptiometry	**FRC**	functional residual capacity
		FSGS	focal segmental glomerulosclerosis

FSH	follicle-stimulating hormone	HRT	hormone replacement therapy
FTD	frontotemporal dementia	HSCT	human stem cell transplantation
FUO	fever of unknown origin	HSP	Henoch–Schönlein purpura
FVC	forced vital capacity	HSV	herpes simplex virus
GABA	γ-aminobutyric acid	5-HT	5-hydroxytryptamine (serotonin)
GBM	glomerular basement membrane	HTLV	human T-cell leukaemia virus
GCS	Glasgow Coma Score	HUS	haemolytic uraemic syndrome
GFR	glomerular filtration rate	IBD	inflammatory bowel disease
GH	growth hormone	ICD	implantable cardiovertor defibrillator
GI	gastrointestinal	ICD-10	International Classification of Diseases version 10
GIST	gastrointestinal stromal tumour	ICH	intracerebral haemorrhage
GN	glomerulonephritis	Ig	immunoglobulin
GnRH	gonadotrophin-releasing hormone	IGF	insulin-like growth factor
GORD	gastro-oesophageal reflux disease	IHD	ischaemic heart disease
Gp	glycoprotein	IL	interleukin
GP	general practitioner	IM	intramuscular
G6PD	glucose-6-phosphate dehydrogenase	INR	international normalized ratio
GPI	glycosyl-phosphatidylinositol	IP	intrathoracic pressure
γ-GT	γ-glutamyl transferase	IPPV	intermittent positive pressure ventilation
GTN	glyceryl trinitrate	IRIS	immune reconstitution inflammatory
GU	genitourinary		syndrome
HAART	highly active anti-retroviral therapy	ITP	immune thrombocytopenic purpura
HAE	hereditary angioedema	ITU	intensive therapy unit
HAIR-AN	hyperandrogenism, insulin resistance and acanthosis nigricans	IUGR	intrauterine fetal growth restriction
HAV	hepatitis A virus	IV	intravenous
Hb	haemoglobin	IVC	inferior vena cava
HBc	hepatitis B core antigen	IVU	intravenous urogram/ureography
HBeAg	hepatitis B e antigen	JC	John Cunningham virus
HBsAg	hepatitis B surface antigen	JVP	jugular venous pressure
HBV	hepatitis B virus	KCl	potassium chloride
HCC	hepatocellular carcinoma	KOH	potassium hydroxide
hCG	human chorionic gonadotrophin	KS	Kaposi's sarcoma
HCM	hypertrophic cardiomyopathy	LA	left atrium
Hct	haematocrit	LAD	left anterior descending
HCV	hepatitis C virus	LBB	left bundle branch
HD	Huntington's disease	LCA	leukocytoclastic angiitis
HDL	high-density lipoprotein	LCIS	lobular carcinoma *in situ*
HER-2	human epidermal growth factor receptor 2	LDH	lactate dehydrogenase
HHV	human herpes virus	LDL	low-density lipoprotein
5-HIAA	5-hydroxyindoleacetic acid	LFT	liver function test
HiB	*Haemophilus influenzae* B	LH	luteinizing hormone
HIV	human immunodeficiency virus	LH-RH	luteinizing hormone-releasing hormone
HLA	human leukocyte antigen	LMN	lower motor neuron
HMG-CoA	hydroxymethyl-glutaryl coenzyme A	LMNOP	lasix (diuresis), morphine, Na^{2+} and water restriction, oxygen and position upright
HMMA	hydroxymethylmandelic acid	LMW	low molecular weight
HNF	hepatocyte nuclear factor	LMWH	low-molecular-weight heparin
HNPCC	hereditary non-polyposis colon cancer	LN	lymph nodes
HONK	hyperosmolar non-ketotic coma	LP	lumbar puncture
HPV	human papillomavirus	LRP	lipoprotein related receptor protein
HR	heart rate	LSD	lysergic acid diethylamide
HRCT	high-resolution computed tomography	LTOT	long-term oxygen therapy

LTRA	leukotriene antagonists
LUQ	left upper quadrant
LV	left ventricle, left ventricular
LVH	left ventricular hypertrophy
MAC	*Mycobacterium avium-intracellulare* complex
MALDI	matrix-assisted laser desorption/ionization
MALT	mucosa-associated lymphoid tissue
MAO	monoamine oxidase inhibitors
MCA	middle cerebral artery
MCH	mean corpuscular haemoglobin
MCHC	mean cell haemoglobin concentration
MCP	metacarpophalangeal
M,C&S	microscopy, culture and sensitivity
MCV	mean cell volume
MDMA	3,4 methylenedioxymetamphetamine (ecstasy)
MDR	multidrug resistant
MDS	myelodysplastic syndrome
MDT	multidisciplinary team
ME	myalgic encephalomyelitis
MELAS	mitochondrial encephalopathy, lactic acidosis, stroke-like episodes
MEN	multiple endocrine neoplasia
MGUS	monoclonal gammopathy of uncertain significance
MHC	major histocompatibility complex
MI	myocardial infarction
MND	motor neuron disease
MODY	maturity-onset diabetes in the young
MR	mitral regurgitation
MRCP	magnetic resonance cholangiopancreatography
MRI	magnetic resonance imaging
MRSA	methicillin-resistant *Staphylococcus aureus*
MS	multiple sclerosis
MSA	multiple system atrophy
MSU	midstream urine
MTP	metatarsophalangeal
MUS	medically unexplained symptom
MV	mechanical ventilation
MVP	mitral valve prolapse
NaCl	sodium chloride
NADPH	reduced nicotinamide adenine dinucleotide phosphate
NEWS	NHS Early Warning Score
NF	nuclear factor
NG	nasogastric
NGU	non-gonococcal urethritis
NHL	non-Hodgkin's lymphoma
NHS	National Health Service
NICE	National Institute for Health and Care Excellence
NIV	non-invasive ventilation
NMO	neuromyelitis optica

NO	nitric oxide
NPV	negative pressure ventilation
NQMI	non-Q wave myocardial infarction
NSAID	non-steroidal anti-inflammatory drug
NYHA	New York Heart Association
OA	osteoarthritis
OCP	oral contraceptive pill
od	*omni die* (once a day)
OGD	oesophago-gastroduodenoscopy
OSA	obstructive sleep apnoea
PA	posteroanterior, pulmonary artery
PAN	polyarteritis nodosa
PARP	poly (adenosine diphosphate ribose) polymerase
PBC	primary biliary cirrhosis
PCI	percutaneous coronary intervention
PCOS	polycystic ovary syndrome
PCP	phencyclidine, *Pneumocystis carinii (jirovecii)* pneumonia
PCR	polymerase chain reaction
PCV	packed cell volume
PCWP	pulmonary capillary wedge pressure
PD	proton density
PDA	patent ductus arteriosus
PE	pulmonary embolism
PEEP	positive end-expiratory pressure
PEFR	peak expiratory flow rate
PEG	percutaneous endoscopic gastrostomy
PET	positron emission tomography
PGE$_1$	prostaglandin E$_1$
PID	pelvic inflammatory disease
PION	posterior ischaemic optic neuropathy
PIP	proximal interphalangeal
PKD	polycystic kidney disease
PM	polymyositis
PML	progressive multifocal leukoencephalopathy
PMR	polymyalgia rheumatica
PND	paroxysmal nocturnal dyspnoea
PNH	paroxysmal nocturnal haemoglobinuria
PNS	peripheral nervous system
PPI	proton pump inhibitor
PR	per rectum
PRL	prolactin
PrP	prion protein
PRV	polycythaemia rubra vera
PS	psychoactive substance
PSA	prostrate-specific antigen
PSC	primary sclerosing cholangitis
PT	prothrombin time
PTH	parathyroid hormone
PTHrP	parathyroid hormone-related protein
PTT	partial thromboplastin time

PUO	pyrexia of unknown origin
PUVA	psoralens and ultraviolet A
PVD	peripheral vascular disease
PVR	post-void residual
RA	rheumatoid arthritis, right atrium
RANK	receptor activator of nuclear factor κB
RANKL	receptor activator of nuclear factor κB ligand
RBB	right bundle branch
RBC	red blood cell
RE	reticuloendothelial
REM	rapid eye movement
RF	rheumatoid factor
RNA	ribonucleic acid
RNP	ribonucleic protein
RP	retinitis pigmentosa
rpm	respirations per minute
RR	respiratory rate
RTA	renal tubular acidosis
RUQ	right upper quadrant
RV	right ventricle, right ventricular
RVF	right ventricular failure
RVH	right ventricular hypertrophy
SA	sinoatrial
SACD	subacute combined degeneration of the cord
SAH	subarachnoid haemorrhage
SARA	sexually acquired reactive arthritis
SBE	subacute bacterial endocarditis
SCC	squamous cell carcinoma
SCID	severe combined immunodeficiency
SCLC	small cell lung cancer
SDH	subdural haematoma
SHBG	sex hormone-binding globulin
SIADH	syndrome of inappropriate antidiuretic hormone secretion
SIJ	sacro-iliac joint
SK	streptokinase
SLE	systemic lupus erythematosus
SMA	smooth muscle antibody
SOB	shortness of breath
SPECT	single photon emission computed tomography
SR	sinus rhythm
SRH	stigmata of recent haemorrhage
STD	sexually transmitted disease
STEMI	ST segment elevation myocardial infarction
SUA	serum uric acid
SUI	stress urinary incontinence
SVC	superior vena cava
SVT	supraventricular tachycardia
T_3	triiodothyronine
T_4	thyroxine
TACS	total anterior circulation syndrome
TB	tuberculosis
tds	*ter die sumendus* (3 times a day)
TED	thromboembolic
TGF	transforming growth factor
TIA	transient ischaemic attack
TIBC	total iron-binding capacity
TIH	tumour-induced hypercalcaemia
TIMP-1	tissue inhibitor of metalloproteinase 1
TIPSS	transjugular intrahepatic portosystemic stent shunt
TLC	total lung capacity
TMJ	temporomandibular joint
TNF	tumour necrosis factor
tPA	tissue plasminogen activator
TRUS	transrectal ultrasonography
TSH	thyroid-stimulating hormone
TT	thrombin time
TTP	thrombotic thrombocytopenic purpura
TURP	transurethral resection of the prostate
UC	ulcerative colitis
U&Es	urea and electrolytes
UFH	unfractionated heparin
UMN	upper motor neuron
URTI	upper respiratory tract infection
USS	ultrasound
UTI	urinary tract infection
UV	ultraviolet
UVB	ultraviolet B
VC	vital capacity
VDRL	venereal disease research laboratory
VEGF	vascular endothelium growth factor
VEP	visual evoked potential
VF	ventricular fibrillation
VIN	vulval intraepithelial neoplasia
VIP	vasoactive intestinal peptide
VLDL	very-low-density lipoprotein
VMA	vanillomandelic acid
$\dot{V}/\dot{Q}$	ventilation/perfusion
VSD	ventricular septal defect
VT	ventricular tachycardia
vWD	von Willebrand's disease
vWF	von Willebrand's factor
VZV	varicella-zoster virus
WCC	white cell count
WG	Wegener's granulomatosis
WHO	World Health Organization
WoB	work of breathing
WPW	Wolff–Parkinson–White

How to use your revision guide

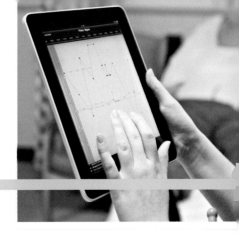

Features contained within your textbook

The overview page gives a summary of the topics covered in each part.

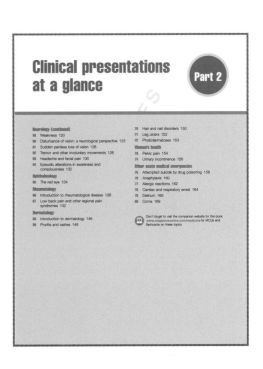

Each topic is presented in a double-page spread with clear, easy-to-follow diagrams supported by succinct explanatory text.

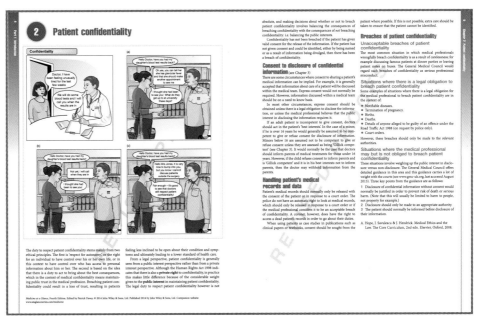

Your revision guide is full of photographs, illustrations and tables.

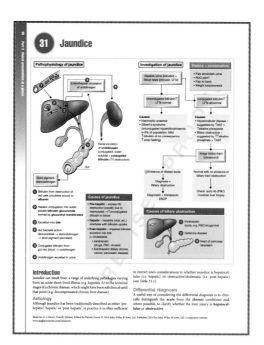

The website icon indicates that you can find accompanying resources on the book's companion website www.ataglanceseries.com/medicine.

The anytime, anywhere textbook

Wiley E-Text

Your book is also available to purchase as a Wiley E-Text: Powered by VitalSource version – a digital, interactive version of this book which you own as soon as you download it.

Your Wiley E-Text allows you to:

Search: Save time by finding terms and topics instantly in your book, your notes, even your whole library (once you've downloaded more textbooks)

Note and highlight: Colour code, highlight and make digital notes right in the text so you can find them quickly and easily

Organize: Keep books, notes and class materials organized in folders inside the application

Share: Exchange notes and highlights with friends, classmates and study groups

Upgrade: Your textbook can be transferred when you need to change or upgrade computers

Link: Link directly from the page of your interactive textbook to all of the material contained on the companion website

The **Wiley E-Text** version will also allow you to copy and paste any photograph or illustration into assignments, presentations and your own notes.

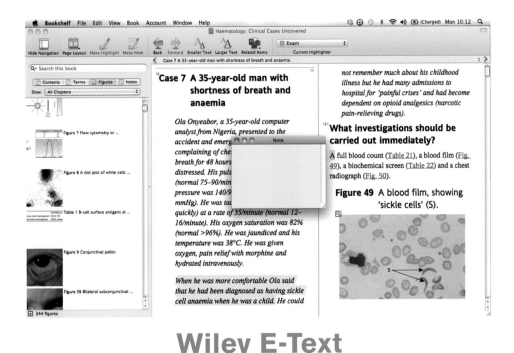

Wiley E-Text
Powered by VitalSource®

To access your Wiley E-Text:

● Visit www.vitalsource.com/software/bookshelf/downloads to download the Bookshelf application to your computer, laptop, tablet or mobile device.

● Open the Bookshelf application on your computer and register for an account.

● Follow the registration process.

CourseSmart

CourseSmart gives you instant access (via computer or mobile device) to this Wiley Blackwell e-book and its extra electronic functionality, at 40% off the recommended retail print price. See all the benefits at: www.coursesmart.com/students.

Instructors . . . receive your own digital desk copies!

CourseSmart also offers instructors an immediate, efficient and environmentally-friendly way to review this book for your course.

For more information visit www.coursesmart.com/instructors.

With CourseSmart, you can create lecture notes quickly with copy and paste, and share pages and notes with your students. Access your CourseSmart digital book from your computer or mobile device instantly for evaluation, class preparation and as a teaching tool in the classroom.

Simply sign in at http://instructors.coursesmart.com/bookshelf to download your Bookshelf and get started. To request your desk copy, hit 'Request Online Copy' on your search results or book product page.

We hope you enjoy using your new book. Good luck with your studies!

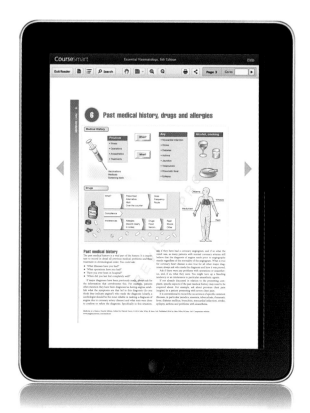

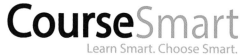

About the companion website

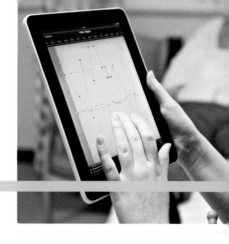

Don't forget to visit the companion website for this book:

www.ataglanceseries.com/medicine

There you will find valuable material
designed to enhance your learning, including:

- Multiple-choice questions for self-test
- Interactive flashcards with on/off label functionality
- A quick reference table of normal values

Scan this QR code to visit the
companion website.

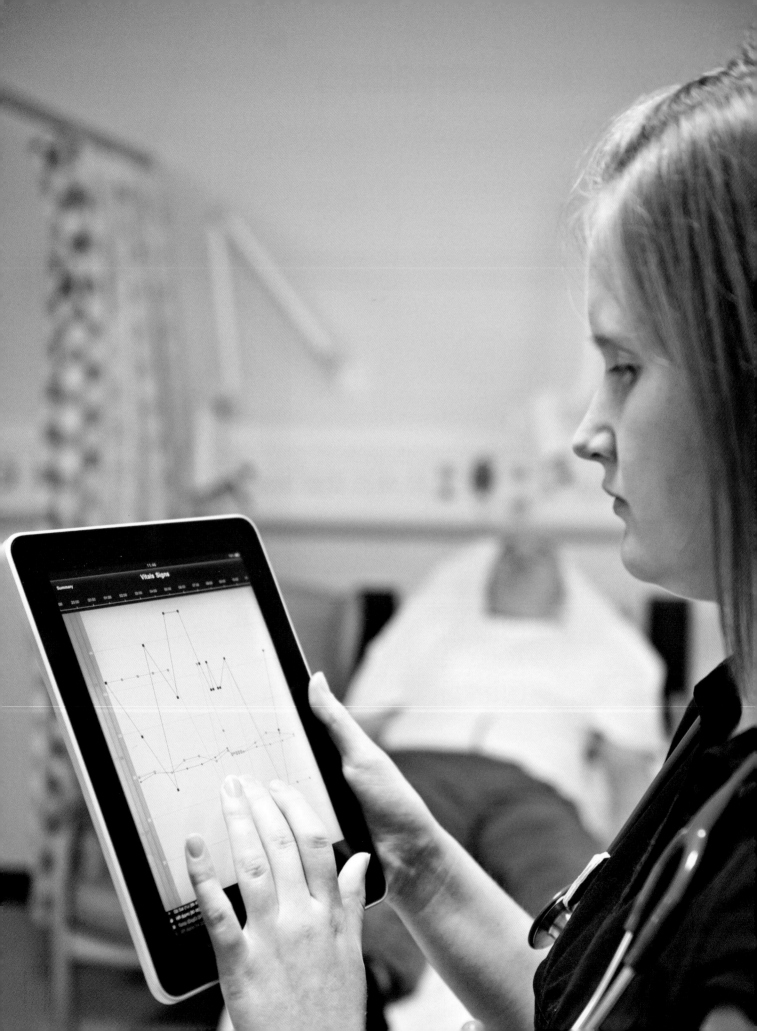

Introduction

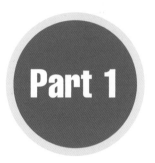

Part 1

Chapters

 Don't forget to visit the companion website for this book www.ataglanceseries.com/medicine for MCQs and flashcards on these topics

1 How to be a medical student

THE HIPPOCRATIC OATH

I SWEAR by Apollo the physician, and Aesculapius, and Health, and All-heal, and all the gods and goddesses, that, according to my ability and judgment, I will heed this oath and this stipulation to reckon him who taught me this Art equally dear to me as my parents, to share my substance with him, and relieve his necessities if required; to look upon his offspring in the same footing as my own brothers, and to teach them this Art, if they shall wish to learn it, without fee or stipulation; and that by precept, lecture, and every other mode of instruction, I will impart a knowledge of the Art to my own sons, and those of my teachers, and to disciples bound by a stipulation and oath according to the law of medicine, but to none other. I will follow that system of regimen which, according to my ability and judgment, I consider for the benefit of my patients, and abstain from whatever is deleterious and mischievous. I will give no deadly medicine to any one if asked, nor suggest any such counsel; and in like manner I will not give to a woman a pessary to produce abortion. With purity and with holiness I will pass my life and practise my Art. I will not cut persons laboring under the stone, but will leave this to be done by men who are practitioners of this work. Into whatever houses I enter, I will go into them for the benefit of the sick, and will abstain from every voluntary act of mischief and corruption; and, further from the seduction of females or males, of freemen and slaves. Whatever, in connection with my professional practice or not, in connection with it, I see or hear, in the life of men, which ought not to be spoken of abroad, I will not divulge, as reckoning that all such should be kept secret. While I continue to keep this oath unviolated, may it be granted to me to enjoy life and the practice of the art, respected by all men, in all times! But should I trespass and violate this oath, may the reverse be my lot.

In 1948 in Geneva the World Medical Association drew up a modern version of the oath.

*A*t the time of being admitted a member of the medical profession:

I solemnly pledge myself to consecrate my life to the service of humanity;

I will give my teachers the respect and gratitude which is their due;

I will practise my profession with conscience and dignity;

*T*he health of my patient will be my first consideration;

I will respect the secrets which are confided in me, even after the patient has died;

I will maintain by all the means in my power, the honour and the noble traditions of the medical profession;

*M*y colleagues will be my brothers;

I will not permit considerations of religion, nationality, race, party politics or social standing to intervene between my duty and my patient;

I will maintain the utmost respect for human life from the time of conception; even under threat I will not use my medical knowledge contrary to the laws of humanity.

I make these promises solemnly, freely and upon my honour.

Good doctors

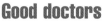

Medicine can seem a large and daunting subject, not only for reasons of intellectual rigour, but also because so many facts need to be learnt. In learning (and practising) medicine, it is vital to realize that facts alone are not enough! Good physicians have the following characteristics:

● A strong humanity, i.e. an interest in human beings.
● An interest in disease, its causation and treatment.
● An ability to communicate with patients, to obtain a correct and full understanding of their problems and, at the same time, to give accurate information sympathetically about the diagnosis, treatment and prognosis. Good physicians are non-judgemental, empathetic listeners.
● An ability to examine patients and elicit abnormal physical signs.
● An ability to marshal the facts into a coherent story and present them clearly to relevant parties, i.e. 'case' presentation of

the history, examination and structured summary, a probable and differential diagnosis, with plans for further investigations, and treatment.
● An up-to-date knowledge base so that appropriate management (diagnosis + treatment) plans can be made.
● An ability to realize when knowledge/skills are deficient and an ability to learn in response to new knowledge, ideas, etc., from the best source available.
● An ability to acknowledge errors and learn from them. It is important to be open with patients and colleagues as soon as errors/misjudgements are recognized.
● Appropriate technical skills in diagnostic and therapeutic procedures.
● An understanding of economic, social and cultural, political and health-care systems so that the best possible help can be delivered to patients in the most timely fashion. If a deficiency in one or other of these systems damages patients, physicians should seek improvements.

Medicine at a Glance, Fourth Edition. Edited by Patrick Davey. © 2014 John Wiley & Sons, Ltd. Published 2014 by John Wiley & Sons, Ltd. Companion website: www.ataglanceseries.com/medicine

- Excellent managerial and interpersonal skills, with personal, financial and intellectual probity.

Hippocratic oath and the modern perspective

High ethical and moral standards are an imperative for good practice – the Hippocratic oath and its modern successors aim to codify behaviour. They are guidelines to best behaviour, although medicine is more complex than implied by such phrases. However, regardless of phrasing, the implication that physicians should have the highest ethical, moral and technical standards stands. Society respects physicians, and consequently physicians face social as well as other penalties if performance is poor.

Health-care systems

Health-care systems are imperfect compromises among society's aspirations, wealth, humanity and individual needs (see Figure 1.2 below and Table 1.1). It is vital to understand how any system works, so that it can be used in a patient's best interests. If individual or organizational failure occurs, this should be highlighted to the appropriate responsible individuals, agencies or, rarely, the media.

How to learn

Becoming a doctor means acquiring a set of skills, knowledge and values. How this is best done depends on the individual and the

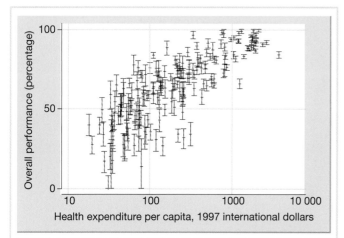

Health care spend related to outcome – different countries can spend the same amounts with very different outcomes, as shown in this graph, where health care expenditure is plotted against health care system performance

Source: The World Health Report 2000.
Reproduced with permission of WHO

Table 1.1 The three fundamental objectives of health systems.

- Improving the health of the population they serve
- Responding to people's expectations (including personal respect from the system to the patient)
- Providing financial protection against the costs of ill health

medical school. However, concentrating on one area/skill to the exclusion of others is counterproductive. Facts alone do not make a physician, and nor do learning or technical skills alone. It is the right combination of the above list that 'maketh the physician'. Students need to determine the right balance for themselves, bearing in mind their individual aptitudes, and their medical school's doctrine. A reasonable approach is the 'patient-centred' one, approached in a 'problem-based' fashion, supplemented by dedicated learning sessions (e.g. seminars, lectures, etc.). Students should:

- See patients, so learning communication skills.
- Ascertain symptoms and signs, so learning clerking and examination skills.
- Formulate a diagnosis or differential diagnosis, so learning diagnostic skills. The first part of this book aims to aid in diagnosis, i.e. the turning of symptoms and signs into diseases with names.
- Present findings to attending physicians, so learning presentation skills.
- Formulate investigation and treatment plans, so refining diagnostic and therapeutic skills. The second part of this book aims to help here.
- Observe patients' progress, so determining whether the original diagnosis and therapy were correct. This feedback is an essential component in improving diagnostic and therapeutic skills.

Deficiencies in knowledge and technique are identified at each stage and corrected using information/skills training obtained from books and libraries, electronic resources, physicians, other health-care professionals, patient groups, skills workshops, learning sessions, etc.

Some medical schools have a structured approach to this process, with substantial guidance at each stage; others are less formalized – which appeals more depends largely on you. Which is better is unclear.

How to behave on the wards

It is particularly important when performing ward work to:

- Introduce yourself to the ward staff as well as the patient, so that they know who you are and why you are there.
- Respect patients' privacy, and their right to refuse to see you.
- Ask for consent before seeing a patient.
- If you undress a patient to examine him or her, help him or her to dress again once you have finished.
- Be courteous to nurses and other members of staff (e.g. physiotherapists, ward cleaners, cooks, etc.) at all times.
- Be punctual in attending teaching sessions – you will find that your teachers, who are often busy clinicians, are often late; this is not deliberately done to infuriate you, rather it reflects how hectic their lives are. It is reasonable to wait for about 10 min, before 'bleeping' to remind them of the session.
- Write in the notes: different medical schools have different policies on this. Often, however, senior medical students are expected to write in the notes. This is a legal document, so write legibly, never use pejorative phraseology, and sign your name, along with your status as student, legibly at the end. *Never* amend the record at a later time, unless you clearly identify who you are and when the alterations occurred.
- Enjoy yourself!

2 Patient confidentiality

Confidentiality

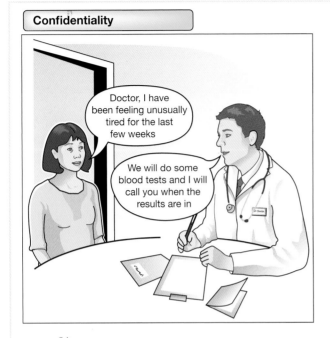

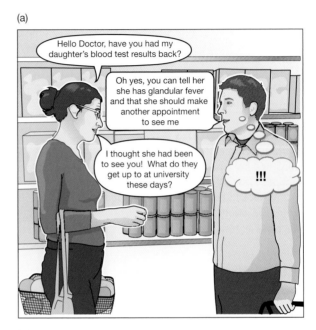

(a)

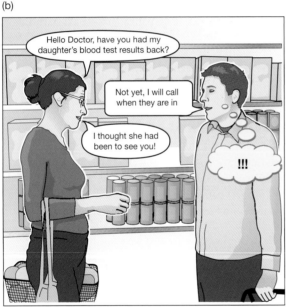

(b)

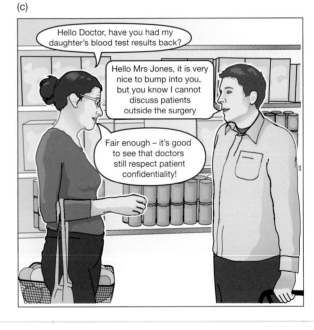

(c)

The duty to respect patient confidentiality stems mainly from two ethical principles. The first is 'respect for autonomy', or the right for an individual to have control over his or her own life, or in this context to have control over who has access to personal information about him or her. The second is based on the idea that there is a duty to act to bring about the best consequences, which in the context of medical confidentiality means maintaining public trust in the medical profession. Breaching patient confidentiality could result in a loss of trust, resulting in patients feeling less inclined to be open about their condition and symptoms and ultimately leading to a lower standard of health care.

From a legal perspective, patient confidentiality is generally seen from a public interest perspective rather than from a private interest perspective. Although the Human Rights Act 1998 indicates that there is also a **private right** to confidentiality, in practice this makes little difference because of the considerable weight given to the **public interest** in maintaining patient confidentiality. The legal duty to respect patient confidentiality however is not

Medicine at a Glance, Fourth Edition. Edited by Patrick Davey. © 2014 John Wiley & Sons, Ltd. Published 2014 by John Wiley & Sons, Ltd. Companion website: www.ataglanceseries.com/medicine

absolute, and making decisions about whether or not to breach patient confidentiality involves balancing the consequences of breaching confidentiality with the consequences of *not* breaching confidentiality: i.e. balancing the public interests.

Confidentiality has not been breached if the patient has given valid consent for the release of the information. If the patient has not given consent and could be identified, either by being named or as a result of information being divulged, then there has been a breach of confidentiality.

Consent to disclosure of confidential information (see Chapter 3)

There are some circumstances where consent to sharing a patient's medical information can be implied. For example, it is generally accepted that information about care of a patient will be discussed within the medical team. Express consent would not normally be required. However, information discussed within a medical team should be on a need to know basis.

In most other circumstances, express consent should be obtained unless there is a legal obligation to disclose the information, or unless the medical professional believes that the public interest in disclosing the information requires it.

If an adult patient is incompetent to give consent, doctors should act in the patient's 'best interests'. In the case of a minor, if he is over 16 years he would generally be assumed to be competent to give or refuse consent for disclosure of information. Minors below 16 are assumed not to be competent to give or refuse consent unless they are assessed as being 'Gillick competent' (see Chapter 3). It would normally be the case that doctors should inform parents of medical treatments for those under 16 years. However, if the child refuses consent to inform parents and is 'Gillick competent' and it is in his best interests not to inform parents, then the doctor may withhold information from the parents.

Handling patient's medical records and data

Patient's medical records should normally only be released with the consent of the patient or in response to a court order. The police do not have an automatic right to look at medical records, which should only be released in response to a court order or if the medical professional considers it to be an acceptable breach of confidentiality. A coroner, however, does have the right to access a dead patient's records in order to go about their duties.

When using patients as case studies in publications such as clinical papers or textbooks, consent should be sought from the patient where possible. If this is not possible, extra care should be taken to ensure that the patient cannot be identified.

Breaches of patient confidentiality

Unacceptable breaches of patient confidentiality

The most common situation in which medical professionals wrongfully breach confidentiality is as a result of carelessness; for example discussing famous patients at dinner parties or leaving patient notes on buses. The General Medical Council would regard such breaches of confidentiality as serious professional misconduct.

Situations where there is a legal obligation to breach patient confidentiality

Some examples of situations where there is a legal obligation for the medical professional to breach patient confidentiality are in the context of:

- Notifiable diseases.
- Termination of pregnancy.
- Births.
- Deaths.
- Details of anyone alleged to be guilty of an offence under the Road Traffic Act 1988 (on request by police only).
- Court orders.

However, these breaches should only be made to the relevant authorities.

Situations where the medical professional may but is not obliged to breach patient confidentiality

These situations involve weighing up the public interest in disclosure versus non-disclosure. The General Medical Council offers detailed guidance in this area and this guidance carries a lot of weight with the courts (see www.gmc-uk.org, last accessed August 2013). Three key points from the guidance are as follows:

1 Disclosure of confidential information without consent would normally be justified in order to prevent risk of death or serious harm. (Note that this will usually be limited to harm to people, not property for example.)
2 Disclosure should only be made to an appropriate authority.
3 The patient should normally be informed before disclosure of their information.

A. Hope, J. Savulescu & J. Hendrick. Medical Ethics and the Law. The Core Curriculum, 2nd edn. Elsevier, Oxford, 2008.

3 Consent

Patient details
on a Patient identifier/label

Patient identifier/label

Name of proposed procedure or course of treatment (include brief explanation if medical term not clear) ....
....
....

Statement of health professional (to be filled in by health professional with appropriate knowledge of proposed procedure, as specified in consent policy)

I have explained the procedure to the patient. In particular, I have explained:

The intended benefits ....
....
Serious or frequently occurring risks ....
....

Any extra procedures which may become necessary during the procedure

☐ blood transfusion...

☐ other procedure (please specify) ....
....

I have also discussed what the procedure is likely to involve, the benefits and risks of any available alternative treatments (including no treatment) and any particular concerns of this patient.

☐ The following leaflet/tape has been provided ....

This procedure will involve:

☐ general and/or regional anaesthesia ☐ local anaesthesia ☐ sedation

Signed:... Date ....
Name (PRINT) .... Job title ....

Contact details (if patient wishes to discuss options later) ....

Statement of interpreter (where appropriate)

I have interpreted the information above to the patient to the best of my ability and in a way in which I believe s/he can understand.

Signed .... Date ....
Name (PRINT) ....

Top copy accepted by patient: yes/no (please ring)

Patient identifier/label

Statement of patient

Please read this form carefully. If your treatment has been planned in advance, you should already have your own copy of page 2 which describes the benefits and risks of the proposed treatment. If not, you will be offered a copy now. If you have any further questions, do ask – we are here to help you. You have the right to change your mind at any time, including after you have signed this form.

I agree to the procedure or course of treatment described on this form.

I understand that you cannot give me a guarantee that a particular person will perform the procedure. The person will, however, have appropriate experience.

I understand that I will have the opportunity to discuss the details of anaesthesia with an anaesthetist before the procedure, unless the urgency of my situation prevents this. (This only applies to patients having general or regional anaesthesia.)

I understand that any procedure in addition to those described on this form will only be carried out if it is necessary to save my life or to prevent serious harm to my health.

I have been told about additional procedures which may become necessary during my treatment. I have listed below any procedures **which I do not wish to be carried out** without further discussion. ....
....
....
....

Patient's signature .... Date............................
Name (PRINT) ....

A witness should sign below if the patient is unable to sign but has indicated his or her consent. Young people/children may also like a parent to sign here (see notes).

Signature .... Date ....
Name (PRINT) ....

Confirmation of consent (to be completed by a health professional when the patient is admitted for the procedure, if the patient has signed the form in advance)

On behalf of the team treating the patient, I have confirmed with the patient that s/he has no further questions and wishes the procedure to go ahead.

Signed:.. Date ....
Name (PRINT) .... Job title ....

Important notes: (tick if applicable)

☐ See also advance directive/living will (e.g. Jehovah's Witness form)

☐ Patient has withdrawn consent (ask patient to sign /date here) ....

In modern health care, it is acknowledged that patient consent is required before any medical intervention is carried out. This would normally be express consent. However, in certain circumstances consent can be implied, for example when a patient holds out his arm for blood to be taken. The importance of consent stems from the ethical concept of autonomy: the right to have control over our own lives. This concept has been incorporated into English law as three criteria that must be met for consent to be valid. These criteria are:

1 That the patient has been **informed** as to the purpose, nature, risks and benefits of the medical procedure.
2 That the patient is **competent** (has capacity) to understand this information.

3 That the patient has given voluntary **consent**, i.e. the patient has not been coerced.

In order to maximize autonomy, patients should be as much in control as possible throughout the course of any medical intervention. This also means that they can withdraw consent at any time. This is important legally in relation to the consent form. The consent form is not a contract. Therefore, it is illegal (battery – see below) to proceed with a medical intervention if the patient withdraws his consent, even if he has previously signed a consent form.

For patients to be 'informed', they should be given general information about the purpose and nature of the proposed course of action. Failure to do this could result in the patient making a

Medicine at a Glance, Fourth Edition. Edited by Patrick Davey. © 2014 John Wiley & Sons, Ltd. Published 2014 by John Wiley & Sons, Ltd. Companion website: www.ataglanceseries.com/medicine

claim for **battery** (touching a person without consent). Information should also be given about any reasonable alternatives, risks and benefits, including common and serious side effects, otherwise a claim could be made for negligence. Even if a patient prefers to know nothing about the proposed procedure, it would be unwise to proceed without informing him or her of the key aspects of the treatment. The General Medical Council offers guidance on the provision of information to patients on their website www.gmc-uk.org (last accessed August 2013).

In English law, a person over the age of 16 is assumed to have capacity, i.e. be competent, unless it can be shown to the contrary.

Mental Capacity Act 2005

The Mental Capacity Act 2005 outlines the procedure for determining capacity and how to act when a patient over the age of 16 lacks capacity. Under the Act (Part 1 Section 3(1)), a person lacks capacity if he is unable to:

- **understand** the information relevant to the decision, *or*
- **retain** that information, *or*
- **use or weigh** that information as part of the process of making the decision, *or*
- **communicate** his decision (by any means).

If a patient is shown to lack capacity, then those caring for him must attempt to enhance his capacity insofar as this is practical (Part 1 Section 1(3)). Note that '**capacity**' refers to the ability of the patient to make a specific decision, not to the patient as a whole. In addition, a patient does not lack capacity simply because he makes an unwise decision (Part 1 Section 1(4)).

Under the Mental Capacity Act, patients who lack capacity (and have not appointed a Lasting Power of Attorney or made an Advance Decision – see below) should be treated in their 'best interests' (Part 1 Section 4). The Act specifies some factors that should be taken into account in making a decision about their best interests. The General Medical Council also offers guidance as to how to determine 'best interests' (see www.gmc-uk.org).

Under the Mental Capacity Act (Part 1 Section 9), a Lasting Power of Attorney can be appointed by a person who has capacity to make medical and non-medical decisions on his behalf at a future time when he no longer has capacity. The Act also allows Advance Decisions to be made, by persons aged 18 or over who have capacity, to refuse treatment at a future time when they lack capacity (Part 1 Sections 24–26). An Advance Decision can relate to life-sustaining treatment if it is in writing and specific to that effect and if it is appropriately signed and witnessed.

In Scotland, although the approach to determining capacity and treatment of those without capacity is similar, the law differs slightly and is covered by the Adults with Incapacity (Scotland) Act 2000.

Consent and minors (<18 years old)

When dealing with minors and consent, it is important to remember that in an emergency situation when the minor and/or those with parental responsibility cannot or will not give consent, the medical professional should normally act to prevent death or serious harm to the patient.

Minors aged 16 or 17 years are presumed to have capacity to consent to medical treatment unless it can be shown otherwise. Those with parental responsibility (usually the parents) can also give consent. If valid consent for the relevant procedure has been given either by the minor or by any person with parental responsibility then the doctor has consent to proceed (without risk of battery). Doctors (and those with parental responsibility) have a legal obligation to act in a minor's best interests. If neither the patient concerned nor a person with parental responsibility consents, and the doctor judges that the treatment is in the patient's best interests, then advice should be sought from the courts.

Children aged less than 16 are presumed not to have capacity to consent unless they demonstrate that they are 'Gillick competent', i.e. have reached a level of intelligence and understanding sufficient to understand what is being proposed. The criteria on this are vague and if there is doubt it would be wise to obtain consent from a person with parental responsibility. The legal position for refusal of treatment by Gillick-competent children is the same as for competent 16- or 17-year-olds.

Consent should be obtained from at least one person with parental responsibility for minors below the age of 16 who are not Gillick competent. If no-one with parental responsibility gives consent and failure to carry out the procedure would be significantly against the child's best interests then doctors should apply to the court for a 'specific issue order'. In an emergency, doctors should act to save the child from death or serious harm.

A. Hope, J. Savulescu & J. Hendrick. *Medical Ethics and the Law. The Core Curriculum*, 2nd edn. Elsevier, Oxford, 2008.

4 Relationship with the patient

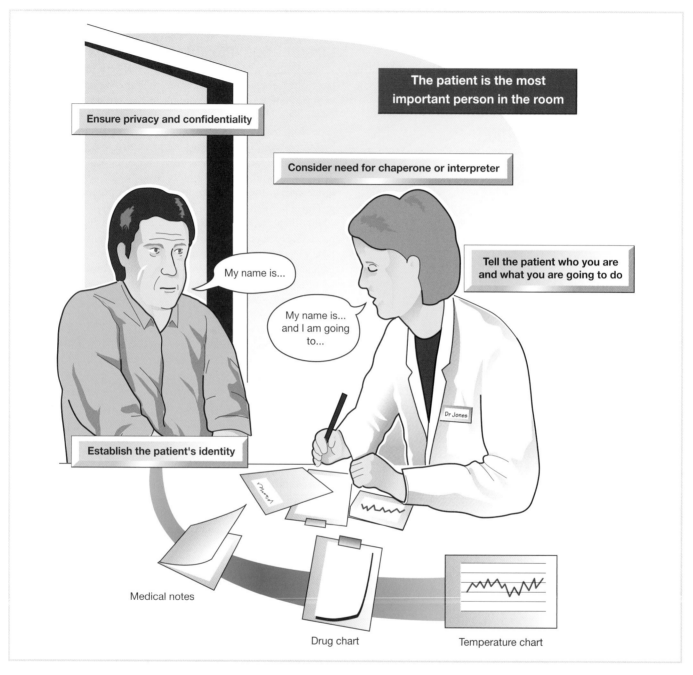

The patient is the most important person in the room

Ensure privacy and confidentiality

Consider need for chaperone or interpreter

Tell the patient who you are and what you are going to do

My name is...

My name is... and I am going to...

Dr Jones

Establish the patient's identity

Medical notes

Drug chart

Temperature chart

Your relationship with your patient is the key determinant of your effectiveness as a clinician. Why is this? You need the patient to give you *all* the information necessary for diagnosis. You must then communicate this decision and any uncertainty surrounding it to the patient in language they understand, and you must convince them that the treatment you recommend is appropriate and effective. None of this will occur unless you have established an effective relationship with your patient. Different patients require different techniques to develop relationships; with some you can be informal and quite chatty, with others you may need to be much more formal, and keep to the point, some appreciate humour, and others find it unprofessional. Develop your style, but modify it for individual patients. So, how do you develop such a relationship? In many ways, though some tips include:

- Listen to your patient, let them do the talking, albeit guided by yourself to elaborate on certain areas and to move on from others.
- Engage in eye contact.
- Appropriate use of non-verbal gestures, such as smiling.
- Minimize the chance of interruptions and other distractions (such as bleeps going off).

Medicine at a Glance, Fourth Edition. Edited by Patrick Davey. © 2014 John Wiley & Sons, Ltd. Published 2014 by John Wiley & Sons, Ltd. Companion website: www.ataglanceseries.com/medicine

- Dress appropriately; in years gone by, most patients expected consultants to wear suits. This era has largely passed – consultants attending patients in the middle of the night often wear jeans, so do adjust your attire according to the setting and time. However, you should be certain your clothes are smart and clean, and that you follow the dress code of your institute (in the UK National Health Service this includes no jewellery and only short sleeve shirts), which is recommended to minimize your risk of transmitting hospital-acquired infection.

When meeting a patient, establish their identity unequivocally (ask for their full name and confirm with their name band, ask for their date of birth, address, etc.) and be certain that all records, notes, test results, etc. refer to that patient, as results can sometimes find their way into the wrong patient's notes. If you are a medical student ensure that the patient understands that and gives their permission for you to talk to them.

Often you may wish to shake their hand and say 'My name is Dr Davey and you are . . .?' Or 'Your name is . . .?', 'Your date of birth is . . .?', 'Your address is . . .?' Tell them your name, your title and job and what you are about to do. For example:

> 'I am Dr Davey, a consultant specializing in heart medicine and I've been asked to try and work out whether your heart is working properly. I'm going to spend about half an hour talking to you about your medical problems, and then I'll examine you thoroughly. After that I'll explain to you what I think the matter is and what we need to do to help you.'

Or you could say, 'I am Patrick Davey, a medical student, and I'd like to ask you some questions about your illness if I may'.

Always be polite, be respectful and be clear. Remember the patient may be feeling anxious, unwell, embarrassed, scared or in pain. If you detect these emotions, ask the patient to elaborate on their fears – unless you know what is really worrying them, you will not have a satisfactory consultation.

You should be gathering information and observing the patient as soon as you meet them: history taking and examination are not distinct, sequential processes, they are ongoing. Your best clues to the presence of thyroid disease, acromegaly, Cushing's syndrome, alcohol dependency and many other conditions, is found from the patient's appearance in the first few seconds of the consultation, so start thinking diagnostically the moment you see the patient, not just at certain times in the consultation.

Sequence of the consultation

Though your diagnostic processes will be working continuously throughout the consultation, the usual order is history, examination, explanation to the patient about their illness and then, crucially, to ask the patient if they have questions they wish to address.

Privacy

Ensure that there is privacy (this is not always easy in busy hospital wards: make sure curtains are properly closed; see if the examination room is free).

Language

Establish whether the patient is fluent in the language you intend to use and, if not, arrange for an interpreter to be present or at least a telephone interpreter. Often a family member will be willing to interpret, but this may subtly distort the history and there may be issues with confidentiality, so you should establish that the patient is happy to discuss their problems via this relative. In the UK, the NHS has issued a guideline stating that relatives should not be used as interpreters as patients may not then divulge key information, for example about abuse that has a particular cultural context. Accordingly, in the UK, use alternatives such as hired translators or other members of staff.

Relatives, friends and chaperones

Establish who else is with the patient, their relationship with the patient and whether the patient wishes for them to be present during the consultation. Ask if the patient wishes for a chaperone to be present during the examination; this may be appropriate in any case.

Remember that **the patient is the most important person in the room**! Remember that all information you gain from your patient or anyone else is **confidential**. This means that information about the patient should only be discussed with other professionals involved in the care of that patient. You must ensure that patient discussions or records cannot be overheard or accessed by others.

Some guidelines for the use of chaperones

- A chaperone is a third person, (usually) of the same sex as the patient and (usually) a health professional (not a relative).
- When asking a patient if they would like a chaperone to be present, ensure they know what you mean; for example, 'We often ask another member of staff to be present during this examination, would you like me have someone present?'
- If either the patient or the doctor/medical student wishes a chaperone to be present then the examination should not be carried out without one.
- Record the presence of a chaperone in the notes – **this is vital if you are to fully protect yourself medicolegally**.
- A chaperone *must* be present for intimate examinations by doctors or students examining patients of the opposite sex (vaginal, rectal, genitalia and female breast examination), and offered for any intimate examinations of either gender.

Hand washing and hospital-acquired infection

In modern health-care systems there is considerable and appropriate concern about hospital-acquired infection; the hands of staff are the commonest vehicles by which microorganisms are transmitted between patients and hand washing is the single most important measure in infection control. So, always ensure your hands are washed, whether using alcoholic rubs or medicated soap is less important than that the hands are actually washed. Hands should be washed before and after each patient contact, and also between wards.

You should also ensure that you minimize the risk of your clothes transmitting infection by not wearing jewellery, long-sleeved shirts or a tie, and ensuring that your stethoscope is disinfected regularly.

5 History of presenting complaint

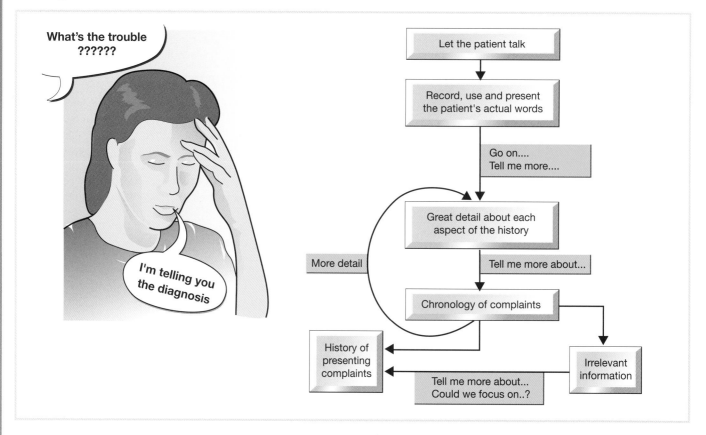

The history of the presenting complaint is the most important part of the history and examination. It provides the information necessary to create the differential diagnosis and also provides vital insight into the features of the complaints most important to the patient. It should receive most time during a consultation.

The history obtained should be recorded and presented in the patient's own words, and not be masked by medical phrases such as 'dyspnoea', 'myocardial infarction', etc., which may disguise the true nature of the complaint and important nuances. As you listen to the presenting complaint, continually ask yourself 'What does this tell me about the diagnosis?' Remember it is the patient's problems that you are trying to understand and record in order to establish diagnoses. Do not force or overinterpret what the patient says to fit into a particular diagnosis or symptom, nor simply record what the patient reports other doctors have said.

If a clear history cannot be obtained from the patient then the history should be sought from relatives, friends or other witnesses. It may be appropriate to seek corroboration of features of the history, such as alcohol consumption or details of a collapse, always bearing in mind the principles of medical confidentiality.

Let the patient talk

The presenting complaint should be obtained by allowing the patient to talk without interruption, if possible. This may be initiated by asking an open question such as:

- 'Why have you come to see me today?'
- 'What's the problem?'
- 'Tell me what seems to be the trouble.'
- 'How long have you been ill for, and what have you noticed over this time?'

The patient should always be allowed to talk for as long as possible without interruption. Small interjections such as 'Go on' or 'Tell me more', may help produce more information from a reticent patient.

It may be possible to enable patients to elaborate on areas of medical interest, without directing the history, by indicating these are areas you are interested in. One way to do this is to repeat the last phrase that a patient has voiced in a questioning way. For example, to 'I'm finding breathing more difficult' you could respond 'Breathing more difficult?' or 'Tell me more' or 'Tell me more about your breathing'.

More specific questioning

After this, open questions should be addressed to reveal more detail about particular aspects of the history. For example, 'Tell me more about the pain', 'Tell me in more detail about your tiredness' or 'You've said that you've been feeling tired?'

More direct questions can then be addressed to gain information about the chronology and other detail of the complaints; for example, 'When exactly did you first notice the breathlessness?',

Medicine at a Glance, Fourth Edition. Edited by Patrick Davey. © 2014 John Wiley & Sons, Ltd. Published 2014 by John Wiley & Sons, Ltd. Companion website: www.ataglanceseries.com/medicine

'Which came first, the chest pain or the breathlessness?' or 'What exactly were you doing when the breathlessness came on?' Sometimes patients find it difficult to accurately recall chronology – in this situation, establish when the patient was last completely well, as this will often tell you for how long they have been ill.

Directed questions can then be addressed to establish diagnostically important features about the complaints; for example, 'What was the pain like?', 'Was the pain sharp, heavy or burning?', 'What made the pain worse?', 'Did breathing affect the pain?' or 'What about breathing in deeply?'

Other aspects of the history (e.g. past medical history or social history) relevant to the presenting complaint, although they are conventionally analysed separately, commonly arise during discussion of the presenting complaint and can receive detailed attention at this point.

In some settings, such as during resuscitation of a very ill patient, very focused or abbreviated questioning may be appropriate.

Premorbid functional status

It is *crucial* to ascertain this. This information is essential in managing the patient, and also for conveying the patient's history to colleagues. This is because:

- Usually, you aim to restore a patient's health to that immediately prior to an illness – knowing their premorbid state means that you know what you are aiming to achieve.
- Functional status is a most important predictor for life expectancy. If a patient's premorbid functional status is poor, then the premorbid life expectancy is usually not good. This information can then be factored into how intensively you should investigate and treat their current illness.

There are many ways to convey premorbid functional status – a good empirical method is to find out how far a patient can walk unaided in one go at a normal pace (e.g. 5 miles, quarter of a mile), if they are housebound or using a zimmer frame for mobility, etc. It is also important to ascertain what symptom limits them. You can do this by asking:

- 'How far can you usually walk?'
- 'What stops you walking this far?'
- 'How do the symptoms interfere with your life (with walking, working, sleeping, etc.)?'

If housebound, ask about mobility within the home, and what carers are needed to support their life (e.g. how many carers are needed to get them up in the morning, wash them, etc.).

Patients' understanding of their illness

You should ask the patient what they think is wrong with them and how the problems have affected them (e.g. ability to work, mood, etc.) and their family.

Focus on the main problems

Some patients devote considerable attention to aspects of their illness that are not helpful in achieving a diagnosis or to understanding the patient and their problems. It may be necessary to interject and divert discussion with phrases such as, 'Could you tell me more about your chest pain?' or 'Could we focus on why you came to the doctor's surgery this time?' Sometimes there may be a very long list of different complaints in which case the patient should be asked to focus on each in turn. Keep in mind the main problems and direct the history accordingly, and for each symptom, obtain and record a precise history.

Summarize your findings

Perhaps the most important aspect to establishing the presenting complaint is to summarize your understanding of the history to the patient, and to ask if you have got it exactly right.

6 Past medical history, drugs and allergies

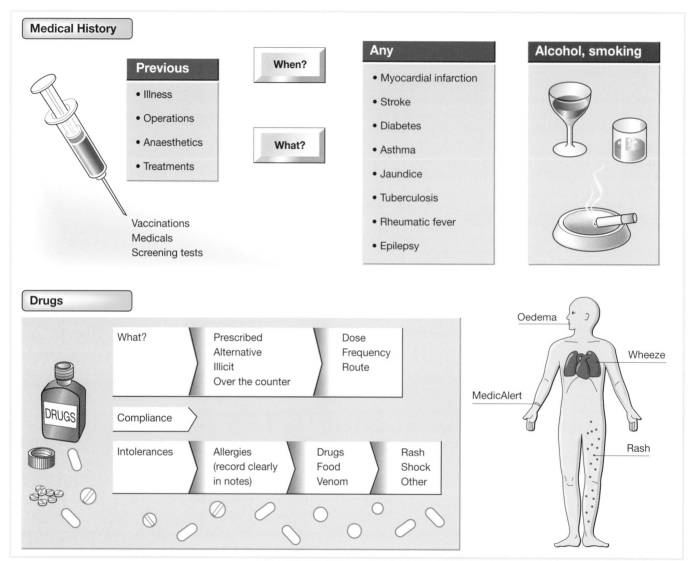

Medical History

Previous
- Illness
- Operations
- Anaesthetics
- Treatments

Vaccinations
Medicals
Screening tests

When?

What?

Any
- Myocardial infarction
- Stroke
- Diabetes
- Asthma
- Jaundice
- Tuberculosis
- Rheumatic fever
- Epilepsy

Alcohol, smoking

Drugs

What?
- Prescribed
- Alternative
- Illicit
- Over the counter

- Dose
- Frequency
- Route

Compliance

Intolerances
- Allergies (record clearly in notes)
- Drugs
- Food
- Venom
- Rash
- Shock
- Other

DRUGS

Oedema

Wheeze

MedicAlert

Rash

Past medical history

The past medical history is a vital part of the history. It is important to record in detail all previous medical problems and their treatment in chronological order. You could ask:

- 'What illnesses have you had?'
- 'What operations have you had?'
- 'Have you ever been in hospital?'
- 'When did you last feel completely well?'

If major diagnoses have been previously made, always ask for the information that corroborates this. For example, patients often mention they have been diagnosed as having angina; establish what the symptoms are that led to this diagnosis (do you think they indicate angina?) who made the diagnosis (clearly, a cardiologist should be the most reliable in making a diagnosis of angina due to coronary artery disease) and what tests were done to confirm or refute the diagnosis. Specifically in this situation,

ask if they have had a coronary angiogram, and if so what the result was, as many patients with normal coronary arteries still believe that the diagnosis of angina made prior to angiography stands regardless of the normality of the angiogram. What is true for coronary heart disease is also true for all other major diagnoses; always ask who made the diagnosis and how it was proved.

Ask if there were any problems with operations or anaesthetics, and, if so, what they were. You might turn up a bleeding tendency or an intolerance to particular anaesthetic agents.

If not already discussed in relation to the presenting complaint, specific aspects of the past medical history may need to be enquired about. For example, ask about previous chest pain (angina) in a patient presenting with severe chest pain.

It is conventional to record the occurrence of specific common illnesses, in particular jaundice, anaemia, tuberculosis, rheumatic fever, diabetes mellitus, bronchitis, myocardial infarction, stroke, epilepsy, asthma and problems with anaesthesia.

Medicine at a Glance, Fourth Edition. Edited by Patrick Davey. © 2014 John Wiley & Sons, Ltd. Published 2014 by John Wiley & Sons, Ltd. Companion website: www.ataglanceseries.com/medicine

The patient should also be asked about vaccinations, medicals, screening tests (e.g. cervical smear) and pregnancies.

Drug history

- What medication is the patient taking?
- What medication is prescribed and what other remedies are they taking (e.g. herbal remedies, 'over-the-counter' tablets)? Ask to actually see the medication and/or the prescription list.
- Do not forget to ask about injections (e.g. insulin), topical treatments and inhalers as patients may not consider them to be drugs.
  - Don't forget oral contraception (patients often do) and other hormone-containing long-acting contraception such as implants.
- What recreational drugs do they or have they taken? It is usually best to come straight out with this question and not 'beat around the bush'. Ask 'Have you ever used any non-prescription drugs?' If the answer is yes, find out what sort, how frequently and how it was taken, e.g. nasally (cocaine), orally or intravenously. If the latter, find out if they shared needles.
- What is the patient's likely compliance with prescribed medication? It is not always easy to know how to assess this. You can ask the patient if you feel they will answer truthfully (clearly, the overwhelming majority of patients). You can find out from their general practitioner how often they renew their prescription. You can ask relatives, who are an extremely useful source of information (always bear in mind the rules on confidentiality).
- Is there supervision? For example, does a relative or the district nurse supervise drug taking? Is a 'dose-it' box used?
- What medication has the patient been intolerant of and why?

Allergies

It is vital to obtain an accurate and detailed description of the patient's allergic responses to drugs and other potential allergens. The patient should be asked if they are allergic to anything. They should be asked specifically whether they are allergic to any antibiotics including penicillin. It is also important to elicit the precise nature of the allergy. Was there true allergy with a full-blown anaphylactic shock, an erythematous rash or an urticarial rash, or did the patient only feel nausea or experience another drug side effect? Many patients label the latter as an allergy, whereas often this is a component of the illness for which they were taking the antibiotic.

Other important allergies may exist to foodstuffs, such as nuts, or to bee or wasp stings.

It is also important to elicit other intolerances, such as side effects, to medication. This is particularly true for drugs used to treat hypertension. If you establish an intolerance, ask what symptoms they noticed, and whether they were present before taking the drug, or after they stopped (in which case it is unlikely to actually reflect a genuine reaction to that drug).

Ensure allergies are clearly recorded in notes, drug charts and, if appropriate, MedicAlert bracelets.

Smoking

Does the patient smoke or have they ever? If so, what type and how many, for how long? Cigarettes, pipe or cigar? Tobacco, cannabis? Have any relatives suffered smoking-related complications (e.g. heart attacks, lung diseases, malignancy)? Establish what the patient's attitude is to giving up; often patients are misinformed about the actual risk of smoking, and giving them the facts, in a polite, digestible manner, helps support them in giving up.

Alcohol

Does the patient drink alcohol? If so, what type of alcohol? How many units and how often? People find it very easy to underestimate their alcohol consumption, so it is often helpful to draw up a list of exactly how much they drink and when. If they stay at home drinking, ask how much beer and how many bottles of wine and spirits (and what size) they buy each week.

Are there/have there been problems with alcohol dependence? There are many ways to assess this, but the CAGE questionnaire is useful:

- Have you ever felt you should *C*ut back?
- Have you ever been *A*ngry when your alcohol intake is commented on?
- Have you ever felt *G*uilty about the amount you drink?
- Have you ever needed an *E*ye-opener (alcoholic drink first thing in the morning)?

Scores of 2 or more are fairly strongly associated with an alcohol problem.

7 Family and social history

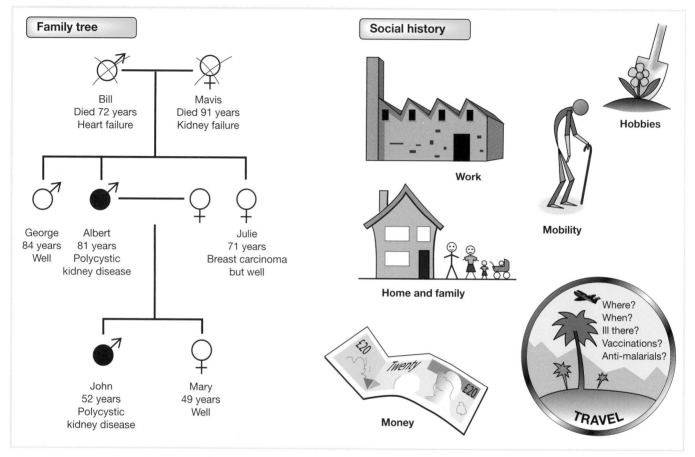

Family history

It is important to establish the diseases that have affected relatives given the strong genetic contribution to many diseases.

- 'What relatives do you have?'
- 'Are your parents still alive? If not, how old were they when they died? What did they die from? Did they suffer from any significant illnesses?'
- 'Have you any siblings, children or grandchildren?'
- 'Are there any diseases that run in the family?' (In rare genetic conditions consider the possibility of consanguinity; you can construct a family tree.)
- 'Are there any illnesses that "run in the family"?'

Social history

It is vital to understand the patient's background and the effect of their illnesses on their life and their family. Particular occupations are at risk of certain illnesses so a full occupational history is important. The following questions should be asked:

- 'What is your job? What does that actually involve doing?'
- 'What other jobs have you done?'
- 'Who do you live with? Is your partner well? Who else is at home? What sort of place do you live in?'

- 'Do you have any financial difficulties?'
- 'Who does the shopping, washing, cleaning, bathing, etc.?'
- 'What have your illnesses prevented you doing?'
- 'How has it affected your spouse and family?'
- 'Do you get out of the house much? What is your mobility like? How far can you walk? Do you have stairs at home?'
- 'What are your hobbies?'
- 'What help do you get at home? Do you have a home help or "meals-on-wheels"? What modifications have been made to the house?'
- 'Do you have pets? Are they well?'

Travel history

Consider the following questions when taking a travel history from the patient:

- 'Have you been abroad? Where? When?'
- 'Where did you stop *en route*?'
- 'Where did you visit? Was it rural or urban?'
- 'Did you stay in hotels, camps, etc.?'
- 'Were you well whilst there?'
- 'Did you have specific vaccinations? Have you taken anti-malarial prophylaxis? If so, what and for how long?'

Medicine at a Glance, Fourth Edition. Edited by Patrick Davey. © 2014 John Wiley & Sons, Ltd. Published 2014 by John Wiley & Sons, Ltd. Companion website: www.ataglanceseries.com/medicine

8 Functional enquiry

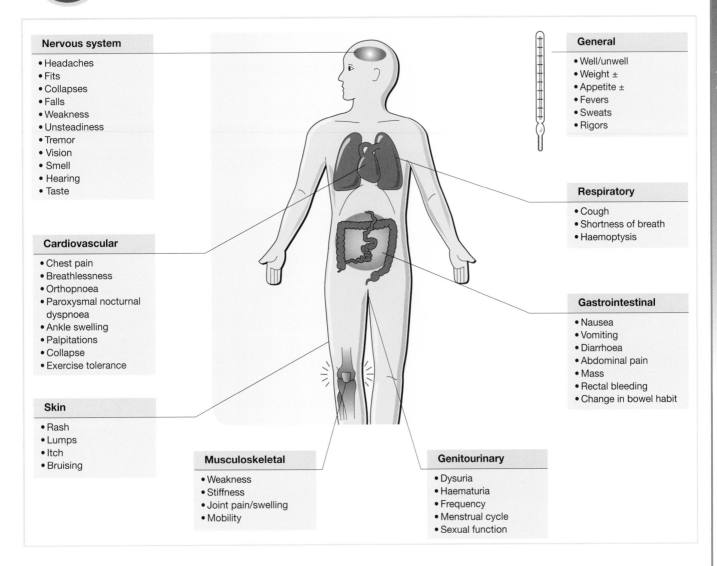

Nervous system
- Headaches
- Fits
- Collapses
- Falls
- Weakness
- Unsteadiness
- Tremor
- Vision
- Smell
- Hearing
- Taste

Cardiovascular
- Chest pain
- Breathlessness
- Orthopnoea
- Paroxysmal nocturnal dyspnoea
- Ankle swelling
- Palpitations
- Collapse
- Exercise tolerance

Skin
- Rash
- Lumps
- Itch
- Bruising

Musculoskeletal
- Weakness
- Stiffness
- Joint pain/swelling
- Mobility

General
- Well/unwell
- Weight ±
- Appetite ±
- Fevers
- Sweats
- Rigors

Respiratory
- Cough
- Shortness of breath
- Haemoptysis

Gastrointestinal
- Nausea
- Vomiting
- Diarrhoea
- Abdominal pain
- Mass
- Rectal bleeding
- Change in bowel habit

Genitourinary
- Dysuria
- Haematuria
- Frequency
- Menstrual cycle
- Sexual function

This part of the history is designed to address any symptoms that have not been elicited from the patient in the history of the presenting complaint. There are obviously a huge number of questions that can be asked. In any given clinical situation these questions will need to be focused depending on the nature of the presenting complaint. The discovery of abnormalities on examination or after investigation may lead to the necessity for further directed questioning. Ask about the symptoms in Figure 8.1.

The overwhelmingly two most important aspects of the functional enquiry are:

1 To establish the exercise capacity of the patient – how far they can walk unaided in one go (flat and hills), and the symptom that stops them. *If you only ask one question ask this one!*

2 To ascertain whether the patient has a systemic illness, the usual manifestations of which are feeling unwell (malaise), loss of appetite and weight loss.

Other general questions that may be appropriate are asking about heat or cold intolerance (thyroid disorders) or whether there has been any recent injury or falls.

You should specifically ask about breathlessness, on effort and at night, wheeze and chest pain. Also, ask about pains anywhere. Ask whether the patient has brought up blood (coughing, vomiting), or passed blood in their urine and stool. Do not forget the gynaecological history: length of the menstrual cycle, period duration, whether periods are heavy, number of pregnancies, age of menarche and menopause.

Ask if the patient has any other symptoms or concerns that have not yet been discussed, e.g. 'Is there anything else bothering you?', 'Do you have any other worries about your health?'

Medicine at a Glance, Fourth Edition. Edited by Patrick Davey. © 2014 John Wiley & Sons, Ltd. Published 2014 by John Wiley & Sons, Ltd. Companion website: www.ataglanceseries.com/medicine

9 Principles of examination

Ensure

Patient's comfort, privacy, confidentiality
Presence of chaperone if appropriate

Optimize examination conditions

- Exposure of relevant area
- Lighting/sound
- Positioning

Then

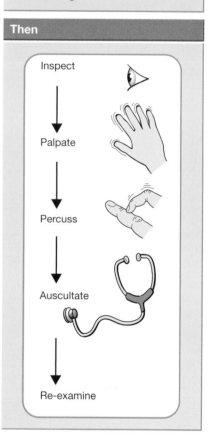

Inspect
↓
Palpate
↓
Percuss
↓
Auscultate
↓
Re-examine

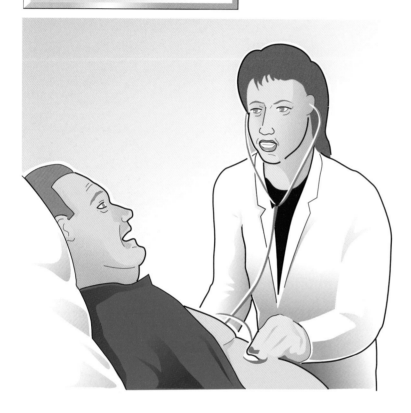

Explain to the patient what you plan to do. Ensure they are comfortable, warm and that there is privacy. Use all your senses: sight, hearing, smell and touch.

Inspect

Stand back. Look at the whole patient. Ensure there is adequate lighting.

- Look around the bed for other 'clues' (e.g. oxygen mask, nebulizer, sputum pot, walking stick, vomit bowl).
- Ensure the patient is adequately exposed (with privacy and comfort) and correctly positioned to permit a full examination.
- Look carefully and thoroughly. Are there any obvious abnormalities (e.g. lumps, unconsciousness, jaundice, cyanosis)? Are there any subtle abnormalities (e.g. pallor, fasciculations)?
- Look with specific manoeuvres, such as coughing, breathing or movement.

Palpate

Seek the patient's permission and explain what you are going to do. Ask whether there is any pain or tenderness. Begin the examination lightly and gently and then use firmer pressure. Define any abnormalities carefully, perhaps with measurement. Check if there are thrills.

Percuss

Percuss comparing sides. Listen and 'feel' for any differences. Ensure that this does not cause pain or discomfort.

Auscultate

Ensure the stethoscope is functioning and take time to listen. Consider the positioning of the patient to optimize sounds; for example, sitting forward and listening in expiration for aortic regurgitation.

If abnormalities are found at any stage, try to compare them with the 'normal'; for example, compare the percussion note over equivalent areas of the chest.

Record findings accurately, measure any abnormality and consider photographic documentation of, for example, a leg ulcer.

Medicine at a Glance, Fourth Edition. Edited by Patrick Davey. © 2014 John Wiley & Sons, Ltd. Published 2014 by John Wiley & Sons, Ltd. Companion website: www.ataglanceseries.com/medicine

10 Basic clinical skills

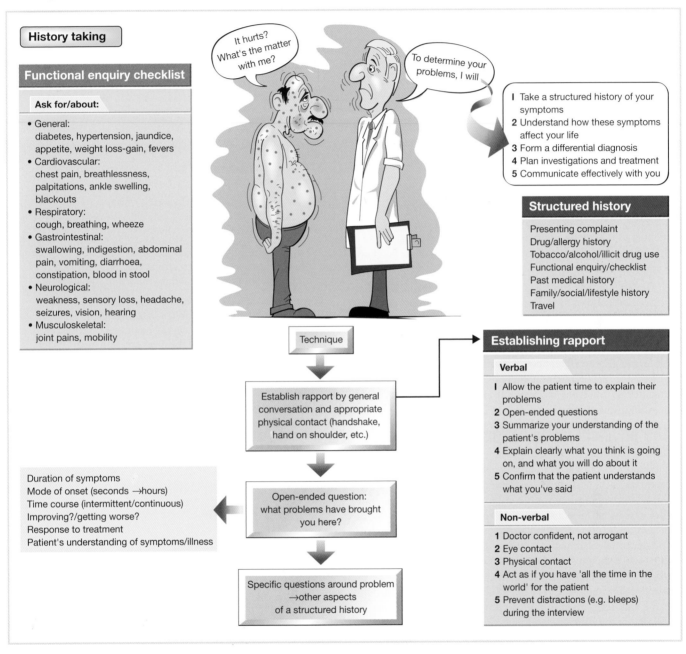

History taking

Functional enquiry checklist

Ask for/about:

- General:
  diabetes, hypertension, jaundice, appetite, weight loss-gain, fevers
- Cardiovascular:
  chest pain, breathlessness, palpitations, ankle swelling, blackouts
- Respiratory:
  cough, breathing, wheeze
- Gastrointestinal:
  swallowing, indigestion, abdominal pain, vomiting, diarrhoea, constipation, blood in stool
- Neurological:
  weakness, sensory loss, headache, seizures, vision, hearing
- Musculoskeletal:
  joint pains, mobility

It hurts? What's the matter with me?

To determine your problems, I will

1 Take a structured history of your symptoms
2 Understand how these symptoms affect your life
3 Form a differential diagnosis
4 Plan investigations and treatment
5 Communicate effectively with you

Structured history

Presenting complaint
Drug/allergy history
Tobacco/alcohol/illicit drug use
Functional enquiry/checklist
Past medical history
Family/social/lifestyle history
Travel

Technique

Establishing rapport

Verbal

1 Allow the patient time to explain their problems
2 Open-ended questions
3 Summarize your understanding of the patient's problems
4 Explain clearly what you think is going on, and what you will do about it
5 Confirm that the patient understands what you've said

Establish rapport by general conversation and appropriate physical contact (handshake, hand on shoulder, etc.)

Duration of symptoms
Mode of onset (seconds →hours)
Time course (intermittent/continuous)
Improving?/getting worse?
Response to treatment
Patient's understanding of symptoms/illness

Open-ended question: what problems have brought you here?

Non-verbal

1 Doctor confident, not arrogant
2 Eye contact
3 Physical contact
4 Act as if you have 'all the time in the world' for the patient
5 Prevent distractions (e.g. bleeps) during the interview

Specific questions around problem →other aspects of a structured history

Clinical assessment of the patient

Competence in the fundamental clinical skills of history taking and physical examination is crucial to being a good doctor. Developing this competence can only be attained by many hours of deliberate practice, and the experience of presenting your findings and thoughts about diagnosis to other doctors: you need to seize every opportunity to do this. Clinical assessment is the foundation of diagnosis and management. History taking should not be skimped as diagnostic gold is most often to be found in the patient's narrative. Your examination should begin while you are taking the history, and you will often need to expand the history in the light of the examination findings.

After the history and examination, you need to be clear about:

- The clinical problems of the patient, i.e. the symptoms and signs placed in coherent groupings (e.g. back pain and progressive weakness of the legs in a man with carcinoma of the prostate).
- The differential diagnosis of these problems (a shortlist of possible diagnoses to account for each clinical problem). As well as the most likely diagnosis (the working diagnosis), you must also

Medicine at a Glance, Fourth Edition. Edited by Patrick Davey. © 2014 John Wiley & Sons, Ltd. Published 2014 by John Wiley & Sons, Ltd. Companion website: www.ataglanceseries.com/medicine

consider those other possible diagnoses that are most serious if missed, and most treatable if found.

● The impact of these problems on the patient as a person (e.g. the ability to work or look after their family; to carry out activities of daily living).

● A plan of action (to include investigation, treatment and what you will say to the patient about the diagnosis and prognosis).

Taking the history

Open the interview with a few friendly words of introduction: establishing rapport with the patient is crucially important to good communication.

● Begin with an open-ended question (e.g. 'Perhaps you would start by telling me the problems that led to you coming into hospital') and *listen* to the patient's story, taking notes as the patient talks.

● After a few minutes of listening, you will usually need to clarify points in the history with the intelligent use of questions. This applies particularly to complaints such as weakness, dizziness, blackouts, collapse and indigestion – words that are applied to a number of different symptoms.

● Cover all the important areas (see Table 10.1) so that you have a complete picture.

Having taken the history, you should summarize the major problems identified, mentally or on paper, and form a provisional differential diagnosis. This will help focus your examination and ensure that you do not miss key physical signs – those which can rule in or rule out possible diagnoses. Do not perform the physical examination on 'autopilot', but rather adjust it in light of the history and ongoing examination findings. You should always be prepared to interrupt the physical examination to ask further questions if necessary.

The physical examination

Before examining the patient, you must obtain his or her consent, and ensure that privacy and dignity will be maintained during the examination. A chaperone, ideally of the same sex as the patient, should be present when you are examining a patient of the opposite sex. For intimate examinations – examination of the female breasts, vaginal examination, examination of the male genitalia and anorectal examination – the chaperone must be a nurse or doctor, you should have the permission of a doctor with responsibility for the care of the patient to carry out this element of the examination, and the patient should confirm consent. Record the name and designation of the chaperone when you write up the clerking in the patient's medical record.

You must adapt your examination method to the circumstances. For most patients, you should examine in detail the system or systems relevant to the clinical problem, and also perform a rapid but thorough general examination. One approach is to perform a general examination by region (e.g. hands–arms–head–neck–chest–abdomen–legs–feet) and then complete a detailed examination of the relevant system or systems. Before you lay hands on the patient, it pays dividends to step back, metaphorically at least, and make a general survey. Does the patient look well or ill and, if ill, in what way? Endocrine disorders (such as hypothyroidism) are easily missed unless you make a point of thinking of them. Table 10.2 gives a checklist for the general examination.

Examination of systems

● **Cardiovascular system**: pulse rate/rhythm; blood pressure; jugular venous pressure (JVP) (height and waveform); carotid

Table 10.1 Checklist for history taking.

● **Age, sex, racial origin and occupation**

● **Main symptoms**

● **History of symptoms**: mode of onset (abrupt/gradual), time course (constant/intermittent; getting better/getting worse/staying the same) and response to treatment

● **Current and previous medication** including over-the-counter and other non-prescribed remedies. Ask women if they are taking the oral contraceptive pill or hormone replacement therapy

● **Allergies to medications and other substances**: clarify the type of allergic response. Also ask about other important adverse effects of medications

● **Tobacco and alcohol use** (and use of recreational drugs if the clinical problem suggests that this may be relevant)

● **Functional enquiry/systems review**: this is your checklist to make sure that no important symptoms have been overlooked or forgotten by the patient

● **Past history**: organized under medical, surgical, obstetric-gynaecological, traumatic (bone fractures and other significant injuries) and psychiatric headings

● **Family history**: establish the age, health or cause of death of parents, siblings and children ('Has anyone in your family had the same problems as you have?'). The family history may be relevant to the diagnosis, and often contributes to an understanding of why certain symptoms may have a particular emotional significance to the patient

● **Social history** including occupational history ('Which job do you do now? Which job did you do before that? Which job have you done the longest?'). In patients with respiratory symptoms, ask specifically about occupational exposure to dusts, fumes and asbestos

● **Personal history**: you need to understand the lifestyle of the patient. If the patient is disabled, who are the main carers? Are services used? Other aspects which may be relevant are: sexual history (begin with an open-ended question such as 'Who are the most important people in your life?'), pets and other contact with animals, and travel history

pulse upstroke and volume; inspection and palpation of the precordium; auscultation of the heart; palpation of the abdominal aorta and peripheral pulses; auscultation for carotid, abdominal and femoral bruits; percussion and auscultation of the lung bases; examination for sacral and peripheral oedema. Recording an electrocardiogram (ECG) can be regarded as part of the examination of the cardiovascular system.

● **Respiratory system**: character of the voice; presence and quality of cough; sputum character and quantity; respiratory rate; presence of stridor or wheeze; examination of the upper respiratory tract (nose, tonsils, pharynx, trachea); inspection, palpation, percussion and auscultation of the chest; bedside spirometry and measurement of peak expiratory flow rate.

● **Alimentary and genitourinary systems**: inspect the lips, tongue, teeth and gums; inspection, palpation, percussion and auscultation of the abdomen (including hernial orifices); examine external genitalia; inspection and digital examination of the anorectum; vaginal examination (anorectal and vaginal

Table 10.2 Examination checklist.

- **General appearance**: well/acutely unwell/chronically unwell?

- **Conscious level and mental state** (e.g. lucid, confused, agitated)

- **Nutritional state**: body mass index (BMI: weight in kilograms/[height in metres]^2) <20 underweight, 20–25 normal weight, 25–30 overweight, >30 obese

- **Temperature**

- **Presence or absence of specific important signs**:

  - *Pallor* (conjunctival pallor is typically present when haemoglobin is <10 g/dL)

  - *Cyanosis* (central cyanosis is usually detectable when arterial oxygen saturation is <90%, unless anaemia is present; however, it is an unreliable sign, and where possible always check oxygen saturation with pulse oximetry)

  - *Jaundice* (detectable when bilirubin concentration is >40–50 micromol/L)

  - *Clubbing* (causes include intrathoracic neoplasms and infection, cyanotic congenital heart disease and inflammatory bowel disease)

  - *Lymphadenopathy* (check supraclavicular, epitrochlear, axillary and inguinal regions)

  - *Breast lump*

  - *Thyroid enlargement and nodules, and clinical thyroid status*

  - *Abnormalities of the skin, nails and subcutaneous tissues* (e.g. rash, pigmentation, surgical and other scars, purpura, bruising, lumps, ulceration)

  - *Metabolic 'flap'* of the hands held outstretched with extension at the wrist (seen in respiratory failure, liver failure and advanced renal failure)

- **Examination of systems**: see text

examination should only be done when specifically indicated); stick testing of the urine.

- **Nervous system**: evaluation of the mental state, speech and other higher cerebral functions; examination of the skull and spine; testing of the cranial nerves; ophthalmoscopy; examination of the motor system – limbs, trunk, stance and gait; examination of the sensory system.
- **Musculoskeletal system**: examination of the limb joints and spine for swelling, deformity, tenderness and restriction of movement; examination of the bones for deformity and tenderness and of the muscles for wasting and tenderness; observation of the patient standing, walking and turning.

Rapid neurological and musculoskeletal examination

If neurological or musculoskeletal disease is not suspected, the minimum examination is to:

- Inspect the hands for wasting of the intrinsic muscles and joint abnormalities, test the power of finger abduction, and check light touch sensation over the hands – gently stroke the skin and ask the patient if this feels normal and equal on both sides.

- Ask the patient to hold the arms outstretched with palms down and fingers abducted, and to make piano-playing movements (upper motor neuron lesions cause the movements to be performed more slowly or clumsily), then to turn the palms up and maintain the posture with the eyes closed (upper motor neuron lesions cause the arm to drift downwards and into pronation).
- Put the wrist, elbow and shoulder joints through their range of movement (to assess muscle tone, and to detect restriction of joint movement) and test the power of shoulder abduction (proximal limb weakness is a feature of myopathies). Ask the patient to put the hands behind the head with the elbows back (to assess the glenohumeral, acromioclavicular and sternoclavicular joints). Check the finger–nose test.
- Check cervical spine movements (ask the patient to touch the ear on to the shoulder).
- Check visual acuity, fields, eye movements and pupils and examine the fundi.
- Put the hip, knee and ankle joints through their range of movement (including rotation of the hip joint with the knee flexed, to assess muscle tone and detect restriction of joint movement); test the power of hip flexion.
- Inspect the feet: test the power of ankle dorsiflexion. Check light touch sensation over the feet – gently stroke the skin and ask the patient if this feels normal and equal on both sides. Check the heel–knee–shin test; test the tendon reflexes and plantar responses.
- Observe the patient standing, walking and turning.

Presenting the case

The cardinal virtues here are brevity, clarity and enthusiasm. Your presentation should last under 5 minutes. If your listener wants more detail, he or she will ask for it. Always include the age and occupation of the patient in your opening remarks. Do not mention the sex and racial origin of the patient if you are presenting the case in his or her presence. Begin with a short summary of the patient's problems; this is especially important in patients with chronic illness who may have multiple medical and social problems. You should then deal, in turn, with information from the history, the findings on examination, your differential diagnosis and the plan of action.

Making the diagnosis

What is diagnosis?

Diagnosis is the central intellectual activity of medicine. It is the process whereby we turn data about the patient into the names of diseases ('diagnoses'). A diagnosis is important because it serves as a guide to action, and it helps us foretell the future ('prognosis'). Providing patients with a diagnosis helps them make sense of what has been happening to their bodies, and to feel they are not alone. The data we bring to the diagnostic process are of many types: elements in the history (e.g. headache), an examination finding (e.g. enlargement of the spleen) or a test result (e.g. microcytic anaemia).

Why can diagnosis be difficult?

So if diagnosis is simply about mapping data onto diseases, why is it difficult?

- Most manifestations of disease are not specific to one diagnosis, e.g. breathlessness can be caused by heart or lung disease, anaemia and many other disorders.
- There are around 5000 clinical manifestations of disease (symptoms, signs, epidemiological data, laboratory and imaging

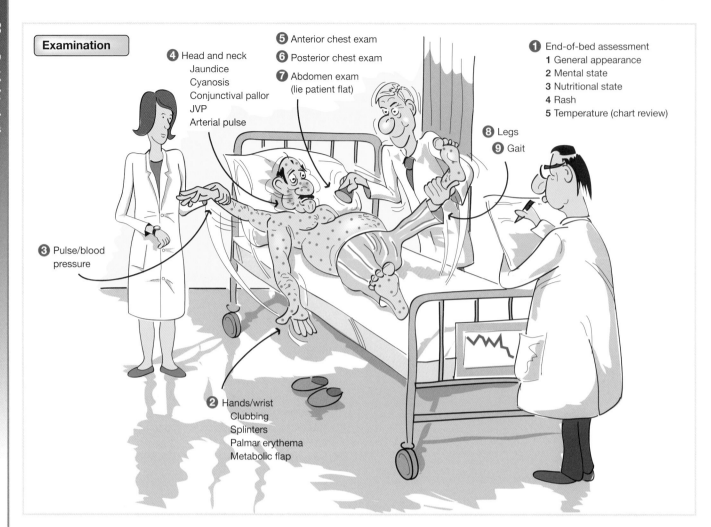

Examination

④ Head and neck
  Jaundice
  Cyanosis
  Conjunctival pallor
  JVP
  Arterial pulse

⑤ Anterior chest exam
⑥ Posterior chest exam
⑦ Abdomen exam
  (lie patient flat)

① End-of-bed assessment
  1 General appearance
  2 Mental state
  3 Nutritional state
  4 Rash
  5 Temperature (chart review)

⑧ Legs
⑨ Gait

③ Pulse/blood
  pressure

② Hands/wrist
  Clubbing
  Splinters
  Palmar erythema
  Metabolic flap

findings), which may occur singly or in combination, and with different time courses, and there are over 10 000 diseases.

● Distinguishing between normal and abnormal may be difficult; for example, is breathlessness due to ageing, physical deconditioning, weight gain or disease?

● The data are often unreliable or partial (e.g. elements in the history may be forgotten by the patient or misinterpreted by the doctor); physical signs may be overlooked or misinterpreted; test results may be misleading (e.g. because the test is not always normal in health and abnormal in disease).

● Patients may have more than one disease (multiple pathology).

● Rare diseases are, in aggregate, common: throughout your professional life you will continue to see patients with diseases that you have not encountered before.

● Some symptoms are medically inexplicable.

● Humans make mistakes in the analysis of data.

How do we go about making a diagnosis?

The presenting complaint is often the key to the diagnosis, because the problem that took the patient to the doctor generally reflects an important manifestation of the patient's illness. Accordingly, the best place to start the diagnostic process is usually with the presenting complaint. How does one analyse the presenting complaint? Several approaches are possible:

● Analysis by body region: this method works well for complaints of pain, e.g. headache, chest pain and abdominal pain.

● Analysis by system: this method works well for functional disorders such as breathlessness or muscle weakness.

● Analysis by organ: e.g. breast lump.

Working towards diagnosis

The road to the diagnosis has several distinct stages. The first is to review the key findings on history and examination, and to put them together in coherent groups. For example, if the patient complains of retrosternal chest discomfort consistently provoked by exercise and relieved promptly by rest, these features can be summarized as typical exertional angina. Having decided on the clinical problem or problems, the next stage is to form a differential diagnosis, a short list of possible diseases that could account for these clinical problems. Lists can be generated from experience, from discussion with colleagues, from reading the medical literature and from other resources such as the internet. A Google search is often a fruitful way of expanding the differential diagnosis. Suggestions from the patient and their family as to the diagnosis may sometimes be very helpful, and should always be considered seriously.

As well as the most likely diagnosis (the working diagnosis), your differential diagnoses should also include those other possible diseases that are most serious if missed, and most treatable if found. To return to our patient with exertional angina, the differential diagnoses includes atheromatous coronary artery disease, aortic stenosis and hypertrophic cardiomyopathy. The clinical and ECG findings will usually allow us to differentiate between these three diseases. If our patient has a slow-rising carotid pulse, a muffled second heart sound and a loud midsystolic murmur at the base of the heart, then angina due to severe aortic stenosis will be the working diagnosis. This is the diagnosis on which you will base your immediate management decisions (e.g. what investigation to do first, what treatment to give). The final diagnosis is the diagnosis made when all the information is in (in this particular case, after the patient has had an echocardiogram, which showed a calcified bicuspid aortic valve with severe stenosis, and an angiogram which revealed no epicardial coronary disease).

A further example would be headache with fever in a 23-year-old medical student just returned from India, with full blood count showing thrombocytopenia. The differential diagnosis includes malaria, typhoid and bacterial or viral meningitis. The additional clinical features in this case make malaria your working diagnosis. Investigation shows malarial parasites on microscopy of a thick blood film, subsequently shown to be *Plasmodium falciparum*. Lumbar puncture reveals normal cerebrospinal fluid, and blood culture is negative. Thus, the final diagnosis is falciparum malaria.

Reasoning about diagnosis

Reasoning about diagnosis is very similar to detective work, or solving problems such as why your car will not start. Having generated a differential diagnosis, you need to work through the diagnoses on the list and ask yourself these questions: 'How well does this diagnosis account for the important positive and negative clinical findings, and the time course of the patient's illness?' 'If this diagnosis is accepted, how many loose ends are left?' You are looking for the diagnosis that has the greatest explanatory power, unifies the largest number of findings and leaves the fewest loose ends. Bear in mind that common diseases do indeed commonly occur. A 60-year-old man with typical exertional angina will usually have atheromatous coronary artery disease. However, if the ECG shows voltage evidence of left ventricular hypertropy with marked ST/T changes, the blood pressure is normal and there is no systolic murmur, hypertrophic cardiomyopathy is the more likely diagnosis – or both disorders are present.

At the end of this process of reasoning, you will have worked through the differential diagnoses, weeded out the diagnoses which do not pass muster, and ranked the others in order of probability. You will be clear as to what additional information will be helpful in discriminating between the diagnoses left on the list.

Coordinating diagnosis with the safe care of the patient

Sometimes one can make the right diagnosis immediately and with confidence. However, often the situation is less than ideal: the diagnosis is unclear, and the tests required to rule in or rule out possible diagnoses are not available (e.g. because it is the middle of the night) or take too long to come back (e.g. blood culture). In this case, you must treat what is probable, and what might be dangerous, while data collection continues. Correction of abnormal physiology is crucial in those with life-threatening disease (e.g. volume replacement in severe gastrointestinal bleeding). Immediate empirical treatment may be needed for illnesses that are dangerous and rapidly progressive (e.g. empirical antibiotic therapy in suspected bacterial meningitis, before lumbar puncture). For patients seen in clinic, with symptoms that do not point to major illness and with reassuring findings on examination, observation over time (with or without further investigation) may be the right course.

Avoiding mistakes in diagnosis

Misdiagnosis is common, and results from:

- Lack of knowledge (e.g. not knowing of rare diagnoses such as oesophageal rupture or cerebral venous sinus thrombosis).
- Inexperience of the 'fuzziness' of many diagnoses (e.g. the many ways in which pulmonary embolism can present).
- Jumping to conclusions, and accepting the 'obvious' diagnosis without considering others (e.g. fever, elevated right hemidiaphragm and right basal lung shadowing after laparoscopic appendicectomy attributed to pneumonia without exclusion of subphrenic abscess).
- Not reconsidering the diagnosis as more data become available.

The best way to improve your skill at diagnosis is repeated practice with new patients seen on-take or in the clinic, attending case presentations (which will enlarge your experience of rare diseases and atypical presentations of common ones) and reading the literature. Remember, 'Clinical diagnosis is an art, and the mastery of the art has no end; you can always be a better diagnostician'.

11 Is the patient ill?

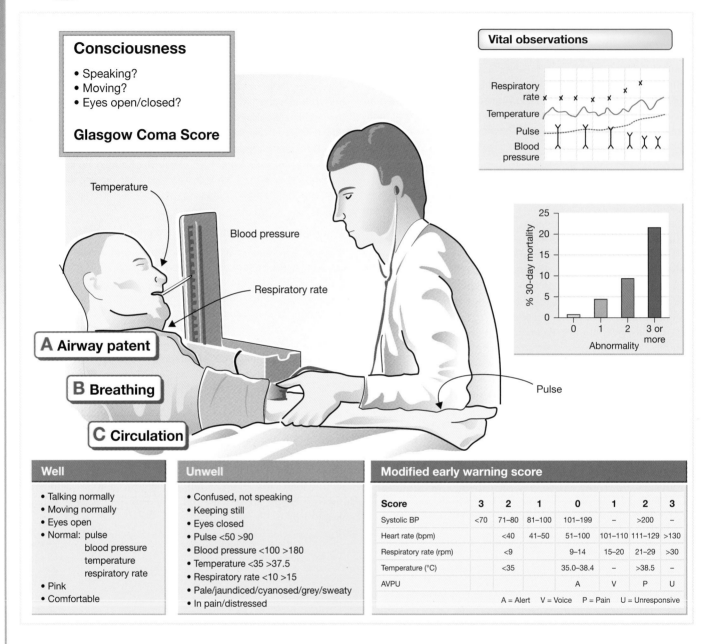

Consciousness

- Speaking?
- Moving?
- Eyes open/closed?

Glasgow Coma Score

Temperature

Blood pressure

Respiratory rate

A Airway patent

B Breathing

C Circulation

Vital observations

Respiratory rate
Temperature
Pulse
Blood pressure

% 30-day mortality

Abnormality

Pulse

Well	Unwell
• Talking normally	• Confused, not speaking
• Moving normally	• Keeping still
• Eyes open	• Eyes closed
• Normal: pulse	• Pulse <50 >90
blood pressure	• Blood pressure <100 >180
temperature	• Temperature <35 >37.5
respiratory rate	• Respiratory rate <10 >15
• Pink	• Pale/jaundiced/cyanosed/grey/sweaty
• Comfortable	• In pain/distressed

Modified early warning score

Score	3	2	1	0	1	2	3
Systolic BP	<70	71–80	81–100	101–199	–	>200	–
Heart rate (bpm)		<40	41–50	51–100	101–110	111–129	>130
Respiratory rate (rpm)		<9		9–14	15–20	21–29	>30
Temperature (°C)		<35		35.0–38.4	–	>38.5	–
AVPU				A	V	P	U

A = Alert   V = Voice   P = Pain   U = Unresponsive

One of the most important skills a doctor can gain is the recognition that a patient is ill. The definition of 'being ill' or 'being sick' is different in hospital medicine when compared to primary care, or from what patients mean by this phrase:

- Patients mean they feel unwell, or, in other words, experience malaise; most inflammatory illnesses cause this, and, in primary care, most of these are benign and self-limiting, with a low mortality risk. This definition is not what doctors mean by the phrase.
- In primary care the phrase usually implies a need for immediate hospital admission; mortality risk exists, but is relatively low, probably around 2–5%.
- In hospital the phrase 'being ill' means that the patient has a high chance of early death or disability. This is largely what most

hospital doctors mean when they say a patient is ill – they think the patient has an appreciable chance of dying, and dying really quite soon.

So, being ill in hospital inevitably leads to the activation of many resources, including specialist wards (coronary care, high dependency unit, critical care), specialist clinicians, and often expensive out-of-hours investigations and treatment. This complex array of therapies is applied to improve an otherwise poor outcome. It is therefore really important to, where possible, diagnose the severity of a patient's illness accurately, so that ill patients can benefit from such resources, avoiding the inappropriate use of these expensive resources, and so that patients and relatives can be prepared for a poor outcome. Once you think the

Medicine at a Glance, Fourth Edition. Edited by Patrick Davey. © 2014 John Wiley & Sons, Ltd. Published 2014 by John Wiley & Sons, Ltd. Companion website: www.ataglanceseries.com/medicine

patient is acutely and seriously ill, get help immediately from other doctors and nurses.

There are several features that experienced clinicians notice instantly as signs that a patient is seriously ill.

Clues from the history

● There are many clues in the history to pick up on – for example, acute severe breathlessness following a long plane journey is likely to constitute a life-threatening pulmonary embolus; or a patient who has just had a very sudden onset of the most severe headache they have ever experienced may have had a critical subarachnoid haemorrhage. In other words, many clinicians will know a patient is ill before they have even seen them!

Laboratory clues

Some patients may have immediately life-threatening illness without any abnormal findings (e.g. severe hyperkalaemia); always check laboratory results on *all* patients shortly after admission in case this applies to your apparently healthy patient.

Observational clues

Experienced nurses and clinicians may also feel that a patient is seriously ill without being able to identify objective abnormalities. Patients who are seriously ill often look ill; picking up on this is an acquired skill, and experienced clinicians are amalgamating information from the history and examination in reaching this diagnosis.

Clues from the charts

However, perhaps the most important means to pick up on sickness is from the vital observations of pulse, blood pressure, temperature, respiratory rate and conscious level. These data can then be picked up in 'early warning scores' (see Figure 11.1), firstly on the early warning score itself and secondly on the relationship between the score and mortality.

Assessment of ill patients

Once you think a patient is ill, go through the following ABC checklist to further assess the patient – this list will essentially tell you that the patient's lungs, cardiovascular system and brain are, at least for the time being, functioning:

● **A for airway.** Is the airway patent? Is the patient breathing easily and talking comfortably? Is there stridor?

● **B for breathing.** Is the patient breathing slowly or rapidly? Noisily? With difficulty, such that they are unable to talk because of breathlessness? Check the respiratory rate, and the pattern of breathing – for example, are there periods of deep breathing lasting half a minute or so interspersed with almost absent breathing, so-called Cheyne–Stokes respiration (found in brainstem lesions and heart failure)? Is there wheeze, and are the accessory muscles being used?

● **C for circulation.** Check there is adequate circulation – are the peripheries warm or cold, is there peripheral (poor cardiac output or vasoconstricted) or central (arterial hypoxaemia) cyanosis? Is the pulse volume low, and what is the heart rate? What is the blood pressure, and is there a postural drop (suggests hypovolaemia)?

General findings

● Is the patient comfortable or uncomfortable?
● What is the patient's colour? Is the patient pale? (Anaemia or shock?)
● What is the temperature? Is the patient pyrexial? Hypothermic?
● Is the patient blue (cyanosed)?
● Is the patient grey? (Combination of cyanosis and pallor?)
● Is the patient clammy? (Sweaty and poor perfusion?)
● Is the patient sweaty?
● Is the patient in pain? Grimacing? Appearing abnormally still?
● Is the patient moving normally, restless or paralysed?

Consciousness

The level of consciousness is well assessed using the Glasgow Coma Score; if significantly impaired, is there abnormal posture, e.g. abnormal extension of limbs (decerebrate) or abnormal flexion of arms (decorticate)? If the Glasgow Coma Score is normal, further assessment of brain function can be picked up by the following:

● Is the patient confused? If so, use the mini-mental state score.
● How does the patient engage with you? Can they talk, smile, make eye contact and answer questions appropriately (are they drowsy, but not actually confused)?

In any patient, significant changes in these observations may indicate serious deterioration.

12 The critically ill patient

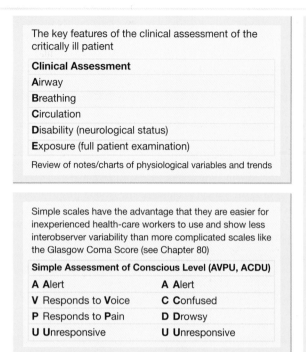

The key features of the clinical assessment of the critically ill patient

Clinical Assessment

Airway

Breathing

Circulation

Disability (neurological status)

Exposure (full patient examination)

Review of notes/charts of physiological variables and trends

Simple scales have the advantage that they are easier for inexperienced health-care workers to use and show less interobserver variability than more complicated scales like the Glasgow Coma Score (see Chapter 80)

Simple Assessment of Conscious Level (AVPU, ACDU)

A **A**lert	**A** **A**lert
V Responds to **V**oice	**C** **C**onfused
P Responds to **P**ain	**D** **D**rowsy
U **U**nresponsive	**U** **U**nresponsive

Clinical response to NEWS triggers

NEWS SCORE	FREQUENCY OF MONITORING	CLINICAL RESPONSE
0	Minimum 12 hourly	• Continue routine NEWS monitoring with every set of observations
Aggregate 1–3	Minimum 4 hourly	• Inform trained nurse who must assess the patient • Trained nurse to decide if increased frequency of monitoring and/or escalation of clinical care is required
Aggregate 4 or more or 3 in one parameter	Increased frequency to a minimum of 1 hourly	• Trained nurse to immediately inform the medical team caring for the patient • Urgent assessment by medical/surgical/critical care outreach team with core competencies to assess acutely ill patients • Clinical care in an environment with monitoring facilities
Aggregate 6 or more	Continuous monitoring of vital signs	• Trained nurse to urgently inform the medical team caring for the patient – this should be at least at Specialist Registrar level • Emergency assessment by a clinical team with core competencies in the assessment of critically ill patients. This team will have critical care competencies and a practitioner/s with advanced airway skills and resuscitation skills • Consider transfer of clinical care to a level 2 or 3 care facility, i.e.higher dependency or ITU

Recognition of the critically ill patient

The severity of illness and associated patient mortality varies widely between individuals (and demographics such as age, and co-morbid illness, such as diabetes, previous infirmity, etc., are all crucial). However, when approaching a potentially sick patient, as in all other patients, taking a history, performing an examination and ordering appropriate investigations are essential in order to make the correct diagnosis and to institute appropriate therapy.

The management of critically ill patients outside the intensive therapy unit (ITU) is often suboptimal, predominantly because there has been a failure to recognize the severity of the patient's illness. Sometimes critical illness is obvious from the end of the bed. Often, however, critical illness is recognized by alterations in key physiological variables rather than 'just' by the patient 'looking' sick.

Maintenance of adequate airway, breathing and circulation are prerequisites for survival. Accordingly, simple physiological observations such as heart rate (HR), systolic blood pressure (BP), oxygen saturations, respiratory rate (RR), level of consciousness, urine output and temperature define inpatient mortality. Mortality can be directly correlated with the number of abnormalities, rising from 0.7% (30-day mortality) with none, 4.4% with one, 9.2% with two, to 21.3% with three or more.

Many patients who suffer a cardiorespiratory arrest or are admitted to intensive care have a documented decline in these physiological variables prior to these events, which often goes unrecognized. It is therefore important to have a system for recognizing critically ill patients, ensuring sufficient monitoring takes place in a designated area, instituting appropriate therapy and calling for additional help or expertise if required. In some cases it might be the realization that the patient is in the process of dying and the patient's symptoms should be palliated.

Examination of the critically ill patient

As the patient is examined, specific immediate life-saving therapies or investigations may be initiated, such as a chest drain in a patient with a tension pneumothorax, before other parts of the examination are undertaken. Adequate monitoring in an appropriate area also needs to be ensured. If the patient is being seen for the first time a full assessment of the notes needs to be undertaken.

Dysfunction of the airway, breathing or circulation can lead to immediate death and so the patient assessment should focus on these systems.

Airway

Obstruction of the airway is an emergency and unless rectified leads to rapid hypoxia and death within minutes. It is therefore pointless making an examination of the circulation in a hypotensive patient with an obstructed airway; indeed the hypotension may be the consequence of airway obstruction.

- **Complete airway obstruction** leads to paradoxical chest and abdominal movements so that the chest moves in on inspiration and the abdomen out (as opposed to both moving out in normal breathing) and vice versa on expiration. Accessory muscle use and a tracheal tug are present. No movement of air is present at the mouth either audibly or by feeling with a hand at the patient's mouth.
- **Partial airway obstruction** leads to noisy breathing with detectable movement of air at the mouth. Stridor indicates obstruction at the larynx or above, while snoring often occurs when the tongue obstructs the pharynx.

In the majority of patients simple measures resolve airway obstruction. Blood, vomit, secretions or foreign bodies may be removed by suction. If consciousness is impaired, loss of muscle tone causes the tongue to fall back and obstruct. A chin lift or jaw thrust opens the airway; occasionally an airway adjunct such as an oropharyngeal (Guedel) or nasopharyngeal airway is required. If these simple methods fail then endotracheal intubation or *rarely* a surgical cricothyroidotomy is required. The use of airway adjuncts, endotracheal intubation or surgical airways should only be performed by appropriately trained staff. These techniques may cause vomiting or laryngospasm if performed by inadequately trained individuals, potentially transforming a partially occluded airway to one that is completely obstructed.

Breathing

Visual examination is extremely informative, with respiratory rate being one of the most important observations. A rate <8 or >20 per minute should alert the examiner to severe illness. Tachypnoea is the most common physiolological abnormality in critical illness so great care should be undertaken to record respiratory rate accurately. Expansion of the chest should be compared bilaterally, as well as depth, abdominal breathing, accessory muscle use and tracheal tugging (respiratory pattern). Abnormal expansion usually accompanies underlying disease (collapse, consolidation, effusion, pneumothorax). The inspired oxygen concentration should be noted and oxygen saturations on pulse oximetry recorded (cyanosis is often a late sign); if indicated, a blood gas is performed. The latter provides information on adequacy of ventilation ($PaCO_2$) and oxygenation (PaO_2 and A-a gradient). Respiratory acidosis (pH <7.3, PCO_2 $>6.0\,kPa$) or failure of oxygenation (SaO_2 $<90\%$ or PaO_2 $<8\,kPa$ on high flow oxygen) requires urgent intervention. Treatment is discussed in Chapters 99, 105 and 106 – all critically ill patients need oxygen saturations maintained above 90%.

Circulation

Important parameters of the circulatory examination are blood pressure, pulse, capillary refill, limb temperature, urine output and level of consciousness. A 'normal' blood pressure may represent hypotension in some patients and it is therefore useful to know the patient's usual pressure. Hypotension may also be a late sign when homeostatic mechanisms fail to compensate and is usually preceded by an abnormal pulse (often tachycardia). Normal capillary refill is less than 2 seconds and prolongation suggests inadequate tissue perfusion. However, this sign is less reliable in elderly patients where normal capillary refill may exceed 2 seconds. An arterial blood gas may be indicated and show metabolic acidosis with a raised lactate if the circulation is inadequate (base excess more than -4 or lactate $>2\,mmol/L$). Treatment of circulatory abnormalities is discussed in Chapters 18 and 237.

Disability

Neurological status is assessed by examining the pupils and the level of consciousness (Glasgow Coma Score (GCS) or simple scales such as AVPU or ACDU; see Figure 12.1). Hypoglycaemia should be excluded in all sick patients.

Exposure

A general examination should be made with particular attention to drains and wound sites. The temperature should be recorded.

Examination of critically ill patients' charts

It is important to examine the patient's charts, which record physiological variables of blood pressure, pulse, temperature, respiratory rate, oxygen saturations, consciousness level and urine output over time. While the absolute values are important, *equal value is attached to the trends and response to treatment.* As emphasized earlier, the number of physiological abnormalities defines mortality. Earlier recognition of patient deterioration would be expected to prevent unexpected cardiac arrests and admissions to intensive care. Many hospitals now utilize severity triggers or modified early warning scoring systems in combination with medical emergency or outreach teams. Some disease-specific scoring systems that define severity of illness and mortality are also in common use and incorporate physiological variables; examples include the CURB-65 (community-acquired pneumonia) and Rockall (upper gastrointestinal bleeding) scores. The Royal College of Physicians has recommended a standardized NHS Early Warning Score (NEWS) be used in all NHS hospitals.

Admission to intensive care

This is a key decision in the management of the sick patient; clearly, patients who benefit from ITU should go there, whereas those who don't shouldn't. However, discriminating these two groups reliably is often not possible, and will require judgement. Obtaining patients' and relatives' views of ITU, in the light of data on outcomes, is crucial to the decision to admit to ITU. Most ITU admissions should be the consequence of discussions between the consultant looking after the patient and the consultant intensivist.

Treatment of the critically sick patient

This is covered in other chapters. Often the crucial question is 'how much treatment', rather than 'what sort of treatment'. This aspect requires great judgement, and excellent communication skills; indeed, in this area perhaps more than any other, the ability to know when to discontinue therapy, when not escalate treatment, and when to implement terminal care at just the right stage are what defines clinical excellence. As relatives often have inappropriately high expectations about the outcome of intensive care therapy, it is important to be realistic (and kind) at all times.

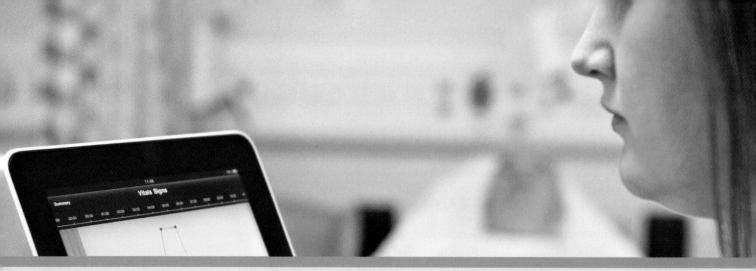

Chapters

Clinical presentations at a glance

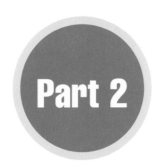

Part 2

Don't forget to visit the companion website for this book www.ataglanceseries.com/medicine for MCQs and flashcards on these topics

13 Chest pain

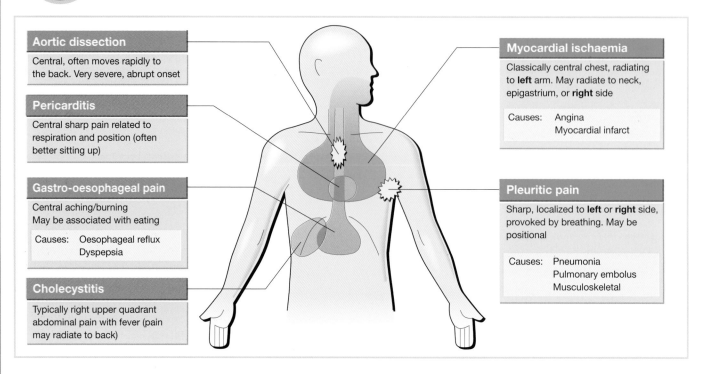

Aortic dissection

Central, often moves rapidly to the back. Very severe, abrupt onset

Pericarditis

Central sharp pain related to respiration and position (often better sitting up)

Gastro-oesophageal pain

Central aching/burning
May be associated with eating

Causes: Oesophageal reflux
Dyspepsia

Cholecystitis

Typically right upper quadrant abdominal pain with fever (pain may radiate to back)

Myocardial ischaemia

Classically central chest, radiating to **left** arm. May radiate to neck, epigastrium, or **right** side

Causes: Angina
Myocardial infarct

Pleuritic pain

Sharp, localized to **left** or **right** side, provoked by breathing. May be positional

Causes: Pneumonia
Pulmonary embolus
Musculoskeletal

Determining the origin of chest pain is a common clinical problem which can present a diagnostic challenge. The greatest concern is whether the pain relates to heart disease. This thought dominates the clinical and investigative approach. Most pains are diagnosed by a full history, sometimes aided by the examination. The diagnostic approach involves determining the nature of the pain, how long it has been present, typical provoking and relieving factors, and the presence of risk factors for heart/lung disease. For patients who are well you should always carry out the full diagnostic process in a thoughtful and methodical manner – history, then examination, then simple investigations, followed by synthesizing the differential diagnosis so as to guide special investigations. However, some patients with chest pain are sick, indeed, sometimes on the edge of death; in such sick patients you will have to act quickly, amalgamating the history with the examination, while simultaneously asking nurses, etc., to organize chest X-rays, and even computed tomography (CT) scans, immediate cath lab access, etc. Tailor your approach to the sickness of the patient.

In the reasonably healthy patient, once a diagnosis has been suggested by the history, perform the physical examination, both to try and obtain data to support the diagnosis (though this is often not forthcoming) and also to exclude other serious illness. Though a full examination should be carried out, the key aspects are to determine:

- Is the patient well; if not (see Chapter 12), you must rapidly work out why and start appropriate therapy as soon as possible.
- What is the haemodynamic status and oxygenation? Check skin perfusion (warm or cold), capillary refill time, heart rate, blood pressure and oxygen saturation; if there is any major upset you must reach a diagnosis quickly and intervene.

- Is there evidence of heart failure (see Chapter 87), especially tachycardia, raised JVP, third heart sound and bibasal pulmonary crepitations.
- Are there features of pulmonary embolus – particularly breathlessness, tachypnoea, increased heart rate, and hypoxia in the absence of lung signs indicating an alternative pathology (e.g. of infection, failure or chronic obstructive pulmonary disease (COPD))? Regardless of how certain you are about the diagnosis, always actively think whether pulmonary embolus could be a component of the illness.
- Are there features suggesting lung sepsis, such as fever, increased heart rate, tachypnoea and areas of bronchial breathing?
- Are there features that suggest major risk factors for coronary disease are present – old age, high BMI (suggesting the metabolic syndrome, the triad of hypertension, diabetes and increased abdominal girth), evidence of smoking (a lined face, nicotine-stained hands, smell of tobacco smoke on clothes), evidence of hyperlipidaemia (look for cholesterol deposits in extensor tendons, and around the eyes).
- Is there any evidence of vascular disease? Examine all peripheral pulses, and listen for bruits over the major arteries, particularly the carotids and femorals.
- Are there features of any important co-morbid illness, such as COPD, dementia, immobility or frailty that will impact on the diagnostic process and influence treatment.

Assimilate all the key historical and examination features so that you have a clear view of what has happened to the patient, what the likely diagnosis is, and what you are going to do about it. The diagnostic process for chronic chest pain versus acute

Medicine at a Glance, Fourth Edition. Edited by Patrick Davey. © 2014 John Wiley & Sons, Ltd. Published 2014 by John Wiley & Sons, Ltd. Companion website: www.ataglanceseries.com/medicine

chest pain differs significantly, in that for chronic chest pain (by which is meant pain that is reasonably long standing, e.g. present for more than 8 weeks, and has not changed in nature recently) the main diagnostic condition to consider is stable effort angina, which, while there can be risks associated with this, is on the whole a condition with a low chance of very early death. This means that for most patients outpatient assessment is appropriate. In acute chest pain, by which is meant chest pain that has been present either for only a few hours or up to a few weeks, the greatest concern is that the cause is immediately life-threatening, either myocardial infarction of one form or another, or something equally dangerous such as pulmonary embolism or aortic dissection. While most patients with chronic chest pain can safely be managed on an outpatient basis, most patients with acute chest pain need at least a period of time of in-hospital assessment, to rule out immediately dangerous conditions.

Diagnostic assessment of acute chest pain

The process is the same as for any other diagnostic process, except that the condition is so common that most hospitals have well-established protocols which you should follow. However your hospital approaches this problem we suggest that the aim of the process should be four-fold:

1 Always yourself *reach either a diagnosis or differential diagnosis using your own skills*; do not be distracted by protocols into ceasing your thought process, and slipping into a syndromic diagnosis, e.g. troponin-negative chest pain, which is not a diagnosis (and includes many serious illnesses), or troponin-positive chest pain (which includes at least three major and quite different diagnoses, including acute coronary syndrome (ACS), pulmonary embolism (PE) and renal failure). Always strive to reach a clear diagnosis.

2 Regardless of what has just been said, you *must* actively exclude an ACS; often this is *entirely possible* on the basis of the exact symptoms (see below) combined with a knowledge of the pre-test probability of coronary disease (which is heavily influenced by demographics (age, sex) and risk factors), with only the simplest tests, e.g. an ECG (and no blood tests). Sometimes you will feel that you cannot exclude an ACS by these simple means outlined above, and you will need some extra investigations – most protocols rely on the fact that most (though crucially not all) patients with an ACS will have (or will develop over a short period of time) an abnormal ECG and/or a rise in a highly selective biomarker of cardiac damage (most commonly, troponin). How long patients need to be observed while having sequential ECGs and troponins is a moot point, but with highly sensitive troponins the time period is probably 3 hours, while with standard sensitivity troponins probably 12 hours is required.

3 You must also actively exclude a pulmonary embolus; how this is done depends on the situation. For patients with low probability symptoms, heart rate, oxygen saturation and an ECG are usually sufficient. Remember that the commonest ECG sign of a PE is not the commonly taught S1Q3T3 changes; rather for almost all patients the commonest sign is tachycardia alone, with the underlying ECG being otherwise unremarkable. For higher risk patients, these data along with a blood gas, chest X-ray and D-dimer may well be required. A small number will need specific radiology imaging. Regardless of how you exclude a PE, always think PE and in your mind exclude it.

4 Always exclude aortic dissection; this immediately life-threatening illness continues to be diagnosed late in A&E, largely as doctors do not think of it – furthermore, if you have made the mistake of slipping into the sloppy habit of labelling patients syndromically (e.g. troponin-negative chest pain) you too will miss this diagnosis, as patients usually have normal ECGs and normal D-dimers and troponins. The clue, as ever, is in the history (see below) and examination. If you have any doubt as to whether dissection is present, order an immediate CT aortogram. The take home message, however, is that you will never diagnosis aortic dissection in time to save your patient unless you routinely think in all patients with chest pain whether this could be the diagnosis.

All patients seen in A&E with chest pain must have a full history, examination (including oxygen saturation), chest X-ray and ECG as a bare minimum.

Typical myocardial ischaemic pain (cardiac pain)

Myocardial ischaemia is a clinical diagnosis, made on the history and supported by finding risk factors for atheromatous coronary disease (see Chapter 84). There are two forms of ischaemic chest pain: angina and myocardial infarction.

Angina

Typical angina is a heavy pain or discomfort felt retrosternally, which may radiate to the neck, and is often associated with heaviness in the left arm. Some patients have atypical symptoms, such as pain in unusual places (e.g. the right chest, shoulder blade), although isolated left-sided chest/submammary pain is rarely angina. A key diagnostic feature is the **relationship of symptoms to effort**. For genuine angina, whatever its location, pain is reliably brought on by effort, and relieved within 1–2 minutes of rest. Angina is described clinically as stable, crescendo or unstable. In **stable angina**, symptoms are only provoked by effort and readily relieved by rest. In **crescendo angina**, the amount of effort required to provoke symptoms decreases rapidly over several weeks, although symptoms do not occur at rest. In **unstable angina**, symptoms come on unpredictably, either with minimal exertion or at rest. Angina is usually the result of ischaemic heart disease, although it may be caused by:

- Aortic stenosis, the signs of which are a slow rising pulse (a difficult sign to reliably elicit), a praecordial thrill (only in a few) and a loud ejection systolic murmer, often best heard in the mid-left sternal edge (quiet if left ventricular function is poor, or if the patient is gravely unwell from heart failure).
- Severe pulmonary hypertension, suggested by a left parasternal lift, and a loud second heart sound (a very difficult sign to reliably ascertain).

In those with coronary artery disease, the occurrence of crescendo or unstable angina means that the underlying coronary obstruction has increased, usually because of thrombus formation. This is associated with a greatly increased risk of myocardial infarction. Most patients with crescendo or unstable angina should be admitted immediately to hospital.

Myocardial infarction

Myocardial infarction (MI) pain typically comes on over a few minutes. Although feeling identical to angina, it is often very severe, and differs from angina in lasting 20 minutes or more and not being relieved by nitrates. Sweating, nausea and vomiting are very common, and when present increase the chance that symptoms are caused by a myocardial infarct rather than angina. Anginal pain suggesting unstable angina or MI, but without definite diagnosis of MI, is termed an **acute coronary syndrome**.

Aortic dissection

Aortic dissection pain is usually unheralded and of abrupt (instantaneous) onset, unlike MI pain which evolves over minutes, is very severe and is described as having a 'tearing' quality. The location of the pain reflects the site of the origin of the dissection and the spread of the pain reflects the propagation of the dissection plane along the aorta. Thus, classically, dissection of the ascending aorta starts in the anterior chest and rapidly (in less than a few minutes) moves into the neck and then the back. Dissections originating in the aortic arch start as neck pain, and those in the descending thoracic aorta as interscapular or shoulder pain.

Pleuritic pain

Pleuritic pain is defined as a 'sharp', 'catching' chest pain, exacerbated by respiration, particularly extreme inspiration. When severe, patients breathe shallowly to avoid pain. There are two causes:

- **Pleural pain**: This is 'pleurisy' localized to one side of the chest, but not position dependent. A pleural rub may be heard.

Achieving a diagnosis depends on defining the associated symptoms and signs. Pleurisy occurs with pneumonia (fever, cough, tachypnoea, bronchial breathing), pulmonary embolus (breathlessness, tachycardia, cyanosis, no bronchial breathing) and pneumothorax (absent breath sounds).

Table 13.1 Clinical features altering the probability of myocardial infarction

Substantial increase in probability (>2-fold increase in risk)
- Radiation to right arm/shoulder
- Radiation to both arms/shoulders
- Associated with exertion
- Radiation to left arm
- Associated sweating

Small increase in probability (<2-fold increase in risk)
- Associated with nausea and/or vomiting
- Worse than previous angina or the same as previous MI
- Described as a pressure

Small decrease in the chance of myocardial infarction (probability reduction 50% or less)
- Inframammary location
- Not associated with exertion

Substantial decrease in the chance of myocardial infarction (probability reduction more than 50%)
- Described as pleuritic
- Described as positional
- Described as sharp
- Reproduced with palpation

Note that these factors can all alter the probability of myocardial infarction, but that none mean that an infarct either must have occurred or could not have occurred. Always use all the information available to reach this diagnosis.

Canadian Cardiovascular Society grading of angina

Grade 1 — Angina on strenuous physical activity

Grade 2 — Angina on ordinary physical activity, e.g. walking uphill or climbing more than one flight of stairs

Grade 3 — Marked limitation on ordinary physical activity, e.g. angina on climbing one flight of stairs

Grade 4 — Angina on any physical activity and also at rest

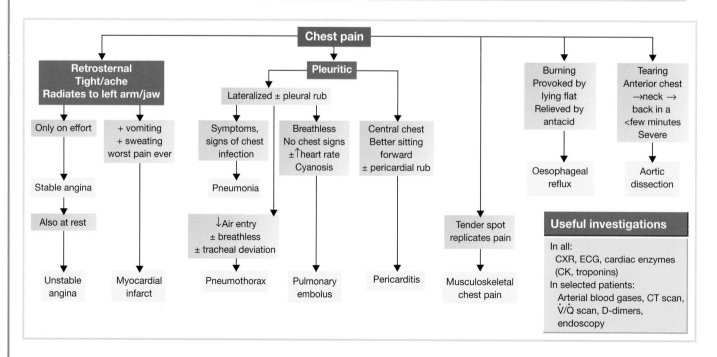

- **Pericardial pain**: As with pleurisy, pericardial pain is worse on deep inspiration, but unlike pleurisy it is located in the centre of the chest, is positional in nature and typically is worse lying down and relieved by sitting. A pericardial rub may be heard on auscultation, which may be positional, quite localized or intermittent. Pericarditis occurs with viral infections, post MI and in autoimmune diseases.

Musculoskeletal chest pain

This is very common. There may be a history of physical injury or unusual exertion, although this is found surprisingly infrequently. Pain is provoked by arm/chest movement and lasts many hours. Although pains may be exacerbated by effort, rest does not reliably relieve them. Examination may show localized tenderness. This diagnosis should be considered only once more serious diagnoses have been excluded, because chest wall pain and coronary disease may coexist.

Gastro-oesophageal pain

Several different gastrointestinal pains can cause diagnostic confusion with cardiac pain:

- **Oesophageal reflux** causes a retrosternal burning, travelling from the epigastrium upwards. There may be frequent belching, odynophagia or, if a stricture has occurred, dysphagia. Reflux is particularly frequent in obese individuals who smoke, just the population in whom coronary disease is found!
- **Oesophageal spasm**, often provoked by oesophageal reflux, can be very difficult to distinguish from cardiac pain, because it causes a retrosternal tightness/heaviness which may be severe. It may, however, be relieved by liquid antacids (e.g. milk) or cold drinks.

The key to the diagnosis of gastrointestinal pain is its clear relationship with food, and the absence of a relationship between the onset of the pain and exertion. Confusingly, some oesophageal reflux (and spasm) can be provoked by exercise, although such pain often resolves only slowly on resting. This can lead to diagnostic confusion with angina – if the risk of coronary artery disease is high, a cardiac origin to the pain should be actively excluded.

Gall bladder disease

Classic biliary colic is felt in the epigastrium and cholecystitis in the right upper quadrant of the abdomen. However, biliary disease may also be felt in the chest and confused with angina. Typically attacks of pain are intermittent, unrelated to exertion and may be severe. Eating certain particularly fatty foods can precipitate them. It is more common in women than in men, and is diagnosed on ultrasonography and by the exclusion of anginal syndromes.

14 Oedema

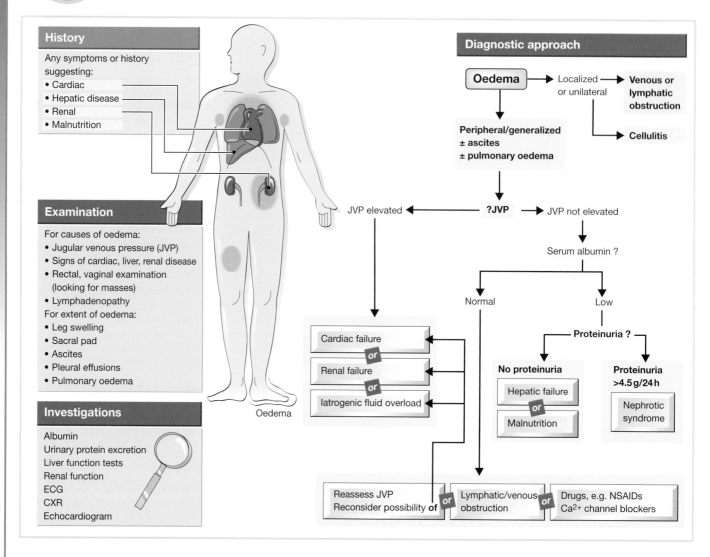

History

Any symptoms or history suggesting:
- Cardiac
- Hepatic disease
- Renal
- Malnutrition

Examination

For causes of oedema:
- Jugular venous pressure (JVP)
- Signs of cardiac, liver, renal disease
- Rectal, vaginal examination (looking for masses)
- Lymphadenopathy

For extent of oedema:
- Leg swelling
- Sacral pad
- Ascites
- Pleural effusions
- Pulmonary oedema

Investigations

Albumin
Urinary protein excretion
Liver function tests
Renal function
ECG
CXR
Echocardiogram

Oedema

Diagnostic approach

Oedema → Localized or unilateral → Venous or lymphatic obstruction
→ Cellulitis

Peripheral/generalized ± ascites ± pulmonary oedema

?JVP

JVP elevated ← → JVP not elevated

Serum albumin?

Normal — Low

Cardiac failure / or / Renal failure / or / Iatrogenic fluid overload

Proteinuria?

No proteinuria — Hepatic failure / or / Malnutrition

Proteinuria >4.5 g/24h — Nephrotic syndrome

Reassess JVP Reconsider possibility of / or / Lymphatic/venous obstruction / or / Drugs, e.g. NSAIDs Ca²⁺ channel blockers

---

Oedema ('an abnormal build up of fluid in the tissues') can be a presenting feature of many serious medical conditions, notably congestive heart failure, liver failure, malnutrition and the nephrotic syndrome. Peripheral oedema can also result from venous or lymphatic obstruction or from excessive administration of salt and water. Agents such as non-steroidal anti-inflammatory drugs (NSAIDs) and calcium channel blockers can also produce peripheral oedema.

Presentation

Patients present complaining of swelling of the legs. In severe cases, oedema extends to cause abdominal swelling (from ascites), sacral oedema, pleural effusions, pulmonary oedema and even facial swelling. Oedema is often, although not always, posturally dependent, and in bed-bound individuals it may be confined to the sacrum.

Diagnosis

Accurate history taking is vital. Symptoms and signs of cardiac, liver and renal disease should be sought. Two questions are the

key to the diagnosis: 'Is the oedema unilateral or bilateral? Is the venous pressure raised or not?' (see Table 14.1). It is also important to determine whether oedema is present in other sites. Oedema diffusely affecting the whole body suggests a low serum albumin, or 'leaky' capillaries, rather than heart failure.

Bilateral leg oedema

In bilateral leg oedema, the diagnosis rests in determining whether the venous pressure is elevated and whether there are signs of liver disease, severe immobility or malnourishment.

- **Heart failure**: leg oedema occurs from right-sided heart failure and is always associated with a high jugular venous pressure (JVP). Hepatomegaly is often seen, as are signs of underlying cardiac pathology. If the oedema is mild in the legs, but severe in the abdomen, pericardial constriction should be considered.
- **Liver failure**: leg oedema is caused by a low serum albumin (usually <20 g/dL). There may be signs of chronic liver disease, such as spider naevi, leuconychia, gynaecomastia, dilated abdominal veins indicating portal hypertension, and bruises (impaired

Medicine at a Glance, Fourth Edition. Edited by Patrick Davey. © 2014 John Wiley & Sons, Ltd. Published 2014 by John Wiley & Sons, Ltd. Companion website: www.ataglanceseries.com/medicine

Table 14.1 Causes of oedema

Bilateral oedema

- Congestive cardiac failure
- Hepatic failure
- Renal failure
- Nephrotic syndrome
- Malnutrition
- Immobility
- Drugs (NSAIDs, calcium channel blockers)

Unilateral oedema

- Lymphatic obstruction
- Venous obstruction (usually DVT; rarely, external compression)
- Venous valve incompetence from previous DVT
- Cellulitis
- Ruptured Baker's cyst
- Localized immobility, e.g. hemiparesis

liver synthetic function). The JVP is not elevated. In severe chronic liver disease (e.g. cirrhosis), liver enzyme tests may be only mildly disturbed, although the prothrombin time is often prolonged (>20 s). In acute liver failure, the patient is usually very unwell, cerebral disturbance is prominent and liver function tests are usually grossly abnormal.

- **Renal failure**: oedema is caused by either a low serum albumin (nephrotic syndrome, where the urine is frothy and contains 3–4+ of protein on dipstick testing; confirmatory tests include estimation of serum albumin (usually <30 g/dL), urinary protein (usually >4 g/24 h) and serum creatinine and urea) or an inability to excrete fluid (nephritic syndrome, associated with hypertension and low urine output).
- **General immobility**: the patient is usually elderly, and obviously immobile from general infirmity or cerebrovascular disease. The JVP is down, and there are no signs of liver or renal disease.
- **Malnutrition**: any chronic illness may be associated with a catabolic state and a degree of malnutrition that can be severe enough to depress serum albumin and cause leg oedema.
- **Inferior vena cava (IVC) compression**: rarely, bilateral leg oedema can be caused by compression on the IVC. This can be diagnosed by ultrasonographic studies of the abdomen, using colour flow Doppler to determine blood flow and computed tomography (CT), and occurs:
  - In extreme obesity.
  - In severe (tense) ascites from whatever cause.
  - With extensive venous thrombosis in the IVC, such as occurs in malignancy, or as a complication of the nephrotic syndrome.

Unilateral leg oedema

A one-sided leg swelling is likely to have a local underlying cause, such as:

- A **deep venous thrombosis** (DVT) in the leg causes a slow onset (more than a few hours) of unilateral leg pain, swelling, skin warmth and possibly tenderness in the calves and along the veins, particularly the great saphenous vein. As symptoms/signs are unreliable for diagnosis, all patients with suspected DVT should undergo definitive investigations (vein ultrasonography or venography) and be examined for complicating pulmonary embolisms (see Chapter 92).

- **Ruptured Baker's cyst**: a Baker's cyst is a knee joint bursa that juts into the popliteal fossa and usually occurs in rheumatoid arthritis. It may rupture and cause sudden-onset leg pain and calf swelling. Ultrasonography is diagnostic.
- **Cellulitis** consists of an intense, spreading skin erythema, sometimes well demarcated, occasionally tracking up the line of the lymphatics. It is often very painful and is associated with a temperature and raised erythrocyte sedimentation rate, C-reactive protein and white cell count. The organism is usually one of the staphylococci or streptococci species, and is occasionally grown from blood cultures, although rarely from skin swabs.
- **Lymphatic obstruction** results in a 'woody' form of unilateral oedema, sometimes described as 'non-pitting'. It is very rare in the West, and when found is usually the result of carcinomatous invasion and obliteration of the draining lymph nodes, e.g. in metastatic melanoma. In Africa, lymph obstruction is very common, often bilateral, and caused by filarial infestation.
- **Pelvic tumours** can unilaterally compress veins, causing unilateral oedema.
- **Localized immobility** can cause unilateral leg oedema, e.g. long-standing hemiparesis.

Investigations

These vary depending on the features established by the history and examination, but determination of serum albumin, urinary protein loss, liver function tests, creatinine, electrocardiogram (ECG), chest X-ray (CXR) and echocardiography are often appropriate.

Treatment

Therapy is directed at correcting the underlying cause. In bilateral oedema diuretics are often used to promote salt and water excretion, although their use should be balanced against the risk of hypovolaemia and worsening renal function, postural hypotension and falls. Several different classes of diuretic agent are used (see Table 14.2). The use of a loop diuretic in combination with a thiazide can produce a pronounced diuretic effect that is useful in resistant oedema. Spironolactone, a competitive aldosterone antagonist, produces a mild natriuresis and potassium retention, and is utilized in conditions with secondary hyperaldosteronism such as liver cirrhosis with ascites. Spironolactone and amiloride are 'potassium-sparing' diuretics, in contrast to the loop and thiazide diuretics which promote potassium depletion.

Table 14.2 Diuretics used in treating oedema

Class	Example	Diuretic potency	Na$^+$/K$^+$ lowering potential
Thiazide	Bendroflumethiazide	+	++/+
Loop	Furosemide (frusemide)	+++	+/+++
K$^+$ sparing	Amiloride	±	±/0
	Spironolactone	±	±/0

15 Palpitations

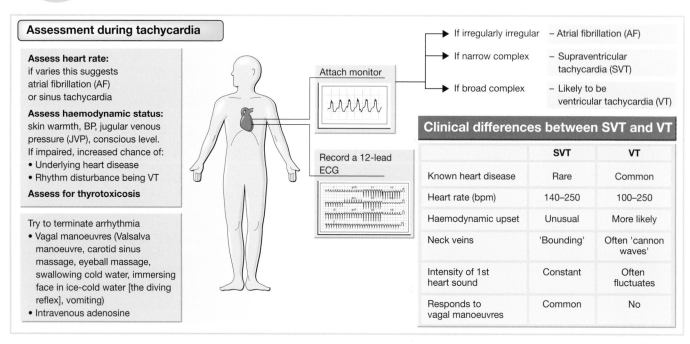

Assessment during tachycardia

Assess heart rate:
if varies this suggests
atrial fibrillation (AF)
or sinus tachycardia

Assess haemodynamic status:
skin warmth, BP, jugular venous
pressure (JVP), conscious level.
If impaired, increased chance of:
• Underlying heart disease
• Rhythm disturbance being VT

Assess for thyrotoxicosis

Try to terminate arrhythmia
• Vagal manoeuvres (Valsalva
  manoeuvre, carotid sinus
  massage, eyeball massage,
  swallowing cold water, immersing
  face in ice-cold water [the diving
  reflex], vomiting)
• Intravenous adenosine

Attach monitor

Record a 12-lead ECG

If irregularly irregular – Atrial fibrillation (AF)

If narrow complex – Supraventricular tachycardia (SVT)

If broad complex – Likely to be ventricular tachycardia (VT)

Clinical differences between SVT and VT

	SVT	VT
Known heart disease	Rare	Common
Heart rate (bpm)	140–250	100–250
Haemodynamic upset	Unusual	More likely
Neck veins	'Bounding'	Often 'cannon waves'
Intensity of 1st heart sound	Constant	Often fluctuates
Responds to vagal manoeuvres	Common	No

Palpitations are an awareness of the heart beat, either due to an abnormal appreciation of the normal heart beat or from a tachyarrhythmia (bradyarrhythmias only very rarely cause palpitations). To establish the diagnosis it is helpful to establish the speed of onset (instantaneous or over several minutes) and the rate and rhythm (ask the patient to tap out the palpitations using their hand).

1 **'Awareness of sinus tachycardia' palpitations**: here the heart rhythm is normal, but the heart beats more rapidly and strongly than usual; this occurs with exercise, fear or psychological distress (e.g. anxiety). The diagnosis is established by finding a characteristic history; palpitations start and stop over many minutes, unlike genuine tachyarrhythmias which start (and stop) instantaneously. They are regular and relatively slow (heart rate <100 bpm). There is often a background of anxiety (work, relationship stress, etc.). Vagal manoeuvres are unhelpful and syncope never occurs.

Causes of a sinus tachycardia include:
• Physiological: exercise, anxiety.
• Common pathologies: sepsis/fever, pain, heart failure, respiratory distress, haemodynamic compromise, anaemia; thyrotoxicosis.
• Rare pathologies: phaeochromocytoma, sinus node re-entrant tachycardia – diagnosed by 'fixed' heart rate on 24-hour taping.

2 **Tachyarrhythmia-associated palpitations**: here the heart beats more quickly than usual as a result of a tachyarrhythmia or extra beats. The characteristic history of a genuine tachyarrhythmia is of sudden (i.e. instantaneous) onset, fast palpitations, which last for a very clearly defined period of time (usually minutes rather than hours) and may (although not reliably) stop as suddenly as they started. Anxiety may occur, but does so during, not before, an attack. Vagal manoeuvres are helpful for supraventricular arrhythmias, and there is often a history of severe heart disease in ventricular arrhythmias. Syncope may

occur. After the event patients may pass abnormally large volumes of urine. A number of different tachyarrhythmias have additional characteristic features:

• **Supraventricular tachycardia (SVT)** (either atrioventricular re-entrant tachycardia (AVRT) or AVNRT (AV nodal re-entrant tachycardia)): these often start during the teenage years. Syncope is very unusual. Post-event polyuria, from atrial natriuretic factor release resulting from atrial stretching during the attack, may occur.

• **Atrial fibrillation**: characteristically the palpitations are felt 'all over the place' or are 'irregularly irregular'. Syncope is very rare (unless the patient has a very fast ventricular response to the atrial fibrillation) but, as this arrhythmia occurs in those with heart disease, breathlessness resulting from associated heart failure is common.

• **Ventricular tachycardia (VT)**: patients are often although not always known to have heart disease. Syncope is common, although not universal. Vagal manoeuvres are unhelpful.

• **Extrasystoles**: patients usually do not feel the extrasystole, but feel the post-extrasystolic beat, which is of increased contraction. They thus feel that the heart misses a beat, then 'restarts' with a thump. Patients often say that they are 'worried that their heart may not restart'.

The most helpful investigation in palpitations is an electrocardiogram (ECG) recorded during an attack, and the aim of investigation should be to obtain this. For lengthy attacks, this is straightforward. If short-lived, then a 24-hour Holter monitor may be useful if attacks are frequent (every 24–48 h). For infrequent attacks, a variety of electronic recorders are available which the patient can apply during the episode. Whatever the cause of the palpitation, patients with a structurally normal heart generally have a good prognosis, whereas impaired ventricular function generally mandates more aggressive investigation and treatment.

16 The painful leg

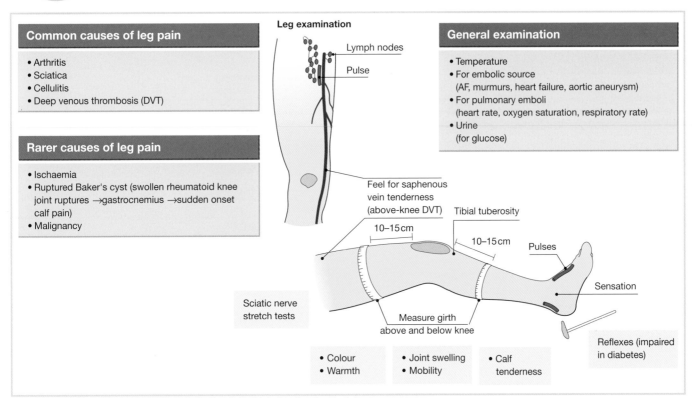

Common causes of leg pain

- Arthritis
- Sciatica
- Cellulitis
- Deep venous thrombosis (DVT)

Rarer causes of leg pain

- Ischaemia
- Ruptured Baker's cyst (swollen rheumatoid knee joint ruptures →gastrocnemius →sudden onset calf pain)
- Malignancy

Leg examination

Lymph nodes
Pulse
Feel for saphenous vein tenderness (above-knee DVT)
Tibial tuberosity
10–15 cm
10–15 cm
Pulses
Sensation
Sciatic nerve stretch tests
Measure girth above and below knee
Reflexes (impaired in diabetes)

- Colour
- Warmth
- Joint swelling
- Mobility
- Calf tenderness

General examination

- Temperature
- For embolic source (AF, murmurs, heart failure, aortic aneurysm)
- For pulmonary emboli (heart rate, oxygen saturation, respiratory rate)
- Urine (for glucose)

As for all symptoms, a clear description of the site, nature and duration of pain, with provoking and relieving factors, along with a careful examination, is usually sufficient to establish the diagnosis. The following are the common causes of leg pain.

- **Deep venous thrombosis (DVT)**: patients notice a gradually increasing (over hours) unilateral calf (more rarely thigh) ache and often calf (or thigh) swelling. Absence of leg swelling does *not* exclude a DVT, although the greater the swelling the more likely it is. Normal D-dimer levels *exclude* the diagnosis. Only those with raised D-dimers should go on to have definitive imaging: venography (painful, but the gold standard) or ultrasonography (less reliable for below-knee DVT). The risk of pulmonary embolism (PE) is very low in below-knee and significant in above-knee DVTs. Accordingly, below-knee DVTs do not mandate anticoagulation, although surveillance imaging every few days is essential to ensure that the clot has not propagated more proximally. All patients may need anticoagulation to relieve symptoms. DVTs may indicate a procoagulant state (see Chapter 190), either genetic or acquired. The incidence of recurrent DVTs/PEs is 10% per annum (i.e. 20% after 2 years, 50% after 5 years, etc.). A case for long-term anticoagulation can therefore be made.
- **Cellulitis** (see Chapter 228).
- **Arterial disease**: chronic arterial insufficiency presents with **intermittent claudication** – pains felt in the calves and/or the buttocks, brought on by exercise and rapidly relieved by rest (i.e. in less than 1 min). Examination shows reduced or absent arterial

pulses, findings confirmed by Doppler measurements. Patients with **critical ischaemia** have pain at rest. Hanging the leg over the edge of the bed relieves symptoms (gravity improves perfusing pressure). **Acute leg ischaemia** presents as a painful leg, and examination shows absent pulses and a bluish discoloration. Causes include *in situ* thrombosis (usually in long-standing claudication) or arterial embolus, from the heart (consider recent myocardial infarction, atrial fibrillation (AF) or mitral stenosis) or a diseased aorta (e.g. abdominal aortic aneurysm; much more rarely from aortic dissection). Doppler measurements and peripheral angiography are diagnostic. Treatment is immediate heparin, removal of any embolic clot (which should be sent for histology, because a few are embolized atrial myxomas or lung tumours) using a Fogarty catheter, arterial reconstructive surgery or amputation, along with diagnosis and treatment of any cardiac problem.

- **Leg ulcers** (see Chapter 71).
- **Arthritis**: symptoms have often been present for months or years. Pain is usually (not always) localized to the affected joint and worse on joint movement or weight bearing, although hip osteoarthritis may cause sufficient nocturnal pain to wake the patient. Septic arthritis presents acutely with systemic symptoms (fever, malaise, shivers) and a hot, red, swollen joint with painful, globally restricted movements. Joint aspiration is diagnostic (see Chapter 215).
- **Nerve root compression**, especially sciatic nerve compression from a prolapsed intervertebral disc ('sciatica'), is common – pain characteristically radiates all the way down the back of the leg (see Chapter 209).

Medicine at a Glance, Fourth Edition. Edited by Patrick Davey. © 2014 John Wiley & Sons, Ltd. Published 2014 by John Wiley & Sons, Ltd. Companion website: www.ataglanceseries.com/medicine

17 Heart murmurs

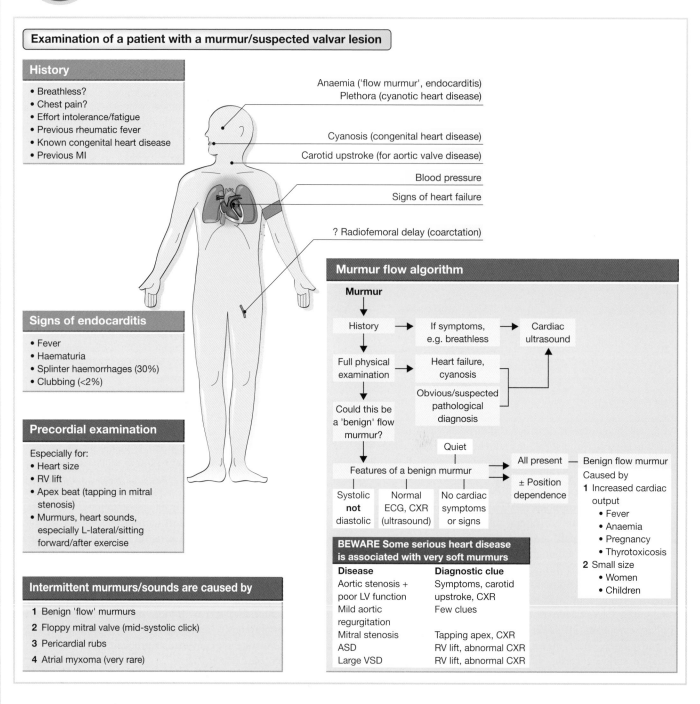

Examination of a patient with a murmur/suspected valvar lesion

History

- Breathless?
- Chest pain?
- Effort intolerance/fatigue
- Previous rheumatic fever
- Known congenital heart disease
- Previous MI

Anaemia ('flow murmur', endocarditis)
Plethora (cyanotic heart disease)

Cyanosis (congenital heart disease)
Carotid upstroke (for aortic valve disease)

Blood pressure
Signs of heart failure

? Radiofemoral delay (coarctation)

Signs of endocarditis

- Fever
- Haematuria
- Splinter haemorrhages (30%)
- Clubbing (<2%)

Precordial examination

Especially for:
- Heart size
- RV lift
- Apex beat (tapping in mitral stenosis)
- Murmurs, heart sounds, especially L-lateral/sitting forward/after exercise

Intermittent murmurs/sounds are caused by

1 Benign 'flow' murmurs
2 Floppy mitral valve (mid-systolic click)
3 Pericardial rubs
4 Atrial myxoma (very rare)

Murmur flow algorithm

Murmur → History → If symptoms, e.g. breathless → Cardiac ultrasound

Full physical examination → Heart failure, cyanosis

Obvious/suspected pathological diagnosis

Could this be a 'benign' flow murmur?

Quiet

Features of a benign murmur

All present → Benign flow murmur

± Position dependence

Systolic **not** diastolic | Normal ECG, CXR (ultrasound) | No cardiac symptoms or signs

Benign flow murmur
Caused by
1 Increased cardiac output
- Fever
- Anaemia
- Pregnancy
- Thyrotoxicosis
2 Small size
- Women
- Children

BEWARE Some serious heart disease is associated with very soft murmurs

Disease	Diagnostic clue
Aortic stenosis + poor LV function	Symptoms, carotid upstroke, CXR
Mild aortic regurgitation	Few clues
Mitral stenosis	Tapping apex, CXR
ASD	RV lift, abnormal CXR
Large VSD	RV lift, abnormal CXR

Murmurs are commonly found on routine physical examination. Although most are benign, not resulting from cardiovascular disease ('flow murmur' – see Figure 17.1), occasionally they are important clues to the presence of heart disease, such as: valvar disease, left ventricular (LV) dysfunction (functional mitral regurgitation), intracardiac shunts (atrial septal defect (ASD) and ventricular septal defect (VSD)). Very occasionally, other malformations, such as an arteriovenous malformation or coarctation of the aorta are responsible for murmurs.

Valvar heart disease is common, important and in most cases associated with murmurs. The characteristics of a murmur depend on the flow velocity, the nature and size of the orifice, and the direction of the flow.

As a rule, narrow atrioventricular (AV) valves cause diastolic murmurs, and leaking AV valves cause systolic murmurs; the reverse is true for the pulmonary and aortic valves. Murmurs radiate in the direction of the blood flow across the diseased valve (e.g. aortic stenosis murmurs radiate to the neck, and mitral

Medicine at a Glance, Fourth Edition. Edited by Patrick Davey. © 2014 John Wiley & Sons, Ltd. Published 2014 by John Wiley & Sons, Ltd. Companion website: www.ataglanceseries.com/medicine

regurgitation caused by anterior mitral leaflet prolapse radiates to the back). The intensity of a murmur is directly proportional to the pressure gradient and the size of the orifice, unless cardiac function is compromised.

Chronic scarring and calcification make a valve orifice smaller (stenosis), whereas destructive disease processes (e.g. endocarditis, vasculitis) make a valve incompetent (regurgitation). Stenosis of a valve causes pressure overload on the cardiac chamber pumping blood through the valve; regurgitation results in volume overload to compensate for the leak.

Aetiology of valvar lesions

- **Congenital**: increasingly common as those with congenital heart disease survive longer, as a result of better childhood surgery and medicines. The most common adult presentation of a congenital lesion is that of a bicuspid aortic valve, which is asymptomatic for many years, but predisposes to early (from 40 years onwards) calcific aortic stenosis.
- **Rheumatic fever** causes scarring, thickening and calcification of valves over subsequent decades. Affects mitral more than aortic valves. Common in elderly people and in developing countries, but rare in developed countries.
- **Degenerative valve disease**: acquired calcific aortic stenosis in elderly people is the best example of a degenerative lesion. Myxomatous degeneration of the mitral valve leads to destruction of leaflets and chordal rupture.
- **Infection**: endocarditis causes destruction of the valve structure and valvar regurgitation, never stenosis.
- **Prosthetic**: artificial valves may degenerate (biological prostheses calcify) or leak as a result of valve dysfunction or dehiscence of the surgical sutures (paraprosthetic leak). Endocarditis is especially high risk with prosthetic valves.

Investigations

- **Chest X-ray** (CXR): shows shape of the heart and identifies chamber enlargement.
- **Electrocardiogram** (ECG): may reveal atrial fibrillation, left atrial enlargement (mitral valve disease) or LV hypertrophy (aortic valve disease).
- **Echocardiography**: this is the most important investigation in (suspected) valvular heart disease, and is used to assess cardiac chamber size and function, valve morphology and opening. Doppler echocardiography measures blood flow velocity, which is then used to calculate pressure gradients across narrow valves and the severity of regurgitation from leaky valves. Colour Doppler turns echo signals from turbulent blood flow into a two-dimensional colour picture, and is particularly useful for assessing valvar leaks. Standard cardiac transthoracic echocardiography with modern equipment produces high-quality images and (usually) sufficient information. Transoesophageal echocardiography (an ultrasound probe is placed in the oesophagus) produces very high resolution images of the heart, because there are no intervening structures (unlike the ribs and lungs for transthoracic echocardiography) and is particularly useful when transthoracic images are inadequate, for left atrial or mitral valve pathology, or for prosthetic valves.
- **Cardiac catheterization**: enables accurate direct measurement of pressure in the cardiac chambers. High-quality echocardiography has largely replaced cardiac catheterization as a routine investigation. However, coronary angiography is still used to diagnose concomitant coronary artery disease when surgery is being considered.

Treatment

The general principles underlying the treatment of all patients with valvar disease involve the following:

- **Monitor for those symptoms** that indicate a need for surgery. It is important to realize that a valve lesion alone is not an indication for valve replacement because many patients live for decades with medically treated valvular disease.
- **Document left ventricular function**, which if it deteriorates may, even in the absence of symptoms, indicate a need for surgery.
- **Maintain left ventricular function**, e.g. using angiotensin-converting enzyme (ACE) inhibitor therapy in regurgitant lesions.
- **Slow progression** of the stenosis/regurgitant leak, e.g. using antihypertensive therapy in the aortic regurgitation associated with hypertension.
- **Treat any complicating rhythm disturbances**, e.g. atrial fibrillation is a very common rhythm disturbance in all forms of valvar heart disease, and can be treated using digoxin and β-blockers to control the ventricular response.
- **Prevent complications** such as endocarditis, e.g. using prophylactic antibiotics when 'dirty' procedures, such as dental work, are carried out (see Table 17.1).
- **Prevent systemic thromboembolism**, e.g. using warfarin in atrial fibrillation.

Surgical treatment

The indications for surgical therapy are intrusive symptoms (breathlessness, exercise limitation), despite medical therapy, or progressive deterioration in LV function occurring in the absence of symptoms (e.g. as in mitral regurgitation). The different forms of surgery are:

- **Commissurotomy** is used for congenital aortic or pulmonary stenosis, and some cases of rheumatic mitral stenosis.
- **Valve repair** is possible in some cases of mitral valve regurgitation.
- **Valve replacement** with a prosthetic valve. There are two sorts of prosthetic valve: first, synthetic **mechanical** valves (usually a composite of metal and other synthetic material), which require lifelong anticoagulation to prevent thromboembolism. They are very durable and last for more than 20 years. The second form of prosthesis is a valve from an animal (**xenograft**) or human (**homograft**). No long-term anticoagulation is needed because the thromboembolic risk is lower, they have better haemodynamic function, although they are less durable, and they may last only 10 years or less.

Table 17.1 Cardiac conditions at higher risk of developing infective endocarditis

- Prosthetic heart valve
- Complex cyanotic congenital heart diseases
- Surgically constructed systemic or pulmonary conduits
- Acquired valvular heart disease
- Mitral valve prolapse with valvular regurgitation or severe valve thickening
- Non-cyanotic congenital heart disease (except for secundum-type ASD)
- Hypertrophic cardiomyopathy
- Previous endocarditis

Endocarditis prophylaxis during 'dirty' surgery was given in years gone by, but is no longer routinely recommended – however, these are guidelines from NICE, and as in all guidelines can be overridden by clinicians if they feel it appropriate.

18 Shock

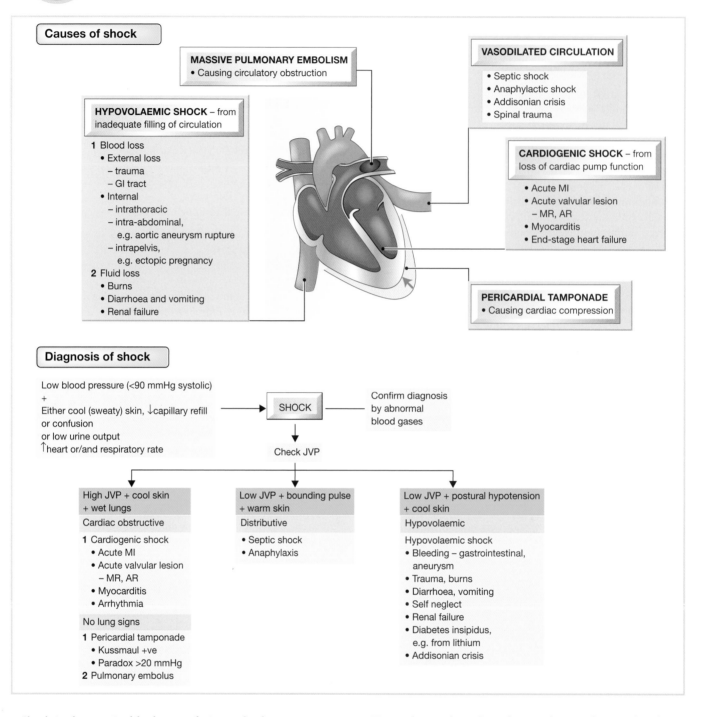

Causes of shock

MASSIVE PULMONARY EMBOLISM
• Causing circulatory obstruction

VASODILATED CIRCULATION
• Septic shock
• Anaphylactic shock
• Addisonian crisis
• Spinal trauma

HYPOVOLAEMIC SHOCK – from inadequate filling of circulation

1 Blood loss
 • External loss
  – trauma
  – GI tract
 • Internal
  – intrathoracic
  – intra-abdominal,
   e.g. aortic aneurysm rupture
  – intrapelvis,
   e.g. ectopic pregnancy
2 Fluid loss
 • Burns
 • Diarrhoea and vomiting
 • Renal failure

CARDIOGENIC SHOCK – from loss of cardiac pump function
 • Acute MI
 • Acute valvular lesion
  – MR, AR
 • Myocarditis
 • End-stage heart failure

PERICARDIAL TAMPONADE
• Causing cardiac compression

Diagnosis of shock

Low blood pressure (<90 mmHg systolic)
+
Either cool (sweaty) skin, ↓capillary refill or confusion
or low urine output
↑heart or/and respiratory rate

→ SHOCK

Confirm diagnosis by abnormal blood gases

Check JVP

High JVP + cool skin + wet lungs

Cardiac obstructive

1 Cardiogenic shock
 • Acute MI
 • Acute valvular lesion
  – MR, AR
 • Myocarditis
 • Arrhythmia

No lung signs

1 Pericardial tamponade
 • Kussmaul +ve
 • Paradox >20 mmHg
2 Pulmonary embolus

Low JVP + bounding pulse + warm skin

Distributive

• Septic shock
• Anaphylaxis

Low JVP + postural hypotension + cool skin

Hypovolaemic

Hypovolaemic shock
• Bleeding – gastrointestinal, aneurysm
• Trauma, burns
• Diarrhoea, vomiting
• Self neglect
• Renal failure
• Diabetes insipidus,
 e.g. from lithium
• Addisonian crisis

Shock is characterized by hypoperfusion and subsequent tissue dysoxia leading to a switch from aerobic to anaerobic metabolism and lactic acidosis. All forms of shock have a high mortality and it is therefore important to make an early diagnosis and institute aggressive treatment. The following types of shock have been characterized:

• **Cardiogenic**: ventricular (usually left) pump failure (myocardial infarction (MI), acute valve dysfunction, acute ventricular septal defect, arrhythmia).

• **Hypovolaemic**: loss of circulating volume with normal cardiac function (trauma, gastrointestinal (GI) bleed, pancreatitis, severe diarrhoea, burns).

• **Distributive**: reduced systemic vascular resistance with normal cardiac function (sepsis, anaphylaxis, Addisonian crisis, spinal trauma).

• **Obstructive shock**: impaired ventricular filling or obstruction of outflow tract (pulmonary embolism (PE), tension pneumothorax, cardiac tamponade).

Medicine at a Glance, Fourth Edition. Edited by Patrick Davey. © 2014 John Wiley & Sons, Ltd. Published 2014 by John Wiley & Sons, Ltd. Companion website: www.ataglanceseries.com/medicine

Clearly more than one form of shock may be present in the same patient. Frequently myocardial depression occurs in the latter stages of other shock states such as sepsis or hypovolaemia, especially if severe acidosis is present.

Successful outcome depends on early diagnosis and treatment. In some patients the cause may be obvious; for example in a patient with acute MI or tension pneumothorax; however, in other cases it may be more subtle, as in massive PE or acute mitral regurgitation (MR). **Tissue hypoperfusion is the hallmark of shock but no single sign or investigation is diagnostic on its own**. Clinical signs of shock such as hypotension, reduced central venous pressure, oliguria and confusion tend to be late features when homeostatic mechanisms can no longer compensate. Tachypnoea, tachycardia, reduced capillary refill and lactic acidosis often occur at a much earlier stage, but are very non-specific. There is an extremely poor correlation between direct measurement of cardiac output and clinicians' ability to estimate whether it is low, normal or high. It is therefore crucial to be able to recognize the acute severely ill patient, consider a diagnosis of shock and institute appropriate investigations early.

Useful investigations in diagnosis and management

- **Electrocardiogram** (ECG): MI (ST elevation), pericardial tamponade (low voltage), PE ($S_1Q_3T_3$, right axis, right bundle branch block).
- **Chest X-ray**: pulmonary oedema in cardiogenic shock, enlarged cardiac silhouette (massive PE, cardiac tamponade), tension pneumothorax.
- **Echocardiogram**: cardiogenic shock due to pump dysfunction (MI, myocarditis), acute valve lesions (colour flow Doppler), PE (pulmonary hypertension, right ventricular dysfunction, clot in transit), pericardial tamponade (effusion and right ventricular collapse in systole), hypovolaemia (left ventricle chamber size).
- **Arterial blood gases**: raised lactate and base deficit, as a consequence of tissue hypoperfusion and anaerobic metabolism, correlate with both severity of shock and mortality. These may be abnormal before hypotension, oliguria or confusion are present. Serial measurements are useful in assessing adequacy of treatment.
- **Central ($ScvO_2$) or mixed venous ($SmvO_2$) oxygen saturations**: true mixed venous saturations (from a pulmonary artery catheter) are 10–15% lower than central mixed venous saturations because of the addition of highly deoxygenated blood from the cardiac veins at the level of the right atrium. When oxygen extraction exceeds delivery, such as in cardiogenic shock, venous saturations are low ($ScvO_2 < 70\%$). However, in septic shock saturations may be normal or elevated because cells are unable to extract the delivered oxygen, or low if there is myocardial depression.
- **Blood tests**:
  - **Haematology**: full blood count (haemorrhage, sepsis/disseminated intravascular coagulation (DIC)), coagulation (haemorrhage and sepsis/DIC), cross-match (haemorrhage).
  - **Biochemistry**: electrolytes: low sodium and raised potassium (Addison's), raised urea (GI haemorrhage, severe diarrhoea); **amylase (panreatitis).**
- **Blood cultures**: to isolate the organism in septic shock and tailor subsequent antibiotic choice.

General principles of management

Resuscitation should be prompt, as should measures specific to the underlying diagnosis such as the insertion of a chest drain in tension pneumothorax. However, general principles of resuscitation should not be forgotten. There must be adequate vascular access; the airway should be patent, oxygen applied and adequate ventilation ensured.

Monitoring

Whether or not mechanical ventilation is required, the patient should be managed in a critical care area with appropriate monitoring and nursing. A minimum requirement is for ECG, pulse oximetry, respiratory rate, central venous pressure, Glasgow Coma Score (GCS), urine output and blood pressure to be monitored. The latter should be continuous through an arterial catheter as both fluid and vasoactive drugs may be required. Furthermore an arterial line will enable serial measurements of pH, lactate and base deficit to be performed, which help guide treatment. Additional haemodynamic monitoring is desirable either in the form of a pulmonary artery catheter (their use is becoming uncommon in the UK outside of cardiothoracic centres), oesophageal Doppler or pulse contour analysis and provides information on cardiac output and vascular resistance.

Supportive treatment

Fluid is, with the exception of cardiogenic shock, requisite in most forms of shock. This may be in the form of crystalloid or colloid (blood products in trauma or haemorrhage); however many UK physicians favour colloid. Colloids containing starch are associated with an increased risk of death and renal failure in septic shock. Fluid should be given rapidly after assessment of intravascular status and the response to a challenge assessed (see Chapter 237). Large volume resuscitation with NaCl-rich fluid may itself cause a metabolic (hyperchloraemic) acidosis. Mechanical ventilation may be required either because of a primary respiratory problem or the inability to protect the airway (GCS <8). The metabolic demand of breathing increases ten-fold in shock and uses one-fifth of cardiac output. Mechanical ventilation therefore reduces metabolic demand, but positive thoracic pressures can have adverse haemodynamic effects if the patient is hypovolaemic.

Renal replacement therapy in the form of haemofiltration may be required if there is anuria, hyperkalaemia, unresolving acidosis or resistant fluid overload (cardiogenic shock).

Following optimization of intravascular volume, vasoactive drugs may be required to ensure an adequate cardiac output and blood pressure. Inotropes such as adrenaline (epinephrine), dobutamine, dopamine or milrinone may be used in low cardiac output states, while vasoconstrictors such as noradrenaline (norepinephrine) are required in forms of distributive shock with low systemic vascular resistance.

Specific treatments

- **Cardiogenic**: inotropes, thrombolytics and/or angioplasty, intra-aortic balloon pump, haemofiltration (fluid removal), surgery (MI, acute valve lesion).
- **Hypovolaemic**: fluids, blood products.
- **Distributive**:
  - Sepsis: fluid, vasoconstrictors (noradrenaline ± vasopressin), steroids, antibiotics, inotropes if reduced cardiac output ($ScvO_2 < 70\%$).
  - Anaphylaxis/Addison's: steroids.
- **Obstructive**: cardiac tamponade (pericardial drain), tension pneumothorax (chest drain), PE (thrombolysis, embolectomy).

Breathlessness, cough and haemoptysis

Cough

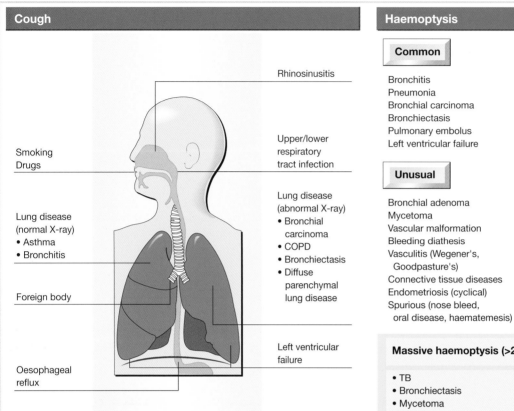

Rhinosinusitis

Upper/lower respiratory tract infection

Smoking
Drugs

Lung disease
(abnormal X-ray)
• Bronchial carcinoma
• COPD
• Bronchiectasis
• Diffuse parenchymal lung disease

Lung disease
(normal X-ray)
• Asthma
• Bronchitis

Foreign body

Left ventricular failure

Oesophageal reflux

Haemoptysis

Common

Bronchitis
Pneumonia
Bronchial carcinoma
Bronchiectasis
Pulmonary embolus
Left ventricular failure

Unusual

Bronchial adenoma
Mycetoma
Vascular malformation
Bleeding diathesis
Vasculitis (Wegener's, Goodpasture's)
Connective tissue diseases
Endometriosis (cyclical)
Spurious (nose bleed, oral disease, haematemesis)

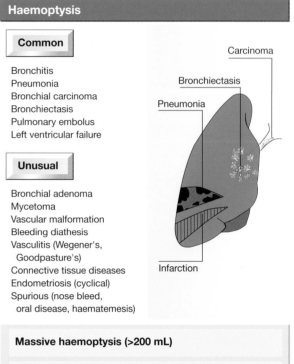

Carcinoma

Bronchiectasis

Pneumonia

Infarction

Massive haemoptysis (>200 mL)

• TB
• Bronchiectasis
• Mycetoma

Breathlessness

NYHA grade*

Unlimited effort capacity   I

Breathless on

severe exercise   II

mild exercise   III

Breathless at rest IV

Mins–hours
Asthma
Pneumothorax
Pulmonary embolism
Pulmonary oedema
Respiratory infection
Psychogenic

Weeks–months
Pleural effusion
Pericardial effusion
Pulmonary fibrosis
Lung cancer
Recurrent pulmonary emboli
Cardiac failure
Neuromuscular disease
Anaemia
Physical deconditioning (from any illness)

Years
COPD
Pneumoconiosis

Recurrent
Asthma
Psychogenic
Exacerbation of COPD | Usually on a background of
Pulmonary oedema | deteriorating breathlessness

Threshold for symptoms
Slow onset ⟶ adaptive response
+ greater tolerance of any symptoms

*NYHA grade = New York Heart Association – usually used for heart failure, can be used for any breathlessness

Medicine at a Glance, Fourth Edition. Edited by Patrick Davey. © 2014 John Wiley & Sons, Ltd. Published 2014 by John Wiley & Sons, Ltd. Companion website: www.ataglanceseries.com/medicine

Table 19.1 Common causes of breathlessness

	Acute breathlessness at rest	Chronic breathlessness on effort
Cardiovascular	Left ventricular failure Acute pulmonary emboli *Mitral stenosis*	Chronic heart failure. 'Angina equivalent' breathlessness Chronic pulmonary emboli
Respiratory	Acute severe asthma Acute exacerbation of COPD Pneumonia Pneumothorax Adult respiratory distress syndrome Acute anaphylaxis *Inhaled foreign body*	COPD Pleural effusion *Interstitial lung disease* Bronchial cancer *Lymphangitis carcinomatosis*
Other	Psychogenic hyperventilation Fever *Metabolic acidosis* *Neurological disease*	Physical deconditioning Obesity Anaemia *Neurological disease*

Rarer causes are in *italics*.

Based on Table 4.5 in *Davidson's Principles and Practice of Medicine*, 18th edn, Churchill Livingstone, Edinburgh, 1999.

Breathlessness

Breathlessness is 'an awareness of the act of breathing' and is a common and frightening symptom. The common causes of breathlessness are listed in Table 19.1.

The rate of onset and the pattern of breathlessness (dyspnoea) may be helpful diagnostically (see Figure 19.1). The characteristic history in some of the different diseases causing breathlessness is outlined below.

Heart failure

- Dyspnoea is not associated with wheeze, a characteristic differentiating it from chronic obstructive pulmonary disease (COPD) (unless 'cardiac asthma', bronchospasm provoked by pulmonary oedema, is present). Symptoms from the underlying heart disease also occur.
- In **mild heart failure** breathlessness occurs only on effort.
- In **more advanced heart failure** breathlessness also occurs on lying flat (**orthopnoea**), promptly (<5–10 min) improved by sitting or standing. When severe, this is called **paroxysmal nocturnal dyspnoea**. There is often ankle oedema – better in the morning, worse at night.

Airway disease

This results in a wheeze when breathless:

- In **COPD**, breathlessness on effort develops progressively over years (often >5 years). Patients often also have **chronic bronchitis** (productive morning cough >3 months/year for 2 years in succession).
- In **asthma**, patients are normal between attacks. Wheezing may be provoked by exercise, pollen (and thus be seasonal), drugs (especially aspirin or β-blockers) or emotion. Symptoms may be worse at night, when a dry cough may occur. Nocturnal

symptoms in asthma, unlike those in heart failure, improve slowly (>30 min) or not at all on sitting/standing.

Respiratory tract infections

Fever and a productive cough are characteristic of respiratory tract infections; sore throat occurs in upper respiratory tract infections. In pneumonia, constitutional upset (fever and malaise) is common and pleuritic chest pain may occur.

Pulmonary embolus

Pulmonary embolus presents with sudden onset, i.e. instantaneous breathlessness, in those predisposed (immobile, obese, oral contraceptive pill, postoperative, cancer). Pleuritic chest pain may occur.

Pneumothorax

Pneumothorax presents with sudden-onset chest pain, often pleuritic in nature, with breathlessness. The diagnosis is made from the physical examination and the chest X-ray.

Lung parenchymal disease

Lung parenchymal disease (interstitial pneumonitis/fibrosis) presents with breathlessness on effort and, with advanced disease, at rest without associated wheeze. Breathlessness, unlike in heart failure, is not strongly dependent on posture. The examination and the chest X-ray are often diagnostic.

Obesity

If severe, obesity can cause breathlessness, both on effort and on lying (orthopnoea, caused by diaphragmatic splinting). Pulmonary embolism, heart failure and obstructive sleep apnoea are all more common in obese individuals.

Physical deconditioning

Physical deconditioning is a potent cause of breathlessness, and often exacerbates breathlessness resulting from other causes. Importantly, most pathological dyspnoea is improved to some extent by physical conditioning. This is helpful therapeutically (rehabilitation).

Rarer causes of breathlessness

There are two much rarer causes of breathlessness:

- **'Angina equivalent' breathlessness**: angina (especially in people with diabetes) is sometimes experienced as breathlessness rather than as chest pain. This is usually caused by severe coronary artery disease.
- **Respiratory failure** can result from a neuromuscular disease, such as motor neuron disease, or related to obesity (Pickwickian syndrome). Physical examination usually reveals the cause and blood gases show type II respiratory failure (see Chapter 100).

Psychological causes for breathlessness

Breathlessness for 'psychogenic' reasons may also occur (**hyperventilation**). The patient complains that they are 'unable to fill the chest' Associated perioral tingling is a specific symptom. Hyperventilation responds to breathing into a paper bag. **Beware**: many patients breathless from organic disease are frightened and appear anxious. Assume that breathlessness within a hospital is the result of organic disease unless there is incontrovertible evidence to the contrary.

Classification of severity of breathlessness

Although there are many ways of classifying the severity of chronic breathlessness (e.g. blood gases, lung volumes, peak oxygen uptake, etc.), the most useful is the **exercise capacity** of the patient at his or her usual pace, without stopping, e.g. is he or she able to walk 50 m, quarter of a mile or several miles? This is the key parameter in understanding the impact of the disease and the severity/extent of the underlying pathology.

Physical examination

The following are diagnostically helpful clues in severe breathlessness. In patients with effort breathlessness alone the signs may be subtle and diagnosis rests on the history and investigations.

- **Skin warmth**: in cardiac dyspnoea (left ventricular (LV) failure, large pulmonary embolus, pericardial effusion) the skin is cool and may be sweaty, whereas in COPD most patients have warm skin with a 'bounding' pulse. A fever may indicate a respiratory tract infection.
- **Heart rate**: severe breathlessness from any cause increases the heart rate. In both LV failure and asthma it can be used as a 'minute-to-minute' guide to the severity of the condition and the effect of treatment.
- **Heart rhythm**.
- **Blood pressure** (BP) itself is rarely diagnostically helpful, but paradox (the difference between inspiratory and expiratory systolic BP: normally $<5\,mmHg$) is. It is increased in asthma, in severe cases to $15–20\,mmHg$, and in pericardial effusion ($>20\,mmHg$).
- **Mucous membranes** for pallor (**anaemia**) and for blueness (**cyanosis**). Patients severely breathless as a result of organic disease are usually centrally cyanosed when breathing air. If not, consider pericardial effusion, anxiety or metabolic acidosis.
- **Jugular venous pressure** (JVP) is a key sign. It is raised in:
  - Heart failure: the most common cause.
  - End-stage COPD (cor pulmonale), when the right heart has failed.
  - Large pulmonary emboli.

  If the JVP is not raised, the breathlessness is less likely to be caused by heart failure, although a normal JVP does not rule out *pure* LV failure.
- **Precordial cardiac examination** may demonstrate a large heart or abnormal LV impulse in most cases of heart failure or a left parasternal lift from right ventricular hypertrophy (in advanced cardiac failure, cor pulmonale and pulmonary embolus). A third heart sound is universal in LV failure, and its absence when breathless suggests that heart failure is not present. Diagnostic murmurs may be heard.
- **Chest examination**:
  - **Respiratory rate** is increased in most patients who are breathless at rest, although not in respiratory failure resulting from neuromuscular disease (which is very rare). A rise in respiratory rate is the most important and often the first sign of any acute illness.
  - **'Hyperinflation'**: a decreased sternal notch-to-trachea distance ('barrel chest') indicates air trapping in the lungs, usually resulting from airway disease (COPD or acute asthma).
  - **'Stony dull' resonance** to percussion occurs in pleural effusions.
  - **Wheeze** (see Chapter 20).
  - **Crepitations**, if 'wet', are often caused by infection (e.g. pneumonia) or fluid (e.g. heart failure), and if 'dry' often indicate pulmonary fibrosis.
  - **Bronchial breathing** indicates consolidation (usually pneumonia).

Investigations

Investigations are directed towards the most likely cause but always include:

- **Chest X-ray**: this is the key investigation in breathlessness, and is always indicated. Often it may not show the cause,

but equally it can sometimes allow a surprising diagnosis to be made.
- **Electrocardiogram** (ECG); again, a key test. A completely normal ECG substantially decreases the chance that heart failure is present
- **Spirometry**; mandatory, unless another diagnosis is obvious.
- **Haemoglobin**.

The following tests help in specific situations:

- **Blood gases**: usually at rest, sometimes on exercise.
- More detailed lung function tests, including measures of gas exchange (e.g. carbon monoxide transfer factor).
- **Computed tomography** (CT): spiral CT is helpful for diagnosis of pulmonary emboli, and high-resolution thin-cut CT for many interstitial lung diseases. Expiratory cuts can reveal gas trapping due to small airways disease.
- **Ventilation/perfusion** ($\dot{V}/\dot{Q}$) (scan to diagnose a pulmonary embolus, though many units now are switching to **CT pulmonary angiograms** as they not only diagnose/exclude pulmonary emboli, but can show other relevant diseases, such as emphysema.
- **Cardiac ultrasonography**.
- **Brain natriuretic peptide** is a small peptide molecule that, despite its name, is released by the atria in response to stretch. A normal level means that symptoms are most unlikely to be due to heart failure; a very raised level means that symptoms are likely to be due to heart failure. A mild or moderate rise means that symptoms *could* be due to heart failure. In other words, this test is most useful in *excluding* heart failure. It is also useful in following the response to treatment in those *known* to have heart failure.

These tests are occasionally helpful:

- **Cardiopulmonary exercise testing**: used before major surgery to assess fitness for anaesthesia and to investigate breathlessness with no clinical clues as to the cause.
- **Exercise ECG** to determine whether myocardial ischaemia is present, and to document exercise capacity objectively.
- **Nuclear cardiology testing**, which is more sensitive than standard exercise testing in determining the presence of myocardial ischaemia. A radioactive isotope is injected at rest, and later after exercise (or a coronary vasodilator). The isotope is taken up by healthy hearts at a rate proportional to blood flow. The rest study allows diagnosis of previous myocardial infarction, the stress study the presence of ischaemic heart.
- **Cardiac catheterization**: to measure intracardiac pressures and perform coronary angiography.

Treatment

Treatment is for the underlying condition (see relevant chapters). Hyperventilation is treated by reassurance, relaxed breathing exercises and encouragement of physical fitness.

Cough

Cough is 'a reflex forced expiration against an initially closed glottis'. The explosive expiration is a protective mechanism for the lung, clearing the lung of harmful substances.

Key points

- Upper respiratory tract infection is by far the most common cause.
- If the chest X-ray is normal, 90% of patients with chronic cough (lasting >6 weeks) have asthma, gastro-oesophageal reflux disease (GORD) or rhinosinusitis. Empirical treatment for asthma and/or GORD is often helpful because cough may be the only symptom and the two may coexist.

- Persistent cough in a smoker raises the possibility of bronchial carcinoma.

Epidemiology

- Extremely common.
- Prevalence is between 5% and 40%.
- May indicate serious underlying pathology but commonly of little significance, not warranting investigation.

Differential diagnosis

Acute cough (<3 weeks)

- Viral upper respiratory infection: most common cause is associated sore throat/rhinitis.
- Other acute infections: pneumonia and infective exacerbations of COPD.
- Foreign body: history of choking and sudden onset.

Chronic cough (>6 weeks)

- Bronchial carcinoma: smoker, weight loss, haemoptysis.
- Asthma: atopy, wheeze, shortness of breath, nocturnal symptoms, variable peak flow.
- GORD: heartburn, symptoms on change of posture, often absent at night.
- Rhinosinusitis: headache, nasal blockage, postnasal drip.
- Bronchiectasis: clubbing, copious mucus production, wheeze.
- Diffuse parenchymal lung disease: clubbing, breathlessness.
- Drugs: β-blockers, angiotensin-converting enzyme (ACE) inhibitors.
- Smoking: 50% of those who smoke >20/day have a persistent cough.

Investigations

A new cough lasting >6 weeks is more likely to be caused by serious disease requiring investigation and treatment. The clinical features often suggest the diagnosis, such as interstitial lung disease, COPD or bronchiectasis.

- **Chest X-ray**: if the cough is chronic or the patient a smoker, this may reveal infection, neoplasm or diffuse lung disease.
- **Spirometry** to diagnose airflow obstruction (peak flow monitoring may be useful in assessing asthma).
- **CT** is used to stage tumours or to diagnose diffuse lung disease.
- **Bronchoscopy** is used to remove a foreign body or for tissue diagnosis of tumours.
- **Oesophageal pH monitoring** is occasionally used to diagnose reflux disease.

In patients with a chronic cough and normal X-ray, sequential empirical treatment with inhaled steroids, antireflux treatment and treatment for rhinosinusitis will provide a 'cure' in a significant percentage of patients.

Haemoptysis

Haemoptysis is the coughing of blood from the lungs.

Causes

Minor haemoptysis is common, often related to respiratory tract infection. This resolves quickly and requires no further investigation. Haemoptysis that persists is more likely to indicate underlying serious pathology. Patients should have a chest X-ray; and many will need CT, bronchoscopy and a specialist respiratory opinion.

Table 19.2 Causes of haemoptysis	
Very common	*Uncommon*
• Bronchitis	• Bronchial adenoma
• Pneumonia	• Mycetoma
Common	*Rare*
• Bronchial carcinoma	• Vascular malformation
• Bronchiectasis	• Bleeding diathesis
• Pulmonary embolus	• Vasculitis (Wegener's granulomatosis, Goodpasture's disease)
• Spurious (nose bleed, oral disease, haematemesis)	• Connective tissue diseases
	• Endometriosis (cyclical)

Clinical approach

Haemoptysis persisting for more than 2 weeks should be investigated (see Table 19.2). A history of smoking (past or present) raises the possibility of lung carcinoma and all patients aged over 40 who smoke should be assumed to have lung cancer until investigation proves otherwise. Serious pathology is more common with increasing age. Associated symptoms or clinical signs may point towards a specific diagnosis.

Routine investigations

- **Plain chest X-ray**, blood count (for anaemia from bleeding or chronic disease), clotting profile.
- **Renal biochemistry** because some diseases produce pulmonary haemorrhage and renal failure – so-called 'pulmonary-renal syndromes' (e.g. Goodpasture's disease, Wegener's granulomatosis).
- **Liver biochemistry** for evidence of metastatic disease.
- **Special investigations** include high-resolution CT (HRCT) of the chest and bronchoscopy. These together achieve a diagnosis in >90% of patients.

Management

The key is to find the underlying diagnosis and treat appropriately, or to exclude serious disease. Most haemoptysis is minor or self-limiting, although on occasions bleeding can be severe and uncontrolled.

- Any **coagulopathy** should be corrected. Antifibrinolytic drugs may help.
- In massive haemoptysis, **bronchoscopy** allows identification and local treatment of the bleeding point.
- **Radiological embolization** or **lung resection** may be necessary in life-threatening haemorrhage.

20 Wheeze (stridor)

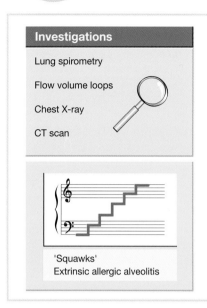

Investigations

Lung spirometry

Flow volume loops

Chest X-ray

CT scan

'Squawks'
Extrinsic allergic alveolitis

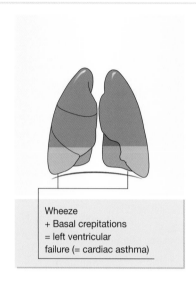

Wheeze
+ Basal crepitations
= left ventricular
failure (= cardiac asthma)

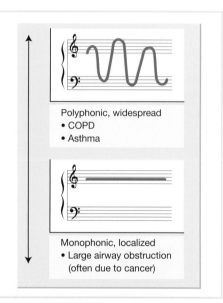

Polyphonic, widespread
• COPD
• Asthma

Monophonic, localized
• Large airway obstruction
  (often due to cancer)

Wheeze is a prolonged sound caused by airway narrowing with apposition of the airway walls. The sound is produced by vibration of airway walls and adjacent tissues. As the airways are generally narrower on expiration, wheeze is more pronounced during the expiratory phase. There are a number of causes of wheeze (see Table 20.1).

Wheeze can be divided according to the timing in the respiratory cycle and the actual sound produced (a single note or multiple notes of different pitches):

● **Polyphonic wheeze**: the most common type of wheeze typical of chronic obstructive pulmonary disease (COPD) and asthma. Multiple simultaneous different pitched sounds occur during expiration and imply diffuse disease of different sized airways.

● **Fixed monophonic wheeze**: a note of single pitch resulting from localized narrowing of a single airway. The sound does not change with coughing and particularly raises the possibility of bronchial carcinoma (see also stridor).

● **Sequential inspiratory wheeze**: otherwise known as 'squawks', caused by vibration after the opening of a previously collapsed airway; they are typical of extrinsic allergic alveolitis.

Table 20.1 Causes of wheeze

- Asthma
- COPD
- Bronchiectasis
- Large airway obstruction
- Pulmonary oedema

● **Stridor**: low-pitched monophonic wheeze heard on inspiration and implying local obstruction to the extrathoracic airways (which tend to collapse on inspiration). Often implies carcinoma or foreign body in the major airways.

Investigations

The cause of most wheezes is readily apparent on clinical grounds, and using straightforward tests such as chest X-ray and simple lung function tests. Occasionally diagnostic difficulty occurs – in these situations flow–volume loops may be helpful, as may computed tomography (CT) and cardiac ultrasonography.

Medicine at a Glance, Fourth Edition. Edited by Patrick Davey. © 2014 John Wiley & Sons, Ltd. Published 2014 by John Wiley & Sons, Ltd. Companion website: www.ataglanceseries.com/medicine

21 Pleural effusion

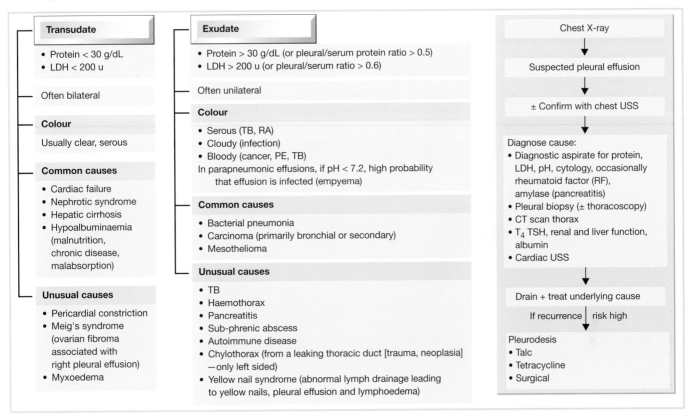

Transudate

- Protein < 30 g/dL
- LDH < 200 u

Often bilateral

Colour

Usually clear, serous

Common causes

- Cardiac failure
- Nephrotic syndrome
- Hepatic cirrhosis
- Hypoalbuminaemia (malnutrition, chronic disease, malabsorption)

Unusual causes

- Pericardial constriction
- Meig's syndrome (ovarian fibroma associated with right pleural effusion)
- Myxoedema

Exudate

- Protein > 30 g/dL (or pleural/serum protein ratio > 0.5)
- LDH > 200 u (or pleural/serum ratio > 0.6)

Often unilateral

Colour

- Serous (TB, RA)
- Cloudy (infection)
- Bloody (cancer, PE, TB)
In parapneumonic effusions, if pH < 7.2, high probability that effusion is infected (empyema)

Common causes

- Bacterial pneumonia
- Carcinoma (primarily bronchial or secondary)
- Mesothelioma

Unusual causes

- TB
- Haemothorax
- Pancreatitis
- Sub-phrenic abscess
- Autoimmune disease
- Chylothorax (from a leaking thoracic duct [trauma, neoplasia] —only left sided)
- Yellow nail syndrome (abnormal lymph drainage leading to yellow nails, pleural effusion and lymphoedema)

Chest X-ray
↓
Suspected pleural effusion
↓
± Confirm with chest USS
↓
Diagnose cause:
- Diagnostic aspirate for protein, LDH, pH, cytology, occasionally rheumatoid factor (RF), amylase (pancreatitis)
- Pleural biopsy (± thoracoscopy)
- CT scan thorax
- T_4 TSH, renal and liver function, albumin
- Cardiac USS
↓
Drain + treat underlying cause
If recurrence | risk high
Pleurodesis
- Talc
- Tetracycline
- Surgical

Definition

A collection of fluid in the pleural space. If the effusion is infected it is called an 'empyema'. If it relates to pneumonia, it is called a 'para-pneumonic effusion'.

Introduction

Pleural effusion is a common problem. The normal parietal pleura produces fluid which is reabsorbed by the visceral pleura. Either excessive fluid production (e.g. as a result of inflammation) or impaired re-absorption leads to an accumulation of fluid. An effusion needs to be at least moderate in size before it produces symptoms of shortness of breath.

Clinical approach

The most common presentation is with breathlessness. Pleural inflammation may cause pain and large effusions may cause cough. The clinical signs are of reduced expansion, stony dullness and reduced breath sounds and vocal resonance. Effusions ≤500 mL are difficult to detect clinically. The chest X-ray will show blunting of the costophrenic angle in small collections and more extensive change in the presence of larger effusions. Large effusions are more commonly the result of malignancy.

Investigations

The main distinction to make in determining the cause of an effusion is between high and low protein content (see Figure 21.1), i.e. exudates versus transudates.

If pleural infection is suspected, the pH of fluid should be measured (pH ≤7.2 suggests complicated para-pneumonic effusion or empyema, which will only resolve with pleural drainage). Fluid should also be sent for biochemistry (lactate dehydrogenase (LDH) – high in rheumatoid effusions and exudates – and protein estimation), microbiology for culture and cytology.

Management

Treatment of the underlying condition, particularly for transudates.

● Therapeutic large volume aspiration will improve symptoms. Formal drainage with intercostal tubes is often necessary with large effusions. Ultrasound guidance is recommended.

● In malignant and other recurrent effusions, agents (generally iodized talc) can be introduced via an intercostal drain to stick the two layers of pleura together and prevent reaccumulation (pleurodesis).

● Thoracoscopy (under local or general anaesthetic) may be useful in some patients to provide access to the pleura for guided biopsies and subsequent pleurodesis.

Medicine at a Glance, Fourth Edition. Edited by Patrick Davey. © 2014 John Wiley & Sons, Ltd. Published 2014 by John Wiley & Sons, Ltd. Companion website: www.ataglanceseries.com/medicine

22 Pneumothorax

Types of spontaneous pneumothorax

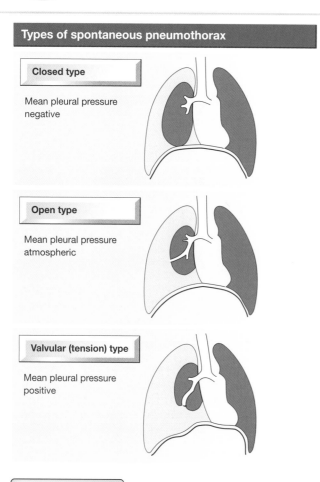

Closed type

Mean pleural pressure negative

Open type

Mean pleural pressure atmospheric

Valvular (tension) type

Mean pleural pressure positive

Management

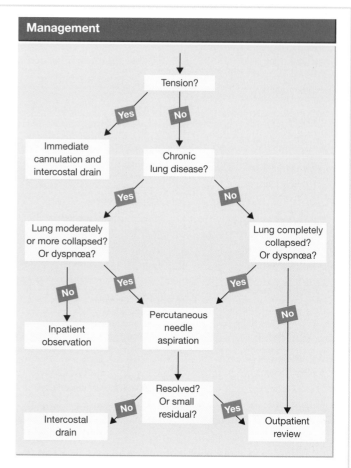

Tension?

Yes → Immediate cannulation and intercostal drain

No → Chronic lung disease?

Yes → Lung moderately or more collapsed? Or dyspnœa?

No → Lung completely collapsed? Or dyspnœa?

Lung moderately or more collapsed? Or dyspnœa? → No → Inpatient observation

Lung moderately or more collapsed? Or dyspnœa? → Yes → Percutaneous needle aspiration

Lung completely collapsed? Or dyspnœa? → Yes → Percutaneous needle aspiration

Lung completely collapsed? Or dyspnœa? → No → Outpatient review

Percutaneous needle aspiration → Resolved? Or small residual?

Resolved? Or small residual? → No → Intercostal drain

Resolved? Or small residual? → Yes → Outpatient review

Drainage

Aspiration

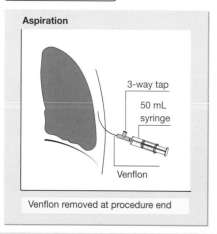

3-way tap

50 mL syringe

Venflon

Venflon removed at procedure end

Tube drainage

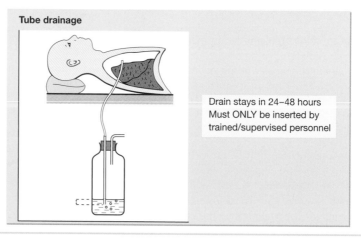

Drain stays in 24–48 hours
Must ONLY be inserted by trained/supervised personnel

Medicine at a Glance, Fourth Edition. Edited by Patrick Davey. © 2014 John Wiley & Sons, Ltd. Published 2014 by John Wiley & Sons, Ltd. Companion website: www.ataglanceseries.com/medicine

Definition

The presence of free gas in the pleural space.

Epidemiology

The incidence is 10/100 000 adults per year, males > females, and it sometimes runs in families. Taller individuals are more prone to primary spontaneous pneumothorax.

Aetiology

- **Primary spontaneous pneumothorax**: implies normal underlying lungs and is caused by rupture of a pleural 'bleb'.
- **Secondary spontaneous pneumothorax** occurs in association with lung disease (chronic obstructive pulmonary disease (COPD), pneumonia, etc.). Rupture of the visceral pleura results in communication between the airway and pleural space.
- **Traumatic** such as stab wounds.

Pathophysiology

The effects of a pneumothorax depend on whether the pleural leak persists or not.

- **'Closed' pneumothorax**: the leak closes as the lung deflates so the amount of air escaping into the pleural space is limited, pleural pressure remains negative and slow resolution will occur even without treatment.
- **'Open' pneumothorax** occurs when persistent communication between the airway and pleural space develops (bronchopleural fistula), seen as a persistent bubbling of the chest drain. The lung cannot re-expand and there is a significant risk of infection developing by transmission of organisms via the airway into the pleural space.
- **A tension pneumothorax** occurs when the leak remains open but acts as a one-way valve between the airway and pleural space. Progressive increase in the volume of gas in the pleural space leads to increase in pressure above atmospheric and compression of the underlying and contralateral lung and the heart and mediastinal shift. Cardiac filling and output decrease and the patient can become extremely unwell and die unless treated urgently.

Clinical features

- **Small pneumothorax** may be asymptomatic.
- **Medium/large pneumothorax**: sudden onset of chest pain with shortness of breath is the most common presentation. There is hyperinflation with reduced expansion and reduced breath sounds.
- **Subcutaneous emphysema**, felt as a crackling feeling in the skin, can occur if there is communication between the pleural space and the skin and subcutaneous tissues. Dramatic facial swelling and airway compromise may occur.
- **Tension pneumothorax** results in pronounced dyspnoea, tracheal deviation, tachycardia and hypotension.

Investigations

- **Chest X-ray** is diagnostic. Mediastinal deviation suggests the presence of tension. The X-ray will also show the presence of any underlying lung diseases.
- **Oxygen saturation** should be measured – usually normal unless there is underlying lung disease.
- **Ultrasonography** or **computed tomography** are both superior to the plain chest X-ray for the detection of small pneumothoraces and are often used after percutaneous lung biopsy.

Management (see Figure 22.1)

- **Drainage (aspiration or tube)** is not required for small (virtually) asymptomatic primary spontaneous pneumothoraces, but is in all symptomatic patients (initial trial of aspiration is often appropriate). Those with underlying lung disease are at greater risk of complications and should be treated as inpatients. Tension pneumothorax is a medical emergency and requires immediate treatment.
- **Surgical treatment**, with pleural abrasion or pleurectomy to obliterate the pleural space, is used for non-resolving pneumothoraces after tube drainage and for recurrent pneumothoraces.
- **Aeroplane travel**: patients with pneumothorax should not fly for 3 months because the pressure changes lead to expansion of the gas in the pleural space and so to a tension pneumothorax.

Prognosis

With adequate drainage, even in the presence of underlying lung disease, resolution can almost always be achieved. After primary spontaneous pneumothorax, 30% of patients have a further episode within 5 years. After a second episode, the recurrence rate rises above 50% and surgical pleurodesis is therefore usually recommended. Recurrence is extremely unusual following pleurodesis.

23 Unintentional weight loss

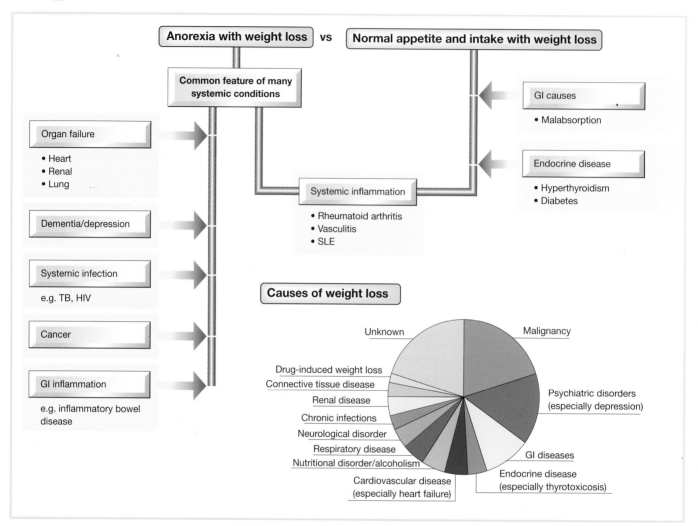

Medicine at a Glance, Fourth Edition. Edited by Patrick Davey. © 2014 John Wiley & Sons, Ltd. Published 2014 by John Wiley & Sons, Ltd. Companion website: www.ataglanceseries.com/medicine

Overall approach

Weight loss is a non-specific symptom, which might relate to a gastrointestinal (GI) condition or to a systemic pathology. Very occasionally it might reflect behavioural or even psychiatric problems.

Epidemiology

Unintentional weight loss is common, affecting up to 8% of elderly patients who seek health care. Severe and rapid weight loss ($\geq$7.5% of usual body weight lost in $\leq$6 months) is relatively unusual.

Differential diagnosis

See Figure 23.1.

Consequences of weight loss

● Weight loss is associated with an increased morbidity and mortality.

● Some of the increased mortality seen in those who unintentionally lose weight is due to the underlying disease process.

● Some of the morbidity and mortality in those with weight loss is due directly to the consequences of malnutrition on vital structures. Skeletal muscle mass may decline rapidly leading to loss of mobility and increased number of falls, which in turn may lead to fractures.

Clinical features

The most important task is to establish the **cause** of the weight loss. It is usually possible on the basis of history, examination and some elemental tests to distinguish between:

● **Dietary insufficiency**: poor diet is not infrequently the cause of weight loss; a full dietary assessment should be carried out; beware, however, as poor diet by itself does not rule out organic disease. It is crucial to determine why the diet is poor: is it due to loss of appetite (which may relate to inflammatory disease including cancer, to depression, to dementia, etc.) or is it due to social factors (poverty, alcoholism, etc.)?

● **Malabsorption**: often a good question to ask patients with weight loss is whether their appetite is preserved; anorexia and subsequent weight loss often relates to inflammatory disease, whereas weight loss in the presence of a good appetite can relate to malabsorption, thyrotoxicosis, etc.

- **'Consumption'**: although the term consumption is historically associated with miliary tuberculosis (TB), any infective, inflammatory or malignant disease can cause weight loss. Similarly weight loss is a feature of the end stage of other disease processes such as dementia, heart failure and emphysema, and features of these should be sought.

History

Important questions to be answered concern the following:

- Try and quantify the weight loss; if weights have not been measured, ask about trouser fit/belt tightening.
- Ask about appetite.
- Ask about gastrointestinal symptoms, e.g. change in bowel habit, nausea and vomiting (steatorrhoea/constipation), rectal bleeding.
- Fever, night sweats, headache (non-specific, intracranial tumour, temporal arteritis).
- Muscle weakness (non-specific or polymyalgia rheumatica).
- Mood and sleep symptoms of depression (diurnal mood variation, early wakening, anhedonia, etc.).
- Smoking increases the risk of most neoplasms (particularly lung and pancreas) as well as Crohn's disease.
- Ask about family history of cancer.
- Alcohol abuse is associated with weight loss.
- Travel history and contact with TB, etc.
- Sexual history and other risks for human immunodeficiency virus (HIV), e.g. intravenous drug use.
- Endocrine symptoms, e.g. thyrotoxicosis.
- If anorexia nervosa is suspected, ask about perception of weight loss and body image.

Examination

Look specifically for:

- Fever.
- Signs of thyroid disease.
- Signs of malnutrition (leukonychia, cheilitis, glossitis, scurvy, pellagra) and objective evidence of weight loss (loose skin, fat and/or muscle loss).
- Lymphadenopathy: generalized as well as Virchow's node (enlarged left supraclavicular node indicating intra-abdominal malignancy).
- Breast examination.

- Abnormalities in respiratory or abdominal examination indicating infection or malignancy.

Investigations

These should be targeted to specific clinical suspicions raised by the history to determine both the cause and the consequence of weight loss:

- **Blood tests**: full blood count (FBC) and raised inflammatory markers (erythrocyte sedimentation rate (ESR)/C-reactive protein (CRP)) often provide non-specific evidence for a worrying cause for weight loss. Also urea and electrolytes (U&Es), liver function tests (LFTs) and albumin, Ca^{2+}, vitamin B_{12}, folate, thyroid function, endomysial antibody for coeliac disease, and HIV test.
- **Chest X-ray**: indicated in all patients regardless of respiratory symptoms (for TB, mediastinal lymphadenopathy, metastases, primary or secondary lung carcinoma).
- **Urine dipstick examination**: for haematuria and glycosuria.
- **Endoscopy**: indicated regardless of upper GI symptoms. Distal duodenal biopsies should be taken if coeliac disease is suspected.
- **Computed tomography** (CT) of the abdomen: pancreatic or ovarian carcinoma is a frequent cause of anorexia and weight loss.
- **Faecal elastase/chymotrypsin** for pancreatic exocrine insufficiency.
- **Nutritional assessment** is very useful where investigations fail to identify a specific cause and where there are no objective markers of disease (e.g. raised ESR, etc.).

Management

Treat underlying the cause (see relevant sections elsewhere). Food supplements may have a role. If no diagnosis is reached and weight loss continues:

- **Repeat baseline investigations**: 'blind' CT (i.e. without clinical pointers) of the abdomen and pelvis (occasionally of the chest) often leads to a diagnosis, or at least excludes many neoplastic lesions.
- **Trial of nutritional support** (sip feeds, nasogastric tube feeding): weight gain with nutritional support can often help rule out sinister causes of weight loss.
- **Therapeutic trials**: in a few elderly patients with elevated inflammatory indices, an empirical trial of steroids is justifiable although a response is not very discriminatory. If the clinical suspicion of TB is high, empirical antituberculous treatment is occasionally justified.

24 Constipation and change in bowel habit

Causes of constipation

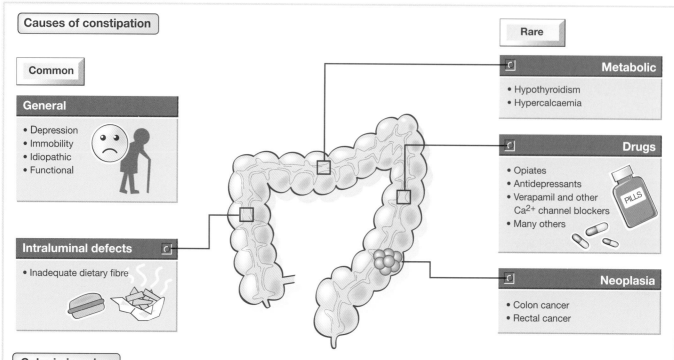

Common

General

- Depression
- Immobility
- Idiopathic
- Functional

Intraluminal defects

- Inadequate dietary fibre

Rare

Metabolic

- Hypothyroidism
- Hypercalcaemia

Drugs

- Opiates
- Antidepressants
- Verapamil and other Ca^{2+} channel blockers
- Many others

Neoplasia

- Colon cancer
- Rectal cancer

Colonic imaging

Barium enema

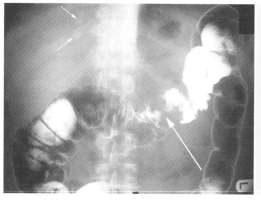

Film from double contrast barium enema in a patient with a large transverse colon carcinoma (see arrow). There is irregular stricturing of the bowel with shouldering apparent. Note lung metastases at lung base (small arrows).

Conventional colonoscopy

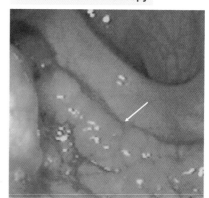

View from conventional colonoscopy confirms irregular morphology of the wall of the rectum. Histological analysis revealed villous adenocarcinoma. Occasionally, very large amounts of fluid are present using a polyethylene glycol preparation and despite supine and prone imaging the entire colonic surface may not be seen.

Virtual colonoscopy

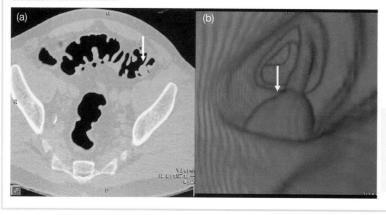

Patient who was unwilling to have conventional colonoscopy. Axial image (a) shows pedunculated polyp (arrow) in sigmoid. Endoluminal image (b) confirms 13mm pedunculated polyp on a stalk (arrow) in the sigmoid colon. When the patient was told of the abnormality he immediately requested endoscopy for removal of the lesion.

Reproduced with permission of Michael Macari

Table 24.1 Differential diagnosis of constipation.

Common
- Idiopathic/dietary
- Drugs, e.g. opioid pain killers, antidepressants, calcium antagonists

Uncommon
- Colorectal neoplasia
- Hypothyroidism
- Hypercalcaemia

Rare
- Hirschsprung's disease

Chronic constipation

Frequency of defecation varies enormously between individuals and in response to dietary and other environmental changes. Patients are often referred when their bowel frequency/habit changes. Although in many circumstances the clinical fear might be the presence of colonic malignancy, benign and functional causes are still more common (see Table 24.1).

Overall approach

It is important to ascertain the exact nature of the patient's problem (i.e. consistency, frequency or both). Does the patient harbour concerns of cancer or are they troubled by symptoms?

Clinical features

A clear history is paramount. Important questions include:

- Over what time period has the patient been constipated? Often a problem dates back many years and many over-the-counter remedies have been tried (often with varying success).
- What exactly is the problem? Has the nature of the problem changed or has the problem become more significantly inconvenient, i.e. needing regular aperients or manual evacuation?
- Past medical history and particularly obstetric history in women: pelvic trauma during protracted labour or assisted delivery may present at a later date with defecatory problems.
- Has there been any rectal bleeding? This may be due to an innocent cause (e.g. haemorrhoids) but may raise considerable anxiety on a background of constipation.
- Dietary history is very important. Patients often take too little regular dietary fibre (e.g. bran) and fluids.
- Drug history: opioids, calcium antagonist, anticholinergics, calcium-containing antacids, iron supplements.

Examination and investigations

This may be unrewarding but a thorough physical examination including rectal examination is important in providing reassurance.

- **Blood tests**: full blood count (FBC), erythrocyte sedimentation rate (ESR), thyroid function and calcium.
- **Computed tomography (CT) colonography**: more useful than colonoscopy in symptomatic constipation. It delineates colonic length and diameter and excludes colorectal neoplasia.
- **Transit studies**: in selected cases the passage of radio-opaque markers may distinguish 'slow transit' from problems of the pelvic floor.
- **Anorectal physiology and defecating proctography**: useful in selected clinical scenarios only.

Management

Management depends largely on the patient's view of the problem.

Reassurance

If the major concern was colorectal cancer, normal investigations may be sufficient.

Diet and hydration

In those with troublesome symptoms, the first line of treatment is to optimize the patient's intake of fibre and fluids.

Laxatives

- Stimulant laxatives (e.g. senna): in general their use should be limited to short-term constipation (such as that associated with hospitalization). Some patients with chronic constipation may come to depend on stimulants.
- Bulk-forming laxatives (e.g. Fybogel, Isogel): these agents are quite safe but they may exacerbate symptomatic bloating.
- Osmotic laxatives (e.g. Movicol, magnesium sulphate): these are generally well tolerated and should be considered first-line treatment. Many of these agents are available over the counter (e.g. Milk of Magnesia, Epsom salts). Although lactulose is effectively an osmotic laxative it is of limited benefit and may cause inconvenient colic and wind.

Surgery

In very resistant/recalcitrant cases surgical intervention (e.g. subtotal colectomy) may be necessary to restore quality of life.

Change in bowel habit in older patients

In the older patient a change in a previously stable bowel habit will often raise specific concerns about the development of colorectal cancer. The following are particular features of the history suggestive of a significant underlying pathology:

- Anorexia and/or weight loss.
- Nocturnal diarrhoea or pain disturbing sleep.
- Rectal bleeding.

Examination

Although often unrewarding, a full physical examination is mandatory. In particular lymphadenopathy, abdominal masses and organomegaly should be sought, and rectal examination performed.

Management

Evidence of serious underlying disease is sought from an FBC, ESR, iron indices, liver function tests, thyroid function and serum calcium; any abnormality here warrants further investigation. Colonoscopy, barium enema or CT colonography are required to exclude colorectal cancer.

American Gastroenterological Association Medical Position Statement. Guidelines on constipation. Gastroenterology. 2000: 119; 1761–78; www.gastro.org (last accessed August 2013).

25 Diarrhoea: acute and chronic

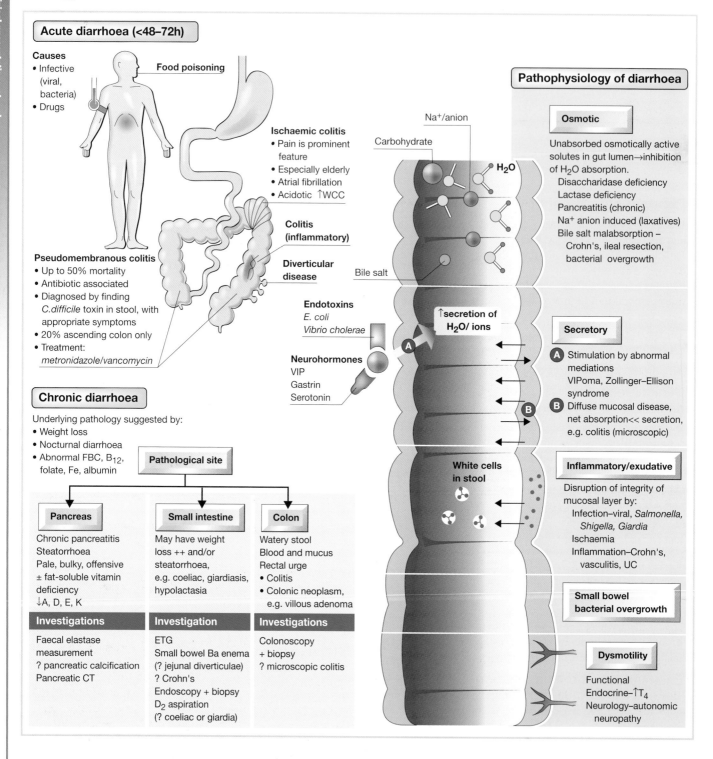

Acute diarrhoea (<48–72h)

Causes
- Infective (viral, bacteria)
- Drugs

Food poisoning

Ischaemic colitis
- Pain is prominent feature
- Especially elderly
- Atrial fibrillation
- Acidotic ↑WCC

Colitis (inflammatory)

Diverticular disease

Pseudomembranous colitis
- Up to 50% mortality
- Antibiotic associated
- Diagnosed by finding *C.difficile* toxin in stool, with appropriate symptoms
- 20% ascending colon only
- Treatment: *metronidazole/vancomycin*

Endotoxins
E. coli
Vibrio cholerae

Neurohormones
VIP
Gastrin
Serotonin

Na^+/anion
Carbohydrate
H_2O
Bile salt

↑secretion of H_2O/ ions

White cells in stool

Pathophysiology of diarrhoea

Osmotic
Unabsorbed osmotically active solutes in gut lumen→inhibition of H_2O absorption.
Disaccharidase deficiency
Lactase deficiency
Pancreatitis (chronic)
Na^+ anion induced (laxatives)
Bile salt malabsorption – Crohn's, ileal resection, bacterial overgrowth

Secretory
A Stimulation by abnormal mediations
VIPoma, Zollinger–Ellison syndrome
B Diffuse mucosal disease, net absorption<< secretion, e.g. colitis (microscopic)

Inflammatory/exudative
Disruption of integrity of mucosal layer by:
Infection–viral, *Salmonella*, *Shigella*, *Giardia*
Ischaemia
Inflammation–Crohn's, vasculitis, UC

Small bowel bacterial overgrowth

Dysmotility
Functional
Endocrine–↑T_4
Neurology–autonomic neuropathy

Chronic diarrhoea

Underlying pathology suggested by:
- Weight loss
- Nocturnal diarrhoea
- Abnormal FBC, B_{12}, folate, Fe, albumin

Pathological site

Pancreas
Chronic pancreatitis
Steatorrhoea
Pale, bulky, offensive
± fat-soluble vitamin deficiency
↓A, D, E, K

Investigations
Faecal elastase measurement
? pancreatic calcification
Pancreatic CT

Small intestine
May have weight loss ++ and/or steatorrhoea, e.g. coeliac, giardiasis, hypolactasia

Investigation
ETG
Small bowel Ba enema (? jejunal diverticulae)
? Crohn's
Endoscopy + biopsy
D_2 aspiration (? coeliac or giardia)

Colon
Watery stool
Blood and mucus
Rectal urge
- Colitis
- Colonic neoplasm, e.g. villous adenoma

Investigations
Colonoscopy + biopsy
? microscopic colitis

Acute diarrhoea

Overall approach

Most acute (<48–72h) diarrhoea is infective and may be viral or related to food poisoning. Other intestinal pathologies (particularly pseudomembranous colitis) may also present acutely. The differential diagnosis is:

- **Common**: viral, food poisoning; colitis; *Clostridium difficile* toxin-related diarrhoea.

Medicine at a Glance, Fourth Edition. Edited by Patrick Davey. © 2014 John Wiley & Sons, Ltd. Published 2014 by John Wiley & Sons, Ltd. Companion website: www.ataglanceseries.com/medicine

- **Uncommon**: inflammatory bowel disease; ischaemic colitis; diverticular change.
- **Rare**: colon cancer.

Clinical features (see Figure 25.1)

History

- Travel, contacts, take-away/restaurant food, sexual history.
- Recent medications: *C. difficile* toxin-related diarrhoea is common 2 days to 1 month after broad-spectrum antibiotics (particularly cephalosporins) in the infirm elderly patient.

Examination

The state of hydration should be determined: even young patients may be considerably volume depleted on admission, with tachycardia and postural hypotension, and may require intravenous saline. Fever generally suggests an infective cause, but may be present in severe colitis. Markers of chronic disease (clubbing, koilonychia, leukonychia, mouth ulcers, weight loss) may reflect an underlying chronic inflammatory bowel disease. Abdominal examination may reveal non-specific tenderness. Sigmoidoscopy and rectal biopsy may be useful although these might not discriminate between the various causes.

Investigations

- **Blood tests**: full blood count (FBC); anaemia or thrombocytosis raise the suspicion of a chronic underlying pathology. A low albumin is a good marker of severity of illness but is non-specific.
- **Stool culture** may identify the responsible organism. *C. difficile* bacteria are found in 5% of normal individuals; diagnosis therefore requires appropriate symptoms in the presence of the toxin rather than the organism alone.
- **Plain abdominal X-ray**: may show features of acute colitis (see Chapter 128).

Management

- **Rehydration**: the initial management involves giving parenteral or enteral rehydration.
- **Treat the underlying cause**: steroids might be indicated if investigations reveal an underlying inflammatory bowel disease. Antibiotics may be indicated in some bacterial food poisoning. Metronidazole is the first-line antibiotic for pseudomembranous colitis. Relapse occurs in up to 20% and is treated with *oral* vancomycin.

Chronic diarrhoea

Overall approach

Most infectious forms of diarrhoea resolve within 2–3 weeks and any diarrhoea that lasts longer than this warrants further investigation. In the outpatient clinic it is important to distinguish diarrhoea from rectal 'frequency' where the number of defecations per day is increased in the absence of an increase in stool weight. The differential diagnosis is: **factitious**: laxatives; **common**: inflammatory bowel disease, coeliac disease, giardiasis, drugs (e.g. proton pump inhibitors); **uncommon**: hypolactasia, colonic neoplasms (including villous adenomas), thyrotoxicosis; **rare**: endocrine tumours (e.g. Zollinger–Ellison syndrome, which results from a gastrin-secreting tumour).

Clinical features

In difficult cases it may be important to confirm that the patient has true diarrhoea (by stool weights) and not a functional bowel disorder (see Chapter 138). The features suggesting a pathological diarrhoea include nocturnal diarrhea, unintentional weight loss and mouth ulcers.

History

The clinical history may give clues about whether the predominant pathology is colonic, small intestinal or pancreatic.

- **Colonic diarrhoea**: watery stool often with blood and mucus. May be associated with urgency of defecation.
- **Small intestinal diarrhoea**: may have features of steatorrhoea (pale, bulky stools that are difficult to flush away) and weight loss.
- **Exocrine pancreatic insufficiency**: steatorrhoea and weight loss are the hallmarks of pancreatic insufficiency. In addition the patient may describe pancreatic pain, which is epigastric (often radiating through to the back) associated with fatty food intolerance.

Examination

- **General appearance**: determine whether the patient looks well or not. If possible, corroborate a history of weight loss (loose clothes or skin, belt notches, etc.).
- **Physical signs of malabsorption**: nail changes such as koilonychia and leukonychia; signs in the tongue and mouth of glossitis, cheilitis and ulcers.
- **Abdominal examination**: this should include rectal examination and preferably rigid sigmoidoscopy.

Investigations

Investigations should be chosen depending on the most likely diagnosis on clinical grounds.

- **Blood tests**: FBC, erythrocyte sedimentation rate and biochemistry, particularly for serum albumin, vitamin B_{12} and folate; thyroid function; tissue transglutaminase antibody for coeliac disease.
- **Stool microscopy and culture** ($\times 3$): negative cultures do not exclude giardiasis.
- **Faecal elastase (or faecal chymotrypsin)** will be low in exocrine pancreatic insufficiency.
- **Abdominal X-ray**: a plain abdominal X-ray may show an empty and oedematous colon. Very rarely pancreatic calcification might be seen although, if pancreatic insufficiency is suspected clinically, this is better investigated by pancreatic computed tomography (CT).
- **Endoscopy and duodenal biopsy**: to exclude coeliac disease and giardiasis.
- **Colonoscopy and biopsies**: lower gastrointestinal endoscopy has the advantage over contrast radiology in that, even if the mucosa looks normal, biopsies might reveal a microscopic colitis (e.g. lymphocytic colitis, collagenous colitis).
- Although now rarely performed **hydrogen breath tests** can confirm a suspicion of hypolactasia (lactose breath test) or small bowel bacterial overgrowth (lactulose breath test).
- **Small bowel imaging** (e.g. CT or magnetic resonance enterography): may show jejunal diverticula *or* intestinal strictures (e.g. Crohn's disease) that might act as a substrate for bacterial overgrowth.
- **Twenty-four-hour stool weights** (repeated when fasting): although this often appears low on the list of investigations, it remains the most useful way of distinguishing osmotic diarrhoea from a secretory one.
- **Fasting gut hormones**: if a hormone-secreting tumour is suspected, fasting hormone levels should be measured. If gastrin levels are measured proton pump inhibitors must be stopped.

Management

Treat the specific cause (see relevant sections).

British Society of Gastroenterology. Guidelines for the investigation of chronic diarrhoea, 2nd edition. *Gut* 2003: 52 (Suppl. V): v1–v15; www.bsg.org.uk (last accessed August 2013).

26 Vomiting and intestinal obstruction

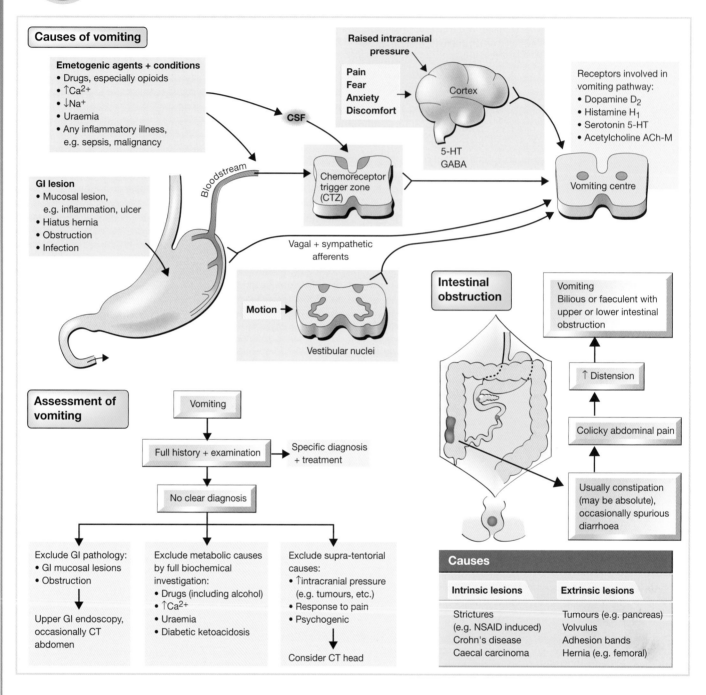

Causes of vomiting

Emetogenic agents + conditions
- Drugs, especially opioids
- $\uparrow Ca^{2+}$
- $\downarrow Na^+$
- Uraemia
- Any inflammatory illness, e.g. sepsis, malignancy

Raised intracranial pressure

Pain
Fear
Anxiety
Discomfort

Cortex

5-HT
GABA

Receptors involved in vomiting pathway:
- Dopamine D_2
- Histamine H_1
- Serotonin 5-HT
- Acetylcholine ACh-M

CSF

Bloodstream

GI lesion
- Mucosal lesion, e.g. inflammation, ulcer
- Hiatus hernia
- Obstruction
- Infection

Chemoreceptor trigger zone (CTZ)

Vomiting centre

Vagal + sympathetic afferents

Motion

Vestibular nuclei

Intestinal obstruction

Vomiting
Bilious or faeculent with upper or lower intestinal obstruction

$\uparrow$ Distension

Colicky abdominal pain

Usually constipation (may be absolute), occasionally spurious diarrhoea

Assessment of vomiting

Vomiting

Full history + examination → Specific diagnosis + treatment

No clear diagnosis

Exclude GI pathology:
- GI mucosal lesions
- Obstruction

Upper GI endoscopy, occasionally CT abdomen

Exclude metabolic causes by full biochemical investigation:
- Drugs (including alcohol)
- $\uparrow Ca^{2+}$
- Uraemia
- Diabetic ketoacidosis

Exclude supra-tentorial causes:
- $\uparrow$intracranial pressure (e.g. tumours, etc.)
- Response to pain
- Psychogenic

Consider CT head

Causes	
Intrinsic lesions	**Extrinsic lesions**
Strictures (e.g. NSAID induced)	Tumours (e.g. pancreas)
	Volvulus
Crohn's disease	Adhesion bands
Caecal carcinoma	Hernia (e.g. femoral)

Intestinal obstruction

Overall approach

The first step in the assessment of vomiting is to consider whether or not there is intestinal obstruction. Intestinal obstruction can be caused by:

- **Intrinsic factors**:
  - Gastrointestinal (GI) neoplasia, e.g. gastric or colonic carcinoma.
  - Crohn's disease.
  - Strictures, e.g. post-surgical; ischaemia; other, including non-steroidal anti-inflammatory drugs (NSAIDs).
- **Extrinsic factors**:
  - Tumour, e.g. pancreas.
  - Incarcerated hernia.
  - Adhesion bands secondary to previous surgery.
  - Volvulus.
- **Pseudo-obstruction**: paralytic ileus/motility disorders.

Clinical features

Key clinical features indicating that vomiting is caused by intestinal obstruction are, first, the presence of colicky abdominal pain and, second, a change in bowel habit (ranging from diarrhoea to absolute constipation).

History

- Ask about the duration of symptoms, anorexia and weight loss (suggests progressive pathology).
- Site of pain (see Chapter 30).
- A sudden onset of pain and vomiting implies a physical/mechanical cause.
- Previous intestinal illness or operations.

Examination

General

Observe the general appearance and presence of lymphadenopathy. It is vital to determine the fluid status of the patient from skin turgor, pulse rate, blood pressure (including postural drop) and urine output.

Abdominal examination

- Scars from previous surgery raise the possibility of obstruction caused by adhesions.
- Abdominal distension may be present. Absent bowel sounds suggest paralytic ileus (pseudo-obstruction), whereas in most other cases of obstruction bowel sounds are increased. A succussion splash suggests gastric outflow obstruction.
- Tenderness and rebound suggest peritonitis (i.e. perforation).
- Palpable inflammatory or neoplastic masses.
- Rectal examination and sigmoidoscopy.

Investigations

- **Blood tests**: full blood count (FBC)/erythrocyte sedimentation rate (ESR) and biochemistry are indicated, partly to determine the effect of vomiting/obstruction on potassium and renal function.
- **Abdominal X-ray**: usually shows features of intestinal obstruction (i.e. dilated fluid-filled loops of bowel) and on occasion may suggest the level of the obstruction (e.g. air absent from the rectum).
- **Endoscopy**: if gastric outflow obstruction is suspected. Beware the risk of aspiration of intestinal contents.
- **Abdominal computed tomography** (CT) with contrast after discussion with radiologist and surgical team.

Management

All cases should be managed in conjunction with a GI surgeon.

Initial management

- **Nil by mouth**: gut rest is probably the best way to relieve symptoms. A large-bore nasogastric tube (Ryle's tube) helps to drain obstructed intestinal contents and in cases of protracted large volume vomiting is imperative in preventing aspiration.
- **Intravenous fluids**: patients may be significantly volume depleted/dehydrated on admission and require substantial fluid resuscitation. Avoid opiate analgesia when possible (as this further inhibits intestinal motility).

Subsequent management

In cases that do not resolve with conservative management, a laparotomy may be necessary even before a definitive diagnosis has been achieved.

Chronic vomiting

Overall approach

In the absence of evidence of mechanical obstruction other causes of vomiting should be considered, such as:

- **Metabolic**:
  - Hypercalcaemia.
  - Hypoadrenalism (Addison's disease).
- **Inflammatory disease**:
  - Visceral inflammation, e.g. pancreatitis.
  - Remote infection, e.g. pneumonia.
- **Drugs**:
  - Cytotoxics.
  - Analgesics (especially opioids).
  - Antibiotics.
- **Neurogenic**:
  - Intracranial tumours.
  - Vestibulocochlear disease.
  - Psychogenic.
- **GI causes**:
  - Obstruction.
  - Gastroenteritis.

History

Ask specifically about:

- Duration of symptoms, and whether the problem is getting worse.
- Drugs, including those bought over the counter.
- Headache or other features of raised intracranial pressure.
- Unusual foods, restaurants, travel.
- Hearing, balance.

Examination

- **General**: check overall appearance and the presence of any relevant pathology. State of hydration, particularly postural blood pressure.
- **Abdominal examination**: usually unrewarding but may reveal signs of intestinal obstruction.

Investigations

- **Blood tests**: FBC, ESR and biochemistry, including renal and liver function, sodium, potassium and calcium, amylase.
- **Cortisol**: short Synacthen test if hypoadrenalism is suspected.
- **Chest X-ray**: for infection (including aspiration pneumonia), neoplasm.
- **Endoscopy** is usually indicated in patients with persistent vomiting when no other cause is found.
- **Small bowel imaging**: may be indicated in difficult cases to exclude occult subacute obstruction.
- **CT or magnetic resonance imaging** (MRI) **scan of the head**: indicated when no other pathology is identified.

Management

- Treat the underlying cause.
- Antiemetics: empirical treatment with antiemetics may be necessary if physical/mechanical obstruction has been excluded. Domperidone does not cross the blood–brain barrier and is useful for long-term 'as needed' treatment. Other agents (e.g. metoclopramide, prochlorperazine) are increasingly being replaced by centrally acting serotonin antagonists (e.g. ondansetron).

27 Haematemesis and melaena

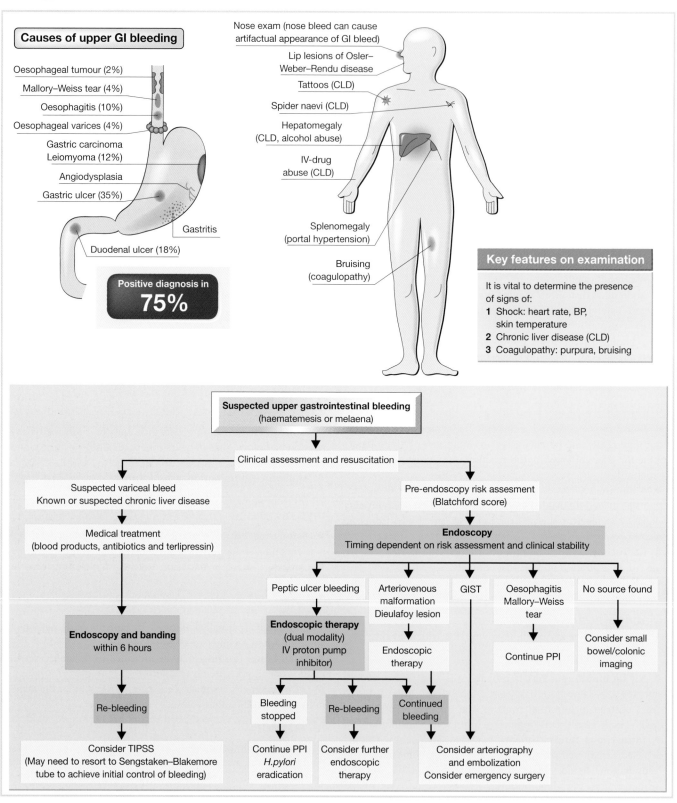

Causes of upper GI bleeding

- Oesophageal tumour (2%)
- Mallory–Weiss tear (4%)
- Oesophagitis (10%)
- Oesophageal varices (4%)
- Gastric carcinoma Leiomyoma (12%)
- Angiodysplasia
- Gastric ulcer (35%)
- Gastritis
- Duodenal ulcer (18%)

Positive diagnosis in 75%

Nose exam (nose bleed can cause artifactual appearance of GI bleed)

Lip lesions of Osler–Weber–Rendu disease

Tattoos (CLD)

Spider naevi (CLD)

Hepatomegaly (CLD, alcohol abuse)

IV-drug abuse (CLD)

Splenomegaly (portal hypertension)

Bruising (coagulopathy)

Key features on examination

It is vital to determine the presence of signs of:
1 Shock: heart rate, BP, skin temperature
2 Chronic liver disease (CLD)
3 Coagulopathy: purpura, bruising

Suspected upper gastrointestinal bleeding
(haematemesis or melaena)

↓

Clinical assessment and resuscitation

Suspected variceal bleed
Known or suspected chronic liver disease

↓

Medical treatment
(blood products, antibiotics and terlipressin)

↓

Endoscopy and banding
within 6 hours

↓

Re-bleeding

↓

Consider TIPSS
(May need to resort to Sengstaken–Blakemore tube to achieve initial control of bleeding)

Pre-endoscopy risk assesment
(Blatchford score)

↓

Endoscopy
Timing dependent on risk assessment and clinical stability

- Peptic ulcer bleeding
- Arteriovenous malformation Dieulafoy lesion
- GIST
- Oesophagitis Mallory–Weiss tear
- No source found

Endoscopic therapy
(dual modality)
IV proton pump inhibitor)

Endoscopic therapy

Continue PPI

Consider small bowel/colonic imaging

- Bleeding stopped
- Re-bleeding
- Continued bleeding

Continue PPI
H.pylori eradication

Consider further endoscopic therapy

Consider arteriography and embolization
Consider emergency surgery

Medicine at a Glance, Fourth Edition. Edited by Patrick Davey. © 2014 John Wiley & Sons, Ltd. Published 2014 by John Wiley & Sons, Ltd. Companion website: www.ataglanceseries.com/medicine

Introduction

- **Haematemesis** refers to the vomiting of blood. Blood may be fresh (clots or bright red liquid) or altered by intestinal acid and enzymes, appearing brown and likened to 'coffee grounds'. Vomiting a small amount of altered blood is often a non-specific feature of protracted retching and does not always reflect a significant upper gastrointestinal (GI) haemorrhage.
- **Melaena** refers to a loose, tarry, jet-black stool, with a deeply offensive smell, which sticks to the pan and indicates brisk upper GI haemorrhage with digestion of the blood in the intestine. Solid dark stool that tests positive for occult blood may indicate intestinal bleeding but is *not* melaena.

Differential diagnosis

- **Common**: peptic ulcer (duodenal, gastric); Mallory–Weiss tear; gastritis, duodenitis, oesophagitis.
- **Uncommon**: oesophageal varices/portal hypertensive gastropathy.
- **Rare**: upper GI malignancy – including gastrointestinal stromal tumours (GISTs).
- **Very rare**: angiodysplasia (including a Dieulafoy lesion); aortoenteric fistula only ever really seen with infected aortic grafts.

Clinical clues to the diagnosis

A history of indigestion may make peptic ulcer more likely but its absence does not exclude this. A history of retching and vomitus initially free from blood suggests a Mallory–Weiss tear. Heavy alcohol consumption suggests gastritis (30–40%) or occasionally varices. Weight loss suggests malignancy. Severe bleeding with clots and treatment-refractory shock raises the probability of varices. Previous abdominal aortic surgery raises the possibility of aortoenteric fistula. In young patients with a history of repeated brisk upper GI bleeding (often with haemodynamic collapse) and 'unremarkable' endoscopies, a Dieulafoy lesion should be considered (a submucosal artery, usually on the lesser gastric curve and situated near the cardia, which intermittently causes large GI bleeds).

- **History**: postural dizziness or loss of consciousness in the context of haematemesis or melaena is significant, implying a 'haemodynamically significant bleed'.
- **Drug history** is relevant both to the underlying diagnosis (e.g. aspirin and non-steroidal anti-inflammatory drugs (NSAIDs) suggest peptic ulceration) and to treatment (β-blockers, warfarin).

Table 27.1 Clinical risk assessment tools: the Blatchford and Rockall scores.

Blatchford score system	Score	Rockall score system	Score			
			0	1	2	3
Blood urea (mmol/L)						
>6.5 <8.0	2	Age	<60	60–79	>80	
>8.0 <10.0	3	Shock	'No shock' BP >100 Pulse <100	'Tachycardia' BP >100 Pulse >100	'Hypotension' BP <100	
>10.0 <25	4					
>25	6	Co-morbidity	No major co-morbidity		Cardiac failure, ischaemic heart disease	Renal failure, liver failure, disseminated malignancy
Haemoglobin (g/dL, men)						
>12 <13	1					
>10 <12	3	Diagnosis	Mallory–Weiss tear, no lesion identified	All other diagnoses	Upper GI malignancy	
<10	6					
Haemoglobin (g/dL, women)						
>10 <12	1	Major SRH	None, or dark spot only		Blood in upper GI tract, adherent clot, visible or spurting vessel	
<10	6					
Systolic blood pressure (mmHg)						
100–109	1					
90–99	2					
<90	3					
Other markers						
Pulse >100	1					
Presentation with melaena	1					
Presentation with syncope	2					
Hepatic disease	2					
Cardiac failure	2					

SRH, stigmata of recent haemorrhage.

27 Haematemesis and melaena (continued)

Mortality vs Risk score*

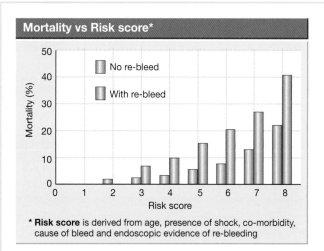

* **Risk score** is derived from age, presence of shock, co-morbidity, cause of bleed and endoscopic evidence of re-bleeding

Management of acute GI bleed

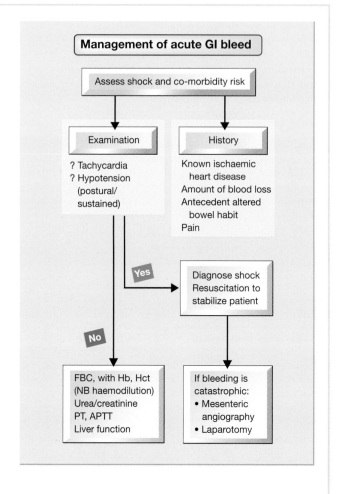

Assess shock and co-morbidity risk

Examination
? Tachycardia
? Hypotension (postural/sustained)

History
Known ischaemic heart disease
Amount of blood loss
Antecedent altered bowel habit
Pain

Yes

Diagnose shock
Resuscitation to stabilize patient

No

FBC, with Hb, Hct (NB haemodilution)
Urea/creatinine
PT, APTT
Liver function

If bleeding is catastrophic:
• Mesenteric angiography
• Laparotomy

Management of haematemesis/melaena

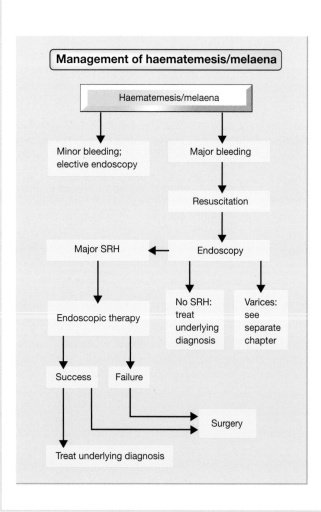

Haematemesis/melaena

Minor bleeding; elective endoscopy

Major bleeding

Resuscitation

Major SRH ← Endoscopy

No SRH: treat underlying diagnosis

Varices: see separate chapter

Endoscopic therapy

Success   Failure

Surgery

Treat underlying diagnosis

Immediate treatment

1 IV access: 2 large bore IV lines
2 Fluid (blood)
3 Endoscopy <12 h or sooner if continued bleeding

Examination

General

- General appearance: is the patient cool and clammy, indicating significant peripheral vasoconstriction?
- Pulse and blood pressure (BP), including postural drop. Documentation of the severity of shock is vitally important.
- Signs of chronic liver disease.
- Signs of neoplasia: lymphadenopathy, organomegaly, weight loss.

Abdominal

This may be uninformative. Epigastric tenderness is most often non-specific. Hepatosplenomegaly and/or abdominal ascites raise the possibility of portal hypertension (i.e. varices).

Predictors of mortality

A number of factors have now been defined as predicting mortality from upper GI bleeding and these form the basis of clinical risk assessment tools (see Table 27.1). The Blatchford score is based upon initial observations and blood test results, whereas the Rockall score incorporates endoscopic finding in predicting risk.

Investigations

- **Blood tests**: full blood count (FBC) and cross-match.
- **Urea and creatinine**: a raised urea relative to creatinine (i.e. raised urea/creatinine ratio) is present in significant upper GI haemorrhage and reflects the protein load of fresh blood within the gut, as well as dehydration ('pre-renal' uraemia, see Chapter 150).
- **K^+**: this may be disproportionately high as a result of absorption from blood in the small bowel.
- **Clotting** should be checked in patients on anticoagulants and those with signs of chronic liver disease (CLD).
- **Endoscopy**: will establish the diagnosis and may allow immediate endoscopic treatment. It also provides prognostic information (i.e. identification of stigmata of recent haemorrhage (SRH)).

Management

All cases should be managed in conjunction with an experienced endoscopist and GI surgeons. If the patient has had abdominal aortic surgery a vascular surgeon should be consulted. Episodes of re-bleeding after admission (as suggested by further haematemesis, melaena, cardiovascular instability or fall in haemoglobin) have a worse prognosis.

Resuscitation

Early volume replacement is vital in patients with shock and coexistent cardiovascular disease.

Central venous pressure monitoring

The benefits of placing a central line include safer resuscitation of patients with heart failure and ischaemic heart disease and early recognition of re-bleeding.

Endoscopic therapy

In addition to providing a diagnosis, endoscopy also allows treatment to bleeding lesions:

- Injection therapy: adrenaline for peptic ulcers with SRH.
- Endoscopic clipping of bleeding vessels.
- Heater probe and argon plasma coagulation of bleeding vessels, tumours and ulcers.
- Band ligation of oesophageal varices.

Medical treatment

In patients with bleeding from peptic ulcers showing SRH, intravenous (IV) proton pump inhibitors (PPIs) increase intragastric pH leading to clot stabilization, which in turn reduces the risk of re-bleeding episodes.

Re-bleeding

Any evidence of re-bleeding after initial therapy carries a poor prognosis and should be addressed by either repeated endoscopic therapy or surgery

Surgery

Although surgery is less common now than in days before the development of endoscopy, it remains a vital treatment. Surgical intervention should be considered in individuals not responding to resuscitation and those with a clinically significant re-bleed, and in those in whom endoscopy has failed or is not feasible. Early consultation with the surgical team always facilitates subsequent management.

NICE Clinical Guideline No. 141. *Acute upper GI bleeding*, June 2012.

28 Rectal bleeding

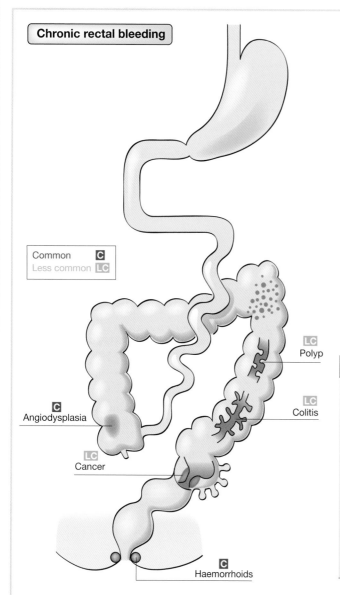

Chronic rectal bleeding

Common **C**
Less common **LC**

LC Polyp

LC Colitis

C Angiodysplasia

LC Cancer

C Haemorrhoids

Outpatient management of chronic GI bleed

History

? Family history/risks for IBD, neoplasia
Nature of blood loss (see text)
Associated symptoms:
change in bowel habit, pain, etc., weight loss

Investigation

Flexible sigmoidoscopy
Colonoscopy

Acute rectal bleeding

Diverticular disease
Angiodysplasia
Ischaemia
Meckel's diverticulum

Clinical differences between upper and lower GI bleeding

	Upper GI source	Lower GI source
Haematemesis	+++	Never
Melaena	++	Never
Dark red blood PR	+	++
Bright red blood PR	Never	+++
Raised urea/creatinine ratio	++	0 – +
Known ulcerative colitis	0 – +	++
Antecedent altered bowel habit	0 – +	++

Distinguish between acute, heavy or lower gastrointestinal (GI) haemorrhage and chronic, persistent, small volume rectal bleeding. The term 'haematochezia' is used in North America to describe rectal bleeding.

Acute lower GI haemorrhage

Sudden large volume rectal bleeding most commonly presents in elderly people as a clinical emergency with varying degrees of cardiovascular compromise.

Differential diagnosis (see Table 28.1)

The common underlying causes are age related and, although they are often in themselves benign, the presence of significant co-morbidity (e.g. ischaemic heart disease) in this group of patients contributes to a significant mortality.

Table 28.1 Differential diagnosis of acute lower GI haemorrhage.

Common

- Diverticular change
- Colonic angiodysplasia
- Ischaemic colitis

Uncommon

- Distal colon/rectal carcinoma
- Inflammatory bowel disease

Medicine at a Glance, Fourth Edition. Edited by Patrick Davey. © 2014 John Wiley & Sons, Ltd. Published 2014 by John Wiley & Sons, Ltd. Companion website: www.ataglanceseries.com/medicine

Clinical features

It can be a challenge to distinguish proximal colonic bleeding from a brisk upper GI bleed. The passage of red blood per rectum (PR) is unlikely to be from an upper GI source. Likewise the passage of classic melaena (jet-black, tarry, smelly) indicates an upper GI tract lesion. The problem arises when blood appears to be neither one nor the other, when upper and lower GI tract investigations are needed.

History

- **Nature of the bleeding**: was it black 'like tar' (i.e. melaena) or black 'like bramble jelly' (i.e. arising from the colon)?
- **Onset**: most commonly the onset of bleeding is sudden, although it is important to elicit whether there had been an antecedent change in bowel habit, which may indicate a colonic neoplasm or colitis.
- **Abdominal pain**: mild colicky pain is a non-specific finding, severe *sudden* pain suggests intestinal ischaemia (i.e. ischaemic colitis).
- **Significant co-morbidity**: the recognition of significant co-morbidity is important in guiding resuscitation and specific interventions.

Examination

- **State of circulation** (pulse, postural blood pressure): any degree of shock must be recognized early and corrected (see below).
- **Abdominal examination**: the absence of a palpable **mass** in the abdomen does not exclude a malignant underlying cause.
- A **bruit** may rarely be heard, indicating mesenteric atheroma and potentially ischaemia.
- **Rectal examination** may identify a low rectal cancer and may be useful in clinically distinguishing lower from upper GI bleeding (melaena = upper).
- **Sigmoidoscopy** will often provide very limited views at the time of a large bleed.

Investigations

- **Blood tests**: a full blood count (FBC) should be taken, although in acute GI bleeding haemodilution takes several hours, so the haemoglobin level may underestimate the severity of the bleed. A clotting profile should be checked if the patient is on anticoagulants or if there are clinical indications of chronic liver disease. Cross-match if shock is present on admission or if there is significant anaemia. A raised urea:creatinine ratio may indicate an upper, not lower, GI source.
- **Abdominal X-ray**: a plain abdominal X-ray may show features of ischaemia (localized area of colonic mucosal oedema, sometimes with 'thumb-printing').
- **Lower GI endoscopy**: once resuscitation has been completed and preferably after the acute bleed has subsided. The timing and extent of the endoscopy (i.e. colonoscopy vs flexible sigmoidoscopy) must be determined on individual clinical grounds. Computed tomography (CT) colonography may be necessary if the upper limit of bleeding is not identified or if total endoscopic examination is prevented by technical limitations (e.g. severe diverticular change, ischaemia, stricture).
- **Upper GI endoscopy**: usually at the time of sigmoidoscopy/colonoscopy for formal exclusion of a significant upper GI pathology.
- **Mesenteric angiography**: in persistent heavy colonic bleeding ($\leq$2–5 mL/min) angiography can identify areas of angiodysplasia or a bleeding vessel that can be embolized.

Management

- **Resuscitation**: early correction of shock is vital.
- **Treat specific pathology**: in most circumstances colonic bleeding will at least temporarily cease, allowing for diagnostic investigations.
- **Laparotomy**: in catastrophic bleeding, a laparotomy, if possible with on-table colonoscopy, and occasionally a 'blind' colectomy may be necessary.

Chronic rectal bleeding

Overall approach

The recurrent/persistent passage of blood PR may present at any age and, in most situations, can be managed as an outpatient.

Differential diagnosis

Although the most common cause of rectal bleeding is benign, appropriate investigations are always indicated in order to make an early diagnosis of colorectal cancer. The differential diagnosis is: **common**: haemorrhoids ('piles'), colorectal neoplasia (polyps, cancer) – more common in the elderly; **rare**: distal colitis, solitary rectal ulcer.

History

The history (particularly the appearance of the blood) often suggests the site of bleeding:
- Bright red 'like tomato ketchup' or dark red 'like bramble jelly' blood suggests, respectively, lower and upper colonic pathology.
- Blood only on the toilet paper and the surface of the stool strongly suggests 'piles' as the source. Blood mixed throughout the stool suggests that the pathology is higher up.
- A change in bowel habit suggests an underlying neoplasm or colitis.
- Bright red bleeding, with mucus discharge, urge and a sense of incomplete emptying (otherwise known as tenesmus) suggest proctitis.
- A family history of colorectal cancer increases the probability (and worry) of this disease.

Examination

Abdominal examination should include the identification of any masses or palpable organomegaly and rectal examination for detection of low rectal tumours. *All* patients should at some point undergo sigmoidoscopy for the detection of rectal polyps/cancer and colitis.

Investigations

- **Blood tests**: FBC, erythrocyte sedimentation rate (ESR), iron indices – iron deficiency anaemia or raised inflammatory markers should *never* be ascribed to haemorrhoids/piles.
- **Lower GI endoscopy**: flexible sigmoidoscopy after an enema should provide good views of the colon as far as the splenic flexure. Total colonoscopy requires full bowel preparation and sedation and is indicated when a proximal colonic neoplasm is suspected clinically, from iron deficiency or the presence of distal colonic polyps.
- **CT colonography** is an alternative to total colonoscopy. This requires full bowel preparation and inflation of the colon with air or CO_2. This technique does not yet have an equivalent sensitivity to colonoscopy and most abnormalities require further evaluation (i.e. colonoscopy). A sigmoidoscopic examination (either rigid or flexible) should be performed in addition to exclude a low rectal neoplasm, which might otherwise be missed on the scan.

Management

- **Treat specific pathology**: see relevant chapters.
- **Haemorrhoids**: often advice on diet and defecatory habits is sufficient to control symptoms. Injection sclerotherapy, banding and excision may be necessary in some circumstances.

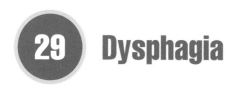

29 Dysphagia

Carcinoma

- Progressive history
- Solids (not liquids)
- Weight loss ++
- Long stricture 'apple core' lesion
- Usually lower ⅓
- Oesophageal or gastric origin

Peptic stricture

- Associated symptoms of reflux
- Short
- Commonest cause of benign strictures
- Other causes: after corrosives after radiotherapy after variceal injection

Neuromuscular dysphagia

- Cause usually obvious, CVA, motor neuron disease, progressive suprabulbar palsy
- If cause unclear, consider myasthenia gravis
- Usually liquids > solids

Systemic disease

- Scleroderma: often associated severe reflux → peptic stricture
- Dermatomyositis
- Connective tissue disorders, especially if Raynaud's present

Extrinsic compression

- Aortic arch aneurysm
- Lymph nodes: lymphoma lung cancer
- Enlarged L-atrium, e.g. mitral stenosis

Achalasia

Progressive dilatation above sphincter

May cause aspiration pneumonia

Local nerve death → Hypertonic sphincter

Prevent any symptoms of reflux

- Rare, 1 in 100,000
- Idiopathic, or Chagas' disease (*Trypanosoma cruzi*)
- Long history of intermittent dysphagia and regurgitation
- Occasionally attacks of severe chest pain due to oesophageal spasm ('vigorous achalasia')

Introduction

Dysphagia relates to difficulty in swallowing which in turn implies oesophageal obstruction. Odynophagia relates to painful swallowing. Globus refers to a patient's description of a sensation 'like a lump in the throat' – this is quite distinct and should not be confused with dysphagia.

Differential diagnosis

See Table 29.1.

Clinical features

Dysphagia is an ominous and frightening symptom and should be investigated at the earliest opportunity.

History

The duration of symptoms and associated heartburn/dyspepsia are useful clinical clues. Progressive symptoms and weight loss are ominous features.

Examination

Examination is often unrewarding. Check for anaemia, weight loss and lymphadenopathy (including Virchow's node behind the head of the left clavicle, indicative of metastatic upper gastrointestinal (GI) cancer).

Investigations

- **General investigations** include a full blood count and erythrocyte sedimentation rate, liver function tests and calcium. A chest X-ray may show either a primary or a secondary lung neoplasia.
- **Endoscopy**: upper GI endoscopy must be performed with great care but allows definitive diagnosis through biopsy and immediate treatment (oesophageal dilatation, placement of stent).
- **Other specific tests** (manometry, pH monitoring, computed tomography) are indicated depending on the results of the above. See sections on reflux and oesophageal carcinoma (see Chapters 123 and 135).

Management

- **Peptic stricture**: strictures associated with reflux oesophagitis occasionally require endoscopic dilatation. Recurrence may be reduced by treatment with proton pump inhibitors.
- **Oesophageal carcinoma**: see Chapter 135.
- **Achalasia**: there are a range of treatments for achalasia. Cardiomyotomy (Heller's operation) remains the definitive procedure and can now be performed laparoscopically. Forced pneumatic dilatation is an alternative for patients in whom surgery is not possible.

Medicine at a Glance, Fourth Edition. Edited by Patrick Davey. © 2014 John Wiley & Sons, Ltd. Published 2014 by John Wiley & Sons, Ltd. Companion website: www.ataglanceseries.com/medicine

Table 29.1 Differential diagnosis of dysphagia.

Common

- Oesophageal carcinoma
- Gastric cancer at the cardia
- Oesophagitis and peptic stricture

Uncommon

- Diffuse oesophageal spasm (intermittent symptoms associated with pain)

Rare

- Achalasia
- Eosinophilic oesophagitis: can only be diagnosed by taking biopsies of distal oesophagus

- **Oesophageal dysmotility**: reassurance after exclusion of a malignant underlying cause for the symptoms often helps patients with oesophageal spasm, together with simple advice about diet and nutrition. Calcium antagonists and nitrates have no role.
- **Eosinophilic oesophagitis**: this recently described but rare condition may be diagnosed on oesophageal biopsy. Treatments that have been tried include both topical and systemic steroids and antihistamines.
- **Neuromuscular dysphagia**: see below.
- **Extrinsic compression** is treated according to the underlying cause.
- **Systemic diseases** producing dysphagia are managed similarly. Scleroderma may produce severe symptoms of reflux, requiring high-dose proton pump inhibition.

Neuromuscular dysphagia

Dysphagia to liquids may occur in motor neuron disease and is an important finding in stroke (it occurs in some 50–70% of stroke patients). Aspiration of food in stroke patients is a crucial mechanism contributing to pneumonia, which itself accounts for some 20–40% of stroke-related deaths.

Neurological disease may interfere with any of the three phases of swallowing:

- The **oral phase**, where food is prepared for swallowing (usually by chewing) and then propelled into the oropharynx (the oral propulsive phase): paralysis of the cranial nerve supplying the tongue, or interference with the cerebellar mechanisms controlling the tongue, may lead to impairment of this phase.
- The **pharyngeal phase**, where food is propelled into the oesophagus, by a complex series of reflex events, involving cranial nerves IX–XII.
- The **oesophageal phase**, where the bolus of food is propelled down the oesophagus by peristaltic motion.

Clinical features

The features of dysphagia in stroke patients include coughing when eating/drinking, recurrent chest infections, weight loss with food avoidance and dehydration. As dysphagia is so frequent in stroke patients, it is crucial to assess swallowing as part of the acute assessment of a stroke. Until this has been done the patient should be 'nil by mouth'.

Examination

Swallowing assessment consists of a full neurological examination, with some additional features:

- Assess cranial nerves V, VII–XII.
- Observe jaw movement, mastication, tongue strength and mobility.
- Test the individual functions of the mouth.
- Test for the gag reflex.
- Assess how strong the cough is, as this determines how good the lung is at protecting against infection.
- If the functions of the mouth are intact, ask the patient to swallow; while doing so, place three fingers on the larynx and assess how it moves during the swallow.
- If all the above are intact, assess how the patient swallows a small amount of water.

If swallowing is impaired, then the patient should not be fed orally; for the very short run, intravenous fluids are appropriate. If swallowing is not satisfactory after a few days, feeding should occur via a nasogastric tube. If swallowing remains impaired after 2–3 weeks, consideration should be given to percutaneous endoscopic gastrostomy (PEG) feeding.

Prognosis

Most patients who have acutely impaired swallowing due to a stroke have recovered by 6 months – only a very small proportion need ongoing PEG feeding.

30 Abdominal pain and dyspepsia

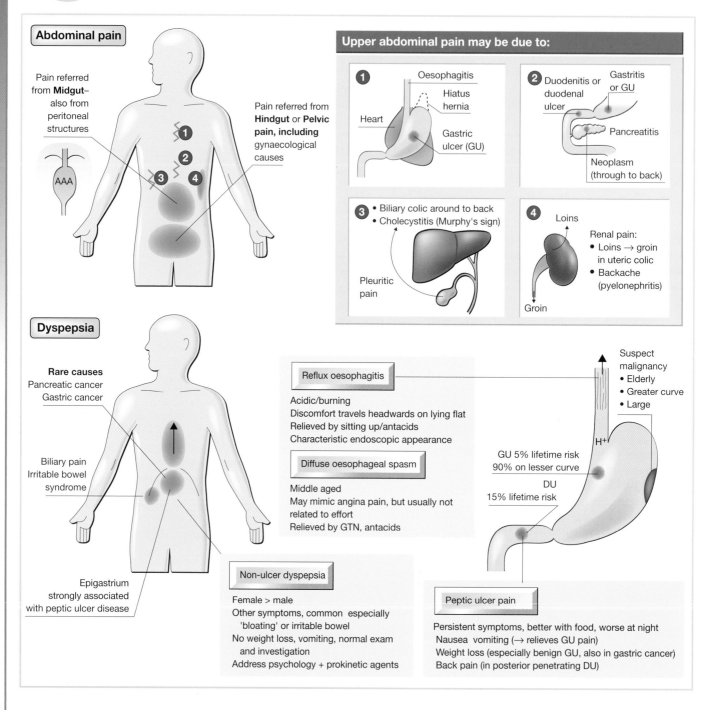

Abdominal pain

Pain referred from **Midgut**– also from peritoneal structures

AAA

Pain referred from **Hindgut** or **Pelvic pain**, including gynaecological causes

Upper abdominal pain may be due to:

1. Oesophagitis
   Hiatus hernia
   Heart
   Gastric ulcer (GU)

2. Duodenitis or duodenal ulcer
   Gastritis or GU
   Pancreatitis
   Neoplasm (through to back)

3. • Biliary colic around to back
   • Cholecystitis (Murphy's sign)
   Pleuritic pain

4. Loins
   Renal pain:
   • Loins → groin in uteric colic
   • Backache (pyelonephritis)
   Groin

Dyspepsia

Rare causes
Pancreatic cancer
Gastric cancer

Biliary pain
Irritable bowel syndrome

Epigastrium strongly associated with peptic ulcer disease

Reflux oesophagitis

Acidic/burning
Discomfort travels headwards on lying flat
Relieved by sitting up/antacids
Characteristic endoscopic appearance

Diffuse oesophageal spasm

Middle aged
May mimic angina pain, but usually not related to effort
Relieved by GTN, antacids

Non-ulcer dyspepsia

Female > male
Other symptoms, common especially 'bloating' or irritable bowel
No weight loss, vomiting, normal exam and investigation
Address psychology + prokinetic agents

Suspect malignancy
• Elderly
• Greater curve
• Large

H+

GU 5% lifetime risk
90% on lesser curve

DU
15% lifetime risk

Peptic ulcer pain

Persistent symptoms, better with food, worse at night
Nausea vomiting (→ relieves GU pain)
Weight loss (especially benign GU, also in gastric cancer)
Back pain (in posterior penetrating DU)

Abdominal pain

A very careful history is critical to formulate a differential diagnosis. Pains usually come from within an organ (midline pain, not often localized to the affected viscus) or from irritation of the peritoneal lining (localized to the site of the inflamed viscus). Patients in pain are often frightened. Patience and perseverance in history taking is rewarded with an earlier and more accurate diagnosis.

History

This is critical to the assessment as physical signs might be limited. Consider the SQITAS questions: Site, Quality, Initiating factors, Time course, Alleviating factors, asSociated symptoms.

Certain patterns point to specific sources of pain although there is considerable overlap.

● **Oesophageal pain** has two forms: 'heartburn' relates to acidic sensations and is commonly related to reflux. Oesophageal spasm

Medicine at a Glance, Fourth Edition. Edited by Patrick Davey. © 2014 John Wiley & Sons, Ltd. Published 2014 by John Wiley & Sons, Ltd. Companion website: www.ataglanceseries.com/medicine

usually manifests as a tightening felt in the chest, and is sometimes indistinguishable from cardiac pain with radiation into the neck.

- **Biliary pain** (biliary tree and gall bladder) is felt in the epigastrium and sometimes the right upper quadrant. It is colicky in nature. Ask about features of cholestasis (pale stools, dark urine, jaundice). Pain from the liver itself is unusual, although it may occur in hepatitis, hepatic metastases or right heart failure as a persistent right upper quadrant discomfort from hepatic capsular distension.
- **Pancreatic pain** is usually epigastric, and typically radiates through to the back. Common precipitants include fatty foods and alcohol.
- **Foregut (gastroduodenal) pain** tends to be acidic (dyspeptic) and situated in the epigastrium. This will be influenced by eating – acid/dyspeptic symptoms may be relieved whilst obstructive/irritative symptoms may be exacerbated.
- **Midgut (small intestinal) pain** is usually colicky and situated periumbilically. It is often associated with bloating, nausea and vomiting.
- **Hindgut (colonic) pain** is usually colicky and experienced below the umbilicus. Other features may include a change in bowel habit and rectal bleeding. Remember that carcinoma of the caecum is more likely to lead to subacute *small* bowel obstruction than colonic dysfunction.
- **Peritonitic pain** is more localized because the parietal peritoneum has a rich sensory innervation. The classic example of this is evolving appendicitis. Initially the pain is periumbilical and colicky, relating to an inflamed midgut viscus. As inflammation progresses there is local peritonism with persistent pain and tenderness in the right iliac fossa. This may progress to perforation and generalized peritonitis with severe global abdominal pain if left untreated.
- **Loin pain** tends *not* to be related to gastrointestinal (GI) tract pathology but is more likely to arise from the kidneys and ureters or to be mechanical and related to the lumbar spine.

Other features of the history

It is useful to determine whether the current pain represents an acute problem or a manifestation of a chronic underlying condition (possibly subclinical until then). Previous GI problems or operations suggest an exacerbation of an old problem. Anorexia and weight loss suggest serious pathology.

Examination

General

Look at general appearance. Assess the circulatory state. Look for markers of chronic disease.

Abdominal

- Areas of tenderness: ask the patient to point to where the pain is maximal. Look for peritonism: guarding and more importantly rebound tenderness.
- Masses, including organomegaly.

Investigations

- **Blood tests**: full blood count (FBC), erythrocyte sedimentation rate (ESR), C-reactive protein, renal function tests; liver function tests, calcium; amylase.
- **Abdominal X-ray**: may show intestinal obstruction, vascular calcification (raising the possibility of ischaemia), loss of psoas outline (implying retroperitoneal pathology), and areas of absence gas pattern (bowel loops displaced by a mass). Look for features of a pneumoperitoneum (e.g. Wriggler's sign).
- **Erect chest X-ray**: look for the presence of air under the diaphragm.

- **Abdominal ultrasonography**: excellent for the biliary and renal tracts. Less good for imaging the pancreas and retroperitoneal structures and less sensitive in obese individuals.
- **Abdominal computed tomography** (CT) produces better images of the retroperitoneal organs. The yield of CT may be enhanced with the use of intraluminal (oral or rectal) contrast.

Management

General measures

- Rest the gut: parenteral rehydration.
- Analgesia: gut-related pain is relatively resistant to simple analgesics. Opioids are effective but are limited by side effects (nausea, constipation, etc.). Antispasmodics (mebeverine, buscopan) might be more effective.
- Treat the underlying cause.

No cause identified

If no cause for persistent pain is identified, a diagnostic laparoscopy/laparotomy is occasionally required. Consider several diagnoses:

- Functional GI disorders.
- Munchausen's syndrome: have a very high index of suspicion when patients not resident to the locality present with severe abdominal pain without convincing clinical or investigative abnormalities. There may be stigmata of multiple previous operations.
- Very rarely myocardial ischaemia presents as upper abdominal pain.
- Rare diseases such as porphyria and familial Mediterranean fever.

Dyspepsia

Dyspepsia refers to symptoms originating from the upper GI tract. These may relate to eating or drinking and include 'heartburn' and 'indigestion' (pain, usually 'acidic', in the upper abdomen/lower chest, as well as 'bloating', anorexia and vomiting). The most common underlying mechanism is gastro-oesophageal reflux. Figure 30.1 shows the differential diagnosis of dyspepsia.

History and examination

Symptoms have often been present for some years. Lifestyle factors (smoking, alcohol, weight, 'stress') are relevant for reflux. Although many patients fear that cancer might account for their long-standing symptoms this is a rare cause of dyspepsia. However, dysphagia and/or weight loss require urgent investigation. Physical examination is usually unrewarding, but may suggest neoplasia (weight loss, lymph nodes, abdominal masses). Abdominal obesity predisposes to reflux.

Investigations

Investigations should exclude serious pathology, principally gastric cancer, as well as establish the diagnosis. In many the cancer risk is low and empirical treatment without endoscopy may be adequate.

- **Blood tests**: a normal FBC and ESR help exclude serious pathology. Positive *Helicobacter pylori* serology might suggest peptic ulcer disease but does not exclude an upper GI malignancy.
- **Endoscopy**: the definitive test for most serious upper GI pathologies (oesophagitis, Barrett's epithelium, peptic ulcer disease). Antral biopsy and urease test for *H. pylori* (CLO test) – see Chapter 124.
- **Barium swallow/meal**: now largely surpassed by endoscopy.

Management

- Treat the underlying cause (see Chapters 123 and 124).
- Treat the symptoms (see Chapters 123 and 124).

31 Jaundice

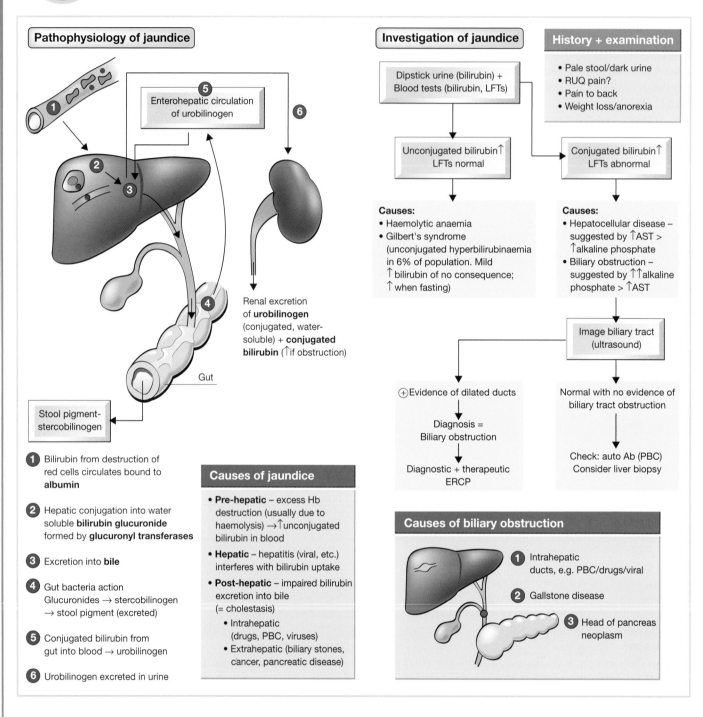

Pathophysiology of jaundice

Enterohepatic circulation of urobilinogen ⑤

⑥

Renal excretion of **urobilinogen** (conjugated, water-soluble) + **conjugated bilirubin** (↑if obstruction)

Gut

Stool pigment-stercobilinogen

① Bilirubin from destruction of red cells circulates bound to **albumin**

② Hepatic conjugation into water soluble **bilirubin glucuronide** formed by **glucuronyl transferases**

③ Excretion into **bile**

④ Gut bacteria action Glucuronides → stercobilinogen → stool pigment (excreted)

⑤ Conjugated bilirubin from gut into blood → urobilinogen

⑥ Urobilinogen excreted in urine

Causes of jaundice

• **Pre-hepatic** – excess Hb destruction (usually due to haemolysis) →↑unconjugated bilirubin in blood
• **Hepatic** – hepatitis (viral, etc.) interferes with bilirubin uptake
• **Post-hepatic** – impaired bilirubin excretion into bile (= cholestasis)
  • Intrahepatic (drugs, PBC, viruses)
  • Extrahepatic (biliary stones, cancer, pancreatic disease)

Investigation of jaundice

Dipstick urine (bilirubin) + Blood tests (bilirubin, LFTs)

Unconjugated bilirubin↑ LFTs normal

Conjugated bilirubin↑ LFTs abnormal

Causes:
• Haemolytic anaemia
• Gilbert's syndrome (unconjugated hyperbilirubinaemia in 6% of population. Mild ↑ bilirubin of no consequence; ↑ when fasting)

Causes:
• Hepatocellular disease – suggested by ↑AST > ↑alkaline phosphate
• Biliary obstruction – suggested by ↑↑alkaline phosphate > ↑AST

Image biliary tract (ultrasound)

⊕Evidence of dilated ducts

Diagnosis = Biliary obstruction

Diagnostic + therapeutic ERCP

Normal with no evidence of biliary tract obstruction

Check: auto Ab (PBC) Consider liver biopsy

History + examination

• Pale stool/dark urine
• RUQ pain?
• Pain to back
• Weight loss/anorexia

Causes of biliary obstruction

① Intrahepatic ducts, e.g. PBC/drugs/viral

② Gallstone disease

③ Head of pancreas neoplasm

Introduction

Jaundice can result from a range of underlying pathologies varying from an acute short-lived illness (e.g. hepatitis A) to the terminal stages of a chronic disease, which might have been subclinical until that point (e.g. decompensated chronic liver disease).

Aetiology

Although jaundice has been traditionally described as either 'pre-hepatic', 'hepatic' or 'post-hepatic', in practice it is often sufficient to restrict one's considerations to whether jaundice is hepatocellular (i.e. hepatic) or obstructive/cholestatic (i.e. post-hepatic) (see Table 31.1).

Differential diagnosis

A useful way of considering the differential diagnosis is to clinically distinguish the **acute** from the **chronic** conditions and, where possible, to clarify whether the liver injury is **hepatocellular** or **obstructive**.

Medicine at a Glance, Fourth Edition. Edited by Patrick Davey. © 2014 John Wiley & Sons, Ltd. Published 2014 by John Wiley & Sons, Ltd. Companion website: www.ataglanceseries.com/medicine

Table 31.1 Aetiology of jaundice.

	Acute	Chronic

Hepatocellular	Acute hepatitis:
	   Viral hepatitides
	   Drug reactions
	   Budd–Chiari
	   syndrome
		Chronic liver disease:
		   Hepatitis B and C
		   Alcoholic disease
		   Autoimmune
		   hepatitis
		   Haemochromatosis

Cholestatic	Biliary obstruction:
	
	   2° biliary disease
	   Pancreatitis
		Chronic biliary
		 disease:
		   1° biliary cirrhosis
		   1° sclerosing
		   cirrhosis

	Pancreatic carcinoma	

Table 31.2 Differences between acute and chronic disease underlying jaundice.

	Acute	Chronic
Preceding ill health	0	0 to ++
Skin signs of chronic liver disease	0	0 to ++
Encephalopathy	0 to +	+ to +++
Ascites	0	++
Varices at endoscopy	0	++
Spleen at ultrasound	0	++
Laboratory tests:		
MCV	→	↑
Urea	→	↓
Albumin	→ or ↓	↓ to ↓↓
Prothrombin	→ or ↓	↑ to ↑↑

Clinical features and history

The two important clinical features to identify are:

- Is this patient's presentation of an acute illness or a chronic disease (see Table 31.2)?
- Is there any clinical evidence of a failing liver?

These questions can often be answered from a careful history:

- What is the duration of the illness and was the patient unwell before the jaundice developed? This is often very revealing and may suggest a long period of subclinical ill health before the jaundice.
- Are there clinical features of cholestasis (i.e. biliary obstruction)? Pale stools, dark urine and pruritis?
- Has the patient experienced any pain? Pain and cholestasis should be considered to be related to gallstones until proved otherwise. The presence of fever and rigors strongly suggests cholangitis (biliary tract infection) as the diagnosis.
- Are there risk factors for chronic liver disease? Alcohol – seek corroborative evidence. Travel/contacts – any favoured sexual practices? Intravenous drug use – ask specifically.
- Are there any features of liver failure? Hepatic encephalopathy (reversal of sleep pattern, reduced attention span, daytime somnolence, constructional dyspraxia)?

Examination

The depth of the jaundice does not actually matter as much as recognizing features of a failing liver and determining whether there is chronic liver disease.

Recognition of liver failure

Encephalopathy is the clinical hallmark of liver failure. Any degree of confusion/delirium in a jaundiced patient should be considered a manifestation of encephalopathy. The specific clinical sign to seek is the metabolic flap (or asterixis). Other bedside measures of encephalopathy include a constructional dyspraxia (e.g. drawing a five-pointed star) or the trail test (i.e. a join-the-dots test against the clock).

Features of chronic liver disease

Typically, features of chronic liver disease are considered to be the peripheral stigmata such as palmar erythema, Dupuytren's contracture, spider naevi and gynaecomastia. In practice, the clinical features of portal hypertension, such as ascites and splenomegaly, often represent 'harder' physical signs.

Investigations

- **Blood tests**: full blood count; a macrocytosis, thrombocytopenia or low urea may indicate chronic liver disease. Hyponatraemia (not caused by diuretics) is a poor prognostic sign.
- **Liver blood tests**: a low albumin may be non-specific. The transaminases give a clue as to whether the jaundice is predominantly hepatocellular (aspartate transaminase (AST) or alanine transaminase (ALT) > alkaline phosphatase) or cholestatic (alkaline phosphatase or γ-glutamyl transferase (γ-GT) > AST), although the picture is often 'mixed'. Normal transaminases suggest the less common conditions of haemolysis or Gilbert's syndrome.
- **Viral hepatitis serology**: hepatitis A IgM is diagnostic of acute hepatitis A. Acute hepatitis B is typified by HBsAg (hepatitis B surface antigen) and detection of hepatitis B DNA. Hepatitis C rarely causes an acute hepatitis but is an increasing cause of chronic liver disease.
- **Autoantibody profile and immunoglobulin** (Ig): anti-double-stranded DNA, antinuclear, antimitochondrial, anti-smooth muscle, anti-liver–kidney microsomal antibodies and serum IgG, IgA and IgM.
- **Liver ultrasonography**: this may help in consolidating a clinical diagnosis. It may show focal liver abnormalities such as metastatic deposits, liver abscesses or vascular abnormalities. It might show evidence of biliary obstruction (i.e. dilated bile ducts) and possibly the underlying cause (e.g. gallstones, pancreatic cancer). It might be normal.
- **Magnetic resonance cholangiopancreatography** (MRCP) and **endoscopic ultrasound** (EUS): increasingly, such non-invasive methods are used to delineate biliary anatomy as a prelude to endoscopic intervention.
- **Endoscopic retrograde cholangiopancreatography** (ERCP): if there is good evidence of biliary obstruction ERCP remains the definitive test in determining whether the obstruction is intraluminal (i.e. gallstones in the common bile duct) or extraluminal (e.g. malignant stricture from carcinoma of the pancreas). It may also allow relief of the obstruction.
- **Liver biopsy**: liver histology remains the definitive investigation for hepatocellular jaundice and also, in some cases, cholestatic jaundice (e.g. primary biliary cirrhosis (PBC), drug-induced intrahepatic cholestasis). The absolute indications vary.

Management

The management of patients with jaundice depends on the underlying cause and if there are clinical features of liver failure. Jaundice itself does not necessarily require hospital admission – many of the underlying conditions and associated complications do.

32 Abdominal mass

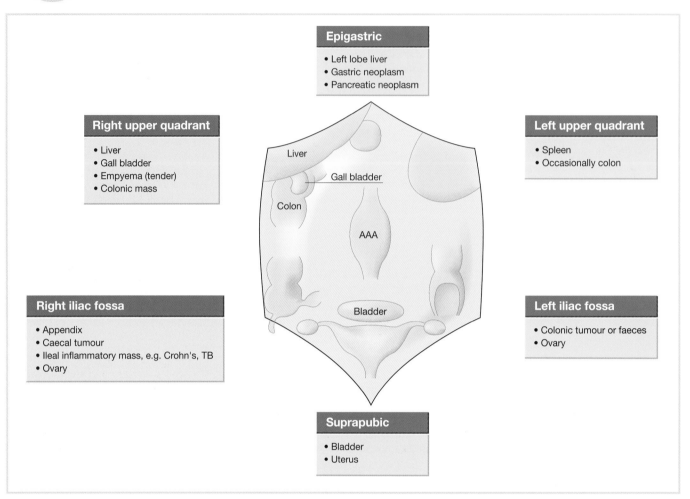

Epigastric
- Left lobe liver
- Gastric neoplasm
- Pancreatic neoplasm

Right upper quadrant
- Liver
- Gall bladder
- Empyema (tender)
- Colonic mass

Left upper quadrant
- Spleen
- Occasionally colon

Right iliac fossa
- Appendix
- Caecal tumour
- Ileal inflammatory mass, e.g. Crohn's, TB
- Ovary

Left iliac fossa
- Colonic tumour or faeces
- Ovary

Suprapubic
- Bladder
- Uterus

It is uncommon for patients to present solely with a palpable abdominal mass. Usually there are other clinical features such as weight loss or pain, or a change in bowel habit.

Differential diagnosis

The differential diagnosis depends largely on the position of the mass (see Figure 32.1).

Investigations

● **Blood tests**: full blood count, erythrocyte sedimentation rate – anaemia, thrombocytosis and raised inflammatory markers suggest an underlying chronic disease process. Biochemistry – abnormal liver blood tests likewise suggest malignancy. The role of tumour markers (e.g. carcinoembryonic antigen, CA19–9, α-fetoprotein) in the diagnosis of malignancy is limited. Their value is greater in monitoring response to treatment and identification of disease relapse.

● **Ultrasonography**: this is very useful as a first-line investigation but has now been largely superceded by abdominal computed tomography (CT).

● **CT scan**: very useful for characterization of retroperitoneal masses and probably more sensitive in identifying intra-abdominal lymphadenopathy. As CT relies on defining tissue planes (i.e. solid tissue against fat), it is more sensitive in relatively obese individuals.

● **Biopsy/aspiration**: if there is doubt about the nature of an intra-abdominal mass, it is usually possible to aspirate cells for cytology or take a percutaneous biopsy under ultrasonic or CT guidance.

● **Laparoscopy/laparotomy**: if the nature of a mass remains obscure, the definitive approach is ultimately a laparotomy and excision. Such interventions are unlikely to be undertaken without shared care with surgeons, radiologists and pathologists through a multi-disciplinary team (MDT).

Medicine at a Glance, Fourth Edition. Edited by Patrick Davey. © 2014 John Wiley & Sons, Ltd. Published 2014 by John Wiley & Sons, Ltd. Companion website: www.ataglanceseries.com/medicine

33 Ascites

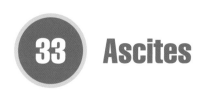

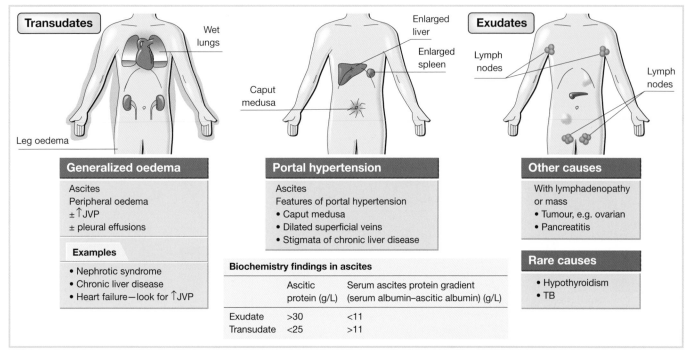

	Ascitic protein (g/L)	Serum ascites protein gradient (serum albumin–ascitic albumin) (g/L)
Exudate	>30	<11
Transudate	<25	>11

Ascites is the pathological accumulation of fluid within the abdominal peritoneal cavity. Ascites frequently reflects the presentation of a chronic disease process that may have been subclinical until that point.

As with other fluid collections ascites is clinically classified as being either an exudate or a transudate (see Figure 33.1):

- **Exudative ascites** has a high protein content and occurs with inflammatory (e.g. infective) or malignant processes.
- **Transudative ascites** occurs in cirrhosis as a result of portal hypertension and alterations in renal sodium clearance.

The differential diagnosis most commonly lies between decompensated chronic liver disease and intra-abdominal malignancy. Other conditions that may present with ascites include heart failure, constrictive pericarditis, nephrotic syndrome, pancreatitis and tuberculosis (TB).

Clinical features and investigations

There are few features in the history and examination that confidently distinguish between the late presentation of liver disease and malignancy. Notwithstanding this, any historical factor pointing to a liver disease is important. Gross ascites may be evident on inspection with pronounced distension of the abdomen, often with eversion of the umbilicus. Lesser degrees of ascites can be demonstrated clinically by eliciting 'shifting dullness'. Helpful investigations include:

- **Examination of the ascitic fluid**: for protein (see above), cell count, bacterial culture and cytology for malignant cells. Ascites may be straw coloured in cirrhosis, bloody in malignancy and cloudy in infection. A leukocyte count of more than >250 polymorphs/mL is considered diagnostic of bacterial peritonitis regardless of whether or not organisms are subsequently cultured. Cytology (large volume and fresh specimen) may be diagnostic of malignancy. Pancreatic disease may present with ascites, and if suspected ascitic amylase should be measured.

- **Ultrasonography of the abdomen**: to measure liver size (small in cirrhosis), signs of portal hypertension (splenomegaly) and patency of the portal and hepatic veins (to exclude hepatic vein thrombosis and Budd–Chiari syndrome). It is also useful for finding focal abnormalities (suggestive of disseminated malignancy) and for the diagnosis of intra-abdominal tumours (e.g. ovarian).
- **Other blood tests**: biochemistry and liver blood tests looking for markers of liver cirrhosis (low albumin, hyperbilirubinaemia, elevated liver enzymes, low platelets, etc.). Tumour markers if malignancy is suspected (especially α-fetoprotein for hepatoma, CA125 for ovarian carcinoma).

Management

Exudative ascites

Treat the underlying cause:

- **Bacterial peritonitis**: antibiotics. In low-protein ascites, prophylactic antibiotics are of benefit.
- **Malignant ascites**: treat underlying malignancy (commonly ovarian). Therapeutic paracentesis is often needed for symptomatic relief.

Transudative ascites

Treat the underlying cause, and consider:

- Fluid and salt restriction: fluid restriction to ≤1–1.5 L/day and a 'no added salt' diet may be sufficient.
- Diuretics: usually spironolactone ± furosemide (frusemide).
- Therapeutic paracentesis for refractory ascites (i.e. ascites not responding to diuretic therapy or only with unacceptable drug side effects – hyponatraemia, encephalopathy, etc.).

K.P. Moore & G.P. Aithal. Guidelines on the management of ascites in cirrhosis. *Gut* 2006: 55; 1–12; www.bsg.org.uk (last accessed August 2013).

34 Polyuria and oliguria

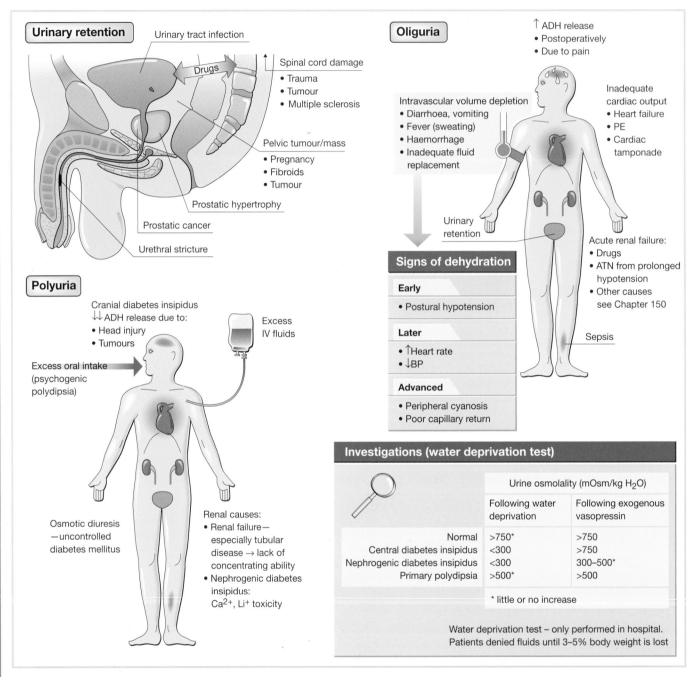

Urinary retention

Urinary tract infection

Drugs

Spinal cord damage
• Trauma
• Tumour
• Multiple sclerosis

Pelvic tumour/mass
• Pregnancy
• Fibroids
• Tumour

Prostatic hypertrophy

Prostatic cancer

Urethral stricture

Polyuria

Cranial diabetes insipidus
$\downarrow\downarrow$ ADH release due to:
• Head injury
• Tumours

Excess oral intake
(psychogenic
polydipsia)

Excess
IV fluids

Osmotic diuresis
—uncontrolled
diabetes mellitus

Renal causes:
• Renal failure—
especially tubular
disease → lack of
concentrating ability
• Nephrogenic diabetes
insipidus:
Ca^{2+}, Li^+ toxicity

Oliguria

↑ ADH release
• Postoperatively
• Due to pain

Intravascular volume depletion
• Diarrhoea, vomiting
• Fever (sweating)
• Haemorrhage
• Inadequate fluid
replacement

Inadequate
cardiac output
• Heart failure
• PE
• Cardiac
tamponade

Urinary
retention

Acute renal failure:
• Drugs
• ATN from prolonged
hypotension
• Other causes
see Chapter 150

Sepsis

Signs of dehydration

Early
• Postural hypotension

Later
• ↑Heart rate
• ↓BP

Advanced
• Peripheral cyanosis
• Poor capillary return

Investigations (water deprivation test)

	Urine osmolality (mOsm/kg H_2O)	
	Following water deprivation	Following exogenous vasopressin
Normal	>750*	>750
Central diabetes insipidus	<300	>750
Nephrogenic diabetes insipidus	<300	300–500*
Primary polydipsia	>500*	>500
* little or no increase		

Water deprivation test – only performed in hospital.
Patients denied fluids until 3–5% body weight is lost

Polyuria

Polyuria is an excessive urine volume, usually ≥ 3 L/day, and may be accompanied by the symptoms of frequency, nocturia, thirst and polydipsia. A presentation with polyuria requires careful investigation as it may be caused by serious underlying disease.

Many conditions can produce polyuria, of which the commonest is **diabetes mellitus** in which increased concentrations of glucose have an osmotic diuretic effect. The causes may be grouped as follows:

1 Excess intake of fluid (primary polydipsia), often associated with psychological disturbance leading to compulsive water drinking. Very rarely, hypothalamic lesions lead to primary polydipsia.

2 An increase in tubular solute load, as with urea in chronic renal failure or glucose from hyperglycaemia caused by diabetes mellitus.

3 Disordered medullary concentration gradient as a consequence of medullary disease (see Chapter 149) or in hypercalcaemia.

4 A reduction in antidiuretic hormone (ADH or vasopressin) production (diabetes insipidus), after trauma to the head, or tumours or infections of the hypothalamus or pituitary (cranial diabetes insipidus).

5 Conditions in which the tubular response to ADH is impaired. These conditions are termed 'nephrogenic diabetes insipidus', and include hypercalcaemia, chronic potassium depletion, lithium toxicity and a rare inherited insensitivity to ADH with X-linked recessive inheritance (due to mutations in the ADH receptor, V2) or autosomal inheritance with mutations affecting the aquaporin-2 water channel.

6 After relief of urinary tract obstruction.

In a patient with polyuria, the history may provide the diagnosis. If blood glucose is normal, creatinine, calcium and potassium should be determined. If diabetes insipidus is suspected, then a water deprivation test should be undertaken with caution; the patient must not become excessively dehydrated. A water deprivation test involves the restriction of water intake until a 3–5% weight loss has been achieved. Measurements of urinary osmolality and change in urinary osmolality in response to exogenous vasopressin will help establish the diagnosis.

It is important to correct any major water deficit and then to treat the underlying cause. Cranial diabetes insipidus can be treated by the intranasal administration of the vasopressin analogue desmopressin.

Oliguria in the hospital setting

Oliguria is defined as a urine output of less than 0.5 mL/kg weight/h. Many patients in hospital develop a reduced urinary output, particularly postoperative or severely ill individuals. Urine output is a sensitive indicator of fluid status and haemodynamic adequacy. It is particularly important because oliguria may progress to acute renal failure. Pain and nausea are very potent stimuli of ADH secretion. In managing the oliguric patient, information can be acquired from the history, examination and investigations. The central issues are whether or not the patient is replete with fluid and excluding urinary retention.

An accurate **history** of fluid intake and output should be obtained. Fluid balance and daily weight charts should be examined; loss of fluid from haemorrhage, diarrhoea, sweating, vomiting, drains and insensible losses all need to be considered. The presence of nausea, pain and thirst should be elicited. Symptoms suggesting urinary retention should be elicited and a urinary catheter passed if there is any doubt.

Examination should include palpation and percussion for a bladder. Signs suggesting fluid depletion or overload should be sought. The signs of fluid depletion include tachycardia, hypotension and, most importantly, postural hypotension, while other signs can include dry mucous membranes, reduced skin turgor, cool peripheries and contracted peripheral veins. Signs of fluid overload can include orthopnoea, tachypnoea, peripheral oedema, pulmonary oedema, elevated jugular venous pressure (JVP) and hypertension. A central venous line provides a direct measurement of central venous pressure (CVP) if the fluid status is uncertain.

Investigations and management

Fluid depletion can be accompanied by elevations in haematocrit, serum albumin and creatinine (with urea often disproportionately raised), whereas in fluid overload a chest X-ray may reveal pulmonary oedema. In the oliguric patient, a urinary catheter should be passed or, if present, flushed to exclude blockage. If the situation suggests fluid depletion then intravenous (IV) fluid (often normal saline) should be given. Replacement fluid should be administered until postural hypotension has been abolished and the JVP or CVP is normal. If there is evidence of haemorrhage, then a blood transfusion may be necessary; the source of blood loss should be identified and treated, and clotting times determined. If the patient appears replete with fluid then other causes of shock need to be considered, such as sepsis, myocardial infarction and pulmonary embolism (PE), and other causes of acute renal failure considered (see Table 34.1). An urgent renal tract ultrasound should be requested, to look for signs of renal tract obstruction (e.g. hydronephrosis), and also to look for kidney size (small in long-standing disease).

It is particularly important to avoid agents that may jeopardize renal perfusion (e.g. NSAIDs, or ACE inhibitors), which could be nephrotoxic (e.g. gentamicin) or accumulate in renal failure (e.g. digoxin).

Urinary retention

Acute urinary retention is a sudden inability to pass urine, usually accompanied by pain, the sensation of bladder fullness and a distended bladder. **Chronic urinary retention** is the presence of an enlarged bladder often without difficulty in micturition, and accompanied by frequency, overflow incontinence, bladder distension and sometimes renal failure. Causes can be grouped into those affecting the lumen of the urethra or the urethral wall, compression of the urethra or neurological dysfunction. Urinary tract infection or pain may precipitate retention. Urinary retention is common in elderly men due to benign prostatic hyperplasia or, more rarely, prostate carcinoma; in young adults serious neurological causes may be responsible and require careful investigation. Rectal examination is crucial to assess both the prostate, and anal tone and sensation. In women, urinary obstruction is more likely to be neurological or gynaecological in origin than urological.

Table 34.1 Typical urine findings in conditions that cause acute renal failure.

Condition	Dipstick test	Sediment analysis	Urine osmolality (mOsm/kg)	Fractional excretion of sodium* (%)
Prerenal failure	Trace or no proteinuria	A few hyaline casts possible	>500	<1
Renal failure				
Tubular injury ischaemia	Mild-to-moderate proteinuria	Pigmented granular casts	<350	>1
Nephrotoxins	Mild-to-moderate proteinuria	Pigmented granular casts	<350	>1
Acute interstitial nephritis	Mild-to-moderate proteinuria; haemoglobin; leukocytes	White cells and white cell casts; eosinophils and eosinophil casts; red cells	<350	>1
Acute glomerulonephritis	Moderate-to-severe proteinuria; haemoglobin	Red cells and red cell casts; red cells can be dysmorphic	>500	<1
Postrenal failure	Trace or no proteinuria; can have haemoglobin, leukocytes	Crystals, red cells and white cells possible	<350	>1

* Fractional excretion of sodium (FENa) = (UNa × PCr)/(PNa × UCr) × 100, where Cr is creatinine, Na is sodium, P is plasma and U is urine.
Data from Thadhani et al. 1996.

35 Dysuria, frequency and urgency

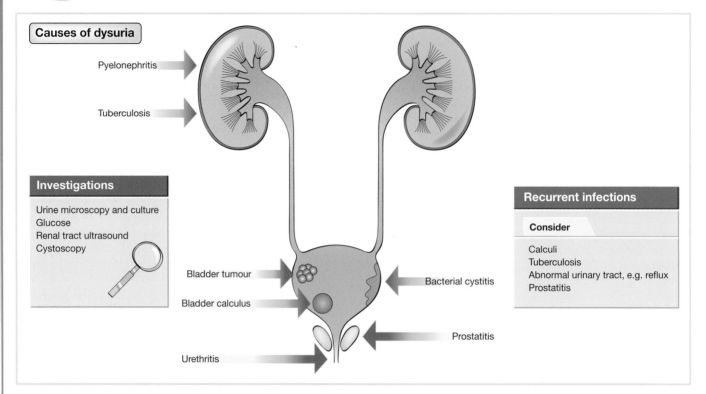

Causes of dysuria

Pyelonephritis

Tuberculosis

Investigations

Urine microscopy and culture
Glucose
Renal tract ultrasound
Cystoscopy

Bladder tumour

Bladder calculus

Urethritis

Bacterial cystitis

Prostatitis

Recurrent infections

Consider

Calculi
Tuberculosis
Abnormal urinary tract, e.g. reflux
Prostatitis

Dysuria is painful micturition. Urinary frequency is the increased frequency of the passage of urine. Urgency is an uncontrollable desire to micturate. In adults the most common cause is urinary tract infection (UTI), a very common diagnosis in both general practice and hospital patients.

Urinary tract infection is commonly looked for in elderly patients (or children) who present with confusion or general deterioration. It is particularly important in all UTIs to ensure that there is pyuria accompanying any bacterial growth from urine, because imperfectly sterile urine collections are common. Bacteriuria is likely to be of clinical significance only when accompanied by pyuria.

Acute pyelonephritis

Urinary tract infection involving the upper urinary tract has systemic features such as fever, which may be very high (>39°C), rigors, malaise, anorexia and flank pain, in addition to the symptoms of dysuria, frequency and urgency. Predispositions include calculi, reflux, obstruction and a neurogenic bladder. Pyelonephritis in an obstructed kidney requires urgent medical attention because of the irreversible loss of renal function that may occur. The key to diagnosis is the microscopy and culture of urine and blood cultures. There should be pyuria (i.e. >100 000 white cells/mL), bacteriuria and often microscopic or even macroscopic haematuria.

Acute cystitis

Urinary tract infection confined to the urinary tract is commonly called acute cystitis. It is more common in women and coliforms are the most common infecting organisms:

- *Escherichia coli* (90% of outpatients, 50% of inpatients).
- *Proteus* and *Klebsiella* species (5% of outpatients, 20% of inpatients).
- Enterococci (2% of outpatients, 7% of inpatients).
- *Pseudomonas* species (0.5% of outpatients, 6% of inpatients).

The symptoms may include dysuria, suprapubic discomfort, frequency, urgency, incontinence and microscopic haematuria. Diagnosis, as in pyelonephritis, requires the growth of a pathogenic organism from a midstream specimen of urine, in a quantity sufficient to cause disease, defined as ≥100 000 colony-forming units/mL.

Urethritis

This is a condition characterized by dysuria and meatal discharge, and is most commonly caused by sexually transmitted diseases such as gonococci or *Chlamydia* species.

Investigations

The microscopy and culture of urine are critical in the management of patients suspected of having a UTI. Other important investigations, particularly with recurrent infections, may include urine or blood glucose, ultrasonography of the renal tract, plain X-rays of the kidney, ureters and bladder, urography or cystoscopy. In recurrent infection, obstruction, prostatitis, renal calculi, diabetes mellitus and bladder dysfunction are potential causes.

Other causes of dysuria, other than acute bacterial infection, are bladder calculi, bladder tumours and tuberculosis (suggested by sterile pyuria in a patient at risk of tuberculosis).

Medicine at a Glance, Fourth Edition. Edited by Patrick Davey. © 2014 John Wiley & Sons, Ltd. Published 2014 by John Wiley & Sons, Ltd. Companion website: www.ataglanceseries.com/medicine

36 Haematuria

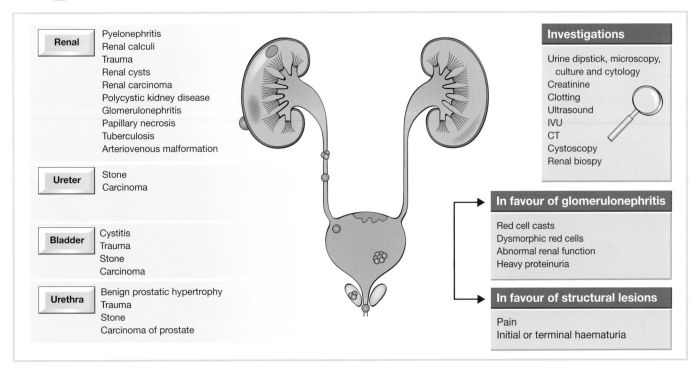

Renal
Pyelonephritis
Renal calculi
Trauma
Renal cysts
Renal carcinoma
Polycystic kidney disease
Glomerulonephritis
Papillary necrosis
Tuberculosis
Arteriovenous malformation

Ureter
Stone
Carcinoma

Bladder
Cystitis
Trauma
Stone
Carcinoma

Urethra
Benign prostatic hypertrophy
Trauma
Stone
Carcinoma of prostate

Investigations
Urine dipstick, microscopy,
  culture and cytology
Creatinine
Clotting
Ultrasound
IVU
CT
Cystoscopy
Renal biospy

In favour of glomerulonephritis
Red cell casts
Dysmorphic red cells
Abnormal renal function
Heavy proteinuria

In favour of structural lesions
Pain
Initial or terminal haematuria

Blood can appear in the urine from pathology at any site in the urinary tract. Even small quantities of blood can produce a significantly pink or red coloration in the urine (although this should not be confused with ingested substances that discolour the urine, such as beetroot or rifampicin antibiotic). The small amount of blood found occasionally in urine from patients with glomerulonephritis can make it 'smoky' in appearance. Urinary dipsticks are very sensitive to even a very few red cells in the urine. False positive dipstick tests for blood can be obtained with the presence of free haemoglobin or myoglobin in the urine and by contamination from menstruation. Haematuria can be confirmed by finding more than three red blood cells per high power field of spun urine. Macroscopic (frank blood) haematuria definitely requires investigation because it may be the first presentation of a carcinoma of the renal tract or a serious renal disorder. The continuing presence of microscopic haematuria (present on dipstick and seen on microscopy) should prompt consideration of the presence of renal disease (is there proteinuria, abnormal creatinine, hypertension?) or a structural lesion of the renal tract but can be detected in a large proportion of asymptomatic normal individuals (from 1% of young adults to 10% in the elderly).

History and examination

The **history** should include the timing of haematuria in the urinary stream; blood on commencing urination suggests a urethral cause, whereas terminal haematuria suggests a bladder or prostatic cause. The presence of painful urination suggests a urinary tract infection or calculus. Episodes of trauma should be sought, as should systemic features that might indicate a disseminated malignancy or a vasculitis.

The **examination** must include palpation for abdominal masses, which might represent renal tumours or cysts, a rectal examination for prostatic malignancy and measurement of blood pressure.

Investigations

Once the presence of haematuria has been established, urinary microscopy may indicate whether the source is likely to be glomerular or from elsewhere in the urinary tract. Red blood cells of glomerular origin tend to be dysmorphic and may be accompanied by red cell casts and significant proteinuria. Glomerular disease can affect renal function (see Chapter 146) which should be assessed with plasma creatinine, and is often accompanied by proteinuria. Abnormal urine cytology can suggest the presence of a urinary tract malignancy. If a structural lesion of the renal tract is suspected, imaging can be undertaken with: plain radiography looking for radio-opaque calculi (although only a small minority of stones are visible on plain X-ray); ultrasonography looking for renal masses or bladder lesions; intravenous urography (IVU), particularly looking for filling defects within the urinary tract; and cross-sectional imaging with computed tomography (CT) or magnetic resonance imaging (MRI). (Remember to be cautious with iodinated contrast media in patients with renal impairment because of the increased risk of contrast nephropathy and the rare skin disorder nephrogenic systemic fibrosis that can be associated with gadolinium.)

If these investigations fail to demonstrate a cause for the haematuria, a cystoscopy should be performed. If a renal source of the haematuria is suspected (usually because there is proteinuria or biochemical evidence of renal impairment), a renal biopsy may be undertaken which could reveal a glomerulonephritis. The most common renal cause of microscopic or macroscopic haematuria is IgA nephropathy. In this condition the haematuria commonly follows a sore throat. Bleeding disorders are a very rare cause of haematuria but should be looked for if the patient has other sites of abnormal blood loss.

37 Sweating, flushing and thyroid swellings

Sweating

Causes

Common
- Anxiety
- Primary dermatological condition
- Self-limiting infections

Rare
- Endocrine disease
- Cardiac disease
- Chronic inflammatory/neoplastic conditions

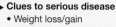

Sweating
↓
Duration? → Long duration suggests a benign diagnosis
↓   Yes
Associated → **Clues to serious disease**
symptoms/   - Weight loss/gain
signs?   - Altered bowel habit
↓ No   - Pain
Anxiety disorder   - Syncope or near syncope
1° dermatological   - Palpitations
condition   Anxiety preceding palpitations
– inflammatory   = anxiety disorder
– excess sweat   Palpitations preceding anxiety
  production   = tachyarrhythmia
                    - Fever

Flushing

Most cases relate to emotion or the menopause

Skin disease
- Acne
- Rosacea
- Photosensitive dermatosis

Drugs
- Alcohol
- Ca^{2+} channel blockers

Food
- Scombroid poisoning

Menopausal flushes
- Affects 80% of females
- Due to oestrogen decline, not absence
- Heat → (1 minute) warmth + sweat upper body
  ↑skin temp (3°C) +
  ↓core temp (0.3°C)

Rare causes
- Medullary thyroid cancer
- Systemic mastocytosis

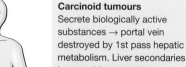

Carcinoid tumours
Secrete biologically active substances → portal vein destroyed by 1st pass hepatic metabolism. Liver secondaries bypass this protection, producing the **carcinoid syndrome**
- Flushing: paroxysmal → fixed
- Watery diarrhoea + abdominal pain
- Right-sided heart valve lesions

Carcinoid tumours arise from **neuroendocrine cells** which:
- Mostly arise in small bowel
- 10% present as appendicitis

Thyroid swellings

Isolated nodule
- 'Colloid cyst'
- Functioning adenoma
- Cancer:
  pain
  rapid enlargement
  local lymphadenopathy

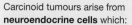

Multiple nodules throughout both lobes
- I_2 deficiency
- Autoimmune disease

Diffuse enlargement
- Graves' disease
  – overlying bruit
- Viral thyroiditis – tender

Complications of a thyroid goitre

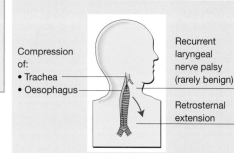

Compression of:
- Trachea
- Oesophagus

Recurrent laryngeal nerve palsy (rarely benign)

Retrosternal extension

Investigations

- Thyroid function test (?hyper-/hypo-function)
- Fine needle aspiration cytology
- ^{131}I scan: if 'hot' (i.e. functioning) – very unlikely to be cancer
- Occasionally ultrasound

Medicine at a Glance, Fourth Edition. Edited by Patrick Davey. © 2014 John Wiley & Sons, Ltd. Published 2014 by John Wiley & Sons, Ltd. Companion website: www.ataglanceseries.com/medicine

Sweating

Sweating is a very common problem, but is very rarely serious. The crucial diagnostic features are: how long the problem has been present (the longer it has been there, the more benign the underlying process); the presence of any associated symptoms (isolated sweating is rarely serious, and usually indicates a dermatological hypersecretory response rather than any underlying disease process); and is there anxiety during the episode (anxiety normally indicates a panic disorder; very rarely it indicates an underlying phaeochromocytoma).

Differential diagnosis

The most common causes are an anxiety state or a primary dermatological condition. Rarely other disease processes are responsible:

- **Endocrine disease**: thyrotoxicosis, acromegaly, phaeochromocytoma, hypoglycaemia (sweating several hours after last eating, relieved by food), hypogonadism (particularly menopausal).
- **Cardiovascular disease**: paroxysmal tachyarrythmias cause paroxysmal sweating, although it is very rare for palpitations not to be felt during the event. Very poor left ventricular function causes sweating on effort, as does marked physical deconditioning.
- **Pain**: if severe enough, pain induces sweating. Some individuals sweat with mild pain.
- **Inflammatory disease**: including cancer (lymphoma or other malignancies) and chronic infection, which may cause sweats, particularly at night (see Chapter 45).

Investigations

The aim of any investigation is to exclude serious diagnoses.

- **Laboratory tests**: thyroid-stimulating hormone (TSH); inflammatory markers; growth hormone/insulin growth factor 1 (for acromegaly); urinary catecholamines (for phaeochromocytoma), fasting glucose and insulin (for hypoglycaemia), follicle-stimulating hormone (FSH)/oestradiol testosterone (for hypogonadism); blood film ± marrow.
- **Other tests**: very rarely a 24-hour electrocardiogram (ECG) recording (for arrhythmias) may be indicated.

Management

Treatment is for the underlying cause. If no cause is found, cleanliness, antiperspirants and physical conditioning are all that can be recommended.

Flushing

Flushing is very common. The usual causes are emotions in youth. Diseases that may have flushing as a prominent component include:

- **Primary dermatological disease**, especially photodermatosis (see Chapter 72), including autoimmune (systemic lupus erythematosus), metabolic (porphyria), plant-related (especially hogweed) and drug-induced (especially amiodarone); rosacea.
- **Drugs**: alcohol (especially in those deficient in alcohol dehydrogenase or on disulfiram – Antabuse) and calcium channel blockers commonly cause flushing, as do spicy foods, food allergy and toxin ingestion.
- **Hypogonadism**: most commonly menopause related (see Chapter 165).
- **Carcinoid syndrome**: carcinoid tumours are rare neuroendocrine tumours that are found in the small bowel and the lung. Many are benign. Malignant ones metastasize to the liver, from where they secrete biochemically active substances (principally 5-hydroxytryptamine (5-HT or serotonin), but also bradykinin, histamine and other peptides) into the systemic circulation, causing paroxysmal flushing which later becomes fixed, with abdominal pain (cramps) and watery diarrhoea – the carcinoid syndrome. Right-sided valve lesions (tricuspid regurgitation or pulmonary stenosis) occur in 50%. The diagnosis is confirmed by finding hepatic metastasis on liver ultrasound examination and high levels of 5-HT metabolites, particularly 5-hydroxyindoleacetic acid (5-HIAA) in the urine. Octreotide and other long-acting somatostatin analogues that inhibit the release of many gut peptides are very useful in controlling symptoms. Hepatic embolization, α-interferon, chemotherapy and therapy with radiolabelled somatostatin analogues are also useful. The tumour is remarkably slow growing and patients live for many years.
- **Medullary thyroid carcinoma**: this rare tumour can present as a neck mass, as Cushing's syndrome or as intractable diarrhoea. However, it can also produce a carcinoid-like syndrome. Of the tumours, 75% are sporadic in elderly individuals, but 25% relate to genetic cancer syndromes – multiple endocrine neoplasia (MEN).
- **Systemic mastocytosis**: overproliferation of mast cells. May be associated with myeloproliferative disorders or lymphomas. Intermittent release of histamine occurs, causing a syndrome much like scombroid poisoning (see below). Hepatosplenomegaly, portal hypertension and malabsorption also occur.
- **Scombroid poisoning**: histamine is produced by certain bacteria (e.g. *Proteus morgani*) acting to decompose the flesh of scombroid (e.g. tuna, mackerel) or non-scombroid (e.g. sardine, pilchard) fish. Symptoms occur 4 hours after ingestion: flushing, urticarial itching, conjunctival suffusion, abdominal colic; vomiting and diarrhoea may also occur. Treatment is supportive, antihistamines may help, and symptoms disappear after several hours.

Investigations

Investigation is indicated only if unusual features are present, suggestive of underlying disease. Laboratory tests include: FSH testosterone/oestradiol, urinary 5-HIAA for carcinoid syndrome; and calcitonin, bone marrow and urinary analysis for histamine excretion in suspected mastocytosis.

Management

Treatment is of the underlying cause.

Thyroid swellings

Thyroid nodules occur in 5% (F:M = 5:1) and may relate to a thyroid goitre (euthyroid or hypothyroid), benign adenomas (associated with hyperthyroidism) or malignancy (2% of goitres). Cancer is suggested by known radiation exposure, a family history or voice change (resulting from recurrent laryngeal nerve palsy). Goitres and cancer can cause tracheal (stridor) or oesophageal (dysphagia) compression. Investigation of any thyroid swelling means assessing the following:

- Thyroid status.
- Fine needle aspiration cytology (FNAC) in outpatients is diagnostic in the majority of cases, and may exclude malignancy, diagnose malignancy or be suspicious of malignancy. Surgical excision is indicated in the latter two categories.
- Ultrasonography of the thyroid gland: if nodules are found, radionuclide scanning may be indicated – cancer appears as a 'cold' nodule. FNAC is indicated for cold nodules to determine whether cancer is present.

Cancer is treated by excision (good prognosis histology), thyroxine (to suppress TSH, which otherwise promotes tumour growth) and radioactive iodine in hormonally active diseases.

Specific thyroid cancers

These account for <1% of all cancers, and affect women more than men, most commonly aged 40–50 years. Exposure to irradiation, particularly at a young age, leads to increased risk. There are five types:

1 Papillary is the commonest thyroid cancer accounting for >80%, affects those aged 30–50 years, spreads via the lymphatics and usually has a good prognosis. For treatment see below.

2 Follicular accounts for 10% of thyroid cancers, usually in those aged 40–50 years, it has a haematogenous spread and usually a good prognosis. Both papillary and follicular thyroid cancers are treated with near total thyroidectomy, postoperative thyroxine to suppress TSH ± radioiodine ablation of the thyroid remnant.

3 Anaplastic is an undifferentiated thyroid cancer accounting for <5%, affects those aged 60–80 years and spreads haematogenously. It has a poor prognosis; the treatment is thyroidectomy ± chemotherapy ± radiotherapy.

4 Medullary cancer (also, see above for flushing) arises from C cells of the thyroid, and accounts for 5–10% of all thyroid cancer, it is usually familial (MEN-2, RET proto-oncogene) and is treated by thyroidectomy.

5 Lymphoma is a rare cancer, associated with Hashimoto's thyroiditis, or systemic non-Hodgkin's lymphoma, treated with radio- and chemotherapy.

38 Obesity

Obesity

Causes

Genetic polymorphisms
Accounts for 30–60% of variation in weight

Diseases < 1% of cases
- Cushing's
- Hypothyroidism
- Polycystic ovary syndrome (Stein–Leventhal)
- Hypothalamic disease
- Genetic disorders, e.g. Prader–Willi syndrome

Environment
- Lack of exercise
- Easy access to food
- High alcohol intake
- Drugs (tricyclics, haloperidol, steroids)
- Poverty

Consequences of obesity

Stroke

Obstructive sleep apnoea (OSA)

Breathlessness
Restrictive defect → type II respiratory failure

Hypertension

Gallstones

Hiatus hernia

Ischaemic heart disease

Type II diabetes

Deep vein thrombosis, varicose veins

Osteoarthritis knee/hip

Increased risk of cancer
- Colorectal
- Gynaecological (breast, ovary, uterus)
- Prostate
- Pancreas
- Liver
- Multiple myeloma

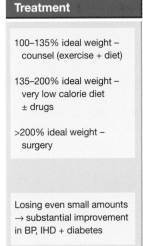

Patterns of obesity

	Centripetal	**Centrifugal**
Waist-hip ratio	♂ >1.0 ♀ >0.9	♂ <0.85 ♀ <0.75
	• Easier to lose weight • Men • Stress, cigarette smoking	• Harder to lose weight • Women
	Stronger link with mortality	

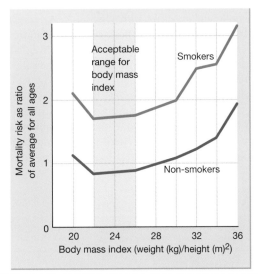

Treatment

100–135% ideal weight – counsel (exercise + diet)

135–200% ideal weight – very low calorie diet ± drugs

>200% ideal weight – surgery

Losing even small amounts → substantial improvement in BP, IHD + diabetes

Medicine at a Glance, Fourth Edition. Edited by Patrick Davey. © 2014 John Wiley & Sons, Ltd. Published 2014 by John Wiley & Sons, Ltd. Companion website: www.ataglanceseries.com/medicine

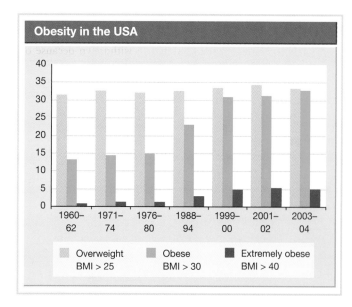

Obesity in the USA

intake and energy expenditure), in association with other neurotransmitters, regulates energy balance, though multiple other pathways are also involved (see Table 38.1).

Assessment of the obese patient

The clinical assessment of the obese patient involves:

- **Confirmation of obesity** from the BMI and assessment of the pattern of body fat distribution: centripetal obesity (waist : hip ratio >0.9 in women, >1.0 in men) is associated with increased cardiovascular risk.
- **Time course of obesity**: whether the obesity is old or new, any previous treatment for obesity and the family history. Explanation of obesity may also be sought by reference to eating habits and physical activity.
- **Secondary causes**: very rare but should be considered if in recent (less than several) years there has been unexplained weight gain and/or if there are abnormal physical signs or biochemical tests. Underlying pathology may include Cushing's syndrome (24 h urinary free cortisol), hypothyroidism (thyroid-stimulating hormone), hypothalamic disorder (uncontrolled appetite), Prader–Willi syndrome (deletion of part of the long arm of chromosome 15, resulting in hypogonadism and obesity) or Lawrence–Moon–Biedl syndrome.
- **Overall cardiovascular risk assessment**: from fasting glucose and lipid profile, and other standard risk factors (age, sex, blood pressure (BP), smoking status, alcohol consumption) and presence of vascular disease.

Complications

- **Metabolic complications**: hyperinsulinaemia and insulin resistance ± impaired glucose tolerance/diabetes mellitus; hypertension; ischaemic heart disease (IHD) (four-fold risk if BMI >29); cerebrovascular disease; hyperlipidaemia.
- **Hepatic complications**: obesity can lead to fatty infiltration of the liver, which can produce a hepatitis, and eventually lead to cirrhosis.
- **Physical problems**: osteoarthritis, varicose veins, hernias (both hiatal hernia and abdominal hernias), hypoventilation (obstructive sleep apnoea, see Chapter 98), operative complications.
- **Increased cancer risk**: breast, ovary, endometrium, prostate, cervix, bowel.

Definition

Obesity is defined as a body mass index (BMI) $>30 \, kg/m^2$ (BMI = weight (kg)/[height^2 (m^2)]); healthy = 18.5–24.9; overweight = 25–29.9; obese >30.

Epidemiology

The prevalence of obesity has doubled in the last decade and is now 21% in the UK adult population and up to 50% in certain racial groups (see Figure 38.2 above for recent US statistics).

Aetiopathogenesis of 'simple obesity'

- **Genetic**: genetic effects are complex and polygenic with a heritability of 30–60%. Monogenic disorders, e.g. leptin deficiency/resistance, and melanocortin 4 receptor deficiency are very rare.
- **Environment**: readily available high-fat, energy-rich diet, associated with a sedentary lifestyle.
- **Neuroendocrine**: ghrelin (released from the fundus of the stomach) increases food intake via hypothamalamic neuropeptide Y release. Neuropeptide Y (hypothalamic hormone that stimulates appetite) and leptin (peptide hormone synthesized in adipose tissue which acts in the hypothalamus to suppress food

Table 38.1 Multiple endocrine and neurological events involved in the regulation of body weight.

	Afferent signals ↓ appetite or ↑ energy expenditure	Afferent signals ↑ appetite or ↓ energy expenditure
Gastrointestinal tract	Glucagon, cholecystokinin, glucagon-like peptide 1, peptide YY, glucose	Opioids, neurotensin, growth-hormone-releasing hormone, somatostatin
Endocrine system	Adrenaline (β-adrenergic effect), oestrogens	Adrenaline (α-adrenergic effect)
Adipose tissue	Leptin	
Peripheral nervous system	Noradrenaline (β-adrenergic effect)	Noradrenaline (α-adrenergic effect)
Central nervous system	Dopamine, γ-aminobutyric acid, serotonin, cholecystokinin	Galanin, opioids, growth hormone-releasing hormone, somatostatin

These afferent signals act on hypothalamic tracts; involving noradrenaline, serotonin, neuropeptide Y, melanocyte-concentrating hormone, glucagon-like peptide I, corticotropin-releasing hormone, orexin A and oxytocin

The hypothalamic tracts effect changes via the sympathetic nervous system, parasympathetic nervous system and thyroid hormone

These systems then affect energy intake and expenditure

Management

Severely obese individuals need treatment to improve prognosis, improve self-image and minimize symptoms, particularly those arising from physical problems. In men, being 10% overweight increases death rates by 13%, and being 20% overweight by 25%.

Behavioural modifications

Behavioural modifications include dietary restriction, exercise and, most importantly, stopping smoking. Alcohol intake should be minimized.

Drugs

- **Fat absorption inhibitor**, Orlistat, inhibits pancreatic lipase reducing fat absorption. It is the only licensed anti-obesity drug in Europe.

- **Appetite suppressants** have been withdrawn.
  - Sibutramine (centrally acting serotonin and noradrenaline (norepinephrine) reuptake inhibitor); withdrawn because of hypertension and tachycardia.
  - Rimonabant (cannabinoid type 1 receptor antagonist reduces appetite); withdrawn because of side effects – depression and risk of suicide.

Amphetamine derivatives (dexfenfluramine, fenfluramine) suppress appetite but have been withdrawn as a result of side effects (cardiac valvulopathy).

Weight loss (bariatric) surgery

Gastric bypass surgery may be useful, e.g. in obese patients with type 2 diabetes mellitus. Sudden profound weight loss has its own complications, including liver dysfunction and QT interval prolongation, which may predispose to an arrhythmic death.

39 Hirsutism and infertility

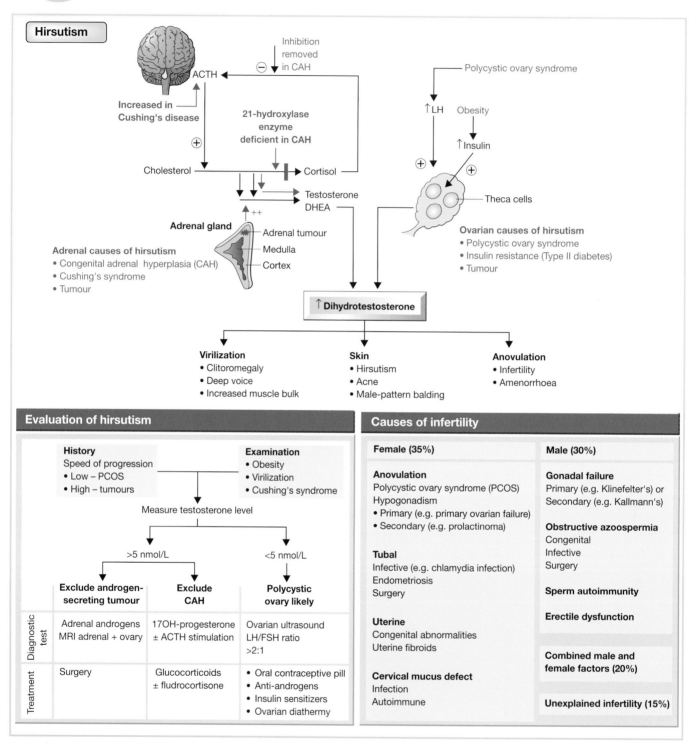

Hirsutism

Inhibition removed in CAH

Increased in Cushing's disease

ACTH

21-hydroxylase enzyme deficient in CAH

Cholesterol — Cortisol

Testosterone
DHEA

Adrenal gland
• Adrenal tumour
• Medulla
• Cortex

Adrenal causes of hirsutism
• Congenital adrenal hyperplasia (CAH)
• Cushing's syndrome
• Tumour

Polycystic ovary syndrome

↑LH   Obesity

↑Insulin

Theca cells

Ovarian causes of hirsutism
• Polycystic ovary syndrome
• Insulin resistance (Type II diabetes)
• Tumour

↑ **Dihydrotestosterone**

Virilization
• Clitoromegaly
• Deep voice
• Increased muscle bulk

Skin
• Hirsutism
• Acne
• Male-pattern balding

Anovulation
• Infertility
• Amenorrhoea

Evaluation of hirsutism

History
Speed of progression
• Low – PCOS
• High – tumours

Examination
• Obesity
• Virilization
• Cushing's syndrome

Measure testosterone level

>5 nmol/L   <5 nmol/L

	Exclude androgen-secreting tumour	Exclude CAH	Polycystic ovary likely
Diagnostic test	Adrenal androgens MRI adrenal + ovary	17OH-progesterone ± ACTH stimulation	Ovarian ultrasound LH/FSH ratio >2:1
Treatment	Surgery	Glucocorticoids ± fludrocortisone	• Oral contraceptive pill • Anti-androgens • Insulin sensitizers • Ovarian diathermy

Causes of infertility

Female (35%)		Male (30%)
Anovulation Polycystic ovary syndrome (PCOS) Hypogonadism • Primary (e.g. primary ovarian failure) • Secondary (e.g. prolactinoma)		**Gonadal failure** Primary (e.g. Klinefelter's) or Secondary (e.g. Kallmann's) **Obstructive azoospermia** Congenital Infective Surgery
Tubal Infective (e.g. chlamydia infection) Endometriosis Surgery		**Sperm autoimmunity**
Uterine Congenital abnormalities Uterine fibroids		**Erectile dysfunction** **Combined male and female factors (20%)**
Cervical mucus defect Infection Autoimmune		**Unexplained infertility (15%)**

Hirsutism

Hirsutism is common, affects 5% of premenopausal women and usually does not indicate a serious underlying illness. It is defined as excess hair growth in women from increased androgen production or skin sensitivity. Hair growth follows a male pattern, being predominantly facial (moustache or beard), thoracic and abdominal. Male pattern baldness may develop. Serious disease should be suspected in thin women, in rapidly progressive hirsutism, in treatment-resistant hypertension or with severe menstrual disruption. If other features of virilization are present (clitoromegaly, deep voice, male muscle pattern), investigations for androgen-secreting tumours are mandatory. The principal

Medicine at a Glance, Fourth Edition. Edited by Patrick Davey. © 2014 John Wiley & Sons, Ltd. Published 2014 by John Wiley & Sons, Ltd. Companion website: www.ataglanceseries.com/medicine

causes of hirsutism are listed below, although it is important to realize that hirsutism is often only a minor feature of these conditions:

- **Obesity** is commonly associated with mild hirsutism. Insulin resistance increases virilization. Acanthosis nigricans occurs in morbidly obese individuals.
- **Polycystic ovary syndrome** (PCOS): in its various forms, this affects 10% of women, commonly causing hirsutism. Sufferers often have marked obesity and mild virilization (male pattern hair growth and loss, with acne).
- **Familial or idiopathic hirsutism**, usually in those of Mediterranean descent.
- **Drugs**, particularly androgenic steroids in athletes.
- **Cushing's syndrome** (<1% of cases): patients rarely present with hirsutism; rather they present with treatment-resistant hypertension and profound hypokalaemia. The physical signs are of thin skin, proximal myopathy and (new and progressive) central obesity.
- **Congenital adrenal hyperplasia** (CAH) is a rare cause of hirsutism (there are 4000 CAH patients in the UK), is more common in Jewish people, and is usually caused by deficiency of 21-hydroxylase – the enzyme responsible for degrading progesterone (via intermediate metabolites) to corticosterone, cortisol and aldosterone. 17-Hydroxyprogesterone accumulates, is turned into androstenedione and, in turn, to testosterone. Symptoms thus relate in part to corticosteroid deficiency and in part to testosterone excess. Hirsutism occurs and there may be a history of acute adrenal failure when physically stressed. High 17-hydroxyprogesterone levels are found, particularly with adrenocorticotrophin hormone (ACTH) stimulation. Treatment is with corticosteroids sufficient to suppress ACTH-mediated 17-hydroxyprogesterone production.
- **Androgen-secreting tumour**: <1% of cases; can arise from the ovary or the adrenals.

The diagnostic approach is to pick up clues from the history and examination (particularly of marked virilization) and to measure luteinizing hormone (LH)/follicle-stimulating hormone (FSH) and androgen levels. Testosterone levels of >5 nmol/L (i.e.

significant elevation) imply that a diagnosis of PCOS is unlikely and that of an androgen-secreting tumour or CAH more likely. These need to be formally excluded by hormonal assessment, including stimulation tests and imaging. Treatment of hirsutism, other than that for the underlying cause, involves weight loss, cosmetic approaches (topical acne treatment, waxing, electrolysis and laser) and insulin-sensitizing drugs (metformin). The combined oral contraceptive pill (OCP), specifically Dianette (an OCP containing the anti-androgen cyproterone acetate), is useful. Androgen receptor blockers (e.g. spironolactone and cyproterone acetate), usually combined with an OCP, are effective.

Infertility

Infertility is defined as failure of pregnancy after 1 year of unprotected intercourse. It affects 10–15% of couples.

Investigation of male and female partners is needed for diagnosis. In men the first investigation is semen analysis: normal sperm motility and numbers exclude the man from further investigation. If abnormal sperm are found, FSH and testosterone are measured to investigate the possibility of gonadal failure. If such investigations are normal, then the possibility of obstruction to the spermatic tract should be considered. In the female, mid-luteal progesterone is measured. Normal levels (>30 pmol/L) imply normal gonadal function. The problem may then be mechanical and laparoscopy for tubal patency is undertaken. Abnormally low progesterone suggests lack of ovulation, e.g. premature ovarian failure or PCOS.

Management

Treatment is for the underlying cause where possible. For anovulation, clomiphene, gonadotrophin-releasing hormone or gonadotrophins are used in low FSH cases (success rate 50–80%), and oocyte donation for raised FSH cases (50% success rate). Complex stimulatory regimens are needed in male pituitary failure. For tubal or obstructive azoospermia, reconstructive surgery is occasionally possible and, for oligospermia, intracytoplasmic sperm injections (success rate 20% per cycle). Unexplained infertility may respond to *in vitro* fertilization (25% success rate/cycle, though rates are much lower in women aged over 40 years).

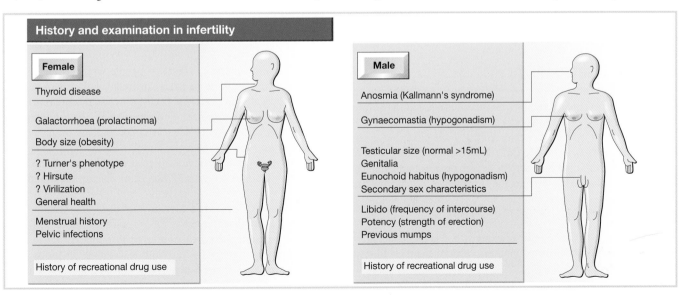

40 Erectile dysfunction and gynaecomastia

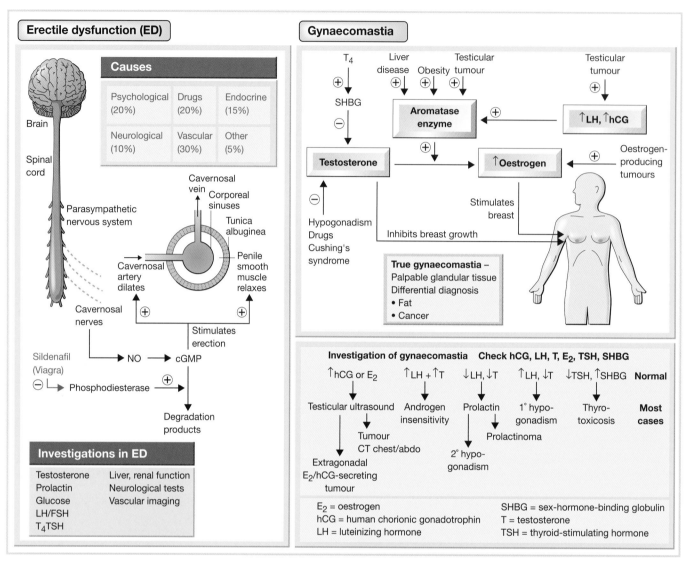

Erectile dysfunction (ED)

Brain

Spinal cord

Causes

Psychological (20%)	Drugs (20%)	Endocrine (15%)
Neurological (10%)	Vascular (30%)	Other (5%)

Parasympathetic nervous system

Cavernosal vein
Corporeal sinuses
Tunica albuginea
Penile smooth muscle relaxes

Cavernosal artery dilates

Cavernosal nerves

Stimulates erection

Sildenafil (Viagra)

NO → cGMP

Phosphodiesterase

Degradation products

Investigations in ED

Testosterone	Liver, renal function
Prolactin	Neurological tests
Glucose	Vascular imaging
LH/FSH	
T_4TSH	

Gynaecomastia

T_4 → SHBG

Liver disease
Obesity
Testicular tumour

Aromatase enzyme

Testosterone → ↑Oestrogen

↑LH, ↑hCG

Testicular tumour

Oestrogen-producing tumours

Stimulates breast

Hypogonadism
Drugs
Cushing's syndrome

Inhibits breast growth

True gynaecomastia –
Palpable glandular tissue
Differential diagnosis
• Fat
• Cancer

Investigation of gynaecomastia   Check hCG, LH, T, E_2, TSH, SHBG

↑hCG or E_2	↑LH + ↑T	↓LH, ↓T	↑LH, ↓T	↓TSH, ↑SHBG	**Normal**
Testicular ultrasound	Androgen insensitivity	Prolactin	1° hypo-gonadism	Thyro-toxicosis	**Most cases**
Tumour CT chest/abdo		Prolactinoma			
Extragonadal E_2/hCG-secreting tumour		2° hypo-gonadism			

E_2 = oestrogen	SHBG = sex-hormone-binding globulin
hCG = human chorionic gonadotrophin	T = testosterone
LH = luteinizing hormone	TSH = thyroid-stimulating hormone

Erectile dysfunction

The normal erection is produced by vasoconstriction of the venous outflow from the penis, resulting in blood distending the corpus cavernosa of the penis. Venous vasoconstriction is the result of activation of sacral autonomic nerves raising levels of venous cyclic adenosine monophosphate (cAMP). Interference with the arterial supply, autonomic nervous system or sex drive (libido) impairs erectile success. Erectile dysfunction (impotence) is defined as an inability to achieve an erection sufficient for sexual intercourse. It affects 10% of males and is caused by the following:

• **Drugs** commonly underlie or exacerbate erectile failure. Particularly important ones are β-blockers, calcium channel blockers and psychotropic agents.

• **Psychological problems**: very common; may cause erectile failure in its own right or complicate a pre-existing medical problem. Impotence is usually variable in severity and morning erections are unaffected.

• **Endocrine disorders**: 30–60% of people with diabetes of 6 years' standing develop some degree of erectile failure, as a result of both neuropathy and vascular disease. Thyroid dysfunction can also impair libido and potency. Androgen deficiency underlies 20% of cases of impotence seen in endocrinology outpatients. Libido is reduced in hypogonadal males.

• **Vascular disease**: peripheral arterial insufficiency involving the terminal aorta is a very common cause for erectile dysfunction. Penis venous insufficiency is, however, a very rare cause of impotence.

• **Neurological disease**: many neurological diseases can be associated with impotence, either directly through damage to the mechanisms involved in erection and ejaculation, or indirectly through psychological mechanisms. Particularly important causes include damage to the sacral nerves, as can occur with radical prostrate or pelvic surgery.

• **Other diseases**: structural penile abnormalities such as Peyronie's disease (which results in a curved penis) and microphallus

Medicine at a Glance, Fourth Edition. Edited by Patrick Davey. © 2014 John Wiley & Sons, Ltd. Published 2014 by John Wiley & Sons, Ltd. Companion website: www.ataglanceseries.com/medicine

may cause erectile dysfunction. Any chronic debilitating disease can also cause impotence.

Diagnosis

The key is to diagnose any underlying disease, which may require specific therapy. Absence of early morning erections is a good clue to the presence of underlying organic disease. Symptoms and signs of hypogonadism must be carefully sought (gynaecomastia, decrease in body hair, fatigue, testicular shrinkage, premature osteoporosis). Arterial disease and the factors closely associated with it should be looked for (intermittent claudication, presence of diabetes, hypertension or smoking, presence of foot and leg pulses). General health needs to be assessed, particularly whether liver, renal or neurological disease is present.

Treatment

Any underlying disease should be treated and any causative drug withdrawn.

- **Androgen treatment** if hypogonadal.
- **Phosphodiesterase inhibitors** (sildenafil (Viagra), vardenafil, tadalafil): inhibit penile phosphodiesterase type 5 and enhance the normal erectile response to sexual stimulation. Contraindicated in recent myocardial infarction/cerebrovascular accident, and if nitrates have been taken in the previous 24 hours (profound hypotension can occur).
- **Intracavernous papaverine or prostaglandin E$_1$ (PGE$_1$) injection**: these are potent vasoconstrictors and, when injected into the penile venous circulation, they prevent venous efflux, so producing erections. Erections may be persistent and painful (priapism).
- **Vacuum devices**: these work but are cosmetically unattractive.
- **Penile prosthesis**: surgically implanted prosthetic devices can stiffen, or mechanically inflate, the penis; they are useful when other forms of treatment are ineffective, undesirable or contraindicated.

Gynaecomastia

This is enlargement of the male breast as a result of hyperplasia of glandular tissue. It affects 30% of men aged <30 years and 50% aged >45 years. It rarely indicates serious underlying disease but if the patient is thin, enlargement is rapid and in particular the glandular tissue is >5 cm, underlying disease should be suspected. Causes include:

- **Obesity**: probably the most common cause. Increased peripheral conversion of testosterone to oestrogen by the aromatase enzyme promotes breast growth.
- **Drugs**: a common cause – digoxin, cimetidine, spironolactone, anti-androgens, alcohol, marihuana, anti-retroviral drugs, etc.
- **Hyperprolactinaemia**: high prolactin levels induce secondary hypogonadism, depressing testosterone levels, allowing for unopposed oestrogen action on the breast.
- **Hypogonadism**: suspect if libido is reduced with erectile dysfunction.
- **Systemic disease**: liver cirrhosis, chronic renal failure.
- **Underlying hormone-secreting tumour**: accounts for 3% of cases of gynaecomastia seen in the endocrine service. The tumour may be testicular (human chorionic gonadotrophin (hCG), oestradiol or aromatase producing), adrenal (oestradiol producing) or a lung/gastrointestinal cancer producing hCG.

Breast cancer, which is rare, may need to be excluded if the breast tissue is hard. Treatment is mainly by reassurance, withdrawal of the offending drug and advice on weight reduction. Drugs may help (anti-oestrogens, or those that inhibit the aromatase enzyme). Surgical resection is occasionally used.

41 Principles of infection

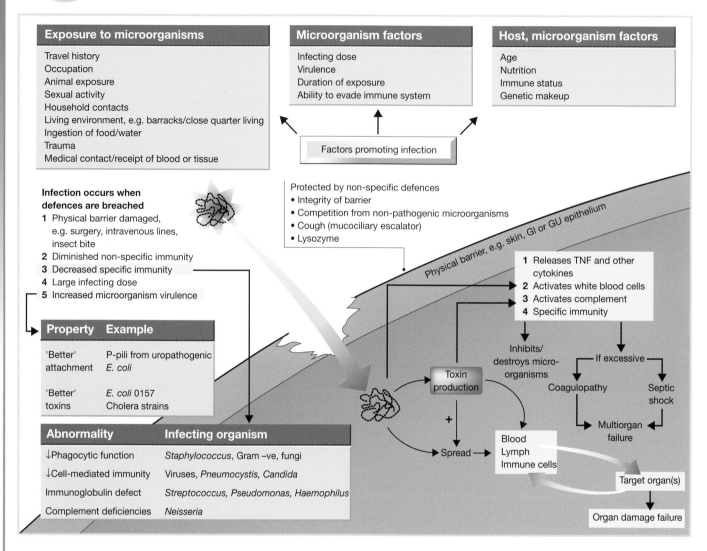

Exposure to microorganisms

Travel history
Occupation
Animal exposure
Sexual activity
Household contacts
Living environment, e.g. barracks/close quarter living
Ingestion of food/water
Trauma
Medical contact/receipt of blood or tissue

Microorganism factors

Infecting dose
Virulence
Duration of exposure
Ability to evade immune system

Host, microorganism factors

Age
Nutrition
Immune status
Genetic makeup

Factors promoting infection

Infection occurs when defences are breached
1 Physical barrier damaged, e.g. surgery, intravenous lines, insect bite
2 Diminished non-specific immunity
3 Decreased specific immunity
4 Large infecting dose
5 Increased microorganism virulence

Protected by non-specific defences
• Integrity of barrier
• Competition from non-pathogenic microorganisms
• Cough (mucociliary escalator)
• Lysozyme

Physical barrier, e.g. skin, GI or GU epithelium

1 Releases TNF and other cytokines
2 Activates white blood cells
3 Activates complement
4 Specific immunity

Property	Example
'Better' attachment	P-pili from uropathogenic *E. coli*
'Better' toxins	*E. coli* 0157 Cholera strains

Abnormality	Infecting organism
↓Phagocytic function	*Staphylococcus*, Gram –ve, fungi
↓Cell-mediated immunity	Viruses, *Pneumocystis*, *Candida*
Immunoglobulin defect	*Streptococcus*, *Pseudomonas*, *Haemophilus*
Complement deficiencies	*Neisseria*

Toxin production

Inhibits/destroys micro-organisms

If excessive

Coagulopathy

Septic shock

Multiorgan failure

+

Spread

Blood
Lymph
Immune cells

Target organ(s)

Organ damage failure

Despite antimicrobial agents being available for over 50 years, infections remain a significant health problem. The burden of infectious disease has shifted as a result of antibacterial resistance, vaccination programmes and the emergence of new diseases (e.g. HIV infection). However, considerable global morbidity and mortality due to infection persists, predominantly driven by continuing poverty. Infections once considered controlled, e.g. tuberculosis (TB), are re-emerging as significant problems in both resource-poor and -rich countries. Infection and the development of clinical disease depend on the interaction of a microbial agent and the host. Both must be considered together, e.g. normally non-pathogenic organisms may cause clinical disease in a severely immunocompromised host.

The host

The host influence can be divided into two categories:

1 Factors determining exposure to microorganisms: assessment of exposure is crucial in evaluating the risk of infection in an individual (or community). One must consider:
• An individual's interaction with his or her environment.
• Particular behaviour that may lead to the acquisition of a potential pathogen.

• Prevalence of infection in a community.
2 Factors influencing infection and development of disease after exposure.

Infection and disease

Non-specific defences
• **Physical barriers**: intact skin and mucosa prevent the entry of microorganisms.
• **Competition** from commensal flora: colonization of body sites by 'normal' bacterial flora prevents colonization with pathogenic microorganisms.
• **Biological barriers**: e.g. oral lysozyme secretion.
• **Chemical barriers**: e.g. acidic environment of the stomach.
• **Physical mechanisms expelling bacteria**: e.g. urine flow through the urinary system, the cough reflex and the action of microcilia in the respiratory tract all reduce the risk of bacterial multiplication.
• **Disturbances in non-specific defences** contribute to the risk of infection in hospital, e.g. urinary catheters or intravenous lines breaching skin/mucosal integrity or the effect of antibiotics on bacterial flora.

Specific defences

These comprise the inflammatory response mounted by:

- Neutrophils and phagocytes.
- The complement system.
- Specific cell-mediated and antibody responses to pathogens.

In any infection, always consider whether a patient has had temporary or permanent changes in any of the defence systems (see Chapters 174 and 175). Age, immunization, chronic illnesses and drug treatment all affect immunity.

Microorganisms

Disease may arise from:

- **Endogenous infection**, i.e. microorganisms that exist on mucosal surfaces or are present in the body as a latent infection. Endogenously acquired infections have become progressively more important in developed countries as populations become more immunocompromised.
- **Exogenous infection** from the environment:
  - Direct exogenous transmission occurs from contact with, or droplet transmission from, an infected host or source (such as soil).
  - Indirect infection may be vector-borne, air-borne or result from transmission via infected blood, blood products or organs.

Disease production

Pathogens have evolved strategies to make transmission and establishment in a host more efficient. Different strategies may be utilized by microorganisms at different points in the establishment of an infection; the following are examples:

- **Mucosal contact**: attachment to epithelial surfaces may be crucial for pathogenesis:
  - Non-specific interactions occur between the hydrophilic bacterial cell surface and the lipophilic endothelial cell surface.
  - Specific interactions also exist: uropathogenic *Escherichia coli* have P-pili (hair-like structures) which adhere to a specific glycolipid receptor on the urothelial cell surface. Influenza virus attaches to cells via the haemagglutinin antigen.
- **Invasion**: pathogens cause damage by invading deeper tissues, either through breaks in the skin or mucosal surface or specific invasion mechanisms:
  - Schistosomal cerceriae are able to penetrate intact skin and subsequently enter the circulation.
  - Enteropathogens utilize a number of different mechanisms to adhere to and then interact with the M cell, leading to transport, invasion and multiplication.
  - *Neisseria meningitidis*, or the measles virus, is able to penetrate epithelium.
- **Immune evasion**: some pathogens produce enzymes or have surface components, which bind or inhibit secretory IgA on mucosal surfaces:
  - The polysaccharide capsule of bacteria such as *Streptococcus pneumoniae* or *Haemophilus influenzae* type B helps to resist phagocytosis.
  - *Leishmania*, *Mycobacterium* or *Salmonella* species are able to survive and multiply within macrophages.
- **Toxin production** is important in the pathogenesis of some diseases:
  - Cholera toxin activates the adenyl cyclase mechanisms of host intestinal cells, thus producing the excretion of large amounts of fluid and electrolytes. The production of toxin transforms asymptomatic carriage of *Clostridium difficile* into a disease-causing pathogen.
- The lipopolysaccharide of Gram-negative bacteria (endotoxin) has an important role in production of the sepsis syndrome.

Potential clinical consequences of infection

Acute consequences

- Cytokine effects: fever, malaise, anorexia, catabolic state, increased white cells and platelets, acute phase response with increased acute phase proteins.
- Circulatory failure (see Chapter 18).
- Disseminated intravascular coagulation.
- Organ damage and failure from shock (e.g. renal failure), direct invasion (e.g. pneumonia producing respiratory failure) or by multiple mechanisms (e.g. adult respiratory distress syndrome).

Chronic consequences

- Muscle wasting and weight loss.
- Anaemia of chronic disease: see Chapter 186.
- Permanent organ destruction: e.g. liver cirrhosis from chronic hepatitis, left ventricular failure after viral myocarditis, permanent paralysis following polio.
- Postinfective phenomena: e.g. lactose intolerance after gastrointestinal (GI) infection.

Autoimmune phenomena

- Generalized syndromes: e.g. poststreptococcal phenomena, such as rheumatic fever.
- System-specific: the following are examples:
  - Neurological: Guillain–Barré syndrome after a viral infection, cerebellar syndromes after chickenpox.
  - Haematological: haemolytic anaemia after *Mycoplasma* infection.
- Rheumatological: arthritis after gut or urinary tract infection in genetically predisposed individuals.
- Dermatological: scarlet fever (rash after streptococcal infection).

Treatment of infection

- Symptomatic support: antipyretics, maintenance of hydration.
- Antimicrobials: either empirical or targeted to identified microorganisms.
- Removal of sources of infection: e.g. draining abscesses or removing infected lines.
- Circulatory and vital organ support in severe infection.
- Many infections (particularly viral) are self-limiting and do not need specific treatment.

Prevention of infection

- Avoidance of exposure to, or contact with, pathogen.
- Altered behaviour,
- Public health measures such as sanitation.
- Infection control within health-care settings.
- Prophylactic measures.
- Before invasive procedures: pre surgery antibiotics.
- Before inducing immunosuppression: treatment of latent TB before transplant.
- After exposure to potential pathogen: post-exposure HIV drugs.
- Immunization, with one of the following:
  - Live attenuated organisms.
  - Killed organisms or components of microbes.
  - Altered toxins from microbes.

42 Diagnosis of infection

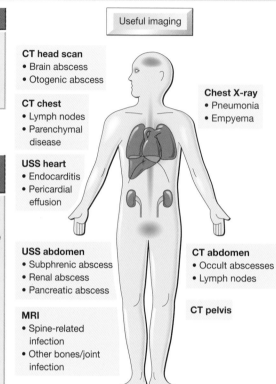

Infective process suggested by:

1 Specific regional syndromes, often pain + fever + specific symptoms
2 Generalized syndromes = unwell + fever ± shock ± haemostatic failure

Helpful tests in suspected infection

1 **Full blood count** (FBC): to look for changes in white cell counts
2 **CRP** and **ESR**. Assess degree of acute inflammatory response:
   • ESR
   • C-reactive protein: acute phase protein with short half-life, rises briskly, falls quickly; particularly useful for assessing response to treatment
3 Tests to assess effect of infection: LFTs, clotting tests, renal function
4 Determination of organism: microscopy/culture/histology of appropriate samples or serological diagnosis
5 Imaging to assess site or extent of infection

Useful imaging

CT head scan
• Brain abscess
• Otogenic abscess

CT chest
• Lymph nodes
• Parenchymal disease

USS heart
• Endocarditis
• Pericardial effusion

USS abdomen
• Subphrenic abscess
• Renal abscess
• Pancreatic abscess

MRI
• Spine-related infection
• Other bones/joint infection

Chest X-ray
• Pneumonia
• Empyema

CT abdomen
• Occult abscesses
• Lymph nodes

CT pelvis

Diagnosis

Rests on proving presence of pathogenic organisms + appropriate clinical presentation.

1 Identification of organism
   • Light microscopy, e.g. Ziehl–Neelson stain for TB
   • Electron microscopy—useful for many viruses
   • Biopsy specimen
2 Identification of microbial antigen
   • e.g. PCR of CSF for viral, bacterial Ag
3 Culture of organism
   • Plating out (various media/ biochemical reactions)
   • Cytopathic effect (viruses)
   • Xenodiagnosis (infection of sterile animal, e.g. trypanosomiasis)
4 Immunological response
   • Antibody response, usually detection of IgM, or rise in IgG titre over time
   • Skin response to antigen, e.g. Mantoux test (TB)

Highly suggestive findings

If organisms are not found, findings highly suggestive of infection are:
1 Classic radiological findings (e.g. 'halo' sign in aspergilloma)
2 Response to specific chemotherapy (e.g. anti-TB treatment)

The initial history and examination usually indicate the most appropriate investigation. In a febrile patient with no obvious source of infection, useful screening investigations include a full blood count (FBC), liver function tests (LFTs), C-reactive protein (CRP) or erythrocyte sedimentation rate (ESR), blood cultures, urine examination and a chest X-ray.

Full blood count

• **Normochromic/normocytic anaemia** occurs in many chronic infections.
• **Raised neutrophil count** or toxic granulation suggests bacterial sepsis.
• **Raised lymphocyte count**: occurs in many viral infections and some bacterial disorders, e.g. typhoid and brucellosis. Atypical lymphocytes suggest Epstein–Barr virus (EBV) or cytomegalovirus (CMV) infection.
• **Low neutrophil count**: iatrogenic immunosuppression or infection with typhoid, brucellosis or rickettsial disease. Bad prognostic indicator in severe sepsis.
• **Low lymphocyte count**: consider human immunodeficiency virus (HIV) but common with other acute infections.
• **Low platelet count**: malaria and dengue fever in particular. May reflect disseminated intravascular coagulation in severe sepsis.
• **Eosinophilia** may occur in schistosomiasis and tissue invasion by other parasites.

CRP and ESR

The ESR is the rate at which red cells settle through plasma. It is dependent on age, sex, serum immunoglobulins, especially IgM, acute phase proteins such as fibrinogen, and the shape and nature of the red cell membrane. It increases with age (the normal ESR is < [age/2] + 10). The ESR is elevated in most infections, but does not reliably discriminate between infective and inflammatory conditions and rises only slowly (over 2 weeks). It is possible to have an acute infection and a normal ESR.

The CRP rises within 4–8 hours after the onset of infection and has a half-life in the circulation of approximately 8 hours. CRP levels are useful in following the response to treatment.

The two tests are not interchangeable. The ESR is sometimes compared to the glycosylated haemoglobin in diabetes (which gives an estimate of the glycaemic control over the previous few weeks), while the ESR gives an average of inflammation over the preceding 2–3 weeks. The CRP, like glucose, gives the picture over the preceding 8 hours.

Liver function tests

Abnormalities in liver function suggest either local infective processes (hepatitis, hepatic abscesses, biliary sepsis) or systemic or disseminated infections. Unrelated causes such as medication or alcohol can change liver function so further evidence is needed to define specific infection.

Microscopy

Direct microscopy of clinical samples allows rapid identification of microorganisms. Wet preparations are used for urine examination or the detection of parasites in the stool.

Fixed stained preparations

- Gram staining: the size, morphology (cocci or bacilli) and staining characteristics (Gram positive or negative) of bacteria give a clue to their species, but definitive identification is rarely possible. Commensal or contaminant organisms in samples make interpretation of microscopy difficult. Microscopy is most useful for samples from normally sterile sites, e.g. cerebrospinal fluid (CSF), joints, etc.
- Specific stains are used to identify some microorganisms: e.g. Ziehl–Neelsen stain for mycobacteria or Giemsa for parasites such as malaria on a blood slide.

Viruses cannot be identified on standard microscopy and although electron microscopy can be used to identify some species, improvements in molecular technology in recent years mean that microscopy has largely been superseded by the polymerase chain reaction (PCR) in clinical practice.

Culture

Culture is the definitive diagnostic method for most bacteria and fungi. Samples are cultured on growth media, whose composition and incubation conditions are varied to isolate particular microorganisms selectively. Organisms are identified by colonial morphology, growth on specific media and in certain conditions, and by biochemical reactions. The use of antibiotic discs on culture plates allows determination of antibiotic sensitivity. These traditional methods are now complemented by molecular techniques, which are used in many laboratories for identification and sensitivity testing.

Contamination of cultures with normal flora, such as non-pathogenic mouth organisms in sputum samples, may make detection of pathogens more difficult.

Blood cultures may identify bacteraemia resulting from infection in many different sites of the body. Repeated blood cultures are necessary to detect organisms that do not grow readily or to determine the significance of an initial isolation of a potential contaminating organism. It is rare to need more than three sets of blood cultures. Blood cultures should ideally be taken before starting antibiotics. In 'difficult to diagnose' infection, it is often appropriate to stop all antibiotics and re-culture all potentially infected sites, e.g. blood, etc.

Serology

Some organisms, particularly viruses, are difficult to identify. Serology measures the host immunological response to an infection. IgM antibodies or a rise in IgG titre over 10–14 days (acute and convalescent titres) can be considered to be diagnostic of recent infection. Serology is particularly useful in infections such as hepatitis or glandular fever.

Histology

Infection can sometimes be diagnosed only by seeing specific pathological features on examination of tissue. These features include:

- Inclusion bodies in tissue suggesting viral infections such as CMV.
- Granulomas: associated with a number of different infections, including tuberculosis (TB).
- Demonstration of fungi in tissues by the use of specific stains.

Tissue biopsy may sometimes be the only way of making a diagnosis in difficult cases.

Molecular methods

Molecular techniques are becoming increasingly important.

- **PCR** uses genetic probes to recognize and amplify the nucleic acid from specific viruses or bacteria that are difficult to culture. For example, nasopharyngeal secretions can be tested using a panel of likely respiratory viruses such as influenza, parainfluenza, coronavirus and syncytial virus. Quantification is also possible and may guide treatment for example in hepatitis B or CMV infection. PCR is also used for the rapid detection of resistance conferred by specific genes in organisms such as *Mycobacterium tuberculosis*.
- **Computerized identification**. In the last few years, use of matrix-assisted laser desorption/ionization (MALDI) combined with mass spectrometry has been developed to improve and speed up microbiological identification. Once a colony has been grown, the signature from ionization of the organism can be compared with a database of known organisms.
  - Automated systems have also been developed that use colourimetry to compare the growth of unknown organisms against a battery of different antibiotics. They decrease the time it takes from initial growth of an organism to identification of its species and antibiotic susceptibility to just a few hours, and are highly accurate.

Imaging

- **Chest X-rays** can show focal lesions, which are undetectable clinically, and are mandatory in those suspected of having an infection in whom the source is not readily apparent.
- **Abdominal and pelvic ultrasonography** may detect hepatic lesions, identify abdominal nodes and locate intra-abdominal or pelvic abscesses as a source of fever or bacteraemia.
- **Computed tomography** (CT) scans are useful in examining all regions of the body in a search for, or to delineate the extent of, infection. They are a useful early investigation in febrile patients with presumed but unidentified infections, and may identify a source in patients who are bacteraemic with gastrointestinal pathogens. CT also allows for diagnostic sampling and therapeutic drainage in many situations.
- **Magnetic resonance imaging** (MRI) is used in the diagnosis of soft tissue and bony/joint infections. X-rays may identify bone changes as a result of long-standing infection but MRI is much more sensitive.
- **Nuclear imaging**: white cell scans are rarely useful because they do not distinguish acute inflammation from infection, nor detect chronic low-grade infections caused by parasites, viruses, mycobacteria or fungi. They are sometimes helpful in identification of the site of pyogenic inflammation.
- **Positron emission tomography** is a relatively new method of functional imaging. It uses a radiolabelled form of glucose (flurodeoxyglucose (FDG)) which is taken up by metabolically active tissues. This information is then mapped onto a CT done at the same time. Its main use is for identification of metastases but can also occasionally be helpful in fevers of unknown origin and occult sources of infection.
- **Cardiac ultrasonography** is indicated in suspected bacterial endocarditis, to look for vegetations and assess valve function. If bacteraemia/septicaemia has occurred caused by *Staphylococcus aureus*, early cardiac ultrasonography is mandatory to exclude endocarditis.

43 Fever and the assessment of the patient with presumed infection

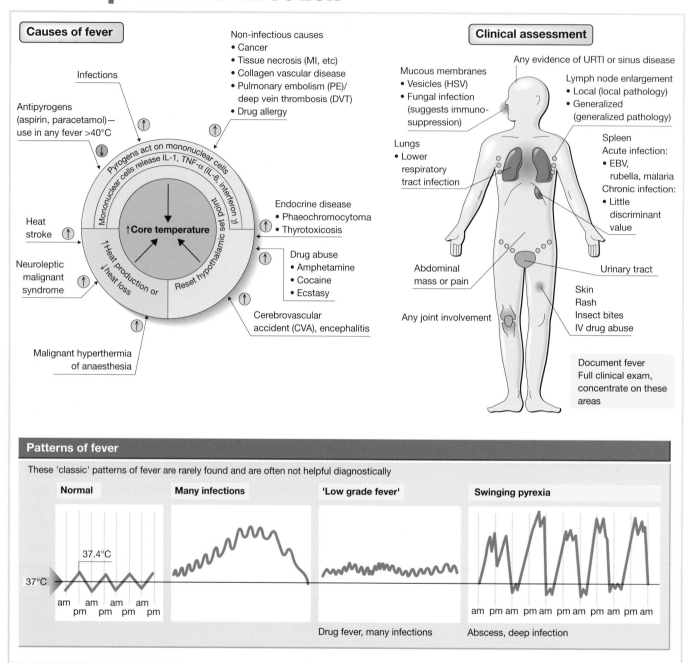

Causes of fever

Non-infectious causes
• Cancer
• Tissue necrosis (MI, etc)
• Collagen vascular disease
• Pulmonary embolism (PE)/ deep vein thrombosis (DVT)
• Drug allergy

Infections

Antipyrogens (aspirin, paracetamol)— use in any fever >40°C

Pyrogens act on mononuclear cells
Mononuclear cells release IL-1, TNF-α (IL-6, interferon γ)

↑Core temperature

↑Heat production or ↓heat loss

Reset hypothalamic set point

Heat stroke

Neuroleptic malignant syndrome

Malignant hyperthermia of anaesthesia

Endocrine disease
• Phaeochromocytoma
• Thyrotoxicosis

Drug abuse
• Amphetamine
• Cocaine
• Ecstasy

Cerebrovascular accident (CVA), encephalitis

Clinical assessment

Any evidence of URTI or sinus disease

Mucous membranes
• Vesicles (HSV)
• Fungal infection (suggests immuno- suppression)

Lymph node enlargement
• Local (local pathology)
• Generalized (generalized pathology)

Lungs
• Lower respiratory tract infection

Spleen
Acute infection:
• EBV, rubella, malaria
Chronic infection:
• Little discriminant value

Abdominal mass or pain

Urinary tract

Any joint involvement

Skin
Rash
Insect bites
IV drug abuse

Document fever
Full clinical exam, concentrate on these areas

Patterns of fever

These 'classic' patterns of fever are rarely found and are often not helpful diagnostically

Normal

37.4°C

37°C

am am am am
pm pm pm pm

Many infections

'Low grade fever'

Drug fever, many infections

Swinging pyrexia

am pm am pm am pm am pm am pm am

Abscess, deep infection

Fever

Fever is a physiological response where the body temperature is increased due to re-setting of the normal hypothalamic set point. Normal body temperature varies considerably between individuals (oral range, 36.0–37.7°C) and varies diurnally (peaks in evening; troughs in early morning).

Hyperthermia

Hyperthermia is an elevated body temperature above the hypothalamic set point. It occurs when there is excessive heat production, reduced heat loss or hypothalamic damage. Temperatures >41°C are rarely the result of infections and usually imply loss of thermoregulation.

Pathogenesis of fever

Fever is produced by the effect of exogenous pyrogens which trigger cytokine and prostaglandin release. Infectious agents and their breakdown products or toxins are the most common triggers of fever. Other molecules, such as immune complexes and lymphocyte products, can also elicit a febrile response. These are

Medicine at a Glance, Fourth Edition. Edited by Patrick Davey. © 2014 John Wiley & Sons, Ltd. Published 2014 by John Wiley & Sons, Ltd. Companion website: www.ataglanceseries.com/medicine

the basis of fever in malignancy, drug reactions and connective tissue disorders.

Assessment of the patient

History
When evaluating those with possible infection, several important questions should be considered:

- Is the illness likely to represent infection, i.e. are other causes of fever absent or at least unlikely?
- Where is the probable site of infection? Symptoms arising from a particular organ are usually reliable guides to the site of infection. Non-specific symptoms (e.g. fever, muscular aches) may occur in generalized infection (septicaemia, viraemia).
- What are the most likely organisms to be involved? This is usually determined by considering the specific symptoms/duration and probable organ affected, and the age, immune status, history of surgical procedures and travel history.
- What organisms has this patient been exposed to? Is there local epidemic disease (e.g. influenza, cholera)?
- Are there reasons why this patient might be prone to infection? An immunocompromised host is more prone to infection, including with normally non-pathogenic organisms.
- Is there evidence of tissue or organ damage (kidney, lung, etc.)? This may indicate whether specific supportive therapy (such as mechanical ventilation, blood pressure support) is needed.

A good clinical history is essential and the systems enquiry is particularly useful to establish a focus of infection.

Symptoms
- Duration (acute or chronic) and fever pattern may help diagnose the organism.
- Rigors are uncommon in non-infective causes of fever.
- Weight loss occurs in most chronic infections (notably tuberculosis, endocarditis, intra-abdominal abscesses).
- Symptoms suggest localization.

Exposure to pathogens
Travel history allows an assessment of exposure to potential pathogens. The occupation may be relevant to pathogen exposure, e.g. leptospirosis in sewage workers. Animal contact is relevant in zoonotic infection. Sexual history and intravenous (IV) drug usage are also important.

Drug history
Recently prescribed medication and herbal or traditional remedies may cause fever. Previous antimicrobial treatment may modify clinical presentation or make isolation of an organism difficult. Drugs may modify immunity (e.g. corticosteroids). Antipyretics may reduce fever response.

Past medical history
- Other underlying illnesses may increase infection risk.
- Frequent infections suggest an underlying immune problem.
- Immunization history is necessary.
- History of transfusions might suggest blood-borne viruses.

Family history
If close contacts are also unwell, this may suggest epidemic transmission. History of infection in family may suggest hereditary immune defects.

Examination and investigations
A careful clinical examination is important, as symptoms can sometimes be subtle or may not be organ-specific. Some areas of the examination warrant particular attention (see Figure 43.1). Routine investigations include:

- Full blood count, inflammatory markers (see Chapters 42 and 186).
- Blood, urine cultures.
- Chest X-ray.
- Serological tests.
- Ultrasonography/computed tomography guided diagnosis and aspiration of any suspected abscesses.

If clinical assessment and early investigations do not reveal a cause, take a wide view. Stop all unnecessary drugs, culture all possible sites frequently, and consider causes of fever other than infection. Do not give empirical antibiotics unless the patient is very unwell, when broad-spectrum parenteral antibiotics are indicated.

Very rare causes of hyperthermia
Other than infections (see relevant chapters), important causes of hyperthermia that need to be distinguished from fever include:

- **Neuroleptic malignant syndrome**: a rare idiosyncratic reaction to antipsychotic agents, promoted by intercurrent illness or dehydration, and characterized by high fever, muscle rigidity, delirium and marked autonomic instability. Muscle enzyme release, e.g. creatine kinase (CK; 'rhabdomyolysis'), which may cause acute renal failure, may occur. Supportive therapy, bromocriptine and dantrolene are all useful. Recurrence is common if major tranquillizers are reintroduced.
- **Malignant hyperthermia of anaesthesia**, with an incidence of 1:15 000 in children and 1:50 000 in adults, occurs in genetically predisposed individuals exposed to suxamethonium or halothane and relates to disordered sarcoplasmic reticulum calcium release. In attacks, cardiac arrhythmias and a rapidly rising core temperature with muscle rigidity develop quickly, leading to coma, profound metabolic acidosis and circulatory collapse. The mortality rate is 30%. Dantrolene, which decreases sarcoplasmic reticulum calcium release, is helpful. Susceptible individuals can be identified between attacks, in 'at-risk' families, by finding elevated CK enzyme levels. In some, the condition relates to an underlying myopathy.
- **Status epilepticus**.
- **Phaeochromocytoma** and **thyrotoxicosis**.
- **Drug abuse**: amphetamines, ecstasy, cocaine.
- **Heat stroke**: can occur in epidemics during hot spells, particularly in people with alcohol problems and people on major tranquillizers, or as a result of exercise when people are fluid deprived or unable to lose heat sufficiently quickly. Patients present with sudden-onset delirium, rapidly progressing to coma. Core temperature is >41°C; sweating may or may not be present. Extreme tachycardia and hyperventilation are common. Pulmonary oedema with shock and multiorgan failure occurs in advanced cases. The diagnosis is clinical, supported by finding elevated muscle enzymes. Treatment involves removing the patient from the hot environment and giving cool fluids, either sprayed on the skin to encourage heat loss or given intravenously. Shivering, which greatly increases heat production, if prominent should be suppressed with major tranquillizers. Specific organ support may be needed.
- **Local hypothalamic damage**: cerebrovascular accidents, head injury, encephalitis and hypothalamic surgery.

44 Fever and infections in hospital patients

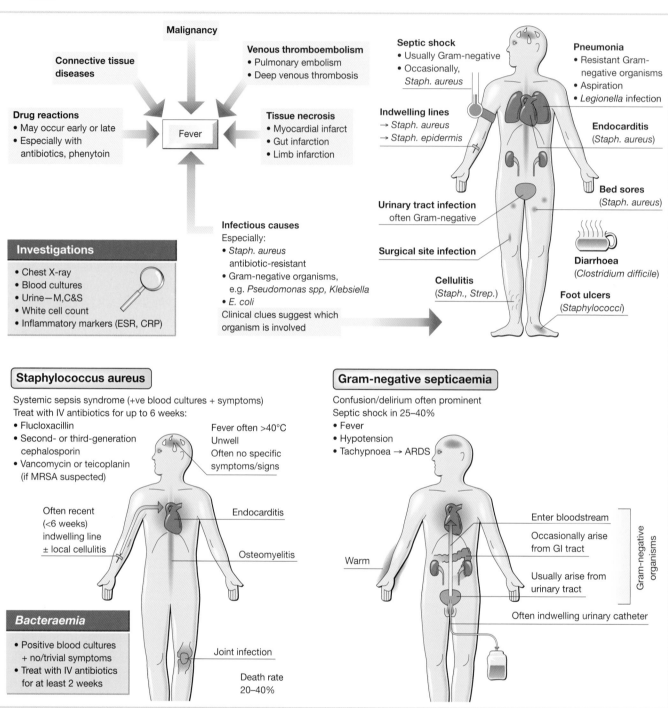

Malignancy

Connective tissue diseases

Venous thromboembolism
- Pulmonary embolism
- Deep venous thrombosis

Drug reactions
- May occur early or late
- Especially with antibiotics, phenytoin

Tissue necrosis
- Myocardial infarct
- Gut infarction
- Limb infarction

Fever

Septic shock
- Usually Gram-negative
- Occasionally, *Staph. aureus*

Pneumonia
- Resistant Gram-negative organisms
- Aspiration
- *Legionella* infection

Indwelling lines
→ *Staph. aureus*
→ *Staph. epidermis*

Endocarditis
(*Staph. aureus*)

Bed sores
(*Staph. aureus*)

Urinary tract infection
often Gram-negative

Surgical site infection

Diarrhoea
(*Clostridium difficile*)

Cellulitis
(*Staph., Strep.*)

Foot ulcers
(*Staphylococci*)

Investigations
- Chest X-ray
- Blood cultures
- Urine—M,C&S
- White cell count
- Inflammatory markers (ESR, CRP)

Infectious causes
Especially:
- *Staph. aureus* antibiotic-resistant
- Gram-negative organisms, e.g. *Pseudomonas spp, Klebsiella*
- *E. coli*

Clinical clues suggest which organism is involved

Staphylococcus aureus

Systemic sepsis syndrome (+ve blood cultures + symptoms)
Treat with IV antibiotics for up to 6 weeks:
- Flucloxacillin
- Second- or third-generation cephalosporin
- Vancomycin or teicoplanin (if MRSA suspected)

Fever often >40°C
Unwell
Often no specific symptoms/signs

Often recent (<6 weeks) indwelling line ± local cellulitis

Endocarditis

Osteomyelitis

Bacteraemia
- Positive blood cultures + no/trivial symptoms
- Treat with IV antibiotics for at least 2 weeks

Joint infection

Death rate 20–40%

Gram-negative septicaemia

Confusion/delirium often prominent
Septic shock in 25–40%
- Fever
- Hypotension
- Tachypnoea → ARDS

Warm

Enter bloodstream

Occasionally arise from GI tract

Usually arise from urinary tract

Gram-negative organisms

Often indwelling urinary catheter

Medicine at a Glance, Fourth Edition. Edited by Patrick Davey. © 2014 John Wiley & Sons, Ltd. Published 2014 by John Wiley & Sons, Ltd. Companion website: www.ataglanceseries.com/medicine

Definition and incidence

Nosocomial means hospital acquired. Hospital-acquired infections affect some 15% of inpatients. Important factors underlying this are:

- Inpatients have underlying conditions that may make their immune system relatively less effective.
- Treatment with antibiotics may select for certain organisms, particularly resistant Gram-negative organisms (e.g. *Pseudomonas* spp.) and *Candida* spp.
- Procedures and care in hospital interfere with the body's natural defences against infection, e.g. intravascular lines, endotracheal tubes.

Significant infection can occur in the absence of fever, particularly in elderly patients, or patients with renal or hepatic disease. Infection should be considered in any patient with changes in clinical state (pulse, blood pressure, mental state).

Nosocomial fever

This may be infectious or non-infectious in origin.

Common infectious causes

- Urinary tract or lower respiratory tract infections, primary and intravascular catheter-associated bacteraemia, sinusitis/middle ear disease in ventilated patients.
- Surgical wound or intra-abdominal sepsis (may not always present with obvious signs), pressure ulcers/skin infections.
- *Clostridium difficile* diarrhoea has a significant mortality and prolongs hospital stay by up to 20 days. Those most commonly affected are:
  - The infirm or very elderly patients (85+ years).
  - Those treated with broad-spectrum antibiotics, particularly cephalosporins.
  - Patients taking proton pump inhibitors.

Diagnosis is by finding *C. difficile* toxin in the stool. Treatment is fluids, oral vancomycin and/or metronidazole and dietary support; 10–20% relapse after treatment.
  - Norovirus and similar viral infections have symptoms that aid transmission, such as vomiting, diarrhoea and cough. Treatment is supportive but effective case recognition and isolation is important to protect other vulnerable patients in health-care settings.

Common non-infectious causes

- Drug fever.
- Venous thromboembolism (deep venous thrombosis or pulmonary embolism), resolving haematoma.
- Myocardial infarction and infarction of other tissue (particularly intestinal).
- Trauma or surgery.

Clinical assessment

- Assessment of immune status.
- History of recent surgical or invasive procedures.
- Examination of lines and catheters.
- Check on new medications and antibiotic therapy.
- Crucial investigations: white cell count, chest X-ray, urinalysis, urine and blood cultures. Other tests are determined by clinical findings. If diarrhoea is present, *C. difficile* toxin should be assayed.

Specific nosocomial infections

Two groups of pathogens are particularly common causes of nosocomial infections (Table 44.1):

Table 44.1 Common organisms causing nosocomial fever.

Gram-positive cocci (60–70%)	Gram-negative rods	Fungi (less common)
Coagulase-negative staphylococci	*Escherichia coli*	*Candida* spp.
Viridans streptococci	*Klebsiella pneumoniae*	*Aspergillus* spp.
Staphylococcus aureus	*Pseudomonas aeruginosa*	

- *Staphylococcus aureus*: often related to indwelling lines. Patients are usually acutely unwell with high fevers and rigors. The mortality rate is 20–30%. Proven staphylococcal bacteraemia requires prolonged (2–6 weeks) intravenous (IV) antibiotic therapy to prevent metastatic infection, especially acute bacterial endocarditis and bone/joint infections, or pulmonary, cerebral and paraspinal abscesses. Persisting blood culture positivity despite appropriate antibiotic therapy may indicate endocarditis, tissue abscesses or an infected device (pacemaker, line, etc.). Methicillin-resistant *S. aureus* (MRSA) infection is an increasingly common hospital-acquired pathogen. It is no more virulent than sensitive strains of *S. aureus*, but invasive infections require treatment with vancomycin or teicoplanin. Asymptomatic skin colonization can be treated using topical antibiotics.
- Gram-negative organisms, particularly *Escherichia coli*, *Pseudomonas* and *Klebsiella* species. These usually arise from the urinary or gastrointestinal (GI) tracts. Around 25–40% of Gram-negative bacteraemias are associated with shock, with a mortality rate of 25%. In addition to fever, chills and hypotension, the earliest sign is often tachypnoea and adult respiratory distress syndrome (ARDS) may develop (see Chapter 120). Mental signs (confusion, delirium) may be prominent. Therapy involves empirical antibiotics, supportive measures and identification, and drainage of any collection.

Bacteraemia and line-related infection

Bacteraemia may accompany infections such as urinary tract and pulmonary infections, but may occur with no obvious source. This is often associated with occult infection of intravascular catheters. Complications such as septic thrombophlebitis or endocarditis or metastatic infection may occur. It is important to determine:

- If blood culture isolates are true pathogens or skin flora. Repeated blood cultures may help; if cultures persistently grow one organism, it is very likely that this is a true infection.
- Whether an existing intravascular device is infected (inflammation at line site – or using line and peripheral blood cultures).

Short-term lines should be removed if they are thought to be infected. Precious semipermanent lines (dialysis or Hickmann's lines) can sometimes be treated with trials of antibiotics without removal.

Fever in the neutropenic patient

This is common after chemotherapy for haematological or other malignancies; it is classically defined as a temperature $\geq 38.3°C$ and ≥ 500 neutrophils/mm^3. Infection is only proven in 50–60% of patients. Drug- and transfusion-related fevers should be considered. The likelihood and seriousness of infection are increased by the duration and severity of neutropenia.

Special attention should be paid to the common sites of infection: skin, lungs, perioral and pharynx, and perianal area.

Signs of inflammation may be subtle; the absence of neutrophils means that the inflammatory response is blunted. Classic signs of infection (e.g. erythema and induration or an infiltrate on a chest X-ray) may not occur. Bacteraemia may occur in the absence of an obvious source.

Profound or prolonged neutropenia and fever unresponsive to broad-spectrum antibiotics for more than 1 week increase the likelihood of fungal infection.

Empirical antibiotic regimens are required in all febrile neutropenic patients as a result of the high mortality in this group. Monotherapy (meropenem) or dual therapy (aminoglycoside and antipseudomonal penicillin) is equally effective.

Vancomycin should be considered in the MRSA-colonized patient, if serious line-related sepsis is suspected, or if prophylaxis against Gram-negative organisms has been used (e.g. ciprofloxacin).

If there is no response, consider:

- Changing antibiotics (e.g. adding vancomycin).
- Further investigation for rarer causes of fever (herpes simplex virus, cytomegalovirus, Toxoplasma spp.).
- Adding antifungal therapy, particularly if no response by 5–7 days.
- Using drugs to increase white cell numbers such as growth colony-stimulating factor.

45 Fever of unknown origin

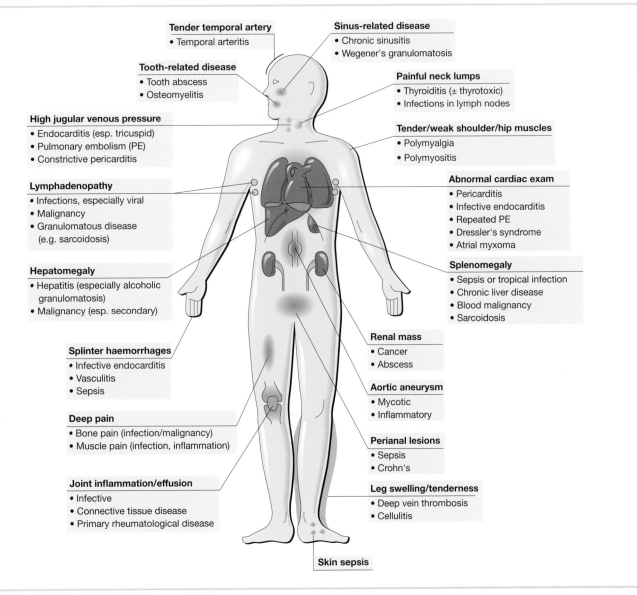

Tender temporal artery
• Temporal arteritis

Sinus-related disease
• Chronic sinusitis
• Wegener's granulomatosis

Tooth-related disease
• Tooth abscess
• Osteomyelitis

Painful neck lumps
• Thyroiditis (± thyrotoxic)
• Infections in lymph nodes

High jugular venous pressure
• Endocarditis (esp. tricuspid)
• Pulmonary embolism (PE)
• Constrictive pericarditis

Tender/weak shoulder/hip muscles
• Polymyalgia
• Polymyositis

Lymphadenopathy
• Infections, especially viral
• Malignancy
• Granulomatous disease
  (e.g. sarcoidosis)

Abnormal cardiac exam
• Pericarditis
• Infective endocarditis
• Repeated PE
• Dressler's syndrome
• Atrial myxoma

Hepatomegaly
• Hepatitis (especially alcoholic
  granulomatosis)
• Malignancy (esp. secondary)

Splenomegaly
• Sepsis or tropical infection
• Chronic liver disease
• Blood malignancy
• Sarcoidosis

Splinter haemorrhages
• Infective endocarditis
• Vasculitis
• Sepsis

Renal mass
• Cancer
• Abscess

Aortic aneurysm
• Mycotic
• Inflammatory

Deep pain
• Bone pain (infection/malignancy)
• Muscle pain (infection, inflammation)

Perianal lesions
• Sepsis
• Crohn's

Joint inflammation/effusion
• Infective
• Connective tissue disease
• Primary rheumatological disease

Leg swelling/tenderness
• Deep vein thrombosis
• Cellulitis

Skin sepsis

Medicine at a Glance, Fourth Edition. Edited by Patrick Davey. © 2014 John Wiley & Sons, Ltd. Published 2014 by John Wiley & Sons, Ltd. Companion website:
www.ataglanceseries.com/medicine

Most patients presenting with fever have a short-lived acute illness, which is rapidly diagnosed. Persisting fever in the face of initial negative investigations is termed 'fever (pyrexia) of unknown origin' (FUO). The classic definition of this is a fever of >38.3°C persisting without diagnosis for 3 weeks including 1 week's investigation in hospital. Most clinicians have modified this definition in the face of an increasing number of immuno-compromised hosts and more rapid diagnostic facilities. Practically, patients with unexplained fever can be divided into categories defined by their immune status:

- Classic FUO (community acquired).
- FUO in hospital patients (see Chapter 44).
- FUO in neutropenic and immunosuppressed patients (see Chapter 44).
- FUO in HIV patients (see Chapter 47).

Classic fever of unknown origin

This may be caused by many different processes (Table 45.1):

- Infections (25–50%).
- Neoplasms (10–30%).
- Connective tissue/collagen vascular diseases (10–25%).
- Miscellaneous (10–20%).
- Undiagnosed (10–25%).

The relative contribution of different categories depends on the geographical location and the age of the patient: infections are more important in the developing world; neoplasia and connective tissue disorders become more important with increasing age.

Infections

Many different infections are implicated in FUO, but consider:

- Systemic infections that are difficult to diagnose, e.g. disseminated mycobacterial disease or culture-negative endocarditis and brucellosis.
- Localized infections and abscesses where the normal inflammatory or immune response is not able to clear organisms, but the diagnosis is difficult because bacteraemia may not occur.

Table 45.1 The most common causes of FUO.

Infections
- Abscess
- Mycobacteria
- Endocarditis

Neoplasms
- Lymphoma
- Solid tumours (gastrointestinal tract, liver, renal cell, sarcoma)
- Leukaemias
- Other haematological tumours

Connective tissue disease
- Temporal arteritis/polymyalgia rheumatica
- Polyarteritis nodosa
- Systemic lupus erythematosus
- Adult Still's disease

Neoplasms

The majority of neoplasms producing FUO are haematological: fever may precede the appearance of lymphadenopathy in lymphoma. In older patients, consider solid tumours, particularly occult gastrointestinal-related neoplasms, such as in the pancreas. In women ovarian cancer should be excluded.

Connective tissue diseases

Adult Still's disease, the commonest cause, is essentially a diagnosis of exclusion. It typically causes myalgia, lymphadenopathy and splenomegaly in addition to fever. In elderly patients, temporal arteritis/polymyalgia rheumatica is common, accounting for up to 20% of FUO presentations, but classic temporal artery tenderness and an extremely high erythrocyte sedimentation rate (ESR) do not always occur. If other investigations have not been productive, a temporal artery ultrasound or temporal artery biopsy should be considered.

Miscellaneous

- Drug fever: can occur with many drugs, particularly antibiotics and anticonvulsants. Eosinophilia and a rash may help in the diagnosis.
- Pulmonary embolism (PE): occasionally, repeated PEs cause fever. Breathlessness with a clear chest X-ray should raise the possibility, which can be pursued with a spiral computed tomography (CT) scan, $\dot{V}/\dot{Q}$ (ventilation/perfusion) scan, etc. The lactate dehydrogenase is often raised in this situation.
- Granulomatous disease of the liver, in the absence of an obvious cause, is not uncommon. It may be steroid responsive. Abnormal liver function tests may reflect a hepatological process, but unfortunately may also be a non-specific response to systemic disease, particularly sepsis.
- Factitious fever: psychiatric disorder, often in women and in paramedical professions.
- Habitual hyperthermia: the hypothalamic set point may be high – exaggerated diurnal variations in temperature may occur. This is of no pathological significance.
- Rare genetic syndromes including familial Mediterranean fever. A family history may give clues, as may chronicity with complete recovery between episodes.

Approach to diagnosis

A comprehensive history and examination are crucial. Establish whether a fever is truly present (a significant proportion of patients have no documented fever at all). The fever pattern may occasionally help. Look for signs accompanying the fever (flushing, sweats, tachycardia, etc.). Determine whether the patient is unwell and whether stable or deteriorating. Stop all non-essential drugs.

Investigations

Use localizing symptoms and signs to target investigations.

Routine

Basic screening tests as previously described (see Chapter 42). High ESR and/or C-reactive protein (CRP) suggests a major systemic disease or infection. Normal ESR makes significant infection or collagen vascular disease unlikely. Immunoglobulins and autoantibody screen (antineutrophil cytoplasmic antibody, antinuclear antibody, rheumatoid factor, complement) may be useful. An abdominal/pelvic CT scan may be helpful, even in the absence of localizing features and should be considered early in the diagnostic process. It may demonstrate abscesses, nodes or malignancy.

Specific

Investigations should ideally focus on abnormalities. Consider:

- Echocardiography.
- Extended blood cultures: brucellosis or fastidious organisms.
- Tissue biopsy: should be aggressively pursued, especially if any organ-specific abnormality is identified. Liver, skin, temporal artery lymph node and bone marrow biopsy can all be helpful.
- 'Blind' CT of the abdomen may be helpful to demonstrate sources such as renal, diverticular or pelvic abscesses.
- Laparotomy is rarely indicated.

Diagnostic trials of therapy

In 5–15% of patients, no cause is found despite extensive investigation. Undiagnosed patients who remain well (no weight loss, stable albumin levels) can be observed. The outcome in this group is extremely good; fever will often spontaneously remit.

A trial of therapy may be indicated in sick or deteriorating patients:

- **Antibiotics**: blind broad-spectrum antibiotics may be indicated if the patient is unwell or conditions such as culture-negative endocarditis are suspected. A trial of anti-tuberculosis (anti-TB) therapy can be justified if the clinical suspicion is high because TB culture confirmation may take several weeks. Defervescence and an increase in weight are good signs of response to anti-TB therapy. Some anti-TB drugs have broad-spectrum antibacterial activity.
- **Corticosteroids**: these are very occasionally helpful, particularly in elderly patients with a possible temporal arteritis/polymyalgia rheumatica syndrome, or in young patients with adult Still's disease. Obvious infection and malignancy must be excluded and the fever and ESR/CRP response followed. An initial response does not always prove a non-infectious aetiology; steroid therapy will blunt fevers caused by some infections and may improve systemic symptoms resulting from malignancy. Therefore, steroids should never be given until repeated blood cultures have come back as negative, likely infections (especially TB) have been excluded, and abdominal CT has ruled out malignancy and intra-abdominal or pelvic sepsis.

46 Fever and rash

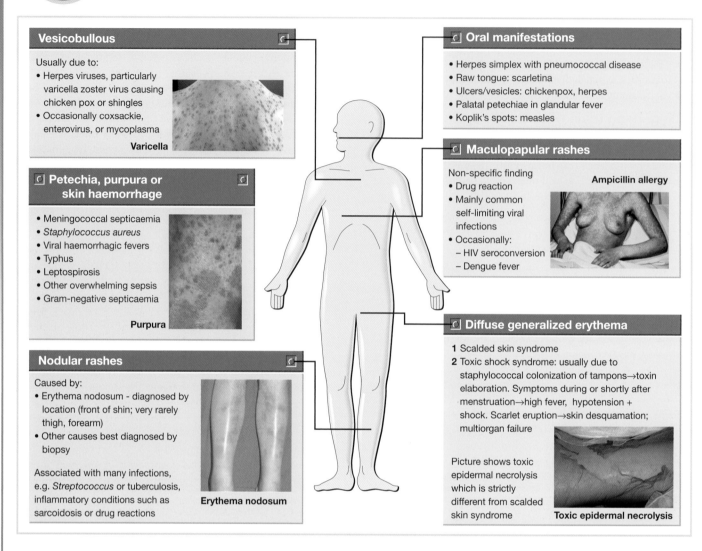

Vesicobullous

Usually due to:
- Herpes viruses, particularly varicella zoster virus causing chicken pox or shingles
- Occasionally coxsackie, enterovirus, or mycoplasma

Varicella

Petechia, purpura or skin haemorrhage

- Meningococcal septicaemia
- *Staphylococcus aureus*
- Viral haemorrhagic fevers
- Typhus
- Leptospirosis
- Other overwhelming sepsis
- Gram-negative septicaemia

Purpura

Nodular rashes

Caused by:
- Erythema nodosum - diagnosed by location (front of shin; very rarely thigh, forearm)
- Other causes best diagnosed by biopsy

Associated with many infections, e.g. *Streptococcus* or tuberculosis, inflammatory conditions such as sarcoidosis or drug reactions

Erythema nodosum

Oral manifestations

- Herpes simplex with pneumococcal disease
- Raw tongue: scarletina
- Ulcers/vesicles: chickenpox, herpes
- Palatal petechiae in glandular fever
- Koplik's spots: measles

Maculopapular rashes

Non-specific finding
- Drug reaction
- Mainly common self-limiting viral infections
- Occasionally:
  – HIV seroconversion
  – Dengue fever

Ampicillin allergy

Diffuse generalized erythema

1 Scalded skin syndrome
2 Toxic shock syndrome: usually due to staphylococcal colonization of tampons→toxin elaboration. Symptoms during or shortly after menstruation→high fever, hypotension + shock. Scarlet eruption→skin desquamation; multiorgan failure

Picture shows toxic epidermal necrolysis which is strictly different from scalded skin syndrome

Toxic epidermal necrolysis

Patients with fever and a rash are challenging; it is vital to identify those with acute bacterial sepsis who require prompt antimicrobial therapy. Although fever and a rash are most commonly caused by an infection, other processes produce similar clinical syndromes:

- Drug reactions.
- Vasculitis (see Chapter 220).

Some rashes are instantly recognizable; others require a systematic approach for diagnosis. Atypical features of a common disease (e.g. appearance modified by an impaired host immune system) are more likely than rare diseases. Factors that are helpful in diagnosis include:

- Time relationship of fever to rash.
- Drug history.
- The presence of: mucosal lesions or conjunctivitis, lymphadenopathy or hepatosplenomegaly, arthropathy.

In addition to standard investigations and blood cultures, the following may be helpful:

- Aspiration of lesions allows Gram smear and culture of organisms in meningococcal, staphylococcal, pseudomonal or systemic fungal infections.

- Punch biopsy may reveal organisms, particularly in fungal infections, or demonstrate specific histological features.
- Polymerase chain reaction (PCR) of body fluids for identification of viruses, including:
  - Vesicle fluid: herpes simplex and zoster infection.
  - Blood: acute viraemias including viral haemorrhagic fevers.
  - Urine: measles.
  - Stool: enterovirus.

Diffuse erythema

Diffuse erythema is the term given to a widespread reddening of the skin. Scarlet fever, caused by a group A streptococci, used to be a common cause of a diffuse blanching erythema. Drug eruptions are currently an important cause of fever with diffuse erythema. Important infective causes that should be excluded include:

- **Toxic shock syndrome**, caused by *Staphylococcus* or *Streptococcus* spp., produces generalized erythema, and later desquamation with multiorgan involvement.
- **Scalded skin syndrome** in children, from staphylococcal toxin, produces diffuse erythema, bulla formation and exfoliation.

Vesiculo-bullous rashes

Vesicles are small fluid-filled blisters, whereas bullae are larger fluid-filled blisters. Varicella-zoster infection has two manifestations with vesiculo-bullous rashes:

- **Varicella** (chickenpox): vesicles produced on a halo of erythema, initially clear and then cloudy. There is successive cropping.
- **Zoster** (shingles): a dermatomal distribution is found, initially maculopapular, then vesicles, bullae and crusting. The rash may be preceded by pain in the same area. Lesions outside the affected dermatome occur in 5% of the immunocompetent and in the immunocompromised.

Rarer causes of vesiculo-bullous rashes are:

- **Disseminated herpes simplex**: may occur from labial/genital lesions with considerable systemic upset in those with eczema or those who are immunocompromised.
- **Hand–foot–mouth** (Coxsackie virus or enteroviruses): small vesicles in the mouth, and on the hands and feet.
- **Bullous erythema multiforma**: classically *Mycoplasma* and herpes simplex infections; many other agents implicated.
- **Staphylococcal infections**: bullous impetigo.

Petechial–purpuric rashes

Bleeding into the skin has a number of terms – petechiae are small bleeds into the skin, <1–2 mm in diameter, whereas purpura describes larger areas of bleeding into the skin (>2 mm in diameter). Skin bleeds larger than about 4 mm are termed ecchymoses. The key purpuric rash to diagnose in acutely sick patients is **meningococcaemia**, which produces a spectrum of rashes from isolated petechiae to multiple purpuric lesions, confluent over the body, associated with complete haemostatic failure and a very high mortality. **Gonococcaemia** typically produces pustular lesions and arthritis, and more rarely mild purpuric rashes; haemostatic failure is unusual and mortality is very low. Other causes of petechial-purpuric rashes include:

- **Staphylococcal endocarditis**: petechiae and purpura may occur, usually immune complex mediated – a 'vasculitic rash'.
- **Disseminated intravascular coagulation** occurs in many severe infections – an important diagnostic clue is spontaneous haemorrhage from old venepuncture sites.
- **Leptospirosis**: conjunctival haemorrhage is common but skin haemorrhage only occasionally develops in those patients who are very unwell.
- **Viral haemorrhagic fevers**: haemorrhages may occur in Lassa, Ebola and Marburg and yellow fever; these patients are very unwell, often jaundiced and very likely to die.
- Petechiae are common in severe dengue infection (**dengue haemorrhagic fever**).

Maculopapular rashes

Macular rashes can be seen, but cannot be felt, i.e. they do not cause any bumps on the skin. The individual spots are usually small – often only a few millimetres in diameter. Papular rashes can be seen and felt, i.e. there are spots a few millimetres in diameter, which cause raised lumps on the skin surface. These rashes are extremely common, and can be produced by many pathogens.

Viral infections

These are the most common cause. Although **rubella** (German measles) and **measles** both produce rashes starting on the face, spreading to the trunk, they differ in that, in rubella, the rash is of discrete pink macules, whereas in measles it is maculopapular with lesions (Koplik's spots) in the mouth. Other common childhood viral rashes are the result of **enteroviruses** (diarrhoea and a rash) and **parvovirus** ('slapped cheeks' syndrome). Rarer causes include:

- **Acute human immunodeficiency virus (HIV) infection**: macules, papules or urticaria.
- **Dengue** (uncomplicated): classically, a transitory rash followed by generalized maculopapular rash in the second febrile phase.

Rickettsial infections

Maculopapular rashes occur in most rickettsial infections, and an eschar (focal necrosis at the site of the antecedent tick bite) is present in infection by some species.

Mycoplasma and chlamydial infections

These infections may cause maculopapular rashes.

Bacterial infections/spirochaetal

- **Secondary syphilis**: macules that may become papular or pustular. There are erosions on the oral mucosa and condylomata lata in intertriginous areas.
- **Leptospirosis**: macules, papules or petechiae occur.
- **Meningococcaemia**: initial lesions may be macules before classic petechiae/purpura.

Nodular lesions

Nodular lesions are seen and can be very easily felt – they differ from papules in that they are larger (and often far fewer in number). The most common nodular lesion is erythema nodosum (EN), an inflammation of small blood vessels in the deep dermis (a panniculitis), usually on the anterior aspect of the lower leg. EN is often preceded or accompanied by systemic upset (fever and malaise) and sometimes with arthralgia. Lesions never scar and normally heal within 2–3 weeks – much longer and other diagnoses should be sought. Common causes for EN in the UK are: streptococcal infections, sarcoidosis, inflammatory bowel disease. Worldwide causes commonly include tuberculosis (TB) and leprosy and, rarely, *Yersinia* spp., hepatitis C, *Histoplasma* and *Coccidioides* spp.

Other nodular rashes are caused by:

- **Disseminated fungal infections**, usually in immunocompromised individuals, most commonly with *Candida*, *Histoplasma* or *Cryptococcus* spp.
- **Mycobacterial disease**: nodular rashes occur occasionally in disseminated TB or atypical mycobacteria.

Other rashes/lesions of importance

- **Typhoid** characteristically results in rose spots (pink papules on the abdomen).
- **Lyme disease** produces a diagnostic lesion (erythema chronicum migrans); the initial macule develops into large, flat, ring-like lesions.
- *Pseudomonas aeruginosa* can cause ecthyma gangrenosum (erythema surrounded by haemorrhages and necrosis) in neutropenic patients.
  - **Necrotizing fasciitis**: mild/minimal skin inflammation with pain out of keeping with the clinical signs or rapidly developing skin inflammation should make one consider this diagnosis; it needs urgent management.

Unusual rashes in tropical disease

- **Cutaneous larva migrans**: caused by larvae of the dog or cat hookworm migrating through the skin, resulting in raised, scaly, erythematous serpiginous lesions in skin that is in contact with ground or sand.
- **Calabar swellings**: transient, non-erythematous, pruritic, subcutaneous swellings found in loiasis.
- **Onchocerciasis**: nodules and pruritic papules or urticaria.
- **Strongyloides infection**: urticaria and 'larva currens' (evanescent urticarial wheals).

47 Fever in HIV-infected patients

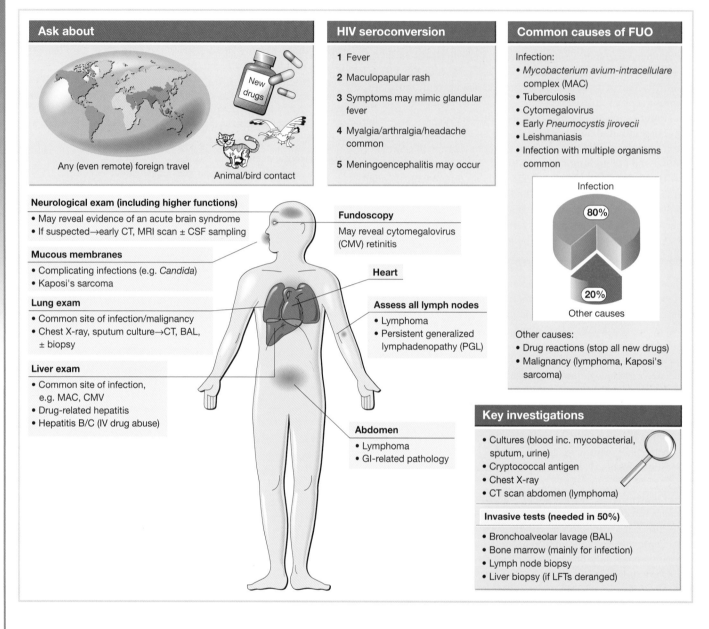

Ask about

Any (even remote) foreign travel

New drugs

Animal/bird contact

Neurological exam (including higher functions)
- May reveal evidence of an acute brain syndrome
- If suspected→early CT, MRI scan ± CSF sampling

Mucous membranes
- Complicating infections (e.g. Candida)
- Kaposi's sarcoma

Lung exam
- Common site of infection/malignancy
- Chest X-ray, sputum culture→CT, BAL, ± biopsy

Liver exam
- Common site of infection, e.g. MAC, CMV
- Drug-related hepatitis
- Hepatitis B/C (IV drug abuse)

Fundoscopy
May reveal cytomegalovirus (CMV) retinitis

Heart

Assess all lymph nodes
- Lymphoma
- Persistent generalized lymphadenopathy (PGL)

Abdomen
- Lymphoma
- GI-related pathology

HIV seroconversion

1 Fever
2 Maculopapular rash
3 Symptoms may mimic glandular fever
4 Myalgia/arthralgia/headache common
5 Meningoencephalitis may occur

Common causes of FUO

Infection:
- *Mycobacterium avium-intracellulare* complex (MAC)
- Tuberculosis
- Cytomegalovirus
- Early *Pneumocystis jirovecii*
- Leishmaniasis
- Infection with multiple organisms common

Infection
80%

20%
Other causes

Other causes:
- Drug reactions (stop all new drugs)
- Malignancy (lymphoma, Kaposi's sarcoma)

Key investigations

- Cultures (blood inc. mycobacterial, sputum, urine)
- Cryptococcal antigen
- Chest X-ray
- CT scan abdomen (lymphoma)

Invasive tests (needed in 50%)

- Bronchoalveolar lavage (BAL)
- Bone marrow (mainly for infection)
- Lymph node biopsy
- Liver biopsy (if LFTs deranged)

Fever is common in human immunodeficiency virus (HIV) infections:

- **Early HIV infection**: fever is a common feature of an acute HIV seroconversion reaction. Appropriate testing should be considered in patients who present with a fever and have risk factors for HIV infection.
- **Fever in established HIV infection**: fever occurs frequently in all patients with reduced CD4 counts: up to half of patients will present with fever at some point. The source of fever is often obvious on initial investigation and is most commonly the result of either standard or opportunistic infections associated with HIV infection, e.g. bacterial pneumonia or *Pneumocystis jirovecii* pneumonia (previously called *Pneumocystis carinii* and still

abbreviated to PCP). However, fever may be difficult to diagnose, particularly in late disease.

Fever of unknown origin (FUO) in HIV-infected patients has been defined as fever >38.3°C lasting more than 4 days in hospital or 4 weeks in outpatients without diagnosis. This usually reflects:

- Systemic infection with few localizing signs or symptoms, e.g. *Mycobacterium avium-intracellulare* complex (MAC) infection.
- Initial stages of an infective process before organ-related signs, e.g. *Pneumocystis jirovecii*, leishmaniasis or cytomegalovirus (CMV) infection.
- A drug reaction: common because of the increased predisposition to drug reactions in HIV and the polypharmacy often associated with the disease.

Medicine at a Glance, Fourth Edition. Edited by Patrick Davey. © 2014 John Wiley & Sons, Ltd. Published 2014 by John Wiley & Sons, Ltd. Companion website: www.ataglanceseries.com/medicine

Table 47.1 Most common infections causing FUO in advanced HIV infection.

- *Mycobacterium avium-intracellulare* complex (MAC)
- *Mycobacterium tuberculosis*
- *Pneumocystis jirovecii* infection (PCP)
- Cytomegalovirus (CMV)
- Leishmaniasis
- HIV infection itself (debated by some)

- Malignancy, most commonly lymphoma, occasionally Kaposi's sarcoma.

In contrast to FUO in other hosts, over 80% of patients will have an infection (see Table 47.1) and up to 20% will have more than one cause for their fever.

History

It is important to assess the stage of HIV infection and degree of immunosuppression, normally measured by the CD4 T-cell count. In earlier stages of HIV with higher CD4 counts (>500 cells/mm^3), infections are usually caused by common organisms and are more easily diagnosed. The profound immunosuppression of advanced HIV disease (CD4 cell counts <100 cells/mm^3) means that fever may be caused by unusual organisms or recrudescence of a previously latent infection. A history of potential exposure to such organisms is crucial. Close note should also be taken of:

- Ethnic origin: affects risk of infections such as tuberculosis (TB) or histoplasmosis.
- Travel abroad, even if in the distant past: Mediterranean travel is associated with risks of visceral leishmaniasis; more exotic infection such as with *Penicillium marneffei* may occur in those who have spent time in the Far East.
- Contact with animals or birds.
- Prophylactic regimens with co-trimoxazole reduce the chance of, but do not exclude, the diagnosis of conditions such as PCP or toxoplasmosis.
- Pre-existing serology for *Toxoplasma* spp. and CMV.
- Recent commencement of anti-retroviral drugs. Immune reconstitution inflammatory syndromes (IRIS) occur as the immune system improves and an inflammatory response occurs to a previously treated or subclinical infection. IRIS most commonly occurs as the CD4 count starts to rise in the first weeks/months after beginning anti-retroviral treatment.

Examination

This should include particularly:

- Skin and mucosal membranes.
- Lungs.
- Examination of the dilated fundi for evidence of CMV retinitis.
- Examination of the lymph nodes.
- Assessment of hepatomegaly or splenomegaly.

Few clinical or biochemical findings are specific for a particular disease process, e.g. abnormal liver function may be found in drug reactions, lymphoma or MAC, and lymph node enlargement may occur in MAC or lymphoma. However, abnormalities warrant further investigation.

Diagnosis

Discontinuing drugs, particularly ones started recently, and watching the fever response may be helpful. Routine cultures should be performed but several specific investigations may be helpful.

Non-invasive methods

- Chest X-ray (CXR).
- Urine, stool and regular blood cultures.
- Mycobacterial and fungal blood cultures: particularly looking for MAC; 60–80% sensitivity using modern techniques.
- Serum cryptococcal antigen.
- CMV viral load by polymerase chain reaction (PCR).
- Examination of induced sputum; diagnosis of PCP in asymptomatic patients, *Mycobacterium tuberculosis* and atypical mycobacteria and other respiratory pathogens.
- Computed tomography (CT) of the abdomen: may show retroperitoneal lymph nodes or masses.

Invasive methods

These are required in up to 50%:

- Bronchoscopy with bronchoalveolar lavage (BAL), in which small aliquots of saline are flushed in and out of the lung, collecting inflammatory cells and organisms from there. Organisms can be identified by culture or specific stains.
- Bone marrow examination: useful for MAC culture and diagnosis of intracellular organisms, e.g. *Histoplasma* spp., cryptococci, leishmaniasis and lymphoma.
- Lymph node biopsy of enlarged nodes: diagnosis of lymphoma or TB.
- Liver biopsy: if there is evidence of liver enzyme abnormality that persists after stopping drug therapy.
- Skin biopsies of unusual rashes should be cultured to exclude fungal diseases.
- Lumbar puncture should be considered if there is altered mentation or neurological function.

Management

Diagnosis is eventually made in about 80% of cases and appropriate therapy should be instituted. Failure of response should lead to searches for other causes because of the high prevalence of multiple conditions. Empirical therapy is sometimes necessary, particularly in very advanced HIV with <50 CD4 cells/mm^3 when MAC is common but cannot always be demonstrated.

48 Fever in the returned traveller

Key questions

- Duration/nature of symptoms
- Countries visited
- Duration of trip
- Lifestyle when abroad including sexual history
- Animal/insect contact
- Malaria prophylaxis used
- Vaccination history

Incubation periods

Short <7 days	Intermediate	Long >21 days
Dengue/other arboviruses	Malaria	Malaria
Enteric infections	Typhoid	Viral hepatitis
Legionella	Typhus	Acute schistosomiasis
Relapsing fever	Leptospirosis	HIV seroconversion
Plague	Brucellosis	Amoebic liver abscess
	African trypanosomiasis	Visceral leishmaniasis
	Haemorrhagic fevers	Brucellosis

Jaundice
- Hepatitis
- Malaria
- Leptospirosis
- Yellow fever

Vomiting
- GI pathogens
- Malaria

Chest signs
- Pneumococcus
- Legionella
- TB

Hepatomegaly
- Amoebic liver abscess (often tender)
- Hepatitis
- Typhoid
- Malaria
- Leptospirosis

Cognitive impairment/delirium
- Malaria
- Fulminant hepatic failure
- Viral encephalitis

Commonest diagnoses
- Malaria (30–50%)
- Hepatitis
- Dengue
- Typhoid
- Diarrhoeal illness
- Respiratory illness
- No cause found

Splenomegaly
- Malaria
- Typhoid
- Brucellosis
- Visceral leishmaniasis (usually extremely marked)
- Rickettsial diseases

Lymphadenopathy (common in many infections)
- Rickettsial infections
- HIV
- Plague (localized, tender)
- Brucellosis
- Filariasis
- Visceral leishmaniasis

?Diarrhoea
- GI pathogens

Key investigations
- Exclude malaria in all cases: 3 thick films
- Cultures (blood, urine, sputum, etc.)
- Microscopy (urine, stool)
- FBC, especially for eosinophils (filaria, schistosomiasis, liver flukes)
- Serology: store for later analysis
- Consider HIV test
- Think about risk of transmission to others

Skin lesions

Rose spots	Typhoid
Eschar	Tick and scrub typhus, anthrax
Petechiae/haemorrhage	Viral haemorrhagic fevers, leptospirosis
Maculopapular	Dengue, tick typhus, syphilis, arboviral infections, leptospirosis, HIV
Chancre	African trypanosomiasis

Medicine at a Glance, Fourth Edition. Edited by Patrick Davey. © 2014 John Wiley & Sons, Ltd. Published 2014 by John Wiley & Sons, Ltd. Companion website: www.ataglanceseries.com/medicine

Incidence

As foreign travel becomes more common, the number of patients presenting with fever following travel has increased considerably. Around 2–3% of travellers report fever during or after a visit to the tropics; 1% of patients have fever after visits to such areas as the Greek islands. Approximately two-thirds of these seek medical advice for fever that persists or first occurs after their return home.

Many of these fevers are not caused by exotic pathogens but reflect ordinary viral, urinary tract or respiratory infections, e.g. infectious mononucleosis (glandular fever, see Chapter 167) is a common final diagnosis in young travellers. However, significant tropical pathogens, particularly malaria, need to be excluded. It is also important to think of potential non-infectious causes, particularly in the elderly.

Most common imported infections

- Malaria (see Chapter 171).
- Hepatitis (see Chapter 132).
- Dengue (see Chapter 173).
- Typhoid (see Chapter 173).
- Diarrhoeal illness (see Chapter 25).

Up to a quarter of fevers settle spontaneously and are undiagnosed.

Diagnosis

Assessing the immune status of the traveller is important. Although most travellers are healthy, increasing numbers of elderly or immunocompromised people are travelling abroad. These individuals may be at particular risk of certain infections. In addition to the presenting symptoms, the history should focus on the time course of the illness, which can include or exclude certain infections on the basis of the incubation period, and on activity and behaviour that can determine potential exposure to pathogens.

Important questions

- Symptoms or illnesses while away.
- Geographical areas visited and length of time away. Names of countries alone are not adequate – the risk of a specific infection can vary considerably within a country (e.g. malaria risk is negligible in Nairobi but considerable on the Kenyan coast). Remember that some people travel extensively and history of exposure during previous (as well as most recent) trips is important.
- Kind of trip: business hotel, tourist, living with local people (incidence of tropical disease is much higher in those who have been travelling rough).
- Level of protection against bites by mosquito, ticks and flies. Full immunization history (appropriate vaccination reduces but does not exclude the chance of a specific infection). Malaria prophylaxis and adherence (need to judge whether choice of prophylaxis was appropriate for area visited).
- Food and water history (enteric infections, hepatitis, exotic parasites).
- Freshwater exposure (schistosomiasis, leptospirosis).
- Sexual activity (studies show a surprisingly high proportion of travellers indulge in risky sexual behaviour).
- Illness in fellow travellers (possible single source exposure) or contact with potentially infected individuals (particularly for health workers with potential exposure to haemorrhagic fevers).
- Animal contact (rabies, brucellosis, histoplasmosis – bats in caves). Subsequent health of animal is particularly important for assessing rabies risk.

Important features of examination

- Physical signs are often rather non-specific.
- Establishing fever and sometimes pattern (biphasic in dengue, tertian in untreated malaria).
- Presence of rash, mosquito bites or ticks. Searching for eschars (necrotic lesions at the site of previous tick bites) necessitates careful examination – they may often be found in skin crevices or under waistbands or straps of underwear.
- Jaundice.
- Hepatosplenomegaly and lymphadenopathy.

Important investigations (guided by symptoms)

- Routine screening tests including blood cultures, chest X-ray, urine dipstick and culture.
- Malaria slide (at least three thick films if malaria is possible). Rapid diagnostic tests are now used by some labs; they detect falciparum malaria but are not so good for other species.
- Consider HIV test and sexual screen if sexually active while away.
- Stool examination for ova, cysts and parasites, and culture.
- Look for eosinophilia (schistosomiasis, filariasis, liver flukes).
- Serology for dengue and other arboviruses, ricketsial diseases and brucellosis. Store serum for later serology if the diagnosis is uncertain.

Management

This depends on the underlying condition. Two major initial aims should be:

1 To exclude malaria: one of the commonest conditions and by far the most potentially dangerous.
2 To consider whether the disease may be transmissible to others, in particular the rare but highly infectious viral haemorrhagic fevers. Tuberculosis (TB) or norovirus are other examples.

Treatment of specific conditions is covered later in this book. Some conditions can be treated on clinical grounds alone; serological confirmation may take several weeks, e.g. the traveller from South Africa with an eschar, maculopapular rash and fever should be treated for African tick typhus. When considering empirical antibiotic therapy in the absence of culture confirmation, patterns of antibiotic resistance in the visited country must be considered – this is particularly important for diseases such as typhoid and TB.

49 Vaginal discharge and urethritis

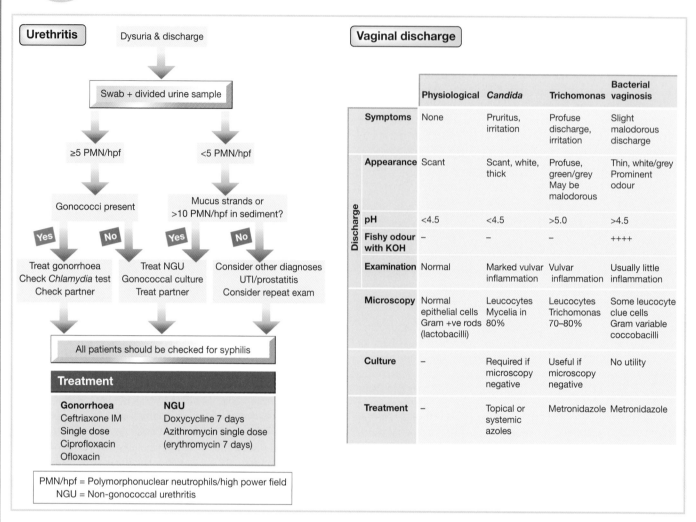

		Physiological	*Candida*	Trichomonas	Bacterial vaginosis
Symptoms		None	Pruritus, irritation	Profuse discharge, irritation	Slight malodorous discharge
Appearance		Scant	Scant, white, thick	Profuse, green/grey May be malodorous	Thin, white/grey Prominent odour
pH		<4.5	<4.5	>5.0	>4.5
Fishy odour with KOH		–	–	–	++++
Examination		Normal	Marked vulvar inflammation	Vulvar inflammation	Usually little inflammation
Microscopy		Normal epithelial cells Gram +ve rods (lactobacilli)	Leucocytes Mycelia in 80%	Leucocytes Trichomonas 70–80%	Some leucocyte clue cells Gram variable coccobacilli
Culture		–	Required if microscopy negative	Useful if microscopy negative	No utility
Treatment		–	Topical or systemic azoles	Metronidazole	Metronidazole

Urethritis — Dysuria & discharge

Swab + divided urine sample

≥5 PMN/hpf → Gonococci present
- Yes → Treat gonorrhoea Check *Chlamydia* test Check partner
- No → Treat NGU Gonococcal culture Treat partner

<5 PMN/hpf → Mucus strands or >10 PMN/hpf in sediment?
- Yes → Treat NGU Gonococcal culture Treat partner
- No → Consider other diagnoses UTI/prostatitis Consider repeat exam

All patients should be checked for syphilis

Treatment

Gonorrhoea
Ceftriaxone IM
Single dose
Ciprofloxacin
Ofloxacin

NGU
Doxycycline 7 days
Azithromycin single dose
(erythromycin 7 days)

PMN/hpf = Polymorphonuclear neutrophils/high power field
NGU = Non-gonococcal urethritis

Vaginal discharge

Vaginal discharge is one the most common symptoms that women present with to their general practitioner, and it accounts for over a quarter of referrals to sexually transmitted disease (STD) clinics. All women have a physiological discharge, which varies considerably between individuals. An abnormal vaginal discharge is most commonly caused by infections, but may also be the result of:

- Chemical and physical irritation (e.g. soaps, spermicides, minipads, etc.).
- Allergy and contact dermatitis.

  Other, much rarer, causes include:

- Cervical polyps and other neoplasms.
- Retained tampons.

Infectious causes

Three conditions account for the vast majority of infectious cases:

- Bacterial vaginosis (40–50%).
- *Candida* spp. (20–30%).
- *Trichomonas vaginalis* (15–20%).

Bacterial infection secondary to a foreign body or atrophic vaginitis may also occur and group A streptococci can cause vaginitis with severe systemic symptoms. The other main sexually transmitted pathogens in women, *Neisseria gonorrhoeae* and *Chlamydia* spp., do not usually cause a profuse vaginal discharge, but may occasionally cause an endocervical or urethral discharge which is noted by the patient.

Pathogenesis

Bacterial vaginosis is caused by an imbalance of the organisms of the normal vaginal flora. Lactobacilli are replaced by an overgrowth of mixed flora, including *Gardnerella* species and anaerobes, leading to clinical symptoms. It is associated with complications in pregnant women or those with other gynaecological disease.

Candida species are frequently found in the genital tract of asymptomatic women; the triggers for progression to clinical disease are not understood. Risk factors for *Candida* carriage and disease include pregnancy, diabetes, steroid therapy and antibiotic therapy.

Medicine at a Glance, Fourth Edition. Edited by Patrick Davey. © 2014 John Wiley & Sons, Ltd. Published 2014 by John Wiley & Sons, Ltd. Companion website: www.ataglanceseries.com/medicine

Trichomonas vaginalis, a flagellated protozoan, is usually acquired from sexual contact and causes epithelial cell damage leading to vaginal and vulval inflammation.

Clinical features

See Figure 49.1. The history and findings on speculum examination sometimes allow a clinical diagnosis, but samples should be taken for microscopy and culture.

Investigations

A wet mount preparation of vaginal secretions is the most useful investigation. This may demonstrate both organisms and polymorphonuclear cells. Culture is useful for *Candida* and *Trichomonas* infection. Bacterial vaginosis is diagnosed on the basis of three of the following four criteria:

1 Adherent white, non-floccular discharge.
2 Vaginal pH >4.5.
3 Fishy odours on addition of 10% potassium hydroxide (KOH) to secretions.
4 Presence of clue cells (vaginal squamous epithelium covered with *Gardnerella vaginalis*).

Management

Oral metronidazole is the drug of choice for both bacterial vaginosis and trichomoniasis: 1-week courses have cure rates of over 90% for both diseases. Partners of patients with trichomoniasis should also be treated. *Candida* spp. can be treated with topical antifungals (e.g. clotrimazole or miconazole) or oral therapy with azoles; good cure rates may be achieved by short courses.

Urethritis in men

Definition and aetiology

Urethritis is a clinical syndrome consisting of a urethral discharge and dysuria. It is the most common STD syndrome in men. Most cases are caused by infection, but chemical irritants, foreign bodies and some inflammatory conditions may cause similar symptoms. There are two main infectious syndromes in men:

- Gonococcal urethritis
- Non-gonococcal urethritis (NGU), caused predominantly by *Chlamydia trachomatis* but also by *Ureaplasma urealyticum* and *Mycoplasma genitalium*.

In the UK, NGU is far more common than gonorrhoea, rates for which have steadily declined over the last 30 years. Co-infection with *Neisseria gonorrhoeae* and agents of NGU occurs in approximately 10–30% of men.

Clinical features

Incubation period

- Short (2–7 days) in gonorrhoea.
- Up to several weeks in *Chlamydia* spp.

Urethral discharge

- Often copious, purulent, yellow or green in gonorrhoea.
- Smaller volume, mucopurulent in *Chlamydia* spp.

Dysuria

- Most marked in gonorrhoea.
- Frequency or urgency (symptoms of cystitis rather than urethritis) are *not* a feature.
- Lymphadenopathy does not occur in either disease.

May need to differentiate from upper urinary tract infection (UTI), other causes of prostatic disease and herpes simplex infection (external vesicles and enlargement of the local lymph nodes is common).

Complications

- Epididymitis (rarely prostatitis).
- Conjunctivitis.
- Reiter's syndrome in NGU (urethritis, uveitis, arthritis).
- Rarely disseminated gonococcal infection (skin lesions, joint swelling).

Examination and diagnosis

Patients should not pass urine for at least 2 hours before examination. Quantity and colour of discharge should be noted. 'Stripping' the urethra by running the thumb along the urethra up to the meatus can often produce discharge. Examine lymph nodes; large or tender nodes make the diagnosis unlikely. Examine epididymis for tenderness or enlargement.

Investigations

A small swab should be passed into the urethra and rolled onto a slide. Gram staining of the slide should be performed to look for polymorphs and Gram-negative intracellular diplococci (*N. gonorrhoeae*). Swabs should be plated out on to a gonococcal culture medium *at the bedside*. Swabs should also be taken for *Chlamydia* detection by DNA amplification techniques, which are now replacing immunoassays for the diagnosis of *Chlamydia*.

Divided urine samples are also useful. The first and second 10 mL aliquots voided after examination should be saved. Mucus threads in the first aliquot suggest urethritis. The sediment after centrifugation of both samples can be examined for cells. The first urine sample should also be examined using DNA amplification.

Management

See Figure 49.1.

Urethritis in women

Urethritis may occur in women, caused by *N. gonorrhoeae* or *C. trachomatis* but the cervicitis is often more marked and a high proportion of both infections are asymptomatic in women. Diagnosis of *Chlamydia* infection, even if asymptomatic, is important because of its association with subsequent infertility. Gonorrhea can be diagnosed by Gram staining and culture of urethral and endocervical swabs; swabs and urine should be send for DNA amplification to detect *Chlamydia* infection.

Management

See Figure 49.1.

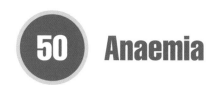

50 Anaemia

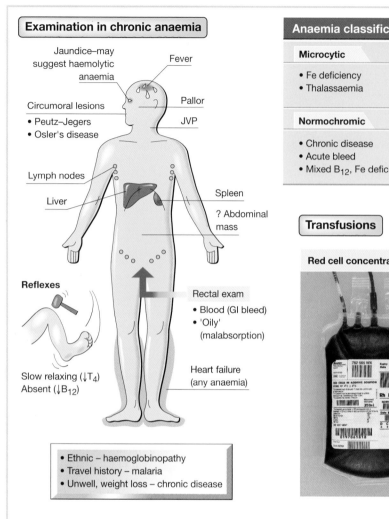

Examination in chronic anaemia

Jaundice–may suggest haemolytic anaemia

Fever

Pallor

JVP

Circumoral lesions
• Peutz–Jegers
• Osler's disease

Lymph nodes

Liver

Spleen

? Abdominal mass

Reflexes

Rectal exam
• Blood (GI bleed)
• 'Oily' (malabsorption)

Heart failure (any anaemia)

Slow relaxing ($\downarrow$T$_4$)
Absent ($\downarrow$B$_{12}$)

• Ethnic – haemoglobinopathy
• Travel history – malaria
• Unwell, weight loss – chronic disease

Anaemia classification

Microcytic
• Fe deficiency
• Thalassaemia

MCV <80 fL

Normochromic
• Chronic disease
• Acute bleed
• Mixed B$_{12}$, Fe deficiency

MCV 80–95 fL

Macrocytic
• Folate/B$_{12}$ deficiency
• Low T$_4$
• Haemolytic anaemias
• Myelodysplasia

Red cell

MCV > 100 fL

Transfusions

Red cell concentrate

Side effects

Acute
• Anaphylaxis
• Mild febrile reactions
• Heart failure
• Infection (e.g. HIV, cytomegalovirus)

In massive transfusions
• Haemostatic failure (Ca^{2+} chelator, lack of clotting factors)
• Electrolyte disturbance (e.g. $\uparrow$Ca^{2+}, $\uparrow$K$^+$)

In multiple transfusions

Fe overload
Sensitization to platelet, WCC antigens $\rightarrow$$\downarrow$ platelet life, transfusion reactions

---

Anaemia is present when the haemoglobin is more than two standard deviations below the mean haemoglobin for that individual. The mean haemoglobin varies with sex and age.

Symptoms

Symptoms depend on the underlying pathology as well as the severity and speed of onset of the anaemia. Mild anaemia often causes no symptoms. Insidious-onset anaemia, even if profound, likewise may cause few symptoms. In more severe or rapid-onset anaemia, the following may occur:

• Fatigue.
• Peripheral oedema, e.g. swollen feet.
• Breathlessness: particularly if heart or lung disease is present. Anaemia is one cause of decompensation in chronic heart failure.
• Angina, if there is underlying coronary disease, which may have been undetected before the anaemia.

Signs

The physical examination in anaemia is usually unremarkable.

• Pallor (palms of the hands, conjunctiva) may occur, although this is an unreliable sign because many pale people are not anaemic, and many anaemic people are not pale.
• A systolic 'flow' murmur is common.

• There may be evidence of the underlying pathology.
• In long-standing iron deficiency anaemia, koilonychia (spoon-shaped nails) may occur.

Classification

Anaemia is a physiological abnormality, not a diagnosis. A final, pathological diagnosis must always be made. The first step in doing this usually involves classifying the anaemia according to red cell size.

• **Microcytic/hypochromic anaemia**: the red cells are smaller than normal (microcytic) and contain less haemoglobin than normal (hypochromic). Common causes are iron deficiency anaemia and thalassaemia trait.
• **Normochromic and normocytic anaemia**: sometimes referred to as the 'anaemia of chronic disease'. The red cells are of normal or just slightly reduced size and have a normal haemoglobin concentration. Common causes include:
  • Chronic infections, e.g. tuberculosis (TB) and osteomyelitis.
  • Inflammatory diseases such as rheumatoid arthritis and connective tissue disorders.
  • Malignant disease.
  • Renal failure.

The anaemia of chronic disease is multifactorial. Erythropoietin deficiency is common in renal impairment. Chronic inflammation leads to an increase in hepcidin levels which reduces absorption of iron from the gut and locks it away in the reticuloendothelial system. Iron deficiency also often complicates chronic diseases and may explain a lower than expected haemoglobin.

- **Macrocytic anaemia**: the red cells are larger than normal. Common causes include:
  - Vitamin B_{12} or folate deficiency.
  - Cytotoxic drug treatment, e.g. azathioprine or cyclophosphamide.
  - Myelodysplasia (see Chapter 185).
  - Haemolytic anaemias.
  - Hypothyroidism: can cause either a normocytic or a macrocytic anaemia.
  - Liver disease and alcohol abuse result in a macrocytosis, but not anaemia, unless there is coincidental bleeding or haematinic deficiency.

Investigations

The clinical features and the morphological characteristics of the red cells drive investigations on the blood film (see diagram of red cell morphology, Chapter 186). The following tests are frequently helpful:

- **Haematinic status** (iron stores, vitamin B_{12} and folate – see Chapter 186): iron status should be evaluated in micro- or normocytic anaemias, and vitamin B_{12}/folate status in macrocytic anaemias. *Beware*: haematinic deficiency is common even when another cause for anaemia is clear (e.g. folate deficiency in haemolytic anaemia, iron deficiency in colon cancer, etc.). Once haematinic deficiency is found, the specific cause (malnutrition, malabsorption, excess use or loss, etc.) should always be determined.
- **Blood film**: often diagnostic in primary haematological disease as well as in many systemic diseases. It is therefore mandatory in all anaemias that have not been diagnosed by more simple investigations. Person-to-person discussion with the haematologist often speeds up the diagnostic process.
- **Blood count**: a blood count for white cells or platelets often helps. A **raised neutrophil count** is common and causes include:
  - Bacterial infection.
  - Underlying chronic inflammatory disease.
  - Myeloproliferative process (leukaemia, etc.) when mature (chronic leukaemias) or immature (acute leukaemias) white cells are found.

A **low white count** is commonly seen in patients with acute infections as well as in primary bone marrow diseases such as myelodysplasia. A **high platelet count** may be reactive to:

- Infection, particularly abscesses.
- Chronic inflammatory disorders such as rheumatoid arthritis.
- Malignancy.
- Bleeding.
- Post splenectomy.
- Or may be a feature of a primary bone marrow disorder such as a myeloproliferative disease.

A **low platelet count** is found in patients with excess consumption of platelets (e.g. idiopathic thrombocytopenic purpura or disseminated intravascular coagulation) or in diseases where bone marrow production of platelets is impaired (e.g. acute leukaemia, myelodysplasia).

- **Other investigations** important in some patients with anaemia are:
  - Bone marrow examination: this is often helpful and should be discussed with a haematologist.
  - Renal and liver biochemistry diagnose underlying organ-specific disease.
  - Markers of inflammation (erythrocyte sedimentation rate or C-reactive protein) are often raised in anaemia of chronic disease, e.g. disseminated malignancy, sepsis or vasculitis.
  - Thyroid status: hypothyroidism can cause a macrocytic or normocytic anaemia.
  - Blood cultures are useful if sepsis is suspected.

Treatment

Treatment is of the underlying disease. In patients with the anaemia of chronic disease, blood transfusion or treatment with recombinant erythropoietin may be of help. There is increasing evidence that intravenous iron may also be beneficial.

Blood transfusion

Donor and recipients need to be blood group 'matched' for successful transfusion.

- **The ABO system**: the A and B genes encode enzymes transforming a cell membrane glycoprotein (substance H) into either A or B antigens. Individuals possess either two A or two B genes (AA or BB), one of each (AB), either A or B (AO, BO) or neither (O), and IgM antibodies to the antigen that they do not possess (i.e. anti-B if AA or AO, and anti-A if BB or BO). To avoid transfusion reactions, patients must receive blood either similar to their own group or from a group 'O' donor (a 'universal donor').
- **The Rh system** comprises three allelic sets of genes: cC; D (Rh positive) and no D (Rh negative); and eE.
- **Other systems**.

Complications of blood transfusion

- **Transfusion reactions** (e.g. acute or delayed haemolytic transfusion reactions): immediate or delayed anaphylaxis (see Chapter 77). Minor reactions (common in those with multiple transfusions) cause (post) transfusion fever and shorten transfused red cell life.
- Large transfusions may provoke **heart or haemostatic failure** (blood preservatives chelate calcium, so inhibiting the clotting cascade).
- **Viral transmission**, especially human immunodeficiency virus (HIV) and hepatitis B or C. Many countries routinely screen all blood for these pathogens.
- **Iron overload** in those receiving multiple transfusions (e.g. hereditary anaemias).
- **Immune suppression**: though there is controversy, there is some evidence that blood transfusion in those with cancer increases the chance of the cancer progressing. This phenomenon is referred to as transfusion-related immunomodulation.
- **Graft-versus-host disease**: this is a rare disease in which the lymphocytes from the donor blood survive in the blood transfusion recipient, and recognize the recipient as being 'foreign'. This results in an illness called 'graft-versus-host disease' characterized by skin rash, diarrhoea and biochemical evidence of liver damage, usually early after transfusion. The illness has a high mortality.
- **Transfusion-related acute lung injury**, which usually occurs 1–6 hours after transfusion. The patient becomes breathless and breathes rapidly, and cyanosis may be evident. Examination may shows inspiratory crackles and decreased air entry. Blood gases confirm hypoxaemia. A chest X-ray reveals widespread 'fluffy' infiltrates, consistent with an acute lung injury. There is no specific treatment; mechanical ventilation may be required.

51 Clinical approach to lymphadenopathy and splenomegaly

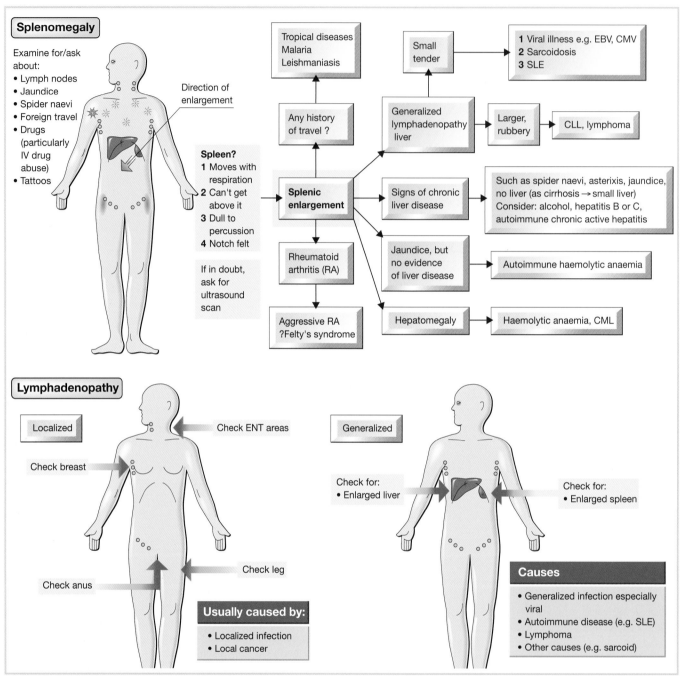

Splenomegaly

Examine for/ask about:
- Lymph nodes
- Jaundice
- Spider naevi
- Foreign travel
- Drugs (particularly IV drug abuse)
- Tattoos

Direction of enlargement

Spleen?
1 Moves with respiration
2 Can't get above it
3 Dull to percussion
4 Notch felt

If in doubt, ask for ultrasound scan

Tropical diseases
Malaria
Leishmaniasis

Any history of travel ?

Small tender → 1 Viral illness e.g. EBV, CMV 2 Sarcoidosis 3 SLE

Generalized lymphadenopathy liver → Larger, rubbery → CLL, lymphoma

Splenic enlargement

Signs of chronic liver disease → Such as spider naevi, asterixis, jaundice, no liver (as cirrhosis → small liver) Consider: alcohol, hepatitis B or C, autoimmune chronic active hepatitis

Jaundice, but no evidence of liver disease → Autoimmune haemolytic anaemia

Rheumatoid arthritis (RA)

Hepatomegaly → Haemolytic anaemia, CML

Aggressive RA ?Felty's syndrome

Lymphadenopathy

Localized

Check ENT areas

Check breast

Check anus

Check leg

Usually caused by:
- Localized infection
- Local cancer

Generalized

Check for:
- Enlarged liver

Check for:
- Enlarged spleen

Causes
- Generalized infection especially viral
- Autoimmune disease (e.g. SLE)
- Lymphoma
- Other causes (e.g. sarcoid)

Lymphadenopathy

Local lymphadenopathy often relates to local infection or malignancy, whereas generalized lymphadenopathy has a wider differential diagnosis, including:

- **Infections** including viral, spirochaetal, rickettsial and protozoal ones.

- **Inflammatory disorders**, such as autoimmune conditions, particularly systemic lupus erythematosus (SLE).
- **Malignancy**, e.g. chronic lymphoblastic leukaemia (CLL), lymphoma.
- **Dermatopathic**: diffuse skin disease such as eczema leads to widespread, small volume lymphadenopathy.
- **Miscellaneous diseases** such as sarcoidosis.

Medicine at a Glance, Fourth Edition. Edited by Patrick Davey. © 2014 John Wiley & Sons, Ltd. Published 2014 by John Wiley & Sons, Ltd. Companion website: www.ataglanceseries.com/medicine

Many patients with lymphadenopathy referred to hospital are worried that they have cancer.

History and examination

The history and examination should focus on possible sites or sources of infection resulting in lymphadenopathy, the presence of inflammatory or connective tissue diseases such as rheumatoid arthritis (RA), SLE or the potentially more sinister symptoms of weight loss, long-lasting malaise or sweats, which might indicate a malignant disease. Lymph node size and texture give some clues:

- Bulky, hard nodes are suggestive of cancer.
- Soft, mobile, tender nodes point towards infection.

These features can be misleading and it is unwise to make a judgement solely on these findings. It is vital to examine the area drained by the lymph node thoroughly, if necessary using radiological techniques, e.g. mammography for axillary lymph nodes.

Investigations

A full blood count (FBC), erythrocyte sedimentation rate (ESR), liver function tests and C-reactive protein estimation are useful screening tests. Other investigations (e.g. computed tomography (CT)) should be tailored to the clinical situation. A biopsy should be undertaken if there is any suspicion of malignancy causing lymph node enlargement. A fine needle aspirate (FNA) is helpful in diagnosing metastatic cancer. If normal, reactive or suggestive of lymphoma, excision of the node (or a core biopsy) should be undertaken. An FNA is not sufficient to diagnose, or exclude a diagnosis of, lymphoma.

Splenomegaly

The differential diagnosis for a mass in the left upper quadrant includes renal or colonic masses and, less commonly, a mass of abdominal lymph nodes. Ultrasonography or CT scan can confirm that the mass is a spleen. The spleen needs to enlarge three-fold before it can be palpated. Thus, a palpable spleen is always pathological and should prompt thorough investigations to establish the cause. The differential diagnosis of splenomegaly includes:

- Infections: e.g. infectious mononucleosis and malaria.
- Lymphoproliferative diseases: especially CLL and lymphoma.
- Myeloproliferative diseases: particularly chronic myeloid leukaemia (CML) and myelofibrosis.
- Haemolytic anaemias, especially autoimmune haemolytic anaemia and hereditary spherocytosis.
- Portal hypertension complicating cirrhosis, or much more rarely without cirrhosis (e.g. portal vein thrombosis, schistosomiasis).
- Autoimmune disease, e.g. SLE.
- Other rarer causes such as sarcoidosis or Gaucher's disease.

The history and physical signs in addition to the splenomegaly often give a strong pointer towards the correct diagnosis:

- Viral infection, often Epstein–Barr virus (EBV) or cytomegalovirus (CMV): several days of flu-like symptoms, sore throat and minor generalized lymphadenopathy, often with mild hepatomegaly.
- Liver cirrhosis: features of chronic liver disease may be noted (see Chapter 133) and, unlike the above disorders, the liver is often small and therefore impalpable.
- Lymphoma: general malaise, weight loss, sometimes night sweats, bulky lymphadenopathy and hepatomegaly.

Investigations

An FBC and film are extremely helpful in ruling many diagnoses in or out:

- **Myeloproliferative disorder**: the haemoglobin is high in polycythaemia rubra vera, the white cell count (WCC) (both mature and immature granulocytes) is high in CML and the platelet count is high in essential thrombocythaemia.
- **Myelofibrosis**: where the bone marrow is replaced by fibrous tissue. Haematopoiesis occurs in extramedullary sites, including the spleen, resulting in massive splenomegaly. The peripheral blood shows leukoerythroblastic features (see Chapter 186) along with misshapen red cells.
- **Haemolytic anaemia**: the blood count shows anaemia and polychromasia (reflecting increased reticulocytes). Other abnormalities (such as spherocytes) may be present depending on the underlying cause of the haemolysis.
- **Viral infection**: reactive lymphocytes in the blood suggest a viral infection.
- **Liver disease**: target cells and a macrocytosis are often seen in liver disease.
- **Lymphoma**: the blood count and film of those with any form of lymphoma may be normal or non-specifically abnormal; it cannot therefore be relied on to rule this diagnosis in or out. However, mild anaemia and rouleaux formation, indicative of a raised ESR, may be present.
- **CLL**: the WCC will be high with $\geq 5 \times 10^9$/L circulating lymphocytes.

Additional investigations, including lymph node or bone marrow biopsy, are sometimes necessary for diagnosis. FNA or biopsy of the spleen is dangerous and is not recommended unless performed by experienced operators. A diagnostic splenectomy is rarely necessary, but should be considered in persistent undiagnosed splenomegaly despite full and thorough investigation. However, CT scanning of the abdomen/thorax in serious conditions associated with splenomegaly often reveals either the diagnosis or lymphadenopathy suitable for percutaneous biopsy. In young patients it is worth sending white cell enzymes to look for the presence of Gaucher's disease as it is a treatable condition.

Complications

Splenomegaly itself is usually asymptomatic, although sometimes a 'dragging' sensation is felt in the left upper quadrant. Occasionally splenomegaly is complicated by:

- **Infarction**, resulting in a 'pleuritic' pain over the spleen, i.e. the lower lateral aspect of the left chest. The differential diagnosis is from other causes of pleurisy (see Chapter 13). Repeated infarction (e.g. in sickle cell disease) or splenectomy causes hyposplenism, which predisposes to overwhelming bacterial (especially pneumococcal) infection (although this is an uncommon complication). Such patients should receive pneumococcal/meningococcal/HiB (*Haemophilus influenzae* B) immunization and life-long prophylactic penicillin (erythromycin in penicillin-sensitive patients).
- **Rupture**: pathological spleens rupture more easily than normal, causing abdominal pain and marked hypotension. Thus, the differential diagnosis of anyone with splenomegaly who becomes hypotensive includes splenic rupture, treated by immediate surgery. A sepsis syndrome should also be considered in hypotensive patients with a large spleen.
- **Hypersplenism**: spleens pool blood in proportion to their size. A normal spleen pools 2% of the blood volume; a very large spleen may pool ≥ 20% of the blood volume, which may result in anaemia, thrombocytopenia (especially in portal hypertension) or even pancytopenia (see Chapter 179). Diagnosis is by excluding other causes.

52 The patient with abnormal bleeding or bruising

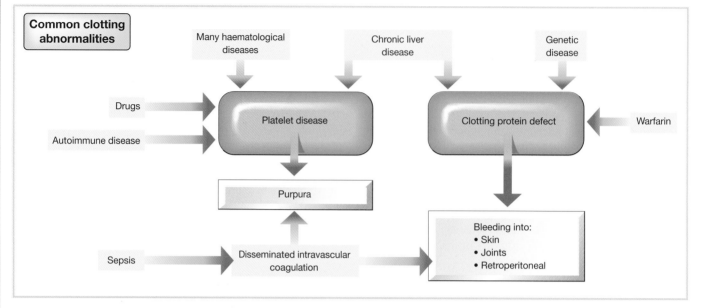

Common clotting abnormalities

The key to assessing a bleeding/bruising problem lies in the history and in particular whether the bleeding has been life-long or is new:

- **Life-long bleeding** suggests an inherited disease, confirmed by ascertaining the bleeding response to remote haemostatic challenges (e.g. operations, dental extractions or postpartum bleeding, although von Willebrand's disease (vWD) improves with pregnancy). The family history and mode of inheritance should be determined (e.g. X-linked for haemophilia A and B).
- **New bleeding** suggests an acquired problem. This often relates to medical problems, either covert (e.g. hypothyroidism) or overt (e.g. septicaemia or disseminated intravascular coagulation).

It can often be difficult to assess the severity of bleeding, and objective findings such as iron deficiency anaemia or the need for a blood transfusion should be recorded. A full drug history must always be taken – aspirin and non-steroidal anti-inflammatory drugs are the most common cause of platelet dysfunction. Other drugs may cause marrow aplasia (see Chapter 179).

Examination

The main purpose of the physical examination is to exclude any underlying medical disease (e.g. sepsis, leukaemia, etc.) and determine the consequences of bleeding (e.g. haemoarthroses, gastrointestinal blood loss), which in themselves need specific treatment. Any bleeding pattern present should be determined because this relates to the underlying defect.

- In **platelet defects** (quantitative or qualitative), purpura/petechiae are common; other manifestations also seen in vWD are epistaxes and, in women, menorrhagia.
- In contrast, in **coagulation factor deficiency** (e.g. haemophilia) bleeding is usually into muscles or joints.

Investigations

First-line investigations (the 'basic clotting screen') include:

- **Full blood count**: particularly the platelet count; the haemoglobin and white cell count provide important clues to the presence of marrow aplasia or leukaemia.

- **Coagulation screen**: a prothrombin time (prolonged when any of factors I, II, V, X or VII are deficient/inhibited), activated partial thromboplastin time (prolonged if any of factors I, II, V, VIII, IX, X, XI or XII are deficient/inhibited) and if indicated a thrombin time (prolonged when fibrinogen is deficient; fibrinogen polymerization is inhibited by fibrin degradation products or if heparin is present). If a prolonged clotting time is found, adding normal plasma (which contains all clotting factors) allows differentiation between bleeding caused by clotting factor deficiency (coagulation corrects) and that caused by inhibition (coagulation does not correct). A common inhibitor is the lupus anticoagulant (see Chapter 190), which paradoxically is associated with a procoagulant state rather than with bleeding.
- **Factor VIII, von Willebrand's factor (vWF) activity and vWF antigen** particularly when inherited disorders are suspected.
- **Bleeding time/PFA 100**: after a skin cut 1 mm deep and 1 cm long, prolonged bleeding occurs with deficient or defective platelets. This bleeding time test has poor sensitivity and specificity and has largely been replaced by *in vitro* alternatives, such as the PFA 100 test. Abnormailities are further investigated by *in vitro* platelet aggregation tests and vWF assays. If bleeding is undeniably abnormal further investigatio is required even if first-line tests are unremarkable (and PFA tesing is often ommitted if platelet aggregation will be perfored in any case). vWD must be specifically looked for because basic screening tests can be normal. Aggregation can be little affected in storage pool disease, so it is routine to also look at the platelet nucleotide content. Factor XIII deficiency is a rare autosomal recessive bleeding disorders that does not affect screening tests, so it should be considered when there is a good history and first-line tests are negative, especially if there is parental consanguinity.

Treatment

This is of the underlying cause. Specific treatments are outlined in Chapters 187 and 188.

53 Leukopenia

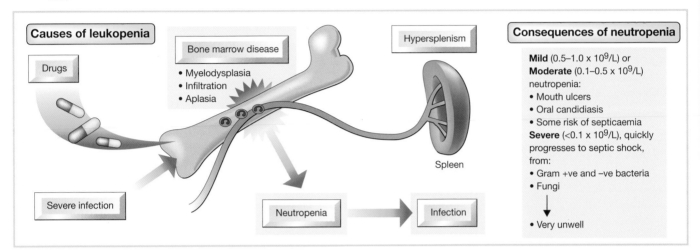

Causes of leukopenia

- Drugs
- Severe infection

Bone marrow disease
- Myelodysplasia
- Infiltration
- Aplasia

Hypersplenism

Spleen

Neutropenia → Infection

Consequences of neutropenia

Mild (0.5–1.0 x 10⁹/L) or **Moderate** (0.1–0.5 x 10⁹/L) neutropenia:
- Mouth ulcers
- Oral candidiasis
- Some risk of septicaemia

Severe (<0.1 x 10⁹/L), quickly progresses to septic shock, from:
- Gram +ve and –ve bacteria
- Fungi

↓

- Very unwell

A decrease in the number of circulating white cells (leukopenia) is common, and may indicate serious disease that needs immediate diagnosis and treatment.

Neutropenia

Neutropenia means decreased circulating neutrophils (total count $\leq 2.0 \times 10^9$ neutrophils/L). In extreme cases there may be no circulating neutrophils – called agranulocytosis. There are many causes of neutropenia:

- **Racial origin**: a mild neutropenia is commoner in negroids than caucasians. This is of no significance and not associated with an increased risk of infection.
- **Drug-induced neutropenia** is the most common cause, and may result in a selective decrease in neutrophils (e.g. carbimazole), or a more general bone marrow depression, a pancytopenia. Examples of the latter include cytotoxic chemotherapy, rheumatological drugs including sulphasalazine, gold and some non-steroidal anti-inflammatory drugs. Many other drugs have been implicated. Alcoholism may underlie neutropenia.
- **Myelodysplastic syndrome**: common in elderly people (see Chapter 185).
- **Severe infection** can cause neutropenia, as in pneumococcal pneumonia with complicating septicaemia, where the low white cell count is associated with a worse outlook. The diagnosis is usually obvious. Typhoid and viral infections likewise can depress neutrophil counts.
- **Bone marrow infiltration**, particularly from haematological malignancy, such as leukaemia. Usually affects all cell lines (pancytopenia) (see Chapter 179).
- **Bone marrow failure** results in pancytopenia, e.g. aplastic anaemia.
- **Hypersplenism** (see Chapter 51), including Felty's syndrome (rheumatoid arthritis with high-titre rheumatoid factor).
- Very rare causes include **cyclical neutropenia**.
- **Autoimmune neutropenia**.

Consequences of neutropenia

Most patients with mild/moderate neutropenia (counts $1.0–2.0 \times 10^9$/L) have no symptoms. However, the lower the count, the greater the risk of infection (neutropenic sepsis); this risk becomes significant when counts are below 0.5×10^9/L and very significant below 0.1×10^9/L.

- Mouth ulceration and oral candidiasis are common in sustained neutropenias.
- Infection can very rapidly (i.e. within hours) become overwhelming, producing severe septic shock (see Chapter 18).
- Organisms may be 'typical' pathogenic bacteria (e.g. *Staphylococcus aureus*, pathogenic streptococci, Gram-negative bacilli), although low-grade pathogens and fungi are also commonly implicated.

Treatment

- Treatment involves establishing which organism is responsible (blood cultures), providing circulatory support (fluids, sometimes vasoconstrictors) and, most importantly, giving high-dose broad-spectrum antibiotics without delay.
- Treatment with granulocyte colony-stimulating factor may sometimes help to shorten a period of neutropenia, depending on the cause (e.g. especially chemotherapy-induced neutropenia).

Lymphopenia

A decrease in the number of circulating lymphocytes is much rarer than neutropenia. Causes other than haematological malignancy and its treatment are uncommon, and include:

- Autoimmune disease, such as systemic lupus erythematosus.
- Viral infections, including acute (e.g. Epstein–Barr virus and cytomegalovirus) or chronic infections (e.g. human immunodeficiency virus).
- Inherited disease (see Chapter 175).

Presentation is with other features of the underlying disease or with infection/malignancy. T-cell deficiency predisposes to infection with intracellular pathogens (especially viruses), pyogenic bacteria (e.g. staphylococcal infection), fungi, *Pneumocystis jirovecii* and protozoa (e.g. *Cryptosporidium* spp.), in addition to increasing the rates of lymphoma and solid organ cancers. B-cell deficiencies predispose to pyogenic bacterial infection.

Medicine at a Glance, Fourth Edition. Edited by Patrick Davey. © 2014 John Wiley & Sons, Ltd. Published 2014 by John Wiley & Sons, Ltd. Companion website: www.ataglanceseries.com/medicine

Oncological emergencies

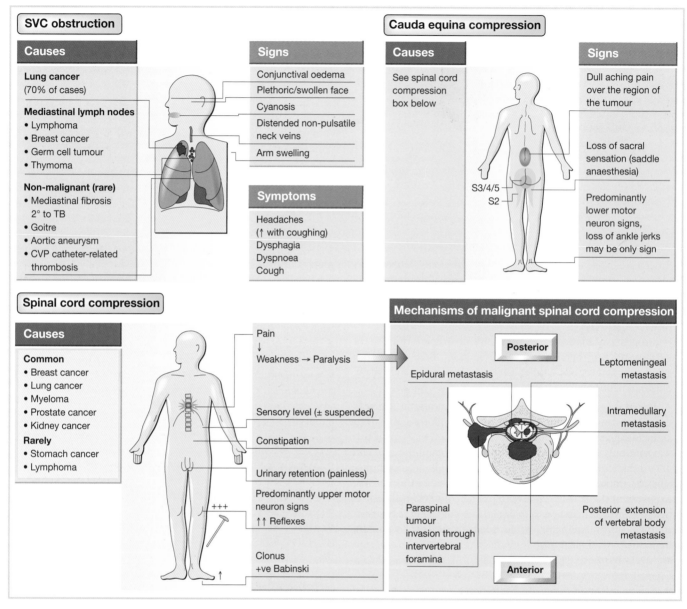

Superior vena caval obstruction

This is a clinical syndrome arising from obstruction of blood flow through the superior vena cava (SVC). This thin-walled vessel may be compressed, invaded or thrombosed.

Aetiology

- **Malignant** (usually): from malignant lymph nodes compressing or invading the SVC. Lung cancer is the cause in 70%. The remainder are the result of lymphoma, and more rarely breast cancer and other tumours.
- **Non-malignant** (rarely): mediastinal goitre, aortic aneurysm, iatrogenic (e.g. thrombosis from indwelling central venous catheters), mediastinal fibrosis (histoplasmosis/tuberculosis (TB)).

Clinical features

Symptoms arise from the increase in venous pressure in the jugular and subclavian veins, and from the local effects of a mediastinal or bronchial tumour; they comprise dyspnoea, facial/arm swelling, headaches (worse on coughing) or head fullness, cough or dysphagia. Signs include non-pulsatile distension of the neck and chest wall veins, oedema of the face, neck and arms, plethoric facies, dilated veins over the upper chest wall, cyanosis and conjunctival oedema (chemosis).

Investigations

SVC obstruction is a medical emergency. Previously, patients received immediate radiotherapy, but modern oncological therapy now makes histological diagnosis vital. However, if patients are acutely ill radiotherapy is still given before histological diagnosis.

Immediate investigations include:

- Chest X-ray: superior mediastinal widening, pleural effusions, right hilar mass.
- CT to confirm diagnosis of SVC obstruction.

Investigations to obtain diagnosis include: sputum cytology, lymph node biopsy (if accessible node is palpable), bone marrow examination, bronchoscopy, mediastinoscopy/thoracotomy, CT-guided, percutaneous, transthoracic fine needle aspiration.

Management and prognosis
Bed rest with head elevated, oxygen and high-dose steroids (e.g. dexamethasone). Additional therapy depends on aetiology:

● **Malignant disease**: chemotherapy for small cell lung cancer (SCLC), lymphoma and germ cell tumours; wire stent insertion followed by radiotherapy for non-SCLC.
● **Non-malignant causes** can be treated by percutaneous angioplasty and wire stent insertion.
● **Thrombotic** SVC obstruction: remove the local precipitant of thrombosis (SVC catheter) and consider thrombolysis. Surgery (bypassing the blocked SVC) is rarely indicated and is reserved for non-malignant cases refractory to other therapies.

Patients with SVC obstruction from non-SCLC often live <6 months. Presentation with SVC obstruction does not affect the prognosis in patients with lymphoma or SCLC. Those with non-malignant causes of the syndrome live much longer – reported average being 9 years.

Malignant spinal cord compression

Malignant spinal cord compression is the second most common neurological complication of malignancy after cerebral metastases. It can be the initial manifestation of malignancy and often arises in the pre-terminal phase of the illness.

Pathophysiology, aetiology and clinical features
In adults, the tip of the spinal cord usually lies at the L1 vertebral level; below this level the lumbarsacral nerve roots form the cauda equina. The pathophysiology of cauda equina compression is similar to the more rostral compression but the clinical signs may differ. The spinal cord and its nerve roots are most commonly compressed anteriorly by posterior extension of haematogenously spread metastases in the vertebral body, extending into the epidural space or through vertebral body collapse. The cord may also be compromised by extension of a paraspinal tumour through the intervertebral foramina, which can occur without evidence of bony involvement. Damage is principally mediated by disruption of small vessel circulation, which is precipitated by the changes in pressure within the spinal canal. There may be multiple epidural metastases causing cord compression at different levels. See Figure 54.1 for the aetiology. Most patients are known to have malignancy. Spinal cord compression is the first manifestation of cancer in 10%. The thoracic spine is the most common site of compression, followed by the lumbosacral and cervical regions.

Symptoms and signs of spinal cord compression

● **Pain**: this is the most common symptom; it may predate neurological signs. Constant, dull, aching pain, which may radiate laterally, and is worse on movement (flexion) or increases with thoracic pressure (sneezing, straining). The involved vertebrae may be tender to percussion.
● **Weakness**: particularly to the proximal muscles of the lower limbs in an upper motor neuron pattern, although the exact distribution of power loss depends on the site of compression. Deep tendon reflexes are increased and the plantar response is extensor.
● **Sensory loss/paraesthesiae**: ascending to or just below the level of the relevant dermatome at the level of compression (suspended level).
● **Ataxia**: loss of proprioception (posterior columns).

● **Urinary retention and constipation**: late symptoms of autonomic dysfunction.

Clinical signs of cauda equina compression include: pain; weakness (lower motor neuron pattern of lower limb weakness); ankle jerks may be lost and Babinski's reflex may be negative; sensory loss (sacral anaesthesia may be present); and urinary retention and constipation.

Investigations
Malignant spinal cord compression is a medical emergency and mandates urgent investigation, i.e. within 24 hours of symptom onset.

● **Plain radiographs** may show vertebral body collapse or pedicle destruction.
● Whole spine **magnetic resonance imaging** is the investigation of choice. It defines the exact location and disease extent. The whole spine must be examined as multiple sites of compression can occur.
● CT-guided **percutaneous biopsy** may be considered if primary is unknown.

Management
● Analgesia and anticoagulation (if no contraindications).
● **High-dose corticosteroids** may improve symptoms and outcome.
● **Surgery**: all patients with spinal cord compression should be discussed with the neurosurgeons. Surgery has significant morbidity and mortality, but has a role in those without a diagnosis, those with a single level of compression and those with spinal instability. Surgery may also be useful in patients with progression of neurological deficit during radiotherapy, compression in a previously irradiated area or in radioresistant disease, and may be associated with better outcome.
● **Radiotherapy** to debulk the tumour is the treatment of choice in those with radiosensitive tumours, if not considered to be surgical candidates or following surgical decompression. It improves pain and there may be some improvement in power, but paraplegia is reversed in only 10–15%. The radiation field includes two vertebrae either side of the site of compression (the site of frequent recurrence).
● **Chemotherapy**: cytotoxic chemotherapy is the treatment of choice in children with chemosensitive tumours, and as an adjunct to radiotherapy in adults with chemosensitive disease. Endocrine therapy may help in prostate and breast cancer.
● **Physiotherapy** is crucial to maximize any return of function.

Prognosis
The three main predictors of outcome are:

1 **Pre-treatment neurological status**: 80% of those ambulant at diagnosis remain so with urgent treatment. Paraplegia is reversed in <15% of cases.
2 **Speed of onset of neurological deficit**: disease progressing gradually is more likely to be reversible.
3 **Tumour type**: radiation- and chemotherapy-sensitive disease responds faster and better to treatment. Radioresistant tumours have a poor outcome.

Some patients presenting with malignant spinal cord compression will not achieve ambulation. They are often pre-terminally ill and face the loss of independence that confinement to a wheelchair brings. Maximizing physical and psychological support in this situation is an important part of the holistic treatment these patients should receive.

For **Hypercalcaemia** see Chapter 162. For **Fever with neutropenia** see Chapter 53.

55 Introduction to neurological diagnosis 1

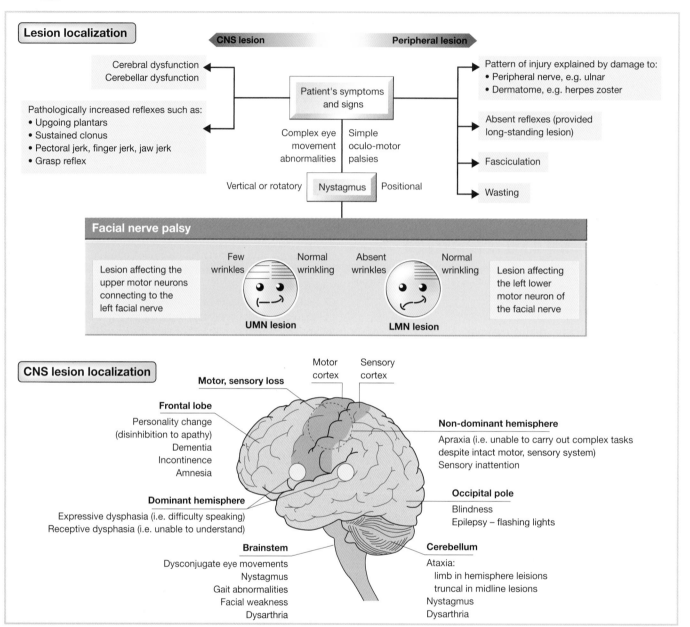

Lesion localization

CNS lesion → | ← Peripheral lesion

Patient's symptoms and signs

Cerebral dysfunction
Cerebellar dysfunction

Pathologically increased reflexes such as:
• Upgoing plantars
• Sustained clonus
• Pectoral jerk, finger jerk, jaw jerk
• Grasp reflex

Complex eye movement abnormalities | Simple oculo-motor palsies

Vertical or rotatory — Nystagmus — Positional

Pattern of injury explained by damage to:
• Peripheral nerve, e.g. ulnar
• Dermatome, e.g. herpes zoster

Absent reflexes (provided long-standing lesion)

Fasciculation

Wasting

Facial nerve palsy

Lesion affecting the upper motor neurons connecting to the left facial nerve

Few wrinkles | Normal wrinkling

UMN lesion

Absent wrinkles | Normal wrinkling

Lesion affecting the left lower motor neuron of the facial nerve

LMN lesion

CNS lesion localization

Motor cortex | Sensory cortex

Motor, sensory loss

Frontal lobe
Personality change (disinhibition to apathy)
Dementia
Incontinence
Amnesia

Dominant hemisphere
Expressive dysphasia (i.e. difficulty speaking)
Receptive dysphasia (i.e. unable to understand)

Non-dominant hemisphere
Apraxia (i.e. unable to carry out complex tasks despite intact motor, sensory system)
Sensory inattention

Occipital pole
Blindness
Epilepsy – flashing lights

Brainstem
Dysconjugate eye movements
Nystagmus
Gait abnormalities
Facial weakness
Dysarthria

Cerebellum
Ataxia:
  limb in hemisphere leisions
  truncal in midline lesions
Nystagmus
Dysarthria

There are many different neurological diseases and it is not always possible to make a firm diagnosis from a particular set of signs and symptoms, e.g. there are numerous causes of ataxia – the combination of peripheral neuropathy and ataxia only narrows this down but still leaves a range of possible underlying diagnoses. Neurologists therefore make an anatomical diagnosis followed by an aetiological or pathological diagnosis.

In addition to acquired diseases, there are also many inherited conditions involving the nervous system. Individually these are rare, but collectively form an important proportion of the burden of neurological disease. Partly, this is because a high proportion of the 20 000 genes in the human genome are expressed in the nervous system. Mutation of these genes may be devastating but not lethal, allowing the survival of individuals with genetic disease. Furthermore, most cells of the central nervous system (CNS) are non-dividing and there is little capacity for regeneration. Therefore the brain is susceptible to the accumulation of damaged protein with ageing and progressive neurodegenerative diseases become an increasing problem as the population ages.

Six steps to neurological diagnosis

1 Knowledge of neuroepidemiology (see Chapter 57). The prior probability of an individual diagnosis depends on the age of the patient and other factors.

2 A neurological diagnosis always depends most of all on a good history, without which the neurological examination and subsequent investigations will be difficult to interpret. Many common neurological diseases are frequently associated with normal scans (e.g. headache, primary epilepsies, many neurodegenerative diseases).

3 Perform a standard, simple examination on every patient. Extend this examination in particular situations.

4 Synthesize the history and examination to decide whether the problem is in the peripheral nervous system (including the muscles) or the CNS, of psychiatric origin, or not due to nervous system disease at all.

5 Only then can you draw up a differential diagnosis, taking into account the location of the problem (brain, spinal cord, nerve, muscle), the onset and progression of symptoms, and the age of the patient.

6 Perform special investigations to confirm your diagnostic hypothesis.

Lesion localization

In clinical practice the key distinction in lesion localization is between the central and the peripheral nervous system (PNS). In diagnostic terms this is far more important than whether the lesion is in a specific brain region.

Cerebral hemispheres

The extent of neurological dysfunction is affected by individual variation, the tempo and nature of the pathological process and cortical plasticity. Hemispheric lesions cause less motor and sensory dysfunction than lesions of equivalent volume in lower structures, and show a less consistent relationship between dysfunction and lesion localization than in the brainstem, spinal cord or PNS:

- **Contralateral hemianaesthesia** arises from damage to the cortical sensory area (see Figure 55.1) or from damage to thalamocortical connections. It is usually incomplete because somatosensory function is partially represented in both hemispheres.
- **Hemiplegia** may be caused by:
  - Lesions of the contralateral primary motor cortex (when conscious level is also often decreased).
  - The descending motor tracts in the corona radiata or the posterior limb of the internal capsule (when conscious level is usually normal).
  - The brainstem (rarely), when there are usually associated cranial nerve signs.
  - The ipsilateral spinal cord if there is a lesion discretely affecting one side. Accompanying sensory disturbance is usual.
- **Bilateral weakness** is unlikely to be the result of a single lesion of the cerebral cortex, except in the context of coma, because the motor pathways for each side of the body are in separate cerebral hemispheres. An extraordinarily rare exception of a single cortical lesion causing bilateral weakness is a midline parasagittal meningioma.

- **Language dominance** is in the left hemisphere in 98% of people (including 60% of left-handed individuals). This is important in deciding whether a lesion is in the left hemisphere.
- **Expressive (Broca's) dysphasia** is caused by lesions of the dominant frontal lobe; patients show a marked decrease in verbal fluency but normal comprehension.
- **Receptive (Wernicke's) dysphasia** is the result of dominant temporal lobe lesions; it is characterized by fluent speech with frequent paraphrasic errors (use of the wrong word) and poor comprehension. Mixed expressive and receptive dysphasia is common.
- **Disorders of spatial awareness**, including neglect, are more common in right posterior hemisphere (parietal) disease.
- **Immediate memory** is dependent on the functional integrity of both hippocampi, which lie adjacent to the temporal lobes. These structures are affected in herpes encephalitis and anoxia (e.g. after cardiac arrest or carbon monoxide poisoning).
- **Executive function** (planning, impulse control, etc.) is probably a diffuse brain function, but selective disorders of executive control have some localizing value for lesions of the frontal lobes.

Cerebellum

The cerebellum functions as a modulator of motor learning and execution to facilitate the smooth integration of movement. Anatomically it is divided into the midline vermis and two hemispheres. The vascular supply of the cerebellum is from the vertebrobasilar system via the posterior inferior cerebellar artery, the anterior inferior cerebellar artery and the superior cerebellar artery:

- Lesions of the vermis cause **truncal ataxia**; lesions of the hemispheres cause **limb ataxia**.
- **Ocular features** of cerebellar disease are usually prominent and include nystagmus, broken smooth pursuit, slow (hypometric) saccadic movement and ocular dysmetria (saccadic overshoot).
- **Cerebellar tremor** is a kinetic tremor with exacerbation at the end of movement, underlining the function of the cerebellum in damping movement.
- Other signs of cerebellar disturbance are **gait ataxia** and **dysarthria**. The latter is characteristically a disorder of loss of prosody with monotonous, slurred speech.

Brainstem

The brainstem consists of the midbrain, pons and medulla oblongata. There is a concentration of anatomically important structures in a small area, so most lesions of the brainstem are complex.

- Typical features of brainstem disease are nystagmus and disorders of conjugate gaze, vertigo, facial weakness, dysarthria, gait disturbance and ataxia. All these can occur as a result of disease in other sites, but the constellation together suggests a brainstem origin.
- Most eponymous vascular brainstem syndromes are rarely seen in pure form – precise localization has been greatly aided by magnetic resonance imaging and angiography.

56 Introduction to neurological diagnosis 2

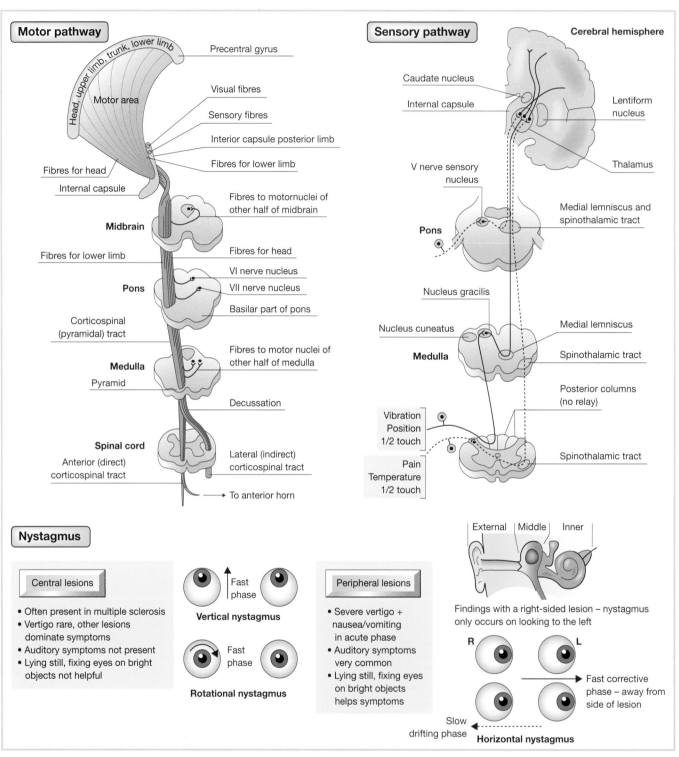

Motor pathway

Head, upper limb, trunk, lower limb

Motor area

Precentral gyrus

Visual fibres

Sensory fibres

Interior capsule posterior limb

Fibres for lower limb

Fibres for head

Internal capsule

Midbrain

Fibres to motornuclei of other half of midbrain

Fibres for lower limb

Fibres for head

VI nerve nucleus

VII nerve nucleus

Pons

Basilar part of pons

Corticospinal (pyramidal) tract

Medulla

Fibres to motor nuclei of other half of medulla

Pyramid

Decussation

Spinal cord

Anterior (direct) corticospinal tract

Lateral (indirect) corticospinal tract

To anterior horn

Sensory pathway

Cerebral hemisphere

Caudate nucleus

Internal capsule

Lentiform nucleus

Thalamus

V nerve sensory nucleus

Pons

Medial lemniscus and spinothalamic tract

Nucleus gracilis

Nucleus cuneatus

Medulla

Medial lemniscus

Spinothalamic tract

Posterior columns (no relay)

Vibration
Position
1/2 touch

Spinothalamic tract

Pain
Temperature
1/2 touch

Nystagmus

External | Middle | Inner

Findings with a right-sided lesion – nystagmus only occurs on looking to the left

Central lesions

- Often present in multiple sclerosis
- Vertigo rare, other lesions dominate symptoms
- Auditory symptoms not present
- Lying still, fixing eyes on bright objects not helpful

Fast phase

Vertical nystagmus

Fast phase

Rotational nystagmus

Peripheral lesions

- Severe vertigo + nausea/vomiting in acute phase
- Auditory symptoms very common
- Lying still, fixing eyes on bright objects helps symptoms

R | L

Fast corrective phase – away from side of lesion

Slow drifting phase

Horizontal nystagmus

Eye movements

Virtually every region of the brain has some influence on the control of conjugate gaze. Voluntary gaze centres in the frontal lobes and parietal cortex initiate volitional eye movement. These send descending pathways to the brainstem nuclei, which receive influences from the cerebellum and basal ganglia, and the ascending influences from the spinal cord. There are important internuclear connections. Thus disorders of conjugate gaze may be:

- Supranuclear.
- Internuclear (see Chapter 60).
- Nuclear.

Eye movements are also affected by disease of the extraocular muscles and the structures of the orbit, and damage to the peripheral segments of cranial nerves III, IV and VI. Examination of eye movements is thus far more than simply the examination of cranial nerves III, IV and VI. It should be directed at describing the abnormality without assumptions about whether the lesion is in the nerve, the brainstem or higher up. Common patterns of abnormality in conjugate gaze are described in Chapters 60 and 61. Nystagmus should be described as:

- Occurring in the primary position (the midline).
- Or occurring on horizontal or vertical gaze.

In practice it is often difficult to localize nystagmus and it is best to consider it in the context of the rest of the history and examination, before deciding if it is arising from peripheral structures (the labyrinth), the brainstem or the cerebellum. The slow phase of nystagmus is the 'pathological' component and the fast phase is corrective.

- **Peripheral (vestibular) nystagmus** is typically associated with severe symptoms of dysequilibrium, nausea and vomiting, and is often unilateral. The fast phase is away from the lesion because the vestibular apparatus functions to stimulate eye movement towards the contralateral side.
- **Central nystagmus**: ipsilateral structures in the brainstem maintain horizontal gaze. Thus, the pathological drift of the eye (the slow phase of nystagmus) is away from the lesion, with a corrective (fast) phase towards the affected side of the brainstem in central nystagmus. Furthermore, central lesions are often bilateral.
- **Cerebellar nystagmus** is similar in that it is probably mediated by cerebellar–brainstem connections.

Spinal cord

The spinal cord is a small structure <1.5 cm in diameter. There is no anatomical boundary between each side, and many pathological processes are therefore bilateral.

The vascular supply to the spinal cord is of clinical relevance. A single spinal artery supplies the anterior portion of the cord, leaving it vulnerable to ischaemic damage (see Chapter 209), whereas the posterior part of the cord has a rich anastomotic supply (from posterior spinal arteries).

Weakness caused by spinal cord disease is therefore usually bilateral and associated with a motor and sensory level. At the level of the lesion, there are lower motor neuron (LMN) signs as evidenced by diminished tendon reflexes and weakness; below the lesion, there are upper motor neuron (UMN) signs, and above the lesion the limbs are normal.

Descending tracts from the motor cortex travel as the lateral corticospinal tract before synapsing on LMNs in the ventral horns. These cells receive descending influences from the basal ganglia, red nucleus and vestibular apparatus. LMNs thus serve as a final common pathway for motor function.

The ascending sensory pathways can be divided into:

- Spinothalamic tracts, which carry pain and temperature in the contralateral lateral spinothalamic tract and light touch in the ventral spinothalamic tract to synapse in the thalamus.
- Gracile and cuneate fasciculi, which carry joint position, sense, kinaesthetic sense, two-point discrimination and light touch on the ipsilateral posterior columns to synapse in the medullary nuclei and on to the thalamus.
- Spinocerebellar tracts.

The vertebral level is not the same as the spinal cord level – the cord ends at L1, so it is safe to perform a lumbar puncture in adults in L2/3, L3/4 and L4/5 spaces.

The cord terminates in the conus medullaris and the cauda equina. Conus lesions are characterized by sphincter dysfunction, sensory loss in the perineum and loss of ankle jerks. Cauda equina lesions can involve the same functions, but sphincter disturbance is a late feature and symptoms and signs are usually asymmetrical.

Nerve roots

The identification of lesions at specific spinal root levels requires knowledge of dermatomes and myotomes:

- Root disease is characterized by radicular pain, and sensory and motor dysfunction.
- Particular diseases (e.g. herpes zoster and Guillain–Barré syndrome) have a predilection for nerve roots.
- The most common levels for intervertebral disc prolapse are between the sixth and seventh vertebrae in the cervical region (C7 root compression) and between the fourth and fifth vertebrae in the lumbar region (L5 root compression).
- The effects of root compression at various levels are as follows:
  - C5: weakness of shoulder abduction (deltoid) and forearm flexion (biceps), sensory loss on the lateral aspect of the arm and loss of the biceps jerk.
  - C6: weakness of forearm flexion, finger and wrist extension, loss of the biceps jerk, sensory loss on the lateral surface of the forearm and first and second digits.
  - C7: loss of the triceps reflex, weakness of elbow extension and wrist extension and flexion, sensory loss in the third and fourth digits.
  - C8: weakness and wasting of intrinsic hand muscles, sensory loss in the fifth digit and the medial forearm; there may be an ipsilateral Horner's syndrome.
  - T1: wasting of the small muscles of the hand and ipsilateral Horner's syndrome.
  - L4: weakness of knee extension, loss of the knee jerk and wasting of quadriceps.
  - L5: weakness of knee flexion, ankle dorsiflexion and plantar flexion.
  - S1: loss of the ankle jerk, weakness of dorsiflexion of the great toe.

Lesion localization in peripheral nerve and muscle

See Chapters 209, 210 and 211.

57 Introduction to neurological diagnosis 3: neuroepidemiology

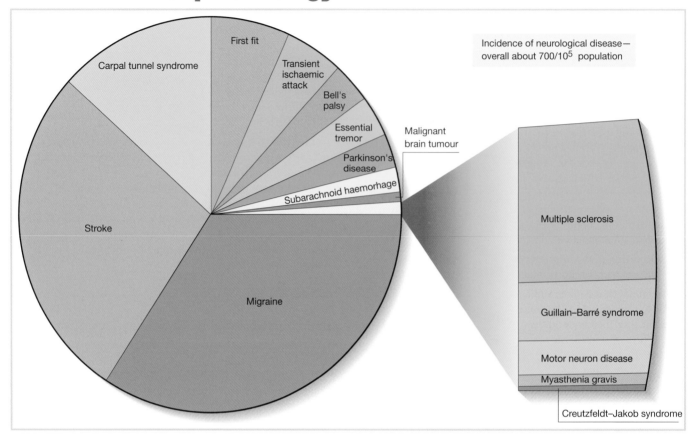

One of the difficulties in learning neurology is that there are apparently a bewildering number of possible conditions and diagnosis for each clinical syndrome, e.g. there are hundreds of different causes of peripheral neuropathy. Therefore, a sensible diagnostician bases the likelihood of a certain diagnosis on the prior probability, or incidence, of that condition. As many conditions are rare, it is reasonable to express this as cases per 100 000 population per year. It will be strikingly apparent from Table 57.1 that the incidence of conditions in general practice is very different from that in a neurology clinic. Although a consultant neurologist (there are one per 140 000 people in the

UK) will see a patient with a first fit in virtually every clinic, a GP may only see one such patient a year. It is also important to remember that it may be the *prevalence* of a disorder that gives a true indication of its impact on society as a whole. For example, multiple sclerosis and Parkinson's disease are disorders that do not significantly shorten lifespan in most patients, but last for decades, and therefore they have a high prevalence and impose a high burden on health and social care systems. It will also be immediately apparent that neurology teaching tends to overemphasize rare conditions that many students may never see again.

Table 57.1 Incidence of neurological conditions in the general population.

Condition	Migraine	Stroke	Carpal tunnel syndrome	First fit	Transient ischaemic attack	Bell's palsy	Essential tremor	Parkinson's disease	Subarachnoid haemorrhage	Malignant brain tumour	Multiple sclerosis	Guillain–Barré syndrome	Motor neuron disease	Myasthenia gravis	Creutzfeldt–Jakob disease
Annual incidence per 100 000 population	250	200	50	50	35	25	25	20	15	5	5	2	1	0.4	0.1
Time between each new case for a GP	10 weeks	12 weeks	6 months	1 years	17 months	2 years	2 years	2.5 years	3.3 years	10 years	10 years	25 years	33 years	125 years	500 years

Source: Warlow C.P. et al. 2001. Reproduced with permission of John Wiley & Sons.

Medicine at a Glance, Fourth Edition. Edited by Patrick Davey. © 2014 John Wiley & Sons, Ltd. Published 2014 by John Wiley & Sons, Ltd. Companion website: www.ataglanceseries.com/medicine

58 Common neurological symptoms

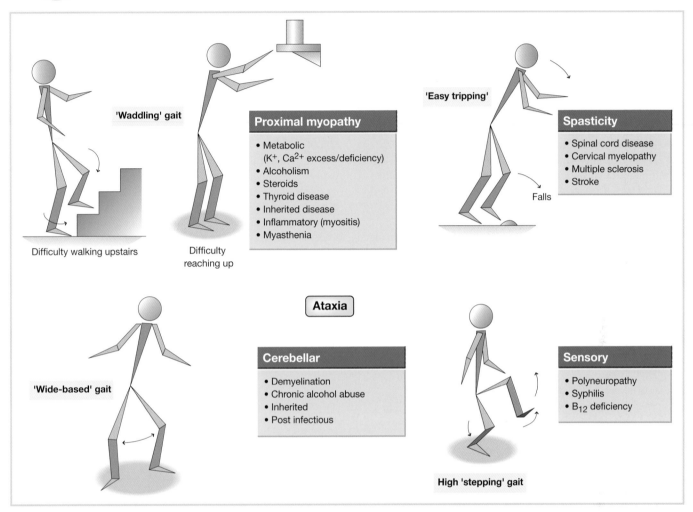

'Waddling' gait

Difficulty walking upstairs

Difficulty reaching up

Proximal myopathy

- Metabolic
  (K^+, Ca^{2+} excess/deficiency)
- Alcoholism
- Steroids
- Thyroid disease
- Inherited disease
- Inflammatory (myositis)
- Myasthenia

'Easy tripping'

Spasticity

- Spinal cord disease
- Cervical myelopathy
- Multiple sclerosis
- Stroke

Falls

Ataxia

'Wide-based' gait

Cerebellar

- Demyelination
- Chronic alcohol abuse
- Inherited
- Post infectious

Sensory

- Polyneuropathy
- Syphilis
- B_{12} deficiency

High 'stepping' gait

Difficulty walking

Both neurological and non-neurological diseases, e.g. joint disease, can cause difficulty in walking. Analysing gait problems in elderly people carries particular difficulties in interpretation and is complicated by:

- Multiple co-morbidities.
- Age-related changes in musculoskeletal function.
- Joint disease.
- Underlying cerebrovascular disease.
- Postural hypotension (see Chapter 64).
- Fear of falling.

A full neurological and rheumatological history and examination are necessary to place all of these contributory factors in context. The most important part of the assessment is to see the patient walking. Invaluable information is obtained by watching the patient get up from the waiting room chair and walk into the consulting room.

Patterns of gait disturbance

Bear in mind that classic gait patterns may be present in their pure form only in advanced disease. Frequently, a non-specific or mixed gait abnormality is observed.

- **Peripheral neuropathies**:
  - Motor nerve damage: foot drop occurs with a 'high stepping' gait.
  - Sensory (proprioceptive) nerve damage: ataxia and sometimes a 'stamping' gait develop.
- **Muscle disease** usually causes proximal muscle weakness and a 'waddling' gait.
- **Spinal cord or upper motor neuron damage**: the earliest symptom is 'easy tripping up' or difficulty walking on rough ground. Subsequently the leg(s) drag. Examination shows a narrow-based gait and brisk reflexes, often with clonus. The gait is described as being 'stiff', and 'spastic scissoring' together of the legs sometimes occurs.
- **Cerebellar disease** causes a wide-based, staggering gait (termed 'ataxic'). Midline cerebellar lesions may cause gait ataxia with relatively few signs in the limbs. For causes of ataxia, see next section.
- **Hemispheric damage** causes a contralateral hemiplegic gait, with the contralateral arm held in flexion. In walking, the leg is swung outwards and forwards, in a circular motion – a movement termed 'circumduction'.

Medicine at a Glance, Fourth Edition. Edited by Patrick Davey. © 2014 John Wiley & Sons, Ltd. Published 2014 by John Wiley & Sons, Ltd. Companion website: www.ataglanceseries.com/medicine

The earliest feature of **Parkinson's disease** is an asymmetrical loss of arm swing. Later, a stooped posture with shuffling footsteps develops. The gait may be 'festinant', which means that there is a tendency to hurrying, and turning is slow resulting in instability.

Diffuse vascular disease causes a variety of gait disturbance, including a form of lower body parkinsonism with a wide-based gait and small steps termed 'marche à petit pas'.

Gait apraxia is an inability to carry out complex tasks, such as walking, as a result of damage to the part of the brain that integrates complex motor function. The gait is disordered and the patient is apparently unable to initiate steps, but individual actions, e.g. making cycling motions on a bed, remain intact. It occurs in a number of different cortical diseases, including diffuse vascular disease and also normal pressure hydrocephalus.

Dizziness: see section on dizziness.

Loss of balance: may relate to inner ear disease (often either continuous or episodic), cerebellar disease, dorsal column loss or peripheral sensory or motor neuropathy.

Differential diagnosis of ataxia

Ataxia is defined as incoordination of complex movement, such as walking in a straight line. Anatomically, ataxia is caused by:

Lesions of the cerebellum ('cerebellar ataxia'): wide-based gait, falling to the side of the lesion. A 'kinetic' or intention tremor (brought out by the 'finger–nose' test) is usually present.

Disorders of proprioception ('sensory ataxia') caused by polyneuropathies (see Chapter 211) or lesions of the dorsal columns (classically, as in subacute combined degeneration due to vitamin B_{12} deficiency or in tabes dorsalis, causing a 'high stepping' or broad-based gait).

The causes of ataxia are legion and include:

- Drugs: anticonvulsants, alcohol, benzodiazepines.
- Multiple sclerosis.
- Cerebellar lesions: tumours or vascular insults.
- Degenerative disease: multiple system atrophy
- Inherited disease: Friedreich's ataxia, spinocerebellar ataxias.
- Metabolic: vitamin B_{12} deficiency, heavy metal poisoning.
- Parainfectious (more common in children): chickenpox, glandular fever, *Mycoplasma* infection, psittacosis and legionellosis.
- Paraneoplastic cerebellar degeneration.

Dizziness

This extremely common problem causes considerable misery to patients, although it rarely has a serious underlying cause. First, establish what is meant by 'dizziness' because this word is used to express a large range of subjective feelings from presyncope or faintness, through vertigo to an odd light-headedness. It is crucial to define the symptom accurately. Although it is always better to let the patient use his or her own words and unwise to put words into patients' mouths, some people have such difficulty describing this symptom that it may be appropriate cautiously to offer some possibilities:

- Do you feel as if you are going to faint? The symptom is likely to represent presyncope (see Chapter 64).

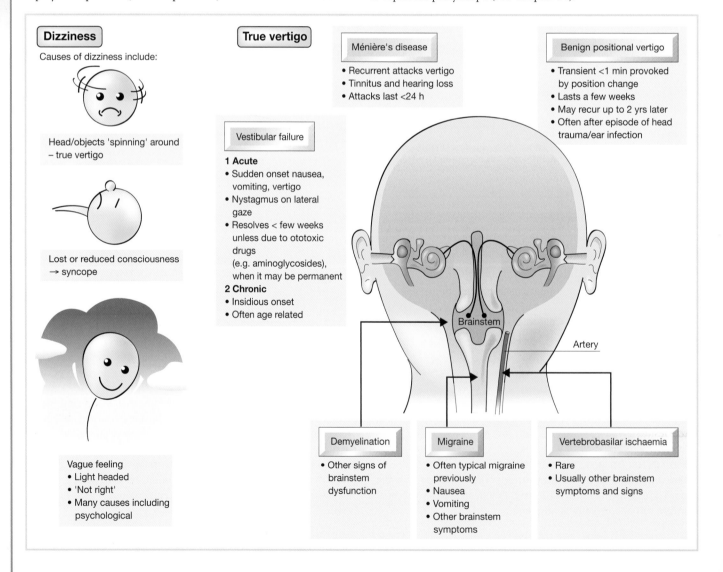

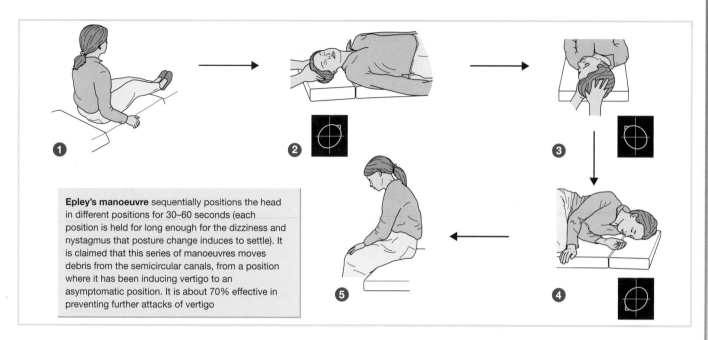

Epley's manoeuvre sequentially positions the head in different positions for 30–60 seconds (each position is held for long enough for the dizziness and nystagmus that posture change induces to settle). It is claimed that this series of manoeuvres moves debris from the semicircular canals, from a position where it has been inducing vertigo to an asymptomatic position. It is about 70% effective in preventing further attacks of vertigo

• Do objects in your vision such as furniture or pictures on the wall actually move around or do you feel as if you are moving? Suggests true vertigo, caused by peripheral pathology affecting the inner ear or cranial nerve VIII, or central pathology affecting the brainstem.

• Do you just have a vague feeling all the time of light-headedness? May represent a variety of problems ranging from hyperventilation through to tension headache. This is sometimes called psychophysical dizziness. It is uncommon to find a clear diagnosis.

• What other symptoms are present? Tinnitus with deafness suggests inner ear pathology. Nausea and vomiting suggest vestibular or brainstem disease. Diplopia suggests brainstem disease. For ataxia, see earlier section.

• What provokes symptoms? If head movement provokes symptoms, then vestibular disease is likely. Provocation on standing suggests postural hypotension.

Once the nature of the symptom has been established, a physical examination should be directed at excluding cardiac arrhythmia or postural hypotension. Then a specific neurological examination should look for evidence of cerebellar and brainstem disease.

Peripheral causes of vertigo

• **Benign paroxysmal positional vertigo** causes recurrent attacks of transient (lasting seconds) dizziness and vertigo associated with changes in head posture, e.g. lying on the pillow at night. Attacks tend to persist for weeks or months before spontaneously resolving, but may recur. Conventional physical examination is normal. Hallpike's manoeuvre is a specific provocation test performed by bringing the patient from a sitting position down onto their back while turning the head briskly in one direction. If positive, there is nystagmus with rotation towards the side of the lesion and the patient's symptoms are replicated. It is caused by debris in the semicircular canals and can be treated by Epley's manoeuvre (see Figure 58.3 above).

• **Acute vestibular failure** is a common clinical problem where patients complain of the sudden onset of nausea, vomiting and severe vertigo. On examination there is nystagmus on lateral gaze and unsteadiness. This condition, which has a good prognosis and tends to resolve over days to weeks, has a variety of synonyms such as 'acute labyrinthitis' and 'vestibular neuronitis' which suggest a possible viral, postviral or inflammatory origin, but betrays our ignorance of the true pathogenesis. It sometimes occurs after an upper respiratory tract infection.

• **Ménière's disease**: recurrent attacks of vertigo, tinnitus and decreased hearing occur in middle life and ultimately may progress to deafness. The attacks build up over minutes, last for hours and then gradually resolve. The key to the diagnosis is to document fluctuating levels of hearing loss.

• **Chronic vestibular failure**: this has a number of causes and presents with a more insidious form of dizziness, which can be rather non-specific in character. Age-related vestibular degeneration is increasingly being recognized.

• **Drugs**, such as high-dose aminoglycosides and furosemide (frusemide) can cause vestibular failure.

Central causes of vertigo

• **Vertebrobasilar ischaemia** is a rarer cause of isolated dizziness than usually thought. Attacks of dizziness of abrupt onset and lasting for several minutes are typical. Most patients with vertebrobasilar ischaemia have other symptoms of brainstem involvement. Brainstem stroke also usually produces other physical signs.

• **Migraine** can cause transient vertigo. Other symptoms of brainstem involvement are usual. A migrainous headache may or may not follow.

• **Brainstem disease**, including multiple sclerosis.

Mixed causes of vertigo

• **Acoustic neuroma**: a benign Schwann cell tumour arising on the vestibular portion of cranial nerve VIII, either isolated or caused by neurofibromatosis type 2 (see Chapter 208), causing deafness and often vertigo. Brainstem compression may cause ataxia and, if severe, aqueduct compression and hydrocephalus. Sensation to the cornea is lost. Magnetic resonance imaging confirms the diagnosis. Surgery may be curative.

59 Weakness

Assessment of weakness

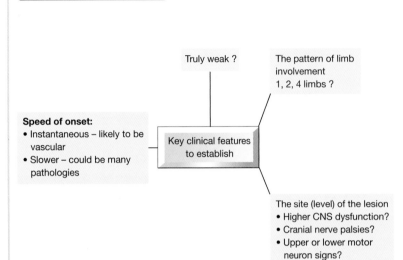

Truly weak ?

The pattern of limb involvement 1, 2, 4 limbs ?

Speed of onset:
- Instantaneous – likely to be vascular
- Slower – could be many pathologies

Key clinical features to establish

The site (level) of the lesion
- Higher CNS dysfunction?
- Cranial nerve palsies?
- Upper or lower motor neuron signs?

Two limbs: Hemiparesis

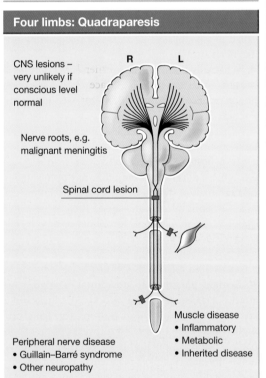

R L

Hemisphere lesion ± language disorder ± neglect

Internal capsule lesion

Brainstem lesion + cranial nerve signs

To arm

To leg

R side affected

One limb: Monoparesis

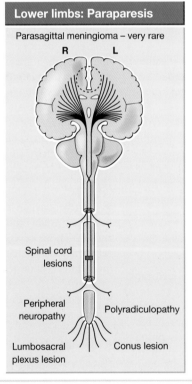

R L

Motor cortex lesion

Internal capsule lesion
No sensory loss, e.g. clumsy hand/ dysarthria syndrome

Plexus lesion, e.g. brachial LMN signs

Motor neuron disease – UMN + LMN signs
L limb affected

Lower limbs: Paraparesis

Parasagittal meningioma – very rare

R L

Spinal cord lesions

Peripheral neuropathy   Polyradiculopathy

Lumbosacral plexus lesion   Conus lesion

Four limbs: Quadraparesis

R L

CNS lesions – very unlikely if conscious level normal

Nerve roots, e.g. malignant meningitis

Spinal cord lesion

Muscle disease
- Inflammatory
- Metabolic
- Inherited disease

Peripheral nerve disease
- Guillain–Barré syndrome
- Other neuropathy

Medicine at a Glance, Fourth Edition. Edited by Patrick Davey. © 2014 John Wiley & Sons, Ltd. Published 2014 by John Wiley & Sons, Ltd. Companion website: www.ataglanceseries.com/medicine

Weakness may be used loosely by patients to include fatigue or tiredness – it is vital to establish that any weakness is genuine, i.e. has led to loss of function (although loss of function may also relate to sensory loss, dyspraxia or incoordination, e.g. as a result of cerebellar disease). It is useful to ask the patient to list the specific activities that cannot be performed (walking, climbing stairs, rising from sitting to standing, reaching above the head, writing, unscrewing lids, etc.). Motor weakness may result from lesions affecting:

- The brain.
- The spinal cord.
- Nerves, neuromuscular junctions or muscles.

In approaching the diagnosis of weakness it is crucial to establish whether the problem is of central or peripheral origin (neuroanatomy, see Chapter 56). Differences between weakness of central (upper motor neuron (UMN)) origin or peripheral (lower motor neuron (LMN)) origin are outlined in Table 59.1. Finally, bear in mind that coexisting medical conditions such as joint disease can lead to difficulties in interpreting neurological weakness.

Weakness of all four limbs

Depending on the evolution and associated physical signs, generalized weakness is most likely to be due to lesions in one of the following structures.

Cerebral hemispheres

It is very unlikely that a patient with a *normal level of consciousness* and generalized weakness has a hemispheric lesion of the brain.

Brainstem

A pontine haemorrhage or other lesion can lead to complete quadriplegia, including the face (locked-in syndrome). Consciousness is usually markedly depressed in the early stages.

Spinal cord

The degree to which weakness is generalized and affects the upper and lower limbs depends on the level of involvement of the spinal cord. Complete weakness affecting all four limbs occurs only if the spinal lesion is above C5. The pathological diagnosis is often suspected from the speed of onset of symptoms:

- Acute: cord compression, anterior spinal artery thrombosis and acute transverse myelitis.
- Subacute: intrinsic spinal cord tumours, vascular malformations of the dura, vitamin B_{12} deficiency and malignant meningeal infiltration.
- Chronic: benign tumours, syringomyelia and inherited conditions – hereditary spastic paraparesis (although this usually affects only the legs), spinocerebellar ataxias (e.g. Friedreich's ataxia) and tropical spastic paraparesis caused by human T-lymphocyte virus 1 infection.

Nerve roots

Inflammation, such as that caused by viral infection (cytomegalovirus, varicella-zoster virus) of the nerve roots can cause weakness in all four limbs, as can malignant infiltration spread through the cerebrospinal fluid (malignant meningitis).

Polyneuropathy

Diffuse nerve damage can cause weakness of all four limbs, such as occurs in Guillain–Barré syndrome (see Chapter 211), chronic inflammatory demyelinating polyneuropathy or inherited neuropathies such as hereditary motor and sensory neuropathy. Other causes include critical illness polyneuropathy, diphtheria, sarcoidosis, Lyme disease, borreliosis and amyloid. In general there is a distal predominant pattern of weakness.

Muscle disease

Inflammatory, metabolic or inherited muscle disease can all produce a diffuse weakness (see Chapter 210).

Table 59.1 Weakness of central and peripheral origin.

	Upper motor neuron (usually pyramidal tract)	Extrapyramidal or basal ganglia disorders	Lower motor neuron	Muscular	Neuromuscular junction
Pattern of weakness	Limb weakness often incomplete, affecting large movements Most marked in the extensors of upper limb and flexors of lower limb	No true loss of muscle power, but failure of integration of agonist and antagonist muscles Generalized throughout a whole limb	Usually marked, affecting specific muscle groups, except in diffuse polyneuropathies Maximal distally in polyneuropathies	Usually generalized, unless one muscle is injured Maximal proximally and usually symmetrical: neck and swallowing and eye muscles may be involved	Variable but fatiguable, ptosis and extraocular muscle weakness common
Tone	Spasticity: velocity-dependent resistance to movement Clasp knife reflex Clonus	Rigidity	Decreased	Normal or decreased	Normal
Reflexes	Brisk	Normal	Reduced or absent	Normal	Normal or depressed (Eaton–Lambert syndrome)
Muscle appearance	Disuse atrophy after prolonged weakness, but no true wasting	Normal	Segmental wasting; fasciculation if lesion at the level of anterior horn cell	Normal or atrophic	Usually normal

Weakness of one limb

This is a difficult problem clinically and can arise from lesions almost anywhere in the nervous system.

Cortical lesions

Cortical lesions affecting the motor pathways to the limbs can start as a problem isolated to one limb. UMN signs are found. Lacunar strokes affecting the basis pontis can give rise to clumsiness and weakness of one hand.

Motor neuron disease

Motor neuron disease not infrequently begins in one limb with foot drop or wasting of the intrinsic hand muscles, although subtle signs can often be seen in other limbs.

Spinal cord lesions

Spinal cord lesions at the appropriate level can give rise to weakness of one leg associated with loss of pain and temperature in the contralateral leg.

Plexopathy

A plexopathy (brachial or lumbosacral) can affect an arm or a leg. Inflammatory diseases such as brachial neuritis or diabetic amyotrophy are examples.

Involvement of multiple large motor nerves (mononeuritis multiplex)

Mononeuritis multiplex can present in one limb or asymmetrically involve several limbs. Mononeuritis multiplex is usually a consequence of an underlying systemic disease process (see Table 59.1). Multiple root lesions can produce a similar pattern.

Isolated mononeuropathy

An isolated mononeuropathy, e.g. femoral, can give rise to isolated weakness of one limb.

Weakness of one side of the body

A hemiparesis can arise in a wide variety of locations.

Contralateral cerebral hemisphere

Damage to the contralateral cerebral hemisphere can cause weakness down one side of the body, when it may be associated with other physical signs (e.g. language dysfunction in the dominant hemisphere, neglect in the non-dominant hemisphere).

Brainstem

Vascular occlusion in this area can cause a number of eponymous syndromes:

- In the midbrain there will be hemiplegia with a contralateral third nerve palsy (Weber's syndrome).
- In the pons, the weakness will be associated with conjugate gaze deviation towards the weak limbs and there may be a contralateral LMN facial weakness.

Spinal cord

See Chapter 209.

Weakness of both lower limbs (paraparesis)

- Spinal cord lesion.
- Peripheral neuropathy.
- Bilateral involvement of the lumbosacral plexus.
- Motor neuron disease.

Rarely, bilateral parasagittal lesions in the brain, classically a meningioma (although this is very rare), or other bilateral pathologies may also be responsible.

Weakness of both upper limbs

- Spinal cord lesion.
- Unusual forms of motor neuron disease.
- Bilateral brachial neuritis.

60 Disturbance of vision: a neurological perspective

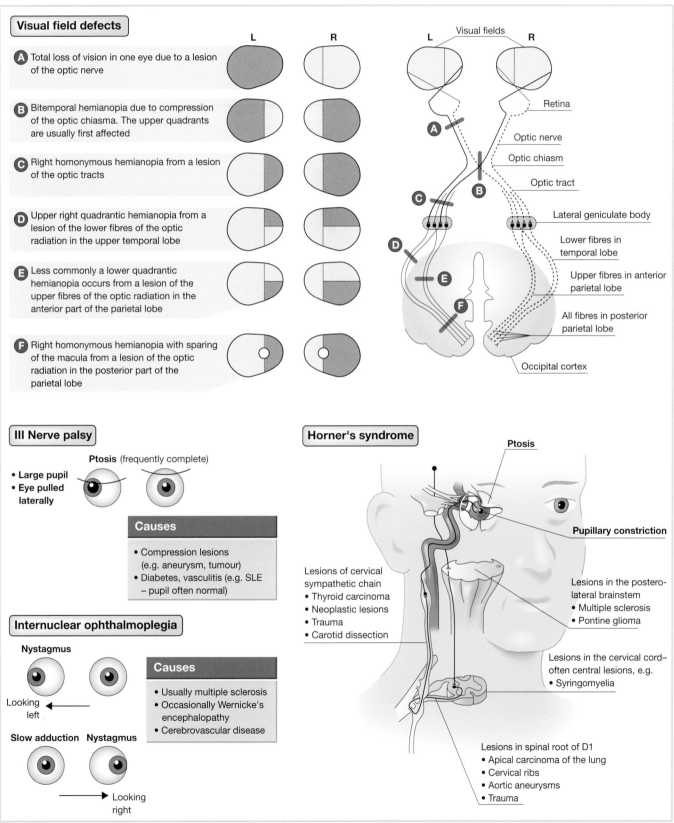

Visual field defects

A Total loss of vision in one eye due to a lesion of the optic nerve

B Bitemporal hemianopia due to compression of the optic chiasma. The upper quadrants are usually first affected

C Right homonymous hemianopia from a lesion of the optic tracts

D Upper right quadrantic hemianopia from a lesion of the lower fibres of the optic radiation in the upper temporal lobe

E Less commonly a lower quadrantic hemianopia occurs from a lesion of the upper fibres of the optic radiation in the anterior part of the parietal lobe

F Right homonymous hemianopia with sparing of the macula from a lesion of the optic radiation in the posterior part of the parietal lobe

Visual fields

Retina
Optic nerve
Optic chiasm
Optic tract
Lateral geniculate body
Lower fibres in temporal lobe
Upper fibres in anterior parietal lobe
All fibres in posterior parietal lobe
Occipital cortex

III Nerve palsy

Ptosis (frequently complete)

- Large pupil
- Eye pulled laterally

Causes

- Compression lesions (e.g. aneurysm, tumour)
- Diabetes, vasculitis (e.g. SLE – pupil often normal)

Internuclear ophthalmoplegia

Nystagmus

Looking left

Slow adduction   Nystagmus

Looking right

Causes

- Usually multiple sclerosis
- Occasionally Wernicke's encephalopathy
- Cerebrovascular disease

Horner's syndrome

Ptosis

Pupillary constriction

Lesions of cervical sympathetic chain
- Thyroid carcinoma
- Neoplastic lesions
- Trauma
- Carotid dissection

Lesions in the postero-lateral brainstem
- Multiple sclerosis
- Pontine glioma

Lesions in the cervical cord– often central lesions, e.g.
- Syringomyelia

Lesions in spinal root of D1
- Apical carcinoma of the lung
- Cervical ribs
- Aortic aneurysms
- Trauma

Medicine at a Glance, Fourth Edition. Edited by Patrick Davey. © 2014 John Wiley & Sons, Ltd. Published 2014 by John Wiley & Sons, Ltd. Companion website: www.ataglanceseries.com/medicine

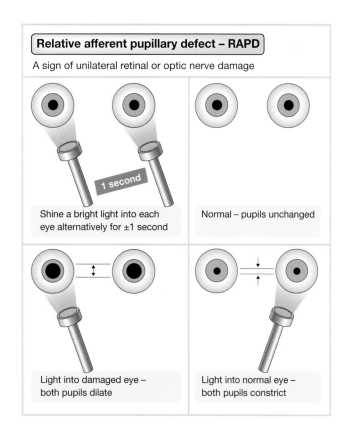

Relative afferent pupillary defect – RAPD

A sign of unilateral retinal or optic nerve damage

1 second

Shine a bright light into each eye alternately for ±1 second

Normal – pupils unchanged

Light into damaged eye – both pupils dilate

Light into normal eye – both pupils constrict

Visual loss

Monocular visual loss

This is a lesion anterior to the optic chiasma:

- The eye: cornea, lens and vitreous, e.g. cataract or vitreous haemorrhage.
- The retina, especially the fovea, e.g. diabetic retinopathy or macular degeneration.
- The optic nerve, e.g. optic neuritis or ischaemic optic neuropathy.

Bilateral involvement of these structures causes bilateral visual loss.

Binocular visual loss

This is a lesion at or behind the chiasma:

- Optic chiasma: classically bitemporal.
- Optic radiation: homonymous – either quadrantanopia (superior: temporal lobe, affecting Meyer's loop; inferior: parietal) or hemianopia.
- Visual cortex: homonymous, often hemianopia.

Typical clinical presentations of 'neurological' causes of visual loss

Brief monocular or binocular visual loss

- Amaurosis fugax: brief unilateral blindness lasting minutes (see Chapter 201).
- Brief transient visual obscurations, caused by idiopathic intracranial hypertension with papilloedema, may occur in one or both eyes. More common in obese young women with headache. The cause is often undefined; some cases are the result of sagittal sinus thrombosis. Acute papilloedema alone has an enlarged blind spot but no visual loss.

Sudden painless loss of vision in one eye

Sudden painless loss of vision in one eye is the result of:

- Anterior ischaemic optic neuropathy: profound, irreversible visual loss with a pale swollen optic disc; caused by atheroma emboli or temporal arteritis (see Chaper 222).
- Established retinal arterial or venous occlusion: visible with the ophthalmoscope.

Rapid progressive monocular visual loss

Rapid and progressive monocular loss of vision as a result of optic neuritis typically comes on over a few days. Symptoms range from clouding of vision with a vague central scotoma to marked monocular blindness. Pain is variable, but characteristically occurs on looking to one side. Signs comprise loss of colour vision, a relative afferent pupil defect, papilloedema early on and optic atrophy weeks/months later. Eyesight improves over a few weeks, although diminished colour vision may be permanent. If the brain shows evidence of demyelinating lesions on magnetic resonance imaging, there is at least an 80% chance of subsequent multiple sclerosis (MS).

Progressive night blindness

Progressive night blindness occurs in retinitis pigmentosa (RP), causes peripheral concentric field loss and spicular pigmentation on fundoscopy. Genetically there are many types, with X-linked or autosomal (dominant or recessive) inheritance. RP is associated with certain neurological syndromes, e.g. Refsum's or Usher's syndromes.

Bitemporal quadrantic or hemianopia

Bitemporal quadrantic or hemianopia is found in a pituitary lesion that compresses the optic chiasma, usually a macroadenoma. This is often slowly progressive and relatively asymptomatic, unless endocrine features are prominent or pituitary infarction occurs (see Chapters 159 and 164).

Homonymous hemianopia

Homonymous hemianopia may indicate a structural lesion of the hemisphere affecting the optic radiation or visual cortex (rarely the optic tract). Common causes include infarct, haemorrhage and tumour.

Visual neglect and visual hallucinations

Visual neglect suggests a parietal lobe lesion, in the presence of intact visual fields. Visual hallucinations, including macropsia or micropsia, result from disease of the visual cortex.

Migraine

See Chapter 63.

Double vision

Double vision may be the result of lesions of the oculomotor cranial nerves, the brain (usually the brainstem), neuromuscular junction or muscles or other disease of the orbit (e.g. Graves' ophthalmopathy, head trauma). It is useful to establish the pattern, e.g. worse in one direction, on near or far vision, or at different times of the day.

Cranial nerve palsies

- In **sixth nerve palsy**, horizontal doubling – worse in the distance and on looking laterally – occurs. Looking straight ahead, there is a convergent squint as the affected eye is held adducted (unopposed medial rectus action). Causes include raised intracranial pressure, compression of the sixth nerve and microvascular disease. In children, sixth nerve palsy can follow a viral infection.

- **Fourth nerve palsy** is rare and causes diplopia on looking down, in and near, i.e. reading, eating and walking down stairs. On examination, there is failure to depress the eye when held in adduction (on abduction the eye is depressed by the inferior rectus).
- In **third nerve palsy** diplopia is complex and occurs in most directions. Ptosis (often complete) and pupil dilatation occur (compare Horner's syndrome which has partial ptosis and pupil constriction). The eye is abducted as a result of unopposed lateral rectus action. It is caused by compressive lesions, e.g. posterior communicating artery aneurysms, tumours and microvascular disease (hypertension, diabetes – pupil usually spared).

Internuclear ophthalmoplegia

Internuclear ophthalmoplegia is caused by medial longitudinal fasciculus damage, which connects the third and sixth nerve nuclei to allow fluent rapid lateral gaze. There is failure of prompt ipsilateral adduction on saccadic movement, and contralateral abducting nystagmus may be seen. Usually a sign of MS (especially if bilateral) but can also occur in other inflammatory lesions and vascular events in the brainstem. It is frequently asymptomatic.

Brainstem lesions

Diplopia with other cranial nerve signs suggests brainstem disease (or cavernous sinus/orbital apex, depending on which nerves are involved). Isolated nuclear cranial nerve palsies may be found, but failure of conjugate gaze is more common. The eyes may be held in skew deviation; there may be gaze instability, nystagmus or failure of upgaze/downgaze. Causes include MS, stroke or tumour, or Wernicke's encephalopathy.

Cerebellar disease

Cerebellar disease may affect conjugate gaze but instability of vision is the usual symptom, rather than diplopia. Nystagmus is common.

Myasthenia gravis

Myasthenia gravis almost always has eye involvement. Diplopia is a common presentation, usually with ptosis. Any muscles can be affected, but the medial rectus is particularly susceptible. The pattern of doubling and the precise signs found are variable and may include fatigue.

Mitochondrial myopathies

Mitochondrial myopathies can present with chronic progressive external ophthalmoplegia and ptosis. They are rarely associated with diplopia, as malalignment is so gradual. Mitochondrial diseases are rare, though important. They can present in multiple different ways (Table 60.1). Damage to the external eye muscles, retina and/or optic nerve is commonly found in the many different forms of mitochondrial disease, and causes defects in vision appropriate for the location of the damage.

Thyroid disease

See Chapter 161.

Table 60.1 Mitochondrial diseases (prevalence is 10–15 per 100 000, i.e. about 6000–9000 in the UK).

Syndrome	Clinical features
MELAS syndrome	Seizures
(*M*itochondrial *e*ncephalomyopathy *lactic acidosis* and *stroke*-like episodes)	Episodes of unconsciousness with lactic acidosis Stroke-like episodes
PEO	Ptosis, external ophthalmoplegia, limb myopathy
(*P*rogressive *external ophthalmoplegia*)	Kearns–Sayre syndrome variant; develops age ≤20 years, + pigmentary retinopathy, ataxia and heart block
MERRF	Myoclonic epilepsy
(*M*yoclonic *epilepsy* with *ragged red fibres*)	Cerebellar ataxia
	Myopathy
NARP (*N*europathy, *ataxia* and *retinitis pigmentosa*)	Proximal muscle weakness, sensory neuropathy, retinal pigmentary degeneration, developmental delay; dementia
	Ataxia, seizures
LHON	Painless subacute visual loss
(*L*eber's *hereditary optic neuropathy*)	Scotomas
	Abnormal colour vision
Others, including aminoglycoside-induced deafness (AID), maternally inherited Leigh's syndrome (MILS), Pearson's syndrome (PS)	Variable, usually suggested by the title; cardiomyopathy and deafness common in AID, sideroblastic anaemia and pancreatic failure in PS

Pupils

Large

- Both pupils enlarge in response to dim lighting, fear, intoxication (e.g. cannabis, deadly nightshade) or death.
- One pupil enlarged may be the result of parasympathetic palsy (e.g. third nerve compression), Adie's pupil or iris paralysis (e.g. dilating drops or trauma).

Small

- Both pupils constrict with bright light, near focus, intoxication (e.g. opiates or cholinesterase inhibitors) or pontine haemorrhage.
- One constricted pupil may be the result of a sympathetic palsy (Horner's syndrome), pilocarpine use or iritis.

61 Sudden painless loss of vision

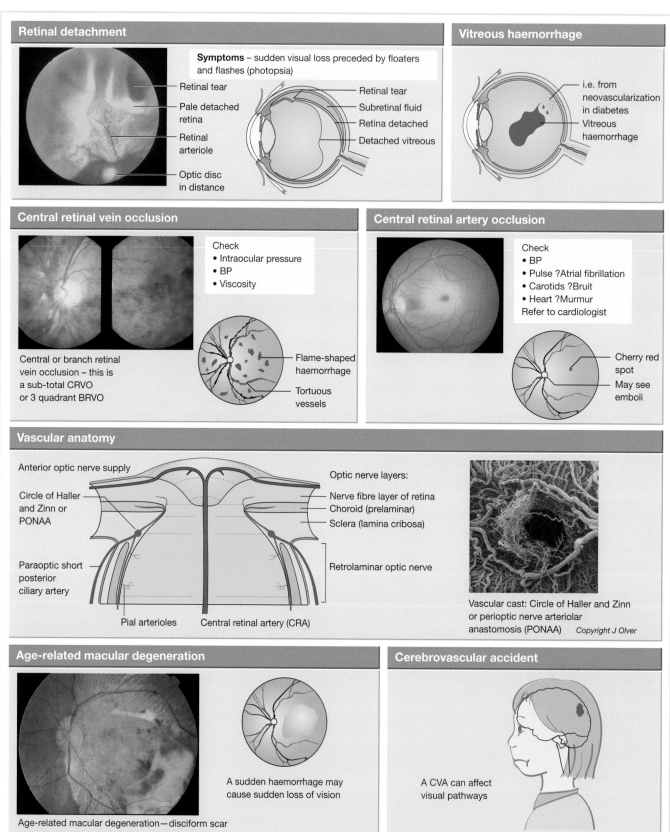

Retinal detachment

Symptoms – sudden visual loss preceded by floaters and flashes (photopsia)

- Retinal tear
- Pale detached retina
- Retinal arteriole
- Optic disc in distance

- Retinal tear
- Subretinal fluid
- Retina detached
- Detached vitreous

Vitreous haemorrhage

i.e. from neovascularization in diabetes
Vitreous haemorrhage

Central retinal vein occlusion

Check
- Intraocular pressure
- BP
- Viscosity

Central or branch retinal vein occlusion – this is a sub-total CRVO or 3 quadrant BRVO

- Flame-shaped haemorrhage
- Tortuous vessels

Central retinal artery occlusion

Check
- BP
- Pulse ?Atrial fibrillation
- Carotids ?Bruit
- Heart ?Murmur
Refer to cardiologist

- Cherry red spot
- May see emboli

Vascular anatomy

Anterior optic nerve supply

Circle of Haller and Zinn or PONAA

Paraoptic short posterior ciliary artery

Pial arterioles   Central retinal artery (CRA)

Optic nerve layers:
- Nerve fibre layer of retina
- Choroid (prelaminar)
- Sclera (lamina cribosa)

Retrolaminar optic nerve

Vascular cast: Circle of Haller and Zinn or perioptic nerve arteriolar anastomosis (PONAA)   *Copyright J Olver*

Age-related macular degeneration

Age-related macular degeneration—disciform scar

A sudden haemorrhage may cause sudden loss of vision

Cerebrovascular accident

A CVA can affect visual pathways

Medicine at a Glance, Fourth Edition. Edited by Patrick Davey. © 2014 John Wiley & Sons, Ltd. Published 2014 by John Wiley & Sons, Ltd. Companion website: www.ataglanceseries.com/medicine

The main causes of painless loss of vision are: vascular occlusion of the retina, optic nerve or brain; acephalgic migraine; vitreous haemorrhage; retinal detachment.

Vascular occlusion

Retinal vein occlusion

Central retinal vein occlusion (CRVO) or branch retinal vein occlusion (BRVO) presents with sudden unilateral painless loss of vision. The diagnosis is made on ophthalmoscopic appearance, which shows multiple blot and flame retinal haemorrhages. It is caused by: systemic hypertension, hyperviscosity, vessel wall disease such as diabetes or inflammation (e.g. sarcoidosis), raised intraocular pressure.

Management

- As CRVO and BRVO are strongly associated with arteriosclerosis, blood pressure (BP) must be checked and evidence sought of arterial disease elsewhere (determine from the history whether there are any symptoms of myocardial infarction, stroke or claudication; feel all the pulses, listen for arterial bruits).
- Check intraocular pressure.
- Check for diabetes and systemic inflammation.

Younger patients presenting with CRVO or BRVO, especially those with a past history or family history of thrombosis, or older patients in whom there is no obvious cause, should be investigated for hyperviscosity syndromes or thrombophilia.

Retinal artery occlusion

Central retinal artery occlusion or branch retinal artery occlusion also present as acute, painless, unilateral loss of vision. The ophthalmoscope shows pale retinal ischaemia, perhaps with a foveal cherry-red spot, and may show a retinal embolus. If unilateral visual loss is profound, a relative afferent pupillary defect will be present.

Aetiology

- Arterial embolus from diseased carotid, left-sided valvular heart disease, left ventricular mural thrombus, or atrial fibrillation with left atrial thrombus.
- Examine the patient carefully, considering that some part of the 'arterial organ' is damaged.

Management

Control risk factors and if appropriate consider carotid endarterectomy, aspirin or cardiac intervention.

Non-arteritic anterior or posterior ischaemic optic neuropathy

This form of occlusion is usually painless, unlike the arteritic form associated with giant cell arteritis, which is usually associated with headache or jaw pain. Visual loss may be altitudinal – loss of the top or bottom half of the visual field – often in stepwise episodes.

- In anterior ischaemic optic neuropathy (AION) the optic disc is swollen. Swelling may be segmental or involve the entire nerve head. There are often associated splinter haemorrhages on the disc.
- In posterior ischaemic optic neuropathy (PION) the optic disc looks normal.

Aetiology

- Occlusion of the small ciliary vessels supplying the optic nerve head (AION) or posterior optic nerve (PION).

- Arteritis must be ruled out with normal erythrocyte sedimentation rate and C-reactive protein. Consider a temporal artery biopsy if in doubt.
- Risk factors include smoking, arteriosclerosis, hypertension, hypotensive episode and 'disc at risk' – a small optic nerve head with no central cup.

Management

Control risk factors. Unlike the arteritic form, corticosteroids have no place in the management.

Cerebrovascular accident

A haemorrhagic or embolic cerebrovascular accident (CVA) affecting the posterior visual pathways – radiation or cortex – will present as acute painless visual loss. Depending on the site of the lesion, the patient will have a corresponding contralateral homonymous hemi or quadrantic field defect to confrontation (see Chapter 60). It is rare for visual loss to be the only symptom.

Acephalgic migraine

This form of migraine presents with transient visual disturbance involving both eyes, in the absence of headache. A homonymous scintillating scotoma evolves over about 20 minutes, and then subsides.

Vitreous haemorrhage

Haemorrhage into the vitreous cavity can result in sudden painless loss of vision. The extent of visual loss will depend on the degree of haemorrhage.

- A large haemorrhage may cause almost total unilateral visual loss.
- A small haemorrhage presents as floaters with normal, or only slightly reduced, visual acuity.

Aetiology

- Proliferative retinopathy with spontaneous rupture of abnormal fragile new vessels that grow on the retinal surface. The most common cause is diabetes.
- Warfarin may predispose.
- Vitreous or retinal detachment: a small retinal blood vessel may rupture when the retinal break occurs.
- Trauma.
- Posterior vitreous detachment can result in vitreous haemorrhage if, as the vitreous separates from the retina, it pulls and ruptures a small blood vessel.

Management

Refer to an ophthalmologist to determine cause and manage accordingly.

Retinal detachment

- Sudden, or rapid, painless loss of vision.
- Often preceded by symptoms of flashing lights (photopsia) and/or floaters and/or visual field defect.
- When the macula is not involved, the visual loss involves the peripheral field and visual acuity may be normal.
- Once the macula is involved, the central vision is lost.

Management

Refer to an ophthalmologist to consider laser to a retinal tear or retinal surgery ± vitrectomy for a full detachment.

62 Tremor and other involuntary movements

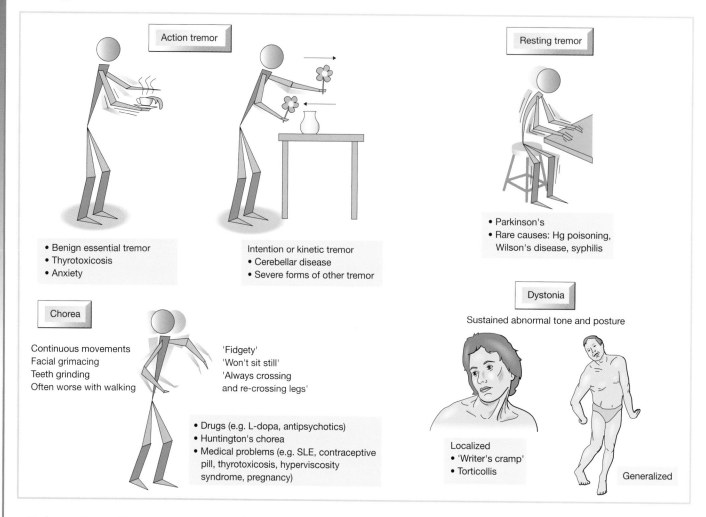

Action tremor

- Benign essential tremor
- Thyrotoxicosis
- Anxiety

Intention or kinetic tremor
- Cerebellar disease
- Severe forms of other tremor

Resting tremor

- Parkinson's
- Rare causes: Hg poisoning, Wilson's disease, syphilis

Chorea

Continuous movements
Facial grimacing
Teeth grinding
Often worse with walking

'Fidgety'
'Won't sit still'
'Always crossing
and re-crossing legs'

- Drugs (e.g. L-dopa, antipsychotics)
- Huntington's chorea
- Medical problems (e.g. SLE, contraceptive pill, thyrotoxicosis, hyperviscosity syndrome, pregnancy)

Dystonia

Sustained abnormal tone and posture

Localized
- 'Writer's cramp'
- Torticollis

Generalized

Understanding and interpreting movement disorders depends on having a precise grasp of the terminology used to describe the phenomenology of abnormal movement and posture.

Tremor is the *involuntary, rhythmical oscillation* of a muscle group around a joint. It should be distinguished from other involuntary movements such as dyskinesia, chorea, myoclonus, tics and mannerisms (defined later). Measuring the frequency of the tremor is not often of value in distinguishing the cause. There are, in clinical practice, only three common types of tremor (see Table 62.1):

1 Resting tremor: if asymmetrical this is almost pathognomonic of idiopathic **Parkinson's disease**.
2 Postural tremor, which is usually the result of **essential tremor**.
3 Action or kinetic tremor, which is a feature of **cerebellar dysfunction**.

Common causes of tremor

Essential tremor
Essential tremor is usually symmetrical and barely present at rest, becomes pronounced on movement and posture (the rattling of a teacup is suggestive of the diagnosis), and can be relieved by small amounts of alcohol, although this effect wanes with time. It is often associated with a family history and is very rarely disabling.

Cerebellar disease
The characteristic feature of cerebellar tremor is that it is brought out at the end of movement. The head may be involved. Isolated tremor is most unusual and usually there are other signs of cerebellar dysfunction.

Parkinsonism
Parkinson's tremor is of asymmetrical onset, is most prominent at rest, and is reduced by voluntary action (see Chapter 212). Head tremor is not characteristic of idiopathic Parkinson's disease, but the jaw is frequently involved.

Dystonic tremor
See section on dystonias.

Drugs and toxins
● Alcohol withdrawal: though tremor is extremely common, and indeed almost universal in alcohol withdrawal, the clinical condition is usually dominated by other features, especially neuropsychiatric ones, including difficult behaviour, acute

Medicine at a Glance, Fourth Edition. Edited by Patrick Davey. © 2014 John Wiley & Sons, Ltd. Published 2014 by John Wiley & Sons, Ltd. Companion website: www.ataglanceseries.com/medicine

Table 62.1 Types of tremor and their features.

	Maximal	Distribution	Response to movement	Involvement of head
Essential tremor	Action and postural	Symmetrical	Worse	If severe
Parkinsonian	Rest, abolished by action	Asymmetrical	Abolished	Never (but does involve jaw)
Cerebellar	Kinetic	Symmetrical, frequently head	Accentuated at end of movement	Frequent

confusional state, hallucinations and seizures. Patients are not infrequently jaundiced, with other stigmata of liver disease, such as spider naevi, ascites, etc.

- Sodium valproate.
- Lithium.
- Caffeine.
- Heavy metal poisoning.

Metabolic

- Thyrotoxicosis.
- Phaeochromocytoma.
- Hepatic encephalopathy.
- Wilson's disease: rare (one in 33 000–100 000), autosomal recessive disease caused by mutations/deletions of the ATP7B gene. Fifty per cent present with movement disorders and neuropsychiatric disturbance (nearly all patients with neurological symptoms have Kayser–Fleischer rings), the remainder with liver disease, anaemia or by proband screening. Screening for Wilson's disease, which is a treatable cause of neurodegeneration, should be considered in any patient presenting with new onset tremor below the age of 50 years.

Other abnormal movements

Myoclonus

This comprises brief, explosive 'electric shock'-like activation of a group of muscles, often involving a whole limb. It is reasonable to think of this as an 'epileptic' phenomenon which can arise from anywhere in the central nervous system, including the brainstem and spinal cord. There are a very large number of causes, ranging from vascular disease, drugs and metabolic derangements to neurodegenerative disease such as spongiform encephalopathies.

Dystonias

These are sustained, abnormal tone and posture of a group of muscles, which can be:
- **Focal**, e.g. writer's cramp, torticollis (now known as 'idiopathic cervical dystonia') and hemifacial spasm.
- **Generalized**, e.g. generalized torsion dystonia, a condition of abnormal writhing movements, which may be genetic (dominantly inherited) or symptomatic of other conditions (drugs, structural lesions of the brain, neurodegenerative disease).

Dystonia frequently presents as a tremor which can be misdiagnosed as either Parkinson's disease or essential tremor. Dystonic tremor commonly affects the upper limb, when it is usually unilateral or markedly asymmetrical, or the head, resulting in a 'no-no' side-to-side tremor.

Chorea

These are continuous, random, flowing or dancing movements of the extremities, which in its mildest form may be turned into semipurposeful movements such that the patient just appears fidgety. The definition of the ad hoc Committee on Classification of the World Federation of Neurology is helpful, and states that chorea is 'a state of excessive, spontaneous movements, irregularly timed, non-repetitive, randomly distributed and abrupt in character. These movements may vary in severity from restlessness with mild intermittent exaggeration of gesture and expression, fidgeting movements of the hands, unstable dance-like gait to a continuous flow of disabling, violent movements.'

There are multiple causes, including:
- **Drug-induced syndromes**: continuous dyskinesia merging into chorea not infrequently complicates long-term Parkinson's disease, where long-term treatment with dopamine and its agonists may be contributory. Similarly, the restless movements complicating long-term treatment with dopamine antagonists, such as the neuroleptic drugs used for major psychosis, can appear choreiform.
- **Huntington's disease** (HD): abnormal movements are the presenting symptom in 50–75% of HD patients. Indeed, choreiform movements can, occasionally, be so profound as to result in severe weight loss due to the high-energy expenditure resulting from nearly continuous motor activity. Chorea is particularly prevalent in those who present at an older age; HD presenting in childhood is dominated by rigidity and cognitive decline. In the majority of patients presenting in mid-adult life, personality change (e.g. impulsivity) may precede chorea with overt cognitive decline occurring later.
- **Sydenham's chorea**: this is a complication of rheumatic fever, which most typically occurs some 1–6 months after an acute attack of rheumatic fever. However, it has been described as occurring up to 30 years after the acute attack. This means that the history is often the vital aspect of the diagnosis, rather than the finding of raised antistreptococcal antibodies. Chorea often occurs in isolation.
- **Systemic lupus erythematosus** (SLE).
- **Oral contraceptive pill**.
- **Hyperviscosity syndromes**.
- **Pregnancy**.
- **Thyrotoxicosis**: while tremor is almost universal in hyperthyroidism chorea, and well described, it is extraordinarily rare. It usually resolves on successfully treating the overactive thyroid.
- **Antiphospholipid syndrome**: most patients (c. 90%) with this syndrome who develop chorea are female, about 25% develop symptoms either on the pill or when pregnant; it is unilateral in 45%, and 35% have abnormalities on brain magnetic resonance imaging.
- There are many **other causes** including Wilson's disease.

Dyskinesias

These are disorders of movement integration, which may have choreiform or dystonic components. The term is usually used for drug-induced movements caused by neuroleptics or Parkinson's disease or its treatment.

Tics

Tics are stereotyped explosive movements, under partial voluntary control, which are recognizably part of the normal movement repertoire (e.g. blinking or winking).

63 Headache and facial pain

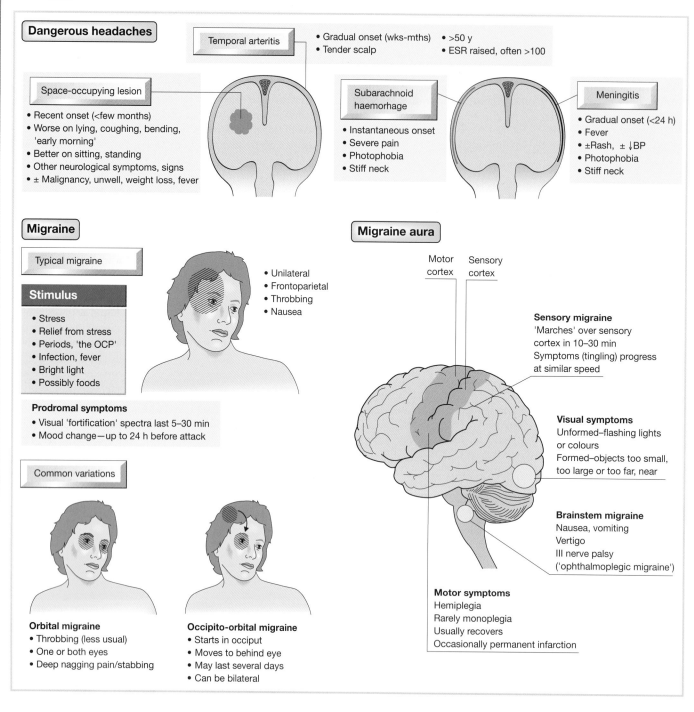

Dangerous headaches

Temporal arteritis
- Gradual onset (wks-mths)
- Tender scalp
- >50 y
- ESR raised, often >100

Space-occupying lesion
- Recent onset (<few months)
- Worse on lying, coughing, bending, 'early morning'
- Better on sitting, standing
- Other neurological symptoms, signs
- ± Malignancy, unwell, weight loss, fever

Subarachnoid haemorhage
- Instantaneous onset
- Severe pain
- Photophobia
- Stiff neck

Meningitis
- Gradual onset (<24 h)
- Fever
- ±Rash, ± ↓BP
- Photophobia
- Stiff neck

Migraine

Typical migraine

Stimulus
- Stress
- Relief from stress
- Periods, 'the OCP'
- Infection, fever
- Bright light
- Possibly foods

- Unilateral
- Frontoparietal
- Throbbing
- Nausea

Prodromal symptoms
- Visual 'fortification' spectra last 5–30 min
- Mood change—up to 24 h before attack

Common variations

Orbital migraine
- Throbbing (less usual)
- One or both eyes
- Deep nagging pain/stabbing

Occipito-orbital migraine
- Starts in occiput
- Moves to behind eye
- May last several days
- Can be bilateral

Migraine aura

Motor cortex   Sensory cortex

Sensory migraine
'Marches' over sensory cortex in 10–30 min
Symptoms (tingling) progress at similar speed

Visual symptoms
Unformed–flashing lights or colours
Formed–objects too small, too large or too far, near

Brainstem migraine
Nausea, vomiting
Vertigo
III nerve palsy
('ophthalmoplegic migraine')

Motor symptoms
Hemiplegia
Rarely monoplegia
Usually recovers
Occasionally permanent infarction

Headache is a subjective sensation, so the patient and not the doctor has to define its presence or absence. The brain is insensate: pain in the head and face arises from the trigeminovascular system, which supplies the meninges, or from bony or ligamentous structures. As an isolated symptom (i.e. no other symptoms or neurological signs), it is almost never indicative of structural brain disease (and is referred to as 'primary headache'). The following isolated headaches are exceptions and may indicate underlying disease:

- 'Thunderclap' headache: may be the result of subarachnoid or intracerebral haemorrhage.
- Headache gradually increasing in severity over several hours with fever, photophobia and neck stiffness (not all components need be present) suggests acute meningitis, a medical emergency. Immediate intravenous antibiotics are given if definitive diagnosis (usually established by lumbar puncture) is unavoidably delayed. Chronic meningitis may cause isolated headache that is progressive over days to weeks.

Medicine at a Glance, Fourth Edition. Edited by Patrick Davey. © 2014 John Wiley & Sons, Ltd. Published 2014 by John Wiley & Sons, Ltd. Companion website: www.ataglanceseries.com/medicine

- Exertional headache, or headache occurring exclusively on coughing, sneezing or stooping: occasionally caused by vascular malformations of the brain or lesions of the foramen magnum, e.g. the Arnold–Chiari malformation.
- Postural headache: may indicate abnormalities of cerebrospinal fluid pressure (high or low).
- Headache waking the patient from sleep: although most often the result of benign conditions, e.g. migraine, this should prompt a search for a structural lesion by careful physical examination (e.g. for hemiplegia) and consideration of neuroimaging.
- New and continuous headache in those aged over 50 years raises the possibility of temporal arteritis. The scalp may be tender. A raised erythrocyte sedimentation rate (ESR) supports the diagnosis (see Chapter 222).

Classification of primary headache

Migraine

The core features of migraine are headache, typically but not exclusively unilateral, nausea and vomiting, and variable constitutional upset (fatigue, carbohydrate craving, diuresis), which usually lasts <48 hours. There are two main types:

- **Migraine with aura**: there is a prodrome of neurological symptoms, evolving gradually over a few minutes, unlike stroke or transient ischaemia where symptoms arise instantaneously. These prodromal symptoms comprise:
  - Visual phenomena: positive (scintillations, fortification spectra, etc.) or negative (scotomata, hemianopia).
  - Altered sensations of the face or limbs.
  - Occasional rare variants such as 'basilar' migraine with double vision and vertigo, and ophthalmoplegic and hemiplegic migraine.
- **Migraine without aura**: there are no accompanying neurological symptoms or signs but nausea and the other constitutional features are still present.

Acute attacks may respond to simple analgesia if given quickly (paracetamol or high-dose aspirin in soluble form; codeine-based preparations are contraindicated because of nausea and rebound headache). Triptans (e.g. sumatriptan) are usually reserved for severe recurrent attacks and ergotamine is now used rarely. Prophylaxis is indicated for debilitating attacks occurring several times a month and propranolol, topiramate, sodium valproate and pizotifen have all been shown to work in selected patients.

Tension-type headache

This is an unsatisfactory term because patients believe that they are being criticized as being tense. The relationship to psychosocial stress is uncertain and variable but the symptoms are still disabling. The key features are:

- A dull generalized headache, usually poorly localized (occasionally localized over the eyes), sometimes referred to as a 'fuzzy head'.
- Poor response to over-the-counter analgesia.
- Worsening throughout the day.
- Duration of days to weeks.

Some neurologists consider this to be a variant of migraine and it is not uncommon to find both types of headache in the same patient or to find a cluster of migraines merging into tension headache. They do not usually respond to antimigraine therapy but some respond to low-dose amitriptyline.

Chronic daily headache

This describes patients who have a non-specific, non-disabling headache on most days (4% of the UK population). It is unresponsive to simple analgesia and difficult to treat.

Cluster headache

This is more common in men (9:1) and characterized by episodes of severe unilateral headache of extreme to excruciating intensity, often arising from sleep. Eye watering may occur; duration is 10–60 minutes. Patients prefer to move around. Occurs in clusters, typically daily for 6–8 weeks before disappearing completely. Acute treatment is with triptan antimigraine therapy; some respond to high-flow oxygen. Prophylaxis is with verapamil or lithium. Once started, clusters can sometimes be aborted with a reducing course of prednisolone.

Indomethacin-responsive headaches

These are a group of unusual headache syndromes, which are defined by the specific response to indomethacin. Paroxysmal hemicrania is a unilateral, lancinating headache of great severity, which continues throughout the day. Patients describe paroxysms of sharp jabbing, lasting for seconds and often localized behind the eye. If it becomes chronic it is known as 'hemicrania continua'.

Facial pain

- Trigeminal neuralgia causes a unilateral, lancinating facial pain in the distribution of the trigeminal nerve (usually maxillary or mandibular), typically arising in middle age. Bilateral symptoms can be the result of multiple sclerosis. Patients usually report that the pain is precipitated by tactile stimulation of the face (shaving, brushing teeth, hot or cold drinks, the wind). The pain can be difficult to control. Most patients respond to carbamazepine but the effect is not always sustained. A minority of patients have vascular compression of the trigeminal nerve shown by magnetic resonance imaging, and may respond to surgical decompression of the artery in the posterior fossa.
- Post-herpetic neuralgia: this troublesome condition affects 30% of people after an episode of shingles. Risk factors are age and late treatment with aciclovir. The most common location is in the ophthalmic trigeminal division, but it can occur anywhere. Although it is difficult to treat, carbamazepine or amitriptyline are worth trying. In many, symptoms abate after several years.
- 'Atypical facial pain', by definition, does not have any of the distinguishing features of the aforementioned conditions. It is most common in young women, and not associated with physical signs. Amitriptyline is the treatment of choice.

Other causes of headache

- Analgesic overuse headache is a major problem.
- Benign paroxysmal headache (triggered by cold, exertion or coughing).
- Temporomandibular joint dysfunction.
- Sinusitis.
- Dental caries.

64 Episodic alterations in awareness and consciousness

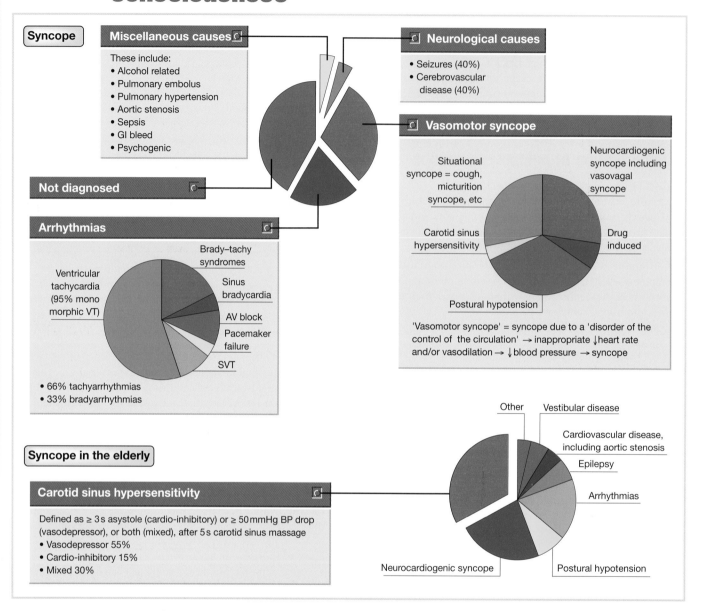

Syncope

Miscellaneous causes

These include:
• Alcohol related
• Pulmonary embolus
• Pulmonary hypertension
• Aortic stenosis
• Sepsis
• GI bleed
• Psychogenic

Neurological causes

• Seizures (40%)
• Cerebrovascular disease (40%)

Not diagnosed

Vasomotor syncope

Situational syncope = cough, micturition syncope, etc

Neurocardiogenic syncope including vasovagal syncope

Carotid sinus hypersensitivity

Drug induced

Postural hypotension

'Vasomotor syncope' = syncope due to a 'disorder of the control of the circulation' → inappropriate ↓heart rate and/or vasodilation → ↓blood pressure → syncope

Arrhythmias

Ventricular tachycardia (95% mono morphic VT)

Brady–tachy syndromes

Sinus bradycardia

AV block

Pacemaker failure

SVT

• 66% tachyarrhythmias
• 33% bradyarrhythmias

Syncope in the elderly

Carotid sinus hypersensitivity

Defined as ≥ 3 s asystole (cardio-inhibitory) or ≥ 50 mmHg BP drop (vasodepressor), or both (mixed), after 5 s carotid sinus massage
• Vasodepressor 55%
• Cardio-inhibitory 15%
• Mixed 30%

Other

Vestibular disease

Cardiovascular disease, including aortic stenosis

Epilepsy

Arrhythmias

Postural hypotension

Neurocardiogenic syncope

Blackouts and near blackouts are frightening experiences. The most helpful diagnostic approach is to obtain a full history from the patient and an accurate witness, because the examination and special investigations may add little. The features of diagnostic value to focus on are:

● What happens immediately before the attack? A prodrome (warning) suggests a vasovagal cause, whereas no warning is a feature of primary generalized epilepsy or Stokes–Adams attacks. Patients with temporal lobe epilepsy (which is rarer than many other causes of loss of consciousness) can have an unusual prodrome, with any form of hallucination, strange epigastric sensations and *deja/jamais vu* ('thoughts of having/never having been here before').

● What does the patient look like during the attack? Abnormal movements suggest epilepsy. Pallor or an appearance 'as if dead'

suggest a cardiovascular cause. These distinctions are not absolute – for example some 40% of patients with vasomotor forms of syncope have some minor twitching during the attack, and a few (especially those kept in the upright position) have more generalized hypoxic seizures (termed 'secondary hypoxic seizures').

● What is the memory of the attack itself? The remembrance of events during the attack suggests that consciousness was not fully lost. This is often so in minor cardiovascular events, in partial epilepsy and, especially, in hyperventilation.

● Did injury occur? Major injury suggests an absence of warning, as well as total loss of consciousness. Attacks with injury are strongly associated with significant underlying pathology.

● What happens immediately afterwards? Post-event confusion suggests epilepsy, whereas post-event flushing or sweating suggests a cardiovascular cause.

Medicine at a Glance, Fourth Edition. Edited by Patrick Davey. © 2014 John Wiley & Sons, Ltd. Published 2014 by John Wiley & Sons, Ltd. Companion website: www.ataglanceseries.com/medicine

- What do witnesses say? This can be the key to diagnosis.
- Are attacks recurrent? If so are they all similar (stereotyped attacks suggest a single underlying aetiology)? Do they all occur in the standing position (which suggests postural hypotension or neurocardiogenic syncope), on effort (see below) or in the same psychological situation (which suggests vasovagal attacks or hyperventilation)?
- The patient's age alters the probability of disease: ≤30 years: vasovagal syncope and epilepsy are more likely; ≥60 years: cardiac causes and micturition syncope are more likely. However, any cause can occur at any age.

Cardiovascular causes of loss of consciousness

Consciousness is disrupted if there is a decrease in the blood supply to the brain, either from a decreased cardiac output or hypotension from inappropriate vasodilatation. Such cardiovascular diseases are characterized by faintness (presyncope, which means that patients feel that they are about to blackout) or actual loss of consciousness (syncope) of brief duration (always less than a few minutes), with pallor during the attack, to the extent that the patient may 'appear dead'. Sweating afterwards is a good clue to a cardiovascular aetiology. Full consciousness returns rapidly. There are different variants of cardiovascular syncope.

Vasovagal syncope This is a common cause of altered consciousness at any age with the following features:
- A coherent account of the events leading up to the attack is given by the patient. Attacks may be precipitated by emotional stimuli and often recur in the same context.
- Loss of consciousness is preceded by: (i) a feeling of lightheadedness or dysequilibrium, which is occasionally prolonged; (ii) ringing in the ears or a progressive alteration in sound quality; (iii) a feeling of warmth or flushing.
- The warning prodrome may be absent in elderly people in whom the picture may be of sudden drop attacks. Younger people often recall slowly falling to the ground before 'blacking out'.
- The patient is fully orientated as he/she comes round, although may feel weak, nauseated and light-headed. Recovery is complete within minutes. Prolonged confusion raises the suspicion that the attack is epileptic.
- Brief, non-sustained jerking of the limbs is common and those who faint with a full bladder may be incontinent. The diagnosis is complicated in those rare patients who faint and have a secondary anoxic convulsive seizure, from maintenance of the upright position.

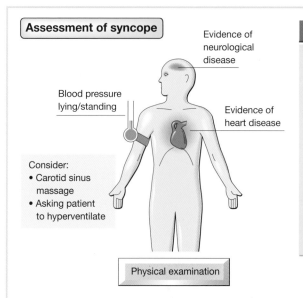

Assessment of syncope

- Evidence of neurological disease
- Blood pressure lying/standing
- Evidence of heart disease

Consider:
- Carotid sinus massage
- Asking patient to hyperventilate

Physical examination

Clinical differences between cardiac and neurogenic syncope

	Cardiac	Neurogenic
Prodrome	0 – +	++
Syncope duration	Secs – mins	Mins – hours
Sweating	++	0
Colour during attack	Pale 'as if dead'	Normal – cyanosed
Abnormal movements	0 (unless 2 fitting)	++
Incontinence	0 – ±	+
Tongue biting	0	+
Time to full recovery	0 – few mins	Hours
Abnormal ECG outside attack	++	0
Abnormal EEG outside attack	0	+
Previous MI	++ (VT likely)	0
Previous CVA	0	+ (epilepsy likely)

Observational tests

Overarching aim is to obtain an ECG **during an attack**

12-lead ECG

- In all
- If abnormal, consider further specialized cardiac investigations

Prolonged ECG monitoring

- 24-hour ECG: 4% chance of diagnosing the cause of syncope. Usually only useful if symptoms occur every 2–7 days
- External loop recorder: useful if symptoms occur every 2–3 weeks
- Implantable ECG recorder – e.g. cardiac reveal device – useful if symptoms occur 2–3 x per year

Provocative tests

Aim to provoke symptoms and monitor ECG, blood pressure, heart rate (occasionally EEG)

Tilt table testing (TTT)

'Circulatory stress test'. Used to diagnose neurocardiogenic syncope. Dark, quiet room. Patient strapped to table and tilted upright (passive TTT), or GTN, isoprenaline given (active TTT). Useful if symptoms atypical, or injury occurs.
Problems with TTT:
- High false-positive, false-negative rates
- Poor reproducibility

Ventricular stimulation study (VSTIM)

Aims to induce the causative ventricular arrhythmia in a controlled manner, by pacing the ventricle, and introducing early extrasystoles. Very useful in ischaemic heart disease (IHD) and syncope with no other cause
- Good predictive accuracy in IHD
- May lead to implantation of implantable defibrillator

Postural hypotension Here the autonomic nervous system fails to prevent blood pressure (BP) falling on standing. Characterized by symptoms of vasovagal syncope on standing, never when sitting or lying:

● Patients are usually elderly. The condition may be provoked or exacerbated by drugs (diuretics, antihypertensives, antipsychotics) and dehydration (e.g. fluid deprivation, diuretics, gastrointestinal (GI) bleed). Autonomic failure is also a common cause, e.g. diabetic neuropathy, Parkinson's disease and related disorders.

● The diagnosis is established by demonstrating a progressive fall in BP on standing over several minutes.

It differs from hypotensive cardioneurogenic syncope in that the BP fall starts immediately, not after a delay, and there is never any absolute bradycardia. Treatment is for the underlying disease (diabetes, dehydration). If this is not possible fludrocortisone may help.

Micturition syncope Patients usually have prostatic hypertrophy. Prolonged straining to initiate micturition decreases venous return to the heart. Cardiac output falls and syncope results. Syncope prevents straining and thus improves cardiac venous return and output, restoring consciousness. A variant of micturition syncope is cough syncope, which occurs in individuals with chronic lung disease and prolonged paroxysms of coughing. The diagnosis is made from the history alone.

Stokes–Adams Attacks describe a specific pattern of syncope, unheralded, with complete loss of consciousness lasting <2–3 minutes. The absence of warning means that patients often fall heavily and sustain significant facial or limb injuries, in contrast to patients who simply faint and are not usually injured. Witnesses state that patients become pale, cyanotic and then reactively hyperaemic on recovery. Afterwards there is a rapid (less than a few minutes) restoration of all mental and physical faculties. Attacks are usually the result of the temporary asystole that accompanies the onset of third degree heart block; if not then they may be caused by ventricular tachycardia (VT).

Syncopal (presyncopal) tachyarrhythmias To cause syncope, tachyarrhythmias must either be very fast or associated with moderately severe, structural heart disease. VT is the most common underlying rhythm disturbance, although atrial fibrillation is occasionally the culprit. Patients complain of fast palpitations before fainting. Total loss of consciousness is unlikely to last for more than a few minutes, although a depressed conscious level can last much longer. The 12-lead electrocardiogram (ECG), 24-hour ECG taping ('Holter monitoring') or specialized cardiac investigation (e.g. ventricular stimulation study) may be diagnostic. If not, and an arrhythmia seems likely, implantation of a solid-state device to continually record the heart rhythm may be appropriate.

GTN syncope Glyceryl trinitrate (GTN) syncope is the result of excess consumption while the patient is standing. Vasodilatation occurs, resulting in syncope. Patients may have failed to understand the role of GTN, and are taking it inappropriately. More usually GTN syncope is associated with severe cardiac disease: either unacceptable angina, such that a coronary intervention is required (see Chapter 85), or impaired left ventricular function or aortic stenosis.

Effort syncope Syncope on effort occurs either because the heart cannot increase the cardiac output as a result of a fixed obstruction (such as in severe aortic stenosis commonly, in hypertrophic obstructive cardiomyopathy less commonly, and in severe pulmonary hypertension rarely) or because exercise provokes an arrhythmia. Cardiac ultrasonography and exercise testing are usually diagnostic.

Cardioneurogenic syncope This is a confusing term applied to an autonomic reflex, activated only in the standing position, whereby either the heart rate or BP or both drop sufficiently to cause syncope. Characteristically patients are standing still, feel faint for 30 seconds to several minutes, and then faint and fall down. Sitting down early on may terminate the attack. The diagnosis is confirmed by replicating symptoms and heart rate/BP changes on tilt table testing.

Carotid hypersensitivity syndrome Patients have hypersensitive carotid baroreceptors, which are activated inappropriately by neck turning (often when looking upwards). Inappropriate bradycardia, sometimes with reflex vasodilatation, occurs and the patient faints. The diagnosis is confirmed by eliciting symptoms and severe bradycardia on carotid sinus massage.

Terminology

Most doctors define syncope as a 'loss of consciousness with loss of postural reflexes'. The definition does not imply any particular mechanism. Thus syncope can occur from a cardiac cause, or equally from a neurological one.

Neurological causes of loss of consciousness

The most common neurological disease underlying loss of consciousness is **epilepsy**, although very occasionally brainstem ischaemia is the cause. Epilepsy resulting in loss of consciousness is classified as generalized epilepsy and is caused by abnormal electrical discharges disrupting the function of the major subcortical structures that maintain consciousness.

● If the abnormal electrical discharges originate in these subcortical structures, unconsciousness occurs immediately and the epilepsy is termed **primary generalized**. Patients have no warning and instantaneous collapse occurs. *Beware*: the absence of a warning is also a feature of some localized seizures that progress unusually rapidly to secondary generalized seizures.

● If these subcortical structures are involved by electrical discharges spreading from a more distant focus it is termed **secondary generalized**. In this situation patients often experience some symptoms referable to the first structure involved, i.e. there is usually an aura or attenuated seizures.

● Seizures without loss of consciousness are termed **partial seizures** and may be simple (normal awareness) or complex (loss of awareness) (for further discussion, see Chapter 205).

Features that are strongly in favour of epilepsy as a cause of loss of consciousness are:

● A good witness account, although this is often absent.

● Post-ictal confusion (ictal = the epileptic attack itself) lasting some time, e.g. often for many hours; post-ictal headache.

● Muscular aching and tongue biting.

● Incontinence, which can also occur in other situations, is suggestive but non-specific.

● Known cerebrovascular disease, i.e. a previous stroke, or a degenerative brain condition increases the probability that a collapse relates to a seizure disorder.

Examination immediately after a seizure may show sleepiness for the first few hours, and bilateral extensor plantar responses for the first day, as well as signs referable to any underlying pathology (see Chapter 56). Generalized seizures cause skeletal muscle fibre damage, so muscle enzymes (e.g. creatine kinase, aspartate transaminase) are often elevated, as are serum prolactin levels for the first day or so. Electroencephalograph (EEG) recordings show abnormal inter-ictal activity in 50% of patients with epilepsy.

Transient loss of consciousness

Brainstem ischaemia can result in falls, with loss of consciousness. Conscious level is usually only transiently disturbed (<1 min). The diagnosis is one of exclusion in a patient with cerebrovascular disease. There are no abnormal movements, the patient does not change colour and no rhythm disturbances are found. The presence of true vertigo (i.e. the external visual world is perceived to 'spin') may be a helpful clue. This syndrome is very rare, and is overdiagnosed.

Prognosis in syncope

Prognosis in syncope varies greatly – in some patients, syncope is due to highly dangerous pathology (e.g. complete heart block) with a very poor natural history (untreated, acquired, complete heart block leads to death within a few weeks or months). At the other extreme, vasomotor syncope is associated with a normal life expectancy (see Figure 64.3 below). It is crucial to determine how likely it is that dangerous pathology underlies the syncope. The clues to this can often be obtained fairly easily:

- If the heart is structurally abnormal (especially left ventricular damage following a myocardial infarction (MI)) or there is a known cardiomyopathy (or complex congenital heart disease) then a high-grade ventricular arrhythmia could underlie syncope (e.g. VT). Patients with syncopal VT are likely to experience further attacks, and the concern is that if the first episode of VT reduced cardiac output enough to cause syncope, the second may reduce myocardial blood flow enough to provoke ventricular fibrillation. Thus syncope from a ventricular arrhythmia is a warning that the patient is at high risk of dying. The clue that VT is the cause of syncope is the presence of damage to the heart, diagnosed from the history (e.g. previous MI, known heart muscle disease, high alcohol intake, or the presence of multiple risk factors for ischaemic heart disease (IHD) – e.g. smoking, age, diabetes, etc.), examination and ECG (most patients with structural heart disease have some ECG abnormality). A cardiac ultrasound can be useful.
- Rarely certain genetic diseases underlie dangerous ventricular arrhythmias; the commonest of these is the still rare Brugada syndrome (prevalence one in 1000); another dangerous genetic disease is hereditary long QT syndrome. Most genetic illnesses cause characteristic abnormalities on the resting ECG; the real clue to their presence is the finding of sudden death in young family members.

Other causes of altered consciousness

- **Hyperventilation** occurs in young adults and there is usually a history of perioral and peripheral paraesthesiae, anxiety and specific provocations.
- **Hypoglycaemia** is associated with sweating, anxiety and confusion before loss of consciousness. Drugs for diabetes are the only common cause. Rarely it may be caused by insulin-secreting pancreatic tumours.
- **Narcolepsy** is not strictly speaking a disorder that leads to loss of consciousness but, because of its curious manifestations, it is often misdiagnosed as epilepsy or patients are labelled as 'functional'. It is fundamentally a disorder of the central nervous system regulation of arousal and the cardinal diagnostic feature is a short rapid eye movement (REM) sleep latency. The four aspects to the full-blown narcolepsy syndrome are: (i) excessive daytime somnolence with an irresistible desire to sleep which cannot be overcome; (ii) cataplexy, a sudden loss of body tone; this may range from full falling to the ground to as mild a feeling as jaw dropping, and is usually precipitated by emotional stimuli such as jokes or arguments; (iii) sleep paralysis; and (iv) hypnagogic hallucinations.
- **Migraine** is often associated with mild, non-specific feelings of dissociation but can very rarely lead to frank coma.
- **Transient global amnesia** is a syndrome of obscure aetiology in which there is complete loss of new memory formation for a period of hours. Patients may appear relatively normal to external observers but are disorientated and ask repetitive and inconsequential questions. It may be a migrainous phenomenon but rarely recurs.
- **Psychogenic disorder** is always a dangerous diagnosis for the non-specialist to make, but psychological illness occasionally underlies blackouts. However, most patients with psychological/psychiatric illness who blackout have genuine organic diseases. Occasionally patients mimic seizures (i.e. have 'pseudoseizures'); this also occurs in psychologically disturbed patients who also have genuine seizures.

Incidence rates of syncope per 1000 person-years of follow-up increased with age among both men and women

Age	Rate per 1000 person-years			Average change
	Men	Women	Average	
20–29 years	2.6	4.7	3.7	-
30–39 years	3.8	3.2	3.5	-0.2
40–49 years	3.2	3.8	3.5	0
50–59 years	5.0	3.9	4.5	+1
60–69 years	5.7	5.4	5.6	+1.1
70–79 years	11.1	11.1	11.1	+5.5
≥80 years	16.1	19.5	17.8	+6.7

Prognosis of syncope according to cause

Follow-up	Probability of survival (P)					Difference between vasovagal and other causes vs cardiac cause
	No syncope	Vasovagal and other causes	Unknown cause	Neurological cause	Cardiac cause	
Year 1	0.99	0.99	0.94	0.92	0.89	–0.1
Year 2	0.92	0.92	0.9	0.88	0.81	–0.11
Year 3	0.91	0.9	0.88	0.81	0.7	–0.2
Year 4	0.88	0.88	0.82	0.79	0.64	–0.24
Year 5	0.85	0.85	0.8	0.7	0.56	–0.29
Year 10	0.7	0.7	0.55	0.48	0.4	–0.3
Year 15	0.51	0.52	0.4	0.25	0.18	–0.34
Year 20	0.38	0.37	0.19	0.14	0	–0.37

Note: The category "vasovagal and other causes" includes vasovagal, orthostatic, medication induced and other, infrequent, causes of syncope

Data from: N Engl J Med 2002; 347; 878–85

65 The red eye

Diagnosis	How common 1 = very common 6 = very rare	Symptoms especially	Signs		Treatment
Conjunctivitis Infective Dry eye Allergic	1 1 2	Sticky Gritty Itchy Stringy discharge		Redness entire surface, eye and two lid linings	Topical chloramphenicol Topical lubricants Topical mast stabilizer
Episcleritis	2	Irritation		Sectorial redness, eye only	None?
Iritis (anterior uveitis)	3	Pain, moderate Photophobia		Redness, eye only around cornea ± small pupil	Topical corticosteroid and dilate
Corneal (keratitis)	4	Pain, sharp Photophobia Watering		Local redness and corneal stain	Topical antiviral
Scleritis	5	Pain, may be severe, may increase on eye movement		Intense redness, eye only	Systemic with corticosteroid and cytotoxic?
Acute glaucoma	6	Pain, aching Vomit		Intense redness, eye only ± large fixed pupil	Topical after diagnosis Acetazolamide also?

Redness of the eye surface is caused by inflammation of its coverings, either the superficial conjunctiva or the underlying episclera, or both.

Is this conjunctivitis?

Do not assume that redness is the result of conjunctivitis, even though this is by far the most frequent cause. If this is a single episode of red sticky eye, the aetiology is usually infective and is most likely to be bacterial, though it could be viral or occasionally chlamydial. It is important to recognize which, because the non-bacterial types need different treatment.

Infective conjunctivitis

The eye is not only red but also sticky, to a variable extent; most sticky with bacterial and least with viral infection. There may be mild discomfort and irritation, but if the patient describes actual pain, consider alternative causes such as iritis or a corneal ulcer. Similarly with vision; in conjunctivitis the vision may be slightly blurred by sticky discharge, which is cleared by blinking or bathing, but the patient usually expects this and should not seem worried about loss of vision.

The straightforward single episode may be treated topically with chloramphenicol drops, hourly for the first day then three times daily for five more days. A meta-analysis of large numbers of cases of aplastic anaemia has shown no significant association with ocular chloramphenicol use.

If the problem fails to settle rapidly or recurs, consider a swab for microbiology, including *Chlamydia* species if the patient is sexually active. If this seems likely, refer to a genitourinary medicine department because the necessary swabs can be taken properly and treatment with oral erythromycin prescribed.

Viral conjunctivitis does not respond to chloramphenicol. It is less sticky, more uncomfortable and takes longer to settle. The patient needs sympathy and explanation, which may be reinforced if adenovirus can be isolated by a swab, which goes into transport medium and takes several days to yield a result.

Medicine at a Glance, Fourth Edition. Edited by Patrick Davey. © 2014 John Wiley & Sons, Ltd. Published 2014 by John Wiley & Sons, Ltd. Companion website: www.ataglanceseries.com/medicine

Dry eye

If symptoms are more chronic and the eyes are described as feeling dry or gritty and worse in heated or smoky atmospheres, the patient may have dryness. In younger patients, especially, this might be a sicca syndrome and related to autoimmunity or even sarcoidosis. Extra signs are revealed by Schirmer's strip test, or staining the cornea and conjunctiva with fluorescein at the slit-lamp.

Allergic conjunctivitis

Certain extra symptoms especially suggestive of allergy, either acute or chronic and possibly seasonal, are itching and a stringy discharge. When the patient tries to remove the offending discharge this emerges from the eye as 'a long string, like melted cheese'.

Could it be episcleritis?

This is relatively common and harmless. The patient notices recurrent redness of part of the eye surface, which settles spontaneously but tends to recur. The eye is uncomfortable, but not painful, and not sticky. Underlying systemic disorders are uncommon and the treatment is usually to do nothing. Referral to the eye department may settle the dilemma if not the condition.

Can I recognize iritis?

This internal inflammation of the anterior chamber is much less common than either conjunctivitis or episcleritis but is very important to recognize because it needs prompt and correct treatment and it might signify an important underlying disorder. Send suspects to the eye department, as definitive diagnosis needs a slit-lamp and treatment is tailored to the intensity of inflammation.

Characteristically the eye is painful and, specifically, often photophobic, so that looking at light hurts. The patient who has experienced attacks before will recognize them early but the inexperienced doctor often delays considering the possibility until several days have passed and the eye is more inflamed. Another clue is a small pupil, which may appear stuck or festooned on dilating. The eye is not sticky and is usually most red around the edge of the cornea. There are a number of causes (see Table 65.1).

Could the cornea be affected?

Keratitis is another uncommon possibility. Characteristic features are photophobia and pain, which may be sharp and, if acute, the eye feels as if scratched; watering may also be present. Redness may be localized to the area adjacent to the affected part of the cornea, and an ulcer, which stains with fluorescein, is sometimes visible to the naked eye. A dendritic, or branching, pattern, seen best with the slit-lamp, suggests herpetic keratitis, typically with herpes simplex virus.

Urgent accurate diagnosis is needed so that effective topical antiviral therapy can be started as early as possible to minimize the risk of corneal scarring and impaired vision. Topical steroids are contraindicated as they promote viral growth and may lead to dramatic deterioration in vision.

Keratitis may also occur in association with graft-versus-host disease, in which corneal malaise is often compounded by dryness. A very rare cause is Cogan's syndrome, associated with deafness, aortitis and raised systemic inflammatory markers; syphilis would be a differential diagnosis.

Is it possible the red eye could be scleritis?

This ischaemic condition of the eye coat is rare but very important. First, it can result in perforation of the eye if not treated correctly and, second, there is often an associated systemic vasculitis that may threaten other organs, especially the kidney. The usual culprit is rheumatoid arthritis, occasionally Wegener's granulomatosis, microscopic polyarteritis or systemic lupus erythematosus, in that order.

Some rheumatoid patients develop necrotizing disease with no pain, but most patients describe an unpleasant ocular ache, which may be severe and characteristically interrupts sleep. The pain is often worse on eye movement. If the posterior part of the eye is involved, the optic nerve may be affected and vision lost as a result.

Treatment for all aspects, including the eye, must be systemic, with corticosteroids and possibly a cytotoxic drug such as cyclophosphamide.

Does the remote possibility of acute angle closure need to be considered?

Very rarely the eye pressure may rise acutely so that the iris becomes ischaemic. Pain is intense and characteristically the patient will vomit, as with acutely raised intracranial pressure. Vision becomes misty with a rainbow halo effect and the congested eye feels like a cricket ball, rather than its usual squash ball tension, with a fixed dilated pupil. This is an ocular emergency and needs to have a slit-lamp examination rapidly; delay of more than an hour dictates immediate intravenous acetozolamide.

Table 65.1 Causes of iritis.

Idiopathic	50% of cases
Systemic disease	Sarcoidosis Ankylosing spondylitis Inflammatory bowel disease Behçet's syndrome Reiter's disease
Infection	Syphilis Tuberculosis Herpes zoster Herpes simplex Lyme disease
Autoimmune	Juvenile inflammatory arthritis

66 Introduction to rheumatological disease

Diagnostic approach

Diagnosis made from the distribution of inflamed joints + pattern of extra-articular involvement

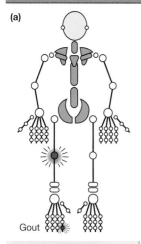

(a)

Gout

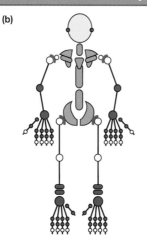

(b)

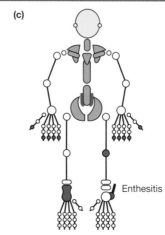

(c)

Enthesitis

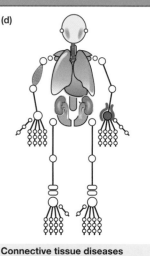

(d)

Acute monoarthritis
- Trauma
- Septic arthritis
- Initial presentation of (b) or more usually (c)
- Gout

Bilateral symmetrical polyarthritis
- Classical RA ± extra-articular manifestations
- Inflammation of:

Lung → + pleura pleuritis effusion basal fibrosis

Pericardium →  pericarditis

Blood vessels: vasculitis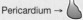

Nodules, e.g. elbow

Asymmetrical oligoarthritis
- The seronegative spondyloarthropathies ± extra-articular inflammation

Iritis

Urethritis

Keratoderma blenorrhagica (soles)

Psoriatic plaques

Connective tissue diseases
- Arthralgia > arthritis
- Major organ involvement:

Pleuritis
Fibrosis

Pericarditis

Glomerulonephritis

Myositis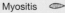

Nail-bed infarcts

Sclerodactyly

Clinical presentations of localized rheumatological disorders

Enthesitis
Tennis elbow
(lateral epicondylitis)

Monoarthritis
Sepsis
Gout
Trauma
or a feature of the seronegative spondyloarthropathies

Olecranon bursitis
Gout
RA

Low back pain
Mechanical trauma
Sacroiliitis

Achilles tendinitis
Trauma
Overuse
Seronegative arthropathies

Key features of inflammation

Symptoms
- **Stiffness**: worst in the early morning, or after prolonged inactivity, progressively easing as the day goes on
- **Pain**: inflammatory pain is usually present at rest as well as on movement
Both are greatly relieved by non-steroidal anti-inflammatory drugs (NSAIDs)

Examination
- Overlying skin is **warm** and may be **red**
- **Tenderness** is elicited all across the joint line
- Swelling is fluid in nature, demonstrated by shifting the fluid within the joint cavity (the bulge or balloon sign)
- **Pain** is elicited throughout the range of both active and passive movement

Laboratory tests
- Acute phase reactants raised (e.g. ESR and C-reactive protein)

Medicine at a Glance, Fourth Edition. Edited by Patrick Davey. © 2014 John Wiley & Sons, Ltd. Published 2014 by John Wiley & Sons, Ltd. Companion website: www.ataglanceseries.com/medicine

Diagnosis in rheumatology largely depends on clinical pattern recognition, because the pattern of joint, periarticular structure and connective tissue involvement is usually highly characteristic for a particular condition. Three patterns are recognized:

1 Localized disorders: involving a single swollen joint/painful area (e.g. gout, low back pain, tennis elbow), of inflammatory, infectious or mechanical origin, and usually presenting as regional pain syndromes (see Chapter 67).

2 Widespread disorders that cause symptoms predominantly in one component of the musculoskeletal system, e.g. rheumatoid arthritis (RA) predominantly affects the joints.

3 Widespread disorders with extra-articular manifestations: involving many components of the musculoskeletal system and connective tissues, e.g. systemic lupus erythematosus (SLE) which affects joints, skin and serosal surfaces as well as major organs such as the kidney and brain.

Definitions of terms used in rheumatology

- **Monoarticular**: single joint involvement.
- **Oligoarticular**: 2–4 joints involved. Usually large joints of the lower limb, but can affect any joint.
- **Polyarticular**: multiple joints involved, but may start with limited joint involvement. Typically affects the small joints of the hands and feet.
- **Periarticular**: involves structures close to but outside the true joint, e.g. enthuses.
- **Extra-articular**: involvement of structures at sites removed from the joints, e.g. rheumatoid nodules in the skin or lung, rheumatoid scleritis or episcleritis (the eye).

Key points in clinical assessment

The impact and consequences (functional impairment, disability, handicap) of the condition to the patient are integral to the clinical assessment.

- Loss of function and pain are key symptoms in rheumatological rheumatic diseases; the severity of disability and distribution and intensity of pain should always be fully assessed.
- Depression is common in rheumatic disease (both as primary and secondary phenomena) and should be specifically sought.
- Inflammation is suggested by pain, swelling, early morning stiffness and tenderness. Assessment of activity of inflammation (i.e. those symptoms reversible with agents that suppress inflammation) is made on the basis of clinical and laboratory findings.
- Distribution of inflamed joints is usually characteristic of particular diseases.
- Extra-articular symptoms may suggest a disease with systemic features and multiorgan involvement.

History

The chronology and impact of symptoms on the patient should be determined. The presenting symptoms usually relate to a joint or area around a joint. Careful questioning should focus on the key areas of:

- Pain.
- Stiffness.
- Swelling and deformity.
- Loss of function and effect of symptoms on normal activities.

These may arise from joints or periarticular structures. Inflammatory characteristics (swelling, pain and duration of early morning stiffness) should be carefully elicited.

Extra-articular symptoms may be diagnostically helpful in pointing to those diseases strongly associated with arthritis:

- **Psoriasis**: skin rash (may be limited to the scalp, umbilicus, nails or natal cleft).
- **SLE**: skin rashes occur in 70% (see Chapter 221) and are classically sun induced, serositis (pain of pericardial or pleural origin; see Chapter 4) and mouth ulcers.
- **Reactive arthritis or seronegative spondylarthropathies** (see Chapter 219): diarrhoea, urethritis, conjunctivitis.
- **Vasculitis**, e.g. Wegener's granulomatosis: sinusitis, mononeuritis multiplex, skin ulcers.

In suspected multisystem diseases specific organ involvement (lung, kidney, nervous system) should be sought on clinical grounds and by special investigations. Constitutional symptoms including fever, malaise, weight loss or fatigue may indicate a widespread inflammatory process.

Examination

Examination of the locomotor system is based on the 'look, feel, move' paradigm.

1 Look for attitude (how the joint/affected part is held), swelling, deformity or asymmetry, muscle wasting around the joint, and redness of the overlying skin. Determine the pattern of joint disease, e.g. small vs large, symmetrical vs asymmetrical. Characteristic patterns of joint involvement in the major arthritides occur (see Figure 66.1). Feel for heat. Determine if swelling is:

- Bony (nodal osteoarthritis).
- Fluid (effusion, synovitis).
- Tissue (rheumatoid nodules).

The site of maximum tenderness elicited by mild/moderate direct pressure (sufficient to blanche the examining finger nail) allows determination of which structures are involved:

- Over joint line: arthritis.
- Over periarticular structure, e.g. enthesitis.

2 Move. Note the pattern and any restriction in joint movement:

- Restriction throughout the range of active and passive motion suggests inflammatory synovitis of the affected joint.
- End-of-range pain and restriction (often with crepitus) suggests osteoarthritis. Crepitus is a 'creaking' sound feeling on passive movement; audible crepitus usually indicates advanced joint destruction.
- Pain only in specific planes or on specific movements suggests a local periarticular or mechanical problem. Active resisted movements that stress the involved structure can aggravate all tendinitis pain arising from tendonitis, enthesitis and bursitis.
- Long-standing disease may produce deformities such as 'fixed flexion' or angular deformities (varus/valgus).

Extra-articular signs

Extra-articular signs may be of diagnostic significance or indicate the extent of multiorgan involvement, particularly in the vasculitides and the other inflammatory connective tissue diseases:

- Systemic: high fever may suggest infection, Still's disease or rheumatic fever but sometimes gout or SLE. Malaise and fatigue are very common but under-recognized features of inflammatory disorders. Weight loss may also occur.
- Skin and appendages: psoriasis, SLE, vasculitis (see Chapter 220), scleroderma and dermatomyositis have characteristic skin changes.
- Mucosa: oral ulcers in SLE, Crohn's disease and Behçet's syndrome. Mucosal dryness in Sjögren's syndrome.
- Major organ involvement: such as renal, heart or lungs, peripheral nerves or central nervous system in the vasculitides, SLE and RA.

On the basis of the history and examination a presumptive diagnosis can be made (see Figure 66.1), which investigations including joint X-rays and specific serological tests and appropriate imaging help to confirm (see individual chapters).

Rheumatoid factor and anti-CCP tests

These immunological tests are useful in the investigation of polyarthritis (see Figure 66.1).

- Rheumatoid factor (RF) is an autoantibody against antigenic determinants of the Fc fragment of IgG; it is usually of the IgM class.
- Positive RF is found in 70% of cases of RA (30% of true RA is RF negative), 40% of SLE and 30% of systemic sclerosis.
- Positive RF in high titre is a poor prognostic factor.
- Positive RF is also found in a number of other systemic conditions (e.g. viral infections such as Epstein–Barr virus (EBV)), chronic inflammatory disease (e.g. tuberculosis or subacute bacterial endocarditis), neoplasia, and in 5% of healthy individuals.
- Anti-CCP (anti-cyclic citrullinated peptide) antibodies are increasingly used in the diagnosis of early RA. These are useful in the diagnosis of early undifferentiated arthritis as the sensitivity of anti-CCP is comparable to RF (50–75%) with a higher specificity (90–95%). The antibodies may be found months to years prior to the onset of clinical disease and may have a role in pathogenesis. They are also associated with erosive disease, and early evidence suggests that they may predict poor prognosis better than RF status.

- Other immunological investigations and inflammatory markers (erythrocyte sedimentation rate (ESR), C-reactive protein (CRP)) are also commonly measured (see Figure 66.2 below, and individual chapters).

Management and outcome

Treatment aims to relieve symptoms, maintain (restore) function and suppress the underlying disease process. The best technique to achieve these aims depends on the disease, its severity and extent. A multidisciplinary approach is required, particularly in the chronic inflammatory disorders. Available techniques include:

- **General measures**, including education and advice, physiotherapy and occupational therapy for joint protection measures, e.g. splinting and local application of heat exercises to maintain strength and the fullest possible range of joint motions. The provision of aids and appliances when function is impaired can help dramatically to improve function.
- Intra- or periarticular **steroid injections**.

Immunology and radiology in rheumatic diseases

Patterns of nuclear staining for antinuclear antibodies can be clinically helpful, though rarely are diagnostic

Pattern appearance	Disease association
Homogeneous (diffuse)	Common pattern
Rim of nucleus (peripheral; annular)	SLE
Nucleolar	Scleroderma, SLE, dermatomyositis/polymyositis
Speckled	SLE, Sjögren's syndrome, mixed connective tissue disease, systemic sclerosis
Centromere (dividing cells only)	Limited systemic sclerosis (CREST syndrome)

Rheumatoid factors are autoantibodies against antigenic determinants of the Fc fragment of IgG
- They may be IgM, IgG or IgA class
- Only measurement of IgM RF is clinically useful
- IgM RF is usually measured by agglutination tests, and expressed as the serum dilution where agglutination still occurs (e.g. 1 in 40, 80, 160, 320, etc.)
- They occur in rheumatic diseases (e.g. in 70% of rheumatoid arthritis, 40% of SLE, 30% systemic sclerosis) – in RA they are of most use in prognosis rather than diagnosis (high titre = adverse prognosis)
- They also are found in:
  – viral infections (e.g. EBV infections)
  – chronic inflammatory diseases (e.g. tuberculosis)
  – neoplasms
  – 5% of healthy individuals

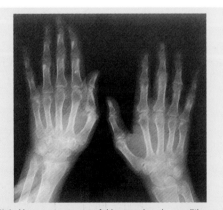

Plain X-rays are very useful in any chronic condition involving joints, and often show characteristic changes. This X-ray of hands with rheumatoid arthritis demonstrates erosive changes in the proximal interphalangeal joints (IPJ) of the thumbs, the metacarpophalangeal joint (MCPJ) of the left thumb, several of the carpal bones and the wrist and distal ulnar joint of the left hand. In addition there is characteristic juxta-articular osteopenia.

Antibodies to different components of extractable nuclear antigens (ENA) can be diagnostically helpful

Antigen	Molecular target	Clinical relevance*
'Smith' (Sm)	Common core proteins of U1, U2, U4, U5, U6—s RNPs	Alone or with RNP antibody—a subset of SLE (20%)
Ribonucleoprotein (RNP)	U1–s RNP	High titre—mixed connective tissue disease (100%)
Ro (SS-A)	60-kDa small RNP-binding Ro RNAs	Primary Sjögren's syndrome, SLE Neonatal lupus and congenital heart block Subacute cutaneous lupus
La (SS-B)	Transcription terminator of Ro RNAs	Primary Sjögren's syndrome
Scl-70	Topoisomerase I	Systemic sclerosis (40–70%)
Jo-1	Histidyl-transfer RNA synthetase	Myositis, arthritis—often with pulmonary fibrosis

*Figures in brackets show percentage of patients in disease category who have demonstrable antibody. U, uridine rich; s RNP, nuclear ribonucleoproteins.

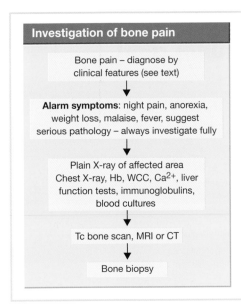

Investigation of bone pain

Bone pain – diagnose by clinical features (see text)

↓

Alarm symptoms: night pain, anorexia, weight loss, malaise, fever, suggest serious pathology – always investigate fully

↓

Plain X-ray of affected area Chest X-ray, Hb, WCC, Ca^{2+}, liver function tests, immunoglobulins, blood cultures

↓

Tc bone scan, MRI or CT

↓

Bone biopsy

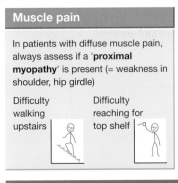

Muscle pain

In patients with diffuse muscle pain, always assess if a '**proximal myopathy**' is present (= weakness in shoulder, hip girdle)

Difficulty walking upstairs

Difficulty reaching for top shelf

Causes of a proximal myopathy

- Alcoholism
- Osteomalacia
- Uraemia
- Polymyalgia rheumatica
- ↑T_4
- Polymyositis
- Dermatomyositis
- Cushing's syndrome
- Carcinomatous myopathy

Causes of generalized muscle pain

- Infection: usually viral, occasionally bacterial
- Drug-induced myositis, e.g. statins
- Autoimmune myositis, e.g. polymyositis
- Other autoimmune disease, e.g. PMR, PAN
- Miscellaneous other causes, e.g. sarcoidosis, fibromyalgia

- **Drugs**, including anti-inflammatory medications and disease-modifying drugs for inflammatory conditions (e.g. methotrexate, sulphasalazine for RA; cyclophosphamide for SLE, renal disease and systemic vasculitis).
- **Biological therapies**: anticytokine therapies and anti-adhesion B-cell molecule therapies. Antitumour necrosis factor therapy is now widely used in RA and inflammatory arthropathies and typically induces remission in a quarter of patients with RA within 3 months. Two-thirds of patients improve by at least 20% and one-quarter by 70% within 6 months.
- **Surgery** (joint fusion, replacement, synovial resection) is useful to highly effective in carefully selected patients to reduce pain, and to stabilize joints and improve function.

Bone pain

Bone pain arises when there is destruction of the integrity of normal bone and is multifactorial. Pain arising from bone has the following characteristics:

- It is deep-seated and intense.
- It is characteristically unremitting and disturbs sleep.
- It is unaffected by movement or posture.
- It is variably responsive to analgesics and non-steroidal anti-inflammatory drugs (NSAIDs).

Differential diagnosis

- **Fracture**:
  - Traumatic.
  - 'Stress' (e.g. related to excess repetitive physical activity, such as marathon running, etc.).
  - Atraumatic low impact (osteoporotic). Uncomplicated osteoporosis does not cause pain.
- **Osteonecrosis** (avascular necrosis).
- **Neoplasia**:
  - Primary tumour: benign or malignant (e.g. osteoid osteoma, osteosarcoma).
  - Secondary tumour: commonly from breast, lung, thyroid and renal or prostate primary. Myeloma can often present as bone pain, commonly from vertebral crush fractures to vertebral bodies.
- **Metabolic**: Paget's disease of bone.
- **Infection**: osteomyelitis.

Investigation of bone pain is shown in Figure 66.3 above.

Muscle pain

Pain arising from muscles is extremely common. Symptoms may be localized (e.g. due to trauma/overuse) or more diffuse (in the context of a systemic process). Muscle pain:

- Is usually felt as a dull ache, i.e. the muscle hurts = myalgia.
- Is often associated with weakness of the affected muscle group. If there is intrinsic weakness of the muscle due to intrinsic muscular disease the process is a myopathic one.
- May be associated with muscle tenderness of the muscles.
- Often affects equivalent groups in the upper and lower limb girdles if due to a systemic process.

Differential diagnosis

Different patterns suggest different illnesses:

- Predominant weakness (usually painless) of muscle groups suggests a myopathy (see Chapter 210).
- Predominant muscular ache and tenderness with stiffness in the proximal muscle groups suggests polymyalgia rheumatica (PMR).
- Predominant pain and tenderness with secondary weakness suggests:
  - Trauma or overuse if symptoms are local.
  - Inflammation (myositis) if there are widespread symptoms, e.g. polymyositis or dermatomyositis.

Management

The aim is to clearly demarcate the symptoms of pain, tenderness, stiffness and weakness and to define as well the extent and distribution of muscle involvement. The physical examination may elicit evidence of muscle tenderness and weakness. Investigations in inflammatory myositis show:

- Elevation of inflammatory markers CRP and ESR (may be >100 in PMR).
- The muscle enzyme creatine kinase may be markedly raised (aldolase and aspartate transaminase are less specific).
- Electromyography may be helpful.
- Diagnostic muscle biopsy with special diagnostic staining.

Treatment is determined by the cause. Trauma/overuse responds to rest and simple analgesics (e.g. paracetamol) or NSAIDs. Most inflammatory diseases require corticosteroids.

67 Low back pain and other regional pain syndromes

Structures which may cause back pain

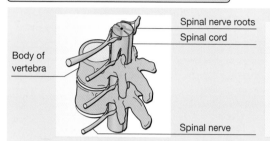

Body of vertebra

Spinal nerve roots
Spinal cord

Spinal nerve

Clinical features of back pain
• Apophyseal joints → pain ↑on back extension
• Disc prolapse → pain ↑ by flexion ± nerve root signs (e.g. 'sciatica')
• Bone disease → constant, severe pain
• Entheses/ligaments → localized pain, no radiation
• Stress fracture of pars interarticularis = spondylolysis
• Bony slip of vertebra on another = spondylolisthesis

Management of low back pain

History + examination suggests

Mechanical origin

Causes
• Prolapsed disc
• Osteoporotic fracture
• Non-inflammatory joint/ligament disease

Clinical features
• Sudden onset
• Eased by rest
• Unilateral symptoms
• ↑ by coughing/sneezing
• Previous episodes

<55 years or previous episodes   New onset >55 or <20 years

Trial of therapy

Review at 3 months

90% well   10% still symptomatic

? Any new/sinister signs or symptoms   Address other factors (see text)

Investigate and treat appropriately

Systemic or inflammatory origin

• Predominant stiffness (>30 minutes in a.m.)
• Gradual onset → progressive
• ↑ Pain with rest
• Disturbs sleep
• Stiff/rigid spine on exam
• Symmetrical restriction SIJ tenderness

Investigations
• Inflammatory markers (CRP, ESR)
• WCC, Hb
• Ca, PO_4, alk phos
• Protein electrophoresis
• Blood cultures if appropriate + image: plain X-ray, CT, MRI

Diagnosis
Sacroiliitis
Neoplasia
Epidural abscess
Paget's disease
(Abdominal visceral origin)

Institute appropriate treatment

Cauda equina syndrome

= compression of cauda equina by posterior disc herniation

• Persistent + progressive
• Leg pain on walking
• Normal leg pulses
• Pain eased by leaning forwards
• Stiff spine on exam
• Neurology is **bladder/bowel** dysfunction + **appears late**

MRI L/S spine

Surgical intervention

Causes of low back pain

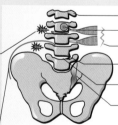

Discitis/epidural abscess (bacterial or spinal TB)

Nerve root compression from postero-lateral disc herniation

Wedge/crush fracture – due to osteoporosis, osteomalacia, Paget's disease/malignancy

Bony neoplasm (1° or 2° – e.g. renal, breast, lung, prostate, colon, cervix, thyroid)

Muscle spasm

Degenerative osteophytosis

Visceral origin – abdominal aortic aneurysm, uterine neoplasia, renal stones, retroperitoneal tumours

Sacroiliitis

Medicine at a Glance, Fourth Edition. Edited by Patrick Davey. © 2014 John Wiley & Sons, Ltd. Published 2014 by John Wiley & Sons, Ltd. Companion website: www.ataglanceseries.com/medicine

Low back pain

Low back pain is common and disabling. The lifetime incidence is 65–80%, representing about 10% of rheumatological problems in general practice. The economic cost in 1990 was $24 billion in the USA and it is much more now.

Aetiology and nomenclature

The different causes of low back pain are:

- **Mechanical** low back pain: arising from an anatomical structures such as muscle, ligament or intervertebral disc or facet joints due to trauma, deformity or degenerative change.
- **Systemic illness** such as inflammatory spondylitis, infection, malignancy, myeloma or Paget's disease.
- **Sciatica**: pain that radiates from the buttock down the back of the leg and into the foot, often accompanied by paraesthesia in the same distribution. It is commonly due to compression of a lumbosacral nerve root by a protruding intervertebral disc or facet joint hypertrophy.

Symptoms

- Mechanical back pain causes localized symptoms, which may be referred to other sites around the pelvic girdle and upper legs. It does not extend below the knee unless there is additional nerve root compression causing sciatica. In this case symptoms and signs in the anatomical distribution of the sciatic nerve occur (see Figure 67.2 below).
- Central canal narrowing stenosis (large central disc prolapse and/or osteophyte formation) may cause compression of the cauda equina, giving rise to distinct symptoms of bilateral leg claudication. Bladder/bowel dysfunction constitutes a medical emergency.
- Lateral recess stenosis may occur as a result of posterolateral protrusion of the disc, osteophytes around a degenerate zygoapophyseal joint, or a combination of the two. Sciatica is prominent on standing or walking for any extended periods of time; nocturnal pain in the leg (with or without paraesthesia) typically wakes the patient in the early hours and may be eased by walking around. Neurological signs may be minor or absent but can sometimes be provoked by activity.
- Features suggestive of systemic/inflammatory illness (malaise, fevers, weight loss, severe pain) or cauda equina compression (paraparesis, bladder involvement) should prompt complete systemic examination and investigations (see algorithm in Figure 67.1 above).

Natural history of low back pain

Most episodes of low back pain are self-limiting and not incapacitating:

- 90% are due to 'mechanical' back pain.
- 50% are better 1 week after onset.
- <10% of patients have pain persistent for more than 6 months. These patients enter a 'chronic pain cycle', are the least likely to return to full employment/activity, and account for 80% of the costs incurred in care.
- 10% are due to underlying systemic or inflammatory illness.

Clinical approach

The aims of the clinical evaluation are:

- To discriminate between mechanical and systemic causes.
- To identify features that suggest the need for advanced imaging studies ± early surgical referral.

Examination

Routine back examination is shown in Figure 67.3 below. Pointers towards serious underlying disease include:

- Patients with systemic or inflammatory features.
- Those >55 or <25 years old with new-onset low back pain.
- Those unresponsive to a 6–8-week trial of conservative therapy for mechanical low back pain.

Management (see Figure 67.1)

Initial treatment consists of reassurance and education; simple analgesia ± non-steroidal anti-inflammatory drugs. Bed rest has a limited role in the acute phase (≤48 h) with early mobilization, followed by a graded exercise programme. Ninety per cent of cases settle.

For unresponsive patients with no new physical findings, the following should be done:

- Identification of occupational, physical and psychosocial contributions. Development of patient-tailored rehabilitation programme, which may include cognitive behavioural approaches.
- Identification of specific anatomical lesions causing the pain (e.g. facet joints, disc lesions, nerve roots, bones).

Where such lesions can be identified, the following **specific measures** may be useful:

- **Facet joint injection** with local anaesthetic and corticosteroids. This is sometimes therapeutic and is particularly helpful in localizing a painful segment prior to considering spinal fusion.
- **Local anaesthetic injections** around nerve roots to confirm compression at specific levels prior to surgical decompression, particularly when there are lesions at multiple levels.
- **Chemonucleolysis** by intradisc injection of chymopapain to relieve compression symptoms from a bulging disc.
- **Surgery** is performed to relieve nerve compression due to disc herniation using the technique of partial laminectomy/discectomy. It is much more effective at relieving sciatica than back pain. It may be combined with spinal fusion at the corresponding level.

Regional pain syndromes

Regional rheumatic pain syndromes are very common. They may be difficult to diagnose with confidence. In particular, pain arising in a localized area, such as the shoulder or hip, presents a clinical challenge. Pain may arise from numerous articular or periarticular structures, or may be referred from a more distant organ or structure site.

Differential diagnosis

The differential diagnosis of regional pain is dependent on a good knowledge of the regional anatomy and a precise history and examination. The differential diagnoses for pain around the hip, shoulder and wrist are shown in Figure 67.4 below.

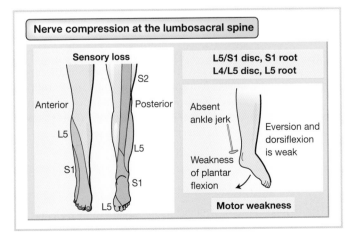

Nerve compression at the lumbosacral spine

Sensory loss

S2

Anterior

Posterior

L5

L5

L5

S1

S1

L5

L5/S1 disc, S1 root
L4/L5 disc, L5 root

Absent ankle jerk

Eversion and dorsiflexion is weak

Weakness of plantar flexion

Motor weakness

Back examination

Examine patient while standing

- **Gait**: look for any abnormality whilst walking and turning, and note whether walking aids are required. Normal gait involves stance (60%) and swing (40%) phases

- **Back**: look for any abnormality including scoliosis, which is described by the side of the vertebral concavity. Cervical lordosis, thoracic kyphosis and lumbar lordosis are normal, i.e. looking at the patient from the side, with the patient facing to the right, a lordosis is a curve shaped like a closing bracket ')', whereas a kyphosis is shaped like an opening bracket '('

- Check for any localized tenderness in the spine (press, and then 'bang' on each of the vertebral processes in turn) – local tenderness may indicate infection

- Look at the progression of the thoracic kyphosis; a useful measure is the distance from the wall to the tragus (ear lobe) when the patient stands with his/her back to the wall

- Forward bending; measure the increase in length between L5/S1 vertebrae and points 10 cm above and 5 cm below (Schober's test) – it should be ≥ 4 cm. (Incidentally, the finger to floor distance on bending forward is not a good measure of spinal stiffness as it may vary with hip mobility)

- Lateral flexion; ask the patient to reach down laterally to the knee joint. This can normally be achieved, but may be restricted in ankylosing spondylitis

- Hyperextension; which is arching the back backwards. Usually 10 from the vertical can be achieved

Examine patients while sitting

- Cervical spine; examine for flexion (i.e. bending the neck forward), extension (i.e. bending the neck backwards), lateral flexion (i.e. tilting the head to one side), and rotation (i.e. moving the head to the left and right). The angle attained is measured from the face forward position – normal ranges are; flexion and extension 70, lateral flexion 40, rotation 80

Pelvis examination

Examine while standing

- Look for asymmetry of the pelvis, which may suggest unequal leg length

- Trendelenburg's test. Ask the patient to stand on one leg – a dropped pelvis on the side of the raised leg (= +ve Trendelenburg test) suggests muscle weakness or hip pathology

Examine while supine

- Sacroiliac tenderness; press the anterior superior iliac spines gently apart. This will cause sacroiliac pain if they are inflamed. With the patient prone, press on the sacrum – this will cause pain if there is sacroiliac joint inflammation

- True and apparent leg lengths. Measure from the anterior superior iliac spine and umbilicus, respectively, to the medial malleolus; an apparent difference may indicate lateral tilting of the pelvis

- Hip flexion; bring the leg in towards the chest with the knees flexed – the normal limit is 110

- Hip extension; with the patient prone, extend the hip – the normal range is 0–30. This will exacerbate the symptoms if there is nerve root irritation, as the femoral nerve will be stretched

- Internal and external rotation, abduction and adduction of the hip. Rotate each hip internally (normal range 25), and externally (normal range 45) with the hip flexed, then measure the range of abduction (normal range 50) and adduction (normal 30)

- Traction manoeuvres. Assess the sciatic nerve by straight leg raising (and record the angle of elevation). Dorsiflex the foot whilst raised (Lasègue's test). This will exacerbate symptoms of lumbosacral root compression

History

- Details of all factors relevant to pain: nature and severity, radiation, factors that relieve or exacerbate, movements that provoke pain.
- Causative factors such as trauma or overuse related to work or leisure.
- Features suggestive of a more widespread inflammatory or systemic condition.

A complete neuromuscular examination is performed. **Look** for swelling, redness, muscle wasting and posture in which the affected part is held. **Feel** carefully to localize where the tenderness is maximal. **Move** carefully and so determine the range of active, then passive, motion around the appropriate joints. Note which movements provoke pain.

Ask the patient to perform these movements against resistance. Lesions such as tendinitis, enthesitis and bursitis are often more painful on movement against resistance.

Principles of management

- Exclude serious systemic disease and infection by appropriate tests, e.g. synovial fluid microscopy for crystals from gouty bursitis or microorganisms from septic bursitis.
- Educate the patient regarding avoidance or correction of mechanical triggers. Reassure.
- Advise on an appropriate level of activity/exercises.
- Splinting (particularly for synovitis and tenosynovitis).
- Analgesia, including intralesional steroid/local anaesthetic.

Prognosis and outcome

Many of these conditions are self-limiting and respond well to simple measures, as above. Most will be asymptomatic within 12–18 months of onset. Those who receive prompt advice and therapy usually do better. A small percentage of cases fail to settle, and it may be necessary to alter work or sporting techniques.

Pain in the shoulder

Referred pain

❶ Cervical spine
- Up into neck
- ± Down into forearm + hand

❷ Myocardial infarction

❸ Diaphragmatic irritation

Local causes

❹ AC joint arthritis

❺ Supraspinatus tendinitis
(painful mid-arc)

❻ Subacromial bursitis

❼ Glenohumeral arthritis

❽ Bicipital tendinitis

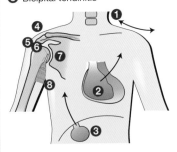

Pain in the hip

Structures giving rise to pain around the hip and buttocks

❶ Sacroiliac joint

❷ Hip joint (OA, RA, sepsis)

❸ Trochanteric bursa
(overuse, mechanical imbalance)

❹ Ischiogluteal bursa (posterior)

❺ Insertion of adductor tendon

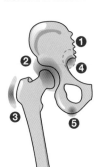

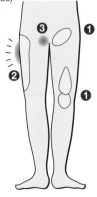

Patterns of pain around the hip

❶ Intrinsic hip **or knee** joint pain

❷ Trochanteric bursitis

❸ Adductor tendinitis

Pain in the wrist/hand

❶ 1st carpometacarpal (CMC) OA

❷ De Quervain's tenosynovitis
(maximal around radial styloid)

❸ Dorsal (extensor) tenosynovitis

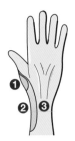

Dorsal view of hand

Origin of pain	Nomenclature and causes	Structures involved in regional pain syndromes	Characteristic features and examples
Synovium (1)	**Synovitis** Inflammatory arthritis Crystal deposition	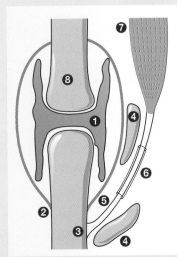	Swelling, heat and tenderness of the joint. Limited passive and active motion at the joint. Pain throughout *all* movements in all planes, e.g. rheumatoid arthritis, gout
Capsule (2) or ligament (enthesis) insertion (3)	**Capsulitis, enthesitis** Trauma Overuse		Localized pain and tenderness Movement restricted in a single plane Pain exacerbated by movement against resistance, e.g. tennis elbow (lateral epicondylitis)
Bursa (4)	**Bursitis** Mechanical Calcific Systemic		Often palpable, with defined limits to swelling Tenderness localized Pressure causes: pre- or infrapatellar bursitis (housemaid's knee) Underlying diseases: olecranon bursitis (gout), sepsis
Tendon (5) / synovial lining of tendon sheaths (6)	**Tendonitis** Overuse **Tenosynovitis** Inflammation		Pain minimal or absent on performing a movement passively which causes pain when performed actively Pain exacerbated by performing the movement against resistance: supraspinatus tendinitis, Achilles tendinitis Tenosynovitis results in swelling and tenderness of the whole tendon sheaths, e.g. extensor tenosynovitis at the wrist in RA
Muscle (7)	**Myositis** Inflammation **Muscle tear** Overuse		See inflammatory muscle diseases
Bone (8)	Fracture/tumour Infection		Persistent pain, wakes at night, unrelated to any specific movement, often not responsive to simple analgesia. See bone pain (Chapter 66)

68 Introduction to dermatology

Dermatological assessment of a rash

1. Take a history 2. Note the distribution of the rash

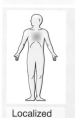
Localized

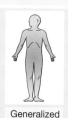
Generalized

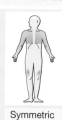
Symmetric

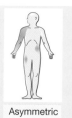
Asymmetric

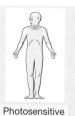
Photosensitive

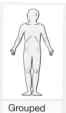
Grouped

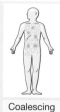
Coalescing

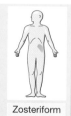
Zosteriform

3. Describe the type of eruption

Erythema
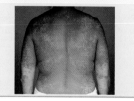

Red and scaly rash
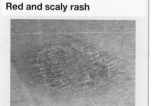

Urticaria
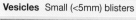

Vesicobullous

4. Examine individual lesions and determine the principal morphologies

Plaques Large elevated lesions
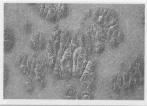

Vesicles Small (<5mm) blisters
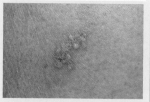

Macules (small) and **patches** (larger) — impalpable lesions
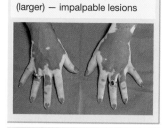

Papules (small) and **nodules** (larger) — palpable lesions

Bullae Large (>5mm) blisters
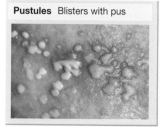

Pustules Blisters with pus
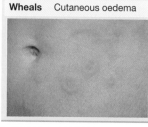

Wheals Cutaneous oedema

Nodule/tumour Large palpable lesion

5. Examine other areas (hair, mouth, nails, genitalia) as indicated: carry out a general examination if appropriate
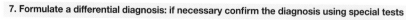

6. Use bedside tests when necessary

Wood's light – in fungal infection and erythrasma (as illustrated)
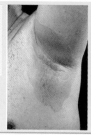
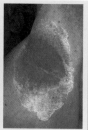

7. Formulate a differential diagnosis: if necessary confirm the diagnosis using special tests

Skin patch tests
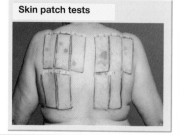

Biopsy
Direct immunofluorescence demonstrating (light green) autoantibodies against intercellular desmosomes in pemphigus vulgaris
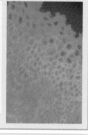

Medicine at a Glance, Fourth Edition. Edited by Patrick Davey. © 2014 John Wiley & Sons, Ltd. Published 2014 by John Wiley & Sons, Ltd. Companion website: www.ataglanceseries.com/medicine

Dermatologists achieve a clinical diagnosis by taking a history (which itself often establishes the diagnosis) and examining the skin.

History

Most patients present with a rash or with a lump/bump. Other symptoms include itch/pruritus (see Chapter 69), flushing (see Chapter 37), pain, hair loss, nail changes (see Chapter 70) and ulceration. It is important to ask about the spatiotemporal characteristics of the presenting symptoms, for example:

- When did the rash or lump appear?
- Where did it spread to?
- When did it ulcerate or bleed?

Determine: age, racial background, occupation, sexual orientation, drug history (could a rash represent an adverse drug reaction?), family history (there is a genetic predisposition in eczema, psoriasis and skin cancer), past medical history and current health, associated symptoms (e.g. joints, genitals) and sun history (easy burning or tanning, lifelong sun exposure, sunburn, sun beds) as sunlight may relieve or exacerbate a rash.

Examination

Skin examination is performed in a good light with the patient lying supine on a couch, using the naked eye first, then a magnifying glass. Undertake a general medical examination (see Chapter 10) when relevant.

- For a rash, ascertain its distribution: asymmetrical (suggests exogenous cause, e.g. local infection), symmetrical (endogenous cause), localized or widespread. Note the morphology: is it an erythema or urticaria, red and scaly (eczematous, psoriasiform or lichenoid), or vasculitis, vesicobullous or erythroderma? Check other sites that may be affected. Complete by examining the scalp, eyes, mouth, hands and nails, breasts, anogenital area and feet. Assess for lymphadenopathy.
- For a lump/bump, note its site and morphology (increasingly a dermascope is used for morphological assessment of pigmented lesions), and the draining lymph nodes and liver (for distant metastases). Note skin phenotypes that predispose to cancer (fair, freckling, degree and type of moles, iris lentigines). A precise clinical diagnosis is often feasible but the prime objective is to differentiate benign from malignant lesions.

Morphology

Important morphological terms include:

- **Macule**: flat, no change in surface markings.
- **Papule**: circumscribed palpable lesion.
- **Nodule**: palpable mass ≥1 cm.
- **Vesicles and bullae** (blisters): visible accumulations of fluid (vesicles are small, bullae are larger).
- Other terms include: telangiectasia, erosion, ulcer, plaque, wheal, comedone, pustule, abscess, cyst, scar, atrophy, purpura and sclerosis.

Special investigations

After physical examination (including urinalysis), the differential diagnosis can be further explored using special investigations:

- Wood's light: ultraviolet radiation of wavelength 360 nm, useful in demonstrating pigmentary diseases and fungal infections.
- Microbiology: swab for bacteria, scrapings for fungi.
- Biopsy for histology: useful in diagnosing many conditions and to exclude malignancy.
- Patch testing: putative allergens are applied to the skin and the resulting reaction is read at 48 and 96 hours.
- Blood tests (e.g. for syphilis, HIV, lupus, iron deficiency).

Dermatological treatment

In the skin a range of pathological processes (inflammation, infection, fibrosis, dysplasia, neoplasia) results in thousands of named diseases, some of which have specific treatments (see individual chapters). Some general principles of management can be outlined.

Supportive treatments

These include:

- Moisturizing the skin and avoiding soap.
- Avoiding the sun and wearing a sunscreen.
- Providing reassurance and psychological support.

Specific treatments

These can be dietary or involve drugs, phototherapy or surgery:

- **Diet**: essential fatty acids (e.g. fish and evening primrose oils) may be useful in inflammatory dermatoses; antioxidants in fruit and vegetables may protect against skin cancer.
- **Drugs** may be applied topically or taken orally:
  - Topical treatments include emollients and soap substitutes, shampoos, sunscreens, antibacterials, antifungals, keratolytics, steroids, calcineurin inhibitors, retinoids and cytotoxics.
  - Systemic treatments include antibacterials, antifungals, antihistamines, anti-inflammatory drugs (e.g. dapsone), antimalarials, retinoids, steroids and 'biological immunomodulators'.
- **Phototherapy**: ultraviolet B and PUVA (psoralens and ultraviolet A) photochemotherapy may be useful in severe dermatoses and mycosis fungoides.
- **Surgery** is used for diagnosis by biopsy and may be curative for skin cancer.

69 Pruritus and rashes

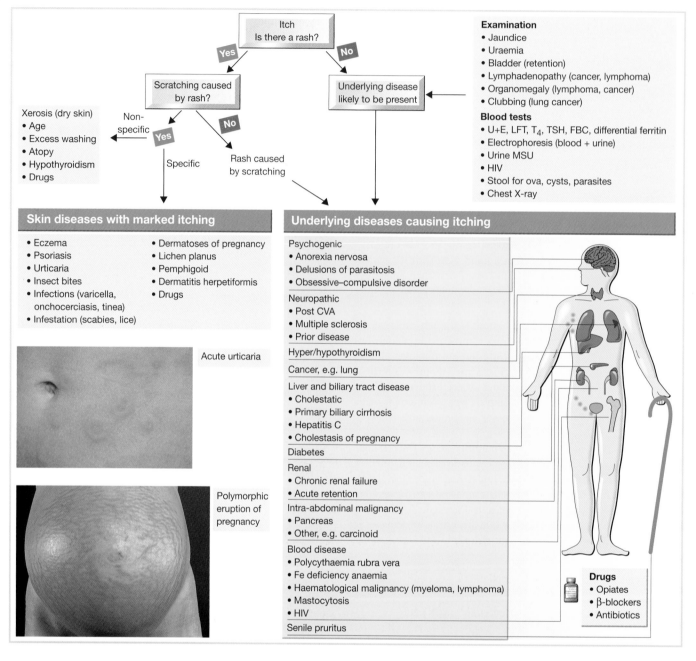

Itch
Is there a rash?

Yes → Scratching caused by rash?

No → Underlying disease likely to be present

Xerosis (dry skin)
• Age
• Excess washing
• Atopy
• Hypothyroidism
• Drugs

Non-specific ← **Yes**

Specific

No → Rash caused by scratching

Examination
• Jaundice
• Uraemia
• Bladder (retention)
• Lymphadenopathy (cancer, lymphoma)
• Organomegaly (lymphoma, cancer)
• Clubbing (lung cancer)

Blood tests
• U+E, LFT, T_4, TSH, FBC, differential ferritin
• Electrophoresis (blood + urine)
• Urine MSU
• HIV
• Stool for ova, cysts, parasites
• Chest X-ray

Skin diseases with marked itching

• Eczema
• Psoriasis
• Urticaria
• Insect bites
• Infections (varicella, onchocerciasis, tinea)
• Infestation (scabies, lice)

• Dermatoses of pregnancy
• Lichen planus
• Pemphigoid
• Dermatitis herpetiformis
• Drugs

Acute urticaria

Polymorphic eruption of pregnancy

Underlying diseases causing itching

Psychogenic
• Anorexia nervosa
• Delusions of parasitosis
• Obsessive–compulsive disorder

Neuropathic
• Post CVA
• Multiple sclerosis
• Prior disease

Hyper/hypothyroidism

Cancer, e.g. lung

Liver and biliary tract disease
• Cholestatic
• Primary biliary cirrhosis
• Hepatitis C
• Cholestasis of pregnancy

Diabetes

Renal
• Chronic renal failure
• Acute retention

Intra-abdominal malignancy
• Pancreas
• Other, e.g. carcinoid

Blood disease
• Polycythaemia rubra vera
• Fe deficiency anaemia
• Haematological malignancy (myeloma, lymphoma)
• Mastocytosis
• HIV

Senile pruritus

Drugs
• Opiates
• β-blockers
• Antibiotics

Pruritus

Pruritus (itching) may be localized or generalized. Primary skin disease, underlying systemic disease or, rarely, a psychological condition must be considered (see Figure 69.1).

History

Localized pruritus suggests a local cause. Generalized pruritus may relate to dermatological or systemic disease. If a rash is present, determine whether the itching occurred before (suggests underlying systemic disorder, with the signs caused by scratching) or after (suggests underlying skin disease) the rash. Undertake a general assessment including a drug history.

Examination and treatment

Excoriations, eczematization and impetiginization are non-specific secondary signs from scratching and infection. Determine whether there are any signs of a primary dermatosis or underlying disease (see Figure 69.1). Treatment is for the underlying cause and includes emollients and antihistamines.

Medicine at a Glance, Fourth Edition. Edited by Patrick Davey. © 2014 John Wiley & Sons, Ltd. Published 2014 by John Wiley & Sons, Ltd. Companion website: www.ataglanceseries.com/medicine

Table 69.1 Causes of erythema.

- Toxic erythema: drug or viral
- Specific viral exanthems
- Erythema chronicum migrans – Lyme borreliosis
- Erythema multiforme (see Chapter 231)
- Erythema nodosum (see Chapter 229)
- Erythema marginatum – very rare reticular erythema
- Still's disease – diurnal angulated macular erythema
- Erythema ab igne – from close contact with heat

Table 69.2 Eruptions that may have red scaly patches.

- Eczema/dermatitis
- Psoriasis
- Lichen planus
- Lichen sclerosus
- Pityriasis rosea
- Lupus erythematosus
- Dermatomyositis
- Tinea
- Pityriasis versicolor
- Mycosis fungoides
- Solar keratosis
- Bowen's disease
- Paget's disease
- Superficial basal cell carcinoma
- Drug eruption

Rashes

Distinguish the distribution, the type of rash and the morphology (see Chapter 68).

Erythemas

The principal causes of erythema in the skin are listed in Table 69.1.

Urticarial lesions

The principal causes are:

- Idiopathic urticaria.
- Drug eruptions.
- Prodromal bullous pemphigoid.
- Henoch–Schönlein purpura.

Red scaly patches

The causes of red scaly patches are listed in Table 69.2.

Erythroderma

Erythroderma is a widespread, confluent, erythematous eruption that may develop acutely or insidiously. Causes, complications and treatment are listed in Figure 69.2 below.

Blistering

Blistering is common and examples include acute eczema, herpes, impetigo and insect bites. Some drug eruptions are bullous, e.g. toxic epidermal necrolysis (see Chapter 227), as are some systemic diseases, e.g. porphyria cutanea tarda and amyloid. Primary bullous disease is discussed in Chapter 227.

Vasculitis

Vasculitis can be localized to the skin or involve internal organs (see Chapter 220). Vasculitic manifestations range from erythema, livedo reticularis and urticaria, to palpable purpuric papules, nodules, necrosis and infarction, depending on the calibre of the vessel involved, the nature of the inflammatory response and the severity of the vasculitic insult.

Flushing (see Chapter 37)

Skin diseases to consider are rosacea (see Chapter 225), urticaria (see Chapter 223) and erythromelalgia.

Pustules

Causes of pustules include acne (see Chapter 225), rosacea, impetigo and autoimmune blistering diseases.

Erythroderma

Complications

- Hypothermia – from heat loss
- Heart failure – from high cardiac output
- Fluid loss
- Increased basal metabolic rate – due to inflamed skin
- Sepsis syndrome – from organisms entering through inflamed skin
- 'Capillary leak syndrome' – very rare – due to inflamed skin releasing cytokines→generalized vascular leakage; can→ARDS
- Hypoalbuminaemia

Causes of erythroderma

Eczema
Psoriasis
Drugs
Mycosis fungoides (Sézary's syndrome)
Photodermatoses (reactions to sunlight)
Toxic erythema
Toxic shock syndrome
Staphylococcal scalded skin syndrome
Toxic epidermal necrolysis
Infestations (scabies and lice)
Congenital disorders

Management

- Establish diagnosis rapidly
- Remove any non-essential drugs
- Keep warm – may need 'space' blanket
- Keep well hydrated
- Treat infection early
- Monitor vital organs, electrolytes regularly
- Guarded prognosis – 10–15% of severe cases may die

70 Hair and nail disorders

Hair loss

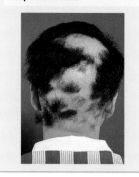

Alopecia areata

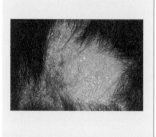

Tinea capitis. Erythema, scale, hair loss and scarring

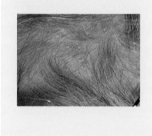

Cicatricial (scarring) Lichen planus

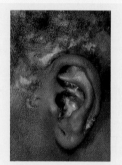

Discoid lupus erythematosus

Hirsutes and hypertrichosis

- **Hirsutes** describes coarse terminal hair in women at sites where it would be normal in a postpubertal male (see Chapter 39). Virilizing tumours of adrenal or ovarian origin are rare (but examine for deepening of the voice and clitoromegaly) as are situations of extreme insulin resistance. Idiopathic hirsutes is common, as is the polycystic ovary syndrome, which may present with other features of cutaneous virilization such as acne, and androgenic alopecia (also obesity, oligomenorrhea and infertility). Late-onset congenital adrenal hyperplasia (CAH) can cause hirsutes alone. CAH is usually due to 21-hydroxylase deficiency (10% due to 11β-hydroxylase or 3β-hydroxysteroid deficiency).
- **Hypertrichosis** is the appearance of excess, usually vellus, hair in non-androgen-dependent sites. Causes include:
  - Localized: Becker's naevus, spina bifida occulta, post inflammatory disorder (trauma, porphyria cutanea tarda, arthritis), occlusion, paraneoplastic hypertrichosis lanuginose (lymphoma).
  - Generalized: hypothyroidism, malnutrition, anorexia, drugs (ciclosporine, corticosteroids, phenytoin, psoralens and ultraviolet A (PUVA)).

Tests in hirsutes and hypertrichosis are listed in Table 70.1. Treatment is directed at the cause; topical eflornithine may be helpful.

Alopecia

Alopecia, or hair loss, is common. It may be subdivided into male pattern, localized or generalized. A *scarring* process must be identified and treated with alacrity. The duration of the process, sites affected and the patient's general condition (pregnancy, nutrition, health) must be ascertained. On examination, elicit local signs (erythema, scarring, pustulosis) and look for signs of a more widespread dermatosis or systemic illness. Helpful investigations include hair microscopy, telogen count, mycology, microbiology, skin biopsy and tests for an underlying systemic illness (full blood count, renal and liver function, iron studies (ferritin), systemic lupus erythematosus (SLE), HIV and syphilis).

- **Diffuse non-scarring alopecia**: the differential diagnosis includes systemic disease, thyroid disorders and other

Table 70.1 Investigations of excess hair growth.

- Thyroid function, glucose
- Luteinizing hormome, follicle-stimulating hormone, testosterone, sex hormone-binding globulin, prolactin
- 0900 cortisol, 17α-hydroxyprogesterone
- Dihydroepiandrosterone, androstenedione
- Pelvic ultrasound

endocrinopathies, iron deficiency anaemia, skin diseases (such as psoriasis, seborrhoeic dermatitis and alopecia areata) and drugs (such as lithium or cytotoxics).
- **Androgenic alopecia**: in men this is physiological and consists of focal frontal and vertical loss with eventual confluence of baldness and occipital sparing. Finasteride 1 mg daily is licensed for treatment. In women the picture is of more diffuse thinning. Minoxidil 2–5% lotion may help some cases. In women the anti-androgen cyproterone acetate given with ethinyl oestradiol to regulate the menstrual cycle has some effect. Other drugs used include spironolactone and metformin (in polcystic ovarian syndrome).
- **Alopecia areata**: this refers to focal areas of complete, non-scarring alopecia. Topical or intralesional corticosteroids help. The prognosis is unpredictable, although patients with nail pits or widespread hair loss do worse. Occasionally patients may have or develop another organ-specific autoimmune disease.
- **Scarring alopecia**: the differential diagnosis includes infection and inflammatory dermatoses (see Table 70.2). Skin biopsy is essential. Diagnosis and treatment must be prompt to save the hair. The principal differential diagnosis is tinea capitis (treat with systemic antifungals), lichen planus (topical/systemic corticosteroids) and lupus erythematosus (topical/systemic steroids and systemic antimalarials).

Nail disorders

The key points in diagnosing nail disorders are to establish whether the signs point to an underlying disease or to a treatable cause of nail dystrophy. The common nail disorders are:

- **Clubbing**: there are many causes for clubbing (see Figure 70.2 below), in practice lung cancer is the most common.
- **Dystrophy** (misshapen, abnormally growing nails): a common cause is fungal infection; exclude by examination of clippings. Peripheral vascular disease or severe Raynaud's phenomenon, psoriasis and trauma are other common causes.
- **Onycholysis** (premature seaparation of the nail plate from the nail bed) occurs commonly in psoriasis, tinea and drug eruptions. Aggressive nail manicure may also be responsible.
- **Nail pits** are found in psoriasis, eczema and alopecia areata.
- **Leukonychia** (white nails) occurs most commonly as small white spots where it is of no significance. Pathological leukonychia occurs mainly in long-standing systemic disease such as cirrhosis, diabetes mellitus, cardiac failure and severe anaemia.
- **Koilonychia** (spoon-shaped nails) may be associated with local nail dystrophy or with a dermatosis such as psoriasis or lichen simplex. Rarely it is a sign of iron deficiency.
- **Splinter haemorrhages** occur with trauma, in autoimmune rheumatic disease and endocarditis.

Table 70.2 Causes of scarring alopecia.

Infections
- Tinea capitis and kerion
- Staphylococcal folliculitis/folliculitis decalvans
- Syphilis
- Herpes simplex and zoster
- Lupus vulgaris (tuberculosis)

Other skin diseases
- Lichen planus
- Lupus erythematosus (especially discoid lupus erythematosus)
- Sarcoid
- Scleroderma
- Basal cell carcinoma
- Acne keloidalis nuchae (keloid reaction to acne)

Clubbing

Normal

<160

Clubbing

>180

- Increased 'bogginess' nail bed
- In severe cases, hypertrophic pulmonary osteoarthropathy
  + Pain around wrist
  + New bone formation at distal radius ulna
- Pathophysiological substrate unclear

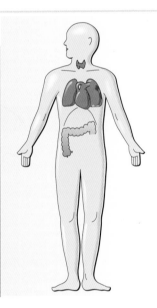

Causes of clubbing

Lung disease
1 Lung cancer: most common (squamous>oat>>alveolar)
2 Chronic lung sepsis
  - Lung abscess
  - Empyema
  - TB (commonest world-wide)
  - Bronchiectasis (either acquired or CF related)
3 Other lung disease
  - Fibrosing alevolitis
  - Asbestosis
NB. Not asthma + not COPD

Cardiac causes
1 Cyanotic congenital heart disease – almost universal
2 SBE: very rare (<5% of cases)

GI causes
1 IBD (Crohn's/UC)
2 Tropical sprue
3 Cirrhosis (particularly autoimmune)

Endocrine disease
Hyperthyroidism (very rare)

Other nail disorders

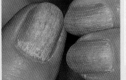
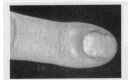

Pits
- Psoriasis
- Alopecia

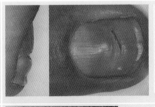

Horizontal lines
Beau's lines (systemic illness)

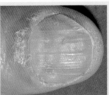

Longitudinal ridges
Single – normal variant
Multiple
- Lichen planus
- Alopecia
- Psoriasis

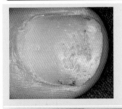

Trachyonychia (rough surface)
- Lichen planus
- Alopecia areata
- Psoriasis

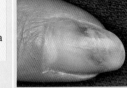

Onycholysis
- Psoriasis
- Trauma

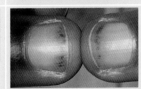

Splinter haemorrhages
- Trauma (RA)
- Vasculitis (SLE)
Nail-fold telangiectasia
- Vasculitis

Paronychia (localized soft-tissue infection)

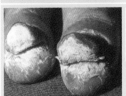

Subungual hyperkeratosis
- Psoriasis
- Hand dermatitis

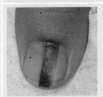

Pigmented streak
- Malignant melanoma
- Normal in dark skins
- Melanocytic naevus

71 Leg ulcers

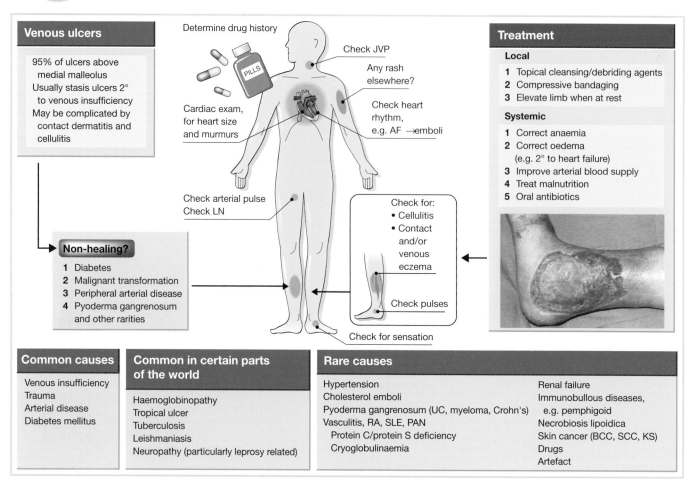

Venous ulcers

95% of ulcers above
medial malleolus
Usually stasis ulcers 2°
to venous insufficiency
May be complicated by
contact dermatitis and
cellulitis

Determine drug history

Check JVP

Any rash
elsewhere?

Cardiac exam,
for heart size
and murmurs

Check heart
rhythm,
e.g. AF →emboli

Treatment

Local

1 Topical cleansing/debriding agents
2 Compressive bandaging
3 Elevate limb when at rest

Systemic

1 Correct anaemia
2 Correct oedema
   (e.g. 2° to heart failure)
3 Improve arterial blood supply
4 Treat malnutrition
5 Oral antibiotics

Check arterial pulse
Check LN

Non-healing?

1 Diabetes
2 Malignant transformation
3 Peripheral arterial disease
4 Pyoderma gangrenosum
   and other rarities

Check for:
• Cellulitis
• Contact
  and/or
  venous
  eczema

Check pulses

Check for sensation

Common causes

Venous insufficiency
Trauma
Arterial disease
Diabetes mellitus

**Common in certain parts
of the world**

Haemoglobinopathy
Tropical ulcer
Tuberculosis
Leishmaniasis
Neuropathy (particularly leprosy related)

Rare causes

Hypertension
Cholesterol emboli
Pyoderma gangrenosum (UC, myeloma, Crohn's)
Vasculitis, RA, SLE, PAN
   Protein C/protein S deficiency
   Cryoglobulinaemia

Renal failure
Immunobullous diseases,
   e.g. pemphigoid
Necrobiosis lipoidica
Skin cancer (BCC, SCC, KS)
Drugs
Artefact

Most leg ulceration is the result of venous disease, although other causes should always be considered. The common causes for acute deterioration in chronic leg ulcers are infection (cellulitis) and allergic contact dermatitis (resulting from a topical medicament or dressing). All chronic ulcers are at risk of malignant transformation (Marjolin's squamous carcinoma), so regular reassessment, especially in elderly people, should occur.

Clinical features

It is important to determine the duration of ulceration, the degree of associated pain (e.g. whether diabetic neuropathy is present), the presence of associated infection and systemic upset (e.g. sepsis), and whether the patient has diabetes, renal failure, arthritis or a connective tissue disease, a haemoglobinopathy or inflammatory bowel disease. Topical agents and dressings may cause contact dermatitis.

Examination

This should be particularly for stasis or contact eczema, venous and arterial insufficiency, inguinal lymphadenopathy and cellulitis.

Investigations

Investigations should be used in selected cases to determine the arterial blood supply to the leg (Doppler studies and/or angiography) and venous drainage (leg and pelvic ultrasonography). Skin biopsy (including immunofluorescence) is necessary when the cause is in doubt.

Treatment

Exclude and treat the different factors (see Figure 71.1). Maximize the arterial blood supply (e.g. angioplasty), and treat anaemia and infection (systemic antibiotics continued long term), heart failure and malnutrition (protein, iron, vitamin C or zinc deficiency).

Encourage regular exercise and weight loss. Elevate the limb at rest and apply compressive bandaging (non-adherent or paraffin gauze), after using a topical cleansing and/or debriding agent to encourage granulation tissue formation. Other measures include mild-to-moderate potency steroids to non-ulcerated eczematous skin. Beware of contact sensitization to topical applications. If a clean granulating ulcer base can be achieved consider 'pinch' skin grafting.

Medicine at a Glance, Fourth Edition. Edited by Patrick Davey. © 2014 John Wiley & Sons, Ltd. Published 2014 by John Wiley & Sons, Ltd. Companion website: www.ataglanceseries.com/medicine

72 Photodermatoses

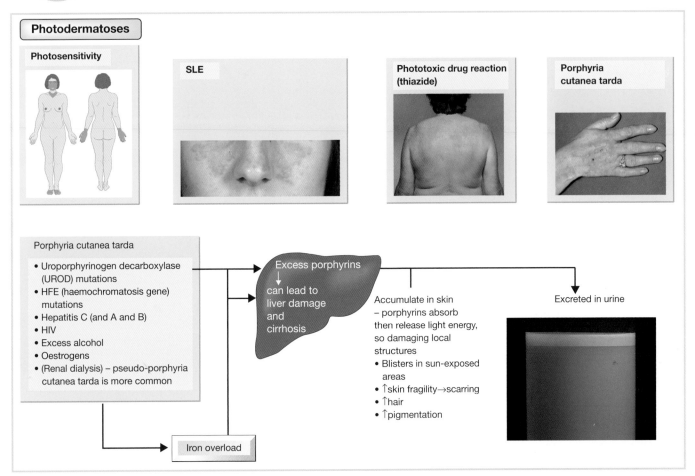

Photodermatoses

Photosensitivity

SLE

Phototoxic drug reaction (thiazide)

Porphyria cutanea tarda

Porphyria cutanea tarda

- Uroporphyrinogen decarboxylase (UROD) mutations
- HFE (haemochromatosis gene) mutations
- Hepatitis C (and A and B)
- HIV
- Excess alcohol
- Oestrogens
- (Renal dialysis) – pseudo-porphyria cutanea tarda is more common

Excess porphyrins ↓ can lead to liver damage and cirrhosis

Accumulate in skin – porphyrins absorb then release light energy, so damaging local structures
- Blisters in sun-exposed areas
- ↑skin fragility→scarring
- ↑hair
- ↑pigmentation

Excreted in urine

Iron overload

A cardinal clue that an eruption is sunlight related (i.e. a photo-dermatosis) is its distribution in sun-exposed areas (forehead, cheeks, ears, nose, chin, anterior chest in a 'V' distribution, hands) with sparing of areas photo-protected by clothes or natural shadows (around the orbit, behind the ears, under the chin). Some primary dermatoses (e.g. psoriasis, acne) can improve with sunlight. Photo-eruptions occur in:

- **Atopic eczema** (this also sometimes improves with sunlight).
- **Systemic lupus erythematosus** (SLE) (see Chapter 221).
- **Lichen planus**.
- **Drug eruptions**:
  - In phototoxic drug eruptions (increased susceptibility to the normal effects of sunlight), sunburn occurs within minutes of sun exposure, e.g. with amiodarone, thiazides or tetracy-cline. Extracts from many plants can act as topical sun sensitizers.
  - Photoallergic drug reactions are idiosyncratic inflammatory reactions (resembling contact dermatitis) to, for example, phenothiazines and angiotensin-converting enzyme inhibitors.
- **Polymorphic light eruption**: this is the most common photoder-matosis. It can cause erythema, papules, urticarial weals and plaques

usually 4–6 hours after (early summer) sun exposure. Topical ster-oids may help short term. Sun avoidance and sunscreens are essen-tial. Prophylactic psoralens and ultraviolet A (PUVA) or ultraviolet B (before holidays) can be used. Gradual exposure to sunlight results in tolerance, which lasts until the following year.

- **Solar urticaria** is rare, but is characterized by an immediate urticarial response to sun exposure. It fades in the shade.
- **Porphyrias** result from deficiencies in the enzymes synthesizing haem. Haem precursors are deposited in the skin, resulting in disease. Porphyria cutanea tarda may be familial or sporadically affect young women (related to alcohol and the contraceptive pill) or middle-aged men (alcoholism). There is an association with hepatitis B/C, HIV and renal dialysis. Skin fragility and photosensitive blister-ing with scarring occurs on exposed sites, especially the hands. Hypertrichosis occurs on the face. Clinical and/or biochemical liver disease may occur. There is a deficiency of uroporphyrinogen decar-boxylase activity and uroporphyrin III is found in the urine and faeces. Treatment is avoidance of alcohol, oestrogen and sunlight, venesection and/or low-dose hydroxychloroquine.
- **Pellagra** (niacin deficiency) may result in a classic tetrad of features (diarrhoea, dementia, dermatitis, death). The classic cutaneous manifestation is an eruption around the neck, 'Casal's necklace'.

Medicine at a Glance, Fourth Edition. Edited by Patrick Davey. © 2014 John Wiley & Sons, Ltd. Published 2014 by John Wiley & Sons, Ltd. Companion website: www.ataglanceseries.com/medicine

73 Pelvic pain

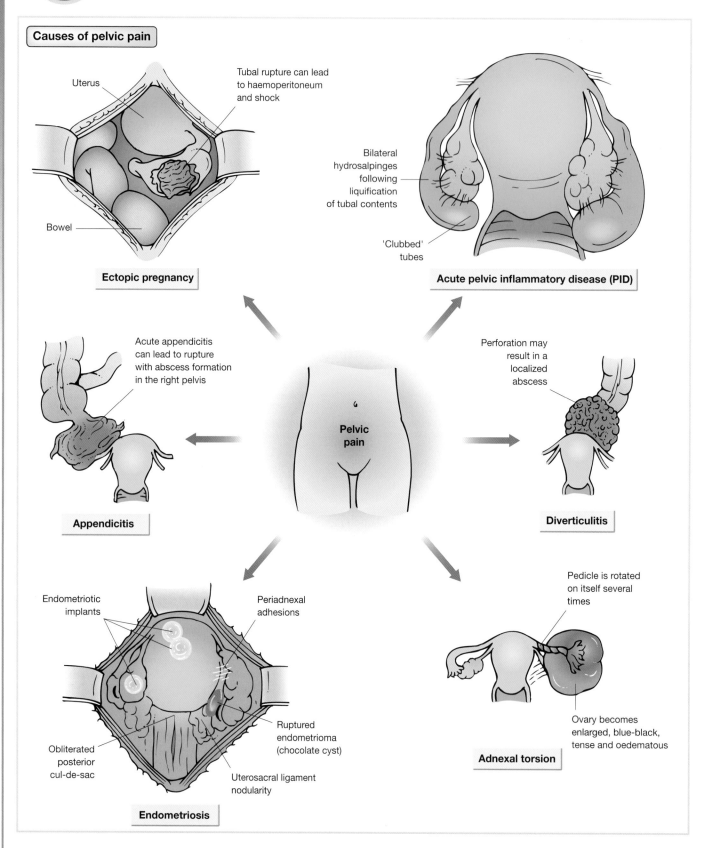

Causes of pelvic pain

Ectopic pregnancy
- Uterus
- Tubal rupture can lead to haemoperitoneum and shock
- Bowel

Acute pelvic inflammatory disease (PID)
- Bilateral hydrosalpinges following liquification of tubal contents
- 'Clubbed' tubes

Appendicitis
- Acute appendicitis can lead to rupture with abscess formation in the right pelvis

Pelvic pain

Diverticulitis
- Perforation may result in a localized abscess

Endometriosis
- Endometriotic implants
- Periadnexal adhesions
- Obliterated posterior cul-de-sac
- Ruptured endometrioma (chocolate cyst)
- Uterosacral ligament nodularity

Adnexal torsion
- Pedicle is rotated on itself several times
- Ovary becomes enlarged, blue-black, tense and oedematous

As pain arising from the pelvis is a subjective perception rather than an objective sensation, accurately determining the aetiology is often difficult. Dysmenorrhea (uterine pain associated with menses) is the most common gynaecological pain complaint.

Clinical approach

- The history provides a description of the nature, intensity and distribution of the pain. However, imprecise localization is typical with intra-abdominal processes.
- Physical examination includes a comprehensive gynaecological examination. Specific attention should be paid to trying to reproduce the pain symptoms.
- Chlamydia/gonorrhea cervical cultures and urinalysis with culture are frequently helpful.
- Ultrasonography and other imaging studies may be indicated.
- Specialized diagnostic studies based on the presumptive diagnosis may require consultation with other specialists in anaesthesiology, orthopaedics, neurology or gastroenterology.

Acute pelvic pain

Potentially catastrophic causes (ruptured appendix) require timely intervention to quickly diagnose and treat.

Gynaecological causes

There are three main categories: rupture, infection and torsion.

- **Ectopic pregnancy**: in all women of reproductive age, the first priority in evaluating acute pelvic pain is to rule out the possibility of a ruptured ectopic pregnancy.
- **Acute pelvic inflammatory disease** (PID) is an ascending bacterial infection that often presents with high fever, severe pelvic pain, nausea and evidence of cervical motion tenderness in sexually active women.
- **Rupture of an ovarian cyst**: intra-abdominal rupture of a follicular cyst, corpus luteum or endometrioma is a common cause of acute pelvic pain. The pain may be severe enough to cause syncope. The condition is usually self-limiting with limited intraperitoneal bleeding.
- **Adnexal torsion** is seen most commonly in adolescents or women of reproductive age. By twisting on its vascular pedicle, any adnexal mass (ovarian dermoid, hydatid of Morgagni) can cause severe pain by suddenly compromising its blood supply. The pain will frequently wax and wane with associated nausea and vomiting.
- **Threatened, inevitable or incomplete miscarriages** are generally accompanied by midline pelvic pain, usually of a crampy, intermittent nature.
- **Degenerating fibroids or ovarian tumors** may cause localized sharp or aching pain.

Non-gynaecological causes

- **Appendicitis** is the most common acute surgical condition of the abdomen, occurring in all age groups. Classically, the pain is initially diffuse and centred in the umbilical area but, after several hours, localizes to the right lower quadrant (McBurney's point). It is often accompanied by low grade fever, anorexia and leukocytosis.
- **Diverticulitis** occurs most frequently in older women. It is characterized by left-sided pelvic pain, bloody diarrhoea, fever and leukocytosis.
- **Urinary tract disorders** (cystitis, pyelonephritis, renal calculi) can cause acute or referred suprapubic pain, pressure and/or dysuria.
- **Mesenteric lymphadenitis** most often follows an upper respiratory infection in young girls. The pain is usually more diffuse and less severe than in appendicitis.

Chronic pelvic pain

Most women, at some time in their lives, experience pelvic pain. When the condition persists for longer than 3–6 months, it is considered chronic.

- It accounts for 10% of all visits to gynaecologists and 20–30% of laparoscopies.
- Frequently there is little correlation between the objective severity of abdominal disease and the amount of perceived pain: a third of women who undergo laparoscopy for chronic pelvic pain will have no identifiable cause.
- 10–20% of hysterectomies are performed for chronic pelvic pain. Postoperatively, 75% of women will experience significant improvement in their symptoms.
- Patients and physicians may both become frustrated because the condition is difficult to cure or manage adequately.

Gynaecological causes

- **Dysmenorrhoea** is the most common aetiology. Primary dysmenorrhoea is not associated with pelvic pathology, and is thought to be due to excessive prostaglandin production by the uterus. Secondary dysmenorrhoea is usually due to acquired conditions (such as endometriosis). Oral contraceptives and nonsteroidal anti-inflammatory drugs are helpful.
- **Endometriosis** has a spectrum of pain that ranges from dysmenorrhoea to severe, intractable, continuous pain which may be disabling. The severity of pain often does not correlate with the degree of pelvic pathology.
- **Adenomyosis** is a common condition that is usually only confirmed by hysterectomy. Most frequently, women are asymptomatic and this is an incidental pathology finding. An enlarged, boggy uterus that is mildly tender to bimanual palpation is suggestive of the diagnosis.
- **Fibroids** are the most frequent (benign) tumuors found in the female pelvis. They may cause pain by either putting pressure on adjacent organs or undergoing degeneration.
- **Ovarian remnant syndrome** is characterized by persistent pelvic pain after the removal of both adnexa. In such cases, a cystic portion of the ovary is usually identified as the source.
- **Genital prolapse** may lead to complaints of heaviness, pressure, a dropping sensation or pelvic aching.
- **Chronic PID** is usually as a result of persistent hydrosalpinx, tubo-ovarian cyst or pelvic adhesions.

Treatment depends on the suspected aetiology, but nonsurgical options may include a discussion of nutritional supplementation, physical therapy modalities, acupuncture/acupressure or antidepressants.

Non-gynaecological causes

- **Gastrointestinal disturbances** such as inflammatory bowel disease.
- **Musculoskeletal problems** such as muscle strain or disc herniation.
- **Interstitial cystitis** (chronic inflammatory condition of the bladder).
- **Somatoform disorders** are characterized by physical pain and symptoms that mimic disease, but are related to psychological factors (e.g. domestic discord, sexual abuse). Patients do not have conscious control over their symptoms and are not intentionally trying to confuse the doctor or complicate the process of diagnosis. Women often have long histories of unsuccessful medical or surgical treatments with multiple different physicians.

74 Urinary incontinence

Diagnosis of urinary incontinence

Simple cystometry

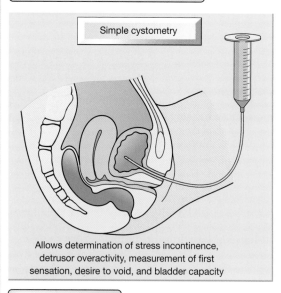

Allows determination of stress incontinence, detrusor overactivity, measurement of first sensation, desire to void, and bladder capacity

Complex urodynamic testing

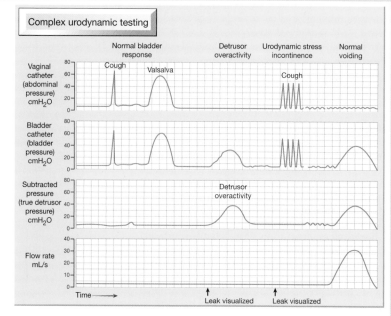

Surgical treatment

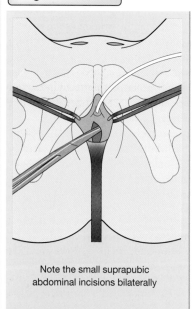

Note the small suprapubic abdominal incisions bilaterally

- Often performed laparoscopically, but also accessible via a Pfannenstiel incision
- A plane is identified beneath the rectus abdominis and dissected to the pubis
- The space of Retzius is opened

Tension-free transvaginal tape (TVT) sling

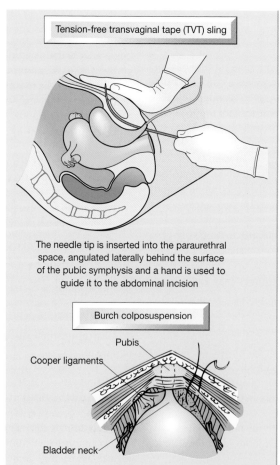

The needle tip is inserted into the paraurethral space, angulated laterally behind the surface of the pubic symphysis and a hand is used to guide it to the abdominal incision

Burch colposuspension

Pubis
Cooper ligaments
Bladder neck

The sling is adjusted to correct tension, the abdominal tape is cut at skin level, and incisions are closed

- A vaginal finger elevates the bladder neck
- 1–3 permanent sutures are placed lateral to the bladder neck and tied to Cooper's ligaments

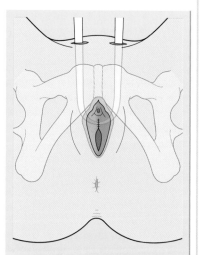

- **Definition**: involuntary leakage of urine that is suffiecient enough in frequency and amount to cause physical and/or emotional distress.

- **Incidence**: highly prevalent in women across their adult lifespan; severity increases linearly with age in women: 4–8% ultimately seek medical attention. One in three women aged >60 years has a bladder control problem.

- **Mechanism**: continence and urination involve a balance between urethral closure and detrusor (bladder smooth muscle) activity. Urethral pressure normally exceeds bladder pressure, resulting in urine remaining in the bladder. Intra-abdominal pressure increases (coughing, sneezing) are normally transmitted to both the urethra and bladder equally, maintaining continence. Disruption of this balance leads to various types of incontinence.

Diagnosis

There are six main steps in diagnosis:

1 History. A detailed history is important to determine the severity of symptoms and rule out medication causes. Emotional distress often does not correlate well with the amount of urine loss that can be demonstrated.

2 Physical examination:
- **General examination** to rule out delirium and atrophic urethritis, restricted mobility or stool impaction.
- **Urogynaecological examination** may reveal severe vulvar excoriation from continual dampness. The vaginal tissue should be inspected for signs of atrophy, stenosis, bladder neck mobility (*Q-tip test*) and atrophic urethritis. The patient is asked to cough repeatedly or undergo a Valsalva manoeuvre with a full bladder in the lithotomy or standing position to induce urine leakage. Rectal examination can evaluate rectal sphincter tone or the presence of faecal impaction.

3 Urinalysis and urine culture. Many relevant metabolic and urinary tract disorders can be screened by a simple urinalysis. A culture is essential to rule out infection before proceeding with further evaluation.

4 Residual urine volume after voiding. A catheterized post-void residual (PVR) urine specimen should be obtained to exclude urinary retention (normal PVR ≤ 100 mL) or infection.

5 Frequency–volume bladder chart. More than seven voids per day suggests a problem with frequency, but this is highly dependent on habit and fluid intake. Patients can be notoriously inaccurate in estimating urinary frequency and should be encouraged to keep a 'urinary diary' for several days as part of their initial evaluation.

6 Urodynamics is a group of tests designed to aid in determining the aetiology of lower urinary tract dysfunction:
- **Simple cystometry** involves placing a catheter and gradually filling the bladder with sterile water. Involuntary 'detrusor' contractions are demonstrated by a rise in water level during filling due to back pressure. Normally, the first sensation to void occurs at 150 mL and bladder capacity is typically 400–600 mL.
- **Uroflowmetry** is used to determine the urinary flow rate and flow time to screen for the presence of outflow obstruction and abnormal detrusor contractility. Normally, women achieve a peak flow rate of 15–20 mL/s with a voided volume of 150–200 mL.
- **Complex urodynamic testing** requires placement of an intravesical catheter to measure detrusor pressures and a vaginal or rectal catheter to indirectly measure intra-abdominal pressures.

Stress urinary incontinence

Patients have loss of small amounts of urine with coughing, laughing, sneezing, exercising or other movements that increase intra-abdominal pressure and thus increase pressure on the bladder.

- **Aetiology**: physical changes resulting from pregnancy, childbirth and menopause often result in weaknesses in the pelvic floor and urethral support structures and nerve damage.

- **Mechanism**: if the fascial support is weakened, the urethra can move downward at times of increased abdominal pressure, causing bladder pressure to exceed urethral sphincter closure pressure (hypermobile urethra). Incomplete urethral closure may be due to scarring or neuromuscular damage, and can cause a more severe form of stress urinary incontinence – intrinsic sphincter deficiency.
- **Diagnosis**: stress urinary incontinence (SUI) is suggested by the history, physical examination and a positive stress test (demonstrable loss of urine while the patient is being examined).
- **Non-surgical treatment** includes pelvic muscle (Kegel) exercises, biofeedback (pressure measurement device notifies the patient when correct muscle contraction is performed and reinforces correct technique) and pessaries.
- **Surgical treatment**:
  - **Tension-free transvaginal tape** or transobturator tape are minimally invasive suburethral sling procedures that are rapidly becoming the 'gold standard'.
  - **Burch colposuspension** involves suture placement at the Cooper ligament. The Marshall–Marchetti–Krantz variation has sutures going through the periosteum of the pubic symphysis.
  - **Anterior colporrhaphy** has a poor long-term success rate.
  - **Collagen periurethral injections** (Coaptite, Macroplastique) are designed as a treatment for SUI resulting from intrinsic sphincter deficiency.

Urge incontinence

Patients experience involuntary leakage for no apparent reason while suddenly feeling an urgent need to urinate. This may be accompanied by urinary frequency and nocturia, and patients often describe their bladder as 'spastic' or 'overactive'.

- **Aetiology**: involuntary detrusor muscle contractions. Detrusor hyperactivity can be due to loss of central nervous system inhibitory pathways, local irritants or bladder outlet obstruction.
- **Mechanism**: frequently idiopathic, but results from damage to the nerves of the bladder, the nervous system (spinal cord and brain) or the muscles themselves.
- **Treatment**: behaviour modification (bladder drills, biofeedback) and/or pharmacological therapy (oxybutynin chloride, imipramine, mirabegron), injection of the detrusor muscle with botulinum toxin A or neuromodulation.

Overflow incontinence

Patients experience continuous, unstoppable dribbling of urine, or continuing to dribble for some time after they have passed urine.

- **Aetiology**: the bladder is always full and overflows, resulting in frequent or continuous urine leakage.
- **Mechanism**: weak bladder detrusor muscles, resulting in incomplete emptying, or a blocked urethra (outflow obstruction) due to advanced vaginal prolapse, or after an anti-incontinence procedure that has overcorrected the problem.
- **Treatment**: catheter drainage, followed by treatment of the underlying condition.

Other types of incontinence

- **Mixed incontinence** usually refers to the common combination of stress and urge incontinence occurring together.
- **Transient incontinence** is often triggered by medications, urinary tract infections, mental impairment, restricted mobility or stool impaction (severe constipation), which can push against the urinary tract and obstruct outflow.
- **Functional incontinence** occurs when a person does not recognize the need to go to the toilet, recognize where the toilet is or get to the toilet in time due to confusion, dementia, poor eyesight or poor mobility.

75 Attempted suicide by drug poisoning

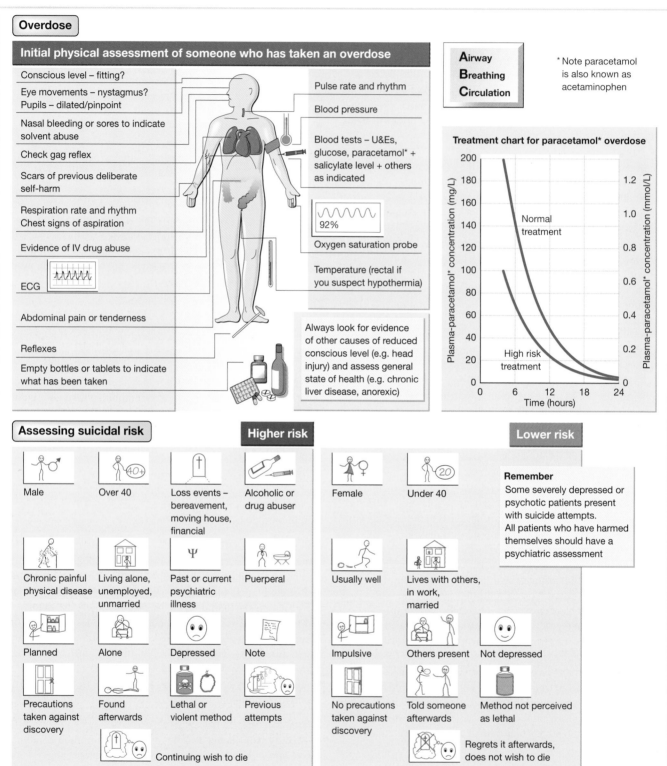

Overdose

Initial physical assessment of someone who has taken an overdose

Airway
Breathing
Circulation

* Note paracetamol is also known as acetaminophen

Conscious level – fitting?

Eye movements – nystagmus?
Pupils – dilated/pinpoint

Nasal bleeding or sores to indicate solvent abuse

Check gag reflex

Scars of previous deliberate self-harm

Respiration rate and rhythm
Chest signs of aspiration

Evidence of IV drug abuse

ECG

Abdominal pain or tenderness

Reflexes

Empty bottles or tablets to indicate what has been taken

Pulse rate and rhythm

Blood pressure

Blood tests – U&Es, glucose, paracetamol* + salicylate level + others as indicated

92%

Oxygen saturation probe

Temperature (rectal if you suspect hypothermia)

Always look for evidence of other causes of reduced conscious level (e.g. head injury) and assess general state of health (e.g. chronic liver disease, anorexic)

Treatment chart for paracetamol* overdose

Normal treatment

High risk treatment

Plasma-paracetamol* concentration (mg/L): 0, 20, 40, 60, 80, 100, 120, 140, 160, 180, 200

Plasma-paracetamol* concentration (mmol/L): 0, 0.2, 0.4, 0.6, 0.8, 1.0, 1.2

Time (hours): 0, 6, 12, 18, 24

Assessing suicidal risk

Higher risk

Male

Over 40

Loss events – bereavement, moving house, financial

Alcoholic or drug abuser

Chronic painful physical disease

Living alone, unemployed, unmarried

Past or current psychiatric illness

Puerperal

Planned

Alone

Depressed

Note

Precautions taken against discovery

Found afterwards

Lethal or violent method

Previous attempts

Continuing wish to die

Lower risk

Female

Under 40

Usually well

Lives with others, in work, married

Impulsive

Others present

Not depressed

No precautions taken against discovery

Told someone afterwards

Method not perceived as lethal

Regrets it afterwards, does not wish to die

Remember
Some severely depressed or psychotic patients present with suicide attempts.
All patients who have harmed themselves should have a psychiatric assessment

Medicine at a Glance, Fourth Edition. Edited by Patrick Davey. © 2014 John Wiley & Sons, Ltd. Published 2014 by John Wiley & Sons, Ltd. Companion website: www.ataglanceseries.com/medicine

Poisoning is a common reason for hospital admission. Most poisonings are deliberate, although some are accidental. Attempted suicide may be the first presentation of psychiatric illness.

History

The key facts to establish are: the circumstances of the attempt, psychiatric history (past and present) and past medical history.

Important points in the history are what was taken, when, how much and in what circumstances? How do they feel about it now? What was their suicide intent and risk? Psychiatric history should include the presence of current or past psychiatric illness and previous attempts; completed suicide rates are higher in patients with previous attempts.

Risk is increased by a history of bipolar disorder, depression, psychotic disorder, personality disorder and substance abuse (particularly alcohol). Anorexia also carries a risk and affects medical treatment. Likewise, medical illness and drug use affects treatment, e.g. liver disease or enzyme-inducing drugs lower the treatment threshold for paracetamol.

Drug information

The national poisons centres can be found in the *British National Formulary* (BNF). They offer invaluable phone advice 24 hours a day.

Examination

Overdose patients may be unconscious, fully alert or anything in between. Assess **a**irway, **b**reathing and **c**irculation (ABC). Look for:

- Hypotension, arrhythmias, e.g. with antiarrhythmics and tricyclics.
- Respiratory depression, e.g. with opiates.
- Aspiration if vomiting with reduced conscious level (unprotected airway).
- Hypothermia with barbiturate or phenothiazine.
- Glucose and electrolyte imbalance should be measured.
- Convulsions and coma: common in severe poisoning with many drugs.

Immediate treatment

- Activated charcoal, which binds poisons in the gastrointestinal tract, preventing absorption, is the treatment of choice for most poisons. It is most effective if used within 2 hours, although for drugs that delay gastric emptying or modified release preparations, it is useful for longer or repeated doses. The only common side effect is constipation (give a laxative). It is not useful for lithium, iron or pesticide ingestion.
- Gastric lavage is rarely used nowadays. It is only helpful within 1–2 hours, in conscious patients, with non-corrosive toxins.
- Ipecacuanha, which induces vomiting, is not used because it does not prevent absorption.
- Haemodialysis may be needed for severe salicylate, phenobarbital (phenobarbitone), methanol or ethylene glycol poisoning. Haemoperfusion can be used for theophylline and barbiturate poisoning.

Some specific commonly ingested poisons

Paracetamol

For paracetamol, 12 g (24 tablets) is a potentially fatal dose in most patients, whereas 7.5 g may be lethal in high-risk individuals. Symptoms are delayed up to 3 days after the overdose, when nausea, vomiting and abdominal pain, and late fulminant hepatic failure, can occur. Paracetamol is metabolized by liver conjugation; when this pathway is saturated a toxic metabolite is formed, usually inactivated by glutathione. When glutathione stores run out, this metabolite binds to cell proteins, causing cell death. Lower doses are toxic in people on enzyme-inducing drugs (e.g. phenytoin, carbamazepine, rifampicin) and undernourished people (anorexia, alcoholism, starvation).

Management

- Activated charcoal.
- *N*-acetylcysteine to increase liver glutathione if the paracetamol level is high 4 hours after ingestion, continued, in high-risk individuals, until paracetamol is no longer detected. Oral methionine is given if *N*-acetylcysteine is unavailable or the patient is allergic.
- Monitor urea and electrolytes (U&Es), glucose, liver function tests and clotting initially and 24 hours after ingestion.
- In severe overdose, patients may require liver support, including transplantation.

Tricyclic antidepressants

Tricyclic overdosage causes drowsiness, dilated pupils, dry mouth, tachycardia and urinary retention (anticholinergic effects), and hypothermia with hyperreflexia. In severe toxicity convulsions, coma, respiratory depression, hypotension, arrhythmias and cardiac arrest may occur. Treatment is activated charcoal and monitoring of heart rhythm (continuous electrocardiogram); intubate ± ventilation if respiration is inadequate or there are convulsions or arrhythmias (hyperventilation and bicarbonate improve arrhythmias). On recovery, delirium, agitation and visual and auditory hallucinations are common and respond to diazepam.

Opiates

Opiates cause respiratory depression, pinpoint pupils and hypotension, vomiting, fits and pulmonary oedema. Naloxone, a specific antidote, is given. The half-life of naloxone is very short (less than opiate), so an intravenous (IV) infusion is often needed.

Salicylates

Salicylates cause restlessness, flushing, sweating and hyperventilation. Nausea, vomiting and tinnitus are common. Confusion, coma and convulsions are rare. Cardiac arrest may occur in severe overdose. Electrolyte abnormalities are common, such as hypokalaemic alkalosis (vomiting), respiratory alkalosis (hyperventilation) or a metabolic acidosis (uncoupling of oxidative phosphorylation). Dehydration and hyperpyrexia occur. Glucose control is impaired causing hypo- or hyperglycaemia. A bleeding tendency may develop. Treat with activated charcoal, repeated activated charcoal and IV saline. A forced alkaline diuresis is rarely used nowadays. Monitor full blood count, U&Es, clotting, glucose and gases; chest X-ray for pulmonary oedema.

Benzodiazepines

In overdose, benzodiazepines cause drowsiness, ataxia, dysarthria and nystagmus. Flumazenil, a specific antidote, is rarely used because it causes fits in those on long-term benzodiazepines, people with epilepsy and when taken with tricyclics.

Alcohol

Alcohol may be taken as part of the attempt or before the attempt, acutely or chronically. Alcoholism affects liver function, and thus affects any drugs or poisons that affect the liver, such as paracetamol. Acute alcohol intoxication depresses the conscious level and respiration – even small quantities of alcohol potentiate central nervous system depressants.

76 Anaphylaxis

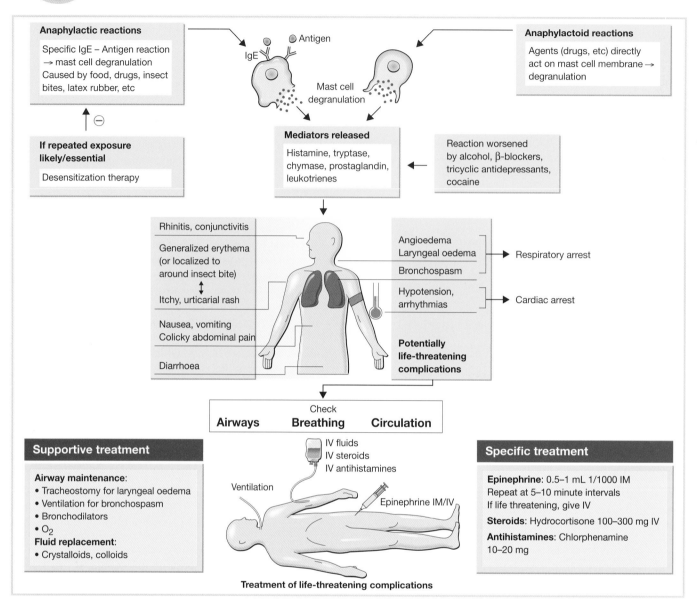

Anaphylactic reactions

Specific IgE – Antigen reaction → mast cell degranulation
Caused by food, drugs, insect bites, latex rubber, etc

If repeated exposure likely/essential

Desensitization therapy

Anaphylactoid reactions

Agents (drugs, etc) directly act on mast cell membrane → degranulation

Antigen
IgE
Mast cell degranulation

Mediators released

Histamine, tryptase, chymase, prostaglandin, leukotrienes

Reaction worsened by alcohol, β-blockers, tricyclic antidepressants, cocaine

Rhinitis, conjunctivitis

Generalized erythema (or localized to around insect bite)
↕
Itchy, urticarial rash

Nausea, vomiting
Colicky abdominal pain

Diarrhoea

Angioedema
Laryngeal oedema → Respiratory arrest

Bronchospasm

Hypotension, arrhythmias → Cardiac arrest

Potentially life-threatening complications

Check
Airways   Breathing   Circulation

Supportive treatment

Airway maintenance:
• Tracheostomy for laryngeal oedema
• Ventilation for bronchospasm
• Bronchodilators
• O₂
Fluid replacement:
• Crystalloids, colloids

Ventilation

IV fluids
IV steroids
IV antihistamines

Epinephrine IM/IV

Specific treatment

Epinephrine: 0.5–1 mL 1/1000 IM
Repeat at 5–10 minute intervals
If life threatening, give IV
Steroids: Hydrocortisone 100–300 mg IV
Antihistamines: Chlorphenamine 10–20 mg

Treatment of life-threatening complications

Anaphylaxis is an acute, generalized, life-threatening allergic reaction, affecting one in 10 000 individuals/year and is the cause of one in every 2700 hospital admissions.

Mechanism

Anaphylaxis results from the rapid systemic release of large quantities of biologically active mediators from mast cells and basophils, triggered by the interaction of the allergen with specific IgE antibodies bound to cell membranes. Cell activation results in the release of preformed mediators stored in granules (including histamine, tryptase and chymase) and of newly formed mediators (including prostaglandins and leukotrienes). These mediators cause capillary leakage, mucosal oedema and smooth muscle contraction.

Anaphylactoid reactions result from the non-specific degranulation of mast cells by drugs, chemicals or other triggers, and do not involve IgE-based sensitivity. These reactions are clinically indistinguishable from anaphylactic reactions. Acutely the discrimination is unnecessary as the management is the same. However, discrimination between IgE-mediated and non-IgE-mediated disease may subsequently be important in identifying the precipitating agent.

Clinical features

Patients present with a range of clinical features:
● Feeling of impending doom.
● Generalized pruritus.
● Erythema and/or urticaria, though some 50% of patients may not experience any rash.
● Angioedema.
● Bronchospasm.
● Laryngeal oedema ± stridor.

Medicine at a Glance, Fourth Edition. Edited by Patrick Davey. © 2014 John Wiley & Sons, Ltd. Published 2014 by John Wiley & Sons, Ltd. Companion website: www.ataglanceseries.com/medicine

- Rhinitis.
- Conjunctivitis.
- Nausea, vomiting, abdominal pain, uterine contractions.
- Palpitations, cardiac arrhythmias.
- Hypotension.
- Cardiorespiratory arrest.

The symptoms are usually of rapid onset, within minutes of exposure, although they may be delayed up to several hours. Route of exposure to the triggering agent, as well as quantity of antigen, rate of administration and coexistent features such as alcohol and exercise, determine the severity of a reaction. Reactions are not always of the same degree of severity, even on exposure to the same allergen.

The immediate symptoms are caused by the release of stored histamine. Occasionally the symptoms of anaphylaxis recur after some hours, a *biphasic reaction*, so all individuals should be kept under observation for at least 6 hours after an anaphylactic episode. Late phase reactions are caused by synthesis *de novo* by the mast cells of leukotrienes, which have similar biological properties to histamine. The late reaction can be blocked by early administration of corticosteroids.

Source of allergen

The commonest causes of anaphylaxis are **foods**. The majority of food reactions are to peanuts (a pea, not a nut!) and to the tree nuts (hazelnut, almond, brazil nut, walnut, cashew, etc.). Peanut-allergic patients often also have allergy to tree nuts as well as other legumes. Peanuts and almonds may be present as a hidden allergen in many different foods. Particular care needs to be taken with oriental food. Shellfish and fish are potent causes of severe allergic reactions, and miniscule levels of exposure may cause severe reactions. Any other food is capable of causing reactions.

Other causes include:

- **Stinging insects** (bees, bumblebees, wasps, hornets, fire ants) can cause severe reactions.
- Severe reactions to **latex** are increasing due to the use of latex in health care. Most patients with latex allergy, however, have type IV delayed hypersensitivity reactions, mainly against the chemicals in the rubber rather than the rubber proteins, leading to contact dermatitis.
- Many **drugs** can cause IgE-mediated reactions including penicillins, muscle relaxants (which are all highly cross-reactive) and other anaesthetic agents and biological products such as vaccines. Opiate drugs such as morphine and codeine cause anaphylactoid reactions due to direct degranulation of mast cells; fentanyl does not seem to have this effect. Non-steroidal anti-inflammatory drugs also cause severe reactions through non-IgE mechanisms. Radiocontrast media, particularly non-ionic media, are potent mast cell degranulating agents.
- **Exercise**, alone or with foods, particularly wheat, can trigger anaphylaxis.
- In some cases **no cause** can be identified despite extensive searching (idiopathic anaphylaxis).

Differential diagnosis

Some clinical features of anaphylaxis are similar to other local or systemic disease. Accurate clinical assessment is essential:

- Shock (see Chapter 18).
- Airway obstruction: status asthmaticus, acute bacterial epiglottitis, acute foreign body upper airway obstruction.
- Mediator release: mastocytosis (excessive collections of mast cells in the gut, skin and bone marrow), carcinoid syndrome.

- Recurrent angioedema: inherited and acquired C1 esterase inhibitor deficiency, drug-induced angioedema; idiopathic angioedema.
- Vasovagal syncope.
- Factitious anaphylaxis (usually occurring in patients with known anaphylaxis).
- Globus hystericus (characterized by a lack of evidence of airway obstruction, despite protestations of swelling in the throat, and no rash or other symptoms).

Management

Acute management
Anaphylaxis is an acute medical emergency, which in the absence of appropriate treatment carries a significant mortality. Resuscitation should follow the normal rules of **a**irway, **b**reathing and **c**irculation (ABC):

- Airway maintenance: look for obstruction (swollen tongue, stridor). Administer high-flow oxygen. Consider a tracheotomy if complete airway obstruction is likely.
- Check breathing: full resuscitation if not breathing.
- Circulation: check pulse and blood pressure. Patients with excess histamine are usually warm and vasodilated with hypotension. Pulse is rapid. Obtain intravenous (IV) access.
- Adrenaline: *early* administration of adrenaline (epinephrine) is essential; 0.5 mL 1/1000 solution intramuscular (0.5 mg IM, Resuscitation Council UK Guideline), repeat after 5 minutes intervals if no response; further doses may be required. Do not administer subcutaneously (poor absorption). In the hospital setting, IV adrenaline may be administered *only* with appropriate electrocardiogram monitoring. It must be given well diluted (10 mL 1/10 000 solution diluted into 100 mL normal saline and administered via an infusion pump).
- Corticosteroids: hydrocortisone 200 mg IV (this prevents late reactions).
- Antihistamines: chlorphenamine 10 mg IV (this is traditional but not of proven value).
- Fluid replacement: use colloid or crystalloid to restore blood pressure.
- Use nebulized salbutamol for bronchospasm.
- Keep under observation for a minimum of 6 hours before discharge, even if there is rapid recovery.
- Do not discharge without a clear plan for further investigation and follow-up.
- If appropriate, discharge with adrenaline for self-administration.

Subsequent management
All individuals who have experienced anaphylaxis should be referred to a clinical immunologist or allergist for further investigation to identify the trigger factor and to educate the patient in avoidance and management of subsequent episodes. Consideration should be given to supplying adrenaline for self-administration. In the specific event of bee or wasp venom-induced anaphylaxis, immunotherapy with graded concentrations of allergen is effective in reducing the risk of further reactions.

Prognosis

The natural history and prognosis of anaphylaxis is variable. There are no predictors of the severity of further reactions. Avoidance remains the mainstay. Anxiety is extremely common and needs to be addressed. If the trigger factor cannot be identified or cannot be avoided, recurrence may be common and should be anticipated. Many children will grow out of early food-induced reactions, although peanut sensitivity is often life-long. Food challenges may be required to prove loss of sensitization.

77 Allergic reactions

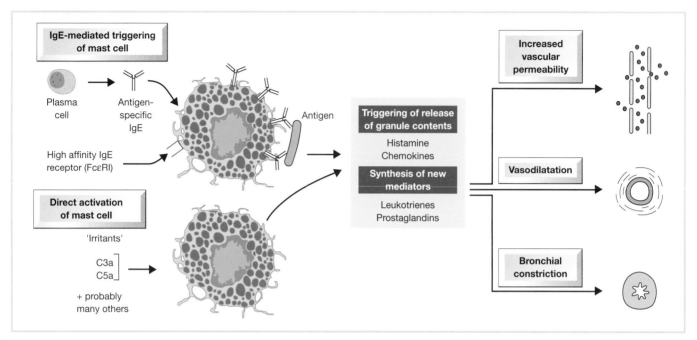

The severity of an allergic reaction depends upon the dose, site of allergen exposure and individual characteristics including medication and previous history. In most the history provides the key to the diagnosis, especially as in non-urgent situations most patients will have few physical signs. Allergic disorders include:

- Summer hayfever (pollen-induced allergic rhinoconjunctivitis).
- Perennial rhinitis (house dust mites, pets).
- Allergic asthma (including occupational asthma).
- Allergy to drugs.
- Food allergy and food intolerance, oral allergy syndrome.
- Allergy to stinging insects.
- Allergic skin disorders, e.g. atopic eczema.
- Anaphylaxis (acute generalized allergic reaction).
- Urticaria (see Chapter 223).
- Angioedema.

Inhalant allergy

Allergy to inhalant allergens such as house dust mite, animal danders and pollens (grasses, trees, weeds) will trigger allergic rhinoconjunctivitis, sinusitis and asthma. Typical features include sneezing, blocked and running nose, headache and sinus pain, and itchy red eyes often with discharge, with or without asthmatic symptoms. Onset is rapid on exposure, but symptoms may be chronic if exposure cannot be avoided. A good history will usually identify the most likely triggers. Diagnosis is by the skin prick test or 'RAST' test. Management is by the use of topical treatments to the eye (sodium cromoglicate, nedocromil sodium), nose (nasal steroid sprays such as beclomethasone, mometasone, triamcinolone, fluticasone) and lung (inhaled bronchodilators such as salbutamol, salmeterol, formeterol and steroids, beclomethasone,

budesonide, fluticasone), accompanied by oral antihistamines (potent non-sedating, long-acting antihistamines such as fexofenadine, cetirizine, levocetirizine). For upper airway allergy, desensitization by immunotherapy is possible for patients whose symptoms cannot be controlled on maximal medical therapy, including oral steroids. Injectable steroids (Kenalog) are no longer recommended.

Food allergy

Food 'allergy' is blamed for a plethora of symptoms, not all of which are related to true, IgE-mediated, food allergy. There is no evidence that irritable bowel symptoms are related to food allergy, although sufferers often complain of bloating with wheat-based products. Excess nasal catarrh is sometimes associated with milk intolerance. Anaphylaxis represents the severe end of the spectrum of disease, but urticaria and angioedema may represent less severe reactions. Eczema is associated with food allergies in children, often to dairy products and wheat, but adult eczema is less commonly helped by dietary manipulation. The oral allergy syndrome is the association of inhalant allergy to birch pollen in association with lip and tongue swelling when eating soft fruits such as peaches, nectarines, apples, almonds and other closely related fruits. This syndrome is rarely associated with anaphylaxis. The allergens are heat labile and destroyed by cooking. Occasionally it may be necessary to undertake an elimination diet with sequential reintroduction of foods to identify foods causing the symptoms. Double-blind, placebo-controlled challenge is the gold standard for investigation of food-related symptoms.

Angioedema

Angioedema relates to deep tissue swelling, which is usually non-itchy. It may occur alone or with urticaria. Bradykinin is the main trigger. It often presents acutely to accident and emergency (A&E) and acute medical services. It must be distinguished from systemic allergic reactions. Hereditary angioedema is extremely rare and is due to deficiency of the complement regulatory protein C1 esterase inhibitor (see Chapter 223). Acquired angioedema caused by autoantibodies against the inhibitor may very rarely be seen in older patients in association with lymphoma and myeloma or in association with other autoimmune disease such as systemic lupus erythematosus. The commonest causes of angioedema, however, are stress, infections and allergic reactions to foods and drugs. The commonest drugs causing angioedema are angiotensin-converting enzyme (ACE) inhibitors, which cause angioedema by preventing the breakdown of bradykinin, non-steroidal anti-inflammatory drugs and statins (cholesterol-lowering drugs). Many cases, particularly of nocturnal angioedema, do not have an identifiable trigger (idiopathic).

Antihistamines are ineffective in many cases of angioedema without urticaria, but tranexamic acid, an antifibrinolytic drug, may be valuable in preventing swelling where there is no avoidable trigger identified. Acute attacks usually require treatment with intravenous or oral corticosteroids. Adrenaline (epinephrine) should be reserved for angioedema where there is clear laryngeal involvement.

Urticaria

The typical rash in urticaria is that of wheal and flare (nettle rash), caused by histamine. The rash may be generalized and patients may feel systemically unwell. Presentation to A&E is common. The causes of acute urticaria are stress, infection, allergy and physical causes (sun, pressure, water, vibration, heat, cold), in association with thyroid disease or haematinic deficiency. However, in many cases there is no identifiable cause. Chronic urticaria, lasting beyond 6 weeks, is rarely associated with allergy (see also Chapter 223).

Acute treatment is with high-dose antihistamine given orally (cetirizine 10–20 mg daily) or intravenously (chlorphenamine 10 mg IV) and 24–48 hours of oral corticosteroid (prednisolone 20 mg/day). Treatment of chronic urticaria is with antihistamines, and it may be necessary to use larger doses than those normally used. Tricyclic antidepressants such as doxepin are valuable as they have potent anti-H1 and -H2 blocking activity. Montelukast may also be helpful. Corticosteroid therapy should be avoided in chronic urticaria apart from emergency management, as the risks of side effects outweigh the benefits.

Investigation of allergic disease

Skin-prick tests are cheap, quick and used to support the diagnosis. The patient is exposed to standardized solutions of allergen extract through a skin prick to the forearm. Positive (histamine) and negative (saline) controls are included. A wheal >2 mm greater than the negative control is a positive test. Testing should be carried out with great caution in patients who have had anaphylaxis. Skin must be normal so this type of testing is inappropriate in patients with eczema.

Antihistamines should be discontinued for 1 week before testing as they abolish the response. Other drugs such as calcium channel blockers (for hypertension) and antidepressant drugs also interfere with the tests.

The 'RAST' test measures specific IgE in a blood sample to the putative antigen. This laboratory test is a useful alternative when skin-prick tests are not available, or if a patient is on antihistamines. The results are similar to skin-prick tests for inhalant allergens and nuts, but are not so useful for drug allergy and certain foods with labile allergens (fruits).

78 Cardiac and respiratory arrest

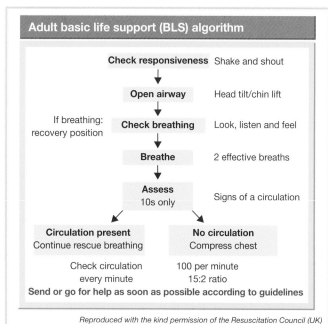

Adult basic life support (BLS) algorithm

Check responsiveness — Shake and shout

Open airway — Head tilt/chin lift

Check breathing — Look, listen and feel

If breathing: recovery position

Breathe — 2 effective breaths

Assess
10s only — Signs of a circulation

Circulation present
Continue rescue breathing

No circulation
Compress chest

Check circulation every minute

100 per minute
15:2 ratio

Send or go for help as soon as possible according to guidelines

Reproduced with the kind permission of the Resuscitation Council (UK)

Cardiac and respiratory arrests are common in the community and in hospital. The common causes of circulatory failure, 'cardiac arrest', are sufficiently severe to cause unconsciousness and compromise life.

Causes of cardiac and respiratory arrest

Cardiac arrest

- **Ventricular arrhythmias**: these can be due to acute coronary occlusions, scar tissue late after a myocardial infarction (MI), heart failure of any aetiology, and metabolic disturbance (e.g. hypo- and hyperkalaemia, hypoxaemia, drugs including tricyclic antidepressants, non-sedating antihistamines, major antipsychotics, macrolide antibiotics, etc.).
- **Bradyarrhythmias**: due to conducting tissue disease, e.g. complete heart block, during MI, following prolonged ventricular arrhythmias or respiratory arrest (see ALS section).
- **Cardiogenic shock**: often caused by large MIs or advanced heart failure.

Electromechanical dissociation

If circulatory failure occurs and QRST complexes are seen on the electrocardiogram (ECG) monitor ('electromechanical dissociation') consider:

- **Hypovolaemia**: e.g. stab wounds, torrential gastrointestinal or retroperitoneal haemorrhage (e.g. ruptured abdominal aortic aneurysm).
- **Pericardial tamponade**: stab wounds, recent MI (where it indicates cardiac rupture), malignancy or immediately after cardiac surgery.
- **Pulmonary embolus**.
- **Tension pneumothorax**: in people with asthma, in chronic lung diseases, especially chronic obstructive pulmonary disease (COPD), or after trauma.

Respiratory arrest

There are a number of common causes of failure to breathe sufficiently to maintain life – 'respiratory arrest':

- **Severe lung disease**: pneumonia, severe airway obstruction (e.g. asthma, exacerbation of COPD, end-stage COPD, etc.).
- **Airway obstruction**: foreign body, or the tongue in a comatose patient.
- **Left ventricular failure**.
- **Brain injury**: stroke, overdose of narcotic drugs (e.g. opiates) or hypnotics (e.g. major tranquillizers, etc.).

Many patients present with combined circulatory and respiratory arrest. This usually means that the initial cardiac or respiratory arrest is far advanced, because one inevitably leads to the other.

Cardiopulmonary resuscitation

Cardiopulmonary resuscitation (CPR) is the term applied for the immediate treatment of cardiac and/or respiratory arrest. CPR constitutes support both for the circulation and respiration, and is a generic treatment applicable to most cases of cardiac/respiratory arrest. However, it does not remove the need to make an accurate diagnosis so that specific therapy, when available, can be given early on when it is most likely to be life saving. Establish the diagnosis using all available tools, e.g. bystander history (nurses, ambulance staff, etc.), finding prescription or street drugs in pockets, physical examination, immediate ECG, chest X-ray, etc.

Key principles underlying CPR

The principles underlying CPR are:

- **Appropriateness**: treatment aims to restore the patient to a high quality of life. If this is not possible, consider whether CPR is inappropriate. 'Do not attempt resuscitation' (DNAR) orders (always clearly recorded in the notes) are made on the basis of:
  - The chance of immediate CPR success (relates to age and disease).
  - The chance of restoring long-term high-quality life (relates to pre-existing quality of life).
  - Patient's and relatives' wishes, which must be established.
- **Speed**: after total circulatory/respiratory failure irreversible hypoxic brain injury follows within 3–4 minutes (unless extreme hypothermia is present). Furthermore, cardiac anoxia develops quickly, preventing successful restoration of the circulation. The penalty for *incorrect and/or late* diagnosis and treatment is the death of the patient!
- **Summon additional help** as soon as possible.

Basic life support

Assess **a**irway, **b**reathing and **c**irculation (ABC) and apply the adult **basic life support** (BLS) algorithm (basic = no equipment available) (see Figure 78.1 above). If victims do not respond to shaking/shouting, turn them on to their back, open and inspect the airway. Remove any obstruction. Determine within 10 seconds whether breathing is normal:

- Look for chest movement.
- Listen at the victim's mouth for breath sounds.
- Feel for air on your cheek.

Medicine at a Glance, Fourth Edition. Edited by Patrick Davey. © 2014 John Wiley & Sons, Ltd. Published 2014 by John Wiley & Sons, Ltd. Companion website: www.ataglanceseries.com/medicine

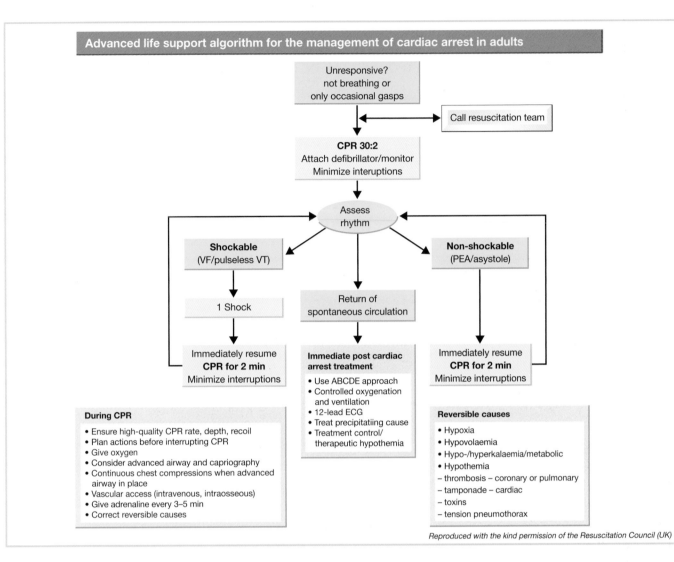

Advanced life support algorithm for the management of cardiac arrest in adults

Unresponsive?
not breathing or
only occasional gasps

Call resuscitation team

CPR 30:2
Attach defibrillator/monitor
Minimize interuptions

Assess
rhythm

Shockable
(VF/pulseless VT)

Non-shockable
(PEA/asystole)

1 Shock

Return of
spontaneous circulation

Immediately resume
CPR for 2 min
Minimize interruptions

Immediately resume
CPR for 2 min
Minimize interruptions

**Immediate post cardiac
arrest treatment**
• Use ABCDE approach
• Controlled oxygenation
  and ventilation
• 12-lead ECG
• Treat precipitatiing cause
• Treatment control/
  therapeutic hypothemia

During CPR
• Ensure high-quality CPR rate, depth, recoil
• Plan actions before interrupting CPR
• Give oxygen
• Consider advanced airway and capriography
• Continuous chest compressions when advanced
  airway in place
• Vascular access (intravenous, intraosseous)
• Give adrenaline every 3–5 min
• Correct reversible causes

Reversible causes
• Hypoxia
• Hypovolaemia
• Hypo-/hyperkalaemia/metabolic
• Hypothemia
– thrombosis – coronary or pulmonary
– tamponade – cardiac
– toxins
– tension pneumothorax

Reproduced with the kind permission of the Resuscitation Council (UK)

If normal breathing is found, turn the victim into the recovery position and seek help. If only weak respiratory efforts occur, give two slow, effective rescue breaths into the mouth (each of 700–1000 mL), with the nose pinched shut, sufficient to make the chest rise and fall. After two effective breaths (use five or more attempts for this), check the circulation (carotid/femoral pulse if you have been trained to do so). If there is no circulation, start chest compressions, pushing the sternum down 4–5 cm each time, at a rate of 100/min, alternating 15 compressions to two breaths. Chest compressions restore 30% of normal cerebral perfusion. Continue this sequence until movement or breathing occurs or expert help arrives.

Advanced life support

Advanced life support (ALS) (i.e. equipment is available; see Figure 78.2 above): apply BLS, attach ECG electrodes and diagnose the heart rhythm:

• **Ventricular fibrillation** (VF) and **pulseless ventricular tachycardia** (VT) are the common, survivable causes of cardiac arrest. Success rates decline by 7–10% for every minute that defibrillation is delayed. Charge the defibrillator and give three shocks with energies of 200, 200 and 360 J. After successful cardioversion, transient ($\geq$10 s) asystole and/or a weak pulse (myocardial

stunning) may occur; accordingly give CPR for 1 minute after the three shocks before re-evaluating the rhythm. If VF/VT persists, secure the airway (endotracheal tube, laryngeal mask airway, Combi-Tube) and ventilate at 12 breaths/min using 100% oxygen. Establish peripheral intravenous (IV) access (central access is unsafe during CPR). Give adrenaline (epinephrine) to improve the efficacy of CPR (α-adrenergic actions cause vasoconstriction, increasing myocardial and cerebral perfusion pressures). Refractory VF/VT may respond to further shocks or IV amiodarone, lidocaine (lignocaine) or procainamide (never give these drugs in combination). Continue until the circulation is restored, or the decision is made to stop. Give bicarbonate if pH is $\geq$7.1, in tricyclic overdose or if hyperkalaemia is present.

• **Asystole** is usually lethal. Consider giving atropine. Complete heart block responds to pacing (external or transvenous) and/or isoprenaline. Beware spurious asystole: VF with a low voltage trace, or incorrectly applied electrodes.

• **Unremarkable ECG tracing**: see section on electromechanical dissociation.

Discontinue CPR, after consultation with other team members, when the situation is irrecoverable, based on duration of CPR and whether a stable circulation was ever attained. Pupil dilatation is an unreliable sign of irreversible brain damage.

79 Delirium

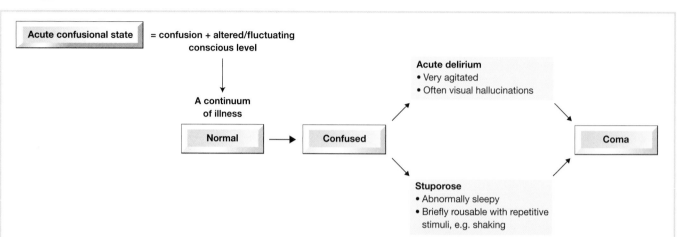

Acute confusional state = confusion + altered/fluctuating conscious level

A continuum of illness

Normal → Confused

Acute delirium
• Very agitated
• Often visual hallucinations

Stuporose
• Abnormally sleepy
• Briefly rousable with repetitive stimuli, e.g. shaking

Coma

Causes of acute confusional state

Infection
• Urinary or respiratory tract infection are commonest causes
• Bacterial meningitis, endocarditis and intra-abdominal sepsis (e.g. cholangitis) should be considered in the febrile patient without localizing signs
• Exclude malaria if there has been recent travel to an endemic region

Drug-related
• Many drugs may cause acute confusional state in older patients, notably benzodiazepines, tricyclics, analgesics (including NSAIDs), lithium, steroids, and drugs for parkinsonism
• Consider poisoning with amphetamine, cocaine and other psychotropic drugs in younger patients with acute confusional state
• Benzodiazepine withdrawal may also cause a confusional state
• Consider neuroleptic malignant syndrome if the patient is taking a neuroleptic

Alcohol-related
• Intoxication or withdrawal (confusional state due to alcohol withdrawal may cause vivid visual or auditory hallucinations)
• Wernicke's encephalopathy, characterized by confusional state, nystagmus, sixth nerve palsy (unable to abduct the eye) and ataxia (wide-based gait; may be unable to stand or walk)

Other systemic disorders
• Hypoglycaemia
• Hyperglycaemic states: ketoacidosis and non-ketotic hyperglycaemia
• Respiratory failure
• Heart failure with low cardiac output
• Acute liver failure
• Advanced renal failure
• Hypernatraemia or hyponatraemia
• Hypercalcaemia
• Hypothermia

Primary neurological disorders
• Head injury
• Post-ictal state
• Meningitis
• Encephalitis
• Non-dominant parietal lobe stroke
• Subdural haematoma
• Subarachnoid haemorrhage
• Non-convulsive status epilepticus (which may be associated with mild clonic movements of the eyelids, face or hands, or simple automatisms)
• Raised intracranial pressure

'Confusion' screen

• Metabolic tests
  – glucose, Na^+, INR (for liver failure), urea, creatinine, T_4, Ca^{2+}, blood gases (for respiratory failure and CO poisoning)

• Full blood count

• 'Septic' tests
  – urine + blood cultures, chest X-ray, C-reactive protein, ESR

• 'Structural' tests
  – CT head scan

+ other 'targeted' tests, including lumbar puncture and EEG

Medicine at a Glance, Fourth Edition. Edited by Patrick Davey. © 2014 John Wiley & Sons, Ltd. Published 2014 by John Wiley & Sons, Ltd. Companion website: www.ataglanceseries.com/medicine

Delirium is a functional brain disorder characterized by clouding of consciousness and impaired cognitive function, which develops over hours or days, and typically fluctuates over the course of the day. Present on hospital admission in around 15% of patients aged over 65, and developing after admission in a further 20%, delirium is a common manifestation of a wide range of systemic disorders (notably infection) or an adverse effect of medications, especially those with an anticholinergic effect. In patients of all ages it may reflect a primary neurological disorder. Common causes of delirium by context are shown in Table 79.1.

Diagnosis of delirium

Delirium is a clinical diagnosis, based on examination of the patient's mental state supplemented by a collateral history from family members, carers or hospital staff.

Table 79.1 Causes of delirium by context.

Patient group	Common causes
Older patient in emergency department	Acute infection (e.g. urinary tract, lower respiratory tract) Adverse effect of medication Electrolyte disorder Stroke
Younger patient in emergency department	Alcohol intoxication Poisoning with psychoactive drug Primary neurological disorder (e.g. encephalitis)
Patient with alcohol dependence or alcoholic liver disease	Alcohol intoxication or withdrawal Liver failure Acute infection (e.g. spontaneous bacterial peritonitis, pneumonia)
Patient with cancer	Brain or meningeal metastases Electrolyte disorder (e.g. hypercalcaemia, hyponatraemia) Adverse effect of medication (e.g. opioid toxicity) Paraneoplastic effect
Older patient after surgery	Acute infection Pain Adverse effect of medication Urinary retention Faecal impaction

Reproduced with permission from the National Institute for Health and Care Excellence (NICE).

Table 79.2a Shortened form of the Mini-Mental Status Examination.

Orientation

1. What is the year / season / month / date / day?

2. Where are we (country / county / town / hospital / ward)?

Registration

3. Name three objects (repeat until all three are learned)

Attention

4. Spell 'WORLD' backwards

Memory

5. Recall the three objects learned in question 3

The duration of the abnormal mental state (developing over hours or days) helps distinguish delirium from dementia, with which it may coexist, as dementia renders the brain vulnerable to delirium. Delirium may be obvious from the patient's behaviour and speech, but you should also suspect the disorder in any older patient labelled as difficult, depressed, uncooperative or a 'poor historian'.

The mental state examination includes tests of attention, orientation and memory, and can be done in a few minutes using the well-known 10-item abbreviated mental status examination or the shortened version of the Mini-Mental Status Examination (see Table 79.2a). The Confusion Assessment Method (CAM) instrument provides a quick and accurate method (when compared to a reference standard) of confirming the diagnosis (see Table 79.2b).

Diagnosing the cause of delirium

Delirium may be due to illness such as respiratory failure that poses an immediate threat to life. You need to make a rapid assessment of the patient, and ensure that the airway, breathing and circulation are stable. Blood glucose should be checked at the bedside to exclude hypo- or hyperglycaemia. You should then complete a focused history and examination (see Figure 79.1), and arrange appropriate investigation. As a general rule, all patients with delirium should have a full blood count, biochemical profile, measurement of C-reactive protein level, urine stick test and chest radiograph. Additional investigations will be guided by the context and clinical findings. Neuroimaging (by computed tomography or magnetic resonance imaging) is indicated: if delirium followed a fall or head injury; if there are new focal neurological signs; if there is papilloedema or other evidence of raised intracranial pressure; if the patient has cancer or HIV-AIDS; if the patient's behaviour prevents adequate neurological

Table 79.2b The Confusion Assessment Method (CAM) instrument for the diagnosis of delirium. Delirium is diagnosed by the presence of features 1 and 2, plus either 3a or 3b.

Clinical feature	Evidence
1. Acute onset and fluctuating course	Is there evidence of an acute change in mental status from the patient's baseline? Does the abnormal behaviour fluctuate during the day (tend to come or go, or increase or decrease in severity)?
2. Inattention	Did the patient have difficulty focusing attention (e.g. easily distractible) or have difficulty keeping track of what was being said?
3a. Disorganized thinking	Was the patient's thinking disorganized or incoherent: such as rambling or irrelevant conversation, unclear or illogical flow of ideas, or unpredictable switching from subject to subject?
3b. Altered level of consciousness	Overall, how would you rate this patient's level of consciousness: alert (normal), vigilant (hyper-alert), lethargic (drowsy but easily aroused), stuporose (difficult to arouse) or comatose? *Positive for any answer other than 'alert'*

Source: S.K. Inouye et al. *Ann Intern Med* 1990; 113; 941–8.

Table 79.3 Prevention and management of delirium.

Clinical factors that can contribute to delirium	Preventative interventions and actions
Disorientation	Provide clear signage, soft lighting, a 24h clock and a calendar, all easily visible to the patient Introduce cognitively stimulating activities Facilitate regular visits from family and friends
Dehydration and/or constipation	Ensure an adequate fluid intake Take advice where necessary when managing fluid balance in patients with co-morbidities such as heart failure or chronic kidney disease Look for and treat constipation
Infection	Look for and treat infection Avoid unnecessary bladder catheterization Implement good infection control procedures
Pain	Find out whether the patient has pain Look out for non-verbal signs of pain, particularly in those with communication difficulties If patients have been prescribed pain relief, ensure they receive it
Polypharmacy effects	Review the medications the patient is taking and stop those which may be contributing to delirium
Poor nutrition	Follow the advice given on nutrition in NICE Clinical Guideline 32 If patients have dentures, ensure they are well-fitting
Restricted or limited mobility or immobility	Encourage patients to carry out active range-of-motion exercises, to walk about if they can, and mobilize early after surgery
Sensory impairment	Ensure hearing and visual aids (in good working order) are available to and used by patients who need them
Sleep disturbance	Promote good sleep patterns and sleep hygiene by scheduling medication rounds to avoid disturbing sleep, and reducing noise to a minimum during sleep periods

Reproduced with permission the National Institute for Health and Care Excellence (NICE).

examination; or if no systemic cause for the delirium is apparent. Examination of the cerebrospinal fluid should be done (assuming no contraindication to lumbar puncture): if meningitis or encephalitis is suspected; if the patient is febrile and no systemic focus of infection is found; or if the cause of delirium remains unclear.

Prevention and management

As well as being highly distressing to patients and their families, delirium is a major threat to health: it predisposes to injury, falls, dehydration, malnutrition, incontinence and pressure ulceration, and may also result in an irreversible worsening of cognitive function. Delirium should therefore be prevented if possible. Multicomponent intervention (see Table 79.3) can reduce the incidence of delirium in patients at risk, such as older patients having major surgery, and should be an integral part of the care of these patients.

In a patient with delirium, the aim is to promptly identify and treat the underlying cause, in a setting where safe care can be delivered: this includes anticipation and prevention of potential complications (see Table 79.3). Physical restraint should be avoided if possible. Short-term (1 week or less) therapy with haloperidol can be used if patients are distressed or are likely to injure themselves or others.

80 Coma

Coma

Causes of coma

Common

- Poisoning with alcohol, psychotropic drugs and other agents
- After cardiac arrest (with hypoxic–ischaemic brain injury)
- After major tonic–clonic seizure (usually lasts 15–30 min after seizure)
- Closed head injury

Less common

- Severe type II respiratory failure
- Stroke and subarachnoid haemorrhage
- Hepatic encephalopathy
- Septic encephalopathy
- Severe hyponatraemia, hypernatraemia or hypercalcaemia
- Bacterial meningitis
- Encephalitis

Glasgow Coma Score

- Scale based on assessment of three clinical signs: eye opening, motor response and verbal response
- To assess motor response, ask the patient to move the limb. If there is no response, apply firm pressure to the nailbed. Test and record for each of the limbs. Test for a localizing response by pressure on the supraorbital notch or sternal rub. For the purpose of assessment of conscious level, the best motor response is taken. Differences between the limbs will be important in identifying any focal neurological lesion
- Sum the scores for eye opening, motor response and verbal response; also record the elements of the score, e.g. E2, M4, V2 (eye opening 2, motor response 4, verbal response 2)
- Coma is defined as a score of 8 or below, and a reduced conscious level as a score of 9–14

Eye opening	None – eyes remain closed	1
	To pain – eyes open in response to painful stimulus applied to trunk or limb (painful stimulus to the head usually provokes closing of the eyes)	2
	To voice	3
	Spontaneous – eyes are open with blinking	4
Motor response	None	1
	Extensor response	2
	Abnormal flexor response	3
	Withdrawal	4
	Localizing – uses limb to locate or resist the painful stimulus	5
	Voluntary – obeys commands	6
Verbal response	None – no sound produced	1
	Incomprehensible – mutters or groans only	2
	Inappropriate – intelligible but isolated words	3
	Confused speech	4
	Oriented speech	5
Total		**3–15**

Assessment and management of the patient with coma

Unconscious patient → Absent carotid pulse? — Yes → Call resuscitation team ALS algorithm

No ↓

Clear airway and secure open airway

↓

Gagging/coughing and respiratory rate > 8/min?

Yes ↓ / No →

Oxygen 60% by mask | Ventilate with oxygen 100% using bag-mask device. Endotracheal intubation if trained. Call resuscitation team

↓

Key observations ECG monitor, IV access

↓

Major arrhythmia? — Yes → see Chapter 78

No ↓

Systolic BP < 90 mmHg and no pulmonary oedema? — Yes → Give IV colloid/saline 500 mL over 15 min

No ↓

Blood glucose < 5 mmol/L? — Yes → Give 50 mL of 50% glucose IV via a large vein

Eye signs in the unconscious patient

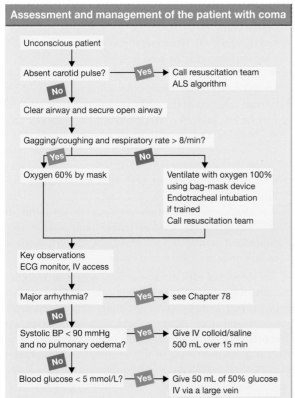

Eyes directed straight ahead. Pupils reactive. Normal oculocephalic reflex (OCR)
- Toxic/metabolic cause (NB: barbiturate, phenytoin and tricyclic poisoning can abolish OCR)

Pinpoint pupils
- Narcotic poisoning (OCR intact)
- Pontine haemorrhage (OCR absent, quadriplegia)

Dysconjugate deviation of eyes (vertical or lateral)
- Structural brainstem lesion (haemorrhage, infarction or compression)

Conjugate lateral deviation of eyes
- Ipsilateral cerebral haemorrhage or infarction (looking away from hemiplegic side)
- Contralateral pontine infarction (looking towards hemiplegic side)

Unilateral dilated pupil
- Supratentorial mass lesion (haematoma/cerebral infarction with oedema) with uncal herniation and compression of IIIrd nerve

Bilateral mid-position, fixed pupils
- Midbrain lesion (haemorrhage infarction, compression)

Medicine at a Glance, Fourth Edition. Edited by Patrick Davey. © 2014 John Wiley & Sons, Ltd. Published 2014 by John Wiley & Sons, Ltd. Companion website: www.ataglanceseries.com/medicine

Coma is a state of unconsciousness from which the patient cannot be roused. It is a medical emergency, because the comatose patient is at high risk of permanent brain injury or death, caused either by the underlying disorder or its secondary effects. Immediate action is needed to stabilize the airway, breathing and circulation, and correct hypoglycaemia, while you diagnose and treat the cause.

The causes of coma you are likely to see in the emergency department (excluding trauma) are shown in Figure 80.1 above. Poisoning, due to ingestion of sedative drugs, often with alcohol, is the cause of non-traumatic coma in 80% of patients under 40, but only 10% of those over 60, in whom stroke is the commonest diagnosis.

Assessment of the level of consciousness

Consciousness is a continuum from full alertness to complete unresponsiveness. It can be graded clinically using the simple four-point AVPU scale (A, alert; V, responds to voice; P, responds to painful stimuli; U, unresponsive). A more detailed scale is the Glasgow Coma Scale (GCS), based on eye opening, motor response and verbal response. How to assess a patient's conscious level using the GCS is summarized in Figure 80.1. The GCS gives a score of 15 (alert) to 3 (unresponsive). Coma is defined as a score of 8 or below, and a reduced conscious level as a score between 9 and 14. On the AVPU scale, A corresponds with a GCS of 15, V with a GCS of around 13, P with a GCS of around 8, and U with a GCS of 3.

Priorities

- **Stabilize the airway, breathing and circulation** (ABC). One of the major risks of impaired consciousness is the loss of the ability to protect the airway. As a general rule, patients with a score on the GCS of 8 or below (P, responds to painful stimuli, or U, unresponsive, on the AVPU scale) should have endotracheal intubation to protect the airway: discuss this with an anaesthetist.
- **Exclude/treat hypoglycaemia.** Check blood glucose by bedside testing.
- If **Wernicke's encephalopathy** is possible (because of coma in the setting of chronic alcohol abuse or malnutrition), give **thiamine** intravenously, before the administration of glucose.
- Give **naloxone** if opioid poisoning is possible, and **flumazenil** if the patient has received benzodiazepine in hospital.
- Treat **generalized seizures** along standard lines.
- **Diagnose and treat the underlying cause.** This is done by clinical assessment and computed tomography (CT) of the brain, together with other investigations.
- **Give supportive care**, with anticipation and prevention of the complications of coma (e.g. airway obstruction, pressure necrosis of skin or muscle, corneal abrasions, inhalation pneumonia).

History

Obtain the history from all available sources: ambulance personnel, family and friends, GP and hospital records, and the patient's belongings. Establish:

- The setting and time course of the loss of consciousness. Was loss of consciousness abrupt (e.g. subarachnoid haemorrhage (SAH), seizure), gradual (e.g. poisoning, bacterial meningitis) or fluctuating (e.g. recurring seizures, subdural haematoma, metabolic encephalopathy)?
- If loss of consciousness was preceded by neurological or other symptoms.
- The co-morbidities of the patient: systemic (e.g. chronic obstructive pulmonary disease, chronic liver disease), neurological (e.g. epilepsy) and psychiatric.

- A complete list of current medications. If the patient was admitted with coma, find out exactly what medications were being taken prior to admission (if necessary, contact the patient's GP to check prescribed medications, and ask a family member to collect all medications in the home).
- If there has been previous or recent alcohol or substance abuse.
- If there has been recent foreign travel (raising the possibility of infectious diseases acquired abroad, such as falciparum malaria).

Examination

Having addressed the ABC priorities above, complete your examination (see Figure 80.2 below). Key questions to be answered are:

- ***Is there evidence of systemic disease?*** Is there fever or hypothermia? Are there signs of chronic liver disease (e.g. spider naevi, ascites) or other organ failure?
- ***Is there neck stiffness?*** Neck stiffness is a sign of meningeal irritation, and may be seen in meningitis, SAH and cerebral or cerebellar haemorrhage with extension into the subarachoid space. If bacterial meningitis or viral encephalitis are possible (e.g. consistent history, fever), take blood for culture and start antimicrobial treatment immediately with cefotaxime (plus ampicillin in patients over 55 or at increased risk of *Listeria* infection) and aciclovir.
- ***Are there focal neurological signs?*** Examine carefully the eyes and the limbs.
    - Check the position of the eyes, the size and symmetry of the pupils and their response to bright light, and examine the fundi. Eye signs that may be seen in the unconscious patient are illustrated in Figure 80.1. With the exception of coma due to opioid poisoning (characterized by pinpoint pupils), normal pupils usually indicate a toxic/metabolic cause.
    - Examine the fundi (you'll save time by carrying your own ophthalmoscope): if you see spontaneous pulsation of the retinal veins, the intracranial pressure is normal. Subhyaloid haemorrhages may be seen in SAH.
    - Check the corneal reflex: a normal response bilaterally (eyelid closure and upward deviation of the eyes) indicates normal function of the midbrain and pons. The corneal reflex may be lost in deep coma due to a toxic/metabolic cause.
    - Provided the cervical spine is stable, check the oculocephalic response: this is a simple test of an intact brainstem. Rotate the head to the left and right. In an unconscious patient with an intact brainstem, both eyes rotate counter to movement of the head.
    - Check limb tone, limb response to a painful stimulus (nailbed pressure), tendon reflexes and plantar responses. Consistent asymmetry between right- and left-sided findings usually indicate a structural cause.

The absence of neck stiffness or focal neurological signs usually indicates a toxic/metabolic cause of coma, but some other brain disorders (e.g. hypoxic-ischaemic injury after cardiac arrest) may not give focal signs. Abnormal eye signs are typically found in structural disorders affecting the brainstem, either a primary event (e.g. haemorrhage) or due to compression/distortion from an expanding supratentorial or posterior fossa mass lesion.

Urgent investigation

- **Computed tomography** (CT) should be done urgently in all patients, unless there is a clear toxic cause of coma in a young patient, with no features to suggest additional pathology. CT is very sensitive for intracranial haemorrhage (>95% positive in SAH and intracerebral haemorrhage) and can identify mass lessions, hydrocephalus, marked cerebral oedema and large

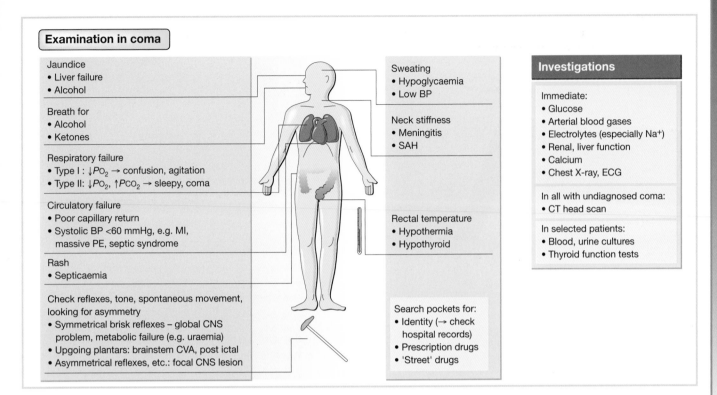

Examination in coma

Jaundice
- Liver failure
- Alcohol

Breath for
- Alcohol
- Ketones

Respiratory failure
- Type I : $\downarrow PO_2 \rightarrow$ confusion, agitation
- Type II: $\downarrow PO_2$, $\uparrow PCO_2 \rightarrow$ sleepy, coma

Circulatory failure
- Poor capillary return
- Systolic BP <60 mmHg, e.g. MI, massive PE, septic syndrome

Rash
- Septicaemia

Check reflexes, tone, spontaneous movement, looking for asymmetry
- Symmetrical brisk reflexes – global CNS problem, metabolic failure (e.g. uraemia)
- Upgoing plantars: brainstem CVA, post ictal
- Asymmetrical reflexes, etc.: focal CNS lesion

Sweating
- Hypoglycaemia
- Low BP

Neck stiffness
- Meningitis
- SAH

Rectal temperature
- Hypothermia
- Hypothyroid

Search pockets for:
- Identity ($\rightarrow$ check hospital records)
- Prescription drugs
- 'Street' drugs

Investigations

Immediate:
- Glucose
- Arterial blood gases
- Electrolytes (especially Na^+)
- Renal, liver function
- Calcium
- Chest X-ray, ECG

In all with undiagnosed coma:
- CT head scan

In selected patients:
- Blood, urine cultures
- Thyroid function tests

---

cerebral hemisphere ischaemic strokes. If CT shows haemorrhage or other structural pathology, an urgent neurosurgical opinion is needed. Non-contrast CT may be normal in early ischaemic stroke especially of the brainstem or cerebellum, hypoxic-ischaemic brain injury and white matter disorders (e.g. central pontine myelinolyis).

- A **chest X-ray** (CXR) should be taken to exclude pneumonia.
- An **electrocardiogram** (ECG) should be recorded in all patients over 50 and in younger patients if there is hypotension, coexistent heart disease or suspected ingestion of cardiotoxic drugs (e.g. antiarrhythmics, tricyclics).
- **Arterial blood gases and pH** should be checked. Respiratory failure may result in coma or complicate coma from other disorders.
- **Key blood tests** are **full blood count**, **coagulation screen** and **biochemic profile**. A **toxicology screen** and **measurement of plasma paracetamol and salicylate levels** shold be done if poisoining is possible. **Blood culture** should be taken if there is fever or hypothermia.

Additional investigation

- **Examination of the cerebrospinal fluid** (assuming no contraindication to lumbar puncture (LP)) should be done if the cause of coma is unexplained by CT and the other tests above, to rule out meningitis and encephalitis.

- **Magnetic resonance imaging** (MRI) is helpful if the diagnosis remains unclear, or you suspect a cause to which CT is insensitive.
- **Electroencephalography** (EEG) should be done if the clinical findings suggest non-convulsive status epilepticus, and can be diagnostically useful if the cause of coma is still unclear after neuroimaging and other tests.
- Other tests that may be helpful in specific circumstances include measurement of **plasma osmolality** (raised in poisoning with ethanol, ethylene glycol, isopropyl alcohol or methanol), **plasma ammonia** (raised in hepatic encephalopathy) and **red cell transketolase** (low in Wernicke's encephalopathy due to thiamine deficiency).

Further management

Patients with coma should be nursed in a high dependency or intensive care unit. Physiological observations and the level of consciousness should be monitored initially every 15–30 minutes. As well as specific treatment directed at the underlying cause, supportive care of the comatose patient includes stabilization of the airway, breathing and circulation, correction of hypoglycaemia or hyperglycaemia, treatment of seizures if present, and anticipation and prevention of the complications of coma. Induced hypothermia should be instituted if coma has followed cardiac arrest, as this improves the neurological prognosis; otherwise, high or low core temperatures should be corrected.

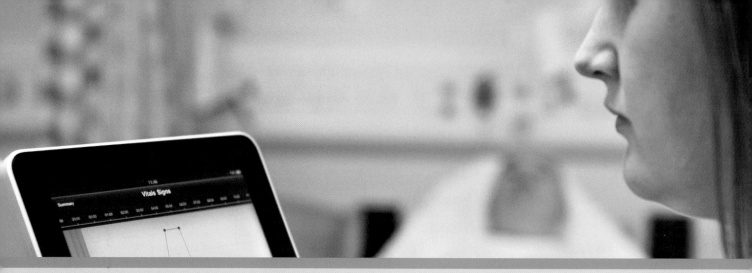

Chapters

Diseases and treatments at a glance

Part 3

Don't forget to visit the companion website for this book www.ataglanceseries.com/medicine for MCQs and flashcards on these topics.

81 Hypertension

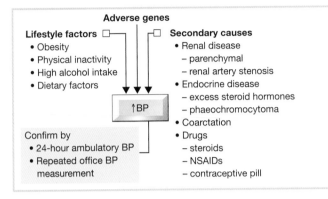

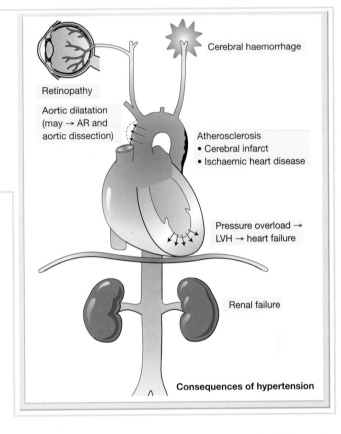

Consequences of hypertension

Definition

Blood pressure (BP) is distributed continuously. The incidence of complications is proportional to BP, so there is no absolute definition of hypertension. Treatment is often beneficial with sustained BPs >140/90 mmHg.

Incidence

Increases with age. Prevalence of mild hypertension is 2% in those aged 25 years or less, rising to 25% in those in their fifties and 50% in those in their seventies.

Pathophysiology

Most (95%) hypertension is **essential hypertension**, a combination of numerous genetic and environmental factors that results in a hypertensive phenotype. **Secondary hypertension**, caused by an identifiable cause, is uncommon, and suggested by:

- Renal dysfunction (look for a raised creatinine and/or dipstick haematuria or proteinurea). If there is ischaemic heart disease (IHD)/peripheral vascular disease (PVD) consider renal artery stenosis.
- Young age (especially 30 years or less); consider coarctation.
- Severe treatment-resistant hypertension.
- Hypokalaemia (in the absence of diuretics), which suggests mineralocorticoid excess (Cushing's or Conn's syndrome).

Clinical features

Hypertension is usually asymptomatic, until end-organ damage occurs. Most headaches in hypertension are *not* related to BP.

Malignant phase hypertension may present with headache and visual loss (papilloedema).

Effects of hypertension

The long-term risk of hypertension is end-organ damage:

- **Cerebrovascular disease**: thrombotic and haemorrhagic stroke.
- **Vascular disease**: coronary artery disease.
- **Left ventricular hypertrophy** (LVH) is a compensatory response to a chronically elevated BP. It is an independent predictor of early death (sudden cardiac death from ventricular arrhythmias, heart failure, myocardial infarction (MI) or cerebrovascular accident). Heart failure in hypertension may relate to the abnormalities in hypertrophied myocyte function (long-standing hypertrophied muscle develops first diastolic and later systolic contractile failure) or to coronary disease, which is more likely in long-standing hypertension.
- **Renal failure**: hypertension leads to renovascular damage and glomerular loss.

Severity

Hypertension is classed according to the presence of end-organ damage and the BP level (Table 81.1).

Investigations

- **Confirm hypertension**: repeated office BP measurement or ambulatory 24-hour recording.

Medicine at a Glance, Fourth Edition. Edited by Patrick Davey. © 2014 John Wiley & Sons, Ltd. Published 2014 by John Wiley & Sons, Ltd. Companion website: www.ataglanceseries.com/medicine

Table 81.1 Classification of hypertension.

Category	Systolic blood pressure (mmHg)	Diastolic blood pressure (mmHg)
Optimal blood pressure	<120	<80
Normal blood pressure	<130	<85
High–normal blood pressure	130–139	85–89
Grade 1 hypertension (mild)	140–159	90–99
Grade 2 hypertension (moderate)	160–179	100–109
Grade 3 hypertension (severe)	≥180	≥110
Isolated systolic hypertension (grade 1)	140–159	<90
Isolated systolic hypertension (grade 2)	≥160	<90

- **Assess for secondary cause**: renal disease (dipstick urine, check creatinine, renal size, non-invasive renal artery imaging by magnetic resonance imaging). Exclude coarctation (clinical examination demonstrating decreased femoral pulse strength, and often 'radiofemoral' delay or 'rib notching' on chest X-ray), hypokalaemia (Cushing's and Conn's syndromes) and phaeochromocytoma (see Chapter 163).
- **Assess end-organ damage**: electrocardiogram, cardiac ultrasonography (for LVH), renal function.

Treatment
Treatment removes the excess stroke risk, and halves the excess coronary risk.

Overall approach
Other cardiovascular risk factors must also be addressed, e.g. smoking, diabetes control, cholesterol (statin therapy is often indicated).

Non-pharmacological measures
Lifestyle modification (weight loss, lower salt and alcohol intake, regular exercise) may be sufficient in mild hypertension. Pharmacological therapy is used if the BP is too high on several recordings or on 24-hour BP monitoring.

Pharmacological treatments
Large long-term clinical trials have shown a clear mortality reduction from treating hypertension, principally from fewer strokes, but also from less sudden cardiac death, heart failure and MI. The benefit of treatment relates to the degree of hypertension, i.e. the more severe the hypertension, the greater the impact of treatment. However, even mild hypertension benefits from treatment when the risk of end-organ damage is high or already present (e.g. elderly people, people with diabetes, previous MI, etc.). The risk reduction is related to the lowering of BP. Except for β-blockers there is *little good evidence that any drug is better than any other*, although individual drugs are particularly suited to some patients:

- **β-Blockers** (e.g. atenolol and metoprolol) reduce heart rate and BP by antagonizing adrenergic signalling. Recent data on atenolol suggest this is not effective in reducing clinical events, though there is good evidence for long-term benefit for some drugs (bisoprolol, carvedilol, nebivolol, metoprolol) in left ventricular (LV) dysfunction. Side effects include lethargy, impotence, cold peripheries, exacerbation of diabetes and hyperlipidaemia. They are contraindicated in people with asthma; use with caution in PVD.

- **Diuretics** (e.g. bendrofluazide) are safe and effective.
- **Calcium channel antagonists** are vasodilators that lower BP. Nifedipine (and possibly amlodipine) causes a reflex tachycardia unless a β-blocker is co-prescribed. Diltiazem and verapamil cause a bradycardia. Side effects include flushing, ankle oedema and worsening heart failure (not with amlodipine).
- **Angiotensin-converting enzyme (ACE) inhibitors** (e.g. captopril, enalapril, lisinopril, ramipril) exert their antihypertensive effects by blocking the formation of angiotensin II. Mortality data are strong for patients with heart failure, impaired LV function or known coronary artery disease. May cause profound hypotension or acute renal failure in those with renovascular hypertension, i.e. bilateral renal artery stenosis. Side effects include dry cough (common) and angioedema.
- **Angiotensin II receptor antagonists** (e.g. losartan, valsartan) antagonize the angiotensin II–renin axis. They have comparable efficacy to ACE inhibitors, although trial data supporting their use are less comprehensive. They are indicated in heart failure or impaired LV function if a cough from ACE inhibitor is troublesome. Effects on renal function in renovascular hypertension are similar.
- **α-Antagonists** (e.g. doxazosin) are vasodilators that lower BP by antagonism of the α-adrenergic receptors in the peripheral vasculature.
- **Other drugs** include centrally acting agents (e.g. methyldopa, moxonidine).

Guidelines in treating hypertension
The choice of antihypertensive therapy is influenced by other diseases/risk factors, e.g. patients with heart failure or coronary disease benefit from a β-blocker and ACE inhibitor. β-Blockers should not be given in asthma. Those with prostatic symptoms find α-blockers relieve these as well as their hypertension. The general paradigm is ACD – standing for ACE inhibitors, calcium channel blockers and diuretics:

- In non-blacks aged <50 years, start with A (angiotensin receptor blocker (ARB) if A intolerant), as such patients often have high renin levels. If this is not sufficient, add in C or D, or both if needed.
- In those >50 years, or black, start with C or D; if this is not sufficient, add in A, then D if needed.
- If hypertension is not controlled with the above approach consider adding in α-blockers or higher dose/alternative diuretics.

• For treatment failure, consider if compliance is an issue, other lifestyle issues (e.g. obesity, lack of exercise) and adverse drug interactions (e.g. non-steroidal anti-inflammatory drugs (NSAIDs) increase BP), as well as underlying secondary diseases driving hypertension.

Malignant or accelerated hypertension

Rarely, patients present with severe, uncontrolled hypertension (e.g. ≥220/120 mmHg) and headache, confusion ('hypertensive encephalopathy') or acute end-organ damage (cerebral haemorrhage, acute renal failure, aortic dissection or heart failure). Malignant phase hypertension is the combination of hypertension, high-grade retinal changes and progressive renal failure; untreated, the 1-year mortality rate is ≥50%.

Treatment

Admit to hospital as a medical emergency because the risks of end-organ damage and life-threatening complications are high. Oral agents are given, unless the patient is critically unwell (repeated hypertensive seizures, severe LV failure, aortic dissection) when cautious intravenous therapy may be given; however, BP lowering must be gradual because sudden falls in BP can precipitate a stroke. Intravenous agents include sodium nitroprusside (a very potent, rapidly acting vasodilator) and labetolol, a β-blocker that also has α-adrenergic antagonist effects.

82 Hyperlipidaemia

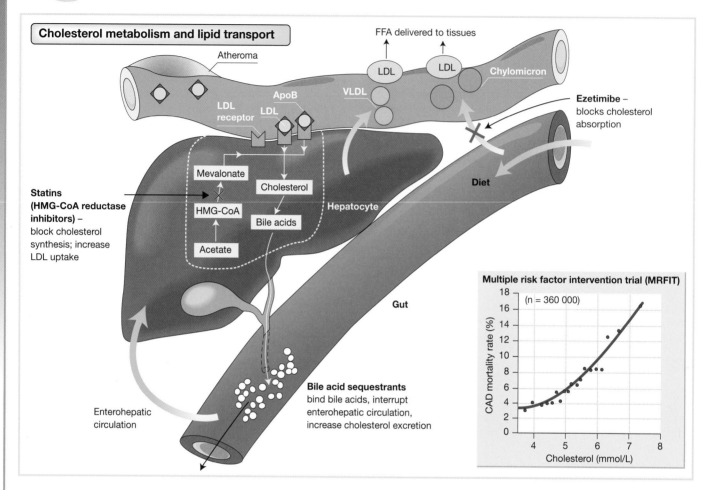

Cholesterol metabolism and lipid transport

FFA delivered to tissues

Atheroma

LDL LDL Chylomicron

ApoB VLDL

LDL receptor LDL

Ezetimibe – blocks cholesterol absorption

Mevalonate Cholesterol

Statins (HMG-CoA reductase inhibitors) – block cholesterol synthesis; increase LDL uptake

HMG-CoA Bile acids

Hepatocyte

Diet

Acetate

Gut

Enterohepatic circulation

Bile acid sequestrants bind bile acids, interrupt enterohepatic circulation, increase cholesterol excretion

Multiple risk factor intervention trial (MRFIT)

(n = 360 000)

CAD mortality rate (%) vs Cholesterol (mmol/L)

Medicine at a Glance, Fourth Edition. Edited by Patrick Davey. © 2014 John Wiley & Sons, Ltd. Published 2014 by John Wiley & Sons, Ltd. Companion website: www.ataglanceseries.com/medicine

Table 82.1 Composition and function of lipoproteins and apoproteins.

	Composition	Function	Major apoproteins
Chylomicrons	Rich in triglyceride (85%) Very large particle (200–500 nm) with low density Very little protein (2%)	Transports lipid from the gut to the liver in the postprandial state	**ApoCII**: activator of lipoprotein lipase enzyme that breaks down triglycerides for delivery to tissues **ApoE** (see below)
VLDL	Rich in triglyceride Size 50–80 nm	Transports lipid from the liver to the tissues	**ApoCII** (see above) **ApoB$_{100}$** **ApoE**: binds to ApoE receptors on hepatocytes, mediates uptake of lipoprotein remnants after catabolism
LDL	Rich in cholesterol Size 20 nm	Produced by catabolism of VLDL, via intermediate-density lipoprotein. Taken up by liver	**ApoB$_{100}$**: the ligand for the LDL receptor on hepatocytes; mediates uptake of LDL **ApoE** (see above)
HDL	Smallest (8 nm) and most dense lipoprotein >50% protein	Carries cholesterol esters back to the liver from tissues and other lipoproteins ('reverse cholesterol transport')	**ApoAI**: activates LCAT enzyme that esterifies cholesterol

Definition and incidence

Hyperlipidaemia is defined as elevated levels of cholesterol and/or triglycerides. Hypercholesterolaemia is common: ≥60% of the UK population have a total cholesterol >5.2 mmol/L and 3% >7.5 mmol/L.

Lipid metabolism and lipoproteins

Cholesterol and triglycerides are transported in the bloodstream complexed with phospholipid and proteins (**apoproteins**) in particles called **lipoproteins**. **Apoproteins** act as signalling molecules or enzymes and play very important roles in controlling lipid transport. The different classes of lipoproteins transport lipids between different tissues and are defined by characteristic composition of lipids and apoproteins (see Table 82.1). Cholesterol is principally metabolized in the liver. Blood levels are controlled by the balance between blood uptake, cholesterol production (activity of cholesterol biosynthetic pathway) and gastrointestinal (GI) excretion (bile acids).

Secondary hyperlipidaemias

Before deciding whether a hyperlipidaemia is primary, diseases producing secondary hyperlipidaemias should be excluded:

- Diabetes.
- Hypothyroidism.
- Chronic renal failure or nephrotic syndrome.
- Chronic liver disease, especially alcoholic.
- Chronic biliary obstruction.
- Drugs: steroids, oestrogens.

Genetic hyperlipidaemias

Single gene defects in lipid metabolism causing extreme hyperlipidaemias are rare. However, common genetic variability or heterozygote status is a very important determinant of cholesterol levels in the general population.

- **Familial hypercholesterolaemia**: a group of single gene disorders affecting the low-density lipoprotein (LDL) receptor and causing deficient or absent uptake of LDL particles, which therefore accumulate in the bloodstream. Homozygotes (1/1 000 000) have extremely high cholesterol levels (10–25 mmol/L) and have extremely high cholesterol levels (10–25 mmol/L) and have coronary artery disease (CAD) in their teens or twenties. Heterozygotes (1/500) have moderately high cholesterol (7–12 mmol/L) and are at risk of premature CAD. Patients may have corneal arcus, xanthelasmas and tendon xanthomas.
- **Polygenetic hypercholesterolaemia and familial combined hyperlipidaemia**: inherited conditions (1/300–600) characterized by moderately elevated cholesterol (7–12 mmol/L) with or without high triglycerides, not caused by a single gene disorder, although in some inheritance is apparently autosomal dominant. Very important cause of increased atherosclerosis risk in the population. Very high triglycerides may cause pancreatitis.
- **Apoprotein E genotype**: genetic variation in the *ApoE* gene results in different isoforms of the ApoE protein. The *ApoE2* isoform binds less avidly to hepatic receptors, resulting in hyperlipidaemia. *ApoE2* homozygotes are uncommon (1/100) but *ApoE2* heterozygotes (15% of the population) appear to have a significantly increased risk of CAD.
- **Lipoprotein lipase deficiency and ApoCII deficiency**: extremely rare. There are very elevated chylomicrons, eruptive xanthomas, hepatomegaly and pancreatitis.

Lipids in atherosclerosis

Studies have identified elevated plasma cholesterol as an important risk factor for the development of CAD:

- Total cholesterol >6.5 mmol/L doubles the risk of lethal CAD; >7.8 mmol/L increases the risk four-fold.
- Reducing total cholesterol by 20% reduces the coronary risk by 10%.
- The strongest association is with LDL cholesterol, whereas high-density lipoprotein (HDL) cholesterol is protective. The LDL:HDL cholesterol ratio is a useful indicator, a ratio of >4 indicating high risk.

Elevated cholesterol (especially oxidized LDL) damages the endothelium early in atherosclerosis and is taken up into the lipid core of established plaques by macrophages (foam cells). Lowering LDL cholesterol reduces cholesterol deposition into atherosclerotic plaques and may reverse this process. Crucially, cholesterol lowering stabilizes plaques, reducing the risk of acute plaque rupture.

Lipid lowering and risk factor modification

- **Lipid lowering by diet**: reducing fat intake, especially high cholesterol foods (red meat, eggs, high fat diet, dairy products) lowers cholesterol by 1 mmol/L and reduces body weight. However, diet alone is *insufficient* in patients with elevated cholesterol and CAD.
- **Lipid-lowering drugs**: statins are effective cholesterol-lowering agents, and should be given to those with a high (>30% risk over 10 years) or medium (>15%) risk of developing cardiovascular disease, as assessed from risk prediction charts (e.g. the Joint British Societies chart found in the *British National Formulary*), which factor in age, systolic blood pressure, cholesterol and smoking/diabetes status.
- **Bile acid sequestrants** ('resins'), e.g. cholestyramine. These lower cholesterol by binding cholesterol in the GI tract, interrupting the enterohepatic circulation, so increasing cholesterol excretion. They are distasteful and may have intolerable GI side effects. They can be effective and remain useful in familial hypercholesterolaemia.
- **HMG-CoA reductase inhibitors** ('statins'), e.g. simvastatin, pravastatin. These are potent agents that inhibit hydroxymethylglutaryl coenzyme (HMG-CoA) reductase, the rate-limiting enzyme in cholesterol biosynthesis. This increases hepatic cholesterol uptake because reduced intracellular cholesterol biosynthesis increases expression of cell surface LDL receptors. For this reason, they are less effective in patients with familial hypercholesterolaemia. Statins typically lower LDL cholesterol 30% or more, and may modestly increase HDL cholesterol. They have relatively little effect on plasma triglycerides.

Large intervention trials (e.g. 4S, WOSCOPS, CARE, LIPID, Heart Protection Study) show that cholesterol lowering with statins significantly reduces the subsequent incidence of coronary events. The benefits are apparent within months, implying that changes in the composition of atherosclerotic plaques occurs rapidly. Angiographic follow-up studies also show that statins can result in regression of established atheroma.

- **Fibric acid derivatives** ('fibrates'), e.g. bezafibrate, fenofibrate. These agents reduce cholesterol moderately, but also reduce triglycerides and increase HDL cholesterol. The mechanism of action is complex but involves stimulation of lipoprotein lipase activity (increases chylomicrons and very-low-density lipoprotein (VLDL) catabolism) and increased cholesterol excretion via bile acids. They are more useful in patients with mixed hyperlipidaemia and/or low HDL.

Multiple risk factor modification

Lipid lowering represents only one aspect of reducing coronary risk, and needs to be considered in the context of the whole coronary risk factor profile for that individual patient. Aggressive lipid lowering is more important in patients who already have an adverse risk factor profile (diabetes, hypertension, smoking) because *multiple risk factors are synergistic in increasing coronary risk*. In contrast, isolated mild hypercholesterolaemia in a patient without other risk factors could be managed by dietary intervention.

83 Acute coronary syndromes

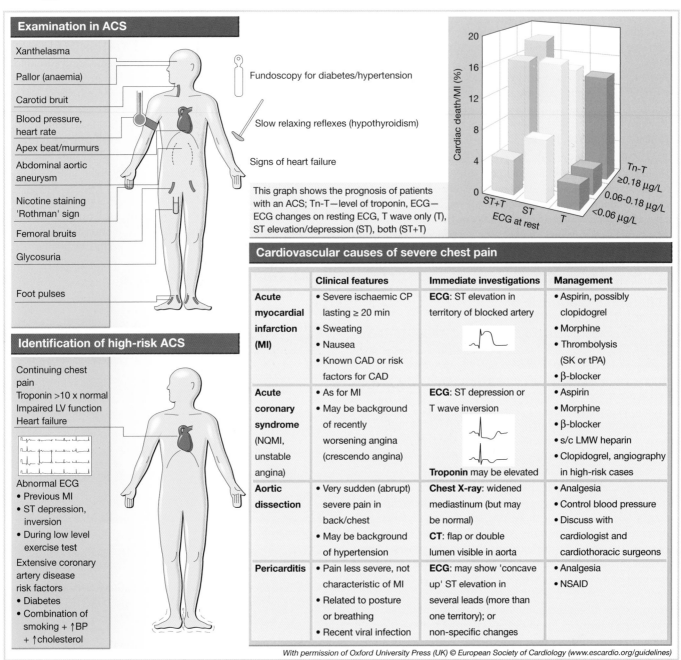

Examination in ACS

Xanthelasma

Pallor (anaemia)

Carotid bruit

Blood pressure, heart rate

Apex beat/murmurs

Abdominal aortic aneurysm

Nicotine staining 'Rothman' sign

Femoral bruits

Glycosuria

Foot pulses

Fundoscopy for diabetes/hypertension

Slow relaxing reflexes (hypothyroidism)

Signs of heart failure

This graph shows the prognosis of patients with an ACS; Tn-T—level of troponin, ECG—ECG changes on resting ECG, T wave only (T), ST elevation/depression (ST), both (ST+T)

Identification of high-risk ACS

Continuing chest pain
Troponin >10 x normal
Impaired LV function
Heart failure

Abnormal ECG
• Previous MI
• ST depression, inversion
• During low level exercise test

Extensive coronary artery disease risk factors
• Diabetes
• Combination of smoking + ↑BP + ↑cholesterol

Cardiovascular causes of severe chest pain

	Clinical features	Immediate investigations	Management
Acute myocardial infarction (MI)	• Severe ischaemic CP lasting ≥ 20 min • Sweating • Nausea • Known CAD or risk factors for CAD	**ECG**: ST elevation in territory of blocked artery	• Aspirin, possibly clopidogrel • Morphine • Thrombolysis (SK or tPA) • β-blocker
Acute coronary syndrome (NQMI, unstable angina)	• As for MI • May be background of recently worsening angina (crescendo angina)	**ECG**: ST depression or T wave inversion **Troponin** may be elevated	• Aspirin • Morphine • β-blocker • s/c LMW heparin • Clopidogrel, angiography in high-risk cases
Aortic dissection	• Very sudden (abrupt) severe pain in back/chest • May be background of hypertension	**Chest X-ray**: widened mediastinum (but may be normal) **CT**: flap or double lumen visible in aorta	• Analgesia • Control blood pressure • Discuss with cardiologist and cardiothoracic surgeons
Pericarditis	• Pain less severe, not characteristic of MI • Related to posture or breathing • Recent viral infection	**ECG**: may show 'concave up' ST elevation in several leads (more than one territory); or non-specific changes	• Analgesia • NSAID

With permission of Oxford University Press (UK) © European Society of Cardiology (www.escardio.org/guidelines)

Acute chest pain is a common presentation in the emergency department and accounts for 10% of medical patients. Management aims to separate out, and treat early, patients with high-risk acute coronary syndromes (ACSs) including acute myocardial infarction (MI), be it ST segment elevation myocardial infarction (STEMI) (see Chapter 84) or non-ST segment elevation myocardial infarction (non-STEMI) from other life-threatening diagnoses such as aortic dissection and from benign causes of pain such as pericarditis or gastro-oesophageal pain.

General approach
The initial assessment of the patient should enable a diagnosis or differential diagnosis that guides immediate management and enables administration of emergency treatment with as little delay

Medicine at a Glance, Fourth Edition. Edited by Patrick Davey. © 2014 John Wiley & Sons, Ltd. Published 2014 by John Wiley & Sons, Ltd. Companion website: www.ataglanceseries.com/medicine

as possible. Rapid clinical assessment by history and examination is combined with simple investigations such as electrocardiogram (ECG) and chest X-ray.

Diagnosis of myocardial ischaemia

Myocardial ischaemia is presumptively diagnosed when a patient at risk of coronary disease experiences:

- Tight retrosternal chest pain, especially if it is severe. Radiation into the neck, or down the left arm, increases the probability of MI.
- Pains occurring for >4 weeks with a strong relationship to exercise. However, if pains are present for <2 weeks, often (surprisingly) there is no/little relationship with effort.
- Pains felt during a previous *unambiguous* episode of MI being similar to the current pains.

If multiple episodes of pain are present over several weeks they should each be of short duration (i.e. <20–30 min). If they are of longer duration, then almost always if they are due to myocardial ischaemia, infarction will have occurred, and leave easily picked up diagnostic clues such as abnormalities on the resting ECG and/or a raised troponin. Put another way, if a patient presents with multiple recent episodes of prolonged chest pain and the ECG is normal and troponin is not raised, then myocardial ischaemia is an unlikely diagnosis.

Differential diagnosis of myocardial ischaemia

The differential diagnosis is broad, and must always be fully considered (see Chapter 13). In essence, all possible causes of chest pain must be evaluated; if you do not, you may miss important disease processes and so fail to treat them. With chest pain par excellence it is easy to slip into sloppy habits; for example, if you assume all chest pain with ST elevation is due to acute thrombotic occlusion of a coronary artery leading to MI, you will miss the cases where coronary occlusion is due to an aortic dissection (and if you miss this diagnosis, you will order the wrong diagnostic tests at the wrong time and also give powerful antiplatelet therapy inappropriately). You will also miss the cases where chest pain is due to myocarditis, and you will miss the cases where chest pain relates to cocaine. All of these have specific treatments, which differ radically from the other. With chest pain, always ask what is going on, and what pathology is driving the process. Never assume that only ACSs can give ECG changes, never assume that the only cause of a raised troponin is an ACS (see Chapter 13), and always consider a broad differential diagnosis. Always test your possible diagnosis against the data you have available on the patient, be it the demographics, the exact symptoms or the easily obtainable investigatory data.

If at the end of this process you are still in doubt about the diagnosis, first ask yourself the question whether greater clarity would change your approach to management? If it would not (e.g. very elderly patient with advanced dementia), then stop investigating. If greater clarity would change management, do the one test that provides you with the answer; in suspected ACS this will often be a coronary angiogram.

Physical examination

This is often unrevealing, but may show evidence of risk factors (nicotine-stained hands, cholesterol deposits around the eyes, hypertension, vascular disease elsewhere) or complications (arrhythmias, heart failure), or suggest other diagnoses. On top of the routine cardiovascular examination, always feel for all pulses (occasionally absent pulses may point to the rare diagnosis of aortic dissection) and measure oxygen saturations (low P_{O_2} is most commonly due to heart failure, but may reflect chronic obstructive pulmonary disease or be the only sign that a pulmonary embolism (PE) is present).

Investigations

The important investigations early on in suspected MI are:

- **ECGs**, repeated whenever there is pain, frequently, and at least daily. The best units will repeat the ECG hourly for the first 3 hours, then at 4, 6, 12 and 24 hours. An ECG must be repeated whenever there is chest pain, as an ACS may at any time suddenly turn into a STEMI, requiring immediate reperfusion therapy (percutaneous coronary intervention (PCI), or less desirably thrombolysis). Make sure that you know how to read an ECG.
- **Chest X-ray** (CXR) to exclude complicating heart failure and alternative pathologies. This must be done in all patients at presentation, the ONLY exception being those with STEMI who are treated with primary angioplasty, in whom nothing should be done that might delay primary PCI. In these patients, the CXR should be done **immediately** following the PCI procedure.
- **Markers** of myocardial necrosis: 'traditional' cardiac markers (creatine kinase (CK), rarely aspartate aminotransferase, lactate dehydrogenase) and especially cardiac-specific troponins. Be aware that there are many causes of a rise in troponin, only one of which is an ACS (see Table 83.1).

Table 83.1 Possible non-acute coronary syndrome causes of troponin elevation. Bold indicates important differential diagnoses.

- **Chronic or acute renal dysfunction**
- Severe congestive **heart failure** – acute and chronic
- **Hypertensive crisis**
- **Tachy- or bradyarrhythmias**
- **Pulmonary embolism**, severe pulmonary hy pertension
- Inflammatory diseases, e.g. **myocarditis**
- Acute neurological disease, including **stroke** or subarachnoid haemorrhage
- Aortic dissection, aortic valve disease or hypertrophic cardiomyopathy
- Cardiac contusion, ablation, pacing, cardioversion, or endomyocardial biopsy
- Hypothyroidism
- Apical ballooning syndrome (Tako-Tsubo cardiomyopathy)
- Infiltrative diseases, e.g. amyloidosis, haemochromatosis, sarcoidosis, sclerodermia
- Drug toxicity, e.g. Adriamycin, 5-fluorouracil, herceptin, snake venoms
- Burns, if affecting >30% of body surface area
- Rhabdomyolysis
- Critically ill patients, especially with respiratory failure or sepsis

Source: Hamm et al. 2011. With permission of Oxford University Press (UK) © European Society of Cardiology (www.escardio.org/guidelines).

- **Haemoglobin**: anaemia is a common provocatant of myocardial ischaemia, and if the patient is anaemic, ask why (cancer, gastrointestinal (GI) bleeding, haematinic deficiency, primary bone marrow problem, etc.) and in particular, might antiplatelet therapy exacerbate the anaemia (e.g. if it is due to GI bleeding from peptic ulceration)?
- **White count and markers of inflammation, especially C-reactive protein**, as an ACS can be complicated by infection (especially lung infection if there is heart failure). A chest infection can also lead to an ACS (the chance of a myocardial infarct rises three-fold in the fortnight following a chest infection).
- **Cholesterol** (on admission, because acute MI artefactually lowers cholesterol from days to months afterwards), triglycerides and glucose. Anyone with elevated cholesterol should have his or her thyroid function checked.
- **Renal function**.

Acute STEMI and acute coronary syndromes

The common pathology underlying acute coronary events is the rupture or erosion of a coronary artery plaque, leading to intracoronary thrombosis. The resulting clinical syndrome depends on whether the coronary artery has occluded totally (producing a STEMI), or whether it is only partially or transiently (<20 min at a time) totally occluded (producing a non-Q wave MI (NQMI) or unstable angina). Damage to the heart can result from the occlusion itself. However, even if the occlusion is not complete, myocardial necrosis can still result from thrombus embolizing down the coronary artery, infarcting distal tissue. So, there are several forms of ACS defined by the ECG and troponin (see Table 83.2):

- **ST elevation MI** (STEMI): here the ECG shows prolonged ST segment elevation, and the troponin is elevated. This is sometimes termed a 'threatened Q wave MI' as, in the absence of treatment, it frequently progresses to a Q wave or full-thickness MI. Therapy aims to prevent this progression and minimize infarction size such that Q waves do not develop, and is discussed further in Chapter 84.
- **Non-ST elevation MI** (non-STEMI): by definition, there must be a troponin rise. Almost any ECG change can occur, the commonest being ST depression/T wave inversion, though transient self-terminating ST elevation can also occur. These were called NQMIs.
- **Troponin-negative acute coronary syndromes**, by definition, do not have a raised troponin. ECG changes are similar to those in non-STEMI patients.

In everyday life, most doctors divide patients with acute coronary events into STEMI patients and ACS patients; the latter comprise non-STEMI and troponin-negative ACS patients.

Table 83.2 Quick guide to acute coronary syndromes.

ECG	Troponin	ACS diagnosis*
ST elevation	+ to +++	STEMI
No ST elevation	+	Non-STEMI
Usually ST depression or T wave inversion	No rise or trivial rise	Unstable angina or troponin –ve ACS

* There is a differential diagnosis for all these ECG/troponin combinations, and only the ACS component is given here.

STEMI and non-STEMI patients have a similar prognosis; of those reaching hospital alive (about 70–80% of those with an ACS, i.e. about 20–30% of ACS patients, die before they can reach hospital), some 10–20% die within the year.

Immediate treatment of ACS

Many patients with ACS are at high risk of early (<10–14 days) adverse events (see Chapter 84 for MI complications, which are the same for STEMI and non-STEMI), and so constitute a medical emergency requiring immediate treatment and close monitoring on a cardiology ward. Non-STEMI/troponin-negative ACS patients do *not* benefit from thrombolytic treatment, and very few benefit from immediate angiography and PCI. Most benefit from:

- Immediate aspirin (chewed), and clopidogrel for most patients. Some units use other antiplatelets, such as prasugrel or ticagrelor.
- Analgesia, with morphine if pain is ongoing.
- β-Blocker, given intravenously, to reduce the resting heart rate to 50 bpm. Mild heart failure (i.e. crepitations less than one-third of the way up the lungs) is *not* a contraindication to β-blockade.
- Subcutaneous low-molecular-weight (LMW) heparin.
- High-dose statin therapy (such as atorvastatin 80 mg od).

Immediate treatment of suspected ACS

This is a difficult problem – you think your patient may have an ACS, but for various reasons you are not sure. What should you do? As in all diagnostic dilemmas – and these are very common in acute medicine – first, do no harm; second, try and clarify the situation as soon as possible using the minimum number of tests; third, always consider the differential diagnosis. Once you have done so, treat the most likely diagnosis in the standard fashion, and if possible the most likely dangerous cause, always bearing in mind that treatment for one condition may excacerbate another one. So, you think the diagnosis is ACS, but clinically you are not sure if a PE is present instead of an ACS. This is easy, give full dose heparin, and either mono-antiplatelet therapy or dual antiplatelet therapy if the ECG is abnormal or troponin raised. Suppose you think ACS is likely, but you are concerned about the possibility of a peptic ulcer. In this case, give no heparin, give aspirin with proton pump inhibitor (PPI) cover and no second antiplatelet agent. If in the latter case you have ECG changes, go for early angiography to clarify what is going on in the coronories prior to giving a second antiplatelet agent, and hence determine the need and benefit from such an agent. You may need an upper GI endoscopy prior to any intervention to clarify in your mind the risk of dual antiplatelet therapy.

There is an almost endless combination of actual and possible diagnoses in chest pain, particularly in the ageing population, and you will have to tailor your approach to the individual. However, the basic principle always remain the same; if more data would change your approach, get the data. It is rarely wrong to perform a coronary angiogram in a patient to determine the state of the coronary arteries, even if they are not on dual antiplatelet therapy, as this greatly clarifies where one might need to go therapeutically, and therefore what the actual need for combination antiplatelet therapy is.

Risk stratification of ACSs

After immediate medical management, further investigation and treatment are determined by the risk of further cardiac events. Factors associated with higher risk include:

- ST segment depression on the presentation ECG or dynamic ST changes later.

- Elevated troponin levels (≥10 times the detectable limit).
- Recurrent episodes of chest pain.
- Diabetes, previous MI, impaired left ventricular (LV) function, heart failure (even if cardiac ultrasonography shows good LV function).

ACS patients without these factors, whose chest pains settle, are mobilized and if they remain pain-free an exercise ECG (or better, nuclear myocardial perfusion scan) is performed. Inducible ischaemia (ST segment depression or angina) at a low workload indicates higher risk. Low-risk patients should be managed medically, though many units will include angiography as part of their formal risk stratification processes.

Higher risk patients should be given dual antiplatelet drugs (aspirin + clopidogrel or similar antiplatelet agent) and undergo early **cardiac catheterization**, as many have critical coronary lesions requiring PCI with intracoronary stenting, or severe multivessel coronary artery disease needing coronary artery bypass graft (CABG) surgery. Coronary angiography should be performed within 72 hours, preferably sooner (see next section).

All ACS patients should have aggressive anti-atherogenic risk factor management:

- Lifestyle changes: no smoking, regular exercise, ideal weight, modest alcohol intake. None of these are easy to do. Doctors must, sympathetically, emphasize the harm that cigarettes do, and should offer nicotine replacement therapy. Exercise should be for a minimum of 20 minutes cardiovascular exercise sufficiently intense to induce some breathlessness at least three times a week. There are no easy approaches to weight reduction; however, if patients are grossly obese (body mass index >40) after recovery from the MI, bariatric surgery may have a role. In most overweight patients, a sympathetic approach, with an understanding that these patients will need considerable support (e.g. as provided by weight loss organizations) is appropriate. Alcohol should be in the 14–21 units per week range for men, and 7–14 for women.
- Cholesterol reduction using statins: initially in high doses, after 1–2 years in more conventional doses.
- Blood pressure (BP) reduced to a target <140/85 mmHg (<130/80 in diabetes or heart failure), using non-pharmacological approaches and drugs as necessary.
- Long-term antiplatelet agents: in troponin-positive ACS the risk of reinfarction (sometimes leading to death) is greatly increased in the months following an ACS, so clopidogrel is added to aspirin for 1 year after an ACS.
- Most benefit from angiotensin-converting enzyme inhibitors, even when LV function is not impaired.
- In those with very severely impaired LV function following revascularization and recovery, there is a role for device therapy (either implantable cardioverter defibrillators (ICDs) or cardiac resynchronization therapy (CRT) – see Chapter 87).

Coronary angiography

Coronary angiography is the definitive investigation to evaluate coronary disease. It is not the only possible coronary investigation (see Chapter 85), though it is by far the most commonly used one in ACS, where a highly accurate and detailed assessment of coronary anatomy is often needed. In chronic chest pain syndromes, other coronary investigations have a role, and these include computed tomography coronary angiography, stress echo, myocardial perfusion imaging and gadolinium cardiac magnetic resonance imaging (cardiac MRI). However, all of these non-coronary angioraphy investigations have limitations that often precludes their use in ACSs.

How coronary angiography is performed

Coronary angiography involves passing a catheter (a small-calibre, long, flexible plastic tube – about 90–120 cm or so long) through a peripheral artery (usually the radial or femoral artery) into the ascending aorta, and then manipulating the catheter so its end sits just in the mouth of the coronary artery. Radio-opaque contrast is injected into the artery (about 2–8 mL over 3–4 s) and an X-ray is taken. These X-rays pass through all the thoracic structures to a greater or lesser extent, but not through any of the contrast contained within the artery. The pictures obtained are therefore a negative image of the lumen of the artery, and any obstruction or occlusion can be seen, as can the general state of the coronary arteries. The procedure takes about 20 minutes, and takes place in a specially constructed and sterile X-ray room, usually one whose sole purpose is the study of coronary arteries. Patients lie flat on the X-ray table, and may be given intravenous sedation (usually a diazepam-type drug, though if the patient is very anxious, sick or in pain, an opiate is used). They are covered in sterile drapes, local anaesthetic is injected over the artery to be entered, and an arterial sheath placed within the artery using a standard Seldinger technique. A small guide wire (a 'J' wire) is passed through the sheath to the ascending aorta, and over this the diagnostic catheter is passed, to the coronaries, as above.

Indications

Indications for coronary angiography include further assessment of angina in its many forms, be it for risk assessment purposes, as a prelude to the invasive treatment of haemodynamically unstable coronary syndromes or to evaluate how best to relieve intrusive symptoms. Other indications include the further evaluation of chest pain of uncertain origin where non-invasive investigations have failed to clarify the diagnosis and as a prelude to valve surgery.

Benefits

Benefits of coronary angiography include a better understanding of the coronary anatomy, which may lead to interventions that prolong life (in ACS and in those with severe coronary disease) and that may also relieve symptoms. Some interventions relieve symptoms but do not prolong life (e.g. PCI in most cases of chronic stable angina).

Risks

Risks of coronary angiography include the provocation of heart attack, stroke, renal failure (usually from the contrast in those with pre-existing impaired renal function) and bleeding, usually but not exclusively around the access site (there is a higher risk of a major bleed with the femoral approach). Any of these severe complications can lead to death. The overall chance of a severe complication is around 1 in 1000, higher in the elderly, those with diabetes or those with renal failure.

Invasive cardiac assessment beyond coronary angiography

Coronary angiography is extraordinarily useful in providing information about the anatomy of the coronary arteries and how diseased they are. Sometimes, indeed quite often, it still remains unclear as to how severe the disease actually is, and what impact it is having on the ability of the artery to work normally and, by extension, what treatment is best. Several diagnostic techniques have been introduced to give additional information:

- **Fractional flow reserve** is a technique used in chronic stable angina (it has not been validated in assessing the unstable plaque), in which a small pressure probe, attached to a tiny wire is passed down the coronary artery beyond the narrowing to be investigated. The pressure drop over the narrowing is measured, first at rest, then when coronary arterial dilatation (and so increased coronary blood flow) is provoked using the coronary vasodilator adenosine. The pressure before (from the catheter tip) and after the narrowing is measured – significant narrowings lose at least 20% of the pre-narrowing pressure over the narrowing. If the narrowing is not significant, then treating the narrowing by PCI or CABG is unlikely to relieve symptoms. The pressure wire used to assess fractional flow reserve can be used to determine other aspects of coronary artery physiology that may be relevant to treatment.

● **Intracoronary vascular ultrasound** is a technique where a very small ultrasound probe is placed on a guide wire, allowing three-dimensional imaging of the lumen of the artery. It can be very useful when the angiogram cannot quite delineate whether a narrowing is significant. It is also used to check whether a stent has been properly deployed, and whether there are any intracoronary complications of PCI, such as coronary dissection.

● **Intracardiac pressure and *P*o$_2$ measurement**: pressures and oxygen saturations can be measured in all the cardiac chambers directly or indirectly (the left atrium), as well as in the pulmonary artery and aorta. This information can be very useful in diagnosing the severity of mitral valve lesions, the presence of pulmonary hypertension and whether it might be relieved by cardiac surgery, the presence of pericardial constriction, and the presence and severity of intracardiac shunts.

Percutaneous coronary intervention

PCI involves passing an angioplasty balloon over a fine guide wire previously steered down the artery and across a coronary lesion. Inflating the balloon opens the artery up. **Stents** (mesh-like stainless steel tube) are usually inserted to help maintain short- and long-term patency (i.e. to lessen restenosis). During PCI, the vessel may **close acutely** if there is an extensive dissection (treated with stenting) or extensive *in situ* thrombus (treated with abciximab, a potent monoclonal antibody drug that blocks platelet action). If the vessel cannot be re-opened, an MI may occur (overall risk is 0.5%). Immediate CABG is only very rarely indicated to treat acute PCI-induced vessel closure, as it does not appear to successfully limit the size of the infarct. Immediate CABG following PCI now only occurs in about 0.2% of cases.

Restenosis of the stented artery can occur from 6 weeks onwards to about 1 year following PCI. Intimal hyperplasia (a process switched on by balloon injury to the vessel wall, and going on for up to a year) impinges on the lumen of the artery sufficient to produce recurrent angina in 10–20% of patients, and is termed 'restenosis'. Further PCI (especially with drug-eluting stents) may establish long-term patency. The introduction of cytotoxic and cytostatic **drug-eluting stents** has greatly reduced the problem of in-stent restenosis by inhibiting vascular smooth muscle cell growth.

Benefits

The technique relieves symptoms in those with angina. In chronic stable angina there is unlikely to be any reduction in the subsequent MI rate, and so prognosis is usually unaffected by PCI in this setting, except for those very few patients who have a tight narrowing in a very large artery proximally, with a lot of still viable tissue beyond the narrowing ('high ischaemic burden'). However, the situation changes radically in unstable coronary syndromes, where PCI does improve prognosis. Those who have the greatest increase in prognosis are those with the most severe expressions of coronary disease, those in cardiogenic shock (early on), those with STEMIs, and those with high-risk non-STEMIs. PCI in STEMI is termed primary PCI (primary indicating the first therapy, as opposed to PCI following thrombolysis, where it could be termed secondary, or for those who do not respond to thrombolysis, termed bail-out PCI). Primary PCI is marginally better than thrombolysis in improving prognosis in STEMIs, and also minimizes symptoms. It is now the preferred treatment for most patients with STEMI in the UK, co-morbidity allowing.

Risks

The risks of PCI are the same complications as for diagnostic angiography, but the overall rate of a major complication goes up substantially as the risk of provoking an MI is much higher. Overall about 1% of patients suffer a major complication.

84 ST segment elevation myocardial infarction

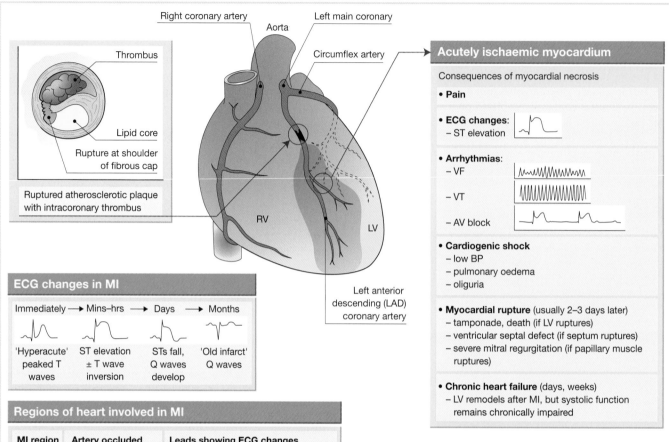

Right coronary artery

Aorta

Left main coronary

Circumflex artery

Thrombus

Lipid core

Rupture at shoulder of fibrous cap

Ruptured atherosclerotic plaque with intracoronary thrombus

RV

LV

Left anterior descending (LAD) coronary artery

Acutely ischaemic myocardium

Consequences of myocardial necrosis

- **Pain**

- **ECG changes:**
  – ST elevation

- **Arrhythmias:**
  – VF
  – VT
  – AV block

- **Cardiogenic shock**
  – low BP
  – pulmonary oedema
  – oliguria

- **Myocardial rupture** (usually 2–3 days later)
  – tamponade, death (if LV ruptures)
  – ventricular septal defect (if septum ruptures)
  – severe mitral regurgitation (if papillary muscle ruptures)

- **Chronic heart failure** (days, weeks)
  – LV remodels after MI, but systolic function remains chronically impaired

ECG changes in MI

Immediately → Mins–hrs → Days → Months

'Hyperacute' peaked T waves | ST elevation ± T wave inversion | STs fall, Q waves develop | 'Old infarct' Q waves

Regions of heart involved in MI

MI region	Artery occluded	Leads showing ECG changes
Anterior	LAD	$V_2 - V_5$: 'anteroseptal chest leads' often I, aV_L as well
Inferior	Right (usually)	II, III, aV_F 'inferior leads'
Posterior	Right or circumflex	Difficult to see: posterior wall infarction causes R wave (not Q wave) in V_1 with ST depression. Often associated with inferior MI
Lateral	Circumflex or diagonal branch of LAD	I, aV_L, $V_{5,6}$ 'lateral leads'

Rare causes of MI

Coronary artery embolism (thrombus, infected vegetation)

Coronary artery spasm (NB drugs, e.g. cocaine)

Spontaneous coronary artery thrombosis (prothrombotic states)

Arteritis (SLE, PAN, Takayasu)

Coronary artery aneurysm (e.g. Kawasaki disease as a child)

Anomalous coronary artery

Spontaneous coronary artery dissection

Medicine at a Glance, Fourth Edition. Edited by Patrick Davey. © 2014 John Wiley & Sons, Ltd. Published 2014 by John Wiley & Sons, Ltd. Companion website: www.ataglanceseries.com/medicine

Demographics

- **Definition**: ischaemic necrosis of the myocardium as a result of acute occlusion of a coronary artery. This results in a typical electrocardiogram (ECG), that showing an ST segment elevation myocaridal infarction (STEMI). The relevance of seperating out STEMI out from other forms of myocardial infarction (MI) is that STEMIs benefit from immediate therapy to open up the occluded coronary artery (either thrombolysis, or in the modern world more likely primary percutaneous coronary intervention (PCI)), treatment that must be applied immediately to be effective. Other forms of MI need immediate *medical* therapy and early angiography (± PCI, coronary artery bypass graft (CABG)) within 72 hours, but not immediate angiography; there is some evidence that immediate angiography and intervention may have some hazards (one interpretation of which is that the antiplatelets have not yet had time to penetrate through the thrombus-laden lesions).
- **Incidence**: very common; 250 000 MIs per year in the UK (one every 2 min), with 100 000 deaths.
- **Pathogenesis**: an MI occurs when a coronary artery occludes, the myocardium supplied by that artery becomes ischaemic and necrosis occurs over several hours; early restoration of blood flow may abort the infarction and limit necrosis. The overwhelmingly common cause is **atheromatous coronary artery disease** (CAD), when an existing coronary atheromatous plaque (not necessarily one severely narrowing the artery) becomes eroded or ruptures, causing a sudden expansion of the plaque and thrombosis of the coronary artery lumen. Other causes of MI occur very occasionally (see Figure 84.1).

Clinical features

- **Classic presentation**: severe, crushing central chest pain ≥20 minutes, unrelieved by nitrates, associated with sweating, pallor and nausea. However, as STEMI is common, atypical manifestations are also common; the intensity of the chest pain may be surprisingly mild (or even absent), the location may be atypical (jaw/arm only, unusual place on the chest, such as left shoulder, only, etc.). Sometimes patients present only with the autonomic features (sweating, vomiting), or just feeling unwell. As acute coronary syndrome (ACS) accounts for a large proportion of acute medical admissions, if you see a patient in this context and the diagnosis is not immediately apparent, always do an ECG to help rule out a STEMI.
- **Other presentations** include arrhythmia, cardiac arrest or acute heart failure.
- May be atypical in **elderly people** (collapse or confusion) and in those with **diabetes**, who may have no chest pain, and develop worsening of metabolic status or heart failure. Up to one-third of patients with MI are 'silent', that is to say, patients do not recognize their symptoms as being due to something serious and do not present to hospital. Such infarcts only come to light later, either when patients have ECGs carried out for other purposes, or when patients present with late complications of MI, such as heart failure or arrhythmias.
- Most patients have risk factors or known CAD; 50% have no preceding angina (and so 50% do!).

Investigations

Initial investigations (especially the ECG) should quickly establish the diagnosis:

- The diagnostic hallmark of acute MI is ST segment elevation. However, not all ST segment elevation is due to acute STEMI – some is due to old infarction, some to pericarditis, some is physiological, some the consequences of bundle branch block (BBB),

hyperkalaemia and rarely Brugada syndrome. The usual clues to ST elevation reflecting STEMI are: (i) the exact nature of the ST elevation (convex upwards); (ii) the regional distribution (reflecting the coronary arteries); and (iii) the clinical context. You should become very familiar with the ECG signs of STEMI, and how to exclude other causes.

- A few patients have BBB. With right BBB it is usually fairly easy to see if there is an underlying STEMI; this is not the case with left BBB, which should always be regarded as concealing a STEMI if the clincial context is appropriate.
- 80% of patients are subsequently shown to have had an MI present with other ECG changes such as ST depression or T-wave inversion. These patients *do not benefit* from thrombolysis, so can safely be treated as having non-ST segment elevation ACSs.

Important differential diagnoses to exclude are **acute aortic dissection** (a wide mediastinum on chest X-ray is regarded as being a classic sign but is of low specificity and sensitivity, loss of pulses, aortic regurgitation) and **pericarditis** (widespread non-specific changes on ECG). **Acute pulmonary embolism** is an extraordinarily common and serious cause of acute chest pain, and is probably the most common condition to be inappropriately diagnosed as an acute MI. Always consider acute pulmonary embolism (PE) in the differential of all chest pain. In general, immediate reperfusion therapy is more commonly withheld from patients who justify therapy, rather than administered inappropriately to patients with other conditions.

Management

Patients with STEMI are usually diagnosed by the emergency first responders (ambulance service) and such patients should be immediately transferred to the primary PCI facility. If the diagnosis is made in A&E, likewise, immediate transfer to the catheter laboratory with primary PCI facilities should occur. Patients with non-STEMI or other actual or potential serious cardiac illness should be moved to a coronary care unit (CCU) for monitoring and further assessment.

- Once STEMI is diagnosed, or considered likely, immediate treatment includes: (i) pain relief with opiate analgesia; (ii) high-dose oxygen (unless there are contraindications, e.g. chronic obstructive pulmonary disease); and (iii) immediate *chewed* aspirin 300 mg (chewed as its antiplatelet action will then be effective within 20 min).
- Immediate coronary angioplasty/stenting (**primary PCI**) is now regarded as the 'gold standard' treatment, provided it can be provided quickly in experienced centres.
- Thrombolysis, usually with tissue plasminogen activator (tPA) or related thrombolytics, was the standard therapy, and remains appropriate for those where timely primary PCI is not available. **'Mandated' angiography/revascularization** should occur ≤24 hours in all those receiving thrombolytic therapy.
- β-Blocker, intravenously, especially if hypertensive or tachycardic without cardiac failure.
- Diuretic for pulmonary oedema.
- Angiotensin-converting enzyme (ACE) inhibitor (day 2 or 3), especially if there is clinical heart failure, or significantly impaired left ventricular (LV) function (anterior MI, large enzyme release, impaired left ventricle on echocardiography).

Complications

Immediate/hours

- **Ventricular arrhythmias** (ventricular tachycardia (VT) or ventricular fibrillation (VF)) occuring within 24 hours or less are the principal cause of pre-hospital death. Patients should be monitored close to a defibrillator. Early VT/VF (provided the patient survives) is not associated with a worse long-term outlook.

- **Atrial arrhythmias**, especially atrial fibrillation (AF), may compromise cardiac output and need immediate cardioversion or, at the very least, heart rate slowing and heparin. AF is more likely in those with more severe and extensive coronary disease, and so is a marker for a worse prognosis.
- **Failed reperfusion** is the failure of treatment to re-establish blood flow in the occluded artery. This was not rare in the thrombolysis era, when immediate PCI was (probably) warrented, and unfortunately remains common, though the mechanism is obscure. It is diagnosed when there is persisting ST elevation, whether or not the infarct-related artery is open. Indeed, many cases are now seen where primary PCI opens the infarct-related artery, but the ST elevation fails to resolve. The mechanism is postulated to be microvascular obstruction, perhaps due to embolizing thrombus, or distal spread of vasoactive substances, and remains a target for therapeutic investigation. `

Hours/days

Cardiac rupture into the pericardium is uncommon, but typically occurs on days 2–5, resulting in fatal cardiac arrest. **Re-infarction** is common after thrombolysis, because a culprit plaque may cause repeat coronary thrombosis, and should be treated by immediate PCI. Re-infarction after primary PCI is rare, but occurs, and is usually treated by further PCI. **Heart failure** with pulmonary oedema results from acute impairment of LV function. **Cardiogenic shock** occurs when cardiac output is inadequate to maintain arterial blood pressure (BP), resulting from:

- **Severe impairment of LV function**: some heart muscle is irreparably damaged, but some is reversibly stunned and may improve its contractile function, provided the patient can be carried over the acute period. If patients develop cardiogenic shock early on during an MI, immediate angiography is often indicated to re-perfuse occluded arteries and in time hopefully improve contractile function and outcome.
- **Infarction of the right ventricle** (usually in inferior MI): in this situation the right heart needs a high (not normal) filling pressure (i.e. right atrial pressure) to operate anywhere like normally. If the filling pressure is normal, or low (dehydration from sweating and inadequate fluid intake is common in acute MI), then right heart output falls, causing inadequate left heart filling. Treatment of cardiogenic shock due to right ventricular infarction is by diagnosing it (inferior infarct and cardiac ultrasound showing a dilated, poorly functioning right heart with reasonable LV function) and then giving intravenous fluids.
- **Mechanical catastrophe** such as: (i) **ventricular septal rupture**, with a new loud pansystolic murmur at the lower left sternal edge; or (ii) **papillary muscle rupture**, with severe mitral regurgitation; murmur may not be loud, but severe pulmonary oedema is out of proportion to apparent LV damage. Both require *immediate* cardiological assessment with a view to surgical repair.

Days/weeks

- **Thromboembolism** (cerebrovascular accident, gut or limb ischaemia): may result from mural thrombus forming at the site of the infarct. Unusual now that antiplatelet agents and heparin are widely used. In the days of single antiplatelet therapy following STEMI, warfarin was commonly given for 3–6 months after large anterior wall MI (when the risk of LV thrombus was quite high) or if there was severe LV impairment. If dual antiplatelet therapy is given, warfarin on top may constitute too high a bleeding risk in many elderly patients.

- **Chronic heart failure**: LV remodelling after MI may worsen rather than improve LV function. Treat with ACE inhibitors, diuretics, cautious β-blockade and spironolactone.
- **Ventricular tachycardia**: occuring after 24 hours implies that the myocardial scar is a substrate for re-entrant circuits. β-Blockers and amiodarone help but, if there is impaired LV function or collapse, the risk of future sudden cardiac death is significant and justifies automatic defibrillator implantation.
- **Dressler's syndrome**: usually self-limiting autoimmune pericarditis occurring several weeks after a full-thickness MI. Occasionally requires steroids, more commonly responds to non-steroidal anti-inflammatory drugs.

Prognosis and rehabilitation

Long-term outlook after MI is governed largely by the extent of **LV damage**, and the severity of the underlying **coronary artery disease**. Most post-MI deaths are caused by heart failure, sudden cardiac death or further MI. Secondary prophylaxis to prevent further MI and other vascular events comprises:

- Aspirin (or another antiplatelet agent such as clopidogrel), β-blockers and ACE inhibitors.
- **Risk factor modification**: stop smoking, reduce cholesterol (diet and statins) and treat hypertension and diabetes.
- **Rehabilitation programme** to increase physical exercise, encourage lifestyle changes and provide psychological support.

Risk stratification

Risk stratification requires a full knowledge of cardiac risk factors, cardiac anatomy and functional capacity. Not all data are relevant in everyone, as much risk factor modification is relevant to all – for example, cholesterol reduction with statins improves outlook regardless of whether the starting cholesterol is very high, high or 'average'. Likewise, exercise is good for all, and this must be emphasized. The important aspects of risk stratification and modification are:

- **Lifestyle measures**: smoking must cease, though there is rarely an easy means to achieve this. Likewise, alcohol consumption should be moderate. Regular high-intensity exercise is vital both to maximize good health and improve prognosis. Achievement of ideal weight is important, both to lessen the atherogenic impact of obesity, which is particularly powerful in the diabetic patient, and to minimize the long-term risk of cancer.
- **Left ventricular function** is a crucial determinant of long-term prognosis, and should be assessed in all patients echocardiographically; this can be done during the MI or, in many, several weeks following the heart attack. Prognosis is worst in those who not only have poor left ventricles but who also have symptoms and signs of heart failure, especially if they have a broad QRS complex on the resting ECG, and ambient complex ventricular arrhythmias on 24-hour ECG recording. Aggressive treatment is with medical therapy, including spironolactone (or the modern equivalent eplerinone), revascularization where appropriate and device therapy, including cardiac resynchronization therapy/ implantable cardiovertor defibrillators.
- **Extent of coronary disease**: those with the most extensive coronary disease have the worst outlook, and gain the most from successful revascularization. Most patients with acute STEMI have had angiography performed during the infarct as part of the primary PCI procedure, and so there is knowledge of the extent of bystander coronary disease (that is, coronary narrowings in

the non-infarct-related artery). Plans can be made for the most appropriate form of revascularization, be it by further PCI or CABG. All elective revascularization must be discussed beforehand by appropriately constituted multidisciplinary teams including cardiac surgeons. If angiography has not been undertaken acutely, many patients will have this electively, though its benefit must be titrated against risk (highest in the very elderly and those with extensive vascular co-morbidity) and benefit (which is limited in those with other disease processes shortening length and quality of life). However, there is a small cohort of patients who are considered low risk, and may not benefit, and this includes: (i) younger patients (increasing age is a powerful adverse risk factor in MI outlook); (ii) completed Q wave infarct (no further heart muscle to save); (iii) no ongoing symptoms of angina (angina suggests there is a significant volume of heart muscle supplied by a stenosed coronary artery); symptomatology can be tested by an exercise stress test, and evidence of silent myocardial ischaemia can also be sought (silent ischaemia may have the same prognostic significance as symptomatic ischaemia); (iv) no preceding angina (which suggests a plaque event rather than fixed high-grade coronary stenosis); and (v) good left ventricular function.

85 Chronic coronary syndromes

Exercise testing

Bruce protocol

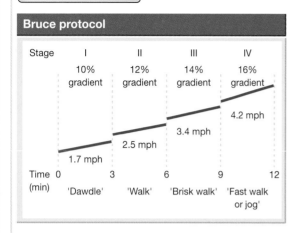

Stage | I | II | III | IV

- 10% gradient
- 12% gradient
- 14% gradient
- 16% gradient

4.2 mph
3.4 mph
2.5 mph
1.7 mph

Time (min) 0   3   6   9   12
'Dawdle' 'Walk' 'Brisk walk' 'Fast walk or jog'

Percutaneous coronary intervention (PCI)

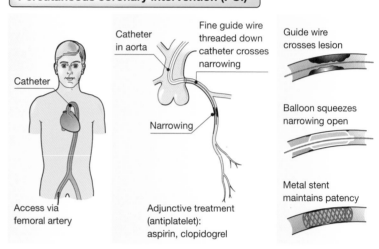

Catheter

Catheter in aorta

Fine guide wire threaded down catheter crosses narrowing

Guide wire crosses lesion

Narrowing

Balloon squeezes narrowing open

Access via femoral artery

Adjunctive treatment (antiplatelet): aspirin, clopidogrel

Metal stent maintains patency

ECG changes on exercise

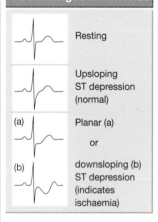

Resting

Upsloping ST depression (normal)

(a) Planar (a)

or

(b) downsloping (b) ST depression (indicates ischaemia)

Typical HR and BP changes

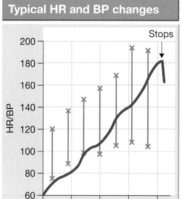

Stops

Coronary artery bypass graft (CABG) surgery

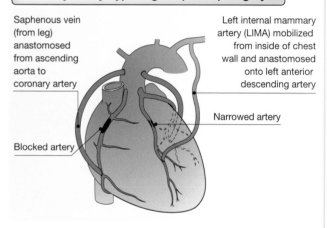

Saphenous vein (from leg) anastomosed from ascending aorta to coronary artery

Left internal mammary artery (LIMA) mobilized from inside of chest wall and anastomosed onto left anterior descending artery

Narrowed artery

Blocked artery

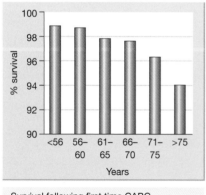

Survival following first time CABG

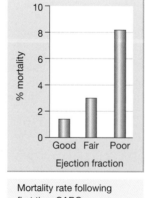

Mortality rate following first time CABG

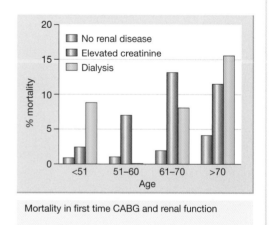

No renal disease
Elevated creatinine
Dialysis

Mortality in first time CABG and renal function

Medicine at a Glance, Fourth Edition. Edited by Patrick Davey. © 2014 John Wiley & Sons, Ltd. Published 2014 by John Wiley & Sons, Ltd. Companion website: www.ataglanceseries.com/medicine

Chronic chest pain is common, as is coronary artery disease (CAD). The key to managing chronic chest pain is to establish whether symptoms relate to coronary disease and, if they do, the risk of an adverse event occurring.

Diagnosis

Chronic stable angina usually relates to CAD, although other pathologies may be responsible (see Chapter 13). It is a common condition, and while the symptoms often are classic, given how common it is it not infrequently presents with atypical symptomatology. The classic symptoms are:

- Retrosternal chest tightness, which may radiate to the jaw or either arm.
- Day-to-day symptoms occur with roughly the same amount of effort and are rapidly (<1 min) relieved by rest/glyceryl trinitrate (GTN). The longer rest/GTN takes to relieve symptoms, the less likely they are to relate to CAD. Effort capacity is decreased by the cold, the wind, on hills or after eating.

Symptoms may be very atypical – the diagnostic clue is the clear provocation with effort and rapid relief by rest, in the presence of appropriate coronary risk factors (age, sex, etc.). Breathlessness, rather than chest pain, may be an 'anginal equivalent' in people with diabetes.

The diagnosis is usually clear from the history alone. If not, exercise testing or other non-invasive investigations often help, although occasionally coronary angiography is needed for diagnostic purposes. Once the diagnosis has been established, risk stratification is vital, and angiography is often used here, though there are equally reliable non-invasive means.

Standard diagnostic tests in chronic chest pain

The central issues in those with chronic chest pain are, firstly, does the pain relate to myocardial ischaemia, some other severe cardiac pathology (e.g. aortic stenosis, hypertrophic cardiomyopathy or very rarely pulmonary hypertension), some other pathology (angina-type symptoms are common in those with airflow restriction) or not to any serious pathology? Secondly, if it relates to coronary disease, how extensive is the coronary disease and what is the prognosis (see section on risk stratification)?

In terms of diagnosing whether chest pain relates to coronary disease, most cardiologists look for two things; firstly, in the history, the strong relationship between effort provoking symptoms and rest relieving symptoms (see Table 85.1). This relationship is almost always present if symptoms have been present long enough (>1–2 months), though for unknown reasons may not be present in the first few weeks of new-onset angina. Beware that inactive people may not show this relationship with effort. Symptoms most typically are retrosternal pain, though some people with angina feel pain symptoms elsewhere, and some feel breathlessness rather than pain. Secondly, cardiologists examining the patient will use the resting electrocardiogram (ECG) to exclude aortic stenosis, hypertrophic cardiomyopathy and pulmonary hypertension. Cardiologists then go on to confirm their diagnosis using simple tests:

- **Exericse stress ECG**: this test has enormous utility when used correctly. It gives excellent data on the relationship between exercise and symptoms, and also good data on prognosis – exercise capacity itself is powerfully related to outcome. Perhaps the least useful data are provided from the ECG itself; while there is broad relationship between patients with severe coronary disease showing ST depression at a low work load, and those with normal hearts not showing any ST changes, the problem in interpreting the test is that some patients with severe coronary disease can have normal ECGs (false negative test) and, conversely, there are quite a few patients (most typically younger women with atypical symtoms) who can manifest substantial ST changes without having any heart disease. These problems with the interpretation of the stress ECG have led various guideline writing committees to recommend using other tests for routine evaluation of chronic chest pain. Nonetheless the fact remains that in well-informed hands the exercise test remains a widely used, cheap and reliable investigation.

Table 85.1 Percentage of people estimated to have coronary artery disease (CAD) according to typicality of symptoms, age, sex and risk factors.

Age (years)	Non-anginal chest pain				Atypical angina				Typical angina			
	Men		Women		Men		Women		Men		Women	
	Lo	Hi	Lo	Hi	L	Hi	Lo	Hi	Lo	Hi	Lo	Hi
35	3	35	1	19	8	59	2	39	39	88	10	78
45	9	47	2	22	21	70	5	43	51	92	20	79
55	23	59	4	25	45	79	10	47	80	95	38	82
65	49	69	9	29	71	86	20	51	93	97	56	84

For men older than 70 with atypical or typical symptoms, assume an estimate >90%. For women older than 70, assume an estimate of 61–90% EXCEPT women at high risk AND with typical symptoms where a risk of >90% should be assumed.

Values are per cent of people at each mid-decade age with significant CAD.

Hi = high risk = diabetes, smoking and hyperlipidaemia (total cholesterol >6.47 mmol/L).

Lo = low risk = none of these three.

The shaded area represents people with symptoms of non-anginal chest pain, who would not be investigated for stable angina routinely.

Note: These results are likely to overestimate CAD in primary care populations. If there are resting ECG ST-T changes or Q waves, the likelihood of CAD is higher in each cell of the table.

Source: National Clinical Guideline Centre for Acute and Chronic Conditions, 2010, http://www.nice.org.uk/nicemedia/live/12947/47931/47931.pdf (last accessed September 2013).

- **Coronary calcium score**: this test involves using the standard computer tomography (CT) scanner to detect and measure the amount of calcium within the coronary artery. Normal coronary arteries have no calcium; calcium is laid done as part of the atherosclerotic process, and the greater the amount of calcium in the coronary artery, the more likely there is to be a significant narrowing. However, one should be clear that the coronary calcium score gives no actual information about coronary narrowings, it merely informs the probability of there being a narrowing. This test is helpful in the assessment of chronic chest pain, and, in particular, the most helpful finding is a low calcium score, making coronary disease very unlikely. If patients have a high calcium score, they usually need additional investigations to determine whether they actually have coronary narrowings, and if so how many and how severe.

- **CT coronary angiography**: this test also uses the CT scanner – however, the difference with coronary calcium score is profound. A bolus of contrast is injected intravenously and after an appropriate delay this passes through the coronary arteries, at which time their presence is detected and outlined by the CT scan. This allows an outline of the lumen of the arteries to be obtained, in essence therefore providing the same information as a standard coronary angiogram, without its attendant invasive risks. This is the main advantage of the CT coronary angiogram. The disadvantages are that:

  - The heart rate must be regular and slow – so patients should be in sinus rhythm and able to have a β-blocker or similar heart rate lowering drug.
  - If there is extensive coronary calcium, it is difficult to accurately image the coronary arteries. Extensive calcification is common in the elderly, the very group most likely to have coronary disease, and the commonest group in whom we search for coronary disease.
  - The radiation dose is the same as a standard coronary angiogram.

Despite these disadvantages, CT coronary angiography has a growing role.

- **Stress echo**: this test involves stressing the heart with increasingly high doses of catecholamines, usually dobutamine, along with atropine. The principle is that a normal heart will increase its contractile performance with such stimulation. However, regions of the heart supplied by narrowed arteries will in the face of this intropic challenge try to contract more, but cannot do so as the blood supply is limited by arterial narrowing. Indeed, they actually contract less in this situation. Thus a marked difference in contractile performance between heart supplied by good arteries and heart supplied by narrowed arteries appears, which can be detected echocardiographically. In the right hands, this is a very good test. However, the accuracy of the test is extremely operator dependent, and unless the operator is highly experienced it is easy for the test to be misinterpreted. The main advantage of the test is that it is radiation free.

- **Myocardial perfusion scintigraphy**, otherwise known as myocardial single photon emission CT or myocardial SPECT. This is an accurate and well-validated test. A radioactive isotope, usually containing technicium 99, is injected intravenously; the isotope is taken up by the hearts tissues proportional to blood flow and can be detected by photomultiplier tubes arranged round the body (the imager is called a gamma camera). The data are then reconstructed into a three-dimensional model of the heart, allowing one to see how much tracer has been taken up in the different coronary artery territories. Injections are made at rest and with stress (either by physical exercise, e.g. treadmill – the preferred modality, or pharmacological, often using a coronary vasodilator such as adenosine or its analogues). Narrowed arteries rarely reduce resting blood flow, so the rest injection allows viable heart to be differentiated from areas of dead heart, i.e. previous myocardial infarction (MI). Narrowed arteries reduce peak blood flow compared to healthy arteries, so leading to less tracer uptake in the supplied territory, which can be imaged using the gamma camera, thus allowing the areas of the heart supplied with narrowed arteries to be determined. This is a good test for assessing the presence of coronary disease, and its severity. The extent of perfusion abnormalities on this test correlates with the prognostic benefit from revascularization. This is useful, as while the test can undercall the presence of coronary disease, if there are no or few perfusion abnormalities then there is no or little prognostic benefit from revascularization.

- **Cardiac magnetic resonance imaging** (cardiac MRI): this test is good for showing cardiac structure, such as previous MI, and cardiomyopathy, even if the changes are subtle. The presence of coronary disease is a more difficult problem for cardiac MRI. Direct visualization of the coronary lumen is not that accurate. The technology has now evolved such that the scans can determine the uptake of gadolinium in the myocardium, which correlates with ischaemia. The test is very useful, particularly if there are concerns about exposing a patient to radiation; the downside of the test is that some 10% of patients cannot complete the test for reasons of claustrophobia. There are also safety concerns about gadolinium in the presence of renal failure.

Risk stratification

Risk stratification is a key component in the assessment of angina. There are several factors associated with a worse outlook in chronic angina:

- Increasing age.
- Exercise intolerance, especially if caused by chest pain/cardiac dyspnoea.
- Impaired left ventricular (LV) function (e.g. previous MI, hypertensive heart disease) or frank heart failure.
- Extensive and severe coronary disease. A non-invasive measure of this can be obtained from the exercise ECG test (or exercise myocardial perfusion imaging using radioisotopes). It is a controversial point as to whether patients with angina should undergo periodic exercise ECG tests; some health care systems promote this, but this is not standard practice in the UK.
- Symptoms and/or ST depression ≥ 2 mm in stage II of the Bruce protocol (see Figure 85.1) correlates with a poorer outcome.
- Exercise-induced hypotension likewise suggests extensive CAD.
- Extensive atherogenic risk factors, particularly diabetes. Indeed diabetes is perhaps the most potent factor influencing prognosis, and its presence mandates the most vigourous approach to management. Ongoing smoking is associated with a worse outlook.
- Vascular disease elsewhere, e.g. peripheral vascular disease.
- Renal failure is associated with a worse outlook in those with angina.

Although some patients with few symptoms benefit from revascularization (and can be identified by non-invasive means), many patients can be identified on clinical criteria:

- Symptomatic angina despite medical therapy.
- Worsening or unstable angina – most patients with acute coronary syndromes (ACSs) benefit from revascularization of the artery with the acute lesion, although there remains debate as to how much bystander disease should be revascularized.

- Post-infarct angina.
- Heart failure with angina.

These patients should undergo coronary angiography to determine the location and severity of coronary stenosis and whether revascularization will reduce subsequent adverse events.

Treatment

- Many patients are managed on medical therapy alone.
- Action should be taken to improve diet (omega-3 fish oils, fruit, decrease animal fats, low cholesterol), lose weight and increase exercise (which lessens blood pressure (BP) by ±10 mmHg and cholesterol by 1.0–1.5 mmol/L).
- Stop smoking – this is vital.
- Treat diabetes and hypertension aggressively (target BP <140/85, unless diabetes is also present, in which case aim for <130/80).
- **Hypercholesterolaemia** (see Chapter 82): all patients should be on statin therapy. If statins cannot be tolerated, try a fibrate. Cholesterol reduction by lifestyle measures is important, but is never a substitute for statin therapy – the dietary intervention trials from 30 years ago were not a success!
- **Angiotensin-converting enzyme inhibitors** have anti-atherogenic actions in those at high risk of vascular events. This is probably through their PB lowering action.
- **Antiplatelet agents**: aspirin has prognostic benefit. In aspirin allergy/intolerance clopidogrel is used (and is marginally superior, a valid difference in higher risk patients). In anyone with a recent (<1 year) ACS, dual antiplatelet therapy with aspirin and clopidogrel (or similar, such as prasugrel, or a drug from another class, such as ticagrelor) for a year from the time of the ACS improves outcome.

Anti-ischaemic therapy

- **Nitrates** are highly effective in relieving angina. Nitrate tolerance develops if they are given throughout the 24 hours. A 'nitrate-free' period of 12–14 h/day is needed. **Nicorandil** is a new drug that acts very much like nitrates do; trials have shown a small survival advantage in patients with angina treated with nicorandil, whereas nitrates themselves do not alter prognosis in angina.
- **β-Blockers** are first-line therapy. They reduce cardiac work, lessen angina and improve prognosis after an MI and in heart failure. **Ivabradine**, a novel drug acting on the sinus node, has heart rate-slowing properties in patients in sinus rhythm, and can be used as an anti-anginal, though its main use is in the treatment of patients in heart failure who are in sinus rhythm but who cannot take a β-blocker.
- **Calcium channel blockers**: second-line therapies are used only when β-blockers are contraindicated. They are contraindicated in heart failure. Only those with heart rate-slowing properties (e.g. diltiazem or verapamil, not nifedipine) can be given as monotherapy in angina. Those without any negatively chronotropic action must be given with a β-blocker.
- **Ranolazine**: this is a new class of drug, a cardiac potassium channel opener, which is an effective anti-anginal, and may have other useful properties also. It is currently used in those with severe symptoms refractory to other treatments.

Revascularization in CAD

Patients benefit from revascularization procedures if their symptoms interfere with their lifestyle, or if they fall into a group known to benefit prognostically from coronary artery bypass graft (CABG), i.e. those with stenoses (>70% luminal narrowing) affecting: (i) all three coronary arteries; or (ii) the left main coronary artery; or (iii) the proximal portion of the left anterior descending artery. Impaired LV function and diabetes magnify

the prognostic benefit of surgery. The extent of coronary disease can be estimated from non-invasive tests (especially myocardial perfusion scintigraphy), but is only confirmed by coronary angiography (see Chapter 83).

Percutaneous coronary intervention (PCI)

PCI is highly effective at relieving symptoms in chronic stable angina, but largely speaking does not prolong life in stable angina. The exception is those few patients who have a tight narrowing right at the start of a large artery supplying a lot of viable heart muscle (this is termed a 'high ischaemic burden'), where the risk of subsequent MI and so death is reduced by successful PCI. PCI can prolong life in unstable coronary syndromes. For further details on PCI see Chapter 83.

Coronary artery bypass surgery

Coronary surgery is highly effective at relieving anginal symptoms and in some cases improves prognosis (see section on risk stratification). In some patients, angioplasty can be safely used to delay the need for CABG, i.e. PCI and CABG are complementary rather than competitive treatments.

In CABG, bypass grafts are connected from the aorta to the coronary artery distal to the stenosis. Usually this requires stopping the heart and supporting the patient by a cardiopulmonary bypass machine (that is to say a machine that takes deoxygenated blood out of the patient, gives it oxygen and also pressurizes it, so acting like the heart and lungs combined). In many patients it is possible to apply grafts without stopping the heart – so-called 'off-pump surgery'. The claimed advantage of off-pump surgery is a lessened 'systemic inflammatory response syndrome' – this is where the membrane in the heart–lung machine activates components of the blood to turn on an inflammatory response throughout the body, which can result in lung damage, kidney failure and a variety of brain syndromes.

There are two forms of bypass graft:
- **Vein grafts** (from leg saphenous veins) are easy to use and quick to apply, but have an annual failure rate of ±8%. Many patients are therefore informed that these grafts should be expected to last no longer than 10 years. When saphenous grafts fail, patients can have any of the following symptoms: none (surprisingly common, the explanation being that the heart has developed internal bypasses), stable angina, an ACS including acute MI, and sudden cardiac death. Most graft failure can be managed medically (with pills), some requires PCI, and for a very few re-do CABG (which is much higher risk than first time CABG) can be undertaken.
- **Arterial grafts** are technically more difficult to apply and have a much better long-term survival rate, and therefore a better medium-term patient survival. The most commonly used arterial graft is the internal mammary artery, usually applied to the left anterior descending (LAD) artery. The application of this graft to the LAD artery is powerfully associated with a prolongation of life. This is by far the most important reason for carrying out CABG.

Elective surgery has, in good hands and in low-risk patients, a ±1% mortality rate. However, in those with damaged left ventricles, renal impairment and other co-morbidities, the risk of surgery goes up substantially, as does the benefit from successful surgery. Deciding which of these high-risk patients should have surgery can be a difficult decision, and most units would routinely pass all these decisions to a multidisciplinary team (MDT) meeting where cardiologists, cardiac surgeons and sometimes cardiac anaesthetists can together decide what approach is in the best interests of the patient. After surgery, anti-atherogenic and antiplatelet measures must continue.

86 Aortic dissection

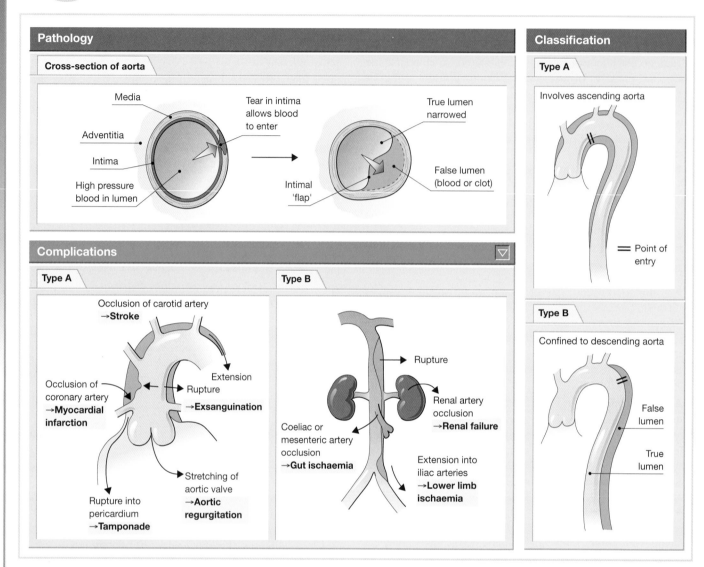

Pathology

Cross-section of aorta

Media

Adventitia

Intima

High pressure blood in lumen

Tear in intima allows blood to enter

Intimal 'flap'

True lumen narrowed

False lumen (blood or clot)

Complications

Type A

Occlusion of carotid artery →**Stroke**

Occlusion of coronary artery →**Myocardial infarction**

Extension

Rupture →**Exsanguination**

Stretching of aortic valve →**Aortic regurgitation**

Rupture into pericardium →**Tamponade**

Type B

Rupture

Renal artery occlusion →**Renal failure**

Coeliac or mesenteric artery occlusion →**Gut ischaemia**

Extension into iliac arteries →**Lower limb ischaemia**

Classification

Type A

Involves ascending aorta

Point of entry

Type B

Confined to descending aorta

False lumen

True lumen

Aortic dissection affects 1/40 000 of the population per year and consists of a tear in the intima of the thoracic aorta, causing bleeding into the aortic wall, and raising a flap. This then propagates distal to the original tear, interrupting vital organ blood supply. Aortic rupture may occur.

Aetiology

- Hypertension.
- Atherosclerosis.
- Marfan's syndrome predisposes to aortic aneurysm formation, dissection and rupture (see Figure 86.2 below).

Pathology

High blood pressure (BP), stretched connective tissues and the presence of diseased intima (atherosclerosis) result in sudden tearing of the intima. Blood enters the layer between the intima and media, and high pressure causes the blood to track longitudinally along the aorta, forwards and backwards from the point of entry, forming a false lumen. Blood in the false lumen may clot,

or remain liquid with some flow. Dissections are classified into one of two types, depending on whether the ascending aorta is involved:

- **Type A**: point of intimal tearing is in the ascending aorta. The dissection usually tracks distally to involve the descending aorta and proximally to disrupt the aortic valve apparatus and into the pericardium.
- **Type B**: point of intimal tearing is in the descending aorta, typically just beyond the origin of the left subclavian artery. It is rare for the tear to propagate proximally.

Clinical features

The clinical presentation is extremely variable because of the diverse consequences and complications of aortic dissection. Symptoms arise from the stripping of the intima away from the aortic wall (presentation symptoms) and from either the interruption of blood supply to vital organs or rupture. The most common presentation is with abrupt onset of extremely

Medicine at a Glance, Fourth Edition. Edited by Patrick Davey. © 2014 John Wiley & Sons, Ltd. Published 2014 by John Wiley & Sons, Ltd. Companion website: www.ataglanceseries.com/medicine

Marfan's syndrome

- 1 in 5000
- In 70% due to mutations in fibrillin-1 gene FBN1 chromosome 15
- Autosomal dominant inheritance

Eyes
- Lens dislocation – 50%, best seen on slit lamp examination
- Myopia
- Retinal detachment (rare)

Narrow high-arched palate

Chest
- Deformity (pectus excavatum carinatum)
- Recurrent pneumothoraces – rare

Skeletal signs
- Tall
- Span > height
- Arachnodactyly (long fingers)
- Scoliosis (rare)
- Joint hypermobility

Aortic disease
- Progressive aortic root dilatation →aortic regurgitation
- Aortic dissection/rupture – often (not always) in those with large aortic roots
- Accounts for most mortality
- β-blockers and prophylactic surgery reduce aortic complications

Mitral valve disease
- Prolapse
- Regurgitation

Dural ectasia
- Seen on pelvic MRI scan
- Can cause backache

severe pain felt in the chest or back (interscapular), particularly in a middle-aged hypertensive man. The complications of dissection are:

- **Rupture**: catastrophic pain, hypotension and collapse. Often fatal, but may be contained as BP falls. Occurs retroperitoneally, in the mediastinum or into the left (although never the right) pleural space.
- **Pericardial tamponade**: rupture of a type A dissection backwards into the pericardium results in haemopericardium and pericardial tamponade, the clinical features of which are hypotension (pulsus paradoxus) and a raised jugular venous pressure (Kussmaul's sign).
- **Aortic regurgitation**: involvement of the aortic root disrupts the aortic valve ring, causing the valve to leak. Early diastolic murmur.
- **Aortic side branch occlusion**: the false lumen compresses the origin of arterial branches as they arise from the aorta. Any branch, at any point along the ascending, descending and abdominal aorta, can be involved. This can lead to a myocardial infarction (MI) (only patients with inferior infarction are seen, because left main coronary dissection is lethal), stroke, upper or lower limb ischaemia, paraparesis caused by spinal artery occlusion, renal failure or gut ischaemia.
- **Extension**: initial dissection may extend along the aorta, typically causing further pain in the direction of the extension.

Investigations

- **ECG**: principally to exclude MI. May show left ventricular hypertrophy from long-standing hypertension.
- **Chest X-ray**: may show widened mediastinum as a result of haemomediastinum, or a pleural effusion, caused by aortic rupture into the (usually left) pleural space.
- **Computed tomography scan**: in most hospitals this is the imaging technique of choice. Its use should *never* be delayed. Cross-sectional images of the aorta show flap and true and false lumina when contrast is given.
- **Echocardiography** rarely shows the dissection flap, but may show complications such as haemopericardium and aortic regurgitation.

- **Transoesophageal echocardiography** is very sensitive in imaging both the ascending and descending aorta. A specialized echo probe is passed down the oesophagus, and positioned behind the heart, allowing imaging of the great vessels and heart, unimpeded by ribs or lungs. Images of a high quality are obtained. The procedure requires a highly skilled operator and is invasive, and patients require sedation; because it may transiently increase the BP, thus provoking extension of the dissection, *it should only be carried out in cardiothoracic centres with access to immediate surgery*.

Management

Aortic dissection is a medical emergency and should be treated with the very highest priority. In both type A and B, the immediate concern is to lower the BP to less than 100 mmHg systolic to prevent further dissection or rupture, using opiate analgesia and intravenous β-blockers. Those with hypotension due to bleeding should be resuscitated to maintain a modest BP only. Specific treatment depends on the site of origination of the flap:

- **Type A dissection**: the risk of catastrophic complications, particularly rupture into the pericardium, is extremely high, with an *hourly* mortality rate of about 2%. Patients should be transferred by blue light/air ambulance to a cardiothoracic centre immediately, whatever the time of day, for immediate surgery to replace the aortic root, with or without a concomitant aortic valve procedure.
- **Type B**: surgery is high risk and therefore not indicated as first-line treatment. Aggressive BP control is indicated, aiming for a systolic BP of <100 mmHg. Surgery is reserved for life-threatening complications, such as threatened rupture. A false lumen may clot and stabilize.

Prognosis

Type A dissection has a very high immediate mortality, but if the patient does not have life-threatening complications (e.g. stroke, paraplegia) the outlook after successful surgery is good. The immediate outlook for type B dissection is better, although there are late complications, including aneurysm formation and rupture.

87 Heart failure

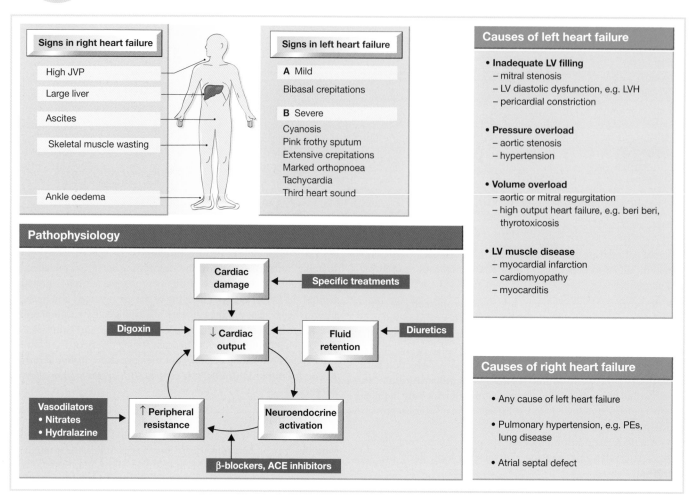

Signs in right heart failure
- High JVP
- Large liver
- Ascites
- Skeletal muscle wasting
- Ankle oedema

Signs in left heart failure

A Mild
Bibasal crepitations

B Severe
Cyanosis
Pink frothy sputum
Extensive crepitations
Marked orthopnoea
Tachycardia
Third heart sound

Causes of left heart failure
- **Inadequate LV filling**
  - mitral stenosis
  - LV diastolic dysfunction, e.g. LVH
  - pericardial constriction
- **Pressure overload**
  - aortic stenosis
  - hypertension
- **Volume overload**
  - aortic or mitral regurgitation
  - high output heart failure, e.g. beri beri, thyrotoxicosis
- **LV muscle disease**
  - myocardial infarction
  - cardiomyopathy
  - myocarditis

Pathophysiology

Cardiac damage ← Specific treatments

Digoxin → ↓ Cardiac output ← Fluid retention ← Diuretics

Vasodilators
- Nitrates
- Hydralazine
→ ↑ Peripheral resistance

Neuroendocrine activation

β-blockers, ACE inhibitors

Causes of right heart failure
- Any cause of left heart failure
- Pulmonary hypertension, e.g. PEs, lung disease
- Atrial septal defect

Cardiac failure is the clinical syndrome resulting from an inability to maintain an adequate cardiac output; it has characteristic clinical and pathophysiological consequences. It affects 1–2% of those aged ≥65 years and 10% of those aged ≥75 years. The prognosis is poor; in severe heart failure ≥50% die within 3 years. Sudden death is a common mode of death in heart failure.

Pathophysiology

Heart failure is a **syndrome** because, despite many different causes, once present the symptoms, signs and pathophysiology are similar. An inadequate cardiac output stimulates compensatory mechanisms resembling the response to hypovolaemia. Initially beneficial, these in turn become maladaptive:

- **Neurohormonal activation** occurs with increases in vasoconstrictors (renin, angiotensin II and catecholamines amongst others, and there are many others) provoking salt and water retention and increasing cardiac afterload. These decrease left ventricular (LV) emptying and depress cardiac output further, producing greater neuroendocrine activation, so increasing afterload, etc., resulting in a vicious downward spiral. Some neurohormones are used to help diagnose the syndrome of heart failure, particularly brain natriuretic peptide. A normal level excludes most heart failure; a very raised level is strongly associated with

heart failure; a mildly or moderately raised level could indicate heart failure, but equally is associated with many other disease processes.

- **Cytokine activation** is increasingly understood as being a hallmark of advanced heart failure, in a manner analogous to cytokine activation occurring in advanced cancer. Cytokines that are rasied include interleukin-6 and tumour necrosis factor α (TNF-α). Such cytokine activation underlies the anaemia of chronic heart failure and the progressive cachexia that is such a distressing feature of advanced heart failure; thus they have important roles in the pathophysiology. They are a target for a number of as yet experimental therapies.

- **Ventricular dilatation**: impaired systolic function (reduced ejection fraction) and fluid retention increase ventricular volume (dilatation). A dilated heart is mechanically inefficient ('law of Laplace'). If energy supply is limited (e.g. coronary disease) this may lead to further contractile failure and neuroendocrine activation.

Classification

The classification of various heart failure syndromes groups together common features dominating the clinical syndrome. This may be useful in diagnosis.

Medicine at a Glance, Fourth Edition. Edited by Patrick Davey. © 2014 John Wiley & Sons, Ltd. Published 2014 by John Wiley & Sons, Ltd. Companion website: www.ataglanceseries.com/medicine

- **Acute heart failure** is largely synonymous with left heart failure and results from a sudden failure to maintain cardiac output. There is insufficient time for compensatory mechanisms to develop and the clinical picture is dominated by acute pulmonary oedema. Such patients are usually quite unwell and require immediate hospital admission.
- **Chronic heart failure** (CHF) is largely synonymous with **right heart failure**. Cardiac output declines gradually, symptoms and signs are less florid, and features relating to compensatory mechanisms dominate. Patients, while unwell, can often be managed on an outpatient basis.

Confusingly both left and right heart failure commonly coexist, usually because chronic left heart failure results in secondary pulmonary hypertension and right heart failure. Chronic biventricular failure is termed 'congestive cardiac failure'. There are other classifications based on the aetiology, or the main problem with the heart, and these include:

- **Systolic heart failure** where the main problem is a failure of the heart to squeeze – this form of heart failure is fairly easy to understand: the heart does not expel enough blood resulting in a reduced ejection fraction and increasingly large intracardiac dimensions. It is relatively easy to diagnose as there are numerous abormalities on standard cardiac investigations.
- **Diastolic heart failure** where the main problem is impaired relaxation of the left ventricle. This form of heart failure is much more difficult to understand, but perhaps the best way to understand it is to imagine that LV relaxation, which is an active energy-requiring process, is impaired, and not enough blood can be sucked into the left ventricle. What gets there can usually be pumped out well (systolic function is good), but not enough blood gets into the left ventricle. This is a common form of heart failure, especially in the elderly, and in those with hypertension and high body mass index. It can be very difficult to diagnose, partly because the symptoms that heart failure presents with (breathlessness and lethargy) are common in the elderly and the overweight, where they have a large differential diagnosis, but also because standard investigations, particularly cardiac ultrasound, can be reported as being normal. Perhaps the best way to diagnose diastolic heart failure is to be certain in your own mind as to whether your patient has heart failure syndrome from the clinical features, perhaps supported by evidence of neuroendocrine activation, before you order the cardiac ultrasound – you can then interpret the ultrasound in the light of your clinical diagnosis, rather than relying on this to make your clinical diagnosis.

Symptoms and signs

- **Left heart failure**: breathlessness, which is worse when lying down (orthopnoea), especially in the middle of the night (paroxysmal nocturnal dyspnoea, PND). Classically when PND occurs patients feel the need to get up and fling open the window to get air. Typically symptoms improve within 15–30 minutes of getting up. Signs comprise tachypnoea, tachycardia, third heart sound ('gallop rhythm') and bibasilar inspiratory pulmonary crepitations. Elevation of the jugular venous pressure (JVP) and peripheral oedema may *not* occur.
- **Right heart failure**: fluid retention in the legs, in severe cases ascites. Signs comprise raised JVP and peripheral oedema. If ascites is more prominent than leg oedema *and the venous pressure is up* (indicating a high probability of a cardiac problem) then consider the very rare diagnosis of pericardial constriction.
- **Chronic heart failure**: in long-standing CHF the heart enlarges (cardiomegaly) and secondary mitral/tricuspid

Table 87.1 New York Heart Association (NYHA) classification.

NYHA class	Breathlessness	Estimated annual mortality
I	None	<5%
II	On strenuous exercise	5–10%
III	On moderate effort	10–15%
IV	At rest	30–40%

Source: www.eperc.mcw.edu/EPERC/FastFactsIndex/ff_143.htm (last accessed September 2013).

Box 87.1 General predictors of worse prognosis.

The following indicators have been independently associated with a limited prognosis in heart failure.

- Recent cardiac hospitalization (triples 1-year mortality)
- Elevated blood urea nitrogen (defined by upper limit of normal) and/or creatinine ≥1.4 mg/dL (120 μmol/L)
- Systolic blood pressure <100 mmHg and/or pulse >100 bpm (each doubles 1-year mortality)
- Decreased left ventricular ejection fraction (linearly correlated with survival at LVEF ≤45%).
- Ventricular dysrhythmias, treatment resistant
- Anaemia (each 1 g/dL reduction in haemoglobin is associated with a 16% increase in mortality)
- Hyponatremia (serum sodium ≤135 mEq/L)
- Cachexia
- Reduced functional capacity
- Co-morbidities: diabetes, depression, chronic obstructive pulmonary disease, cirrhosis, cerebrovascular disease, cancer and HIV-associated cardiomyopathy

regurgitation occurs. Skeletal muscle loss ('cardiac cachexia') may be substantial and responsible for fatigue, tiredness and weakness. The New York Heart Association classification grades severity (see Table 87.1). Prognosis relates to many factors, but symptom severity is an important predictor (see Table 87.1 and Box 87.1).

Aetiology

Any disease that damages or overloads the pumping ability of the heart can result in cardiac failure (see Figure 87.1). Common diseases include coronary disease, hypertension, age, obesity and alcohol-related disease. Valvar heart disease can be either age related (aortic stenosis) or rheumatic. HIV is common worldwide as a cause of cardiac failure, and in some countries other infections are relevant (e.g. South American trypanosomiasis in Brazil).

Provoking/exacerbating factors

It is vital to consider whether there are contributory factors in any patient presenting with new-onset or decompensated heart failure:

- **Arrhythmias** (e.g. atrial fibrillation (AF)), which can often provoke symptoms of heart failure in someone with a previously asymptomatic damaged heart – for example, patients with hypertensive heart disease not infrequently present out of the blue with heart failure provoked by new-onset AF.
- **Drug issues** (non-compliance, fluid-retaining drugs, e.g. nonsteroidal anti-inflammatory drugs): these are all very common.

- **Anaemia**: mild anaemia is common in severe heart failure, but more profound anaemia can provoke symptoms in heart failure.
- **Infection**, e.g. pneumonia, urinary tract infection.
- **Thyroid disease**.

Investigations

The aims of investigations are to confirm the diagnosis of the heart failure syndrome, to ascertain the underlying cause, to assess severity and guide and monitor treatment:

- **Echocardiography**: essential, simple, non-invasive tool in diagnosing aetiology and severity and in ruling out important valvar heart disease. However, you should be aware that there are limitations to the technique:
    - In obese subjects, and in some other patients, it may not be possible to obtain good views of the heart and the study therefore may not be of diagnostic quality (after checking the name of the patient, the next most important aspect to check is the echocardiographers assessment of the adaquacy of the views, and you will find this information on the echo report).
    - An apparently normal echo does not rule out heart failure – the standard study may miss pericardial constriction (a rare but important cause of heart failure) and, much more importantly, diastolic heart failure. Many patients with diastolic heart failure have one or more of the following three important clues: they are elderly, have hypertension and/or have left ventricular hypertrophy (LVH) echocardiographically – there are, however. many exceptions to this.
    - An abnormal cardiac ultrasound does not mean that a patient inevitably has heart failure! Heart failure is the syndrome that results from a cardiac abnormality – just having a cardiac abnormality does not neccesarily mean that symptoms inevitably have accrued from this. Put another way, always be clear in your own mind as to whether the symptoms you are exploring are heart failure, and use the test to evaluate causation, rather than use the test to explore directly whether symptoms are heart related. If you don't follow this rule, you will find a heart abnormality, label this as the cause of the patient's symptoms and so miss the serious pathology that is causing the symptoms, such as severe chronic obstructive pulmonary disease (COPD), pulmonary emboli, interstitial lung disease, anaemia, etc.
- **Electrocardiogram (ECG)**: look for old myocardial infarction, LVH (e.g. hypertension, aortic stenosis), T-wave changes that are associated with critical coronary disease (e.g. symmetrical pan–anterior T-wave inversion) or cardiomyopathy (asymmetrical widespread T-wave inversion). A normal ECG makes CHF unlikely. Look for arrhythmias (e.g. AF).
- **Chest X-ray**: large heart, pulmonary congestion (Kerley B lines) or pulmonary oedema. Be aware that most reports labelling obese patients as having cardiomegaly are wrong – the cardiac silhoutte is increased by pericardial fat, rather than by the heart genuinely being enlarged. The cause of most breathlessness in obese patients is physical deconditioning compounded by a restrictive lung defect rather than cardiac illness.
- **Biochemistry**: electrolytes must be measured as a common mode of death in heart failure is sudden cardiac death due to ventricular fibrillation, the probability of which is greatly increased by hypokalaemia, which itself occurs readily with diuretic therapy. Potassium-sparing diuretics lessen mortality in heart failure. Monitor renal function and haematology (anaemia). Check thyroid function.
- **Nuclear isotope scanning**: useful for accurate measurement of the ejection fraction (isotope ventriculography or multiple-gated acquisition scans) or the presence of hibernating myocardium – living heart muscle, currently not contracting as a result of a tight coronary stenosis in the nutrient artery, which will contract if the blood flow is improved by percutaneous coronary intervention or coronary artery bypass graft.
- **Cardiac catheterization**: in all unexplained heart failure to exclude critical coronary artery disease (CAD), or to assess CAD severity and treatment options in those with known ischaemic heart disease.
- **24-hour ECG** recording to investigate arrhythmias.

Treatment

- **General measures**: treat the underlying cause and any arrhythmias. Reduce salt and water intake, and monitor treatment by daily weights. Treat hypertension and CAD risk factors vigorously – aim for a blood pressure (BP) not above 130/80.
- **Specific measures**: if possible, treat the cause – valve surgery for valve disease, meticulous heart rate control for any rate-related cardiomyopathies (this is where heart failure has resulted from an uncontrolled arrhythmia driving the heart too fast for too long, e.g. an atrial tachycardia for 2–3 months with a heart rate of >140 bpm), teetotal status in those with alcohol-related heart disease, HIV therapy in HIV cardiomyopathy, etc. Revascularization is a complex issue in CHF due to coronary disease, but if large areas of the heart either with reversible ischaemia or hibernation are found, revascularization may be appropriate and may improve LV function and outlook.
- **Diuretics** are the mainstay of symptomatic treatment. The dose should be sufficient large to remove pulmonary and/or peripheral oedema. The principal side effect is hypokalaemia (give potassium supplements or sparing diuretic, e.g. amiloride). **Spironolactone**, a potassium-sparing diuretic (aldosterone antagonism), improves prognosis in severe CHF.
- **Angiotensin-converting enzyme (ACE) inhibitors** block conversion of angiotensin I to II, interrupting the maladaptive neuroendocrine response, vasodilating and lowering BP. Several large, randomized, controlled trials show they improve symptoms, quality of life and prognosis in overt heart failure or impaired LV function. They may provoke renal failure in bilateral renal artery stenosis (check urea and electrolytes). The most common other side effect is a persistent dry cough in 5%.
- **Angiotensin II receptor antagonists** (e.g. losartan) block angiotensin II by direct antagonism of its receptor. They have similar effects and benefits to ACE inhibitors.
- **β-Blockers** (e.g. bisoprolol, metoprolol, carvedilol) were previously felt to be contraindicated in heart failure. However, high circulating catecholamines and downregulation of adrenergic receptors are detrimental in heart failure. β-Blockers (started *only in stable patients*, at very low doses, and increased slowly) reverse these abnormalities and improve functional status and prognosis. They reduce both pump failure and arrhythmic sudden deaths.
- **Digoxin** has a positive inotropic effect in sinus rhythm and results in symptomatic improvement and a reduction in hospital admissions, although it has no mortality benefit.
- **Multisite ventricular pacing**: in advanced heart failure, not infrequently, 'dyscoordinate' ventricular contraction occurs. This means that, instead of the physiological situation, where the conducting tissue ensures that all parts of the ventricle contract fairly simultaneously, different parts of the ventricle contract at different times. This leads to a loss of cardiac output, as blood can move around the ventricle, as one segment contracts against a segment yet to contract, rather than contributing to cardiac output. This condition is suspected by finding a broad QRS complex on the

standard ECG, and confirmed by measuring the difference between the onset of the QRS complex to pulmonary and aortic blood ejection (easily done from the cardiac ultrasound). Patients with dyscoordinate contraction benefit from complex pacemakers; in addition to the standard atrial lead, leads are place in the apex of the right ventricle and the lateral wall of the left ventricle (via the coronary sinus). Thses two ventricular leads allow simultaneous activation of two widely separated parts of the ventricle, so minimizing dyscoordinate contraction and maximizing cardiac output. Cardiac resynchronization therapy improves symptoms and lowers mortality. It can be combined with implantable cardiovertor defibrillator (ICD) therapy.

Complications

- **Thromboembolism**: the risk of venous clot (deep venous thrombosis and pulmonary embolism (PE)) and of systemic emboli is high, especially in severe CHF. It may be reduced by warfarin, which is mandatory in anyone with heart failure and AF, and is sometimes used in advanced heart failure and sinus rhythm. Part of the differential diagnosis in any patient with known heart failure developing sudden worsening of breathlessness is PE.
- **Atrial fibrillation** commonly complicates CHF, when it can provoke a dramatic deterioration. Rate control (digoxin/β-blocker) and warfarin are indicated.
- **Progressive pump failure** may respond to increasing doses of diuretics. Heart transplantation is an option in selected patients.
- **Ventricular arrhythmias** are common, and may cause syncope or **sudden cardiac death** (25–50% of deaths in CHF). In those successfully resuscitated, amiodarone, β-blockers and ICDs have a role. ICDs also have a prophylactic role in those with severe systolic dysfunction.

88 Aortic valve disease

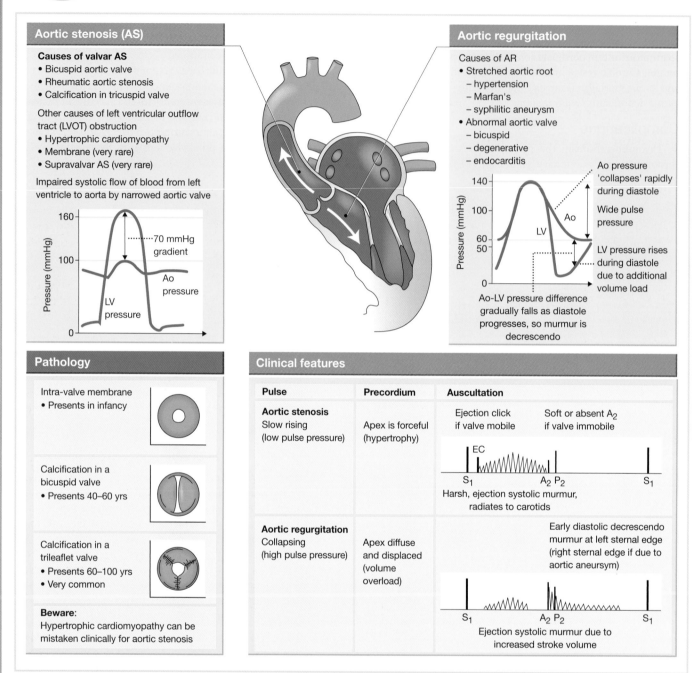

Aortic stenosis (AS)

Causes of valvar AS
- Bicuspid aortic valve
- Rheumatic aortic stenosis
- Calcification in tricuspid valve

Other causes of left ventricular outflow tract (LVOT) obstruction
- Hypertrophic cardiomyopathy
- Membrane (very rare)
- Supravalvar AS (very rare)

Impaired systolic flow of blood from left ventricle to aorta by narrowed aortic valve

70 mmHg gradient

LV pressure

Ao pressure

Aortic regurgitation

Causes of AR
- Stretched aortic root
  - hypertension
  - Marfan's
  - syphilitic aneurysm
- Abnormal aortic valve
  - bicuspid
  - degenerative
  - endocarditis

Ao pressure 'collapses' rapidly during diastole

Wide pulse pressure

LV pressure rises during diastole due to additional volume load

Ao-LV pressure difference gradually falls as diastole progresses, so murmur is decrescendo

Pathology

Intra-valve membrane
- Presents in infancy

Calcification in a bicuspid valve
- Presents 40–60 yrs

Calcification in a trileaflet valve
- Presents 60–100 yrs
- Very common

Beware:
Hypertrophic cardiomyopathy can be mistaken clinically for aortic stenosis

Clinical features

Pulse	Precordium	Auscultation	
Aortic stenosis Slow rising (low pulse pressure)	Apex is forceful (hypertrophy)	Ejection click if valve mobile	Soft or absent A₂ if valve immobile
		EC S₁ ... A₂ P₂ S₁ Harsh, ejection systolic murmur, radiates to carotids	
Aortic regurgitation Collapsing (high pulse pressure)	Apex diffuse and displaced (volume overload)	Early diastolic decrescendo murmur at left sternal edge (right sternal edge if due to aortic aneursym)	
		S₁ ... A₂ P₂ ... S₁ Ejection systolic murmur due to increased stroke volume	

Aortic stenosis

There are three causes of aortic stenosis:

1 **Congenital aortic stenosis**: this is very rare, and may be the result of a bicuspid valve, or a subaortic membrane, constricting the left ventricular (LV) outflow tract.

2 Premature calcification of a congenitally **bicuspid aortic valve**: patients typically develop symptoms from age 40 years onwards.

3 **Calcific aortic stenosis** of a normal valve: this is an exceptionally common valve lesion, occurring from age 65 years onwards. At aged 80 years, about 10% of the population have aortic stenosis. Calcification occurs earlier in those with renal failure or hypercholesterolaemia, where it can be found in those aged 20 years.

Symptoms

There is a classic triad of symptoms associated with aortic stenosis. All are exertional and progressive:
- **Effort dyspnoea**.
- **Effort angina**.
- **Effort dizziness or syncope**.

Medicine at a Glance, Fourth Edition. Edited by Patrick Davey. © 2014 John Wiley & Sons, Ltd. Published 2014 by John Wiley & Sons, Ltd. Companion website: www.ataglanceseries.com/medicine

- **Sudden cardiac death**: this is very rare in those without any of the above symptoms, but becomes increasingly likely as other symptoms develop. It is for this reason that asymptomatic patients are followed up, whereas symptomatic patients undergo valve replacement surgery.

Angina at rest is caused by concomitant coronary disease, not aortic stenosis. Syncope at rest is usually the result of atrioventricular (AV) block (e.g. complete heart block) because concomitant conducting tissue disease is very common.

Signs

Ejection systolic murmur is often harsh and loud. The area where the murmur is heard loudest varies – usually it is the middle of the left sternal edge, sometimes in the 'aortic' area (second right intercostal space) and occasionally in the 'mitral' area, i.e. at the apex (fifth intercostal space, midclavicular line). The murmur often radiates into the carotids. A slow rising pulse, absent second heart sound and signs of LV hypertrophy (LVH) indicate severity. Signs of complicating heart failure may also be present.

Investigations

Echocardiography allows assessment of LV function and valve structure (e.g. bicuspid or tricuspid, calcified or not) and severity of stenosis. Stenosis severity is usually quoted as the peak velocity of blood (determined from the Doppler ultrasonic probe) through the valve (a value of 3.5 m/s indicates that the aortic stenosis may be sufficiently severe to cause symptoms). This peak velocity is used to estimate the (instantaneous) pressure drop over the valve, using the formula:

$$\text{Pressure drop (mmHg)} = 4 \times (\text{Peak velocity})^2$$

Occasionally, the valve area is estimated, especially if LV function is poor. Cardiac catheterization is rarely used to measure valve function, but is used before surgery to determine whether there is coronary disease that may need bypass grafting at the same time. A chest X-ray is not useful in making the diagnosis, although it is if complicating heart failure is suspected. An electrocardiogram (ECG) may show LVH, and occasionally conducting tissue disease (calcium from the valve 'burrows' down into the interventricular septum, interfering with electrical impulse propagation).

- **Creatinine**: impaired renal function is an important predictor of increased surgical risk.
- **Cholesterol and glucose**: aortic valve disease may be a marker for other atherosclerotic vascular disease.
- **Full blood count**: there is an association between angiodysplasia and aortic stenosis. As aortic stenosis can induce functional von Willebrand's disease, iron deficiency may complicate the natural history of this valve lesion.

Treatment

In the absence of symptoms, medical therapy monitors LV function and the severity of the stenosis. When symptoms occur or the left ventricle deteriorates, there is a high risk of deterioration due to heart failure or sudden death, and early valve replacement is indicated.

Aortic regurgitation

There are two pathologies that give rise to aortic regurgitation (AR). They can usually be distinguished echocardiographically:

- **Disease processes affecting the aortic valve** (including rheumatic heart disease, endocarditis, systemic lupus erythematosus). Calcific aortic stenosis is often associated with significant AR.
- **Diseases resulting in dilatation of the aortic root** and thus the aortic valve ring (including aortic aneurysm caused by hypertension, Marfan's syndrome, ankylosing spondylitis or syphilis, or the rarer annulo-ectasia, which is idiopathic dilatation of the aortic root). Aortic dissection disrupts the aortic root, causing acute AR.

Symptoms

With gradual-onset AR, even if the leak is severe, symptoms are often mild or absent. If the leak worsens, or if LV decompensation occurs, exertional dyspnoea can develop, which when severe may happen at rest.

Signs

Collapsing pulse with a volume-overloaded left ventricle (hyperdynamic apex beat). The diastolic blood pressure (BP), which relates directly to how much blood has leaked back from the aorta into the left ventricle, is a good guide to the severity of chronic AR (low diastolic BP = severe AR). Wide pulse pressure may cause:
- Corrigan's sign (visible carotid pulsations).
- De Musset's sign (head bobbing).
- Quinke's sign (nail-bed pulsations).
- Pistol shot femorals (also known as Traube's phenomenon): auscultation over the femoral arteries reveals a loud sound during systole, likened to a pistol shot, due to the large forward stroke volume.
- Duroziez's murmur, a to-and-fro murmur heard when the femoral artery is auscultated, and slight pressure is placed on the stethoscope, relates to the large forward and backward flow in the aorta from the AR.

An early diastolic murmur is heard along the left sternal edge (with the patient leaning forward in end-expiration), unless the AR is caused by an aortic root aneurysm, when the murmur is loudest along the right sternal edge. The murmur may be surprisingly loud in mild AR, and is often quiet in very severe AR, or if the lesion is acute, e.g. endocarditis.

Investigations

Echocardiography is useful for monitoring LV function, determining whether the regurgitation is the result of a valve or aortic root problem, and determining its severity. Although the aortic root diameter can be measured, if there is substantial enlargement computed tomography or magnetic resonance imaging of the thoracic aorta is needed to determine how much of the aortic arch (and descending aorta) is enlarged. A chest X-ray may show an enlarged heart, or aortic aneurysm; an ECG usually shows LVH. Coronary angiography is useful to assess for concomitant coronary disease once surgery has been decided on.

Treatment

Angiotensin-converting enzyme (ACE) inhibitors (and possibly other vasodilators such as calcium channel blockers) and diuretics may maintain LV function for many years in the face of significant AR. Increasing LV dimensions and symptoms are indications for AV replacement. If AR is the result of dilatation of the aortic root, valve and root replacements are necessary.

Aortic valve replacement

- **Conventional surgery**: used for low-/medium-risk patients. Under general anaesthesia, via a midline sternotomy, the heart–lung machine is connected, the aorta clamped, cut open, and under direct vision the old damaged aortic valve is cut out, and a artificial one sewn in. Operative mortality is 2–5%.
- **Percutaneous valve replacement**: this is an emerging and promising technology, whereby a new aortic valve is placed over the old one, either via the femoral artery or the apex of the left ventricle. Its use is currently restricted to high-risk patients only.

89 Mitral valve disease

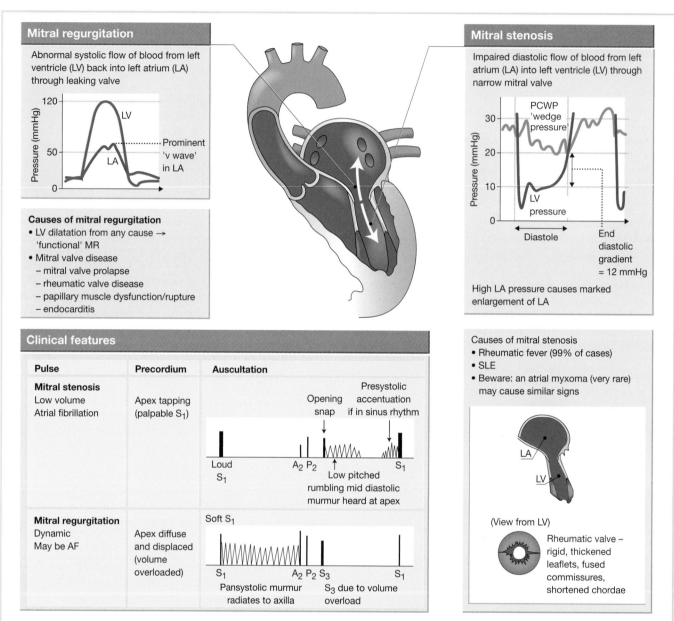

Mitral regurgitation

Abnormal systolic flow of blood from left ventricle (LV) back into left atrium (LA) through leaking valve

Causes of mitral regurgitation
- LV dilatation from any cause → 'functional' MR
- Mitral valve disease
  - mitral valve prolapse
  - rheumatic valve disease
  - papillary muscle dysfunction/rupture
  - endocarditis

Mitral stenosis

Impaired diastolic flow of blood from left atrium (LA) into ventricle (LV) through narrow mitral valve

High LA pressure causes marked enlargement of LA

Causes of mitral stenosis
- Rheumatic fever (99% of cases)
- SLE
- Beware: an atrial myxoma (very rare) may cause similar signs

(View from LV)

Rheumatic valve – rigid, thickened leaflets, fused commissures, shortened chordae

Clinical features

Pulse	Precordium	Auscultation
Mitral stenosis Low volume Atrial fibrillation	Apex tapping (palpable S_1)	Low pitched rumbling mid diastolic murmur heard at apex
Mitral regurgitation Dynamic May be AF	Apex diffuse and displaced (volume overloaded)	Pansystolic murmur radiates to axilla. S_3 due to volume overload

Mitral stenosis

Although on a worldwide basis mitral stenosis is still very common, this is now a rare lesion in the developed world, because of the decline in the incidence of rheumatic valve disease. In practice, all mitral stenosis relates to previous rheumatic fever.

Symptoms

Half of those diagnosed have documented/remembered childhood rheumatic fever. Symptomatic mitral stenosis develops within a few years in deprived communities, but may take decades in the West. Typically there is the gradual onset of progressive exertional dyspnoea, as a result of chronic heart failure, in those aged 40–50 years. Sudden and severe symptoms occur with the onset of atrial fibrillation (AF). Mitral stenosis with AF is a very potent substrate for systemic thromboemboli (e.g. a stroke) that are sometimes the first manifestation of the lesion.

Signs

- Female > male.
- Mitral facies (malar flush).
- May be signs of chronic heart failure: elevated jugular venous pressure, oedema.
- Usually AF.
- Right ventricular 'heave' if there is secondary pulmonary hypertension.

Medicine at a Glance, Fourth Edition. Edited by Patrick Davey. © 2014 John Wiley & Sons, Ltd. Published 2014 by John Wiley & Sons, Ltd. Companion website: www.ataglanceseries.com/medicine

- 'Tapping' apex beat (palpable S_1), which is undisplaced in the absence of significant mitral regurgitation.
- Low-pitched, rumbling, mid-diastolic murmur, best heard with the bell in a left lateral position.
- Opening snap (rigid valve opening) precedes murmur.

Investigations

Echocardiography confirms the diagnosis and follows disease progression. The valve may be 'rheumatic' (thickened and distorted). The velocity of the blood flow during diastole through the mitral valve can be measured using the Doppler probe. In normal individuals this starts high, and then declines rapidly as diastole proceeds. A much slower velocity decline is found in mitral stenosis, and the severity can be deduced from the rate of velocity decline ('pressure half-time'). Pulmonary hypertension can also often be diagnosed from Doppler measurements of regurgitant blood through the tricuspid valve. Concomitant mitral regurgitation (MR) and aortic valve disease likewise can be diagnosed and followed up. An electrocardiogram (ECG) may show left atrial enlargement (when in sinus rhythm) or AF. In pulmonary hypertension, a dominant R wave may appear in chest lead V_1. A chest X-ray may show left atrial enlargement (cardiomegaly, 'splayed' tracheal bifurcation).

Treatment

- **Medical therapy** (with diuretics, digoxin and warfarin) maintains good functional status for decades. The only indication for surgery is when symptoms are not controlled by drugs.
- **Surgical treatment**: there are two approaches:
  - **Mitral valvotomy**: this can be carried out percutaneously in some, using a balloon, or at thoracotomy (often made over the left lung, so as to gain easy access to the valve through the left atrium).
  - **Mitral valve replacement**: this is a common operation. Usually a mechanical valve (rather than a biological one) is used because warfarin is already indicated on account of the AF.

Differential diagnosis

Very rarely, similar symptoms and signs are caused by an atrial myxoma, a benign tumour, usually found in the left atrium attached to the interatrial septum, which grows sufficiently to impede mitral diastolic blood flow. It causes episodic or progressive breathlessness, and occasionally fever and weight loss with an elevated erythrocyte sedimentation rate. Cardiac ultrasonography is diagnostic. Immediate surgery is usually curative.

Mitral prolapse

In mitral valve prolapse (MVP) (Barlow's syndrome), the mitral valve is larger than usual and/or the chordae attached to the mitral valve are too long. As a consequence of this, a component of the mitral valve 'prolapses' back into the left atrium during ventricular systole. There may or may not be MR (see next section). In MVP without MR, the usual signs are of a 'click', heard in early mid-systole. The 'click' of MVP can be a rather intermittent phenomenon. There is some controversy about whether MVP without MR causes symptoms; most cardiologists feel that it probably does not. MVP with MR predisposes to bacterial endocarditis (see Chapter 93).

Mitral regurgitation

Mitral regurgitation is an extremely common valve lesion. Like aortic regurgitation, there are two underlying pathologies:

- Those caused by **intrinsic valve disease** (e.g. myxomatous degeneration, rheumatic heart disease, infective endocarditis) or disease of the valve-related apparatus (e.g. chordal rupture, as in some cases of floppy mitral valve) or of the papillary muscles (e.g. dysfunction/rupture resulting from ischaemia/infarction, usually of the circumflex artery).
- **Secondary** (also termed 'functional') caused by stretching of the valve ring when the left ventricle is dilated, as in many cases of left heart failure. The MR murmur may become dramatically quieter as the heart failure responds to treatment.

Symptoms

Patients are often asymptomatic for many years, unless the lesion has occurred/progressed over a very short time span. Unfortunately, during this asymptomatic period left ventricular (LV) function may be permanently damaged. Symptoms when they occur are those of heart failure, such as breathlessness, effort intolerance and fatigue.

Signs

- Displaced, diffuse apex resulting from volume overload.
- Loud pansystolic murmur at apex.
- Functional MR may not be pansystolic.
- The murmur radiates up the LV outflow tract (i.e. is heard along the left sternal edge/aortic area) in posterior leaflet mitral valve prolapse, and is heard in the back in anterior mitral valve leaflet prolapse.

Investigations

Echocardiography can be helpful in establishing both the presence of MR and its mechanism. Often, transthoracic echocardiography provides a good estimate of the severity of the MR, but this is not always true, and sometimes transoesophageal echocardiography is needed to determine severity more accurately. This is particularly true if an artificial mitral valve is present (i.e. previous mitral valve replacement). Cardiac ultrasonography is also useful in monitoring LV function, although this can easily be overestimated. Chest X-ray is useful for diagnosing heart failure. An ECG often shows LV hypertrophy, and may show AF.

Treatment

Initially medical therapy with diuretics and angiotensin-converting enzyme inhibitors are used; they can control symptoms and maintain the systolic function of the left ventricle for years in the face of severe MR. In intrinsic valve disease, when symptoms are intrusive or if the left ventricle enlarges progressively, surgery is indicated. Prognosis after mitral valve repair is better than after mitral valve replacement.

90 Cardiomyopathies

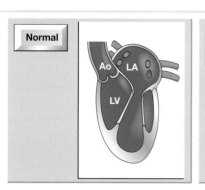

Normal

Ao · LA · LV

Hypertrophic cardiomyopathy

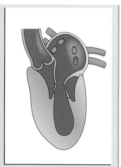

- Thick myocardium (especially septum)
- LV outflow tract obstruction
- Diastolic dysfunction

Restrictive cardiomyopathy

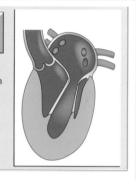

- Rigid myocardium
- Diastolic dysfunction

Dilated cardiomyopathy

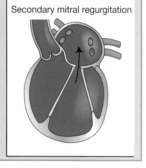

Secondary mitral regurgitation

- Dilatation
- Large volume heart
- Systolic dysfunction

Causes of dilated cardiomyopathy (DCM)

Toxins	Alcohol, drugs (anthracyclines)
Endocrine	Hypothyroidism, thyrotoxicosis, phaeochromocytoma
Infection	Viruses (Coxsackie), Trypanosoma species (Chagas' disease)
Dietary	Beri-beri (thiamine)
Infiltrative	Sarcoid, iron overload (haemochromatosis, excess blood transfusions)
Genetic	Familial DCM, muscle dystrophies (Duchenne, myotonia, mitochondrial)

Cardiomyopathies are **primary heart muscle diseases**. They are uncommon but not rare, e.g. dilated cardiomyopathy (DCM) underlies 5–10% of heart failure. Cardiomyopathies are classified according to the echocardiographic findings.

Dilated cardiomyopathy

DCM causes left ventricular (LV) (and often right ventricular (RV)) enlargement, and often massive and global hypokinesia (rather than regional, which would suggest coronary artery disease). Clinically, LV or congestive cardiac failure occurs, often severe and progressive, with displacement of the apex beat and prominent S_3. Functional mitral regurgitation (MR) and atrial fibrillation are common. There is a high risk of thromboembolism. The chest X-ray shows a large heart. Several illnesses can cause **secondary DCM**, the most common of which is **excess alcohol**. 'Idiopathic' or 'primary' DCM is a diagnosis of exclusion. One-third of cases have a family history, suggesting a significant genetic contribution.

Treatment is standard heart failure therapy. **Cardiac transplantation** is an important option for younger patients with severe refractory heart failure.

Hypertrophic cardiomyopathy

Hypertrophic cardiomyopathy is a genetic disease characterized by asymmetrical hypertrophy of the LV myocardium, especially the septum. The myocardial structure is abnormal (**myocyte disarray** and **interstitial fibrosis**). Gross hypertrophy results in a small LV cavity, diastolic dysfunction and secondary MR. Septal hypertrophy results in dynamic LV outflow tract obstruction. Often asymptomatic, but severe, hypertrophy and outflow tract obstruction may cause exertion breathlessness, chest pain or dizziness. The greatest risk is of collapse or sudden death as a result of ventricular arrhythmias, which may be unheralded and occur in otherwise fit patients. Hypertrophic cardiomyopathy is most commonly caused by mutations in genes encoding a variety of contractile proteins including myosin, actin, troponins and myosin-binding protein C. Different mutations in different genes are associated with variations in the phenotype, including the age of onset, severity of hypertrophy and risk of sudden death from arrhythmias.

Treatment is with:

- **β-Blockers** or **calcium channel antagonists**: these are used to treat exertional symptoms.
- **Amiodarone**: used in those at high risk of ventricular tachycardia. Implantable cardiovertor defibrillators (ICDs) may be justified in patients with high risk and/or a strong family history of sudden death.
- **Genetic counselling** and **screening** of asymptomatic family members by echocardiography are important aspects of management.

Restrictive cardiomyopathy

Restrictive cardiomyopathy results in a rigid, stiff and thickened myocardium, usually as a result of myocardial infiltration by abnormal materials or of fibrosis. It causes congestive cardiac failure resulting from diastolic dysfunction, which is manifest predominantly as RV failure. They are rare. The most common is amyloid (primary amyloid AL type, e.g. multiple myeloma/paraproteinaemia or in secondary amyloid AA type, e.g. chronic inflammatory conditions). Other causes include sarcoid, scleroderma, endomyocardial fibrosis and hypereosinophilic syndromes.

Restrictive cardiomyopathy is usually refractory to treatment. Symptomatic cardiac amyloid has a very poor prognosis. Treatment is usually limited to diuretics to reduce features of right heart failure.

91 Pericardial disease

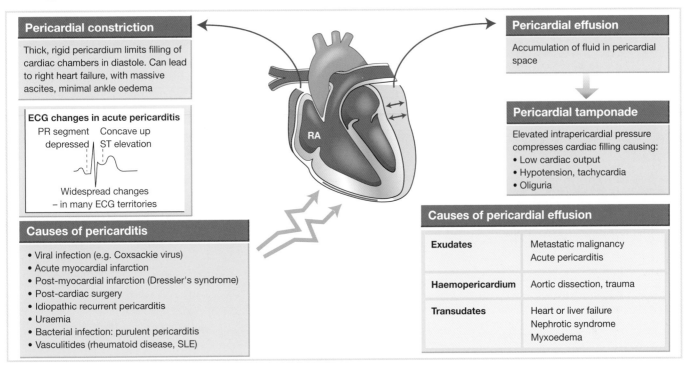

Pericardial constriction

Thick, rigid pericardium limits filling of cardiac chambers in diastole. Can lead to right heart failure, with massive ascites, minimal ankle oedema

ECG changes in acute pericarditis

PR segment depressed   Concave up ST elevation

Widespread changes – in many ECG territories

Causes of pericarditis

- Viral infection (e.g. Coxsackie virus)
- Acute myocardial infarction
- Post-myocardial infarction (Dressler's syndrome)
- Post-cardiac surgery
- Idiopathic recurrent pericarditis
- Uraemia
- Bacterial infection: purulent pericarditis
- Vasculitides (rheumatoid disease, SLE)

Pericardial effusion

Accumulation of fluid in pericardial space

Pericardial tamponade

Elevated intrapericardial pressure compresses cardiac filling causing:
- Low cardiac output
- Hypotension, tachycardia
- Oliguria

Causes of pericardial effusion

Exudates	Metastatic malignancy Acute pericarditis
Haemopericardium	Aortic dissection, trauma
Transudates	Heart or liver failure Nephrotic syndrome Myxoedema

RA

Pericardial disease presents as one of four syndromes. **Pericarditis** describes inflammation of the pericardium, either acute or chronic. The accumulation of fluid within the pericardial space, **pericardial effusion**, can result in **pericardial tamponade**. Chronic or recurrent pericarditis may result in fibrosis of the pericardium, adherence of the visceral and parietal layers and **pericardial constriction**.

Acute pericarditis

Pleuritic chest pain, often positional, is classically relieved by sitting forwards. Many patients experience only a dull central ache without any specific features. A **pericardial rub** may be heard, often only in one position or on inspiration. There may be fever or systemic features. An electrocardiogram (ECG) shows **ST segment elevation** which is concave upwards, typically *affecting leads in multiple territories*, not just one territory as in myocardial infarction. Echocardiography may demonstrate a small pericardial effusion. Specific tests may demonstrate the cause. Non-steroidal anti-inflammatory drugs reduce the pain and inflammation.

Pericardial effusion

Pericardial effusion refers to the accumulation of fluid within the pericardial space. The effusion is categorized according to the protein content of the fluid into **transudates** (high protein), **exudates** (low protein) or bloody (**haemopericardium**). Occasionally the effusion is **purulent** as a result of bacterial infection. **Cardiac tamponade** is caused by the accumulation of a pericardial effusion to the point where elevated intrapericardial pressures compromise cardiac filling. Slowly enlarging pericardial effusions allow the pericardium to stretch to accommodate the fluid; they may be very large (>1 L) before tamponade occurs. Rapidly growing effusions

cause tamponade early on (the pericardium does not comply). A pericardial rub does not exclude tamponade.

Clinical features and treatment of cardiac tamponade

- Low output state (tachycardia, low blood pressure (BP), cold peripheries, oliguria – sometimes the most prominent sign of tamponade is progresive renal failure).
- Greatly elevated jugular venous pressure (JVP) (Kussmaul's sign: JVP increases further rather than falls with inspiration).
- Pulsus paradoxus: BP falls with inspiration. The radial pulse may disappear in severe tamponade. Quiet heart sounds, no gallop.
- Large 'globular' heart on chest X-ray, but no pulmonary congestion. Echocardiography confirms the presence of large pericardial effusions and evidence of tamponade (diastolic collapse of the atrium early on, and of the right ventricle in advanced cases). A simple pericardial effusion without haemodynamic compromise does not need drainage. In contrast, pericardial tamponade is a medical emergency requiring immediate percutaneous or surgical drainage.

Constrictive pericarditis

Acute, chronic or relapsing pericarditis (often caused by tuberculosis or radiotherapy) may cause pericardial fibrosis sufficient to constrict the heart, impede cardiac filling and decrease cardiac output. Progressive **exertional dyspnoea**, peripheral **oedema** and **ascites** occur.

A greatly elevated JVP and pericardial knock (loud diastolic heart sound) are seen. Computed tomography/magnetic resonance imaging suggests, and cardiac catheterization proves, the diagnosis. Diuretics relieve symptoms. Surgery may help.

Medicine at a Glance, Fourth Edition. Edited by Patrick Davey. © 2014 John Wiley & Sons, Ltd. Published 2014 by John Wiley & Sons, Ltd. Companion website: www.ataglanceseries.com/medicine

92 Pulmonary embolism

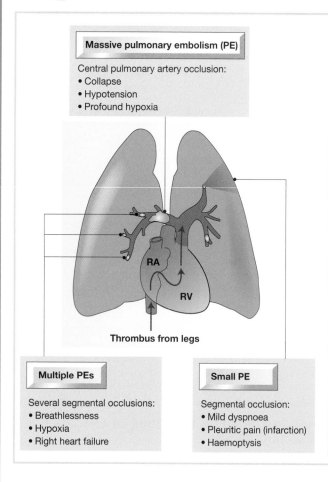

Massive pulmonary embolism (PE)

Central pulmonary artery occlusion:
• Collapse
• Hypotension
• Profound hypoxia

RA

RV

Thrombus from legs

Multiple PEs

Several segmental occlusions:
• Breathlessness
• Hypoxia
• Right heart failure

Small PE

Segmental occlusion:
• Mild dyspnoea
• Pleuritic pain (infarction)
• Haemoptysis

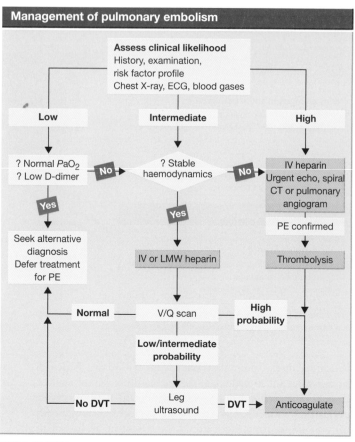

Management of pulmonary embolism

Assess clinical likelihood
History, examination,
risk factor profile
Chest X-ray, ECG, blood gases

| Low | Intermediate | High |

? Normal PaO_2
? Low D-dimer — **No** → ? Stable haemodynamics — **No** → IV heparin
Urgent echo, spiral CT or pulmonary angiogram

Yes ↓ **Yes** ↓ PE confirmed

Seek alternative diagnosis
Defer treatment for PE

IV or LMW heparin

Thrombolysis

Normal V/Q scan **High probability**

Low/intermediate probability

No DVT → Leg ultrasound → **DVT** → Anticoagulate

Definition
Pulmonary embolisms (PEs) result when thrombi (often from the deep veins of the thigh or pelvis) embolize via the right heart into the pulmonary arteries.

Risk factors
Predisposing factors are found in 90% of patients and are an important clue to diagnosis. They comprise:

● Surgery less than 12 weeks ago.
● Immobilization for more than 3 days in the last 4 weeks.
● Previous deep venous thrombosis (DVT)/PE or family history.
● Lower limb fracture.
● Malignancy.
● Postpartum.
● Long distance travel, especially in cramped conditions.

Clinical features
The clinical presentation of PE can be varied, so a high degree of clinical suspicion is required. PEs cause hypoxia from ventilation/perfusion ($\dot{V}/\dot{Q}$) mismatch and interrupt pulmonary blood flow, causing pulmonary infarcts (so inflaming the pleura) and lowering cardiac output. These features are responsible for the three distinct clinical syndromes with which pulmonary thromboembolic disease presents:

1 Pleurisy and/or haemoptysis: small or moderate-sized PEs cause pulmonary infarction. Dyspnoea is absent or minor.
2 Dyspnoea with hypoxia in the absence of other causes: this suggests a moderate or large PE or repeated PEs over a period of time. There may be signs of cardiopulmonary disturbance (tachycardia, tachypnoea, elevated jugular venous pressure (JVP), left parasternal lift from acute right heart strain). Pleurisy/haemoptysis is often absent.
3 Circulatory collapse: large or massive PE. Typically a high-risk patient (e.g. post-surgery) with unheralded collapse or unexplained clinical deterioration, and with hypotension, tachycardia and hypoxia.

Investigations
An assessment of the likelihood of PE, based on clinical, blood gas and chest X-ray (CXR) parameters, remains central to the diagnosis of PE, and directs early therapy. Later therapy is guided by more specific tests, e.g. $\dot{V}/\dot{Q}$ scans, although these often suggest rather than confirm the diagnosis.

● **Chest X-ray**: excludes other conditions, e.g. pneumonia, pneumothorax, pulmonary oedema. In PE, the CXR abnormalities are minimal/minor in relation to the degree of cardiorespiratory compromise.

Medicine at a Glance, Fourth Edition. Edited by Patrick Davey. © 2014 John Wiley & Sons, Ltd. Published 2014 by John Wiley & Sons, Ltd. Companion website: www.ataglanceseries.com/medicine

- **Arterial blood gases**: haemodynamically significant PE causes $\dot{V}/\dot{Q}$ mismatching and hypoxia. Compensatory hyperventilation results in a reduced $PaCO_2$. The alveolar–arterial gradient is increased (see Chapter 100). *In hypoxaemia with a normal/near normal CXR, always consider the diagnosis of PE.*
- **Electrocardiogram (ECG)**: abnormalities are common, but are usually non-specific and not diagnostically useful, e.g. sinus tachycardia, minor ST and T-wave abnormalities (especially in $V_{1–3}$). In large or massive PE, the more classic ECG features of acute right ventricular strain (S_1, Q_3, T_3), right bundle branch block or atrial fibrillation may occur.
- **D-dimers** are cross-linked fibrin degradation products. A normal D-dimer level implies a very low probability of PE. High D-dimers are found in many conditions (e.g. recent surgery, malignancy and inflammatory states) including PE.
- **Echocardiography**: occasionally detects large thrombi in the pulmonary artery, or the right atrium or ventricle. More commonly, echocardiography shows right heart dilatation and strain (i.e. poor systolic contractile function).
- **$\dot{V}/\dot{Q}$ scanning**: isotope $\dot{V}/\dot{Q}$ scanning relies on the fact that a significant PE results in regional hypoperfusion of a segment or lobe of the lung without a corresponding defect in ventilation. To simplify the procedure, a normal CXR is sometimes used as a surrogate to imply normal ventilation. It is widely used, but with significant diagnostic limitations:
  - Strengths: a high probability scan or a normal scan is diagnostically powerful (>95%), especially in the setting of high or low clinical suspicion.
  - Limitations: 75% of scans are in the low or intermediate categories, which are less useful in confirming or excluding the diagnosis. Even a high probability $\dot{V}/\dot{Q}$ scan fails to detect >50% of PEs.
- **Pulmonary angiography**: historically the 'gold standard' investigation for the diagnosis of PE. It is invasive and costly. It is useful when rapid diagnosis critical, e.g. in critical illness.
- **Computed tomography (CT)**: spiral CT ('CT pulmonary angiography') allows imaging of the pulmonary arteries to detect thrombi with high sensitivity and specificity. It is increasingly replacing $\dot{V}/\dot{Q}$ scanning and invasive pulmonary angiography, and is especially useful when the CXR is abnormal, for any reason. Another reason why it is taking over from conventional $\dot{V}/\dot{Q}$ scanning is that it may well allow the cause of symptoms to be diagnosed even if they are not due to pulmonary emboli – for example, interstitial lung disease, heart failure and even coronary disease (whose probability can be partly estimated from the degree of coronary calcification seen).

Treatment (see Table 92.1)

- **Oxygen**: should be given to all patients with suspected PE.
- **Heparin**: should be administered when there is clinical suspicion of PE, while investigations are completed. Intravenous (IV) heparin should be used for large or massive PE, and subcutaneous low-molecular-weight (LMW) heparin in small or moderate PE.
- **Thrombolysis**: streptokinase or tissue plasminogen activator (tPA) dissolves thrombi. It is indicated for confirmed PE with hypotension, severe hypoxia or other evidence of marked haemodynamic compromise.

Table 92.1 Management of pulmonary embolism.

Small PE	Subcutaneous heparin if PE suspected. Warfarin after confirmation of diagnosis with $\dot{V}/\dot{Q}$ scans
Large or massive PE	Immediate high-dose O_2; IV heparin and IV fluids if chest X-ray and ECG exclude myocardial infarction/pulmonary oedema Consider echocardiography, spiral CT or pulmonary angiography if clinical conditions and local availability allow If haemodynamic compromise or deterioration, thrombolysis with tPA, then continued IV heparin For massive PE, surgical embolectomy is an alternative if immediately available
Multiple chronic PE	Warfarin. Refer for cardiological assessment

- **Warfarin**: initial treatment with heparin should be followed by oral anticoagulation with warfarin once the diagnosis of PE is confirmed, aiming for an international normalized ratio (INR) of 2.5–3.0. If there is a remediable underlying cause (e.g. surgery, immobility), anticoagulation for 6 weeks is adequate. If not, the incidence of recurrent PE is high, so anticoagulation should be continued for longer, often indefinitely.

Chronic thromboembolic disease

Although the usual mode of presentation of PE is with an acute illness, occasionally patients present with a more chronic picture. The typical history is of several months' progressive breathlessness, markedly limiting the time of presentation. The physical signs are of cyanosis with marked pulmonary hypertension (left parasternal lift, raised JVP, sometimes peripheral oedema). Investigations show marked hypoxaemia; $\dot{V}/\dot{Q}$ scanning is usually floridly abnormal and CT often shows large thrombi in the central pulmonary arteries. Echocardiography allows determination of the pulmonary artery pressure, often 70–80 mmHg. Treatment is problematic. Much thrombus is endothelialized and only rarely regresses on standard anticoagulant therapy. In a few selected patients, surgical pulmonary thromboembolectomy has a role, although the operative mortality rate of >10% restricts this to highly selected cases.

Thrombophilia

Rare disorders of blood coagulation predispose to thromboembolism, and should be considered in the following:

- Patients aged <40 years with no other risk factors.
- Those with first-degree relative with a history of venous thromboembolism.
- Patients with previous episodes of venous thromboembolism.

Deficiencies of proteins S, protein C or antithrombin III are the most common of these rare disorders (see Chapter 190). Other procoagulant states include lupus anticoagulant (anticardiolipin antibodies) and homocystinuria. More common are genetic polymorphisms in genes encoding clotting proteins – these increase thromboembolic risk, e.g. factor V Leiden.

93 Cardiac infections

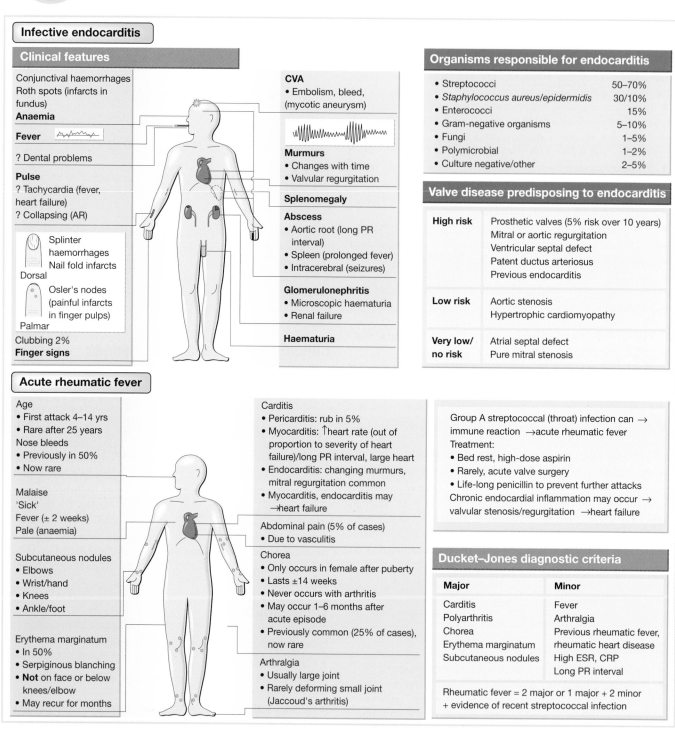

Infective endocarditis

Clinical features

Conjunctival haemorrhages
Roth spots (infarcts in fundus)
Anaemia

Fever

? Dental problems

Pulse
? Tachycardia (fever, heart failure)
? Collapsing (AR)

Splinter haemorrhages
Nail fold infarcts
Dorsal

Osler's nodes (painful infarcts in finger pulps)
Palmar

Clubbing 2%
Finger signs

CVA
• Embolism, bleed, (mycotic aneurysm)

Murmurs
• Changes with time
• Valvular regurgitation

Splenomegaly

Abscess
• Aortic root (long PR interval)
• Spleen (prolonged fever)
• Intracerebral (seizures)

Glomerulonephritis
• Microscopic haematuria
• Renal failure

Haematuria

Organisms responsible for endocarditis

• Streptococci	50–70%
• *Staphylococcus aureus/epidermidis*	30/10%
• Enterococci	15%
• Gram-negative organisms	5–10%
• Fungi	1–5%
• Polymicrobial	1–2%
• Culture negative/other	2–5%

Valve disease predisposing to endocarditis

High risk	Prosthetic valves (5% risk over 10 years) Mitral or aortic regurgitation Ventricular septal defect Patent ductus arteriosus Previous endocarditis
Low risk	Aortic stenosis Hypertrophic cardiomyopathy
Very low/ no risk	Atrial septal defect Pure mitral stenosis

Acute rheumatic fever

Age
• First attack 4–14 yrs
• Rare after 25 years
Nose bleeds
• Previously in 50%
• Now rare

Malaise
'Sick'
Fever (± 2 weeks)
Pale (anaemia)

Subcutaneous nodules
• Elbows
• Wrist/hand
• Knees
• Ankle/foot

Erythema marginatum
• In 50%
• Serpiginous blanching
• **Not** on face or below knees/elbow
• May recur for months

Carditis
• Pericarditis: rub in 5%
• Myocarditis: ↑heart rate (out of proportion to severity of heart failure)/long PR interval, large heart
• Endocarditis: changing murmurs, mitral regurgitation common
• Myocarditis, endocarditis may →heart failure

Abdominal pain (5% of cases)
• Due to vasculitis

Chorea
• Only occurs in female after puberty
• Lasts ±14 weeks
• Never occurs with arthritis
• May occur 1–6 months after acute episode
• Previously common (25% of cases), now rare

Arthralgia
• Usually large joint
• Rarely deforming small joint (Jaccoud's arthritis)

Group A streptococcal (throat) infection can → immune reaction →acute rheumatic fever
Treatment:
• Bed rest, high-dose aspirin
• Rarely, acute valve surgery
• Life-long penicillin to prevent further attacks
Chronic endocardial inflammation may occur → valvular stenosis/regurgitation →heart failure

Ducket–Jones diagnostic criteria

Major	Minor
Carditis	Fever
Polyarthritis	Arthralgia
Chorea	Previous rheumatic fever,
Erythema marginatum	rheumatic heart disease
Subcutaneous nodules	High ESR, CRP
	Long PR interval

Rheumatic fever = 2 major or 1 major + 2 minor + evidence of recent streptococcal infection

Infective endocarditis

This is infection of the lining of the heart, usually the heart valves, which are commonly diseased or prosthetic. There are 3000 cases/year in the UK.

Aetiology and pathogenesis

Blood-borne organisms settle on a heart valve. Fibrin deposits together with microorganisms form **vegetations** on a valve leaflet or cusp. The clinical manifestations are from valve damage (heart failure), embolization of infected material from the heart (abscesses, infarction of vital organs) or the immune response to chronic infection (renal failure). The most common source of infection is the mouth after dental procedures or a tooth abscess. Skin infections (*Staphylococcus aureus*) and the gastrointestinal tract are also common sources. Intravenous drug abusers are at risk of tricuspid valve endocarditis and infection with unusual organisms (coliforms, fungi, etc.). Prosthetic valves are at high risk of infection <3 months after surgery from skin-related organisms (e.g. *S. epidermidis*, *S. aureus*), and later from the same organisms as native valves.

Clinical features

Presentation is typically non-specific, so a high clinical suspicion is required. The duration of symptoms before diagnosis is often weeks or months.

- **Systemic features**: these are common, especially with low virulence organisms, e.g. *Streptococcus viridans*. There is fatigue, fever, anaemia or weight loss. A common and surprising symptom is back pain of obscure origin.
- **Valve destruction** by infection causes valvular regurgitation, not stenosis, leading to heart failure, and new or changing heart murmurs; 99% of endocarditis patients have a murmur.
- **Systemic complications** result from 'seeding' of infection caused by bacteraemia or embolism of infected vegetation fragments, leading to new infection or abscess formation at distant sites, and/or manifestations of thromboembolism:
  - Cerebrovascular accident (CVA) from embolism, or haemorrhage resulting from ruptured mycotic aneurysm.
  - Finger/toe gangrene caused by embolism ± vasculitis.
  - Renal or splenic abscess or infarction.
  - Mesenteric embolism (ischaemic bowel and an acute abdomen).
  - Joint infection.
  - Bone infection: this is quite a common occurrence in infective endocarditis, and often affects the vertebrae. The most common symptom is back pain, though sometimes persistent sepsis is the diagnostic clue. The investigation of choice is bone magnetic resonance imaging; treatment is usually medical, though rarely surgical debridement is needed.
- **Acute renal failure**: this may occur from immune complex disease, haemodynamic upset (acute heart failure), damage during cardiac surgery and nephrotoxic antibiotics. Close monitoring of renal function throughout the illness is mandatory.

The physical examination often only reveals evidence of fever (temperature), mild weight loss, murmurs and sometimes complicating heart failure. Rarely (<2%) clubbing is found. Splinter haemorrhages are more common (50%). More substantial hand infarcts (Osler's nodes) are very rare but pathognomonic. Splenomegaly is common. Dipstick haematuria is almost universal.

Investigations

- **Blood tests**: the most important investigation is blood culture, three sets of which detect bacterial endocarditis in 97% of cases.
  - Systemic inflammatory markers: erythrocyte sedimentation rate (ESR) and C-reactive protein (CRP) are usually elevated.
  - Anaemia of chronic disease and elevated white cell count.
  - Urine dipstick and microscopy (haematuria).
- **Echocardiography**: important, but only rarely makes the diagnosis, and *can never exclude endocarditis*. Echocardiography is more important in assessing the degree and consequences of valvular damage and guiding subsequent management.
- **Transoesophageal echocardiography**: useful when transthoracic images are unclear or with prosthetic valves, because higher resolution allows more detailed imaging. It is also useful in assessing complications of endocarditis (abscess formation or acute valvular destruction) before surgery.

Treatment and prognosis

Antibiotic therapy is the mainstay of treatment, based on blood culture findings and organism sensitivities. This requires close collaboration with microbiologists. Antibiotics are usually intravenous, often in drug combinations in order to attain the best antibacterial killing and tissue penetration. Treatment commonly continues for 4 or 6 weeks. **Surgery** to remove and replace the infected valve is sometimes indicated for:

- Severe valvular destruction causing heart failure.
- Abscess formation.
- Failure to eradicate infection despite prolonged antibiotic therapy.
- Prosthetic valve endocarditis.

Prognosis is variable, but overall mortality rate is 10–20%.

Antibiotic prophylaxis to prevent infective endocarditis

Patients with known valvular disease or prosthetic valves should have antibiotics before undergoing procedures that provoke bacteraemia (dental procedures involving the gums and other invasive procedures, e.g. lower gastrointestinal endoscopy). Further details can be found in the *British National Formulary*.

Myocarditis

Myocarditis is inflammation of the heart muscle caused by:

- **Viral infections**, e.g. Coxsackie, mumps and influenza. Subclinical infection is common in HIV infection.
- **Bacterial infection**: may occur in severe septicaemia, although other features dominate the clinical picture.
- **Radiation exposure**: much commoner before targeted beam therapy.
- **Autoimmune disease**: the commoner myocarditis on a worldwide basis is rheumatic fever (see Figure 93.1).
- **Toxin damage** such as from diphtheria infection.

The clinical features depend on the severity and duration of the inflammation. In **acute myocarditis** the dominant feature is acute heart failure. The patient may be severely unwell, breathless and in a low output state. The clue that myocarditis is present is that the tachycardia is out of proportion to the severity of the heart failure. A particularly distressing manifestation of acute myocarditis is **sudden cardiac death**, which may be more prevalent in athletic sufferers. In **chronic myocarditis**, e.g. South American trypanosomiasis (*Trypanosoma cruzii*) infection, patients may present with chronic heart failure. Investigations include:

- **Echocardiography**: shows impaired systolic contractile function, and in chronic processes dilatation of the left ventricle and atrium.
- **Cardiac enzymes**: elevated and, unlike myocardial infarction, often stay high for many days or weeks before declining.
- **Inflammatory markers**: CRP and ESR are usually high.
- **Serological tests**: may reveal the responsible organism.

Treatment and prognosis

There is rarely any specific treatment. Standard anti-heart failure therapy is given (see Chapter 87). The prognosis in acute severe myocarditis is good provided that life can be maintained; this may require circulatory support with an implantable left ventricular assist device. In refractory cases cardiac transplantation should be considered.

Pericarditis

See Chapter 91.

Rheumatic fever

See Figure 93.1.

94 Tachyarrhythmias

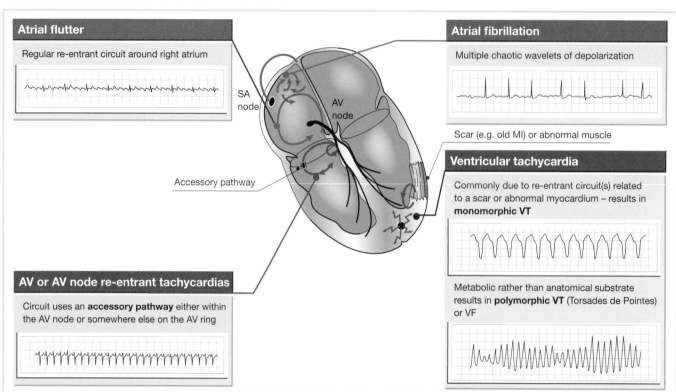

Atrial flutter

Regular re-entrant circuit around right atrium

Atrial fibrillation

Multiple chaotic wavelets of depolarization

SA node

AV node

Accessory pathway

Scar (e.g. old MI) or abnormal muscle

Ventricular tachycardia

Commonly due to re-entrant circuit(s) related to a scar or abnormal myocardium – results in **monomorphic VT**

Metabolic rather than anatomical substrate results in **polymorphic VT** (Torsades de Pointes) or VF

AV or AV node re-entrant tachycardias

Circuit uses an **accessory pathway** either within the AV node or somewhere else on the AV ring

Arrhythmias are abnormal heart beats, either fast (tachyarrhythmias) or slow (bradyarrhythmias). Minor arrhythmias are universal. The most common sustained arrhythmia, atrial fibrillation (AF), occurs in 1% of those aged 50 years or more, and 10% of the over eighties. Sudden cardiac death is often the result of arrhythmias (usually ventricular tachycardia (VT) and ventricular fibrillation (VF)) and causes 15–40% of deaths in coronary artery disease or heart failure.

Clinical features

Arrhythmias may be asymptomatic, cause intermittent minor palpitations, or be the cause of blackouts, severe cardiovascular compromise or cardiac arrest. **Palpitation** is the symptom that describes an abnormal awareness of the heart beat; however, it does not necessarily mean that the heart rhythm is abnormal.

Key facts for understanding arrhythmias

The heart beat is controlled by the fastest pacemaker focus. During a tachyarrhythmia, the normal sinus node depolarizations are 'suppressed' by the faster depolarizations of the abnormal focus. The surface electrocardiogram (ECG) is a 'superimposed' graph of both atrial and ventricular activity. Atrial and ventricular activity are not necessarily linked during arrhythmias, so they need to be considered separately. Arrhythmias are categorized according to where the initial depolarization originates:

- **Supraventricular arrhythmias** originate in the atria or around the atrioventricular (AV) node.
- **Ventricular arrhythmias** originate in the ventricles.

In the normal heart, the only communication between the atria and ventricles is the AV node, so the ventricular rate during arrhythmias arising in the atria is governed not just by the arrhythmia itself, but by conduction through the AV node. The normal AV node acts as a 'turnstile', because it conducts depolarizations slowly and is refractory for a relatively long period after each depolarization. Abnormal additional conducting pathways between the atria and ventricles ('accessory pathways') are common, and in some people may allow depolarizations to spread from the atria to ventricles, or from the ventricles to atria, without necessarily passing fully through the AV node. This allows re-entry circuits to be set up, and in some circumstances bypasses the normal 'safety valve' of the AV node.

Supraventricular tachyarrhythmias

AV-reciprocating tachycardias (paroxysmal supraventricular tachyarrhythmias)

Pathogenesis

A re-entrant circuit is set up by the presence of an accessory pathway, an additional conducting pathway:

- Between the atria and ventricles, causing AV re-entrant tachycardia (AVRT). This additional pathway may be seen in the ECG during normal sinus rhythm (see next section).
- Between the atrium and AV node to form a complete circuit within the AV node: this is the most common additional pathway and underlies AV nodal re-entrant tachycardia (AVNRT).

Medicine at a Glance, Fourth Edition. Edited by Patrick Davey. © 2014 John Wiley & Sons, Ltd. Published 2014 by John Wiley & Sons, Ltd. Companion website: www.ataglanceseries.com/medicine

ECG diagnosis

A regular, narrow QRS complex tachycardia, usually at a rate of 150–200 bpm is found. Regular P waves may be visible interspersed between the QRS complexes. Often the P waves are of an abnormal shape, as they are activated retrogradely, either by impulses passing up an accessory pathway from the ventricle as in orthodromic tachycardia complicating Wolf–Parkinson–White (WPW) syndrome, or more commonly by impulses passing up from the AV node, as during an episode of AVNRT. In the latter, the P wave is upside down, and follows closely just after the QRS complex.

Clinical features

They usually present as recurrent attacks of rapid palpitations, lasting from a few minutes to hours or even days.

Treatment

Slowing conduction through the AV node may stop the tachycardia:

- **Vagotonic manoeuvres** that increase vagal tone (e.g. Valsalva manoeuvre, swallowing cold drinks or carotid sinus massage); patients may discover these themselves.
- **Drug treatment**: slows or blocks conduction in the AV node.
  - Intravenous (IV) adenosine transiently (≤4 s) blocks AV node conduction, terminating any tachycardia using the AV node as part of the circuit (i.e. both AVRT and AVNRT), so restoring sinus rhythm.
  - β-Blockers (e.g. verapamil, flecainide) are useful as long-term oral prophylaxis or intermittent therapy.
- **Radiofrequency ablation**: the treatment of choice if symptoms are severe enough for long-term medication. During an electrophysiological study, applying radiofrequency energy through a catheter destroys the accessory pathway. Successful ablation cures the patient.

Accessory pathways, pre-excitation and WPW syndrome

An accessory pathway, which conducts atrial depolarizations directly into the ventricular myocardium, bypassing the AV node, characterizes the WPW syndrome; pre-excitation, AV reciprocating tachycardias and pre-excited AF may occur.

- **Pre-excitation**: atrial impulses are propagated more quickly to the ventricle by the accessory pathway than by the normal AV node. The part of the myocardium into which the accessory pathway is inserted depolarizes earlier (i.e. is pre-excited) than the part of the ventricle depolarized by the normally conducted beat. This shortens the PR interval. Electrical activity propagates slowly from the pre-excited ventricular myocardium by myocyte-to-myocyte transmission, not through specialized conducting tissue, so slurring the first part of the QRS complex (δ wave).
- **Atrial fibrillation in WPW syndrome**: normally the AV node acts as a 'safety valve' preventing an over-rapid ventricular response in AF. Some (about 5–10%) accessory pathways conduct impulses more frequently than the normal AV node, allowing AF to be conducted to the ventricles at ≤250 bpm, shortening diastole, impairing ventricular filling and lessening cardiac output, so that haemodynamic collapse or VF ('sudden cardiac death') occurs. It is one of the aims of treatment in the WPW syndrome to prevent such sudden cardiac death. The ECG in 'pre-excited' AF has very abnormal, wide QRS complexes, because ventricular depolarization is largely from the impulse conducted down the accessory pathway. Pre-excited AF is treated with immediate direct current (DC) cardioversion. As a result of the tendency for fast pre-excited AF, all patients with WPW syndrome *must* have formal electrophysiological studies to ascertain the conducting potential of the accessory pathway. If it is high then the pathway is ablated. It should be emphasized that AF in patients without WPW syndrome is not in itself a cause of sudden cardiac death.

Atrial fibrillation (see Figure 94.2 below)

Pathophysiology

The atria depolarize spontaneously in a rapid (frequently >300 bpm), uncoordinated fashion, bombarding the AV node continuously with electrical impulses. Conduction to the ventricles is limited by AV node refractoriness (often to <200 bpm) and occurs unpredictably, causing a completely irregular ventricular response. Heart rates in AF can vary widely, but in untreated AF are typically around 100–150 bpm.

Classification

There are several different forms of AF:

- **Paroxysmal AF**, where attacks terminate spontaneously without intervention.
- **Persistent AF**, where attacks do not terminate spontaneously and require medical intervention.
- **Permanent AF**, where AF is considered to be permanent, and medical intervention either will not re-establish sinus rhythm or cannot hold the patient in sinus rhythm for long and the AF is therefore accepted as permanent.

ECG diagnosis

The QRS rate is usually fast and irregularly irregular. No P waves are visible; the baseline may be flat or show fast, small depolarizations. The key diagnostic feature is that no other cardiac rhythm is truly irregularly irregular.

Clinical features

There are many possible different symptoms in AF:

- Most patients present with **fast irregular palpitations** that are typically cardiac (i.e. sudden onset, defined duration, sudden offset, as opposed to non-arrhythmic palpitations, which are of slow onset, ill-defined duration and slow offset). The duration of palpitations varies greatly; some patients only experience symptoms for a few minutes, some for several days.
- Some patients present with additional symptoms of **breathlessness**. In the vast majority of patients who are breathless with AF, there is a cardiac pathology beyond AF, most commonly impaired left ventricular (LV) function, occasionally cardiomyopathy or coronary disease. Breathlessness is not a feature of uncomplicated AF and should always prompt an alert that the patient may have severe underlying heart disease.
- Many patients present with vague and **ill-defined symptoms of loss of good health** – only recognized as being due to AF once the AF is terminated and they feel better – or effort intolerance, due to the marked tachycardia during exercise in AF impairing cardiac efficiency and so limiting exercise capacity.
- In some patients, distressingly, the first sign of AF is a **stroke** (see Treatment section). These are most commonly patients who have not felt palpitations, or have not recognized palpitations as being a possible sign of a cardiac illness.
- In a very few patients, **syncope** occurs. This is very rare, and the only situation is where there is underlying sinus node disease. The sinus node disease itself can predispose to AF. During an episode of AF sinus node function is suppressed, and when the AF terminates, due to the sinus node disease it takes unusually long for sinus node function to restart, and a period of asystole

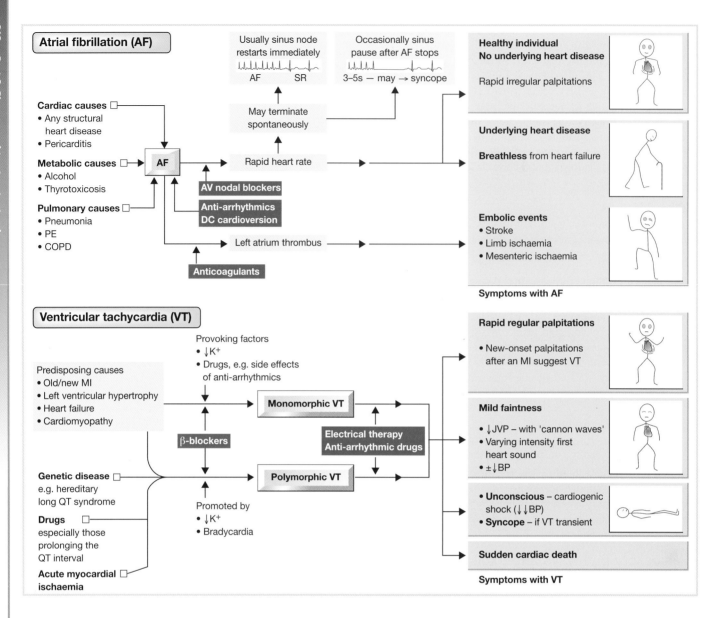

Atrial fibrillation (AF)

Cardiac causes
- Any structural heart disease
- Pericarditis

Metabolic causes
- Alcohol
- Thyrotoxicosis

Pulmonary causes
- Pneumonia
- PE
- COPD

AF

AV nodal blockers

Anti-arrhythmics
DC cardioversion

Anticoagulants

Usually sinus node restarts immediately

AF   SR

Occasionally sinus pause after AF stops

3–5s — may → syncope

May terminate spontaneously

Rapid heart rate

Left atrium thrombus

Healthy individual
No underlying heart disease

Rapid irregular palpitations

Underlying heart disease

Breathless from heart failure

Embolic events
- Stroke
- Limb ischaemia
- Mesenteric ischaemia

Symptoms with AF

Ventricular tachycardia (VT)

Predisposing causes
- Old/new MI
- Left ventricular hypertrophy
- Heart failure
- Cardiomyopathy

Provoking factors
- ↓K⁺
- Drugs, e.g. side effects of anti-arrhythmics

β-blockers

Monomorphic VT

Polymorphic VT

Electrical therapy
Anti-arrhythmic drugs

Genetic disease
e.g. hereditary long QT syndrome

Drugs
especially those prolonging the QT interval

Acute myocardial ischaemia

Promoted by
- ↓K⁺
- Bradycardia

Rapid regular palpitations
- New-onset palpitations after an MI suggest VT

Mild faintness
- ↓JVP – with 'cannon waves'
- Varying intensity first heart sound
- ±↓BP

- **Unconscious** – cardiogenic shock (↓↓BP)
- **Syncope** – if VT transient

Sudden cardiac death

Symptoms with VT

can occur, occasionally lasting tens of seconds, sufficient to cause syncope. It must be emphasized that this is rare, and for the vast majority of patients who come to hospital with a blackout and are found to be in AF, the AF is not relevant to their blackout.

- In a very few patients the AF itself does not give rise to symptoms of palpitations, or, initially, any other symptoms. The heart rate can then be 140–160 bpm for several months, and the patient can develop a '**rate-related cardiomyopathy**', a condition where after several months of rapid heart rate LV function falls dramatically. Patients then present with symptoms and signs of congestive heart failure (see Chapter 87). With meticulous heart rate control LV function almost always returns to normal.

- In many patients with AF **no symptoms** are present, and the condition is only picked up during a medical examination for another condition. These patients must have formal thromboembolic risk evaluation carried out to minimize the long-term risk of stroke.

Aetiology

There are many causes of AF, and it is vital to determine which one(s) are present in any individual, as many need specific therapy:

- **Cardiac**: ischaemic heart disease, hypertensive heart disease (LV hypertrophy), mitral valve disease (especially mitral

stenosis), pericarditis and cardiomyopathy or heart failure (any cause).

- **Metabolic**: thyrotoxicosis and alcohol (acute or chronic). Alcohol is an extraordinarily common cause of AF and a very careful history should be taken from *all patients with AF regardless of background*.

- **Pulmonary**: pulmonary embolism (PE), pneumonia, chronic obstructive pulmonary disease (COPD) and cor pulmonale.

- **Idiopathic**: in some no cause is found – idiopathic or 'lone AF'. This is quite common, perhaps accounting for +40% of cases. AF incidence increases with age, and at any age is commoner in men than women.

Treatment

- **Rate control**: the ventricular rate should be decreased by reducing conduction through the AV node using digoxin, β-blockers or certain calcium channel antagonists. Rate control does not terminate the AF, this continues. Most patients require digoxin (which slows the ventricular response to AF at rest, but not during exercise) and β-blockers (to slow the ventricular rate during exercise).

- **Reversion back to sinus rhythm**: drugs (amiodarone, flecainide, sotalol) can convert AF back to sinus rhythm and/or prevent further episodes of AF. DC cardioversion under anaesthesia/deep sedation is very effective in restoring sinus rhythm provided that AF has been present <1 year, and the heart is not that abnormal. If ongoing episodes of AF are troublesome despite anti-arrhythmic drugs, or there is actual or possible concern over drug side effects, ablation of certain electrical structures in the left atrium can greatly reduce AF incidence. There are several different techniques; all use ablating catheters inserted into the left atrium via the femoral vein, right heart and across the interatrial septum. The ablation circuits can isolate the pulmonary veins, often the initial source of the abnormal electrical impulses in AF, or channel the electricity within the left atrium preventing self re-entering AF circuits. Anti-AF catheter ablation is a rapidly expanding field. The procedure has great success, at least for several years, and the risk is low (though up to 2% of patients may have a major complication).

- **Anticoagulation**: systemic thromboembolism (stroke, embolic occlusion of a limb or visceral artery) is a significant risk in AF. All patients with AF, unless there is a clear cut and reversible non-recurring cause must be evaluated for their stroke risk and *this is probably the most important aspect of caring for patients with AF*. Systemic emboli arises from thrombus in the left atrium. The risk is especially high in those with structural cardiac disease (especially mitral stenosis), large left atria ($\geq 40\,mm$) and in those aged 65 years or over. The risk of systemic emboli in AF can be estimated using predictive charts, of which the most common is the CHA_2DS_2-VASc score (see Figure 94.3 below). Those with a score ≥ 2 are anticoagulated with warfarin (target international normalized ratio (INR) = 2.5 – 3.0) or one of the more modern antithrombotic agents, such as dabigatran or rivaroxaban. The benefit from anticoagulants must always be titrated against the risk of bleeding, and this may be high in the frail elderly, the confused and those falling over. A score (HASBLED) sumarizes some of these risk factors (**H**ypertension, **A**bnormal renal/liver function, **S**troke, **B**leeding history or predisposition, **L**abile INR, **E**lderly, **D**rugs/alcohol concomitantly); for a score ≥ 3 risk is high, and great caution should be used with anticoagulants. If the risk is high and anticoagulants are contraindicated, closing the left atrial appendage with a device (e.g. the watchman device) may reduce stroke risk sufficiently to justify its use. The thromboembolic risk is the same in paroxysmal or permanent AF, and remains high regardless of the frequency of symptoms. Following cardioversion, if a patient's CHA_2DS_2-VASc is high, they should remain on anticoagulants for at least 2–3 years, as the risk of recurrent AF remains high.

Atrial flutter

Pathophysiology

The atria depolarize in a rapid coordinated fashion, as a result of a macro re-entry circuit moving anticlockwise around the right atrium. Atrial depolarizations occur at a rate of 300/min; conduction to the ventricles is limited to every second, third or fourth depolarization, because of AV node refractoriness.

ECG diagnosis

The QRS rate is exactly 150/min if alternate flutter waves are conducted ('atrial flutter with 2-1 block') – or can be other divisibles of the flutter rate, e.g. 100 (3-1), 75 (4-1), sometimes varying every few beats. Continuous sawtooth 'flutter waves' are visible instead of P waves, most obviously in leads II, III, aVf and V1. *If a regular tachycardia has a constant rate of exactly 150/min, always think of atrial flutter* even if flutter waves are not obvious – they may be obscured by the QRS/T waves.

Clinical features

The pulse rate is usually 150 and regular. The patient may be asymptomatic, experience rapid palpitation or breathlessness, or be in heart failure. The incidence and causes of atrial flutter are similar to those of AF; these two arrhythmias commonly occur in the same patient.

Treatment

This is similar to AF. As atrial flutter is the result of a macro re-entry circuit, radiofrequency ablation of the critical part of the circuit in the right atrium may be curative. It is indicated if drug therapy fails or in patients in whom long-term drug treatment is not a good option (e.g. the young). Thromboembolic risk is considered to be the same as in AF.

Ventricular tachycardias (see Figure 94.2 above)

Pathogenesis

Rapid depolarizations arise in the ventricular myocardium, as a result of:

- Re-entrant circuit(s) in an anatomically abnormal substrate such as myocardial infarction (MI) scar tissue. The ECG shows monomorphic VT.
- Abnormal triggered activity in ventricular myocardium, resulting from electrophysiological/metabolic disturbances that often prolong the QT interval, such as acute ischaemia and drugs. The ECG shows polymorphic VT.

The most powerful stimulus to VT is myocardial damage, e.g. in heart failure VT is common. For each 10% decrease in ejection fraction, the chance of an arrhythmic death occurring increases by 65%. If patients with impaired LV function develop syncope, unless there is clear evidence for an alternative diagnosis, VT should be strongly suspected.

ECG diagnosis

The QRS complexes are broad with an abnormal shape. VT should *always be suspected* when patients known to have heart disease (especially recent or remote MI) present with a regular tachycardia with broad QRS complexes:

- In monomorphic VT the QRS morphology is uniform; typically the rate is 120–190 bpm. There may be evidence of independent atrial activity, i.e. dissociated P waves.
- Polymorphic VT (see Table 94.1) is less regular, more chaotic and sometimes with a characteristic phasic variation in the QRS morphology – 'torsades de pointes'. Polymorphic VT is inherently unstable and often degenerates early on into VF.

Clinical features

The pulse rate is fast or may be weak, or there may be no pulse palpable. The patient may be in acute cardiac failure, be severely compromised, suffer cardiac arrest (pulseless VT) or be relatively well, except for rapid palpitation or breathlessness. A good clinical state to a patient does not exclude VT, and the risk of haemodynamic deterioration remains.

Treatment

This is of individual episodes:

- **Pulseless VT, or impending cardiovascular collapse**: DC cardioversion, either immediate or after urgent anaesthesia/sedation.
- **Haemodynamically stable VT**: IV lidocaine (lignocaine) or drugs such as amiodarone. Never use multiple drug combinations. If drugs are unsuccessful, use DC cardioversion.

Condition	Points		Annual stroke risk	
C – Congestive heart failure (or left ventricular systolic dysfunction)	1		CHA_2DS_2VASc score	Stroke risk %
H – **Hypertension**: blood pressure consistently above 140/90 mmHg (or treated hypertension on medication)	1		0	0
A_2 – Age ≥75 years	2		1	1.3
D – Diabetes mellitus	1		2	2.2
S_2 – Prior **stroke** or **TIA** or **thromboembolism**	2		3	3.2
V – Vascular disease (e.g. peripheral artery disease, myocardial infarction, aortic plaque)	1		4	4.0
			5	6.7
A – Age 65–74 years	1		6	9.8
Sc – Sex category (i.e. female gender)	1		7	9.6
			8	6.7
			9	15.2

Causes of sudden death

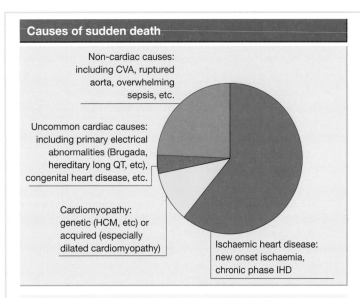

The role of ejection fraction in predicting death at 4 years following an acute MI. Ejection fraction is the proportion of blood ejected from the heart with each cardiac cycle, i.e. the (end-diastolic – end-systolic volume) /end-diastolic volume. Ejection fraction is plotted against % dying; the highest risk of death is in those with the lowest ejection fraction (affects a rather small proportion of the post MI population)

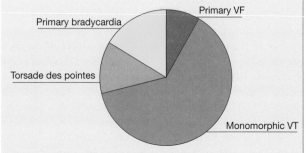

Arrhythmias underlying sudden cardiac death

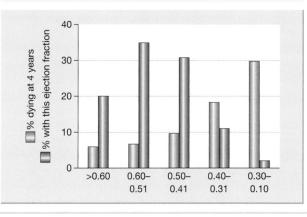

Table 94.1 Causes of polymorphic ventricular tachycardia.

- Acute ischaemia

- Drugs (cause prolongation of the QT interval): quinidine, sotalol, amiodarone, tricyclic antidepressants, antihistamines

- Hypokalaemia

- Hypomagnesaemia

- Hypocalcaemia

- Bradycardias (any cause)

- Congenital QT prolongation syndromes (ion channel mutations): Jervell–Lange–Nielsen syndrome, Romano–Ward syndrome

Source: Eur Heart J. 2010. Reproduced with permission of Oxford University Press.

- **Polymorphic VT**: DC cardioversion, IV magnesium, correction of the underlying metabolic or electrophysiological abnormality. Slow heart rates prolong the QT interval and may worsen polymorphic VT. Increasing the heart rate by pacing often prevents or dramatically reduces the incidence of polymorphic VT.

Prevention of future episodes

- **Long-term drug therapy**: β-blockers, amiodarone, angiotensin-converting enzyme inhibitors and spironolactone to improve LV function and maintain K^+.
- **Revascularization** (coronary artery bypass graft or percutaneous coronary intervention): for severe coronary disease.
- **Implantable cardiovertor defibrillators** (ICDs): monitor the cardiac rhythm and deliver antitachycardic therapy (overdrive pacing and/or intracardiac shocks) if VT or VF is detected. They are indicated for survivors of cardiac arrest, and in symptomatic VT with impaired LV function.

Ventricular fibrillation

VF is often lethal, especially out of hospital, but provided patients can be resuscitated (see Chapter 78) without major neurological damage, it is important to determine the underlying cause, and this usually needs full cardiac and coronary imaging:

- **Ischaemic heart disease** (IHD): either acute MI, which is then treated in the standard fashion, or critical coronary stenosis, treated with complete revascularization. If there is no new ischaemia, and the problem relates to an old MI-related scar, the treatment is an ICD.

- **Other structural heart disease**: especially cardiomyopathies. Many patients in these categories need an ICD.
- **Channelopathies**: these are usually genetically mediated proarrhythmic conditions, and include hereditary long QT syndrome and Brugada's syndrome.
- **Other rare conditions**: including WPW syndrome with complicating AF and very high heart rates, and acquired long QT syndromes (including starvation-related syndromes).

95 Bradyarrhythmias

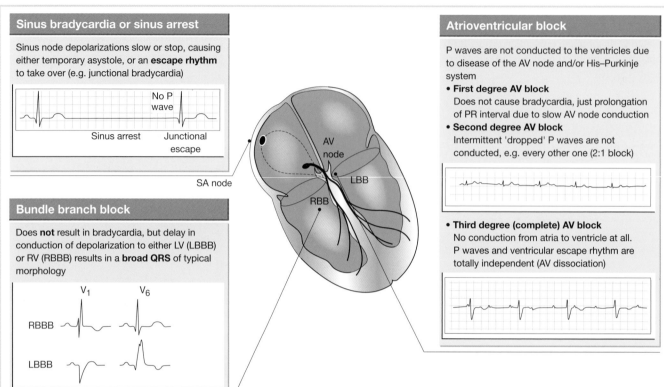

Sinus bradycardia or sinus arrest

Sinus node depolarizations slow or stop, causing either temporary asystole, or an **escape rhythm** to take over (e.g. junctional bradycardia)

No P wave
Sinus arrest   Junctional escape

SA node

AV node
LBB
RBB

Bundle branch block

Does **not** result in bradycardia, but delay in conduction of depolarization to either LV (LBBB) or RV (RBBB) results in a **broad QRS** of typical morphology

V₁   V₆
RBBB
LBBB

Atrioventricular block

P waves are not conducted to the ventricles due to disease of the AV node and/or His–Purkinje system

- **First degree AV block**
  Does not cause bradycardia, just prolongation of PR interval due to slow AV node conduction
- **Second degree AV block**
  Intermittent 'dropped' P waves are not conducted, e.g. every other one (2:1 block)

- **Third degree (complete) AV block**
  No conduction from atria to ventricle at all. P waves and ventricular escape rhythm are totally independent (AV dissociation)

Type of AV block	ECG features	Site/cause of impaired conduction	Natural history/treatment
First degree	Prolonged PR interval only	AV node May be functional, due to drugs or high vagal tone	If functional – progression unusual If due to AV node disease, progression common Usual treatment is observation only
Second degree	Some P waves are not conducted		
Mobitz I (Wenckebach)	Progressive PR interval prolongation leads to 'dropped' beat	AV node. May be functional, due to drugs or high vagal tone	May be benign, BUT often needs a pacemaker
Mobitz II	Only every second or third P wave is conducted	Usually structural AV node/His bundle disease	Always progresses to CHB Early permanent pacemaker
Third degree (complete) **Complete heart block (CHB)**	No P waves are conducted P waves and ventricular escape rhythm are completely independent (AV dissociation)	Structural disease of AV node and/or conducting system	Untreated death ≤ 6 weeks Urgent pacemaker Immediate pacemaker if any history of syncope, or heart rate <35 bpm

Definition and clinical features

Bradyarrhythmias are abnormally slow heart beats (<60/min). Mild or transient bradyarrhythmias may be asymptomatic or even physiological, e.g. sinus bradycardia during sleep or in a healthy athlete. Symptomatic bradycardias commonly cause dizziness or syncope, or less commonly fatigue or heart failure. Palpitations are not a feature of bradyarrhythmias. The classic syncopal episode caused by a bradyarrhythmia is a **Stokes–Adams attack**. The characteristics are:

- Sudden onset without warning (within a few seconds). A warning, typically lasting up to a minute, is not typical for Stokes–Adams attacks, and rather suggests that the diagnosis is a form of fainting

(vasomotor syncope), or just possibly an epileptiform seizure.
- Immediate collapse with loss of consciousness.
- Pale and still 'as if dead'.
- Duration a few seconds to 1 or 2 minutes.
- Rapid recovery back to normal, only transient disorientation at most for a few minutes, and no focal neurological symptoms or signs. Prolonged time to full recovery suggests some form of epilepsy, or that a secondary anoxic seizure has complicated the attack.

Aetiology

Bradyarrhythmias arise either from the failure of the sinoatrial (SA) node to provide regular depolarizations (**sinoatrial disease**), or by failure of the conducting system to convey the depolarizations into the ventricles (**atrioventricular (AV) block** or **complete heart block**). The total absence of any depolarizations (**asystole**) is usually prevented for more than a few seconds by the emergence of an **escape rhythm**, arising from the next most active intrinsic cardiac pacemaker. When the sinus node stops, this is usually the AV node (**junctional escape rhythm**); when AV conduction is blocked, a **ventricular escape rhythm** arises either from the conducting tissues or from the ventricular myocardium itself. The 'lower' (i.e. further away from the SA node) the escape rhythm, the slower it is.

Sinoatrial node disease

This is a dysfunction of the sinus node that manifests either as inappropriate **sinus bradycardia** or by periods of **sinus arrest**. It may be one aspect of the **sick sinus syndrome**, where patients experience both episodes of bradyarrhythmias and episodes of atrial tachyarrhythmias such as atrial fibrillation (AF). The bradycardias in SA node disease may be exacerbated by drugs used to control tachyarrhythmias, such as β-blockers or digoxin. Another manifestation of SA node disease is 'fainting' (syncope) or feeling faint (pre-syncope), occurring at the moment that an episode of AF stops. The usual mechanism for this is a prolonged sinus pause before the intrinsic SA node pacemaker starts up (see Chapter 94). SA node disease often has no particular cause, though it can relate to coronary disease, drugs (particularly long-term amiodarone) and occasionally to hypothyroidism. It can also complicate many forms of heart disease, especially congenital. The prognosis of SA node disease not associated with any heart disease is good.

Atrioventricular block

Disease of either the AV node and/or the conducting system results in failure of transmission of the P waves to the ventricles. AV block is classified according to the extent of the failure of transmission, seen on the electrocardiogram (ECG), and this is broadly related to the site and extent of the disease in the AV node/His–Purkinje system (see Figure 95.1). The signs depend on the type of AV block. First-degree block is difficult to detect clinically: the first heart sound may be quiet. Second-degree block usually has a heart rate of <40 bpm. In third-degree block the atria, which beat independently of the ventricles, occasionally contract on a closed tricuspid valve. Blood cannot leave the atria for the ventricle and instead will be propelled into the neck veins, seen as a prominent jugular venous pressure (JVP) pulsation – 'cannon' waves.

Investigations

Distinguishing Stokes–Adams attacks from other causes of dizziness or syncope (e.g. vasovagal episode, seizure, transient ischaemic attack (TIA)) is often difficult. The clinical history and additional information from a witness are extremely important, and may be the only information on which to base management decisions. The diagnostic investigation is an ECG during an attack – this is often not possible to obtain. If this is so, inter-attack investigations may be helpful:

- **12-lead ECG**: this may show circumstantial evidence of bradyrhythmias, e.g. first-degree AV block or bundle branch block (BBB). The risk of intermittent complete heart block (CHB) is increased by extensive conducting tissue disease. The left bundle is a much larger structure than the right bundle; thus, isolated left BBB is more likely to give rise to intermittent CHB than right BBB. However, extensive conducting tissue disease on the 12-lead ECG is only a guide that symptoms arise from CHB, e.g. patients with ischaemic heart disease (IHD) and extensive conducting tissue disease may blackout either from CHB or ventricular tachycardia.

- **24-hour ECG recording (Holter monitor)**: this is commonly used to detect the occurrence of both tachyarrhythmias and bradyarrhythmias, but is often not useful unless the patient experiences a typical episode during the recording. Furthermore, minor rhythm disturbances are commonly detected on Holter monitors and may not necessarily be related to the symptoms.

- **Reveal device**: this is implanted if it is crucial to obtain an ECG during an attack, for instance if there is high suspicion that either high-grade AV block or ventricular tachyarrhythmias underlie the attack, as these are both associated with early death if untreated. The usual 'danger' signals are: blackouts occurring without warning (i.e. unlike simple faints), known structural heart disease, conducting tissue disease, especially if major, or an ECG known to be associated with tachyarrhythmias (when other tests have been non-diagnostic). The reveal device is a very small, implantable ECG machine, about $1 \times 4 \times 0.5\,cm$, implanted under the skin on the left side of the chest, which continually records the ECG. It is most usefully interrogated just after an attack.

Treatment

Minor arrhythmias that do not cause symptoms do not require specific treatment. SA node disease requires treatment only if symptomatic or if a potentially exacerbating medication cannot be stopped. First-degree AV block, BBB and Wenckebach block also do not require treatment. However, higher degrees of AV block (Mobitz II and complete) should always be treated even if not symptomatic, because there is a high risk of future syncope or even of sudden death.

- **Pacemaker implantation** is the preferred treatment for symptomatic bradyarrhythmias. A permanent pacemaker is a small electronic device that generates regular pulses to depolarize the heart through an electrode inserted into the right side of the heart through the venous system. A **single-chamber pacemaker** has an electrode in either the right ventricle or the right atrium. A **dual-chamber pacemaker** paces both the atrium and the ventricle through two electrodes, and can pace the ventricle synchronously after each P wave that is sensed in the atrium. This provides a close approximation to the physiological depolarization of the heart, and allows the heart beat to change rate in track with the sinus node.
    - **Pacemaker nomenclature**:
    - First letter: chamber paced (V, ventricle; A, atrium; D, both).
    - Second letter: chamber sensed (V, A or 0 for none).
    - Third letter: pacemaker response to the detection of cardiac electrical activity (I, inhibited; T, triggered; D, both).
    - Fourth letter: relates to whether the pacemaker stimulates quicker on physical activity (R, rate responsive, e.g. VVI-R).
    - Fifth letter: relates to whether the device has any antitachycardic functions, such as whether it can defibrillate or overdrive the pace.

So, using this system, typical pacemakers are VVI, which means that the ventricle is paced, and sensed, and if electricity is detected (i.e. the ventricle has fired normally) then the system is inhibited (i.e. is silent).

Another common pacemaker is a DDD one, where D stands for both atrial (A) and ventricular (V) leads. So, A and V can be paced, A and V are sensed, and the response can either be inhibited (I, as above) or triggered (T).

96 Congenital heart disease

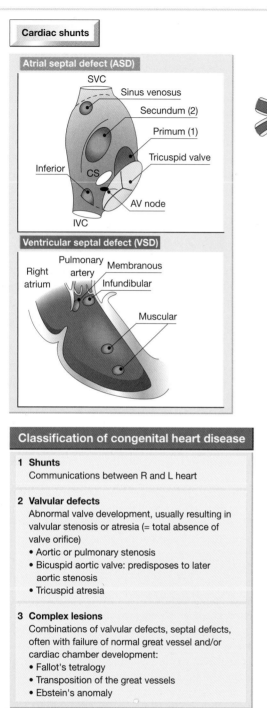

Cardiac shunts

Atrial septal defect (ASD)
- SVC
- Sinus venosus
- Secundum (2)
- Primum (1)
- Tricuspid valve
- Inferior
- CS
- AV node
- IVC

Ventricular septal defect (VSD)
- Right atrium
- Pulmonary artery
- Membranous
- Infundibular
- Muscular

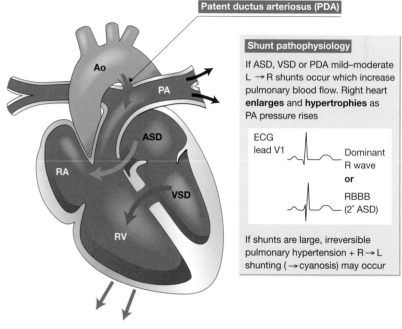

Patent ductus arteriosus (PDA)

- Ao
- PA
- ASD
- RA
- VSD
- RV

Shunt pathophysiology

If ASD, VSD or PDA mild–moderate L →R shunts occur which increase pulmonary blood flow. Right heart **enlarges** and **hypertrophies** as PA pressure rises

ECG lead V1 — Dominant R wave

or

RBBB (2° ASD)

If shunts are large, irreversible pulmonary hypertension + R→L shunting (→cyanosis) may occur

Classification of congenital heart disease

1 Shunts
Communications between R and L heart

2 Valvular defects
Abnormal valve development, usually resulting in valvular stenosis or atresia (= total absence of valve orifice)
- Aortic or pulmonary stenosis
- Bicuspid aortic valve: predisposes to later aortic stenosis
- Tricuspid atresia

3 Complex lesions
Combinations of valvular defects, septal defects, often with failure of normal great vessel and/or cardiac chamber development:
- Fallot's tetralogy
- Transposition of the great vessels
- Ebstein's anomaly

Syndromes associated with congenital heart disease

Maternal factors
- Rubella infection in 1st trimester
- Consanguinity
- Drugs – phenytoin, thalidomide, ethanol, retinoic acid, lithium

Chromosomal abnormalities

Cardiac defects common in most aneuploidies, deletions, duplications
- Down's syndrome (Tris.21) — Septal defects
- Turner's syndrome (XO) — Aortic coarctation
- Klinefelter's syndrome (XXY) — Septal defects

Single gene disorders

Usually transcription factors that are involved in regulating cardiac embryonic development, or genes encoding structural proteins:

Syndrome	Gene	Cardiac defects
Noonan's syndrome	Unknown	Pulmonary stenosis, HCM
William's syndrome	Elastin	Supravalvular aortic stenosis
Rubenstein–Taybi syndrome	CBP	Endocardial cushion defects
Holt–Oram syndrome	TBX 5	ASD
Di George syndrome	TBX 1	VSD, pulmonary atresia

Definition and incidence

Congenital heart disease (CHD) is an abnormal embryological cardiac development, or persistence of some parts of the fetal circulation after birth resulting in structural cardiac defects. The conditions discussed here (along with congenital aortic and pulmonary stenosis) account for 80% of CHD. The incidence of major defects is 8/1000 live births. Minor defects are more common, e.g. bicuspid aortic valve affects 2%.

Classification
See Figure 96.1.

Medicine at a Glance, Fourth Edition. Edited by Patrick Davey. © 2014 John Wiley & Sons, Ltd. Published 2014 by John Wiley & Sons, Ltd. Companion website: www.ataglanceseries.com/medicine

Ventricular septal defect

Ventricular septal defect (VSD) comprises 25% of CHD. A defect in the interventricular septum allows systolic blood flow from the left to right ventricle.

- **Small defects** produce high velocity jets and a loud murmur (maladie de Roger) that is not of haemodynamic significance.
- **Large defects** may have a quiet murmur and a large left-to-right shunt. Untreated, this may cause pulmonary hypertension and Eisenmenger's syndrome. Treatment is surgical closure before pulmonary hypertension develops.

There is a high risk of endocarditis (especially in small defects), so antibiotic prophylaxis is essential.

Atrial septal defect

Atrial septal defect (ASD) comprises 10% of CHD. A defect in the interatrial septum allows shunting of blood from the left to right atrium.

- Secundum ASD: 70%.
- Primum ASD: 30%; often involves the atrioventricular (AV) valves with mitral or tricuspid regurgitation. May be associated with other defects including VSD.

Left-to-right shunting increases pulmonary blood flow, producing a systolic pulmonary flow murmur, wide fixed splitting of the second heart sound and right ventricular hypertrophy (RVH). An electrocardiogram (ECG) shows right bundle branch block (RBBB) with right axis deviation and RVH (secundum) or left axis deviation with RVH (primum). Supraventricular tachycardias, e.g. atrial fibrillation, are common. ASDs may be undetected until adult life when they present with exertional dyspnoea and fatigue. The diagnosis is confirmed by transoesophageal cardiac ultrasonography. Treatment is closure of the defect, either by surgery or by a percutaneous closure device.

Patent ductus arteriosus

Patent ductus arteriosus (PDA) comprises 15% of CHD. The ductus arteriosus fails to close after birth, resulting in left-to-right shunting from the aorta to pulmonary artery and a continuous (machinery) murmur. A large duct with a significant shunt leads to left ventricular hypertrophy (LVH) and heart failure, or pulmonary hypertension and Eisenmenger's syndrome. Duct endocarditis is a significant long-term risk.

Treatment in neonates involves indomethacin blockade of prostaglandin production, which may provoke duct closure. Ducts remaining open require surgical ligation or percutaneous closure (coil or umbrella devices).

Eisenmenger's syndrome

This describes irreversible pulmonary hypertension (from the high pulmonary blood flow of large left-to-right shunts) with shunt reversal (from left to right to right to left) resulting from the high right-sided heart pressures. Patients experience worsening symptoms with breathlessness; there is cyanosis, clubbing and signs of severe pulmonary hypertension. Surgical closure of left-to-right shunts must be undertaken before Eisenmenger's syndrome develops; the only surgical treatment for established Eisenmenger's syndrome is heart–lung transplantation.

Coarctation of the aorta

This comprises 5% of CHD. A developmentally hypoplastic segment of the aorta causes narrowing of the aorta and a significant pressure gradient, usually (98%) immediately distal to the origin of the left subclavian artery. Sixty per cent also have a bicuspid aortic valve. Blood flow to the lower body is maintained by an increase in collateral flow (which may be huge) via the mammary arteries and intercostal arteries. Usually presents as (upper limb) hypertension with absent or weak femoral pulses and radial–femoral delay. There are features of LVH and palpable collaterals around the scapulae. There may be signs of bicuspid aortic valve and systolic murmur from the coarctation. The diagnosis is by echocardiography, computed tomography or magnetic resonance imaging. Treatment is surgical correction of the narrowing, preferably in older childhood (allows a sufficient increase in aortic calibre). Percutaneous dilatation using a balloon is sometimes a viable alternative.

Complex congenital heart disease

In complex CHD there are abnormal relationships of the arteries, ventricles and great vessels, abnormalities of chamber development, often with septal defects, and/or valvular lesions.

Fallot's tetralogy

This is the most common 'complex' CHD (10% of CHD), involving a combination of VSD with right-to-left shunting, due to:

- **Pulmonary stenosis**, either infundibular or valvar.
- **Right ventricular overload** and hypertrophy
- **Dextro position** of the aorta so that it overrides the VSD.

There is cyanosis, clubbing, signs of RVH and a pulmonary systolic murmur (the large VSD does not generate a murmur). Children with Fallot's tetralogy experience exertional breathlessness, dizziness and growth retardation. Squatting kinks the femoral arteries, increases systemic resistance and reduces the right-to-left shunt.

Surgery aims to:

- Totally **correct the defects**, if the pulmonary arteries are large enough.
- Alternatively, **pulmonary blood flow is increased** using systemic to pulmonary artery shunts:
- **Blalock–Taussig shunt**: subclavian artery to pulmonary artery.
- **Waterston's shunt**: ascending aorta to right pulmonary artery.
- **Potts' shunt**: descending aorta to left pulmonary artery.

Ebstein's anomaly

The tricuspid valve is displaced downwards into the right ventricle, resulting in a very small right ventricular cavity and a very large right atrium. There is tricuspid regurgitation and usually an ASD; 20% have accessory pathways (Wolff–Parkinson–White syndrome).

Transposition of the great arteries

There is ventriculo-arterial discordance: the aorta arises from the right ventricle and the pulmonary artery from the left ventricle. In isolation, this is incompatible with life (totally separate pulmonary and systemic circulations); an associated ASD usually allows shunting. Surgical treatments include:

- **Balloon septostomy** (Rashkind): increases shunting and reduces cyanosis.
- **Interatrial shunt** (Mustard or Senning operation): directs systemic venous return from the right atrium across the ASD into the morphological left ventricle; pulmonary venous return passes in the opposite direction and into the aorta.
- **Arterial 'switch' operation** totally corrects the defect by reconnecting the aorta to the left ventricle and the pulmonary artery to the right ventricle.
- **Congenitally corrected transposition**: the right and left ventricles and AV valves are interchanged (venous return drains via the right atrium into a morphological left ventricle, which ejects blood into the pulmonary artery). Usually well tolerated in childhood but heart failure may occur in adult life (the morphological right ventricle cannot sustain systemic pressures long term).

97 Lung function tests

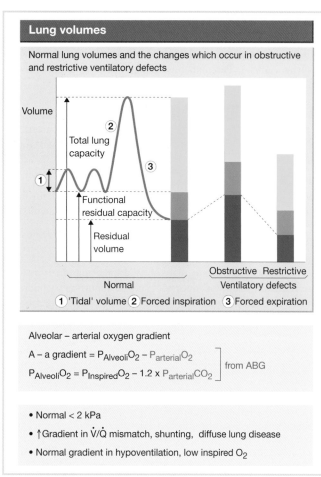

Lung volumes

Normal lung volumes and the changes which occur in obstructive and restrictive ventilatory defects

Volume

② Total lung capacity

③

① 'Tidal' volume ② Forced inspiration ③ Forced expiration

Functional residual capacity

Residual volume

Obstructive Restrictive
Normal   Ventilatory defects

Alveolar – arterial oxygen gradient

$A - a$ gradient $= P_{Alveoli}O_2 - P_{arterial}O_2$

$P_{Alveoli}O_2 = P_{Inspired}O_2 - 1.2 \times P_{arterial}CO_2$ $\Big]$ from ABG

• Normal < 2 kPa

• ↑Gradient in $\dot{V}/\dot{Q}$ mismatch, shunting, diffuse lung disease

• Normal gradient in hypoventilation, low inspired O_2

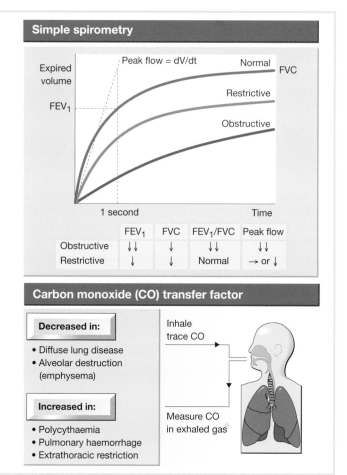

Simple spirometry

Peak flow = dV/dt

Normal FVC

Restrictive

Obstructive

Expired volume

FEV_1

1 second   Time

	FEV_1	FVC	FEV_1/FVC	Peak flow
Obstructive	↓↓	↓	↓↓	↓↓
Restrictive	↓	↓	Normal	→ or ↓

Carbon monoxide (CO) transfer factor

Decreased in:

• Diffuse lung disease
• Alveolar destruction (emphysema)

Increased in:

• Polycythaemia
• Pulmonary haemorrhage
• Extrathoracic restriction

Inhale trace CO

Measure CO in exhaled gas

Spirometric tests of airway function

These are simple, cheap and reproducible:

• **Forced expiratory volume in 1 second** (FEV_1).
• **Forced vital capacity** (FVC): the total volume of air expelled by a forced expiration after maximal inspiration.
• **FEV_1/FVC ratio** (%): the percentage of FVC exhaled in 1 second during forced expiration. These measures allow for the classification of lung diseases into restrictive or obstructive. In obstructive disease the ratio is less than 70% and in restrictive disease there is reduction of both FEV_1 and FVC with a normal or high ratio.
• **Peak expiratory flow rate** (PEFR): fastest flow rate attained at the start of a forced expiration after maximal inspiration. Useful for monitoring changes in airflow obstruction. This is effort dependent and can be reduced in restrictive disease so it is not useful in isolation as a diagnostic test.
• **Reversibility testing**: measurement of airway function before and after an inhaled bronchodilator. An improvement of $\geq 20\%$ and 300 mL represents a positive test.

Lung volumes

Total lung capacity (TLC) is measured by dilution of an inert gas such as helium or in an enclosed box (total body plethysmograph):

• TLC: the total amount of gas in the lungs at maximal inspiration. Residual volume is the amount of gas left in the lung after maximal expiration and is derived from the TLC and vital capacity (VC).
• Functional residual capacity (FRC): the amount of gas left in the lung at end expiration during tidal breathing, derived by helium dilution during tidal breathing.

Tests of gas exchange

• Carbon monoxide transfer factor (K_{CO}): measured by inhalation of a trace of CO, which is avidly taken up by haemoglobin. Assesses the size and efficiency of the gas-exchanging area.
• Pulse oximetry: measured by the absorbance of light by haemoglobin; used to assess hypoxaemia and in particular the response to oxygen therapy. CO_2 is not measured.
• Blood gas analysis (see Chapters 99 and 100).

Other investigations

• **Flow–volume loops** are useful for diagnosing large airway obstruction of both intra- and extrathoracic airways.
• **Tests of respiratory muscles**: muscle power is measured by breathing against a closed orifice or by a sniff. Maximal inspiratory pressure is measured at FRC and expiratory pressure at TLC. Values <60 cmH$_2$O are abnormal.

Medicine at a Glance, Fourth Edition. Edited by Patrick Davey. © 2014 John Wiley & Sons, Ltd. Published 2014 by John Wiley & Sons, Ltd. Companion website: www.ataglanceseries.com/medicine

98 Sleep apnoea

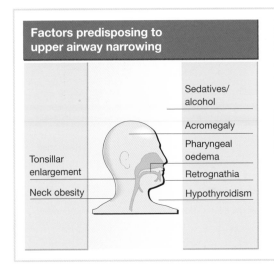

Factors predisposing to upper airway narrowing

Sedatives/alcohol

Acromegaly

Pharyngeal oedema

Retrognathia

Hypothyroidism

Tonsillar enlargement

Neck obesity

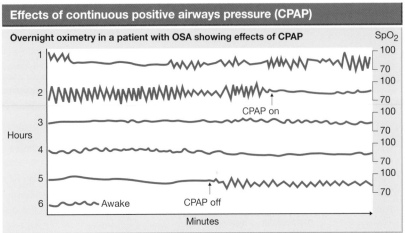

Effects of continuous positive airways pressure (CPAP)

Overnight oximetry in a patient with OSA showing effects of CPAP

SpO₂

CPAP on

Hours

Awake   CPAP off

Minutes

Sleep apnoea may relate to conditions disturbing the control of breathing, although most relates to obstruction to the upper airways – obstructive sleep apnoea (OSA). Pathological episodes of nocturnal apnoea or desaturation often occur during rapid eye movement (REM) sleep in:

- Brainstem disease, either as a result of hypnotics or as a pre-terminal event in many conditions.
- Motor weakness, most commonly motor neuron disease, occasionally from previous poliomyelitis.
- OSA.
- Chronic obstructive pulmonary disease (COPD).

Apnoea leads to hypoxaemia, sometimes profound, arousal and waking. Frequent episodes disturb sleep, resulting in daytime sleepiness. Severe sleep apnoea may lead to nocturnal arrhythmias (and death) or right-sided heart failure.

Obstructive sleep apnoea

A syndrome of upper airway collapse leading to sleep disruption, which results in symptoms, usually of daytime sleepiness. It is very common: 5% of middle-aged adult men are affected. It is more common in men but increasingly recognized in women.

Aetiology

OSA is caused by upper airway narrowing and obstruction due to reduction in muscle tone during sleep. Arousal from sleep results. Sleep fragmentation causes the predominant symptom of excessive daytime sleepiness. Factors leading to upper airway narrowing predispose to OSA:

- Neck obesity, retrognathia and tonsillar enlargement.
- Endocrine abnormalities, including acromegaly, amyloidosis and hypothyroidism predispose to upper airway obstruction by enlarged tissues around the oropharynx.
- Neuromuscular disease or myopathy.
- Alcohol, sedatives and sleep deprivation worsen the effects of an anatomically narrow airway.

Clinical features

Classic symptoms are snoring in association with excessive daytime sleepiness. A partner may describe the episodes of obstruction with apnoea, terminating with a sudden loud gasp. Sleepiness may impair performance at work and there is a seven-fold increased risk of motor accidents. Potential symptoms are of morning headache, poor concentration and impotence. Examination reveals factors predisposing to upper airway narrowing (see Figure 98.1). Hypertension is a common finding.

Investigations

Occasional obstructions are common in snorers and do not require investigation unless associated with sleepiness. Overnight sleep studies including video and pulse oximetry confirm the diagnosis. Apnoea typically decreases oxygen saturation by ≥4%; such episodes may occur many times each hour (see Figure 98.1). Full polysomnography studies include electroencephalography and measurement of airflow, ribcage and abdominal movement, as well as recording snoring and continuous oximetry. Endocrine or neurophysiology studies are occasionally appropriate.

Treatment and prognosis

Avoid alcohol and sedatives. Treat any underlying illness.

- **Severe cases**: continuous positive airway pressure (CPAP) delivered overnight by a tight-fitting nasal mask splints the upper airway open, prevents obstruction and arousal, and results in rapid improvement in symptoms. NICE guidance recommends CPAP for severe OSA and moderate OSA when associated with significant sleepiness. Treatment of severe OSA with CPAP improves 24-hour mean blood pressure significantly.
- **Milder cases**: weight loss and/or mandibular advancement devices may be sufficient.
- **Surgery**: tonsillectomy may be curative, particularly in young patients with significant tonsillar enlargement. Palatal surgery may help but, if unsuccessful, can make future application of CPAP difficult.

Effective treatment results in rapid improvement of symptoms.

Medicine at a Glance, Fourth Edition. Edited by Patrick Davey. © 2014 John Wiley & Sons, Ltd. Published 2014 by John Wiley & Sons, Ltd. Companion website: www.ataglanceseries.com/medicine

99 Respiratory failure

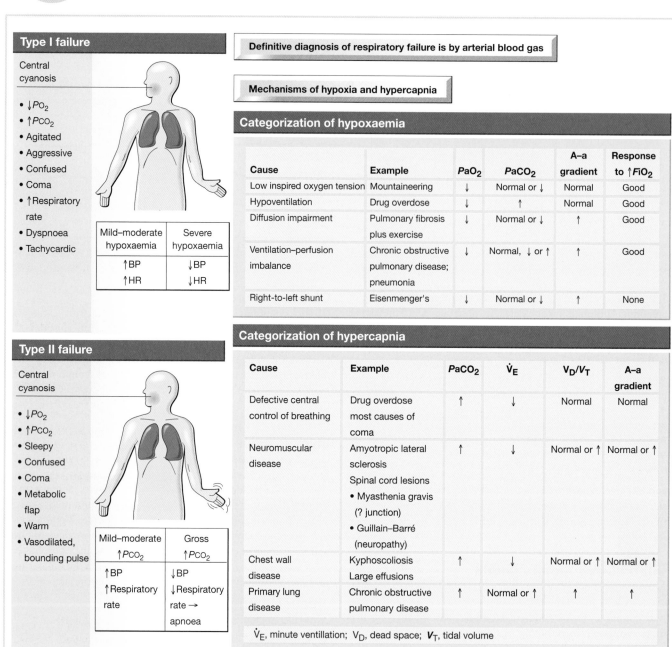

Type I failure

Central cyanosis

- $\downarrow PO_2$
- $\uparrow PCO_2$
- Agitated
- Aggressive
- Confused
- Coma
- $\uparrow$ Respiratory rate
- Dyspnoea
- Tachycardic

Mild–moderate hypoxaemia	Severe hypoxaemia
$\uparrow$ BP	$\downarrow$ BP
$\uparrow$ HR	$\downarrow$ HR

Type II failure

Central cyanosis

- $\downarrow PO_2$
- $\uparrow PCO_2$
- Sleepy
- Confused
- Coma
- Metabolic flap
- Warm
- Vasodilated, bounding pulse

Mild–moderate $\uparrow PCO_2$	Gross $\uparrow PCO_2$
$\uparrow$ BP	$\downarrow$ BP
$\uparrow$ Respiratory rate	$\downarrow$ Respiratory rate $\rightarrow$ apnoea

Definitive diagnosis of respiratory failure is by arterial blood gas

Mechanisms of hypoxia and hypercapnia

Categorization of hypoxaemia

Cause	Example	PaO_2	$PaCO_2$	A–a gradient	Response to $\uparrow FiO_2$
Low inspired oxygen tension	Mountaineering	$\downarrow$	Normal or $\downarrow$	Normal	Good
Hypoventilation	Drug overdose	$\downarrow$	$\uparrow$	Normal	Good
Diffusion impairment	Pulmonary fibrosis plus exercise	$\downarrow$	Normal or $\downarrow$	$\uparrow$	Good
Ventilation–perfusion imbalance	Chronic obstructive pulmonary disease; pneumonia	$\downarrow$	Normal, $\downarrow$ or $\uparrow$	$\uparrow$	Good
Right-to-left shunt	Eisenmenger's	$\downarrow$	Normal or $\downarrow$	$\uparrow$	None

Categorization of hypercapnia

Cause	Example	$PaCO_2$	$\dot{V}_E$	V_D/V_T	A–a gradient
Defective central control of breathing	Drug overdose most causes of coma	$\uparrow$	$\downarrow$	Normal	Normal
Neuromuscular disease	Amyotropic lateral sclerosis Spinal cord lesions • Myasthenia gravis (? junction) • Guillain–Barré (neuropathy)	$\uparrow$	$\downarrow$	Normal or $\uparrow$	Normal or $\uparrow$
Chest wall disease	Kyphoscoliosis Large effusions	$\uparrow$	$\downarrow$	Normal or $\uparrow$	Normal or $\uparrow$
Primary lung disease	Chronic obstructive pulmonary disease	$\uparrow$	Normal or $\uparrow$	$\uparrow$	$\uparrow$

$\dot{V}_E$, minute ventillation; V_D, dead space; V_T, tidal volume

---

Respiratory failure may be acute, chronic or acute-on-chronic (e.g. a patient with an exacerbation of chronic obstructive pulmonary disease (COPD) and pre-existing hypoxia). Abnormal levels of arterial oxygen (PaO_2 <8 kPa) or carbon dioxide ($PaCO_2$ >6.0 kPa) are used to define the presence of respiratory failure, which is thus divided into:

- Hypoxaemic (type I): failure of oxygenation.
- Hypercapnic (type II): failure of ventilation to remove CO_2.

Generally hypercapnic failure is the result of a disorder with respiratory muscles ('pump failure'), whereas hypoxaemic failure is usually due to pulmonary pathology. However, type II respiratory failure often supersedes type I failure as the patient becomes exhausted.

What is the A–a gradient?

Alveolar O_2 and CO_2 levels are interdependent and a high alveolar partial pressure of carbon dioxide results in a lower partial pressure of oxygen. The alveolar–arterial oxygen gradient (A–a gradient) is calculated from the alveolar gas equation and is a measure of ventilation and perfusion mismatch (reflecting the severity of lung disease).

Medicine at a Glance, Fourth Edition. Edited by Patrick Davey. © 2014 John Wiley & Sons, Ltd. Published 2014 by John Wiley & Sons, Ltd. Companion website: www.ataglanceseries.com/medicine

$$A - a \text{ gradient} = FiO_2 \text{ (atmospheric pressure} - \text{water pressure)}$$
$$- PaO_2 - 1.25(PCO_2)$$
$$= 0.21 (101 \text{ kPa} - 6.3 \text{ kPa}) - PaO_2 - 1.25(PCO_2)$$
$$= 19.9 \text{ kPa} - PaO_2$$
$$- 1.25(PCO_2) \text{ (on air } - 21\% \text{ oxygen)}$$

A normal A–a gradient is 2–4 kPa; it increases with age and at $FiO_2 > 0.28$ (FiO_2 = fraction of O_2 in inspired air). Certain disease processes also increase the A–a gradient (see Figure 99.1); measuring the A–a gradient is thus helpful in ruling in or out these diseases in patients with respiratory failure.

Causes of hypoxaemia

- **Shunt**: the lung is perfused but not ventilated (the opposite of dead space). A right-to-left shunt leads to hypoxaemia that does not respond to 100% oxygen.
- **Ventilation/perfusion mismatch** ($\dot{V}/\dot{Q}$ mismatch): *this is by far the commonest form*, even in diseases like pulmonary fibrosis where one might expect diffusion block. Poorly ventilated alveoli contribute to hypoxaemia, which is overcome by an increase in FiO_2.
- **Diffusion block**: a thickened interstitium between alveolus and capillary (uncommon). Only important during exercise when erythrocytes have insufficient time to equilibrate for gas exchange.
- **Low FiO_2 at altitude**.
- **Hypoventilation**: ventilation is inversely proportional to $PaCO_2$. The interdependence of PaO_2 and $PaCO_2$ thus leads to hypoxaemia in hypoventilation.

All causes of hypoxaemia other than true shunts improve with an increase in FiO_2.

Causes of hypercapnia

This is a failure of ventilation, which may be caused by central nervous system, neuromuscular, chest wall or primary lung diseases. There is either insufficient respiratory drive or ineffective (increased dead space) ventilation.

Symptoms and signs of respiratory failure

See Figure 99.1.

Treatment of respiratory failure

It is important to establish whether the onset of respiratory failure is acute, chronic or acute-on-chronic, and the underlying aetiology. Patients need to be appropriately monitored in a critical care area. Ideally monitoring should include respiratory rate, continuous electrocardiogram (ECG), oximetry, arterial line (blood pressure (BP), arterial blood gas (ABG) analysis) and Glasgow Coma Score (GCS). Although, as discussed below, one can treat the consequences of respiratory failure (hypoxaemia and hypercapnia) the **cornerstone of management is treating the underlying disease process**. This is considered in the following chapters on specific respiratory diseases.

Hypoxaemia

Oxygen may be delivered by variable or fixed performance devices.

Variable performance devices Air is entrained during breathing whilst oxygen is delivered from a reservoir. The latter may be the nasopharynx, mask or reservoir bag. The FiO_2 delivered to the lungs therefore depends on the oxygen flow rate, the patient's inspiratory flow, respiratory rate and the amount of air entrained. Examples include:

- **Nasal cannulae**: oxygen flow rates up to 4 L/min (higher rates dry the nasal mucosa). The nasopharynx acts as a reservoir. FiO_2 varies between breaths for a given flow rate depending on the patient's respiration; delivers between 24% and 34%.
- **Facemask**: flow rates must exceed 5 L/min to stop rebreathing of CO_2. Mask provides additional reservoir to oro/nasopharynx. FiO_2 can be 50–60% at 15 L/min.
- **Non-rebreathing masks**: these have a reservoir bag, which should be full before placing on the patient. A one-way valve stops exhaled air entering the oxygen reservoir. High flow rates of 10–15 L/min provide $FiO_2 > 60\%$ (often approaching 100%).

Fixed performance devices These are independent of the patient's pattern of breathing and use the Venturi device to entrain air into the mask, exceeding inspiratory flow and thus deliver a fixed oxygen concentration. Typically colour-coded and deliver 24% (blue), 28% (white), 35% (yellow), 40% (red) or 60% (green) FiO_2 for a prescribed flow rate.

- **Continuous positive airway pressure** (CPAP): uses a tight-fitting mask and a flow generator to delivery a positive pressure throughout the respiratory cycle (5–15 cmH$_2$O). This increases functional residual capacity, thereby recruiting more alveoli and improving oxygenation.
- **Intubation and mechanical ventilation**: may be required if hypoxia does not respond to treating the underlying disease, oxygen therapy and/or CPAP.

What is adequate oxygenation?

Generally one should aim for oxygen saturations exceeding 90% as this puts the patient on the flat part of the oxygen dissociation curve. Further increases in PaO_2 will have only small effects on oxygen delivery (as almost all oxygen in blood is bound to haemoglobin). The British Thoracic Society have issued guidelines for emergency oxygen use in adults and recommend saturations of 94–98% for most acutely ill patients or 88–92% for those at risk of hypercapnia. However, caution should be exercised about relying too much on oxygen saturations alone. Despite adequate oxygen the patient may continue to deteriorate and require invasive ventilation. Furthermore oximetry gives no information on the patient's CO_2 or pH. Some patients (e.g. many with COPD) with chronic hypoxia depend on hypoxaemia rather than hypercapnia to drive respiration, and oxygen therapy may remove this drive and stop them breathing (whilst initially being well oxygenated!). It is essential to continue to monitor patients when supplemental oxygen is prescribed and ideally an ABG should be performed.

Hypercapnia

Any sedative drugs should be reversed or avoided (opiates, benzodiazepines). If hypercapnia and respiratory acidosis persist, despite treating the underlying condition, artificial ventilation should be considered. Non-invasive ventilation is now widely available and can be delivered via nasal, face, full face or helmet interfaces. It is not a substitute for invasive ventilation, which should be adopted if this method fails.

Indications for intubation and mechanical ventilation in respiratory failure

- Apnoea.
- ↑ Acidosis, $PaCO_2$.
- $PaO_2 < 8$ kPa despite $FiO_2 > 0.5$ (±CPAP).
- GCS <8.
- Unable to clear pulmonary secretions by conventional methods.
- Tiring; ↑ respiratory rate, tachycardia, dyskinetic respiratory pattern.

100 Arterial blood gas analysis

Arterial blood gas analysis

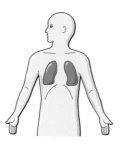

An arterial blood gas from a patient having taken an overdose of opiate shows a pH of 7.29, PaO_2 8 kPa and $PaCO_2$ 8 kPa on room air. The patient has a respiratory acidosis and is hypoxaemic because of hypoventilation, but has a normal A-a gradient as the lungs are normal

$PaO_2 = FiO_2$ (atmospheric pressure – water vapour pressure) – (1.25 x $PaCO_2$)

$PaO_2 = 0.21$ (101–6.3) – (1.25 x 8)

$PaO_2 = 19.9 - 10 = 9.9$ kPa

A-a gradient ($P_AO_2 - PaO_2$) = 9.9 – 8 = 1.9 kPa (normal 2–4 kPa)

Henderson–Hasselbach equation

The bicarbonate buffer system

Carbonic anhydrase

$$CO_2 + H_2O \leftrightarrow H_2CO_3 \leftrightarrow HCO_3^- + H^+$$

The Henderson–Hasselbach equation

→ $K = [HCO_3^-] \times [H^+] / [H_2CO_3]$

From the law of mass action
K = dissociation constant

→ $K_A = [HCO_3^-] \times [H^+] / [H_2CO_3]$

At equilibrium $[CO_2] \alpha [H_2CO_3]$
K_A = corrected dissociation constant

→ $\log K_A = \log [H^+] + \log ([HCO_3^-] / [CO_2])$

→ $-\log [H^+] = -\log K_A + \log ([HCO_3^-] / [CO_2])$

→ $pH = pK_A + \log ([HCO_3^-] / [CO_2])$

(Henderson–Hasselbach equation)

Respiratory acidosis

$PaCO_2$ increases, pH falls: compensation kidneys retain HCO_3^-
- Central nervous system depression: sedatives, CNS disease
- Lung disease: COPD, pneumonia, asthma, pulmonary oedema, ARDS
- Musculoskelatal disorders: kyphoscoliosis, chest trauma, Guillain–Barré, myasthenia gravis

Metabolic acidosis

HCO_3^- falls, pH falls: compensation $PaCO_2$ falls
Increased anion gap
- Ketoacidosis: diabetic ketoacidosis, alcohol, starvation
- Poisons: methanol, ethylene glycol, salicylates
- Renal failure
- Lactic acidosis: sepsis, cardiac failure, metformin
Normal anion gap
- GI loss of HCO_3^-: diarrhoea, ileostomy
- Renal loss of HCO_3^-: proximal renal tubular acidosis, carbonic anhydrase inhibitor

Respiratory alkalosis

$PaCO_2$ falls, pH increases: compensation kidneys excrete HCO_3^-
- Catastrophic CNS event
- Altitude
- Drugs: salicylates
- Anxiety

Metabolic alkalosis

HCO_3^- increases, pH increases: compensation minute volume falls and $PaCO_2$ rises (this is the least complete form of compensation because of the effect of hypercapnia and hypoxia on respiratory drive)
- H^+ ion loss: vomiting, diuretics, hypokalaemia
- Bicarbonate administration
- Cushing's and Conn's syndrome

The ability to correctly interpret arterial blood gas (ABG) samples is essential for the management of critically ill patients. Blood gas analysers have three electrodes which measure pH, PaO_2 and $PaCO_2$ at 37°C. Values for bicarbonate (HCO_3^-), base excess (BE) and oxygen saturations (SaO_2) are then *calculated* from these variables. Some blood gas analysers used in critical care or the emergency department have a co-oximeter and also *measure* SaO_2, carboxyhaemoglobin, methaemoglobin and haemoglobin content. They also measure lactate. An ABG provides information about the patient's oxygenation (PaO_2 and SaO_2), ventilation ($PaCO_2$) and acid–base balance (pH, $PaCO_2$, bicarbonate, BE). It is only possible to interpret whether the patient is oxygenating normally if the inspired oxygen fraction is recorded; it is therefore essential that the concentration of oxygen the patient receives is written down.

Although the vast majority of blood gas samples are arterial, occasionally these samples are venous or capillary. Venous samples should generally not be used; however in critical care, a central venous oxygen saturation (ScvO$_2$) may be obtained

in shock states to assess if global oxygen delivery has been adequate (see Chapter 18). In respiratory clinics the application of a topical vasodilator to the earlobe allows a capillary sample to be drawn, which approximates closely to an arterial sample. To avoid spurious measurements of PaO_2 and $PaCO_2$, once the sample is drawn any air should be expelled, and if the measurement is not performed immediately the sample should be transported on ice.

Blood gas values

Normal values for an ABG are as follows:
- pH 7.35–7.45.
- $PaCO_2$ 4.5–6 kPa.
- PaO_2 10–13 kPa.
- HCO_3^- 22–26 mmol/L.
- BE −2 to +2.

The arterial partial pressure of oxygen (PaO_2) is lower than the alveolar partial pressure (P_AO_2) because of imperfections in ventilation/perfusion ($\dot{V}/\dot{Q}$) matching, even in normal lungs.

Medicine at a Glance, Fourth Edition. Edited by Patrick Davey. © 2014 John Wiley & Sons, Ltd. Published 2014 by John Wiley & Sons, Ltd. Companion website: www.ataglanceseries.com/medicine

This alveolar–arterial (A–a) gradient is approximately 2–4 kPa in normal lungs (at the higher end of the range with increased age). Gas in the alveolus differs from inspired air in that the partial pressure of carbon dioxide is much higher and therefore within the alveolus the partial pressures of oxygen and carbon dioxide are interdependent. This relationship is defined by the alveolar gas equation:

$$P_AO_2 = FiO_2 \text{ (atmospheric pressure – water vapour pressure)} - (1.25 \times PaCO_2)$$

The alveolar gas equation enables one to deduce the P_AO_2 and hence the A–a gradient (see Chapter 99). Any significant cardiopulmonary disease can increase the A–a gradient and in effect this represents increased $\dot{V}/\dot{Q}$ mismatch. Simple hypoventilation (with normal lungs) will result in hypercapnia and hypoxia but the A–a gradient remains normal (see Figure 100.1).

The $PaCO_2$ is inversely proportional to effective minute volume. Acute changes in $PaCO_2$ lead to predictable changes in pH. Thus pH falls by 0.1 for a 2.6 kPa rise, and rises by 0.1 for a 1.3 kPa fall in $PaCO_2$ with respect to normal. Changes in pH outside this range have a metabolic contribution.

pH is the negative log of the hydrogen ion concentration and homeostatic mechanisms generally keep this value within a narrow range. Since this is a logarithmic scale a change in pH of one unit represents a ten-fold change in hydrogen ion concentration. Bicarbonate (actual and standard) (and BE) are calculated from the pH and $PaCO_2$ using the Henderson–Hasselbalch equation (see Figure 100.1). The actual bicarbonate is the calculated bicarbonate using the $PaCO_2$ measured in the sample, whilst the standard bicarbonate is the calculated value using a 'normal' $PaCO_2$ (usually 5.3 kPa). The purpose of the two values is to help differentiate the components of acid–base disturbance. For example, in a pure respiratory acidosis (low pH and high $PaCO_2$) actual bicarbonate will be low, but standard bicarbonate will be normal. BE is a measure of the amount of acid or alkali that must be added under standard conditions (37°C and $PaCO_2$ 5.3 kPa) to return the pH to 7.4 and is thus a measure of the metabolic component of acid–base abnormalities.

Acid–base homeostasis

The body tightly regulates pH within a narrow range by the use of buffers and the excretion of acid by the kidneys and lungs. Buffers bind or release hydrogen ions and limit sudden changes in pH. The principal buffers in blood are haemoglobin, plasma proteins and bicarbonate; however it is the latter which is the most important. Carbon dioxide combines with water to form carbonic acid, which then dissociates into a hydrogen ion and bicarbonate. The Henderson–Hasselbalch equation describes the relationship between pH, $PaCO_2$ and bicarbonate. Since $PaCO_2$ and bicarbonate can be controlled independently by the lungs and kidneys, respectively, these organs regulate changes in pH. Thus when a metabolic acidosis develops, minute ventilation increases to reduce $PaCO_2$ and to return pH towards normal. Similarly during hypoventilation (reduced minute volume) $PaCO_2$ rises and an acute respiratory acidosis develops. If this situation persists over several days the kidneys retain bicarbonate and pH returns towards normal. Compensation by the lungs can occur quickly as minute volume is regulated instantaneously, whereas renal compensation occurs over days. In any case where compensation occurs it is rarely complete, in other words the pH returns towards normal but not quite to the previous level. Disorders of acid–base homeostasis can therefore be defined as respiratory acidosis, metabolic acidosis, respiratory alkalosis and metabolic alkalosis (see Figure 100.1 and Chapter 143).

The **anion gap** is used in the differential diagnosis of metabolic acidosis; it is:

$$([Na^+] + [K^+]) - ([Cl^-] + [HCO_3^-]) = 8-16 \text{ mmol/L}$$

Since electrical neutrality always exists, the gap represents unmeasured cations (Ca^{2+}, Mg^{2+}) and anions (PO_4^{2-}, sulphates, albumin, organic acids). In some diseases the gap is increased because of other unmeasured anions, e.g. ketones in diabetic ketoacidosis, ethylene glycol or salicylate in poisoning (see Figure 100.1).

A practical approach to blood gas interpretation

- Note the inspired fraction of oxygen; is the patient hypoxaemic, in other words is the PaO_2 low? Does the patient have an oxygenation problem? The PaO_2 may be normal (say 12 kPa), but if this is taken on 60% oxygen there is an oxygenation problem. This will be manifested by an increase in the A–a gradient (see Chapter 99 for what represents adequate oxygenation).
- Is the pH normal or is the patient acidotic (<7.35) or alkalotic (>7.45)?
- Examine the $PaCO_2$ and standard bicarbonate to see if the problem is respiratory or metabolic.
- Check to see if there is compensation.
- In a metabolic acidosis calculate the anion gap.

101 Chest X-ray anatomy

Normal adult male chest X-ray

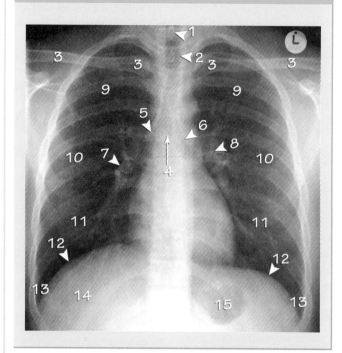

Normal adult female chest X-ray

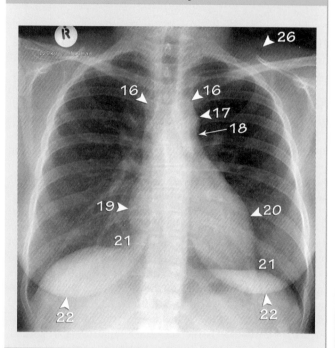

Normal adult male chest X-ray

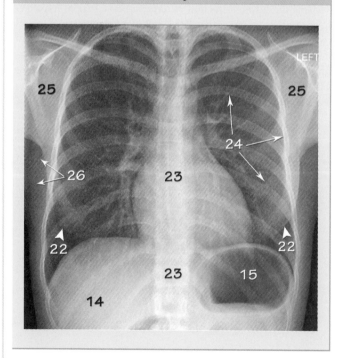

Key

1	Spinous process	14	Liver
2	Trachea	15	Stomach bubble
3	Clavicle	16	Sternum
4	Carina	17	Aortic knuckle
5	Right main bronchus	18	Aorto-pulmonary window
6	Left main bronchus	19	Right atrial edge
7	Right pulmonary artery	20	Left ventricular edge
8	Left pulmonary artery	21	Cardiophrenic angles
9	Upper lung zone	22	Breast
10	Middle lung zone	23	Spine
11	Lower lung zone	24	5th rib (left)
12	Diaphragm	25	Scapula
13	Costophrenic angle	26	Fat in soft tissue

Medicine at a Glance, Fourth Edition. Edited by Patrick Davey. © 2014 John Wiley & Sons, Ltd. Published 2014 by John Wiley & Sons, Ltd. Companion website: www.ataglanceseries.com/medicine

Chest anatomy seen on posteroanterior view

The five principal densities seen on plain imaging should be used as reference points to identify anatomical and pathological structures.

- **Black** – air/gas
- **Dark grey** – fat
- **Light grey** – soft tissue/fluid
- **White** – bone and calcified structures
- **Bright white** – metal

It is important to remember that adjacent structures of different densities form defined edges.

Important anatomical landmarks and structures on a normal chest X-ray

Airways and lungs

These are dark areas due to their high air content:

- **Trachea**: seen as a central vertical lucent tubular structure overlying the vertebral column. The right edge of the trachea, otherwise known as the right paratracheal stripe, is usually thin and well defined because it lies adjacent to the air-dense lung. The left edge, however, lies adjacent to the oesophagus (posterior to the trachea) and great vessels (left of the trachea) and therefore blends in due to their soft tissue density.
- **Carina**: the bifurcation of the trachea.
- **Right main bronchus**: shorter, wider and more vertical than the left main bronchus. This increases the chance of aspiration affecting the right lung.
- **Left main bronchus**: more horizontal due to its passage over the left atrium of the heart.
- **Left lung**: the upper, lingula and lower lobes are not clearly demarcated on a posteroanterior (PA) chest X-ray (CXR). It is therefore best to describe the location of a lesion in terms of upper, middle and lower lung 'zones'. Each zone can then be compared with its counterpart in the contralateral lung.
- **Right lung**: the upper and middle lobes are delineated by the horizontal fissure, which is often visible. The lower lobe cannot be clearly demarcated from the other lobes. Displacement of the horizontal fissure may help determine the location of a disease process.

Mediastinum

The mediastinum is the middle part of the chest and includes all the organs *except the lungs*, i.e. the heart, great vessels, trachea, oesophagus, thymus, lymph nodes, phrenic and vagus nerves.

Due to the similar soft tissue densities of these adjacent structures it may be difficult to clearly identify individual structures. The contours of the heart, aorta and trachea are, however, usually identifiable.

Heart

The heart appears as a large soft tissue density structure. The heart borders are made up of the following:

- **Left border** (superior to inferior): aortic knuckle/arch, aorto-pulmonary window, left atrial appendage, left ventricle.
- **Right border** (superior to inferior): superior vena cava, right atrium.
- **Inferior border** (in contact with diaphragm): right ventricle.

Hila

The hila are seen as concave structures formed by the configuration of the divergent pulmonary vessels and bronchi. The *left hilum is usually slightly higher* than the right.

Hemidiaphragms

The highest point of the *right hemidiaphragm is slightly higher* than that of the left to accommodate the liver. A dark rounded area is usually seen under the left hemidiaphragm, which is the *gastric air bubble*. This should not be confused with free intra-abdominal gas, which forms a dark crescent under the diaphragm (pneumoperitoneum).

Costophrenic and cardiophrenic angles

Each hemidiaphragm forms a sharp angle at the point of contact with the thoracic wall, known as the costophrenic angle. Loss or blunting of this angle may be due to lung pathology or fluid accumulation in the pleural space (pleural effusion). Each hemidiaphragm also forms an angle at the point of contact with the pericardium, known as the cardiophrenic angle.

Bones and soft tissues

The bones visible on a CXR include:

- **Spine**: lower cervical spine to upper lumbar spine.
- **Sternum**.
- **Ribs**.
- **Clavicles**.
- **Scapulae**.
- **Upper left and right humerus**.

The soft tissues visible on a CXR include:

- **Breasts**: may mimic lung shadowing, particularly if large or asymmetrical.
- **Normal soft tissues of the neck and thoracic wall**: may be separated by layers of well-defined fat tissue, which appear darker.

102 Basic chest X-ray interpretation

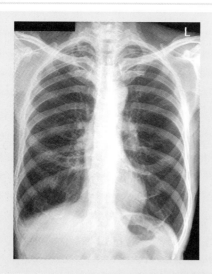

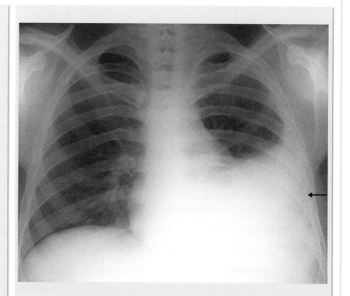

Typical chest X-ray in COPD; the lungs are hyperinflated. There are several radiological signs for this; counting the posterior ribs (i.e. the ribs just as they leave the spinal column) – normal is 8–9, so ≥10 is abnormal. Alternatively, count the number of the last rib that can be seen crossing the diaphragm. The 8th rib can be seen here, ≥7 is abnormal. The diaphragms are flat, and the heart shadow is 'thin'. BEWARE that though COPD can be strongly suggested from the chest X-ray, it cannot really be diagnosed from the chest X-ray. Always confirm the presence of COPD by lung function tests, and its functional impact by, among other tests, blood gases. As pneumothoraces are common in COPD these should always be looked for (they can 'hide' in the lung apexes); as cigarette smoking is almost universal, always look for radiological evidence of lung cancer in these patients

This chest X-ray shows a large left pleural effusion. Instead of the normal appearance, with the lung clearly visible to the diaphragm, only the top half of the lung is visible. It is not possible to see the left border of the heart, nor the left diaphragm, unlike normal. This is because both these structures have pleural fluid abutting against them; clearly defined edges in X-rays rely on there being differences in composition between adjacent structures, e.g. air (lungs) and fluid (heart). These edges disappear when the composition becomes identical, as with a pleural effusion

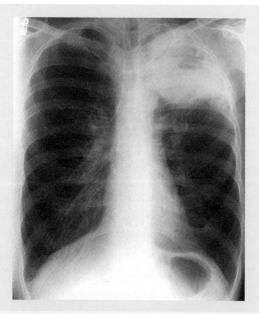

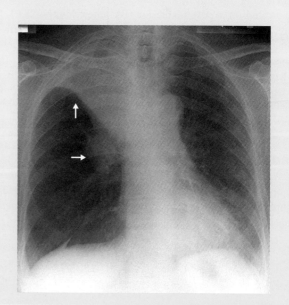

This chest X-ray shows an obvious abnormality at the top (apex) of the left lung. There is a roughly circular structure, quite large, white (so fluid filled) for which there is a differential diagnosis, including consolidation and even tumour. It has a 'fluid level' within it, in other words, about half way up, there is a line, above which one can see an air-filled space (darker area); this is a typical appearance of an area of consolidation, with abscess formation, in this case, due to tuberculosis (the clue to this diagnosis being the apical position)

Right upper lobe collapse. There is a wedge-shaped opacification radiating out from the hilum. The horizontal fissure has been pulled up, implying that whatever is going on has led to loss of upper lobe lung volume, and hence the compensatory fissure movement. Inspection of the right hilum reveals a mass, hence the diagnosis here is a tumour (almost certainly malignant) in the right hilum obstructing the bronchus leading to the right upper lobes, resulting in collapse of this lobe

Medicine at a Glance, Fourth Edition. Edited by Patrick Davey. © 2014 John Wiley & Sons, Ltd. Published 2014 by John Wiley & Sons, Ltd. Companion website: www.ataglanceseries.com/medicine

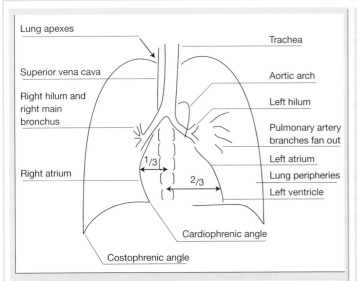

Structure seen in the normal chest X-ray. An abnormality may be obvious, but if not, check the apexes (lung cancer or tuberculosis are commonly restricted to this area), the bases (small pleural effusions can easily be missed), behind the mediastinal contents for, amongst others, signs of left lower lobe collapse (the sail sign). If the patient is genuinely in respiratory failure (confirmed by blood gases), and the chest X-ray is normal, think of: 1) pulmonary emboli (common) – a cardiac ultrasound may help early management (expect some right heart dilatation and decrease in function); 2) *Pneumocystis jirovecii* pneumonia (rare in the UK) – reviewing the history may help; 3) early pneumonia; 4) early ARDS – for 3&4 repeating the chest X-ray after a few hours may help (treat empirically in the mean time)

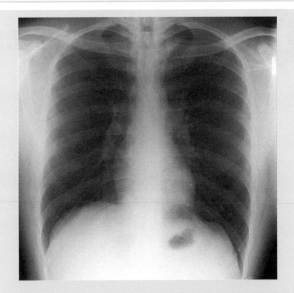

This is a normal chest X-ray. How do we recognize normality here? Largely, by experience; always look at the X-rays of your patients, and interpret them before you have seen the official report. You should check the X-ray systematically; check name, date of birth, date of X-ray, then look at the lungs, are they normal, the hilar regions, then the cardiac silhouette, for shape and size. Next look at the mediastinum, for masses and tracheal shift, then the diaphragms (are they too high, too flat?) and also ensure that the costophrenic angles are clear, sharp and deep. Finally check the bones for abnormalities, such as rib fractures, malignant deposits, etc., and the soft tissues (has there been a mastectomy, etc?)

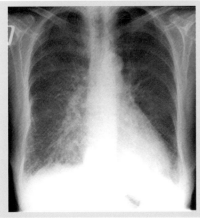

A chest X-ray from a patient with left heart failure (=pulmonary oedema). There are a number of characteristic findings: 1) the heart is enlarged (the normal cardiothoracic ratio is ≤50%; 2) there is interstitial pulmonary oedema ('fuzzy' shadows), especially in the mid and lower zones (where the pulmonary venous pressure is highest – provided the patient has been upright!); 3) the upper lobe veins, which are usually smaller than the lower lobe ones, have become enlarged (upper lobe venous diversion, otherwise known as pulmonary venous imbalance). There is fluid in the lymphatics, seen as Kerley B lines (short horizontal lines 1–2 cm in length, extending horizontally from the lower outer lung fields; heart failure is the commonest cause, though malignancy and infection rarely can underlie them); 4) there are small bilateral pleural effusions (shadowing at both lung bases). The shape of the heart usually gives no clues as to the cause of the heart failure; occasionally, enlargement of the left atrium, seen as: 1) great splaying of the left and right bronchi to ≥ 90°, 2) a large 3rd bulge down the left heart border – the aorta is the 1st, the pulmonary artery the 2nd, and the ventricle the 4th – leads one to suspect mitral valve disease

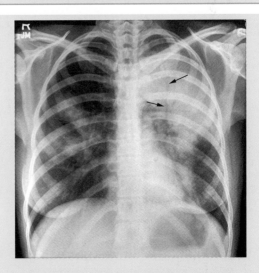

A chest X-ray from a patient with pneumococcal pneumonia. There is extensive shadowing of the left upper zone, within which an air bronchogram (arrows) is seen. An air bronchogram is a pathognomonic sign of consolidation – and by far the commonest cause of consolidation is an infective process. There is also some patchy shadowing in the right mid zone. Respiratory failure is unusual in otherwise well patients who develop pneumonia, but can occur if the infection is severe, or if there is underlying lung disease, such as COPD (which the chest X-ray may underestimate). BEWARE also that patients immobile from septic processes can also develop pulmonary emboli, which can contribute to hypoxaemia. Clinical deterioration in a patient known to have pneumonia may relate to worsening of the infective process, but also may be due to PEs

103 Chest X-ray cases 1

(a) Cardiomegaly

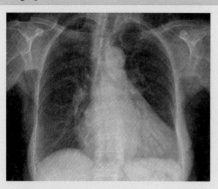

The heart is abnormally large. It takes up greater than 50% of the internal width of the thorax. The patient was known to have left ventricular failure

(b) Pulmonary oedema

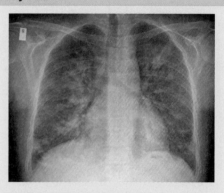

The heart is not enlarged but there are signs of pulmonary oedema with shadowing spreading from the hila. The patient was diabetic and presented with acute myocardial infarction and left ventricular failure

(c) Kerley B lines

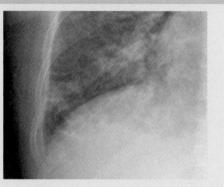

Close-up of costophrenic angle of pulmonary oedema (b). Here septal 'Kerley B' lines are seen. These are horizontal lines that reach the pleural surface. They are caused by fluid between the interlobular septa and are a specific sign of pulmonary oedema

(d) Pleural effusions

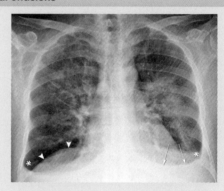

This patient with heart failure has pulmonary oedema and fluid is filling the pleural cavities forming pleural effusions (arrows). The costophrenic angles (*) are blunted. The dome of the diaphragm is still visible (arrowheads)

(e) Prosthetic heart valves

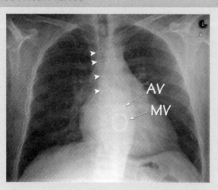

The heart is enlarged due to left ventricular failure. There is evidence of previous cardiac surgery with midline sternotomy wires (arrowheads) and metallic replacements of both the aortic valve (AV) and the mitral valve (MV)

(f) Asbestos plaques

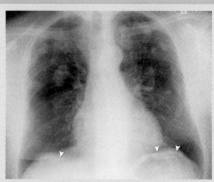

There are multiple dense irregular-shaped opacities over both lungs. These are typical appearances of asbestos plaques. The give-away sign is the layering of dense material over the diaphragm (arrowheads)

Medicine at a Glance, Fourth Edition. Edited by Patrick Davey. © 2014 John Wiley & Sons, Ltd. Published 2014 by John Wiley & Sons, Ltd. Companion website: www.ataglanceseries.com/medicine

Cardiomegaly

Cardiomegaly is an abnormal enlargement of the heart where the *maximum width of the heart shadow is greater than 50% of the maximum internal width of the thorax*. The causes include:

- **Hypertrophy**: caused by an increase in afterload of a particular chamber (e.g. aortic stenosis, hypertension).
- **Dilatation**: secondary to toxic, metabolic or infectious agents causing myocardial damage.

Hypertrophy of either ventricle does not usually enlarge the heart shadow unless there is synchronous dilatation. Cardiomegaly is usually abnormal, except in athletes, and is associated with other cardiovascular pathology. The shape of an enlarged heart on a chest X-ray (CXR) will depend upon the chamber affected and it may point to the cause:

- A 'globular' shape occurs with pericardial effusion or generalized cardiomyopathy.
- Left ventricular (LV) dilatation causes lengthening and rounding of the left heart border and a downward extension of the apex.
- Right ventricular dilatation lifts the apex off the hemidiaphragm.
- Left atrial enlargement causes a double density along the right heart border, comprising the left and right atrial edges. Other signs include left atrial appendage prominence and bronchial splaying of the bronchi at the carina.

Pulmonary oedema

Pulmonary oedema occurs when fluid leaks into the lung interstitium from the pulmonary vasculature, leading to impairment of gaseous exchange. It is caused by either an *increase in vascular hydrostatic pressure* (e.g. cardiogenic causes – LV dysfunction, mitral stenosis), a *decrease in plasma oncotic pressure* (e.g. liver failure, renal failure) or an *increase in pulmonary capillary membrane permeability* (e.g. adult respiratory distress syndrome, aspiration, inhalation injury, neurogenic pulmonary oedema, multiple blood transfusions).

The CXR features of pulmonary oedema include:
- **Absence/presence of cardiomegaly**: cardiomegaly is often seen with cardiogenic causes although it may be normal in size in the early stages. The heart is usually normal in size with non-cardiogenic causes.
- **Upper lobe blood diversion**: the upper lobe blood vessels are normally narrower than the lower lobe vessels. In cardiogenic pulmonary oedema, lower zone alveolar hypoxia causes arteriolar vasoconstriction, diverting blood to the upper lobes to optimize gaseous exchange.
- **Alveolar shadowing**: this represents oedema in the alveoli. It predominates in the lower zones if the cause is cardiogenic, and more diffusely if non-cardiogenic. In acute cardiogenic cases, alveolar shadowing spreads out from the hila in the shape of bats' wings.
- **Kerley lines**: these represent interstitial oedema. They are thin linear shadows caused by interstitial fluid or cellular infiltration.
- **Kerley A lines**: these represent distension of channels between peripheral and central lung lymphatics. They are unbranching lines (over 2 cm long) extending from the periphery towards the hilum.
- **Kerley B/septal lines**: these represent oedema of the interlobular septa and are characteristic of pulmonary oedema. They are 1 cm long, thin, horizontal and parallel and seen peripherally above the costophrenic angles.
- **Pleural effusions**: pleural fluid causes blunting of the costophrenic angles.

Pleural effusion

Pleural effusion is excess fluid in the pleural space. Aspiration allows biochemical division into transudates (<30 g/L of protein) and exudates (>30 g/L of protein). Transudates are caused by LV failure, pulmonary embolism and cirrhosis. Exudates are causes by infection, neoplasia and inflammatory conditions, e.g. rheumatoid arthritis or systemic lupus erythematosus. CXR is the primary diagnostic tool for detecting pleural effusions and may point to the cause, e.g. an enlarged heart shadow, lung mass, parenchymal disease, apical fibrosis or bone metastases. Effusions collect in gravity-dependent areas (lung bases when positioned upright). The CXR appearances of pleural effusions include:
- Small effusions, which *blunt the costophrenic angles with a meniscus*.
- Large effusions, which can cause complete *'white-out'* of the lungs, lung collapse and push the mediastinum away from the side of the effusion.

Prosthetic heart valves

Normal heart valves may become dysfunctional due to acute and chronic disease, e.g. bacterial endocarditis, aortic stenosis or rheumatic fever. Replacement valves are designed to restore normal function and may be mechanical or biological tissue grafts. *Mechanical valves are radio-opaque*, appearing as white artefacts within the heart shadow on CXR. The major classes of mechanical valves include 'caged ball', 'tilting disk' and 'bileaflet'. A prosthetic mitral valve is larger and aligned more anteroposteriorly than a prosthetic aortic valve, which is smaller and aligned more obliquely on a posteroanterior (PA) CXR.

Pleural plaques

Pleural plaques are focal areas of pleural fibrosis caused by *previous exposure to asbestos*. Pleural calcification is a late sign, occurring in approximately half of those with asbestos-related disease. It is most easily seen along the diaphragmatic pleura. The CXR features include:
- **Widespread distribution**: commonly mid-lung, paravertebral, diaphragmatic, peripheral and bilateral.
- **Peripheral pleural thickening**: appears as a thickened white line, often non-uniform around the edge of the lung.
- **Calcified plaques**: mimic the appearance of a 'holly leaf' with dense, irregular, rolled edges and relatively lucent centres.

Plaques evolve slowly and previous CXRs should be reviewed for comparison.

Table 103.1 Classic chest X-ray features 1.

- **Cardiomegaly**	Heart shadow greater than 50% of thoracic cage width
- **Pulmonary oedema**	
Cardiogenic	Bilateral alveolar shadowing, bats' wings, upper lobe blood diversion, Kerley A lines, Kerley B lines, cardiomegaly, effusion, cardiac pathology signs (sternotomy wires, prosthetic valve, pacemaker/defibrillator)
Non-cardiogenic	Normal heart size, diffuse alveolar shadowing
- **Pleural effusion**	Costophrenic angle blunting, meniscus, 'white-out'
- **Pleural plaques**	Peripheral pleural thickening, pleural calcific deposits

104 Chest X-ray cases 2

(a) Simple pneumothorax

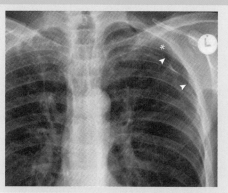

The edge of the left lung can be seen as a thin well-defined line (arrowheads). Beyond this line there are no further lung markings because air is collecting in the pleural cavity (*)

(b) Chest drain

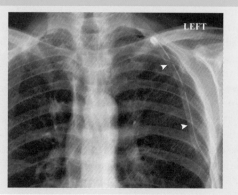

A tube has been inserted to drain air from the pleural cavity. It has been placed appropriately with its tip pointing high up towards the apex of the hemithorax. (Same patient as in (a).)

(c) Tension pneumothorax

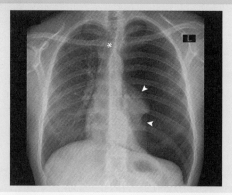

The left lung (arrowheads) is being compressed, the left hemidiaphragm is depressed, and the trachea (*) is pushed towards the right. Immediate aspiration is required

(d) Hydropneumothorax

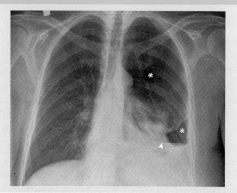

This patient has both a pneumothorax (*) and a pleural effusion (arrowhead) due to an oesophageal rupture. The fluid level does not have the curved meniscus sign of a simple effusion. Note the presence of a chest drain. Haemopneumothorax has identical appearances and is often associated with rib fractures

(e) Lower left lobe collapse

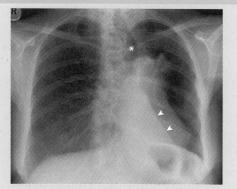

The left lower lobe bronchus is occluded with collapse of this lobe. The edge of the collapsed lobe forms the 'sail sign' (arrowheads). The trachea (*) is pulled towards the side of volume loss

(f) Right upper lobe collapse

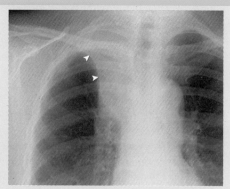

The horizontal fissure (arrowheads) has been pulled upwards due to volume loss of the right upper lobe. The patients in both (e) and (f) had an occluding bronchial carcinoma

Medicine at a Glance, Fourth Edition. Edited by Patrick Davey. © 2014 John Wiley & Sons, Ltd. Published 2014 by John Wiley & Sons, Ltd. Companion website: www.ataglanceseries.com/medicine

Pneumothorax

Pneumothorax is the presence of air in the pleural cavity. During normal ventilation, the thoracic volume increases to create relative negative intrathoracic pressure for lung inflation. However, in the presence of a pleural defect, air enters the potential pleural space and breaks this pressure potential, thereby compromising lung inflation. This impairs gaseous exchange and may cause breathlessness.

- **Simple pneumothorax** is common and occurs in healthy chests, especially in tall, slim, young males. Secondary pneumothoraces can arise in individuals with underlying disease, e.g. chronic obstructive pulmonary disease, asthma, barotrauma, penetrating chest trauma and pneumonia.
- **Tension pneumothorax** is a medical emergency where air accumulates under pressure in the pleural space due to the formation of a one-way valve at the point of injury, permitting air to enter but not to escape. It can develop from a simple pneumothorax, often following traumatic injury, and requires emergency decompression.

Chest X-ray (CXR) features include:
- **Linear pleural shadow with absence of lung markings** beyond this linear shadow in the peripheral thorax.
- **Air in the pleural cavity will rise to the apices** in an upright CXR. It is therefore vital to review the apical areas.

Haemothorax

A haemothorax is a pleural effusion due to the accumulation of blood within the pleural cavity. It most commonly arises from blunt or penetrating chest trauma. Non-traumatic haemothorax is less common and can result from malignancy, blood dyscrasias, pulmonary infarction and tuberculosis. CXR is the primary diagnostic investigation and the typical appearances on *upright* imaging are *identical to a pleural effusion* (meniscus, blunting of the costophrenic angle, 'white-out' and/or mediastinal shift with a large haemothorax).

Approximately 200–300 mL of blood is required to obliterate the costophrenic angle on an upright CXR. In the acute trauma setting, however, a portable supine CXR is often the first and only view available upon which management decisions are based. Unfortunately, the presence and size of haemothoraces is extremely difficult to evaluate on supine images. In blunt trauma cases, there may be other associated injuries, e.g. rib fractures, pneumothorax or damage to the great vessels. These should be excluded on the CXR.

In the context of a traumatic pneumothorax, the presence of a pleural effusion is almost always due to the accumulation of blood in the pleural cavity (haemopneumothorax). There is no meniscal sign due to a direct interface between the pleural air and blood.

Lobar collapse

Collapse of a single lobe causes characteristic patterns on CXR:
- **Right upper lobe collapse**: the horizontal fissure is pulled up and there is a soft tissue shadow in the right upper zone. The remainder of the lung expands to fill the void.
- **(Right) middle lobe collapse** (there is no left middle lobe): the horizontal and oblique fissures are pulled closer and there is loss of interface between the right heart border and the lung (*silhouette sign*). The lateral CXR demonstrates a wedge-shaped opacity stretching from the hilum anteroinferiorly.
- **Right lower lobe collapse**: there is a soft tissue shadow in the right lower zone and loss of interface between the right hemidiaphragm and lung (*silhouette sign*). The collapsed lobe appears as a triangular opacity behind the right heart border without

obscuring it. The lateral CXR demonstrates increased density over the lower thoracic spine caused by the shadow of the collapsed lobe.
- **Left upper lobe collapse**: there is a 'veil-like' shadow cast over the entire left lung due to the anteriorly lying collapsed lobe. Interposition of the lower lobe between the collapsed lobe and aortic arch may be seen as a crescent of air, known as the *Luftsichel sign*.
- **Lingula lobe collapse**: there is loss of interface between the left heart border and the lung (*silhouette sign*).
- **Left lower lobe collapse**: the collapsed lobe is displaced medially and lies behind the heart. A triangular opacity is seen through the heart shadow with a straight left lateral border (*sail sign*). There is also loss of interface between the medial part of the left hemidiaphragm and lung (*silhouette sign*).

Tubes, lines and prostheses

CXR is the usual method for confirming correct positioning of tubes and lines in the chest. On CXR:
- *The tip of an endotracheal tube should be mid-tracheal, 2–3 cm above its bifurcation* at the level of the fourth to fifth thoracic vertebrae. The tip has a radio-opaque marker to enhance its visibility on CXR. If inserted too far, it may enter a bronchus and inflate only one lung causing contralateral collapse.
- *The tip of a central venous catheter should be in the superior vena cava (SVC), just above the right atrium.* If it is inserted too far, it may cause arrhythmias through direct contact with the heart. It may also erode through the SVC or right atrium causing haemorrhage and tamponade.
- *The nasogastric tube should follow the central vertical descent of the oesophagus and continue below the left hemidiaphragm into the stomach.* If incorrectly placed, it may enter the trachea or bronchi, perforate the oesophagus or penetrate into the brain through the ethmoid bone.
- *Chest drain*: this tube passes through the chest wall via an intercostal space and its tip lies in the pleural space.
- *Pacemakers and implantable cardioverter defibrillators (ICDs)*: these are usually sited below the lateral left clavicle. Pacing wires connect the pacemaker and/or ICD to the heart muscle. Pacemakers may pace one or more heart chambers. ICDs are used in patients at risk of sudden death from arrhythmia.

Table 104.1 Classic chest X-ray features 2.

- **Haemothorax**	Costophrenic angle blunting, meniscus, 'white-out'
- **Pneumothorax**	Linear pleural shadow with absent lung markings in the periphery beyond
- **Collapse of:**	
Right upper lobe (RUL)	Superiorly displaced horizontal fissure, upper zone shadowing
(Right) middle lobe (R)ML	Right heart silhouette sign, wedge-shaped opacity on lateral CXR
Right lower lobe (RLL)	Right hemidiaphragm silhouette sign, lower zone shadowing, increased lower thoracic spine density on lateral CXR
Left upper lobe (LUL)	Veil-like' shadow, Luftsichel sign
Lingula	Left heart silhouette sign
Left lower lobe (LLL)	Left hemidiaphragm silhouette sign, sail sign

105 Non-invasive ventilation

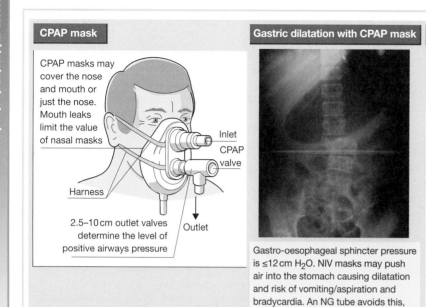

CPAP mask

CPAP masks may cover the nose and mouth or just the nose. Mouth leaks limit the value of nasal masks

Harness

Inlet

CPAP valve

2.5–10 cm outlet valves determine the level of positive airways pressure

Outlet

Gastric dilatation with CPAP mask

Gastro-oesophageal sphincter pressure is ≤12 cm H_2O. NIV masks may push air into the stomach causing dilatation and risk of vomiting/aspiration and bradycardia. An NG tube avoids this, but mask leaks can occur

Benefits and limitations of positive pressure NIV

Benefits	Limitations
• Avoids complications associated with intubation and mechanical ventilation – pulmonary infection – pressure-induced damage • Avoids ETI complications – mini-aspiration – upper airway trauma • Allows rest periods • Preserves cough • Allows oral nutrition • Speech (and decision-making) • Allows earlier mobilization • Allows time to decide if MV is appropriate	• Lack of airways protection • No endotracheal suction • Less complete correction of blood gases than with MV • Mask discomfort; eye damage – prolonged use difficult • Ulceration over nasal bridge • Gastric dilatation and vomiting – may need NG tube • Limited ventilatory capacity • Increased nursing time • Continual patient reassurance • Intolerance and distress • Impedes sputum clearance

CPAP = continuous positive airways pressure,
ETI = endotracheal intubation,
MV = mechanical ventilation, NG = nasogastric,
NIV = non-invasive ventilation

Non-invasive ventilation (NIV) is provided by machines that support ventilation and assist gas exchange through the patient's upper airway by means of a mask or similar interface. Continuous positive airway pressure (CPAP) is applied in the same way but is not a mode of ventilation. It is most successful in alert, cooperative, self-ventilating, haemodynamically stable patients who are able to protect and clear their airways.

Indications

One of the commonest uses of NIV is in acute exacerbations of chronic obstructive pulmonary disease (COPD) where a respiratory acidosis (pH <7.35) persists despite optimal medical therapy. It is also used in respiratory failure due to chest wall or neuromuscular disease and cardiogenic pulmonary oedema. It has a role, on occasion, in pneumonia, asthma and as an aid to weaning from mechanical ventilation in the intensive care unit. It is important to make a decision, prior to initiating NIV, whether, if this modality fails, escalation to invasive mechanical ventilation is indicated. Ideally, this should be discussed between the patient, the patient's consultant and the consultant intensivist. There should also be a clear plan of what to do if NIV fails and the patient is not to be intubated.

NIV should be avoided in refractory hypoxaemia, copious pulmonary secretions, undrained peumothorax, reduced Glasgow Coma Score, facial trauma, recent upper gastrointestinal surgery and vomiting. A nasogastric tube prevents gastric distension and reduces the risk of aspiration (see Figure 105.1).

Continuous positive airways pressure

CPAP is maintained throughout inspiration and expiration (typically c. 5–10 cmH$_2$O) by a flow generator, although many non-invasive ventilators have a CPAP mode. All the work of breathing (WoB) is provided by the patient; however the addition of CPAP reduces WoB by increasing lung compliance. CPAP recruits collapsed lung units and keeps them open during expiration. Consequently ventilation/perfusion ($\dot{V}/\dot{Q}$) relationships improve and oxygenation increases. Functional residual capacity inceases as a result of alveolar recruitment and inflation occurs on the more compliant steep part of the pressure–volume curve; this reduces WoB. CPAP is used in cardiogenic pulmonary oedema, pneumonia and in obstructive sleep apnoea where it helps prevent upper airways collapse.

Negative and positive pressure ventilation

NIV can be divided into negative and positive pressure ventilation:

• **Negative pressure ventilation** (NPV) was originally developed to support victims of poliomyelitis-induced respiratory paralysis. Patients were placed in **tank ventilators** sealed at the neck. Lowering tank pressures expanded the chest causing inspiration. Expiration was passive. However, these 'iron lungs' were limited by difficulties with nursing access, poor CO_2 clearance and secretion retention, which caused airways obstruction or pneumonia. NPV has largely been superseded by the development of positive pressure ventilators, which are particularly successful in the management of acute respiratory failure. NPV is now rarely used except in patients with chronic hypoventilation (e.g. kyphoscoliosis) or as part of rehabilitation programmes (e.g. spinal injury). Current NPV techniques include: (i) **jacket (cuirass) ventilators**, which only produce a negative pressure around the chest but leaks often limit effectiveness; and (ii) **rocking beds**, which utilize gravity to enhance diaphragmatic movement.

Medicine at a Glance, Fourth Edition. Edited by Patrick Davey. © 2014 John Wiley & Sons, Ltd. Published 2014 by John Wiley & Sons, Ltd. Companion website: www.ataglanceseries.com/medicine

- **Positive pressure NIV** is delivered through tight-fitting interfaces which may be nasal, face mask, full face masks or a helmet (see Figure 105.1). Interfaces come in a variety of sizes and should be carefully matched to individuals to ensure comfort and compliance. Figure 105.1 also lists the potential benefits and disadvantages. Numerous ventilators are available for NIV, they range from ventilators used in intensive care with sophisticated monitoring to small, cheap, lightweight ventilators designed for home ventilation. However, it is more important for staff to be familiar with a single type rather than a specific ventilator. Ventilators may be volume or pressure (more common) preset and operate in: (i) triggered mode (also called spontaneous or assist); (ii) assist/control mode (spontaneous or timed) where breaths are triggered by the patient but there is a back-up controlled rate if the patient fails to trigger a breath; and (iii) control mode (mandatory breaths). Bilevel pressure support ventilators are in most frequent use because they are cheap and simple to use. Successful use requires well-trained staff, gradual introduction to a cooperative patient and careful synchronization of breathing with the ventilator. Several modes of ventilation exist and terminology varies between manufacturers; the commonest are:

- **Pressure support ventilation**: delivers an inspiratory pressure (c. 10–30 cmH$_2$O) triggered by the patient and adjusted according to the patient's requirements. It augments tidal volume, clears CO$_2$ and reduces WoB. Modern NIV ventilators also provide adjustable expiratory positive airway pressure which has the same effects as CPAP.
- **Bilevel positive pressure ventilation**: alternates between two levels of CPAP whilst allowing spontaneous respiration. The difference in the two pressures augments alveolar ventilation and CO$_2$ clearance; the lower pressure maintains alveolar recruitment.

106 Mechanical ventilation

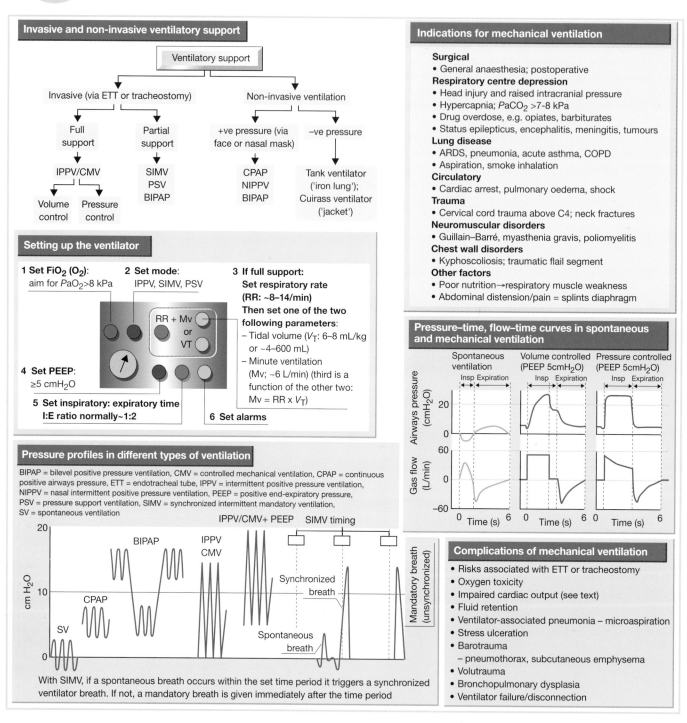

Invasive and non-invasive ventilatory support

Ventilatory support
- Invasive (via ETT or tracheostomy)
  - Full support
    - IPPV/CMV
      - Volume control
      - Pressure control
  - Partial support
    - SIMV
    - PSV
    - BIPAP
- Non-invasive ventilation
  - +ve pressure (via face or nasal mask)
    - CPAP
    - NIPPV
    - BIPAP
  - –ve pressure
    - Tank ventilator ('iron lung'); Cuirass ventilator ('jacket')

Setting up the ventilator

1 Set FiO$_2$ (O$_2$): aim for PaO_2>8 kPa

2 Set mode: IPPV, SIMV, PSV

3 If full support: Set respiratory rate (RR: ~8–14/min)
Then set one of the two following parameters:
– Tidal volume (V_T: 6–8 mL/kg or ~4–600 mL)
– Minute ventilation (Mv; ~6 L/min) (third is a function of the other two: Mv = RR x V_T)

RR + Mv or VT

4 Set PEEP: ≥5 cmH$_2$O

5 Set inspiratory: expiratory time I:E ratio normally~1:2

6 Set alarms

Pressure profiles in different types of ventilation

BIPAP = bilevel positive pressure ventilation, CMV = controlled mechanical ventilation, CPAP = continuous positive airways pressure, ETT = endotracheal tube, IPPV = intermittent positive pressure ventilation, NIPPV = nasal intermittent positive pressure ventilation, PEEP = positive end-expiratory pressure, PSV = pressure support ventilation, SIMV = synchronized intermittent mandatory ventilation, SV = spontaneous ventilation

With SIMV, if a spontaneous breath occurs within the set time period it triggers a synchronized ventilator breath. If not, a mandatory breath is given immediately after the time period

Indications for mechanical ventilation

Surgical
- General anaesthesia; postoperative

Respiratory centre depression
- Head injury and raised intracranial pressure
- Hypercapnia; $PaCO_2$ >7-8 kPa
- Drug overdose, e.g. opiates, barbiturates
- Status epilepticus, encephalitis, meningitis, tumours

Lung disease
- ARDS, pneumonia, acute asthma, COPD
- Aspiration, smoke inhalation

Circulatory
- Cardiac arrest, pulmonary oedema, shock

Trauma
- Cervical cord trauma above C4; neck fractures

Neuromuscular disorders
- Guillain–Barré, myasthenia gravis, poliomyelitis

Chest wall disorders
- Kyphoscoliosis; traumatic flail segment

Other factors
- Poor nutrition→respiratory muscle weakness
- Abdominal distension/pain = splints diaphragm

Pressure–time, flow–time curves in spontaneous and mechanical ventilation

Complications of mechanical ventilation
- Risks associated with ETT or tracheostomy
- Oxygen toxicity
- Impaired cardiac output (see text)
- Fluid retention
- Ventilator-associated pneumonia – microaspiration
- Stress ulceration
- Barotrauma
  – pneumothorax, subcutaneous emphysema
- Volutrauma
- Bronchopulmonary dysplasia
- Ventilator failure/disconnection

Invasive mechanical ventilation (MV) is frequently required during critical illness to maintain gas exchange and reduce the work of breathing (WoB). This is delivered through an endotracheal tube or tracheostomy (if prolonged ventilation is required) and provides complete or partial respiratory support. Non-invasive ventilation, which uses an interface attached to the patient's face, also provides respiratory support and is discussed in Chapter 105.

Indications

Outside the operating theatre, one of the main indications for MV is respiratory failure. However, it is also used in circulatory failure, neurological disease, trauma, poisoning and following prolonged major surgery. MV may also be required to facilitate investigations (such as a computed tomography scan in a head-injured patient who is unable to cooperate) or bronchial toilet. The decision to intubate and mechanically ventilate a patient requires careful

Medicine at a Glance, Fourth Edition. Edited by Patrick Davey. © 2014 John Wiley & Sons, Ltd. Published 2014 by John Wiley & Sons, Ltd. Companion website: www.ataglanceseries.com/medicine

thought as this modality only provides organ support. There needs to be some treatable or reversible cause for why MV is indicated. Generally, such decisions need to be made between the patient's consultant, the consultant intensivist and either the patient (if possible) or family members. It is often difficult to decide exactly when to ventilate a progressively deteriorating patient. There are no simple guidelines. However, hypoxaemia (PO_2 <8kPa on FiO_2 >0.4), hypercapnia (PCO_2 >7.5kPa), respiratory/metabolic acidosis (pH <7.2) and other factors such as confusion, exhaustion, poor cough and sputum retention usually indicate the need for MV. *Trends in these variables and any response or failure to treatment are often more helpful than absolute values.*

Ventilator set-up

Typical initial adult intermittent positive pressure ventilation (IPPV) settings would be: tidal volume (V_T) *c.* 6–8 mL/kg; respiratory frequency (f) *c.* 8–14bpm; and minute ventilation ($M_V = V_T \times f$) *c.* 6 L/min. FiO_2 and M_V are adjusted to maintain PaO_2 >8kPa and $PaCO_2$ <7kPa, respectively, but acceptable values depend on individual disease processes. Initially positive end-expiratory pressure (PEEP) is set at around 5 cmH$_2$O and the inspiratory:expiratory time (I:E ratio) at *c.* 1:2. Inappropriate ventilation can itself contribute to lung injury or other mechanical complications and generally the ventilator needs to be set by an experienced critical care practitioner.

Mode of ventilation

The terminology concerning modes of ventilation is often confusing; they describe whether a breath is: (i) fully or partially supported; (ii) volume or pressure controlled; (iii) mandatory (delivered by the ventilator regardless of patient respiratory effort); or (iv) spontaneously triggered (see Figure 106.1). Modern ventilators with microprocessor controls are sophisticated devices and provide considerable flexibility, allowing a change from mandatory (all the WoB performed by the ventilator) to partial support modes that minimize sedation requirements and allow patients to be conscious but comfortable. PEEP is generally applied to all modes of invasive mechanical ventilation.

- **Full (mandatory) support modes** (e.g. IPPV or controlled mechanical ventilation): the ventilator iniates, delivers and terminates the breath. The breaths themselves, which are time triggered, may be targeted to a set pressure or volume. In a pressure-controlled mode, inspiratory pressure does not exceed the set value, however V_T may vary according to airway resistance and lung compliance. In volume control the delivered V_T does not exceed the set value but inspiratory pressures may vary for the same reasons. Controlled mechanical ventilation is uncomfortable if the patient makes any respiratory effort and requires heavy sedation or even neuromuscular blockade. It is used in severe respiratory disease, in circulatory instability or when respiratory drive is absent.

- **Partial support modes** reinforce spontaneous ventilation and are preferred when possible, to allow a reduction in sedation. Breaths are initiated by the patient and detected by sensitive flow/pressure triggers in the ventilator, which then provides inspiratory support.

  - **Synchronized intermittent mandatory ventilation** delivers a set number of mechanically imposed breaths (pressure or volume controlled) which are triggered by the patient. In between mandatory breaths, spontaneous breathing can occur and these may be pressure-supported breaths. The mandatory rate is reduced as the patient becomes ventilator independent during weaning.

  - **Pressure support**: a preset pressure supports every spontaneous breath. The triggering, respiratory rate, V_T and length of inspiration are all determined by the patient. Gradual pressure reductions make it a comfortable and effective mode of weaning.

- **PEEP** describes a positive pressure, maintained throughout expiration, that increases functional residual capacity (i.e. alveolar recruitment), prevents alveolar collapse at end expiration, reduces $\dot{V}/\dot{Q}$ mismatch and decreases alveolar oedema by increasing lymphatic drainage. PEEP improves oxygenation and oxygen delivery for any given mode of ventilation, provided that the cardiac output is not significantly reduced by the associated increase in intrathoracic pressure (IP).

Physiological responses to mechanical ventilation

- **Cardiovascular effects** are due to increased IP and alveolar overdistension. Increased IP has two effects on the heart:

  - **Right ventricular (RV) preload reduction** is due to increased right atrial pressure, which reduces venous return and RV cardiac output. However, fluid infusion rapidly restores venous return and cardiac output.

  - **Left ventricular (LV) afterload reduction** is due to reduced LV transmural pressure, which decreases LV work. In the normal heart, any beneficial effect of LV afterload reduction is offset by reduced venous return. However, in the failing heart, cardiac output is relatively insensitive to preload changes but very sensitive to afterload reduction. Consequently, MV may increase cardiac output in heart failure, a useful therapeutic effect.

The overall response to raised IP depends on the state of the heart, vasomotor tone and fluid status (e.g. hypovolaemia). MV also increases lung volumes. Overinflated alveoli compress alveolar blood vessels, increasing pulmonary vascular resistance and causing pulmonary hypertension. Subsequent RV distension displaces the septum into the LV cavity, reducing LV filling and cardiac output, an effect known as interventricular dependence.

- **Respiratory effects**: MV reduces WoB, which increases the proportion of cardiac output going to other potentially ischaemic organs. Re-expansion of collapsed lung segments also improves oxygenation. Unfortunately, supine position, reduced surfactant production and ventilation of poorly perfused lung increases $\dot{V}/\dot{Q}$ mismatch.

- **Fluid retention** is due to antidiuretic hormone secretion.

Complications

Mechanical ventilation may itself cause or exacerbate lung injury. This so-called ventilator-induced lung injury may be as a consequence of barotrauma (high airway pressures), volutrauma (overdistention of alveoli) and alectotrauma (repeated opening and closing of lung units). Air leaks may develop causing a pneumothorax or pneumomediastinum; these complications are more frequent when the lungs are stiff (poor compliance) such as in adult respiratory distress syndrome (ARDS). This has led to the concept of a lung protective strategy where V_T does not exceed 6 mL/kg of ideal body weight and peak inspiratory pressure is kept below 30 cmH$_2$O. This strategy frequently leads to respiratory acidosis and is often referred to as permissive hypercapnia. PEEP should also be optimized and inspired oxygen kept to the minimal amount to achieve adequate oxygenation.

The presence of an endotracheal tube circumvents many of the airway's host defense mechanisms and also provides an artificial surface, which can be colonized by bacteria. Thus intubation predisposes individuals to ventilator-associated pneumonia which is the commonest nosocomial infection in intensive care and has a substantial impact on length of stay and cost. Rates of ventilator-associated pneumonia may be reduced by daily sedation breaks and elevating the head of the bed.

107 Lower respiratory tract infection: pneumonia

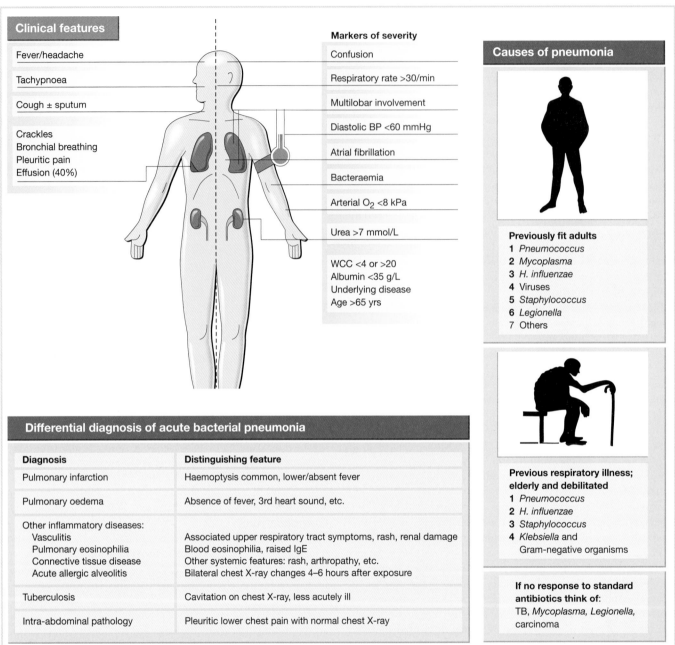

Clinical features

Fever/headache

Tachypnoea

Cough ± sputum

Crackles
Bronchial breathing
Pleuritic pain
Effusion (40%)

Markers of severity

Confusion

Respiratory rate >30/min

Multilobar involvement

Diastolic BP <60 mmHg

Atrial fibrillation

Bacteraemia

Arterial O₂ <8 kPa

Urea >7 mmol/L

WCC <4 or >20
Albumin <35 g/L
Underlying disease
Age >65 yrs

Causes of pneumonia

Previously fit adults
1 *Pneumococcus*
2 *Mycoplasma*
3 *H. influenzae*
4 Viruses
5 *Staphylococcus*
6 *Legionella*
7 Others

**Previous respiratory illness;
elderly and debilitated**
1 *Pneumococcus*
2 *H. influenzae*
3 *Staphylococcus*
4 *Klebsiella* and
  Gram-negative organisms

**If no response to standard
antibiotics think of:**
TB, *Mycoplasma, Legionella,*
carcinoma

Differential diagnosis of acute bacterial pneumonia

Diagnosis	Distinguishing feature
Pulmonary infarction	Haemoptysis common, lower/absent fever
Pulmonary oedema	Absence of fever, 3rd heart sound, etc.
Other inflammatory diseases:	
Vasculitis	Associated upper respiratory tract symptoms, rash, renal damage
Pulmonary eosinophilia	Blood eosinophilia, raised IgE
Connective tissue disease	Other systemic features: rash, arthropathy, etc.
Acute allergic alveolitis	Bilateral chest X-ray changes 4–6 hours after exposure
Tuberculosis	Cavitation on chest X-ray, less acutely ill
Intra-abdominal pathology	Pleuritic lower chest pain with normal chest X-ray

Pneumonia is an acute infective respiratory illness causing radiological shadowing. It is classified according to the setting in which it is acquired, because this influences the likely microbial pathogens and therefore the best empirical treatment:

- Community acquired.
- Hospital acquired (nosocomial).
- Aspiration pneumonia.
- Pneumonia in immunocompromised individuals.

Community-acquired pneumonia

Epidemiology and pathophysiology

Very common. Community incidence is 1–3/1000 in adults. A quarter of cases require hospital admission. M = F, although Legionnaires' disease is more common in males. Pneumonia tends to occur at the extremes of age, but it remains an important cause of morbidity and even mortality in young adults.

Medicine at a Glance, Fourth Edition. Edited by Patrick Davey. © 2014 John Wiley & Sons, Ltd. Published 2014 by John Wiley & Sons, Ltd. Companion website:
www.ataglanceseries.com/medicine

Causes and specific features of community-acquired pneumonia

Pathogen	% cases	Specific features
Streptococcus pneumoniae	60–75	Commonest in winter months
		Lobar involvement >> bronchopneumonic pattern
		Rapid onset, high fever, herpes labialis, vomiting. Mortality 5–10%
Mycoplasma pneumoniae	5–18	Mainly in autumn. Epidemics every 3–4 years
		Complications (20%): myocarditis, meningo-encephalitis, rash, haemolytic anaemia (cold haemagglutinin)
Haemophilus influenzae	4–5	Bronchopneumonia. Usually underlying lung disease
Legionella	2–5	Commonest in autumn in previously healthy individuals, from contaminated air conditioning. Key features: confusion, hepatitis, renal impairment, ↓Na+
Chlamydia psittaci	2	From infected birds. Protracted illness. 50% hepato-splenomegaly
Staphylococcus aureus	1–5	During influenza A epidemics. Rapid progression and high mortality (30%)
		Cavitation in 50%, pleural effusion/empyema in 15%, pneumothorax
Gram-negative pneumonia	10	Underlying illness, often chronic. Increased chance in nosocomial infections. Often severe pneumonia, with septic shock. *Klebsiella, Pseudomonas, E. coli*
Influenza	5–8	Preceding myalgia + severe prostration. Epidemic
Other	2–8	

CURB-65 criteria for severity of pneumonia

1 point for each of the following:

C onfusion

U rea (>7 mmol/L)

R espiratory rate (>30/min)

B lood pressure (systolic BP <90 or diastolic BP <60 mmHg)

65 age ≥ 65 years

Risk of ITU admission or death:

0 : 0.7%

1 : 3.2%

2 : 13.0%

3 : 17.0%

4 : 41.5%

5 : 57.0%

Infection occurs by droplet spread. Organisms multiply in the lung and, if local defence mechanisms are overcome, pneumonia develops. Tobacco smoke impairs local defences by depressing ciliary function. The causes of pneumonia are listed in Figures 107.1 and 107.2 above.

Clinical features

Fever and cough (initially non-productive) are common symptoms. Chest pain and breathlessness may also occur. Systemic features (more common but not specific to atypical pneumonia) include headache, confusion, myalgia and malaise. A prolonged prodrome is more specific to the atypical organisms. Examination may reveal local signs of consolidation and crackles over the affected lobe. Tachypnoea, hypotension, confusion and cyanosis all suggest severe disease. For the differential diagnosis of pneumonia see Figure 107.1.

Investigations

- **Confirm diagnosis**: this is usually done radiologically using a plain chest X-ray (CXR).
- **Define cause**: microbiological diagnosis is achieved by a diagnostic Gram stain, by growing the organism, by demonstrating a characteristic antigen from the organism or serologically (or other diagnostic blood test). All these tests have advantages and disadvantages and a combined approach may be necessary.
- **Assess severity**: see markers of severity in Figure 107.1.
- **Identify complications**: complications can be detected by CXR, computed tomography (CT) and bronchoscopy, and include pleural effusion and empyema, lobar collapse (sputum retention), pneumothorax (in cavitating pneumonia) and organizing pneumonia.
- **Exclude cancer**: bronchoscopy should be considered in all people aged ≥50 years who smoke presenting with pneumonia, to exclude underlying lung cancer.

Management and prognosis

- **General supportive measures**: intravenous (IV) fluid, oxygen and physiotherapy.

- **Antibiotic therapy**: severe pneumonia – IV co-amoxiclav and macrolide (clarithromycin). In less severe cases, ampicillin is substituted for the co-amoxiclav and in mild cases, amoxicillin alone is adequate.

The outcome is generally good. Mortality is higher in the elderly. Overall mortality is 5% but increases to 20% if hospital admission is required and 50% if intensive care is needed. Following improvement, particularly in smokers, radiological resolution should be confirmed to exclude underlying pulmonary abnormality, including lung cancer.

Hospital-acquired pneumonia

This is pneumonia occurring ≥2 days after admission to hospital. Infection before this is classified as community acquired.

- Causative organisms are predominantly Gram negative.
- Broad-spectrum antibiotics are necessary.
- High mortality associated with co-morbid factors.

Epidemiology and aetiopathogenesis

This is more common in elderly people, complicates 2–5% of all hospital admissions and accounts for 10–15% of hospital-acquired infections. Several factors predispose patients to the development of pneumonia in hospital – principally increased aspiration risk, reduced host defences and lung/skin instrumentation breaching the normal defences. Although those organisms that cause community-acquired pneumonia also cause infections in hospital, Gram-negative bacteria, *Staphylococcus aureus* and anaerobic organisms are far more likely to be found. Patients with underlying lung disease who develop postoperative pneumonia are still most likely to have pneumococcal or *Haemophilus* infection.

Clinical features and investigations

These are as for community-acquired pneumonia. The severity of illness is often greater as a result of the presence of underlying disease.

Management

- **General supportive treatment**: oxygen, fluids and physiotherapy.

- **Specific antibiotic treatment** needs to cover Gram-negative organisms that are resistant to the antibiotics given in community-acquired pneumonia. Antibiotics for nosocomial pneumonia include:
  - Third-generation cephalosporin (e.g. cefotaxime) + aminoglycoside.
  - Thienamycin (imipenem, meropenem).
  - Antipseudomonal penicillin (piperacillin/tazobactam).
  - Consider antistaphylococcal ± methicillin-resistant *Staphylococcus aureus* (MRSA) cover (flucloxacillin/vancomycin).

The prognosis depends on the causative organism and underlying disease severity. Pneumonia is often the cause of death in elderly hospital patients. In ventilated patients in intensive care, pseudomonas pneumonia has a 50% mortality rate.

Lung abscess

A lung abscess is localized infection of the lung parenchyma with associated cavitation caused by necrosis. It is an uncommon problem occurring mainly in elderly people.

- Certain specific pneumonic agents are more likely to cavitate: *S. aureus*, *Klebsiella* spp. and anaerobic infection.
- Aspirated gastric contents, typically in those who have lost consciousness, who have bulbar palsy or who have problems with alcohol. Infected sinuses also predispose to anaerobic infection.
- IV drug abusers with right-sided endocarditis can develop multiple lung abscesses.
- Tuberculosis (TB) also causes cavitation, although the presentation is generally less acute.

Clinical features

These are of severe infection with fever and systemic upset. Large amounts of purulent and offensive sputum are produced if an abscess drains into an airway. Rapid weight loss and finger clubbing occur, and make the distinction from cavitating bronchial carcinoma important. Localized clinical signs in the chest may be minimal or there may be signs of consolidation and a pleural rub if there is pleural inflammation.

Investigations

These are as for pneumonia to confirm the diagnosis, the cause and assess the severity of the illness. By definition, the CXR will show signs of cavitation, although this must be distinguished from the cavitation found in cancer, TB, vasculitis (Wegener's granulomatosis) and other rarer causes.

Management and prognosis

Prolonged (6 weeks) antibiotics – e.g. amoxicillin, or co-amoxiclav if unwell, and metronidazole to cover *Klebsiella* spp. and anaerobes – are usually adequate. Drainage of the abscess usually occurs via the airway and this may be encouraged at bronchoscopy, which will also exclude an underlying obstructing lesion. Percutaneous drainage is not employed because there is a risk of introducing infection into an otherwise sterile pleural cavity.

With adequate drainage and appropriate antibiotics, the prognosis is generally very good.

Pneumonia in the immunocompromised

Definition and epidemiology

This is pneumonia occurring in patients with a deficiency of cellular or humoral immune mechanisms. The incidence is increasing as a result of the use of immunosuppressive drugs (transplantation, vasculitis), chemotherapy (malignancy) and HIV infection. Effective anti-retroviral treatment and prophylaxis against *Pneumocystis jirovecii (carinii)* has significantly reduced the incidence of pulmonary infections complicating HIV (see Chapter 168).

Pathophysiology

Pulmonary infection is normally prevented by a combination of mechanical elements (epiglottis, cough and gag reflexes, the mucociliary escalator) and specific immunological mechanisms (macrophage/neutrophils, antibodies produced by B lymphocytes, cellular immunity effected by T lymphocytes). Defects in any of these mechanisms lead to increased risk of infection. Infection with multiple organisms is common. Infections associated with immunosuppression are:

- **Neutropenia**: Gram-negative bacteria, *S. aureus*, fungi (*Candida*, *Aspergillus* spp.).
- **Reduced immunoglobulins**: bacteria (pneumococci, *Haemophilus influenzae*).
- **T-cell defects**: bacteria (pneumococci, *H. influenzae*, *S. aureus*), fungi (*Candida*, *Pneumocystis* spp.), viruses (herpes group, cytomegalovirus, adenovirus) and mycobacteria.

Clinical features and investigations

The diagnosis may be clear with fever, cough and breathlessness with focal clinical signs – symptoms that suggest bacterial infection. Symptoms are often more vague when infection is with opportunistic organisms. Onset may be over several weeks and fever may be absent. A high index of suspicion is necessary in patients known to be immunosuppressed.

- Investigation of the underlying immunological defect may be necessary. Full blood count, immunoglobulin levels and other tests including for HIV.
- Plain CXR may reveal focal changes. CT may reveal alternative pathology but cannot provide a microbiological diagnosis.
- Standard microbiological investigation includes culture of sputum, blood and pleural fluid. If doubt exists, bronchoalveolar lavage may be necessary, but this has risks and should be reserved for those in whom initial investigation does not achieve a diagnosis. In those who fail to improve or where diagnostic doubt remains, lung biopsy may be necessary.
- At all stages in investigation, close liaison with microbiologists is necessary because specific culture techniques are necessary to identify likely organisms, particularly mycobacteria, viruses and fungi. DNA amplification techniques are used increasingly, particularly for diagnosis of viral infection.

Management and prognosis

A microbial diagnosis is often not known before treatment is started. In general, broad-spectrum antibacterial agents are necessary while the results of cultures are awaited. Combinations should cover Gram-negative bacteria, including *Pseudomonas* spp., and staphylococci. A combination of antipseudomonal penicillin or third-generation cephalosporin with an aminoglycoside is often used as empirical treatment. Treatment can subsequently be changed according to the results of microbiological investigation. Treatment for viral and fungal infections will include specific antiviral and antifungal agents such as ganciclovir and amphotericin.

Infections often progress rapidly in immunocompromised patients. Achieving an accurate diagnosis to guide treatment is therefore important. Despite full supportive treatment and antibiotics, pulmonary infection in these patients accounts for up to 50–60% of the mortality.

108 Upper respiratory tract infection

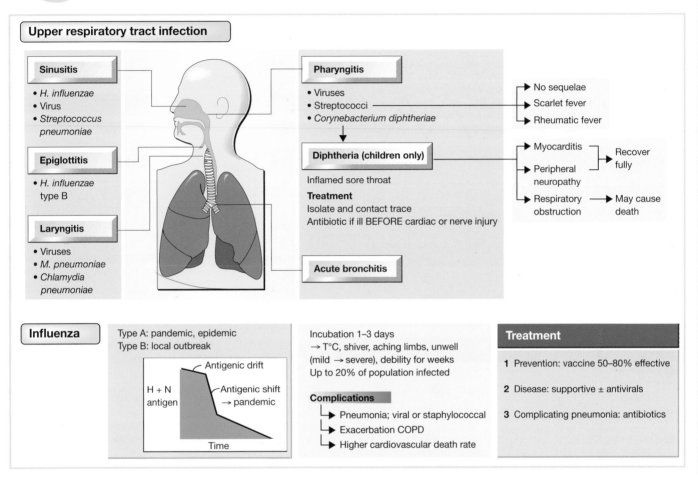

Table 108.1 The common causes of upper respiratory tract infection, their features and management.

	Cause	Features	Investigation	Management	Prognosis
Common cold (coryza)	Viruses	Sneezing, nasal blockage and discharge	None	Symptomatic	Remits in days
Pharyngitis (all ages)	Viral; occasionally streptococcal	Fever, sore throat	Throat swab ASO titre	Antibiotics if bacterial; surgery if abscess develops	Remits in 1 week if viral
Laryngitis (adults)	Viral; occasionally pneumococci or *Haemophilus* spp.	Fever, hoarse voice	Throat swab	Antibiotics, humidification	Remits in about 1week
Epiglottitis (children)	*Haemophilus influenzae* (occasional pneumococci)	Fever, sore throat, stridor, upper airway obstruction	Throat swab blood cultures, lateral neck X-ray	Intravenous antibiotics, humidification, facilities for intubation Prevention by HiB vaccination	Slow improvement with treatment, risk of death from airway obstruction
Bronchitis (all ages)	Viral; occasional pneumococci or *Haemophilus* spp.	Dry cough, retrosternal soreness, wheeze; sputum if bacterial	Sputum culture	Usually resolves but antibiotics often given	Improves over a week
Sinusitis (all ages)	Various bacteria 15% viral	Headache, facial pain, nasal congestion	None; sinus X-ray if severe	Antibiotics; decongestants may help; sinus washout or surgery if persistent	Remits if acute; chronic problems are common

ASO, antistreptolysin O; HiB, *Haemophilus influenzae* B.

Medicine at a Glance, Fourth Edition. Edited by Patrick Davey. © 2014 John Wiley & Sons, Ltd. Published 2014 by John Wiley & Sons, Ltd. Companion website: www.ataglanceseries.com/medicine

109 Asthma

Asthma

Asthma is an inflammatory condition causing reversible airway obstruction and symptoms of:

- Cough ⎤
- Wheeze ⎤ All, or
- Chest tightness ⎤ any one
- Breathlessness ⎦

Symptoms respond to β_2 agonists

Peak flow chart showing classical morning dipping

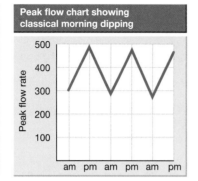

Consider underlying disease when asthma bad, adult onset, abnormal laboratory tests or chest X-ray

1 Allergic bronchopulmonary aspergillosis
2 Churg–Strauss
3 Bronchiectasis

I. Intrinsic

- Adults
- Fewer have ↑IgE or +ve skin tests

II. Extrinsic

- Children
- Atopic ↑IgE
- +ve skin tests

Triggers (may be multifactorial)

Drugs
- Aspirin
- β-blockers

Allergens
- Dust mite
- Cat/dog dander
- Pollens

Occupational
- Isocyanates
- Drugs/enzymes
- Wood resin
- Dyes

Environment
- Cold air
- Exercise
- Emotion

Clinical features

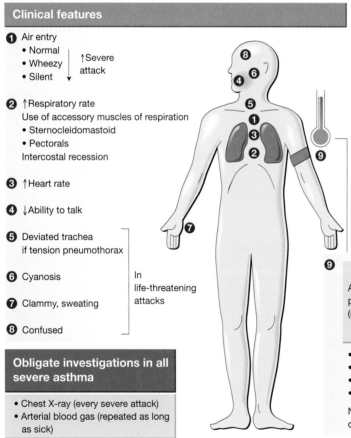

❶ Air entry
- Normal
- Wheezy ⎤ ↑Severe
- Silent ⎦ attack

❷ ↑Respiratory rate
Use of accessory muscles of respiration
- Sternocleidomastoid
- Pectorals
Intercostal recession

❸ ↑Heart rate

❹ ↓Ability to talk

❺ Deviated trachea if tension pneumothorax

❻ Cyanosis

❼ Clammy, sweating

❽ Confused

In life-threatening attacks

Obligate investigations in all severe asthma

- Chest X-ray (every severe attack)
- Arterial blood gas (repeated as long as sick)

In between attacks	Moderate	Severe	Life threatening
Normal exam Normal lung function tests	PEFR <65% predicted ↓ Admit to hospital	PEFR <50% Pulse rate >110 Respiratory rate >25 Can't complete sentences Wheezy chest Alert → mild confusion	PEFR <33% Bradychardia Exhaustion Can't talk at all Silent chest Confusion →coma
PO_2	↓	↓↓	↓↓↓
PCO_2	↓	→	↑
pH	Ⓝ or ↑	Ⓝ	↓

Alert ITU

❾ Pulsus paradoxus

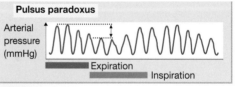

- Normal <5 mmHg
- Moderate 5–10 mmHg
- Severe 10–20 mmHg
- Life threatening >20 mmHg

NB Large paradox may also arise from tension pneumothorax or from pericardial tamponade

Medicine at a Glance, Fourth Edition. Edited by Patrick Davey. © 2014 John Wiley & Sons, Ltd. Published 2014 by John Wiley & Sons, Ltd. Companion website: www.ataglanceseries.com/medicine

Methods of delivering bronchodilators

Dry powder device	Spacer devices	Nebulizer treatment

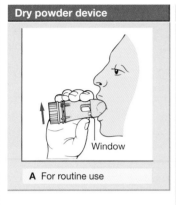

Window

A For routine use

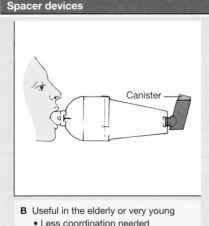

Canister

B Useful in the elderly or very young
- Less coordination needed
- Lower pharyngeal deposition of drug

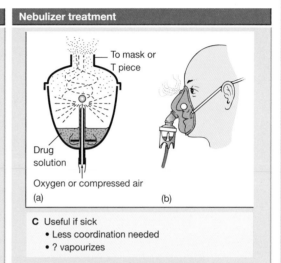

To mask or T piece

Drug solution

Oxygen or compressed air

(a)   (b)

C Useful if sick
- Less coordination needed
- ? vapourizes

Definition

There is no universally accepted definition. Asthma is present if a combination of cough, wheeze or breathlessness with *variable* airflow obstruction is present.

Epidemiology

Asthma is the single most important cause of respiratory disease morbidity and causes 1500 deaths/year in the UK. The prevalence, currently 10–15%, is increasing in western societies. The incidence of wheeze is highest in childhood (one in three children wheeze and one in seven schoolchildren have a diagnosis of asthma). Asthma is classified as:

- **Extrinsic**: childhood asthma, associated with atopy (atopy = familial allergic diathesis, manifest as childhood eczema and hay fever). Often remits by teenage years, although it may recur during adult life.
- **Intrinsic**: develops in later life, is less likely to be caused by allergy, may be more progressive and does not respond as well to treatment.
- **Occupational**: relates to industrial/work place allergens (e.g. photocopier material, baking, soldering, welding, paint spraying, etc.).

Aetiology

Genetics

Asthma runs in families in association with atopy. Genetic studies show linkage to the high-affinity IgE receptor and the T-helper (Th2) cytokine genes (chromosome 5).

Environmental factors

Specific bronchial stimuli include house-dust mite, pollen and cat dander; 3% of people with asthma are sensitive to aspirin.

- **Occupational exposure** to irritants or sensitizers is an important cause of work-related asthma.
- **Non-specific stimuli**: viral infections, cold air, exercise or emotional stress may also precipitate wheeze. High atmospheric levels of ozone (e.g. as found during a thunder storm) or particulate matter predispose to exacerbations of pre-existing asthma.
- **Other environmental factors**, including dietary ones (high Na^+, low Mg^{2+}), reduced incidence of childhood infections (partly as a result of immunization) and increased environmental load of allergens (dust mite) are responsible for increasing prevalence.

Pathology

Airway remodelling occurs with smooth muscle hypertrophy and fibrosis. Histology shows inflammatory cell infiltrate (particularly eosinophils) in airway walls.

Clinical features

Asthma presents with symptoms of cough, wheeze and breathlessness, which vary over time. An obvious trigger such as exercise or allergen exposure may be present. Examination may be normal or may reveal expiratory wheeze.

Investigations

Lung function tests may show airflow obstruction or may be normal. Serial peak flow measurements can be useful in making the diagnosis, and often show a classic pattern of morning dipping. In people with known asthma, peak flow measurements are useful markers of severity. Allergy testing, serum IgE and eosinophil count are useful in some patients.

Management

The objective of treatment is to keep patients free of symptoms on the minimum therapy.

- **Patient education**: vital for successful management, particularly explanation of the triggers, use and role of medication, and how to detect and react to a deterioration. All patients should be given a written self-management plan.
- **Avoidance of environmental triggers or allergens** is important, especially of cigarette smoke.
- **Chronic asthma**: a stepped care approach is recommended (see Figure 109.2 above). For severe persistent allergic asthma, anti-IgE therapy can be useful.
- **Acute asthma**: oxygen, systemic corticosteroids, inhaled β-agonists, anticholinergics and intravenous magnesium or theophyllines if necessary.

Prognosis

Asthma is a chronic disease requiring maintenance treatment. With appropriate treatment many individuals are symptom-free. If asthma is not adequately treated with inhaled corticosteroids, lung function is liable to deteriorate over time and airflow obstruction may become irreversible. Risk factors for death from asthma include poor treatment compliance, intensive therapy unit (ITU) admissions and hospital admission despite steroid treatment.

Management of chronic asthma

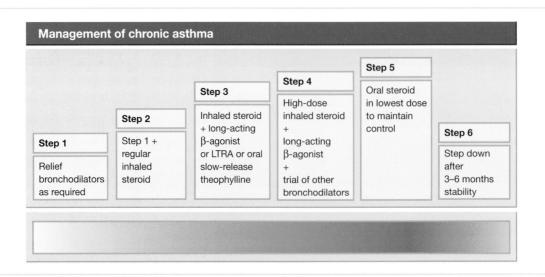

Step 1

Relief bronchodilators as required

Step 2

Step 1 + regular inhaled steroid

Step 3

Inhaled steroid + long-acting β-agonist or LTRA or oral slow-release theophylline

Step 4

High-dose inhaled steroid + long-acting β-agonist + trial of other bronchodilators

Step 5

Oral steroid in lowest dose to maintain control

Step 6

Step down after 3–6 months stability

Deaths from asthma

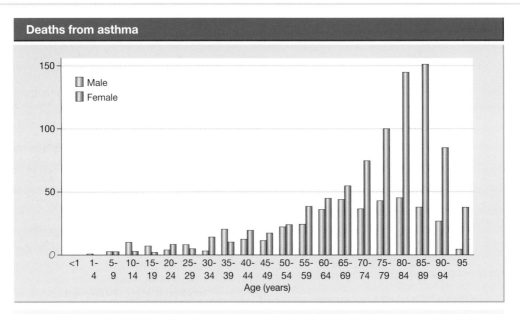

The graph shows the age-specific deaths from asthma in the United Kingdom in 2003. It can be seen that rather more women than men died from asthma, and that the elderly were particularly affected.

110 Chronic obstructive pulmonary disease

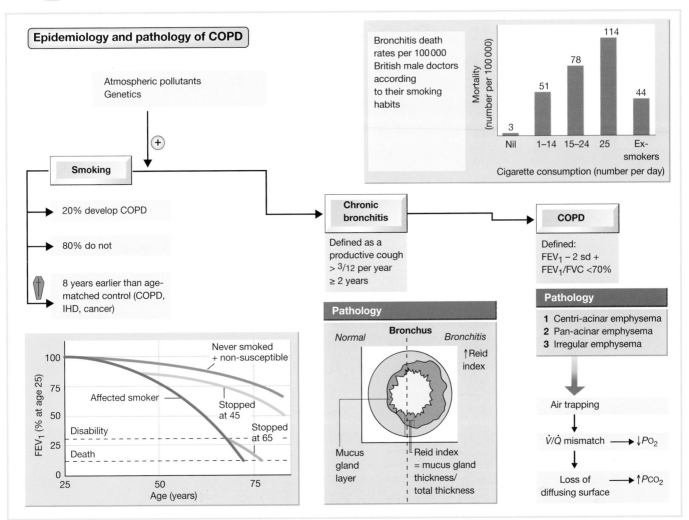

Epidemiology and pathology of COPD

Atmospheric pollutants
Genetics

Bronchitis death rates per 100 000 British male doctors according to their smoking habits

Smoking

20% develop COPD

80% do not

8 years earlier than age-matched control (COPD, IHD, cancer)

Chronic bronchitis

Defined as a productive cough > 3/12 per year ≥ 2 years

COPD

Defined:
$FEV_1 - 2$ sd +
$FEV_1/FVC < 70\%$

Pathology

1 Centri-acinar emphysema
2 Pan-acinar emphysema
3 Irregular emphysema

Air trapping

$\dot{V}/\dot{Q}$ mismatch ⟶ $\downarrow PO_2$

Loss of diffusing surface ⟶ $\uparrow PCO_2$

Pathology

Normal   **Bronchus**   Bronchitis

↑Reid index

Mucus gland layer

Reid index = mucus gland thickness/total thickness

FEV1 graph: Never smoked + non-susceptible, Affected smoker, Stopped at 45, Stopped at 65, Disability, Death. FEV$_1$ (% at age 25) vs Age (years).

Definition
Chronic obstructive pulmonary disease (COPD) and chronic obstructive airway disease are interchangeable terms. It is a chronic, slowly progressive disorder characterized by fixed or partially reversible airway obstruction, unlike the reversible airway obstruction seen in asthma (see Chapter 109).

Epidemiology
COPD is a major public health problem from which 25 000 people die per year in the UK (5% of all deaths). The prevalence is about 3 000 000. Rates are higher in industrialized countries, in inner city areas, among lower income groups and in elderly people. Rates have plateaued in men but are still rising in women.

Aetiology
● **Environmental factors**: cigarette smoking is the major cause, with additional risk from atmospheric pollutants in the workplace or in the inner city. Some patients have chronic, undiagnosed and untreated asthma.

● **Genetics**: α_1-antitrypsin deficiency predisposes to early development of COPD.

Pathology
Smoking causes bronchial mucus gland hypertrophy and increased mucus production, leading to a productive cough. In chronic bronchitis ('productive cough' >3 months/year for >2 years) the early changes are in the small airways. In addition, destruction of lung tissue with dilatation of the distal airspaces (emphysema) occurs, leading to loss of elastic recoil, hyperinflation, gas trapping and an increase in the work of breathing, causing breathlessness. As the disease progresses CO_2 levels rise and the drive to respiration switches from CO_2 to hypoxaemia. If supplementary oxygen corrects hypoxaemia, the drive to respiration may also be reduced, provoking respiratory failure.

Clinical features
Slowly progressing symptoms of cough and shortness of breath over several years in a smoker or ex-smoker suggests the

Medicine at a Glance, Fourth Edition. Edited by Patrick Davey. © 2014 John Wiley & Sons, Ltd. Published 2014 by John Wiley & Sons, Ltd. Companion website: www.ataglanceseries.com/medicine

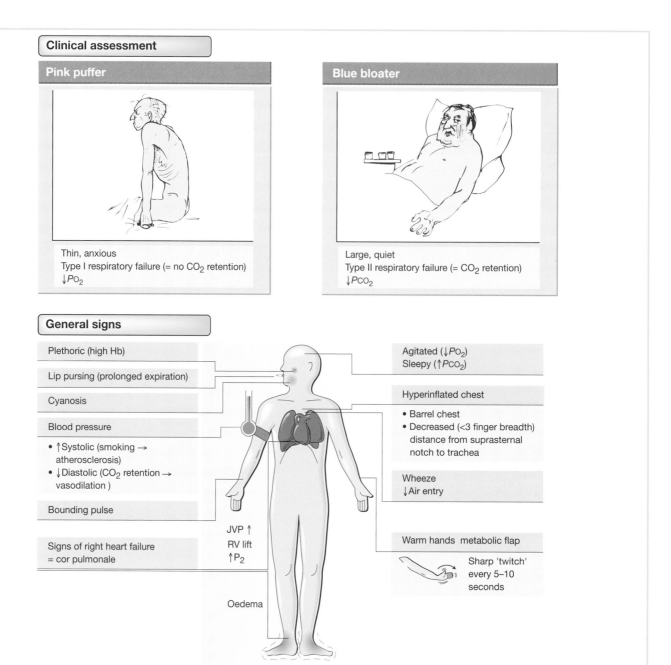

Clinical assessment

Pink puffer

Thin, anxious
Type I respiratory failure (= no CO_2 retention)
$\downarrow PO_2$

Blue bloater

Large, quiet
Type II respiratory failure (= CO_2 retention)
$\downarrow PCO_2$

General signs

Plethoric (high Hb)

Lip pursing (prolonged expiration)

Cyanosis

Blood pressure

• ↑Systolic (smoking →
  atherosclerosis)
• ↓Diastolic (CO_2 retention →
  vasodilation)

Bounding pulse

Signs of right heart failure
= cor pulmonale

JVP ↑
RV lift
↑P_2

Oedema

Agitated ($\downarrow PO_2$)
Sleepy (↑PCO_2)

Hyperinflated chest

• Barrel chest
• Decreased (<3 finger breadth)
  distance from suprasternal
  notch to trachea

Wheeze
↓Air entry

Warm hands metabolic flap

Sharp 'twitch'
every 5–10
seconds

diagnosis. Severity of disease is defined according to the degree of airflow obstruction (forced expiratory volume in 1 s (FEV_1); see Chapter 97):

• Mild: FEV_1 80% or higher of age/sex predicted – cough, minimal dyspnoea and normal examination.
• Moderate: FEV_1 50–79% – cough, breathless on moderate exertion, wheeze, hyperinflation and reduced air entry.
• Severe: FEV_1 30–49% – cough, breathless on minimal exertion, signs of moderate COPD and possibly of cor pulmonale.
• Very severe: FEV_1 <30% or <50% with respiratory failure.

Investigations

• **Pulmonary function tests** show airflow obstruction and reduced gas transfer as a result of destruction of lung tissue. Total lung capacity may be normal, or increased as a result of gas trapping. Twenty per cent of patients derive benefit from bronchodilators. Response to bronchodilator treatment is not predicted by reversibility testing, which is therefore not recommended.

• **Chest X-ray** (CXR) may be normal but, in emphysema, will reveal hyperinflation with loss of lung markings and a small heart.
• **Computed tomography** (CT) may confirm emphysematous bullae.
• **Blood gases** should be analysed if there is any suspicion of respiratory failure. In chronic hypoxaemia the haemoglobin may be increased.

Management

• **Smoking cessation** is a priority.
• **Bronchodilators** (β-agonists or anticholinergics) are used in the 20–40% who benefit. In severe disease up to 10% of patients derive more benefit if high doses are delivered by nebulizer rather than metered dose inhaler. A 2-week trial of oral steroids should be considered to determine reversibility (from serial peak flow or spirometry) of airway obstruction if a diagnosis of untreated asthma is suspected. Long-acting bronchodilators are

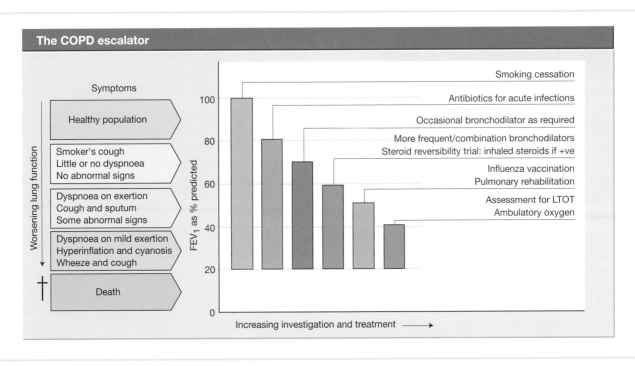

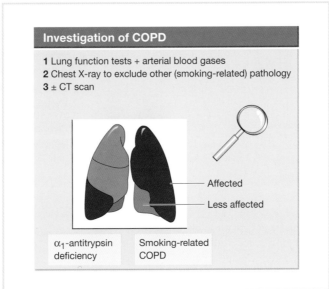

recommended in patients who are still symptomatic on short-acting drugs and in patients with two or more exacerbations per year.

- Long-term **oxygen therapy** (LTOT) for >16 hours daily prolongs life in patients with chronic respiratory failure (i.e. those with a PaO_2 of <7.3 kPa and FEV_1 of <1.5 L).
- In an acute exacerbation, treatment may need to be increased. **Antibiotics** have not been shown to improve outcome, although short-course antibiotics shorten symptom duration of purulent sputum and respiratory deterioration. **Oral steroids** improve recovery from acute exacerbations. Long-term **inhaled steroids** reduce the frequency of exacerbations in those with moderate disease and should be used in those with an FEV_1 of <50% and at least one exacerbation per year.

- **Pulmonary rehabilitation** (especially exercise training) produces significant symptomatic benefit in patients with moderate to severe disease.
- **Resection of large bullae** enables adjacent areas of the lung to reinflate. **Lung volume reduction surgery** may also produce improvement by improving elastic recoil, so maintaining airway patency. Selection of patients is important – currently there are no clear criteria. **Lung transplantation** is used rarely.

Prognosis

This is variable. With continued smoking, decline in lung function will be more rapid than after smoking cessation. LTOT is the only treatment shown to improve life expectancy.

111 Bronchiectasis

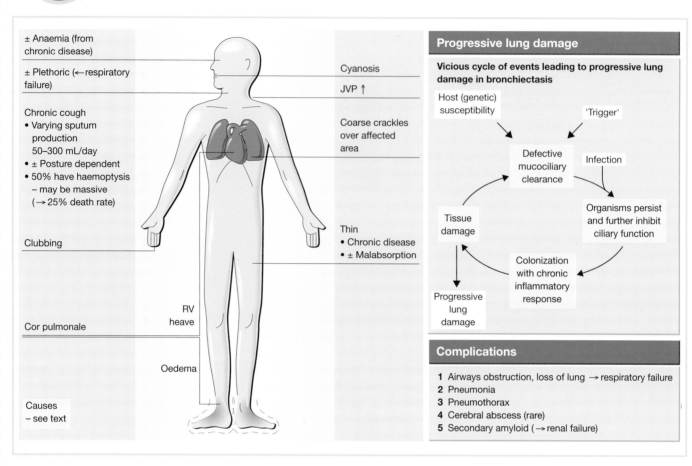

± Anaemia (from chronic disease)

± Plethoric (←respiratory failure)

Chronic cough
• Varying sputum production 50–300 mL/day
• ± Posture dependent
• 50% have haemoptysis – may be massive (→25% death rate)

Clubbing

Cor pulmonale

RV heave

Oedema

Causes – see text

Cyanosis

JVP ↑

Coarse crackles over affected area

Thin
• Chronic disease
• ± Malabsorption

Progressive lung damage

Vicious cycle of events leading to progressive lung damage in bronchiectasis

Host (genetic) susceptibility → Defective mucociliary clearance

'Trigger' → Infection → Organisms persist and further inhibit ciliary function → Colonization with chronic inflammatory response → Tissue damage → Progressive lung damage

Complications

1 Airways obstruction, loss of lung → respiratory failure
2 Pneumonia
3 Pneumothorax
4 Cerebral abscess (rare)
5 Secondary amyloid (→ renal failure)

Definition and epidemiology

This is a disease characterized by bronchial wall dilatation, often with superadded pulmonary infection. The incidence is unknown. Prevalence is 1/1000 and falling (less childhood whooping cough and tuberculosis). The disease has generally been less severe since the introduction of antibiotic therapy.

Aetiology

This depends on the distribution:

• **Localized bronchiectasis** follows severe pneumonia, or occurs distal to endobronchial (foreign body, tumour) or extrabronchial (tuberculous hilar nodes – Brock's syndrome) obstruction.
• **Generalized bronchiectasis**: cystic fibrosis (see Chapter 112), ciliary dyskinesia (Kartagener's syndrome), mucus abnormality (Young's syndrome) and immune defects (immunoglobulin or complement deficiency, chronic granulomatous disease) cause persistent infection and bronchial wall damage, as do immune complexes (allergic bronchopulmonary aspergillosis, rheumatoid arthritis, inflammatory bowel disease). Underlying pulmonary fibrosis can lead to traction on bronchial walls causing traction bronchiectasis. Rare disease associations are yellow nail syndrome, α_1-antitrypsin deficiency and Marfan's syndrome (see Table 111.1).

Pathophysiology

Retention of bronchial secretions occurs and lung infection results, which is not cleared so the lungs become colonized. In addition, certain bacteria further reduce sputum clearance (e.g. *Pseudomonas aeruginosa*). A 'vicious cycle' is set up and the chronic inflammatory response in the airways leads to tissue damage and bronchial wall dilatation (see Figure 111.1).

Clinical features

These are extremely variable. Minor bronchiectasis can be found on computed tomography (CT) scanning during investigation of patients with cough as the only symptom. Some patients have no symptoms or signs. The classic symptoms are of chronic cough and production of large volumes of mucopurulent sputum. Unpleasant breath ('foetor') is common. Haemoptysis occurs in 50% of patients at some stage; 30–40% of patients have associated chronic sinusitis.

• Anaemia, from chronic illness (see Chapter 186), or polycythaemia, from respiratory failure in late disease, may occur.
• Clubbing is found in severe disease.
• Cyanosis and signs of cor pulmonale are present at a late stage in generalized disease.
• Crackles are present in affected areas, particularly during exacerbations and a significant number of patients have airflow obstruction with wheeze.

Other symptoms and signs relate to the underlying cause (e.g. sinusitis, infertility and dextrocardia in Kartagener's syndrome; bronchial carcinoma, etc.).

Complications

The complications are all uncommon:

Table 111.1 Diseases associated with bronchiectasis.

	General clinical features	Frequency
Cystic fibrosis (CF)	Due to malfunction of the gene coding for the CF transmembrane conductance regulator (CFTR) protein. Usually diagnosed at a young age; lung disease often dominates the clinical pictures. Malabsorption very common; cirrhosis, azoospermia, etc.	1 in 400 (Scotland) 1 in 2000–4000 (most white populations) 1 in 15 000–20 000 (African Americans) 1 in 30 000–100 000 (Asians)
Kartagener's syndrome	Due to mutation in gene coding for dynein protein, causes ciliary dysmotility, resulting in sinusitis, situs inversus and infertility in men	1 in 30 000–70 000
Young's syndrome	Triad of bronchiectasis, rhinosinusitis and decreased fertility (obstructive azoospermia) due to abnormally viscous mucus	Rare 15–40% of men with obstructive azoospermia
Immune defects	IgA deficiency: repeated respiratory tract infections, 25% develop autoimmune conditions (e.g. RA, SLE, coeliac disease) IgM deficiency: recurrent infancy/childhood infections with encapsulated organisms. Later on, autoimmune illnesses and malignancy	1 in 600 (Europe) 1 in 250 (Nigeria) 1 in 4000
Allergic bronchopulmonary aspergillosis (ABPA)	Usually complicates long-standing asthma, leading to worsening of asthma symptoms and transient pulmonary infiltrates on CXR often with eosinophilia	ABPA occurs in 10% of those with long-standing asthma
Rheumatoid arthritis (RA)	Bronchiectasis can occur before overt arthritis, though more common during overt RA	Clinically relevant bronchiectasis in 1–3% of RA sufferers; occult occurrence in 30%
α_1-Antitrypsin deficiency	Chest disease, especially in smokers, at a young age. Symptomatic liver disease (cirrhosis) occurs at a young age	1 in 3000–5000
Marfan's syndrome	Family history of premature sudden cardiac death, due to aortic dissection; aortic root enlargement ± dissection; tall, joint hypermobility, lens dislocation	1 in 5000–10 000 Bronchiectasis is a rare complication

CXR, chest X-ray; SLE, systemic lupus erythematosus.

- Respiratory failure.
- Brain abscess from haematogenous spread of infection.
- Amyloid, with renal failure in long-standing severe disease (see Chapter 147).

Investigations

- The **chest X-ray** usually shows ring shadows or 'tram lines', representing thickened bronchial walls, although it is normal in 10%.
- **High-resolution CT chest scan** will confirm the diagnosis. The typical finding is the 'signet ring' sign – a thick-walled bronchus larger than the adjacent blood vessel.
- **Investigation of the cause**: immunoglobulin estimation, *Aspergillus* precipitins and IgE and relevant tests for cystic fibrosis. CT and/or bronchoscopy can demonstrate localized bronchial obstruction.
- **Saccharin test**: if ciliary abnormalities are suspected the time taken for saccharin placed in the nose to reach the taste buds is measured. If prolonged, electron microscopy of cilia confirms the diagnosis.
- **Lung function testing**: may reveal airflow obstruction, which is often reversible.
- **Blood gases**: in severe disease if respiratory failure is suspected.
- **Sputum microscopy and culture**: common bacterial pathogens include *Haemophilus* spp., pneumococci and *Pseudomonas* spp. Atypical organisms, including mycobacteria and fungi, may also cause infection and these should be specifically sought.

Management

- **Physiotherapy**: patients should perform twice daily postural drainage themselves to remove secretions. Supervised physiotherapy is useful during exacerbations.
- **Bronchodilators**: β-agonists, anticholinergics and inhaled steroids are used if reversibility has been demonstrated by formal testing.

Specific treatments

- **Immunoglobulin** replacement in hypogammaglobulinaemia reduces infections.
- Inhaled α_1-antitrypsin has not been shown to benefit deficient patients.
- **Antibiotics**: in high doses and for longer duration than standard courses (10–14 days) are used for infective exacerbations, guided by sensitivity from sputum cultures. Some patients with frequent exacerbations benefit from continuous/rotating antibiotic courses. *Pseudomonas* infection requires the simultaneous use of two antibiotics from different generic groups for a prolonged course ($\geq$14 days).
- **Oxygen**: for symptom relief in hypoxic patients. Patients with chronic hypoxia and cor pulmonale should be prescribed long-term oxygen therapy.
- **Surgery**: resection of localized disease is sometimes effective in single lobar involvement and to control bleeding in massive haemoptysis, but is not useful in widespread disease. Lung transplantation should be considered in young patients with severely impaired lung function (FEV$_1$ <30% predicted).

Prognosis

Depends on severity. Some patients have few symptoms and lead a normal life with normal life expectancy. Patients with cystic fibrosis or the ciliary dyskinesias that lead to generalized disease tend to progress into respiratory failure.

112 Cystic fibrosis

Clinical features

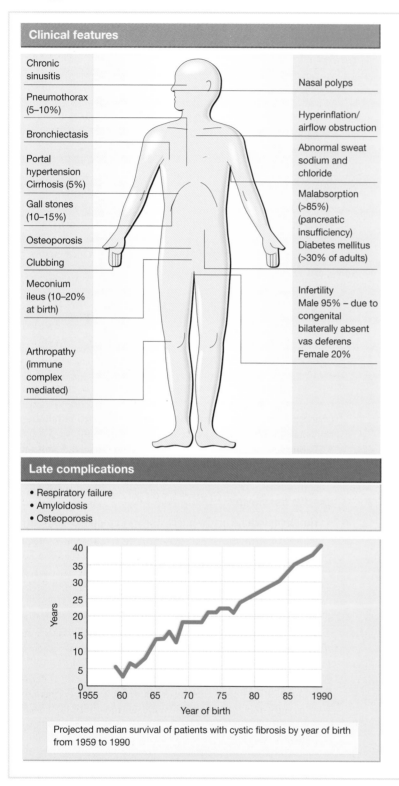

Chronic sinusitis

Nasal polyps

Pneumothorax (5–10%)

Hyperinflation/ airflow obstruction

Bronchiectasis

Abnormal sweat sodium and chloride

Portal hypertension Cirrhosis (5%)

Malabsorption (>85%) (pancreatic insufficiency)
Diabetes mellitus (>30% of adults)

Gall stones (10–15%)

Osteoporosis

Clubbing

Infertility
Male 95% – due to congenital bilaterally absent vas deferens
Female 20%

Meconium ileus (10–20% at birth)

Arthropathy (immune complex mediated)

Late complications

- Respiratory failure
- Amyloidosis
- Osteoporosis

Projected median survival of patients with cystic fibrosis by year of birth from 1959 to 1990

Pathogenesis of cystic fibrosis

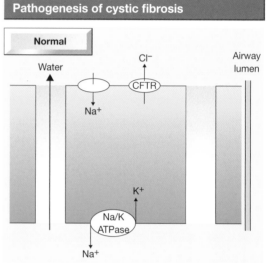

Normal

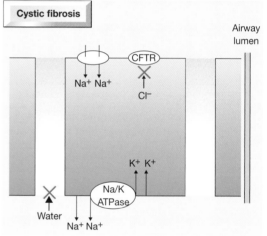

Cystic fibrosis

The cystic fibrosis transmembrane conductance regulator (CFTR), in health, acts as a channel allowing chloride ions out of the cell. This in turn keeps sodium in the mucus, which then by osmotic forces drags water into the mucus. In cystic fibrosis, the CFTR fails to allow the passage of chloride ions out of the cell. Sodium is retained intracellularly; this minimizes the osmotic forces that previously dragged water into the airway mucus. The mucus then becomes short of water, and accordingly very viscous

Medicine at a Glance, Fourth Edition. Edited by Patrick Davey. © 2014 John Wiley & Sons, Ltd. Published 2014 by John Wiley & Sons, Ltd. Companion website: www.ataglanceseries.com/medicine

Definition

Cystic fibrosis is a multisystem genetic disease leading to recurrent respiratory infections, pancreatic insufficiency and abnormal sweat sodium and chloride concentrations.

Epidemiology

Cystic fibrosis is the most common autosomal recessive condition in white people, with a carrier frequency of one in 25–30 and incidence of one in 3000 live births. The incidence is one in 20 000 in Africans/Caribbeans and one in 100 000 in Asians.

Aetiology

The abnormal gene is found on the long arm of chromosome 7 and encodes the cystic fibrosis transmembrane conductance regulator (CFTR), a cellular chloride channel that regulates the movement of salt and water across membranes. Though there are more than 800 known mutations of the gene; the DF508 mutation accounts for 70% of cases in Europeans and causes more severe disease with pancreatic insufficiency. Generally, the genetic mutation correlates only weakly with disease severity. Genetic screening is available for several of the common mutations. Functionally, the defective channel excretes less chloride into the airway lumen and has a three-fold increase in sodium absorption. Water follows sodium uptake, making airway secretions more 'sticky'.

Pathophysiology

The abnormal CFTR results in high concentrations of sodium chloride in sweat and in other secretions, which leads to an increase in the viscosity of bronchial mucus and secretions from the pancreas, liver and reproductive tract. In the lung, mucus clearance is reduced and this predisposes to infection. DNA released from infecting bacteria increases viscosity and exacerbates the problem. Recurrent infection eventually leads to generalized bronchiectasis. Pancreatic secretions are water depleted and therefore more viscid. This leads to reduced secretion of pancreatic enzymes and also local damage to pancreatic tissue, including islet cells. This further worsens secretory function and also results in diabetes mellitus.

Clinical features

- **Pulmonary features**: the lungs are normal at birth but recurrent infections in childhood lead to early-onset bronchiectasis, initially in the upper lobes, and a progressive decline in lung function with airflow obstruction, hyperinflation and breathlessness. In the later stages, clubbing, cor pulmonale and respiratory failure are common. Less severe mutations may result in bronchiectasis presenting in adulthood.
- **Pancreatic features**: pancreatic dysfunction leads to steatorrhoea, malnutrition and deficiency of fat-soluble vitamins. Diabetes is common with increasing age, occurring in more than one-third of patients by their late teens.

Investigations

- **Sweat test**: this is the routine diagnostic test of choice. Sweat sodium and chloride levels are both elevated above 60 mmol/L.
- **Genetic testing**: polymerase chain reaction (PCR) on blood is useful if the genetic mutation is known. Screening using PCR looking for the most common mutations will identify over 90% of cases.
- **Radiology**: early on, the chest X-ray reveals upper lobe bronchiectasis, although later this becomes more diffuse. If there is doubt, computed tomography will confirm this.
- **Lung function tests**: these reveal airflow obstruction with increased residual volume. There is often significant reversibility and this should be assessed. On average, lung function deteriorates by about 3% per year. Lung function impairment correlates well with mortality in late disease.
- **Sputum microbiology**: infection with common respiratory pathogens occurs with increased frequency. Most patients eventually become colonized with *Pseudomonas aeruginosa* which requires more intensive treatment. *Burkholderia cepacia* has also been found with increasing frequency and is important because transmission between patients occurs and it can lead to rapid decline in lung function. Segregation of affected individuals may be necessary. Other important respiratory pathogens include atypical mycobacteria, methicillin-resistant *Staphylococcus aureus* (MRSA) and *Stenotrophomonas maltophilia*.
- **Other routine tests**: full blood count, urea and electrolytes, liver function test, glucose, glycosylated haemoglobin (HbA1c) and glucose tolerance test for diabetes. Abdominal ultrasonography for portal hypertension. Tests for malabsorption (see Chapter 129).

Management

Patients require regular review in specialist units.

- **Lung disease**: this is managed as for bronchiectasis with regular physiotherapy, bronchodilators and aggressive treatment of infection with antibiotics. Resistant organisms such as *Pseudomonas* spp. require prolonged treatment with at least two antibiotics. Indwelling central venous lines may be required if regular courses of antibiotics are required, and patients or relatives can be trained to administer these at home.
- **Recombinant DNase** is used to improve sputum viscosity and aid clearance by breaking down bacterial DNA in the sputum. One-third to a half of patients demonstrate improved lung function with this treatment.
- **Influenza immunization** as for all patients with severe lung disease.
- **Nutrition**: nutritional supplements to provide high calorific intake are often required and may require feeding enterostomy for overnight supplements in severe disease. Pancreatic enzymes are taken by mouth to improve digestion and reduce malabsorption. Fat-soluble vitamin supplements are also given, and insulin for diabetes.
- **Lung transplantation**: patients with an FEV_1 (forced expiratory volume in 1 s) $\leq$30% predicted should be considered for lung or heart–lung transplantation. Survival after transplantation is approximately 55% at 5 years and 35% at 10 years.
- **Gene therapy**: so far, this has not proved a clinically effective treatment. CFTR can be transfected into respiratory epithelium, but currently only at low levels insufficient to reverse the abnormality in airway secretions. In the future, it is hoped that gene therapy may provide a cure for the disease.

Prognosis

Early diagnosis, improved nutrition and effective treatment of respiratory infections have all led to an improved prognosis. Currently median survival is until age 31 years. Patients diagnosed currently have a better prognosis, with 85% anticipated to survive to age 50 years.

113 Sarcoidosis and other granulomatous lung diseases

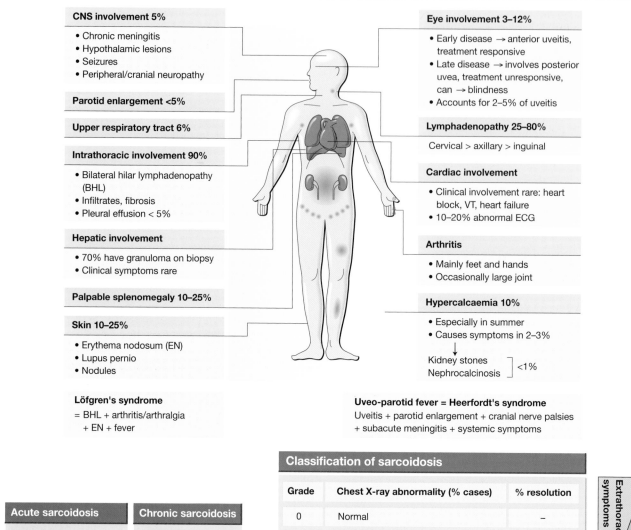

CNS involvement 5%

- Chronic meningitis
- Hypothalamic lesions
- Seizures
- Peripheral/cranial neuropathy

Parotid enlargement <5%

Upper respiratory tract 6%

Intrathoracic involvement 90%

- Bilateral hilar lymphadenopathy (BHL)
- Infiltrates, fibrosis
- Pleural effusion < 5%

Hepatic involvement

- 70% have granuloma on biopsy
- Clinical symptoms rare

Palpable splenomegaly 10–25%

Skin 10–25%

- Erythema nodosum (EN)
- Lupus pernio
- Nodules

Löfgren's syndrome

= BHL + arthritis/arthralgia + EN + fever

Eye involvement 3–12%

- Early disease → anterior uveitis, treatment responsive
- Late disease → involves posterior uvea, treatment unresponsive, can → blindness
- Accounts for 2–5% of uveitis

Lymphadenopathy 25–80%

Cervical > axillary > inguinal

Cardiac involvement

- Clinical involvement rare: heart block, VT, heart failure
- 10–20% abnormal ECG

Arthritis

- Mainly feet and hands
- Occasionally large joint

Hypercalcaemia 10%

- Especially in summer
- Causes symptoms in 2–3%
  ↓
  Kidney stones ⎤
  Nephrocalcinosis ⎦ <1%

Uveo-parotid fever = Heerfordt's syndrome

Uveitis + parotid enlargement + cranial nerve palsies + subacute meningitis + systemic symptoms

Acute sarcoidosis

Erythema nodosum
Bilateral hilar adenopathy
No pulmonary fibrosis

Chronic sarcoidosis

No EN
No BHL
Lung fibrosis

Steroid responsiveness

Need for treatment

Classification of sarcoidosis

Grade	Chest X-ray abnormality (% cases)	% resolution
0	Normal	–
1	BHL (65%)	80%
2	BHL and pulmonary infiltrate (22%)	50%
3	Pulmonary infiltrate without BHL (13%)	25%

Extrathoracic symptoms

Chest symptoms

Sarcoidosis

Definition

This is a multisystem disease of unknown aetiology characterized by the presence of non-caseating granulomas in the affected organs. It may relate to dust inhalation and a significant genetic contribution is suggested by an increased incidence in monozygotic twins. Association with the human leukocyte antigen HLA-B8 has been demonstrated, particularly with the combination of arthritis and erythema nodosum. There is no evidence that the disease is the result of tuberculosis although the histology can be similar.

Epidemiology

Females > males. Usually presents in early adult life. Incidence in the UK is 5/100 000. The clinical pattern of sarcoidosis is racially determined, in part caused by the ethnic variation in HLA-B8 incidence (see Table 113.1). Sarcoid is 15 times more common in Africans/Caribbeans.

Pathophysiology

The organs most commonly involved are: the skin, eyes (see Chapter 65) and respiratory tract. The cause is unknown but the pathological lesion is the non-caseating granuloma. In the

Medicine at a Glance, Fourth Edition. Edited by Patrick Davey. © 2014 John Wiley & Sons, Ltd. Published 2014 by John Wiley & Sons, Ltd. Companion website: www.ataglanceseries.com/medicine

Table 113.1 Clinical features (%) of sarcoidosis in different ethnic groups.

Clinical feature	White	Black	Asian
Abnormal chest X-ray	34	7	10
Respiratory symptoms	25	57	55
Systemic symptoms	5	57	55
Erythema nodosum	20	8.5	17
Eye symptoms	7	12	3
Superficial lymphadenopathy	3	34	17

lung, a lymphocytic alveolitis is present initially. Subsequent T-lymphocyte-stimulated recruitment of macrophages occurs and these organize into granulomas, which mediate inflammation and long-term damage. A syndrome clinically and histologically indistinguishable from sarcoidosis is found occasionally in patients with underlying malignancy. This should be considered when sarcoidosis presents in older patients.

Clinical features

This is a multisystem disease and features depend on the organs involved. Intrathoracic involvement is most common. There are two typical patterns:

1 **Acute presentation** with erythema nodosum, arthralgia and bilateral hilar lymphadenopathy is most common and carries a good prognosis (80% resolution in 1 year).

2 **Chronic presentation** with slowly progressive breathlessness has a worse prognosis and is associated with progressive pulmonary fibrosis.

Investigations

- **Laboratory tests**: a full blood count may show lymphopenia in active disease. Thrombocytopenia is described. The erythrocyte sedimentation rate is raised in active disease. Serum and urinary calcium are raised in 10%, more commonly so in the summer months, as a result of abnormal vitamin D metabolism. Hypercalcaemia can progress to nephrocalcinosis. Immunoglobulins are diffusely raised in active disease. Serum angiotensin-converting enzyme levels are raised in two-thirds of cases, although this is not specific for sarcoidosis.
- **Chest X-ray** findings are traditionally divided into stages that influence prognosis.
- **High-resolution computed tomography** (HRCT) reveals typical findings of mediastinal nodal disease. Pulmonary parenchymal changes include nodules in a bronchovascular, subpleural and fissural distribution.
- **Pulmonary function tests** are often normal. In fibrotic disease, reduced lung volumes and gas transfer are typical. Obstructive pulmonary function with gas trapping may be found.
- **The Kveim test** involved intradermal injection of a preparation of splenic tissue from a patient with sarcoidosis and subsequent skin biopsy. It is no longer used because of concerns over the risk of transmitting infection. Tuberculin tests are negative in two-thirds of patients.
- **Histology** is the best diagnostic test and a tissue diagnosis should always be sought if there is diagnostic doubt or if immunosuppressive treatment is to be used. Transbronchial biopsy is positive in 80%.

Management

- **No treatment**: sarcoidosis with a good prognosis (erythema nodosum and bilateral hilar lymphadenopathy) requires no treatment. Non-steroidal anti-inflammatory drugs are used for pain.

- **Oral steroids** are used in symptomatic pulmonary disease, cardiac and neurological sarcoid. Patients with pulmonary disease and radiological changes that persist for longer than 6 months have a better long-term outcome if given oral steroids (prednisolone 30–40 mg daily, discontinued after a month if no improvement) for 6 months. Other immunosuppressive drugs (most commonly methotrexate) have been used with some reported benefit.
- **Topical steroids**: for uveitis. Sometimes oral prednisolone is needed.
- **Chloroquine** can be useful in cutaneous and progressive pulmonary disease.

Prognosis

This is worse with older age of onset, more widespread disease and in Africans/Caribbeans. Two-thirds of white and one-third of black patients recover with no treatment. Fewer than 3% of patients die from sarcoidosis.

Beryllium disease

Beryllium is a heavy metal used in the manufacture of fluorescent lighting tubes. Lung disease resulting from exposure is rare.

- **Acute exposure** to fumes leads to an alveolitis, but industry precautions should prevent this occurring.
- **Chronic low level exposure** can lead to a systemic disease similar to sarcoidosis. Non-caseating granulomas appear in the skin or lungs. Radiologically, there may be nodularity in the lung fields and bilateral hilar lymphadenopathy. The pulmonary abnormality progresses to fibrosis with small lung volumes, impaired gas transfer and respiratory failure. Early treatment with corticosteroids can result in improved lung function. Workers who have been exposed to beryllium undergo regular screening with chest X-rays to detect development of asymptomatic pulmonary disease. They should of course report the development of respiratory symptoms.

Histiocytosis X (Langerhans' cell histiocytosis)

Epidemiology

This is a rare multisystem disorder of unknown aetiology occurring more often in males and usually presenting in early adult life. The vast majority of patients are smokers.

Pathophysiology and investigation

Initially there is infiltration of lung tissue with eosinophils and Langerhans' cells. This progresses to granuloma formation, which breaks down to form cystic areas, particularly in the upper zones. Ultimately pulmonary fibrosis develops. Pneumothorax is common. The diagnosis can be made radiologically. Plain X-rays and HRCT show diffuse nodularity with cyst formation in the characteristic distribution. Lung volume is often well preserved. Pulmonary function tests often reveal a restrictive defect with high residual volume and normal total lung capacity as a result of gas trapping.

Clinical features

Most patients are breathless but 25% are asymptomatic with an abnormal X-ray. Spontaneous pneumothorax is the presenting feature in 10%.

Management

Smoking cessation is essential and complete resolution with no additional treatment is possible. A variety of immunosuppressive regimens have been used. Oral corticosteroids remain the mainstay of treatment in patients with symptomatic disease. Long-term survival is commonly reported.

114 Extrinsic allergic alveolitis (hypersensitivity pneumonitis)

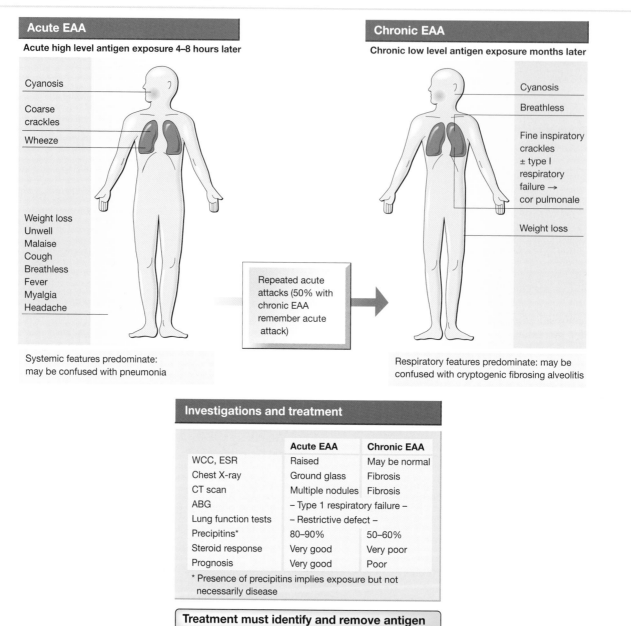

Acute EAA

Acute high level antigen exposure 4–8 hours later

- Cyanosis
- Coarse crackles
- Wheeze

- Weight loss
- Unwell
- Malaise
- Cough
- Breathless
- Fever
- Myalgia
- Headache

Systemic features predominate: may be confused with pneumonia

Repeated acute attacks (50% with chronic EAA remember acute attack)

Chronic EAA

Chronic low level antigen exposure months later

- Cyanosis
- Breathless
- Fine inspiratory crackles ± type I respiratory failure → cor pulmonale
- Weight loss

Respiratory features predominate: may be confused with cryptogenic fibrosing alveolitis

Investigations and treatment

	Acute EAA	Chronic EAA
WCC, ESR	Raised	May be normal
Chest X-ray	Ground glass	Fibrosis
CT scan	Multiple nodules	Fibrosis
ABG	– Type 1 respiratory failure –	
Lung function tests	– Restrictive defect –	
Precipitins*	80–90%	50–60%
Steroid response	Very good	Very poor
Prognosis	Very good	Poor

* Presence of precipitins implies exposure but not necessarily disease

Treatment must identify and remove antigen

Definition
This is a condition caused by hypersensitivity to inhaled organic dusts, leading to an inflammatory reaction in the distal airspaces.

Epidemiology
Uncommon: 1–2 per 100 000 in the UK. Mainly in middle-aged people.

Aetiology
Inhalation of a number of antigens may result in a pulmonary inflammatory response. For some causes, see Table 114.1.

Pathophysiology
Extrinsic allergic alveolitis (EAA) is a granulomatous reaction to a variety of organic dusts, including animal proteins (particularly from birds) and microbial spores.

- Occupational or environmental exposure to these dusts results in an immunological response, with inflammatory cell (neutrophil and lymphocyte) activation in the bronchioles extending distally into the alveoli. Accumulation of giant cells leads to granuloma formation in a bronchocentric distribution.

- Progressive fibrosis results if there is persistent inflammatory cell activation. The formation of granulomas implies that T-cell

Medicine at a Glance, Fourth Edition. Edited by Patrick Davey. © 2014 John Wiley & Sons, Ltd. Published 2014 by John Wiley & Sons, Ltd. Companion website: www.ataglanceseries.com/medicine

Table 114.1 Some causes of extrinsic allergic alveolitis – there are many other reported causes.

Disease	Cause	Agent
Farmer's lung	Mouldy hay	Thermophilic actinomycetes
Bird fancier's lung	Pigeon, budgerigar, poultry	Bloom/excreta
Wood worker's lung	Wood	Wood dust
Byssinosis	Cotton dust	? Agent
Suberosis	Cork dust	*Penicillium frequentens*
Humidifier fever	Air humidification units	Variety of agents
Malt worker's lung	Whisky maltings	*Aspergillus clavatus*
Coffee worker's lung	Coffee bean dust	Coffee

activation is involved in the pathogenesis of EAA. The presence of IgG serum precipitins implies exposure to an antigenic dust with the formation of immune complexes, but does not relate to the pathology in the lung.

Clinical features

EAA may present as acute or chronic alveolitis:

● **Acute allergic alveolitis**: 4–8 hours after exposure to high doses of antigen, systemic features of fever, myalgia and headache develop, with cough and breathlessness. Persistent exposure over weeks can produce considerable weight loss. Examination reveals inspiratory crackles and squeaks.
● **Chronic allergic alveolitis**: presents with progressive exertional breathlessness as a result of pulmonary fibrosis. Prolonged low level antigen exposure is the cause and there may be a history of acute episodes. Examination reveals inspiratory crackles typical of pulmonary fibrosis.

Investigations

● **Laboratory tests**: in acute alveolitis, a neutrophil leukocytosis may be present. The presence of circulating precipitating antibodies implies antigen exposure but not necessarily disease.
● **Chest X-ray** reveals subtle diffuse ground-glass change with small nodules, which can be confirmed by **high-resolution computed tomography** (HRCT). In chronic alveolitis, fibrosis,

typically in the mid and upper zones, is present on the chest X-ray and HRCT.
● **Pulmonary function testing**: shows a restrictive pattern in both acute and chronic disease with impaired gas transfer. Respiratory failure with hypoxaemia may be present in severe acute or chronic fibrotic disease.

The combination of symptoms, radiology, pulmonary function abnormality and the relevant exposure (presence of precipitins) is usually sufficient for a diagnosis. If doubt remains, lung biopsy may be necessary.

Management

This is aimed at optimizing lung function and preventing the development of pulmonary fibrosis. The key is antigen avoidance or reduction of exposure by the use of respiratory protection equipment. Oral corticosteroids (prednisolone 40–60 mg daily for 3–6 months) accelerate the rate of recovery, but do not improve long-term outcome. They should be reserved for patients with acute alveolitis or significant respiratory compromise.

Prognosis

● **Acute disease**: usually full recovery after cessation of exposure.
● **Chronic disease**: progressive and permanent lung damage may occur.

115 Pulmonary fibrosis

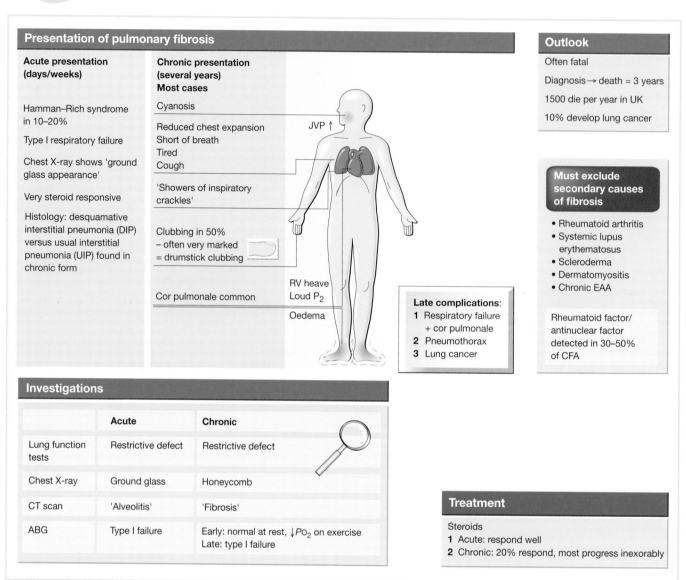

Presentation of pulmonary fibrosis

Acute presentation (days/weeks)

Hamman–Rich syndrome in 10–20%

Type I respiratory failure

Chest X-ray shows 'ground glass appearance'

Very steroid responsive

Histology: desquamative interstitial pneumonia (DIP) versus usual interstitial pneumonia (UIP) found in chronic form

Chronic presentation (several years) Most cases

Cyanosis

Reduced chest expansion
Short of breath
Tired
Cough

'Showers of inspiratory crackles'

Clubbing in 50%
– often very marked
= drumstick clubbing

Cor pulmonale common

JVP ↑

RV heave
Loud P$_2$
Oedema

Late complications:
1 Respiratory failure + cor pulmonale
2 Pneumothorax
3 Lung cancer

Outlook

Often fatal

Diagnosis → death = 3 years

1500 die per year in UK

10% develop lung cancer

Must exclude secondary causes of fibrosis

- Rheumatoid arthritis
- Systemic lupus erythematosus
- Scleroderma
- Dermatomyositis
- Chronic EAA

Rheumatoid factor/antinuclear factor detected in 30–50% of CFA

Investigations

	Acute	Chronic
Lung function tests	Restrictive defect	Restrictive defect
Chest X-ray	Ground glass	Honeycomb
CT scan	'Alveolitis'	'Fibrosis'
ABG	Type I failure	Early: normal at rest, ↓PO_2 on exercise Late: type I failure

Treatment

Steroids
1 Acute: respond well
2 Chronic: 20% respond, most progress inexorably

Definition

This is a condition involving inflammation and fibrosis of the distal airspaces, defined histologically. The combination of clinical features, restrictive pulmonary function and typical radiological changes suggests the diagnosis, often making a tissue diagnosis redundant.

Aetiology

Unknown, but an identical disease can be caused by several agents, including asbestos, hard metals, drugs and radiation. This suggests that an inhaled or environmental agent is responsible. A number of autoimmune diseases are also associated with pulmonary fibrosis. A few cases are familial, suggesting genetic influence.

Epidemiology

More frequent with increasing age. Prevalence is increasing and is currently 30/100 000. Cryptogenic fibrosing alveolitis (CFA) is more common in males. The median survival from diagnosis is only 3 years despite intervention. In some individuals, lung function may remain stable for many months.

Pathology

Histologically, alveolar walls become progressively thickened as a result of organizing inflammatory cell infiltrate with fibroblast proliferation. Two main types are recognized:

1 **Usual interstitial pneumonia** where inflammatory cells are present in the airspaces and fibrosis leads to the contraction of lung tissue and honeycombing.
2 **Desquamative interstitial pneumonia** in which the predominant infiltrate is mononuclear cell and fibrosis is less prominent.

Lung volume is reduced, diffusion impaired and respiratory failure eventually develops. There is an increased risk of lung cancer (occurs in 10% of patients).

Medicine at a Glance, Fourth Edition. Edited by Patrick Davey. © 2014 John Wiley & Sons, Ltd. Published 2014 by John Wiley & Sons, Ltd. Companion website: www.ataglanceseries.com/medicine

Clinical features

Gradual onset of breathlessness is typical. Cough is very common and is usually non-productive. In 5%, pulmonary fibrosis is an incidental finding and no symptoms are present. Examination reveals clubbing in 50%. Showers of fine, late, inspiratory crackles are present on auscultation. Respiratory distress, cyanosis and signs of cor pulmonale may develop. The Hamman–Rich syndrome is a predominantly inflammatory alveolitis of acute onset and more frequently shows a better response to treatment.

Investigations

- **Laboratory tests**: routine blood tests are normal. Blood gases may show hypoxaemia. Weakly positive titres of antinuclear antibodies and rheumatoid factor are present in a quarter.
- **Pulmonary function tests** show reduction in all lung volumes with impaired gas transfer. Gas transfer, total lung capacity and alveolar volume are used as markers of disease progression. The change in forced vital capacity (FVC) in the 6 months following diagnosis is useful in predicting prognosis. A <10% change predicts more stable disease with a better prognosis and a >10% fall in FVC suggests deteriorating disease with a poor prognosis.
- **Chest X-ray** may show diffuse predominantly basal and peripheral ground-glass change with loss of definition of the heart borders and hemidiaphragms. This may progress to reticulonodular changes and honeycombing.
- **High resolution computed tomography** (HRCT) reveals subpleural reticulation (usual interstitial pneumonia) and ground-glass change (desquamative interstitial pneumonia), with progression to honeycombing and traction bronchiectasis (usual interstitial pneumonia).
- **Histological** examination may show typical cellular infiltrate or fibrosis. The changes are patchy and transbronchial biopsy may therefore be inadequate.

Frequently the combination of clinical features and radiological changes is sufficient for the diagnosis to be made.

Management

Oral corticosteroids are the mainstay of treatment. High doses (40–60 mg prednisolone) are often used in patients with severe disease and an acute presentation. In less acutely unwell patients a lower dose (2 mg prednisolone on alternate days) may be used to reduce treatment side effects. Additional immunosuppressive drugs have been used to reduce the required steroid dose. The most commonly used is azathioprine at a dose of 2 mg/kg. A response in terms of improved lung function is reported in 10–20%, with improvement in symptoms in more. Oral N-acetyl cysteine (an anti-oxidant) has also been reported to improve lung function in some patients. Current guidelines suggest that the above three treatments should be considered in patients with pulmonary fibrosis. A recent clinical trial was stopped early as this treatment combination was associated with worse clinical outcome than placebo.

For advanced disease, supportive treatment is required. Long-term oxygen for the relief of breathlessness, diuretics for fluid retention in cor pulmonale and antibiotics for infection may all be useful. In young patients with advanced unresponsive disease, lung transplantation should be considered.

Prognosis

The 5-year survival rate is only 50%. Current treatment has not influenced this figure. In the UK, 1500 people die annually from fibrosing alveolitis.

116 Pulmonary eosinophilia and vasculitis

Causes of pulmonary eosinophilia

Common
- Asthma
- ABPA
- Drugs
- Parasites

Rare
- Churg–Strauss
- Chronic eosinophilic pneumonia
- Polyarteritis nodosa
- Hodgkin's disease

Löffler's syndrome
= eosinophilia + transient chest
X-ray infiltrate lasting 4–6 weeks
Often related to
- Drugs
- Parasitic worms

Pulmonary eosinophilia

Disease	Features	Investigations	Treatment
Acute eosinophilic pneumonia	Fever, dry cough, dyspnoea, myalgia, chest pain Crackles or wheeze	Eosinophilia Segmental infiltrates; peripheral ground glass on CT Restrictive lung function	Prednisolone 30–40 mg/day Reduce rapidly following improvement
Chronic eosinophilic pneumonia	Cough, fever, dyspnoea, weight loss	Eosinophilia Bilateral peripheral infiltrates Restrictive lung function	Prednisolone 30–40 mg/day Reduce slowly over 6 months
Hypereosinophilic syndrome	Cough, malaise Cardiac failure (myocardial infiltration)	Eosinophilia $<20 \times 10^9$/L Chest X-ray; pulmonary infiltrates and effusions	Prednisolone 30–60 mg/day May require long-term treatment Anticoagulants
Churg–Strauss syndrome	Asthma, sinusitis, multisystem involvement	Eosinophilia, raised IgE ↑pANCA in 50% Pulmonary infiltrates Pleural effusion in up to 30% Vasculitis on biopsy	Prednisolone 40–60 mg/day reducing over a year Other immunosuppressives in severe disease

Immunologically mediated lung disease

Disease	Features	Investigations	Treatment
Goodpasture's syndrome	Pulmonary haemorrhage (breathless, haemoptysis) Renal failure	Anti-GBM antibody positive ↑ANCA (in some) Pulmonary infiltrates Renal failure – diagnostic renal biopsy	Plasma exchange Prednisolone Other immunosuppressives in severe disease Renal replacement if necessary
Wegener's granulomatosis	Nose bleeds, sinusitis, cough, haemoptysis, dyspnoea, malaise, weight loss Multisystem involvement	Anaemia, leucocytosis, renal failure Active urine sediment Pulmonary nodules (may cavitate) ↑cANCA in almost all cases Biopsy shows necrotizing granulomatous vasculitis	Prednisolone 40–60 mg/day Cyclophosphamide Renal replacement if necessary

Pulmonary eosinophilia

This is a group of rare diseases, mainly of unknown aetiology, which cause chest X-ray (CXR) abnormalities associated with a raised eosinophil count in peripheral blood. Diseases included in this category include: (i) acute eosinophilic pneumonia; (ii) chronic eosinophilic pneumonia; (iii) hypereosinophilic syndrome; and (iv) Churg–Strauss syndrome.

Other diseases that cause pulmonary disease in association with eosinophilia are: (i) asthma; (ii) fungal diseases (including allergic bronchopulmonary aspergillosis (ABPA)); (iii) parasitic infection (e.g. to the filarial parasite *Wuchereria bancrofti*); (iv)

Medicine at a Glance, Fourth Edition. Edited by Patrick Davey. © 2014 John Wiley & Sons, Ltd. Published 2014 by John Wiley & Sons, Ltd. Companion website: www.ataglanceseries.com/medicine

drug reactions (see Chapter 119); (v) polyarteritis nodosa; and (vi) Hodgkin's disease.

Epidemiology and prognosis

- **Acute and chronic eosinophilic pneumonia** are more common in women; peak incidence is 40–50 years. Fifty per cent of patients have asthma. Eosinophilic pneumonia responds well to treatment and recurrence is uncommon. Chronic disease responds less well to treatment and recurrence may require long-term steroid treatment.
- **Hypereosinophilic syndrome** is very rare, is usually of unknown cause (although it occurs more often in the tropics where it may relate to parasitic infection) and often responds poorly to treatment. Complicating cardiac failure can occur and carries a poor prognosis.
- **Churg–Strauss syndrome** is a rare form of pulmonary vasculitis (incidence about one per million) affecting small and medium-sized vessels. It occurs in patients with asthma. Antineutrophil cytoplasmic antibody (ANCA) is commonly positive. Untreated vasculitis has a poor prognosis (renal involvement). Vasculitis often responds well to treatment and relapse is unusual.

Vasculitis without eosinophilia

Several vasculitides affect the lung without provoking eosinophilia:

- **Rheumatoid arthritis**: pleural disease (thickening, effusion) is the most common manifestation. Localized nodules or more diffuse fibrosing alveolitis can occur. Extensive nodular fibrosis, called Caplan's syndrome, occurs in those with pneumoconiosis (now rarely seen).
- **Systemic lupus erythematosus**: pleural inflammation ('pleurisy') is very common. Fibrosing alveolitis occurs but is rare.
- **Wegener's granulomatosis** (WG).

Wegener's granulomatosis

General features

- WG is a multisystem vasculitis (see Table 116.1), involving small and medium-sized vessels, associated with ANCA.
- Aetiology is unknown, but may involve an infectious agent.
- Prevalence is about one per 100 000. Men and women are equally affected (i.e. 600 in the UK).
- >90% of WG patients first seek attention due to symptoms arising from the upper or lower respiratory tract.

Upper airways

- Nasal/sinus disease → congestion and nose bleed. Nasal septum perforation → saddle nose; occurs in up to 30%.
- Subglottic stenosis occurs in 20% → breathlessness (which may be severe), voice change and cough. The diagnosis of subglottic stenosis is suggested by flow–volume loops; this responds very poorly to systemic therapy but may respond to mechanical dilatation and local injection of corticosteroids.

Lower airways

- Parenchymal disease: two-thirds of those with parenchymal involvement have symptoms, one-third only have asymptomatic CXR abnormalities.
- Variable changes: bilateral nodular infiltrates, cavitatary disease and pulmonary haemorrhage.
- 15% have inflammation/stenosis of endobronchial airways → cough, wheezing, breathlessness, haemoptysis or lung collapse.
- Major cause of morbidity, but rare cause of mortality.

Renal disease

Glomerulonephritis may rapidly progress to renal failure with no or few symptoms. Renal failure is common (affecting up to 40–50%), and end-stage renal failure requiring dialysis occurs in some 10%. It is detected by dipstick testing of urine (red cells, casts, ↑ creatinine). Common cause of death.

Table 116.1 Profile of organ involvement at presentation and during the course of the disease in Wegener's granulomatosis.

	Involvement at presentation (%)	Involvement during the disease course (%)
Upper airways	73	92
Lower airways	48	85
Kidneys	20	80
Joint	32	67
Eye	15	52
Skin	13	46
Nerve	1	20

Source: Langford 1999. Reproduced with permission of BMJ Publishing.

Other features

- Eye disease: many possible manifestations, including (epi)scleritis, conjunctivitis, anterior or posterior uveitis and optic neuritis. Some 8% of patients develop permanent visual loss.
- 15% have mononeuritis multiplex; 8% have central nervous system involvement.

Diagnosis

The diagnosis is made from a biopsy showing a necrotizing vasculitis, with granuloma formation in a clinically relevant setting. Antibodies against neutrophil cytoplasm are found, in two staining patterns:

- **Cytoplasmic ANCA** (cANCA): the antigen is proteinase-3 (PR3), a 2 kDa serine proteinase found in the azurophilic granules of neutrophils. cANCA is found in 70–90% of WG. Though cANCA has a high specificity and sensitivity for WG, it should not be relied on in isolation from the clinical situation and appropriate histology, as many patients with WG do not have cANCA. In some patients, cANCA titre relates to disease activity, though in many it does not.
- **Perinuclear ANCA** (pANCA): the antigen is usually myeloperoxidase. Found in 5–10% of WG, but also many other conditions, so it has a low sensitivity and specificity for the diagnosis of WG.

Treatment and prognosis

Untreated WG has a very high mortality. Treatment with cyclophosphamide and prednisolone dramatically reduces morbidity and mortality: 75% achieve complete disease remission, and the 2-year survival rate is 80%.

Drug-related side effects (sepsis from immunosuppression, late malignancy) are common. *Pneumocystis jirovecii (carinii)* pneumonia is so common as to justify septrin prophylaxis.

Other immunologically mediated disease of the lung

- **Goodpasture's syndrome**: results from immune attack by an antibody against the lung and renal glomerular basement membrane (GBM). Pulmonary haemorrhage (causing anaemia, haemoptysis and respiratory failure) occurs usually some days to months before acute renal failure. Anti-GBM antibodies are found, and less frequently a positive ANCA. Treatment is with immunosuppression and plasma exchange.
- **Idiopathic pulmonary haemosiderosis**: a similar disease to Goodpasture's (though renal involvement is uncommon) occurring in young children (>7 years).

117 Fungi and the lung

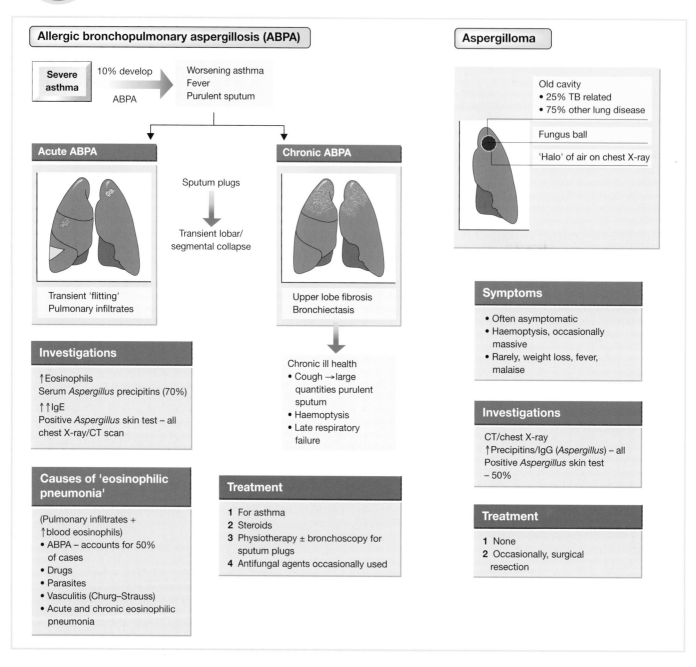

Allergic bronchopulmonary aspergillosis (ABPA)

Severe asthma → 10% develop ABPA → Worsening asthma / Fever / Purulent sputum

Acute ABPA

Transient 'flitting' Pulmonary infiltrates

Sputum plugs → Transient lobar/segmental collapse

Chronic ABPA

Upper lobe fibrosis
Bronchiectasis

Chronic ill health
- Cough → large quantities purulent sputum
- Haemoptysis
- Late respiratory failure

Investigations

↑Eosinophils
Serum *Aspergillus* precipitins (70%)
↑↑IgE
Positive *Aspergillus* skin test – all
chest X-ray/CT scan

Causes of 'eosinophilic pneumonia'

(Pulmonary infiltrates +
↑blood eosinophils)
- ABPA – accounts for 50% of cases
- Drugs
- Parasites
- Vasculitis (Churg–Strauss)
- Acute and chronic eosinophilic pneumonia

Treatment

1 For asthma
2 Steroids
3 Physiotherapy ± bronchoscopy for sputum plugs
4 Antifungal agents occasionally used

Aspergilloma

Old cavity
- 25% TB related
- 75% other lung disease

Fungus ball

'Halo' of air on chest X-ray

Symptoms

- Often asymptomatic
- Haemoptysis, occasionally massive
- Rarely, weight loss, fever, malaise

Investigations

CT/chest X-ray
↑Precipitins/IgG (*Aspergillus*) – all
Positive *Aspergillus* skin test – 50%

Treatment

1 None
2 Occasionally, surgical resection

Common fungal lung infections

Fungal lung infection develops in the immunologically incompetent and in those with chronic lung disease. Infection is usually localized in the immune competent, but those with immune deficiencies develop invasive fungal pneumonia, which has a very high mortality, caused by *Pneumocystis* spp. (see Chapter 168), *Aspergillus* spp., *Candida* spp. and cryptococcosis (see Chapter 169).

Aspergillosis

Aspergillus fumigatus is the most important human pathogen, and disease occurs in immunosuppressed individuals and in those with underlying lung disease. There are three pathologies in lung disease: allergy, colonization and invasion (see Table 117.1).

Asthma

Some patients with asthma are allergic to *Aspergillus* spp. Asthma attacks occur when fungal spores are inhaled. They have positive

Medicine at a Glance, Fourth Edition. Edited by Patrick Davey. © 2014 John Wiley & Sons, Ltd. Published 2014 by John Wiley & Sons, Ltd. Companion website: www.ataglanceseries.com/medicine

Table 117.1 Pathologies of aspergillus lung disease.

Allergic	Asthma
	Allergic bronchopulmonary aspergillosis (ABPA)
	Allergic *Aspergillus* sinusitis
	Allergic alveolitis
	(Bronchocentric granulomatosis)
Colonizing	Aspergilloma
Invasive	Invasive *Aspergillus* pneumonia

skin tests, but such positive reactions are not associated with worse disease, unless allergic bronchopulmonary aspergillosis (ABPA) is also present.

Allergic bronchopulmonary aspergillosis

Epidemiology, aetiology and pathophysiology

This uncommon complication of asthma is found in 10% of difficult asthma cases and underlies some 50% of UK pulmonary eosinophilia. Inhalation of *Aspergillus* spores leads to an IgG- and IgE-mediated hypersensitivity immune reaction, which in turn leads to dense eosinophilic infiltration of lung tissue, mucus plugging and distal collapse. A chronic inflammatory response in the airway wall causes tissue destruction and bronchiectasis. It is not clear why only some patients with asthma develop ABPA, but a genetic predisposition has been suggested.

Clinical features

ABPA patients are usually people with known asthma. Symptoms are of deteriorating asthma with purulent sputum, fever and breathlessness. Transient infiltrates on the chest X-ray (CXR) occur. In chronic bronchiectatic disease, copious purulent sputum production and haemoptysis are present.

Investigations

ABPA should be considered in people with asthma who have an abnormal CXR and high blood eosinophil count.

● **Skin tests**: a positive skin test to *Aspergillus* spp. (or raised serum-specific IgE) is required for diagnosis.
● **Blood tests**: the eosinophil count is raised, particularly in acute episodes. Total serum IgE is markedly elevated. Precipitating antibodies (IgG) are present in 70%.
● **Sputum examination**: fungal hyphae may be present in the sputum.
● **Chest X-ray**: transient ('flitting') perihilar infiltrates are present during acute attacks. Lobar or segmental collapse may occur as a result of bronchial occlusion. In chronic disease upper lobe contraction, fibrosis and bronchiectasis may occur.

Management and prognosis

Oral corticosteroids (prednisolone) are the mainstay of treatment. They improve asthma control and reduce the growth of *Aspergillus* spp. Inhaled steroids do not affect *Aspergillus* spp. but are used, along with bronchodilators, as part of the overall treatment of asthma. Physiotherapy and sometimes bronchoscopy are necessary for removal of mucus plugs. The antifungal agent itraconazole may reduce the dose of steroids required. ABPA usually progresses to bronchiectasis.

Aspergillus sinusitis

Sinusitis unresponsive to medical treatment in patients with nasal polyps has been found occasionally to be caused by *Aspergillus*

spp., and may coexist with ABPA. The histology and immunology are identical to ABPA.

Allergic alveolitis caused by *Aspergillus* spp.

This rare disease found in malt workers is caused by *A. clavatus* from mouldy barley. The pathology, clinical features and management are as for extrinsic allergic alveolitis of any cause (see Chapter 114).

Aspergilloma

A mycetoma or fungus ball is a collection of fungus.

Aetiology and pathogenesis

The causative organism is *A. fumigatus* in the UK and *A. niger* in the USA. Spores seed a pre-existing lung cavity, often (25%) as a result of previous tuberculosis (TB), and thus in the apex of the lung. Twenty per cent of cases are multiple. Spores germinate and a ball of fungus grows to fill the cavity. An immunological reaction to this process occurs. Precipitating antibodies (IgG) are universally present and a positive skin test to *Aspergillus* spp. is found in 50%.

Clinical features

Often asymptomatic and found incidentally on a CXR. The most common symptom is haemoptysis, occurring in 75%, occasionally massive, requiring embolization or surgery. Rarely, systemic features of weight loss, fever and malaise occur. Symptoms of the underlying lung disease are often present.

Investigations

The combination of the radiological features (a dense opacity with surrounding halo or crescent) and the presence of precipitating antibodies suggest the diagnosis. In patients with severe underlying lung disease, a computed tomography (CT) scan will define the mycetoma more clearly.

Management and prognosis

Antifungal therapy is ineffective. Corticosteroids have been used for systemic symptoms but increase the risk of invasion (see Chapter 169). In fit patients with systemic symptoms or significant haemoptysis, surgical resection of the mycetoma or a whole lobe is used. Ten per cent cause no problems and resolve. Death occasionally occurs as a result of massive haemoptysis. Invasive disease worsens outcome.

Aspergillus pneumonia

See Chapter 169.

Other fungal lung infections

Histoplasmosis

Histoplasma capsulatum is found worldwide and particularly in the USA, in soil contaminated by bird and bat droppings. Histoplasmosis is not found in the UK. Infection usually causes no symptoms but may lead to a febrile illness with cough, chest pain and dyspnoea, followed by resolution. Ten per cent of cases become chronic. In the acute illness, there are bilateral CXR infiltrates with enlarged mediastinal lymph nodes. Calcification of multiple pulmonary nodules can occur sometimes with cavitation. Diagnosis is either made by culture of blood or biopsy specimens or by serological tests, which usually become positive within 3 weeks of acute infection. Treatment is with amphotericin in severe disease. Itraconazole has been used for chronic disease.

Candida spp.

See Chapter 169.

Cryptococcosis

See Chapter 169.

118 Industrial lung disease

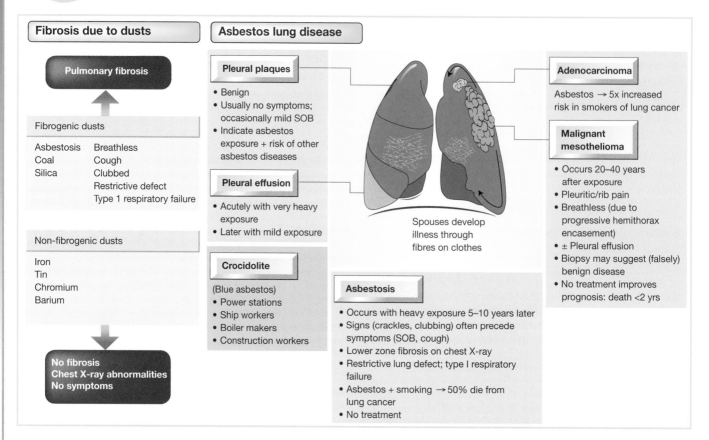

Inhalation of dusts may lead to pulmonary fibrosis or asthma (see Chapter 109).

Dust inhalation diseases

- **Fibrogenic dusts** (asbestos, coal, silica) can impair pulmonary function.
- **Non-fibrogenic dusts** (iron, tin, chromium, barium) lead to a nodular appearance on a chest X-ray (CXR) but do not impair lung function.
- **Organic dusts** can cause extrinsic allergic alveolitis (see Chapter 114).

Asbestosis

Asbestosis is lung fibrosis resulting from asbestos exposure.

Epidemiology

Asbestos-related diseases are industrial diseases (men > women), found in those exposed to blue asbestos (crocidolite). The greater the asbestos exposure, the higher the asbestosis and mesothelioma rates. Symptoms occur decades after exposure. Rates for asbestos-related diseases will increase for some years because effective legal regulation occurred relatively recently and there is often a long delay between exposure and development of disease.

Pathology

Asbestos fibres are small and penetrate distally into the lung. Fibres are engulfed by macrophages that release cytokines, so producing an inflammatory reaction, which leads to progressive fibrosis, mainly in the lower lobes. Pleural plaques are usually also present. Cigarette smoke acts synergistically with asbestos to increase pulmonary fibrosis and lung cancer rates.

Clinical features

Occupational exposure is usually present. Typical symptoms are:

- Progressive breathlessness.
- Cough.

Clinical signs are of bibasal end-inspiratory crackles, and finger clubbing in 50%. Haemoptysis suggests the development of lung cancer.

Investigations

- **Chest X-ray** reveals symmetrical basal parenchymal changes, and 75% have pleural plaques.
- **High-resolution computed tomography** (HRCT) may be abnormal when the CXR is normal and reveals subpleural changes progressing to honeycombing. Beneath areas of pleural fibrosis, nodular areas of collapse may develop (rounded atelectasis, Blesovsky's syndrome) which on CXR appear as a mass. HRCT distinguishes these appearances from those of carcinoma.
- **Pulmonary function tests** reveal a restrictive defect with reduced lung volumes and gas transfer. Blood gases show respiratory failure in end-stage disease.

Medicine at a Glance, Fourth Edition. Edited by Patrick Davey. © 2014 John Wiley & Sons, Ltd. Published 2014 by John Wiley & Sons, Ltd. Companion website: www.ataglanceseries.com/medicine

Management

- **Prevention**: risk of progression increases with cumulative dose. Prevention by reduction of exposure has reduced the incidence and severity of disease.
- **Treatment** is ineffective.
- **Prognosis**: 20% of patients with asbestosis die from the disease and 50% from an associated malignancy (lung cancer or mesothelioma).
- **Medicolegal advice**: all patients with asbestosis (and any asbestos injury caused as a result of employment) should be advised to take legal advice on whether they should make a claim for damages against the employer responsible for the asbestos exposure.

Other asbestos-related diseases: mesothelioma

This is a malignant growth arising in the pleura or occasionally in the peritoneum or pericardium; more common in males. Incidence is increasing (predicted peak 2010–2020). Develops 20–40 years after exposure as a local mass often associated with pleural effusion (>80%), which progressively encases the lung and hemithorax. Histological distinction from benign pleural disease can be difficult even with large biopsies and special staining techniques.

Clinical features

Breathlessness caused by pleural effusion is usual at presentation. Local tumour effects include severe pain due to chest wall invasion, and worsening breathlessness as a result of encasement of the lung.

Investigations

- **Chest X-ray** may reveal pleural nodularity or effusion, and pleural plaques.
- **CT** appearances suggestive of malignancy include pleural nodularity, thickening >1 cm and extension of pleural thickening over the mediastinal pleural surfaces.
- **Pleural aspiration** shows blood-stained fluid (30%). Cytology is often negative. Closed pleural biopsy is positive in 50%. Thoracoscopic biopsy is positive in 90%.

Management

For patients who are fit for chemotherapy, a combination of pemetrexed and cisplatin is licensed for treatment. Surgery may be used in early disease and can be combined with chemoradiotherapy. Clinical trials of this treatment option are currently under way. Treatment is often symptomatic: pleural aspiration for effusion causing breathlessness, often combined with pleurodesis (see Chapter 21). Alternatively, indwelling pleural catheters allowing regular drainage at home can provide symptom relief. Tumour invasion at drainage sites is common and is prevented by local radiotherapy.

Prognosis

Relentless progression occurs with increasing symptoms. Median survival is 12–18 months. Prognosis is better for epithelioid than sarcomatous mesothelioma.

Pleural plaques, pleural thickening and pleural effusion

- **Pleural plaques** are an incidental finding on CXR, implying asbestos exposure and therefore increased risk of other asbestos-related diseases. In themselves they are a benign problem and of no clinical consequence. They occur in 50% of asbestos-exposed people. Compensation is no longer available for pleural plaques.
- **Diffuse pleural thickening** occurs in 5% of asbestos workers exposed to high doses, and may cause symptoms as a result of restriction of chest wall movement. Lung function tests reveal reduced lung volumes. Such high-level exposure increases the risk of other asbestos-related diseases.
- **Pleural effusion** occurs either at the time of high level exposure or early after exposure. A blood-stained exudative effusion is typical. Resolution is normal but some patients are left with pleural thickening.

Coal worker's pneumoconiosis

Definition, epidemiology and aetiopathogenesis

This is now a rare lung disease, presenting in elderly men, and caused by inhalation of coal dust. Inhalation of small particles (0.5–7 μm) that are toxic to macrophages initiates the process. Total dose of exposure correlates with disease severity. There are three forms:

- **Simple coal worker's pneumoconiosis** (CWP): inhaled dust is enveloped by inflammatory cells resulting in small nodules. Simple CWP produces no symptoms.
- **Complicated CWP**: aggregates of small nodules lead to larger nodules >1 cm in diameter. Surrounding emphysema develops. Cavitation of nodules may occur (termed 'progressive massive fibrosis'). Complicated CWP causes progressive breathlessness; cough with black sputum (melanoptysis) may occur, as may cor pulmonale.
- **Caplan's syndrome**: large nodules may develop in coal workers with positive rheumatoid factor.

Management

- **Diagnosis** is by CXR (small or large nodules) and pulmonary function tests in complicated CWP (reduced lung volumes with airflow obstruction).
- There is no specific treatment. Avoidance of exposure has reduced the incidence. Disability from CWP is compensatable.
- **Prognosis**: as a result of control of dust levels, severe disease is rare. Respiratory failure develops in patients with progressive massive fibrosis.

Silicosis

This is a rare, restrictive, fibrotic lung disease caused by inhalation of silicon dioxide (quartz) particles (mining, sand blasting, pneumatic drilling). Inflammation and damage to local and hilar lymph node structures occur. There are two forms:

- **Acute silicosis** results from high level exposure and causes rapidly progressive breathlessness with death within months.
- **Lower level exposure** causes more slowly progressive symptoms and **predisposes to tuberculosis** (TB).

CXR shows small (1–3 mm) nodules mainly in the upper zones and larger nodules later in the disease. 'Eggshell' calcification of the hilar lymph nodes is pathognomonic. Management involves reducing dust levels, the use of respiratory protection and regular screening for TB. With avoidance of exposure, prognosis is usually good. Progressive disease or acute silicosis results in death from respiratory failure.

119 Lung disease caused by drugs

Radiological features

Lung disease	Typical pattern
Pulmonary fibrosis	Diffuse bilateral infiltrates Usually predominantly basal
Pulmonary eosinophilia	Bilateral subpleural opacities Predominantly basal in 50%
Organizing pneumonia (BOOP)	Patchy bilateral opacities Asymmetrical distribution May aggregate and form nodules Variation in distribution over time
Non-cardiogenic pulmonary oedema (ARDS)	Diffuse bilateral alveolar shadowing
Alveolar haemorrhage	Diffuse alveolar shadows
Pleural disease	Effusion ± pleural thickening Occasional pericardial effusion

Drug effects

Cough
ACE inhibitors
(10% of patients)

Pulmonary haemorrhage
Anticoagulants
Penicillamine
Carbamazepine
Nitrofurantoin

Asthma
β-blockers
NSAIDs
Cholinergic drugs
(pilocarpine)
Histamine release
(atracurium)

Pleural effusion
Bromocriptine
Amiodarone
Methotrexate
Drugs causing SLE:
• Hydralazine
• Isoniazid

ARDS
Aspirin/opiate overdose
Hydrochlorothiazide

BOOP
Amiodarone
Amphotericin
Bleomycin
β-blockers
Gold salts
Sulfasalazine

Eosinophilic pneumonia
NSAIDs
Penicillin
Septrin
Sulfasalazine
Penicillamine
Tricyclics
Captopril
Chlorpromazine

Pulmonary fibrosis
Methotrexate
Amiodarone
Nitrofurantoin
Penicillamine
Cyclophosphamide
Bleomycin
Busulfan
Other cytotoxics

The effects of drugs on the lung are extremely variable. Figure 119.1 shows common drug effects on the lung and their major causes. It is by no means exhaustive: virtually any lung disease may be drug related and thus the differential diagnosis should always include drugs as the cause.

Clinical features

These depend on the nature of the resulting lung disease. Some symptoms relate to a predictable pharmacological effect (e.g. asthma caused by β-blockers). Others may be dose related (e.g. amiodarone) or idiosyncratic. For patients on drugs commonly associated with pulmonary side effects (amiodarone, cytotoxic chemotherapeutic agents), baseline pulmonary function tests are helpful to determine whether new symptoms relate to new lung abnormalities.

Radiological features

See Figure 119.1.

Investigations

These are driven according to the nature of the respiratory symptoms. A detailed drug history, including current and previous treatment, should always be sought in any patient with respiratory symptoms. In patients with suspected pulmonary drug toxicity, diagnosis should be based on:

• The likelihood of a drug reaction to the drug(s) being taken and exclusion of alternative pathology; this may involve bronchial lavage or biopsy techniques to look for infection or confirm lung pathology.

• Consideration of which drug is responsible. If a drug reaction is confirmed, this will usually result in withdrawal of the agent concerned. Often no specific treatment is necessary. The consequences of stopping treatment need to be weighed against the likely adverse effects of continuation. Alternative treatment may need to be given to replace the effects of the drug being withdrawn.

• **Reporting to the Committee on Safety of Medicines**: all patients with drug-induced lung disease should be reported to the committee.

Medicine at a Glance, Fourth Edition. Edited by Patrick Davey. © 2014 John Wiley & Sons, Ltd. Published 2014 by John Wiley & Sons, Ltd. Companion website: www.ataglanceseries.com/medicine

120 BOOP and ARDS

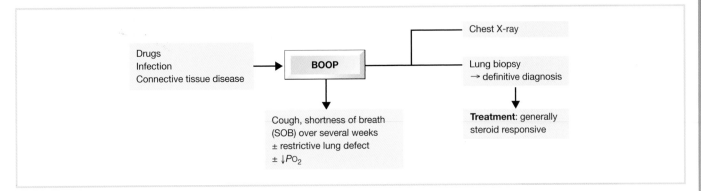

Bronchiolitis obliterans organizing pneumonia

Epidemiology
This rare disease, also known as cryptogenic organizing pneumonia, is of unknown aetiology but may present after infection or drug treatment, or as part of a connective tissue disease. Preponderance in the spring suggests an inhaled agent in some instances. There is no sex difference and no obvious geographical variation; the incidence is 6–7 per 100 000.

Pathophysiology
This is a histological diagnosis. Bronchiolitis obliterans organizing pneumonia (BOOP) is a specific way in which the lung may respond to an inflammatory stimulus. The histology reveals the changes of a pneumonitis with organization of inflammatory cells into granulation tissue. The disease originates in the alveoli with a variable amount of extension into the airways.

Clinical features
BOOP presents with systemic upset, usually over a period of a few weeks. Cough and breathlessness are present in the majority. Fever and weight loss are common. Crackles are often present.

Investigations
Chest X-ray (CXR) and computed tomography (CT) scanning show infiltrates which are often multifocal. The erythrocyte sedimentation rate is almost invariably raised and the eosinophil count is normal. Pulmonary function tests may be normal or show a restrictive defect with impaired gas transfer. In severe disease, blood gases may reveal hypoxaemia. Transbronchial biopsy may be helpful but samples are often inadequate. Open lung biopsy is diagnostic.

Management
If a causative drug can be identified, this should be discontinued. Oral corticosteroids (prednisolone 30–40 mg daily) will achieve a rapid improvement in symptoms over days in most patients. Radiological changes resolve over months and the steroid course should be reduced over an extended period (several months), as relapse is common. Relapse is likely to respond well to further steroid courses.

Acute respiratory distress syndrome

Acute respiratory distress syndrome (ARDS) is a relatively common complication of conditions that activate inflammatory mediators (see Table 120.1), resulting in diffuse lung injury, damaged pulmonary vasculature and non-cardiogenic pulmonary oedema. After several days, the inflamed lungs may fibrose, which can interfere with long-term lung function. Key points are:

- ARDS usually occurs in patients already 'sick' for other reasons. Often multiple pathologies underlie ARDS, e.g. sepsis with hypotension.
- Impaired gas exchange occurs, causing breathlessness and central cyanosis. The first indication of ARDS is usually unexplained breathlessness in an already sick patient. Signs include tachycardia, cyanosis (often with confusion and/or agitation) and inspiratory crackles throughout the lung fields.
- CXR may initially be fairly unremarkable, but later shows diffuse 'patchy' infiltrates, which can progress to a 'white out'. The differential diagnosis includes pneumonia, heart failure and interstitial lung diseases. CT scanning may help differentiate these if doubt exists.
- Intravascular capillary obstruction occurs, causing pulmonary hypertension.
- Treatment involves removing the cause (e.g. sepsis), supporting gas exchange (ventilation, which may be difficult, as the lungs are 'stiff') and other failing organs, and minimizing pulmonary oedema (keeping the patient 'dry' without provoking renal failure).
- Mortality is high at around 30–60%.

Table 120.1 Causes of ARDS.

- Sepsis, especially if shock present
- Pneumonia including influenza
- Chemical lung injury, e.g. toxic gas inhalation, gastric aspiration
- Hypotension, especially if prolonged, or with trauma
- Blood transfusion, especially if massive
- Pancreatitis
- Systemic inflammatory response syndrome (SIRS)
- Disseminated intravascular coagulation
- Obstetric causes; amniotic fluid embolism, pre-eclampsia
- Adverse drug reaction (both prescribed and 'street' drugs, e.g. heroin)
- High-altitude-related lung injury

Medicine at a Glance, Fourth Edition. Edited by Patrick Davey. © 2014 John Wiley & Sons, Ltd. Published 2014 by John Wiley & Sons, Ltd. Companion website: www.ataglanceseries.com/medicine

121 Primary tumours of the lung

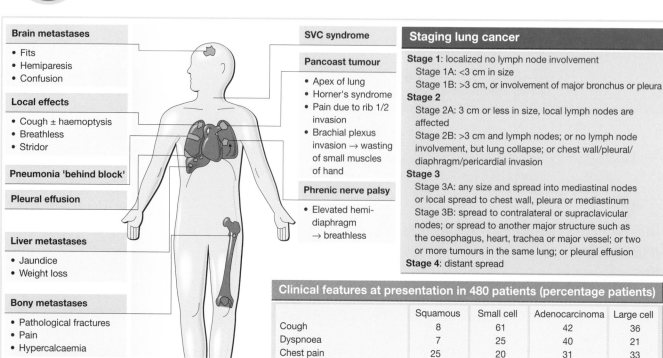

Brain metastases

- Fits
- Hemiparesis
- Confusion

Local effects

- Cough ± haemoptysis
- Breathless
- Stridor

Pneumonia 'behind block'

Pleural effusion

Liver metastases

- Jaundice
- Weight loss

Bony metastases

- Pathological fractures
- Pain
- Hypercalcaemia

SVC syndrome

Pancoast tumour

- Apex of lung
- Horner's syndrome
- Pain due to rib 1/2 invasion
- Brachial plexus invasion → wasting of small muscles of hand

Phrenic nerve palsy

- Elevated hemi-diaphragm → breathless

Staging lung cancer

Stage 1: localized no lymph node involvement
Stage 1A: <3 cm in size
Stage 1B: >3 cm, or involvement of major bronchus or pleura
Stage 2
Stage 2A: 3 cm or less in size, local lymph nodes are affected
Stage 2B: >3 cm and lymph nodes; or no lymph node involvement, but lung collapse; or chest wall/pleural/diaphragm/pericardial invasion
Stage 3
Stage 3A: any size and spread into mediastinal nodes or local spread to chest wall, pleura or mediastinum
Stage 3B: spread to contralateral or supraclavicular nodes; or spread to another major structure such as the oesophagus, heart, trachea or major vessel; or two or more tumours in the same lung; or pleural effusion
Stage 4: distant spread

Non-metastatic manifestations

- Weight loss: universal
- Endocrine: 10% often → confusion
- Neurologic: 10% often → weakness

Clinical features at presentation in 480 patients (percentage patients)

	Squamous	Small cell	Adenocarcinoma	Large cell
Cough	8	61	42	36
Dyspnoea	7	25	40	21
Chest pain	25	20	31	33
Haemoptysis	31	29	16	6
Weight loss/anorexia	88	56	55	
Hoarse voice	5	13	4	3
Bone pain	7	13	11	6
Clubbing	20	0	14	24
Supraclavicular nodes	26	39	28	42
Pleural effusion	12	13	33	12
Hepatomegaly	10	20	9	6
Neurological symptoms/signs	4	18	21	12

Cellular types of lung cancer

Cell type	% cases	Features
Squamous	40–60	Large airways Slow growth Late metastasis Cavitation occurs
Adenocarcinoma	10–20	More often peripheral lung More common in non-smokers Slow growth Metastases earlier than squamous Alveolar cell subtype grows slowly and spreads via airways Association with mutations of epidermal growth factor receptor (EGFR) which can affect response to some chemotherapy treatments
Small cell	20–25	Often central Rapid growth Early metastases (often presents with extensive disease)
Large cell	5–15	Intermediate type: progression/spread between that of squamous and small cell

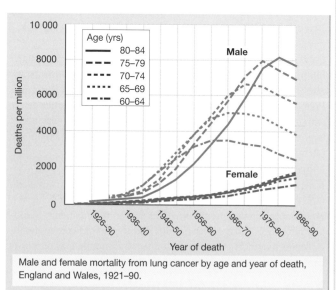

Male and female mortality from lung cancer by age and year of death, England and Wales, 1921–90.

Medicine at a Glance, Fourth Edition. Edited by Patrick Davey. © 2014 John Wiley & Sons, Ltd. Published 2014 by John Wiley & Sons, Ltd. Companion website: www.ataglanceseries.com/medicine

Epidemiology

Nearly all primary lung tumours are malignant. Lung cancer is the most common malignancy in the western world, occurring in one in 13 men and one in 20 women, with 35 000 cases/year in the UK. Most (60–65%) occur in men and are the result of cigarette smoking. Women now smoke more and accordingly their lung cancer rates are rising.

Aetiology

- **Tobacco** causes 85% of lung cancers (not adenocarcinoma). Cancer is rare in never-smokers. The more cigarettes smoked and the higher the tar content, the higher the cancer rates. After smoking cessation, lung cancer risk only falls back to that of never-smokers over the next 40 years.
- **Other risk factors**: passive smoking, occupational exposure to asbestos, silica and nickel, and pulmonary fibrosis. Genetic factors play a part.

Clinical features

New or persistent respiratory symptoms in a current or ex-smoker should always raise the suspicion of lung cancer. Symptoms may be absent or non-specific (40%: lack of energy, anorexia, weight loss), as a result of the primary cancer or caused by local spread, distant metastases or non-metastatic manifestations.

- **Effects of the primary cancer**: cough ($\geq$50%); breathlessness resulting from bronchial obstruction, lobar collapse or pleural effusion; haemoptysis ($\geq$35%). Fixed wheeze or stridor suggests large airway narrowing.
- **Effects of local spread**: local pain from chest wall involvement. Apical (Pancoast's) tumours invade the brachial plexus (pain radiating down the arm) and cause Horner's syndrome (see Chapter 60). Mediastinal invasion causes recurrent laryngeal nerve palsy (hoarseness), superior vena cava (SVC) obstruction (plethora, facial swelling), phrenic nerve palsy (breathlessness) and oesophageal compression (dysphagia).
- **Effects of distant metastases**: metastases occur in the bone (pain or hypercalcaemia), liver (asymptomatic, capsular pain) or brain (headache, confusion, seizures).
- **Non-metastatic manifestations**: endocrine – syndrome of inappropriate release of antidiuretic hormone (SIADH) (hyponatraemia especially with small-cell lung cancer; see Chapter 142) or hypercalcaemia (parathyroid hormone-related peptide in 6% of squamous carcinoma). There is ectopic adrenocorticotrophic hormone (ACTH) secretion in 30% of small cell tumours, although Cushing's syndrome rarely has time to develop; gynaecomastia occurs in $\leq$1% of squamous carcinoma.
- **Neurological symptoms**: usually relate to metastases; non-metastatic manifestations include the Lambert–Eaton myasthenic syndrome with small cell lung cancer (SCLC) (see Chapter 197). Cerebellar degeneration, peripheral neuropathy, encephalopathy, and mixed and sensory neuropathies all occur relatively infrequently.
- **Finger clubbing**: mainly in squamous carcinoma. Advanced clubbing is associated with hypertrophic pulmonary osteoarthropathy, which presents with pain and swelling in the long bones.
- **Other symptoms**: dermatomyositis and the nephrotic syndrome rarely occur.

Investigations

These should confirm the diagnosis, the cell type and stage the disease to determine treatment.

- **Chest X-ray**: usually abnormal by the time symptoms develop.
- **Paraneoplastic syndromes**: diagnosed from the full blood count, urea and electrolytes, and calcium.
- **Lung function tests**: low FEV$_1$ (forced expiratory volume in 1 s) or gas transfer preclude surgery, radical radiotherapy and percutaneous biopsy.

- **Bronchoscopy or percutaneous biopsy**: bronchoscopy produces diagnostic histology in 70% of central lung cancers. Transbronchial needle aspiration can be used to stage positive mediastinal nodes. For peripheral tumours, a computed tomography (CT)/ultrasound-guided percutaneous approach is used. If the radiological features are highly suggestive of early stage carcinoma, excision biopsy is preferable. If lymph node or liver metastases are present, biopsy of these is preferable.
- **Sputum cytology**: only used when invasive procedures are inappropriate (poor pulmonary function, co-morbid factors).

Staging investigations

For **non-SCLC**:

- **Thoracic CT**: to include the common sites for metastases – the liver and adrenal glands (4%). Small mediastinal nodes <1 cm are not malignant in 25% and, unless 'on-table' mediastinoscopic staging is positive, should not preclude surgery.
- **Isotope bone scanning** for bony metastases (bone pain or hypercalcaemia).
- **Brain CT**: for neurological disease.
- **Positron emission tomography scanning**: can reveal nodal or distant metastases not revealed by other staging methods. Should be used to confirm localized disease in all patients prior to radical treatment (surgery or radical chemo-radiotherapy). Will not reveal brain metastases.

Staging for **SCLC** differs, as metastases are often present at presentation:

- **Limited disease**: confined to one hemithorax and the ipsilateral supraclavicular fossa.
- **Extensive disease**: all other patients (70% of cases).

Management

- **Surgery** offers the best chance of cure, but <25% are operable and only 25% of these (5% of all patients) are alive at 5 years. Perioperative mortality rate is 3% for lobectomy and 6% for pneumonectomy.
- **Radical radiotherapy** is used for inoperable non-SCLC. Radical treatment is suitable for anatomically localized disease, and cures only a few.
- **Palliative radiotherapy** for haemoptysis, cough, breathlessness or local pain. Brain metastases are treated with steroids and radiotherapy.
- **Chemotherapy** is used for SCLC, because surgery is *never appropriate* with this histology. Response occurs in 60–85%; survival gain is approximately 4 months. In limited disease, radiotherapy after chemotherapy reduces local recurrence rates from 75% to 30%. Chemotherapy is recommended in non-SCLC for fit patients with metastatic disease. Chemotherapy is used increasingly preoperatively to downstage tumours and improve postoperative survival.
- **Endobronchial treatments** such as cryotherapy, laser treatment or the use of stents can provide rapid relief of symptoms in patients with significant symptomatic endobronchial disease.
- **Palliative care**: opiates are helpful for pain and dyspnoea. Steroids help non-specific symptoms and improve appetite. Support from carers, family and palliative care specialists is extremely important.

Prognosis

This depends partly on cell type. Overall survival rate at 1 year is 27% in men and 30% in women. At 5 years this falls to 7% and 9% respectively. Even after apparently successful surgical resection, the 5-year survival rate is only 40–50%. Median survival in small cell disease without treatment is 2–3 months and, with extensive disease at presentation, survival is 4 weeks without treatment. With treatment 25% of patients with limited disease at presentation survive 2 years. In extensive disease 2-year survival falls to less than 5%.

122 Food poisoning and gastrointestinal infections

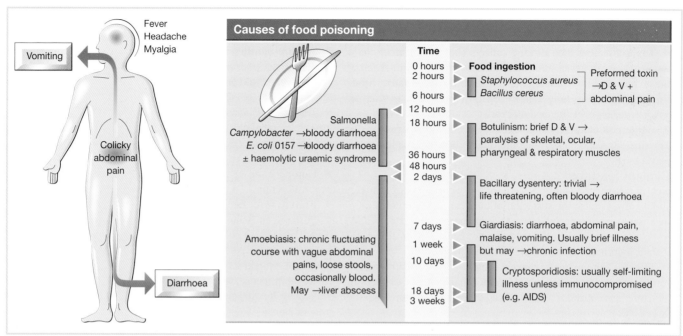

Causes of food poisoning

Time	
0 hours	Food ingestion
2 hours	*Staphylococcus aureus* / *Bacillus cereus* — Preformed toxin →D & V + abdominal pain
6 hours	
12 hours	
18 hours	Botulinism: brief D & V → paralysis of skeletal, ocular, pharyngeal & respiratory muscles
36 hours	
48 hours	
2 days	Bacillary dysentery: trivial → life threatening, often bloody diarrhoea
7 days	Giardiasis: diarrhoea, abdominal pain, malaise, vomiting. Usually brief illness but may →chronic infection
1 week	
10 days	Cryptosporidiosis: usually self-limiting illness unless immunocompromised (e.g. AIDS)
18 days	
3 weeks	

Fever / Headache / Myalgia

Vomiting

Colicky abdominal pain

Diarrhoea

Salmonella
Campylobacter →bloody diarrhoea
E. coli 0157 →bloody diarrhoea
± haemolytic uraemic syndrome

Amoebiasis: chronic fluctuating course with vague abdominal pains, loose stools, occasionally blood. May →liver abscess

Acute gastroenteritis

Acute and short-lived diarrhoea (with vomiting (D&V) or without) is now a very common complaint. In many cases the management is empirical and based on history rather than positive cultures. Important causes include:

- **Common**: culture negative (viral), *Campylobacter* spp., *Salmonella* spp., cholera (developing countries).
- **Uncommon**: *Shigella* spp.
- **Rare** but important: *Escherichia coli* O157, *Staphylococcus aureus*, *Vibrio para-haemolyticus*, *Clostridium botulinum*.

Clinical features

Symptoms are usually of sudden onset: diarrhoea with or without vomiting, abdominal pain and fever, headache or myalgia. There may be a history of travel or suspect food, and other individuals may also be affected.

Investigations

Most cases settle spontaneously and do not require investigation. In patients sufficiently ill to warrant admission to hospital, investigations should be considered, including stool and blood cultures, full blood count, electrolytes and plain abdominal radiology.

Management and prognosis

Mild cases require no more than an encouragement for oral rehydration. More severe cases may require intravenous fluids. Antibiotics are indicated in septicaemia (i.e. fever, positive blood cultures). Ciprofloxacin is a good first-line agent, active against the common bacterial pathogens (*Salmonella*, *Shigella* and *Campylobacter* spp.).

If diarrhoea persists for more than 3 weeks the patient will need further investigation (e.g. colonoscopy) and should be referred to a gastroenterologist. Common causes of persistent diarrhoea include hypolactasia, postinfective irritable bowel and

giardiasis, but consideration should be given to the presence of an unrelated underlying pathology (colitis, coeliac disease).

Chronic infections

Giardiasis

Infection with *Giardia lamblia* may cause a persistent infection. Making a positive diagnosis on culture may prove difficult (even with culture of duodenal aspirates). Empirical treatment with tinidazole or metronidazole is effective.

Tuberculosis

Gastrointestinal tuberculosis (TB) is a rare but important diagnosis. The diagnosis should be considered in patients from developing countries who have chronic abdominal symptoms. There are a number of possible clinical presentations:

- **Ileocaecal TB**, which mimics Crohn's disease (fever, abdominal pain, weight loss, diarrhoea). The chest X-ray is usually normal and TB is not found elsewhere in the body.
- **Tuberculous peritonitis**: exudative ascites. May require peritoneal biopsy to make the diagnosis.
- **Mesenteric lymphadenopathy**, which may cause right iliac fossa pain and subacute obstructive symptoms. Lymph nodes elsewhere (cervical, mediastinal, peritoneal) are also usually affected.

Treatment is the same as for pulmonary TB.

Amoebiasis

Infection with *Entamoeba histolytica* may cause a variety of clinical presentations: asymptomatic excretion of cysts is the most common finding, amoebic dysentery, non-dysenteric colonic disease and invasive disease/hepatic abscess also can occur. The diagnosis may be made by microscopy of 'hot' stool looking for ova cysts and parasites or by histology of colonic biopsies and/or serology. Treatment is with metronidazole followed by diloxanide furoate.

Medicine at a Glance, Fourth Edition. Edited by Patrick Davey. © 2014 John Wiley & Sons, Ltd. Published 2014 by John Wiley & Sons, Ltd. Companion website: www.ataglanceseries.com/medicine

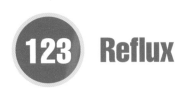

123 Reflux

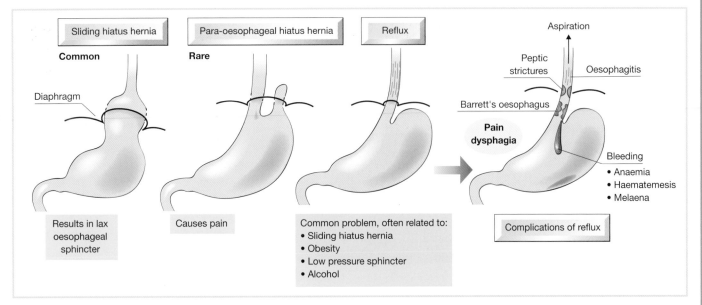

| Sliding hiatus hernia | Para-oesophageal hiatus hernia | Reflux |

Common

Rare

Diaphragm

Aspiration

Peptic strictures

Oesophagitis

Barrett's oesophagus

Pain dysphagia

Bleeding
• Anaemia
• Haematemesis
• Melaena

Results in lax oesophageal sphincter

Causes pain

Common problem, often related to:
• Sliding hiatus hernia
• Obesity
• Low pressure sphincter
• Alcohol

Complications of reflux

Incidence
Symptoms of gastro-oesophageal reflux are very common in the western world (20–40% of the population).

Pathophysiology
• Laxity of the lower oesophageal sphincter predisposes to episodic reflux of acid and other gastric contents back into the oesophagus.

• Symptoms of reflux will be exacerbated by **lifestyle factors**. Obesity increases intra-abdominal pressure. Smoking, stress and dietary factors (e.g. fatty foods, pastry, alcohol, chocolate) all reduce the pressure in the lower oesophageal sphincter and promote reflux. Symptoms might also be provoked by postural factors, e.g. eating late at night.

• Some patients with symptomatic reflux might be shown to have a hiatal hernia but the two are not synonomous.

Clinical features
Symptomatic reflux is diagnosed on the basis of a good clinical history and many patients will have unremarkable investigations.

• **Heartburn**: reflux most commonly presents with heartburn and occasionally nausea (see Chapter 30). Effortless regurgitation (to be distinguished from vomiting) and belching ('northerly wind') will often be present and the symptoms may have a marked postural element.

• **Chest pain** may be the presenting symptoms and results from reflux-precipitated oesophageal spasm. This may be indistinguishable from angina. Cardiac pain should be excluded (often by exercise testing) before the upper gastrointestinal tract is investigated.

• **Transient dysphagia** may be experienced in severe oesophagitis. More predictable dysphagia with food bolus impaction or vomiting suggests the development of a secondary complication such as a peptic oesophageal stricture or even carcinoma.

Investigations
• **Upper gastrointestinal endoscopy** may be useful in reflux. In many this is normal or it may demonstrate oesophagitis.

• **24-hour oesophageal manometry and pH recording**: patients with persistent and troublesome symptoms may benefit from manometry and pH recording, which is used to select those patients who might benefit from antireflux surgery.

Management and prognosis
• **Lifestyle changes**: most patients with reflux symptoms will experience a significant improvement by:
  • Limiting chocolate, coffee and alcohol intake.
  • Maintaining a reasonable body mass index.
  • Eating regular meals (especially breakfast) and avoiding late night eating.

• **Antacids**: over-the-counter antacids (often with an alginate) are used intermittently by many reflux sufferers.

• **Proton pump inhibitors** (e.g. omeprazole, lansoprazole) are the most potent treatment for reflux symptoms. Clinical response to a therapeutic trial of acid suppression often proves informative – if not diagnostic.

• **Pro-kinetics**: patients with more regurgitation than heartburn may be better treated with a pro-kinetic agent (e.g. domperidone) to aid gastric emptying.

• **Surgery**: antireflux surgery (laparoscopic Nissen's fundoplication) is beneficial in those whose symptoms are resistant to medical therapy, who have unacceptable side effects on proton pump inhibitors (usually diarrhoea) or those with a rolling hiatal hernia and a high risk of incarceration/volvulus. Endoscopic antireflux procedures may become an alternative option for some patients.

Barrett's oesophagus
Barrett's epithelium is present in up to 15% of patients with reflux symptoms. This is potentially a premalignant condition, predisposing to lower third oesophageal adenocarcinoma. The incidence of cancer in patients with Barrett's is now recognized to be lower than initially feared (0.5%) and although regular surveillance endoscopy and oesophageal biopsies to identify dysplasia has been widely advocated the benefit of such strategies remains unproved.

American Gastroenterological Association. Medical position statement on the management of Barrett's esophagus. Gastroenterology 2011: 140; 1084–91.

124 Peptic ulcer disease

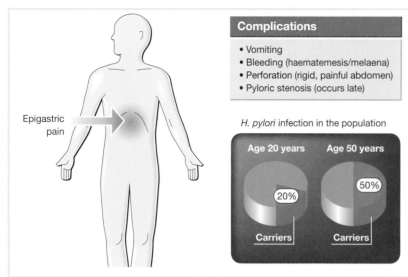

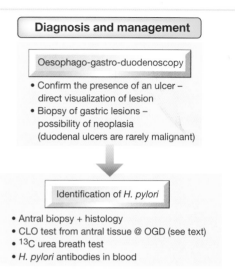

Complications

- Vomiting
- Bleeding (haematemesis/melaena)
- Perforation (rigid, painful abdomen)
- Pyloric stenosis (occurs late)

H. pylori infection in the population

Age 20 years — 20% Carriers

Age 50 years — 50% Carriers

Diagnosis and management

Oesophago-gastro-duodenoscopy

- Confirm the presence of an ulcer – direct visualization of lesion
- Biopsy of gastric lesions – possibility of neoplasia (duodenal ulcers are rarely malignant)

Identification of *H. pylori*

- Antral biopsy + histology
- CLO test from antral tissue @ OGD (see text)
- ^{13}C urea breath test
- *H. pylori* antibodies in blood

Epigastric pain

Peptic ulceration of the upper gastrointestinal (GI) tract may occur in either the duodenum or the stomach.

Duodenal ulcer

Duodenal ulcers occur predominantly when gastric acid production exceeds the buffering capacity of the alkali secreted from Brunner's glands and the pancreas. There is a very strong association with the presence of *Helicobacter pylori* and the use of nonsteroidal anti-inflammatory drugs (NSAIDs).

Clinical features

- **Gastrointestinal haemorrhage**: now the most common presentation of peptic ulceration (see Chapter 27).
- **Dyspepsia**: abdominal pain has historically been considered to be the classic symptom of a duodenal ulcer but many patients presenting with acute GI bleeding deny indigestion symptoms.
- **Vomiting**: may be the presenting feature if long-standing duodenal ulceration results in pyloric stenosis.
- **Perforation** with peritonitis is occasionally a presenting or complicating feature.

Investigations

- **Endoscopy** is the first-line investigation for patients with dyspepsia and for upper GI bleeding (for diagnosis and endoscopic therapy in bleeding).
- **Testing for *H. pylori***: various tests allow the identification of this organism, which is characteristically very difficult to culture:
  - **Serology**: measurement of *H. pylori*-specific IgG antibodies in blood.
  - **Urease breath test**: ^{13}C radiolabelled urea is ingested, which is split by bacterial urease producing $^{13}CO_2$, which is then exhaled and detected in the breath.
  - **CLO test** (*Campylobacter*-like organism test), from endoscopically obtained gastric antral biopsy: this test also detects the presence of bacterial (i.e. *H. pylori*) urease causing a colour

change in a pH-sensitive gel indicator (changing from yellow to red).
  - **Faecal antigen testing**: possibly more specific and sensitive than serology.

Detection of *H. pylori* alone is not sufficient for a diagnosis of duodenal ulceration, because 20% (aged 20 years) to 50% (aged 50 years) of the population are carriers.

Gastric ulcer

Although there is considerable overlap in the pathophysiology of duodenal and gastric ulcers, the latter commonly occur in circumstances of impaired mucosal defence (e.g. NSAID use). Distinguishing between benign and malignant gastric ulcers can be extremely difficult endoscopically. Biopsies should always be taken and endoscopic follow-up arranged to ensure healing.

Clinical features and investigations

The clinical presentation is similar to duodenal ulcers and GI bleeding is now as common a presentation as indigestion. As newly identified gastric ulcers may represent early gastric cancer, biopsy of the ulcer edge and interval re-endoscopy after 6 weeks of medical therapy are mandatory.

Management and prognosis

- **Medical therapy** with proton pump inhibitors with or without *H. pylori* eradication results in ulcer healing after 4–6 weeks. Wherever possible NSAIDs should be stopped.
- ***H. pylori* eradication**: ulcer recurrence is common without eradication of *H. pylori*. Eradication regimens consisting of high doses of a proton pump inhibitor in combination with two different antibiotics are 70–80% successful. Success should be documented using the urease breath test. In failed eradication, re-endoscopy with culture of organisms for antibiotic sensitivity is occasionally indicated.
- **Surgery**: required in those with perforation and recurrent or persistent bleeding. Elective surgery is an infrequent option for persistent ulceration and/or intolerance of medical therapy.

Medicine at a Glance, Fourth Edition. Edited by Patrick Davey. © 2014 John Wiley & Sons, Ltd. Published 2014 by John Wiley & Sons, Ltd. Companion website: www.ataglanceseries.com/medicine

125 Diverticular disease

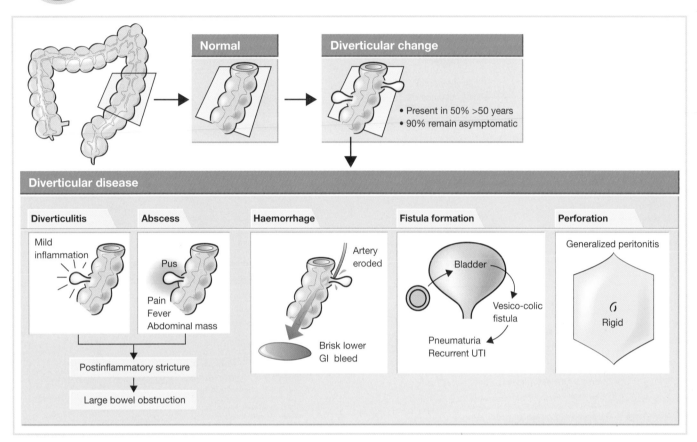

Diverticulosis represents a degenerative change in the colon resulting in the formation of out-pouches or pockets of colonic mucosa extruding through the muscular wall of the bowel. In many elderly people this may be asymptomatic and the terms 'diverticular change' or 'diverticulosis' may be more appropriate than the more commonly used term diverticulitis.

Incidence
The prevalence increases with age and is 5% at 40 years rising to 50% at 80 years.

Pathophysiology
There may be an underlying genetic predisposition to diverticular disease but it is best considered to be an acquired condition.

Clinical features
Diverticular change itself is asymptomatic and it is the common complications that lead to symptomatic presentation.

● **Diverticulitis**: an associated inflammation of the colon – considered to be precipitated by impaction of faeces within a diverticulum. This may evolve into a diverticular abscess with abdominal pain, fever and a left-sided abdominal mass.

● **Colonic bleeding**: this is a frequent presentation of diverticular disease, possibly because diverticula form at the point of maximal weakness in the colon, i.e. at the point where blood vessels penetrate the muscle coat.

● **Repeated infective episodes** may result in the formation of either a diverticular stricture presenting with symptoms of colonic obstruction or a colovesical fistula presenting with recurrent urinary tract infections (UTIs) or the characteristic symptom of pneumaturia.

Investigations
● **Colonoscopy** or computed tomography (CT) colonography: asymptomatic diverticular change may be demonstrated as an incidental finding at colonoscopy or on other colonic imaging.

● **Abdominal CT**: the best way to demonstrate abscesses. Colovesical fistulae require a high index of suspicion (recurrent UTIs, pneumaturia, etc.), and may need to be looked for specifically (i.e. using rectal contrast).

Management and prognosis
The management of diverticular disease is conservative, though surgery is occasionally required.

● **Avoidance of symptomatic constipation**: may reduce the risk of complications.

● **Treatment of complications**: acute diverticulitis requires intravenous fluids, antibiotics and analgesics. Diverticular abscess may require drainage in addition to the above. Bleeding usually settles with supportive treatment.

● **Surgery**: this is usually reserved for complicated diverticular disease (i.e. bleeding, abscess, stricture).

Medicine at a Glance, Fourth Edition. Edited by Patrick Davey. © 2014 John Wiley & Sons, Ltd. Published 2014 by John Wiley & Sons, Ltd. Companion website: www.ataglanceseries.com/medicine

126 Iron deficiency

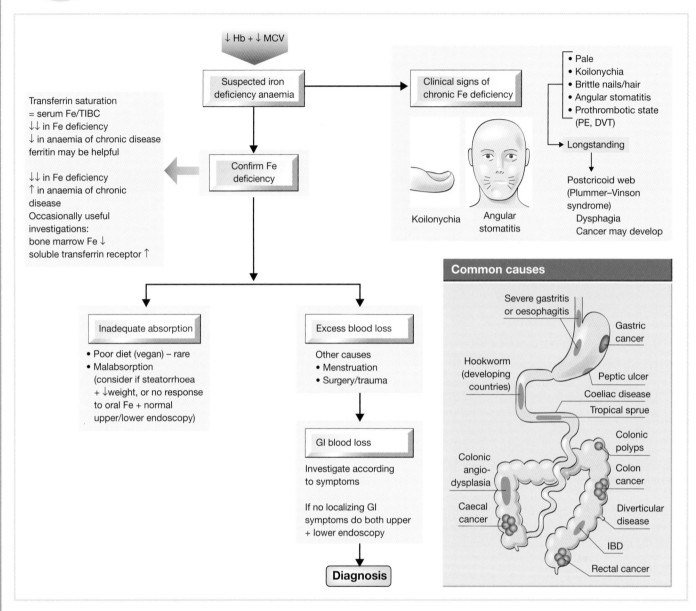

Iron is absorbed in the proximal small intestine. There is no physiological route of iron excretion in humans. Hence there are two potential reasons for iron deficiency:

1 **Reduced iron absorption** from the gastrointestinal (GI) tract, as a result of mucosal disease (coeliac disease) or duodenal bypass (polyagastrectomy).
2 **Chronic blood loss**, the most common cause, resulting from: (i) menstrual bleeding (pre-menopausal women); (ii) GI neoplasia (colonic adenomatous polyps, caecal/gastric carcinoma); or (iii) intestinal angiodysplasia.

Clinical features

Many patients do not have GI symptoms, although any symptoms found may prioritize the subsequent investigation.

History

In pre-menopausal women, a menstrual history should be taken. Previous gastric surgery may predispose to iron deficiency through duodenal bypass (i.e. gastroenterostomy) or gastric cancer.

Examination

In elderly people, an underdiagnosed cause of iron deficiency is intestinal angiodysplasia – small angiodysplastic lesions may be seen on the lips or buccal mucosa. Lymphadenopathy should be sought (i.e. Virchow's node). An abdominal mass may be present and each iliac fossa should be carefully palpated. Even without altered bowel habit or rectal bleeding, a rectal examination and sigmoidoscopy are mandatory.

Medicine at a Glance, Fourth Edition. Edited by Patrick Davey. © 2014 John Wiley & Sons, Ltd. Published 2014 by John Wiley & Sons, Ltd. Companion website: www.ataglanceseries.com/medicine

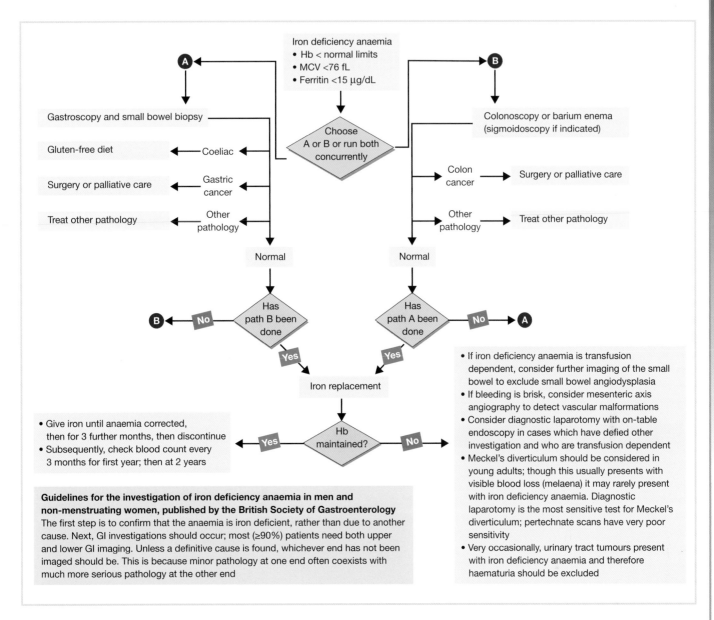

Iron deficiency anaemia
- Hb < normal limits
- MCV <76 fL
- Ferritin <15 μg/dL

Choose A or B or run both concurrently

Gastroscopy and small bowel biopsy

Gluten-free diet ← Coeliac

Surgery or palliative care ← Gastric cancer

Treat other pathology ← Other pathology

Colonoscopy or barium enema (sigmoidoscopy if indicated)

Colon cancer → Surgery or palliative care

Other pathology → Treat other pathology

Normal

Normal

Has path B been done — No → B

Has path A been done — No → A

Yes

Yes

Iron replacement

Hb maintained? — Yes / No

- Give iron until anaemia corrected, then for 3 further months, then discontinue
- Subsequently, check blood count every 3 months for first year; then at 2 years

- If iron deficiency anaemia is transfusion dependent, consider further imaging of the small bowel to exclude small bowel angiodysplasia
- If bleeding is brisk, consider mesenteric axis angiography to detect vascular malformations
- Consider diagnostic laparotomy with on-table endoscopy in cases which have defied other investigation and who are transfusion dependent
- Meckel's diverticulum should be considered in young adults; though this usually presents with visible blood loss (melaena) it may rarely present with iron deficiency anaemia. Diagnostic laparotomy is the most sensitive test for Meckel's diverticulum; pertechnate scans have very poor sensitivity
- Very occasionally, urinary tract tumours present with iron deficiency anaemia and therefore haematuria should be excluded

Guidelines for the investigation of iron deficiency anaemia in men and non-menstruating women, published by the British Society of Gastroenterology
The first step is to confirm that the anaemia is iron deficient, rather than due to another cause. Next, GI investigations should occur; most (≥90%) patients need both upper and lower GI imaging. Unless a definitive cause is found, whichever end has not been imaged should be. This is because minor pathology at one end often coexists with much more serious pathology at the other end

Investigations

- **Blood tests**: a full blood count shows a microcytic anaemia.
- **Ferritin and transferrin saturation** (serum iron divided by total iron-binding capacity (TIBC)) are low. Ferritin is an acute phase reactant and may be raised (or inappropriately 'normal') in the presence of any coexisting inflammation. A microcytic anaemia should always be confirmed as being caused by iron deficiency before treatment/GI investigation.
- **Tissue transglutaminase** antibodies: persistent or recurrent iron deficiency in the absence of obvious loss requires investigation for malabsorption and tissue transglutaminase antibody to exclude coeliac disease.
- **Faecal occult blood**: chemical tests for haem oxygenase (haemoccult) are very sensitive – persistently strongly positive results suggest significant GI blood loss; these tests are rarely used other than in the context of bowel cancer screening (see Chapter 193).
- **Colonoscopy and endoscopy**: most patients with iron deficiency require examination of both upper and lower GI tracts. At upper endoscopy, duodenal biopsies should be taken to exclude

coeliac disease. Polyps identified at colonoscopy are snared and removed.
- **Computed tomography colonography**: may be considered a suitable alternative to colonoscopy in elderly and frail patients.
- **Small bowel imaging**: if no source is identified, consideration should be given to small bowel imaging, preferably with wireless capsule endoscopy.

Management

- **Treat underlying cause**: GI angiodysplasia can be managed by continuous oral iron replacement (for gastric and colorectal cancer, see Chapters 135 and 136).
- If **no source of GI blood loss is identified**, consideration should be given to either continuous oral iron replacement or a course of replacement, and repeat investigation should the problem recur.

British Society of Gastroenterology. *Guidelines for the Management of Iron Deficiency Anaemia.* www.bsg.org.uk (last accessed September 2013).

127 Abnormal liver function tests

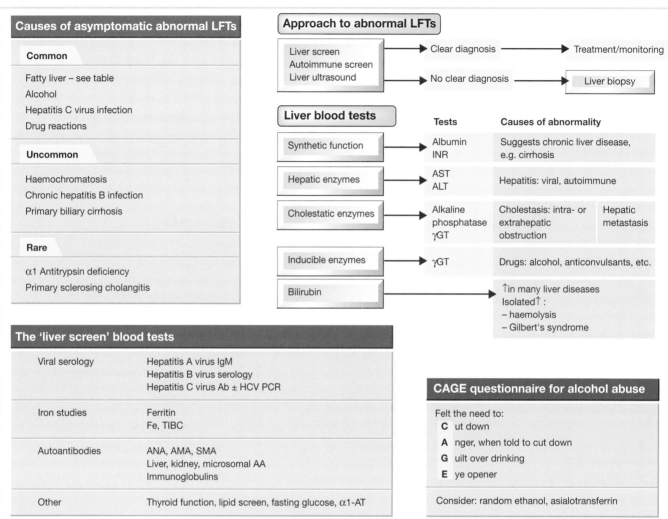

Causes of asymptomatic abnormal LFTs

Common

Fatty liver – see table
Alcohol
Hepatitis C virus infection
Drug reactions

Uncommon

Haemochromatosis
Chronic hepatitis B infection
Primary biliary cirrhosis

Rare

α1 Antitrypsin deficiency
Primary sclerosing cholangitis

Approach to abnormal LFTs

Liver screen / Autoimmune screen / Liver ultrasound → Clear diagnosis → Treatment/monitoring

Liver screen / Autoimmune screen / Liver ultrasound → No clear diagnosis → Liver biopsy

Liver blood tests

	Tests	Causes of abnormality	
Synthetic function	Albumin INR	Suggests chronic liver disease, e.g. cirrhosis	
Hepatic enzymes	AST ALT	Hepatitis: viral, autoimmune	
Cholestatic enzymes	Alkaline phosphatase γGT	Cholestasis: intra- or extrahepatic obstruction	Hepatic metastasis
Inducible enzymes	γGT	Drugs: alcohol, anticonvulsants, etc.	
Bilirubin		$\uparrow$in many liver diseases Isolated$\uparrow$: – haemolysis – Gilbert's syndrome	

The 'liver screen' blood tests

Viral serology	Hepatitis A virus IgM Hepatitis B virus serology Hepatitis C virus Ab ± HCV PCR
Iron studies	Ferritin Fe, TIBC
Autoantibodies	ANA, AMA, SMA Liver, kidney, microsomal AA Immunoglobulins
Other	Thyroid function, lipid screen, fasting glucose, α1-AT

CAGE questionnaire for alcohol abuse

Felt the need to:
C ut down
A nger, when told to cut down
G uilt over drinking
E ye opener

Consider: random ethanol, asialotransferrin

Overall approach

Abnormalities in liver function tests (LFTs) accompanied by symptoms are described in the relevant chapters. Abnormalities of LFTs in asymptomatic individuals are a frequent reason for outpatient hospital referral. Although these individuals are often not ill at the time of the consultation, the abnormal test may herald an underlying disease and an attempt is made to reach a diagnosis to make prognostic and therapeutic decisions. For differential diagnosis, see Figure 127.1 and Table 127.1.

Often there is little in the clinical history, although there are many features that should be specifically sought:

● *Alcohol intake is commonly understated/under-reported by the patient.* Many patients quote the national recommendations of 14 units/week (women) and 21 for men. It is more informative to know whether or not the patient takes alcohol daily and what the patient drinks. Remember that the alcohol concentration of beers varies considerably. The CAGE questionnaire may be useful (see Figure 127.1); a positive answer to two or more questions has a 90% correlation with alcohol dependence.

● Features suggesting hepatitis B or C, including foreign travel (Far East and Africa), sexual preferences and intravenous drug use (past or present).

● Full current and recent medication history, including antibiotics, over-the-counter drugs, herbal and alternative medicines.

● Family history of liver disease or multiorgan pathology such as alcohol, diabetes (e.g. haemochromatosis) or emphysema (e.g. α_1-antitrypsin (α_1-AT) deficiency).

● Other illnesses.

Examination

Look for signs of chronic liver disease, although these may be sparse. Record the patient's weight and body mass index (see Chapter 38).

Investigations

Blood tests

A predominant rise in alanine transaminase (ALT) represents a hepatocellular injury, whereas a predominant rise in alkaline phosphatase indicates a 'cholestatic' or biliary pattern. Random ethanol levels may help diagnose occult alcoholic liver disease (and this may also be suggested by increased γ-glutamyl transferase (γ-GT) levels and erythrocyte mean red cell volume). Other routine tests include:

● **Viral serology**: hepatitis A does not cause persistently abnormal LFTs, although hepatitis B and C can.

Table 127.1 Non-alcoholic steatosis: common cause of abnormal liver function tests.

	Non-alcoholic fatty liver disease (NAFLD)	Non-alcoholic steatohepatitis (NASH)	Cirrhosis due to NASH
Epidemiology	• Also known as simple steatosis • Affects 10–25% of the population • Found in 70% of obese subjects • Increasing rates in older subjects	• May affect 2–3% of US population • Found in 25% of those undergoing anti-obesity surgery • 40% overweight/obese • 20% diabetic • 20% dyslipidaemic • 50% men	• Occurs in a variable number with NASH; ±3% at 10 years with simple steatosis or non-specific inflammation on biopsy • Occurs in 25–30% at 8–10 years in those with NASH and hepatocyte necrosis on biopsy • 80% of those developing cirrhosis have fibrosis on preceding biopsy for NASH
Clinical features	• Usually asymptomatic • Small proportion 'tired', upper abdominal discomfort	50% have persistent fatigue and/or upper abdominal discomfort	Features of chronic liver disease: • Tired • Other features (see Figure 133.1)
Cause	Relates to 'the metabolic syndrome' (insulin resistance)	Primary NASH: • Obesity; especially central pattern Secondary NASH: • Drugs, including amiodarone, methotrexate • Sudden weight loss (e.g. jejunoileal bypass surgery) or weight-cycling • Wilson's disease, lipodystrophy	• Genetic factors may promote progression from NASH to cirrhosis • Cytokines, and reactive oxygen species may also promote cirrhosis
Laboratory data	Biochemistry usually normal	• ALT and AST raised. ALT:AST ratio >1 (in EtOH-related disease ratio usually <1) • TNF-α may promote progression from simple steatosis to NASH • 20–50% have ↑ ferritin levels	• Features in common with other cirrhosis patients • Liver enzymes may be normal ↔ abnormal • ± ↓ albumin; ± ↑ INR
Imaging	Ultrasound, CT and MRI can diagnose moderate–severe steatosis	Imaging cannot distinguish NAFLD from NASH	Liver often small, spleen large
Histology	Normal liver architecture + lipid accumulation in hepatocytes (lipids comprise 5–10% by weight)	• Steatosis + some inflammation ± fibrosis • BMI >28; ALT >2× normal; age >50 years; triglycerides >1.8; hypertension and diabetes predict fibrosis (confirmatory biopsy needed) • Biopsy shows liver inflammation + variable fibrosis	• Frank cirrhosis
Treatment	• Weight loss (must be gradual) • Exercise	• Control hyperglycaemia • Remove any contributor drugs • Possibly probiotics to reduce gut-derived cytokines, LPS. Possibly vitamin E, etc.	• Standard care for chronic liver disease • Accounts for 3% of liver transplants
Prognosis	Excellent; probably the same as for age-matched controls	Reasonable, though some increase in mortality	• Poor; 15% of hepatomas may relate to NASH or NASH-related cirrhosis

ALT, alanine transaminase; AST, aspartate transaminase; BMI, body mass index; EtOH, ethyl alcohol; INR, international normalized ratio; LPS, lipopolysaccharide; TNF-α, tumour necrosis factor α.

• **Soluble markers of liver fibrosis**: a number of blood tests have be identified as indicators of liver fibrosis (pro-collagen III peptide, hyaluronidase, TIMP-1 (tissue inhibitor of metalloproteinase 1)). These are probably best employed in combinations.

• **Autoantibodies and immunoglobulins**: primary biliary cirrhosis may present with non-specific malaise and pruritus. Antimitochondrial antibodies will be present in 95% and will often be accompanied by an elevated IgM. Autoimmune hepatitis is usually accompanied by autoantibodies to double-stranded DNA, smooth muscle, soluble liver antigen, liver cytosol and liver–kidney microsomes. The IgG and IgA are usually elevated. Primary sclerosing cholangitis is associated with atypical antineutrophil cytoplasmic antibody (ANCA).

• **Iron studies** to detect haemochromatosis: the early identification of this common inborn error of metabolism is very important.

• **α₁-AT levels**: the relationship between α_1-AT deficiency and liver disease is very complex but patients should not smoke.

• **Fasting glucose**: diabetes can cause abnormal LFTs, as can obesity and, paradoxically, starvation.

• **Depressed albumin or prolonged prothrombin time** indicates impaired liver function.

• The **lipid profile** is often deranged in significant chronic liver disease and should be measured.

• **Liver ultrasonography**: this is mandatory to exclude focal liver abnormality, such as malignancy, and may occasionally identify features suggesting chronic liver disease (e.g. splenomegaly, ascites, intra-abdominal varices). Doppler examination of the portal vein may indicate portal hypertension.

• **Liver elastography** (e.g. FibroScan): measurement of liver elasticity (or 'stiffness') with low amplitude ultrasound has been demonstrated in many liver conditions to correlate with fibrosis and cirrhosis.

• **Liver biopsy** remains the definitive way of determining prognosis (i.e. the presence of fibrosis), even if a formal diagnosis is not possible.

Management

Management depends on the underlying pathology. Often the need is for qualified reassurance and an opinion about prognosis.

128 Inflammatory bowel disease

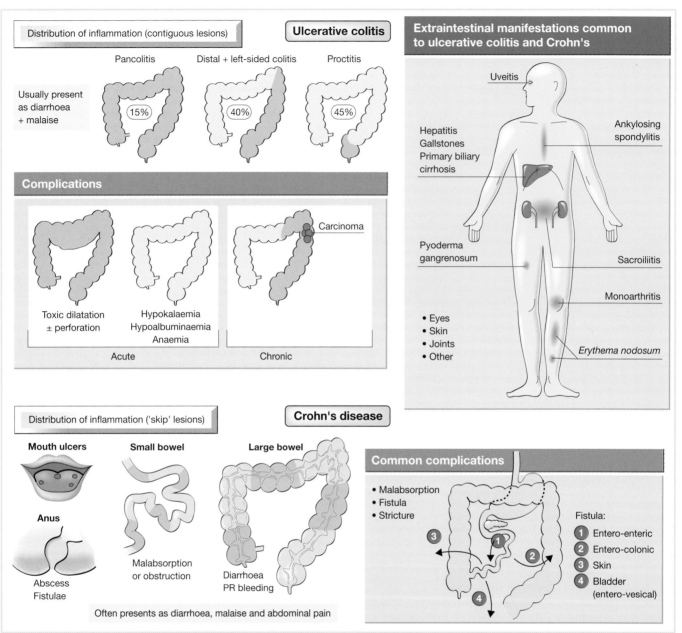

Distribution of inflammation (contiguous lesions)

Ulcerative colitis

Pancolitis   Distal + left-sided colitis   Proctitis

Usually present as diarrhoea + malaise   15%   40%   45%

Extraintestinal manifestations common to ulcerative colitis and Crohn's

Uveitis
Hepatitis
Gallstones
Primary biliary cirrhosis
Ankylosing spondylitis
Pyoderma gangrenosum
Sacroiliitis
Monoarthritis
Erythema nodosum
• Eyes
• Skin
• Joints
• Other

Complications

Toxic dilatation ± perforation   Hypokalaemia Hypoalbuminaemia Anaemia   Carcinoma

Acute   Chronic

Distribution of inflammation ('skip' lesions)

Crohn's disease

Mouth ulcers   **Small bowel**   **Large bowel**

Anus

Malabsorption or obstruction   Diarrhoea PR bleeding

Abscess Fistulae

Often presents as diarrhoea, malaise and abdominal pain

Common complications

• Malabsorption
• Fistula
• Stricture

Fistula:
1 Entero-enteric
2 Entero-colonic
3 Skin
4 Bladder (entero-vesical)

Idiopathic inflammatory bowel disease (IBD) comprises ulcerative colitis (UC), Crohn's disease and the microscopic colitides (lymphocytic and collagenous colitis). In some patients the distinction between these conditions may prove difficult and the term 'indeterminate colitis' may be used.

Ulcerative colitis

This is the most common form of IBD, affecting 80–160 per 100 000 of the population. It commonly presents in young adults. No unifying cause has been identified, although genetic factors play a major role with 15% of cases having a clear family history. Smoking appears to protect against UC for unknown reasons. After the first attack, 5% die within <1 year, 10% have continually active disease, 75% intermittently active disease and 10% a long-lasting (>15 years) remission. There is a 20% risk of colon cancer after 30 years.

Pathophysiology and clinical features

The pathological hallmarks of UC are: inflammation is always present in the rectum, it extends a variable distance proximally in the colon, is continuous and is limited to the mucosa of the bowel (i.e. it is superficial).

● 'Total' colitis (pancolitis) presents with chronic diarrhoea (>6 weeks), sometimes with constitutional upset and objective biochemical markers of inflammation.

● 'Distal' UC (left-sided colitis, proctosigmoiditis, proctitis) more often presents with rectal bleeding associated with urge and a sense of incomplete rectal emptying (tenesmus). Constitutional disturbance is less frequent.

With either presentation there may be extraintestinal manifestations of disease (arthralgia, iritis, skin lesions). Pain is an infrequent feature.

Investigations

The diagnosis is made on the basis of history, histology and imaging. It is crucial to recognize severe colitis early and treat vigorously.

- The **Truelove–Witts criteria** for severe colitis are:
  - Stool frequency >6/day – plus one of the following:
  - Temperature >37.8°C.
  - Pulse >90 bpm.
  - Haemoglobin <10.5 g/dL.
  - Erythrocyte sedimentation rate (ESR) >30 mm/h.
- **Rectal biopsy** may differentiate a short-lived infective colitis (hallmarks of chronicity being distortion of colonic crypts and depletion of goblet cell stores of mucus).
- **Flexible sigmoidoscopy or colonoscopy** is used to delineate the disease extent. Long-standing total colitis carries a risk for colonic carcinoma. Reassessment of the extent of the disease by colonoscopy is recommended 8–10 years from diagnosis. Surveillance colonoscopy with biopsies of the colon looking for dysplasia may be appropriate and should occur every 2 years initially. In some patients yearly surveillance may be necessary (those with coexistent primary sclerosing cholangitis and those with a disease history of over 20 years).
- **Abdominal X-ray**: in severe acute colitis a plain abdominal X-ray confirms the extent of disease (inflamed bowel being empty) and excludes 'toxic dilatation' – a life-threatening complication with a high risk of perforation, which requires consideration of emergency surgery.
- **Stool culture**: to exclude infective diarrhoea.

Management

- **Steroids**: severe acute colitis requires hospital admission and intravenous (IV) steroids. Less severe attacks require oral or topical steroids depending on disease *extent.*
- **Ciclosporin**: may be of benefit for severe acute colitis that fails to respond to initial treatment.
- **5-Aminosalicylic acid** compounds: effective in mild attacks and reduce the risk of subsequent episodes.
- **Azathioprine** (or related compound 6-mercaptopurine): used in those experiencing frequent relapses.
- **Infliximab**: some studies have demonstrated a benefit of tumour necrosis factor α (TNF-α) antibodies such as infliximab in UC. The exact role of such therapies remains to be fully defined.
- **Surgery**: for a colon that is *life-threatening* (i.e. perforation, cancer or severe dysplasia) or one that is *life limiting* (i.e. incompatible with a reasonable quality of life despite maximal medical therapy).

Crohn's disease

A chronic granulomatous inflammatory disease affecting the gut. Pathological features that distinguish it from UC include:

- It affects any part of the gut from the mouth to the anus.
- The inflammation is discontinuous with 'skip lesions'.
- The inflammation is deep and sometimes transmural, resulting in gut stenosis and penetrating ulcers leading to abscesses and fistulae.
- Uncommon; UK prevalence is 40–80 cases per 100 000 population.

Clinical features

The cardinal symptoms are abdominal pain and systemic upset with weight loss and fever. Bloating and vomiting will be present when stricturing disease is present. Diarrhoea is reported by most patients but has numerous different mechanisms (colonic inflammation, bile salt malabsorption, small bowel bacterial overgrowth). The combination of symptoms will depend upon:

- **Site of disease**: small bowel disease is more likely to present with malabsorption and features of small bowel obstruction than colonic disease, which causes diarrhoea.
- **Extent and severity of inflammation** are easily underestimated in young adults – many patients present with pronounced fatigue, anorexia and poor general health.
- **Secondary complications**: such as abscess, stricture and fistulae.
- **Extraintestinal manifestations** may be related to disease activity (e.g. aphthous ulceration, erythema nodosum, acute arthropathy, eye complications) or occur independently from disease flares (sacroiliitis, ankylosing spondylitis).

The differential diagnosis includes *Yersinia* infection and intestinal tuberculosis.

Investigations

- **Systemic markers of inflammation**: the ESR and C-reactive protein are useful in monitoring disease activity.
- **Intestinal imaging**: small bowel Crohn's disease can be demonstrated on a small bowel enema or barium follow-through study. This type of examination is being increasingly replaced by computed tomography (CT) and magnetic resonance imaging (MRI), which not only give important information about the extent of small bowel disease and the degree of intestinal obstruction but also delineate extraintestinal complications (abscesses, fistulae).
- **Endoscopy**: allows for diagnostic biopsy. Colonoscopy with terminal ileoscopy is useful for delineating the extent and severity of colonic disease.
- **Wireless capsule endoscopy**: may be of use in identifying subtle mucosal inflammation but the presence of intestinal strictures is a contraindication (risk of capsule impaction).
- **Ultrasonography/CT of abdomen**: useful for excluding abscess formation in sick patients with a palpable abdominal mass. MRI is useful for the investigation of perianal and pelvic Crohn's disease.

Management and prognosis

Multidisciplinary, involving physicians, surgeons, radiologists and nutritionists. Crohn's disease is an incurable illness, which follows a remitting/relapsing course, causes considerable morbidity and has a 15% mortality rate.

- **Steroids**: remain the most potent medical treatment. Other than in isolated distal colonic disease, these must be administered systemically (e.g. oral prednisolone or IV hydrocortisone), with the attendant long-term risks of adrenal suppression and osteopenia.
- **5-Aminosalicylic compounds**, such as sulfasalazine and mesalazine, are used as maintenance treatment of colonic Crohn's disease.
- **Other immunosuppressive agents**: azathioprine, 6-mercaptopurine and methotrexate are effective maintenance treatments and are used in those with frequent or severe relapses:
  - 'Biologicals': antibodies to TNF-α are used for steroid-resistant disease and perineal fistulae.
  - Other monoclonal antibodies are under evaluation.
- **Surgery**: given the patchy and recurrent nature of Crohn's disease, surgery tends to be conservative and reserved for symptoms due to structural disease (i.e. strictures) not responding to medical therapy and other specific complications (e.g. abscesses, fistulae).
- **Nutrition**: nutritional support presents specific challenges, given the combination of the high metabolic demand of acute inflammation with small intestinal dysfunction. Liquid diets are very effective. An 'elemental diet' is a liquid diet in which the nitrogen source is in the form of amino acids. A 'polymeric diet' provides short peptides.

129 Malabsorption

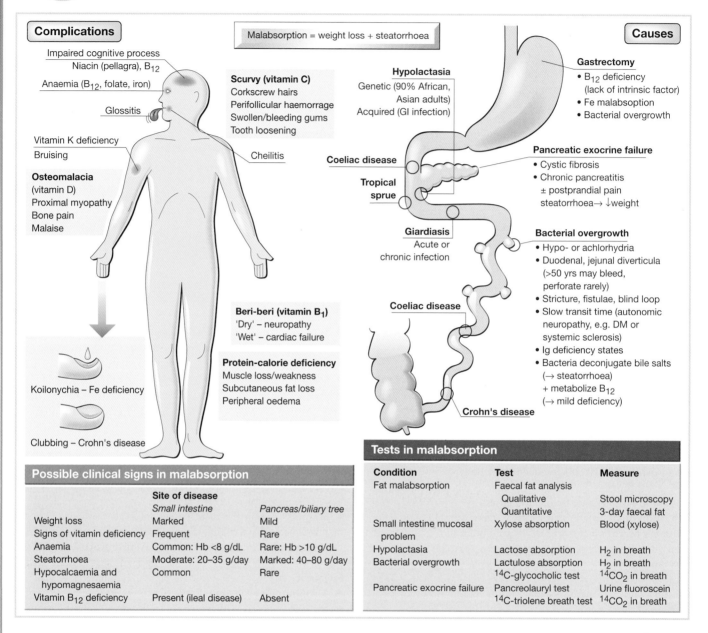

Complications

Impaired cognitive process
Niacin (pellagra), B_{12}
Anaemia (B_{12}, folate, iron)
Glossitis
Vitamin K deficiency
Bruising

Osteomalacia
(vitamin D)
Proximal myopathy
Bone pain
Malaise

Koilonychia – Fe deficiency

Clubbing – Crohn's disease

Malabsorption = weight loss + steatorrhoea

Scurvy (vitamin C)
Corkscrew hairs
Perifollicular haemorrage
Swollen/bleeding gums
Tooth loosening

Cheilitis

Beri-beri (vitamin B_1)
'Dry' – neuropathy
'Wet' – cardiac failure

Protein-calorie deficiency
Muscle loss/weakness
Subcutaneous fat loss
Peripheral oedema

Hypolactasia
Genetic (90% African,
Asian adults)
Acquired (GI infection)

Coeliac disease

Tropical sprue

Giardiasis
Acute or
chronic infection

Coeliac disease

Crohn's disease

Causes

Gastrectomy
• B_{12} deficiency
  (lack of intrinsic factor)
• Fe malabsoption
• Bacterial overgrowth

Pancreatic exocrine failure
• Cystic fibrosis
• Chronic pancreatitis
  ± postprandial pain
  steatorrhoea→ ↓weight

Bacterial overgrowth
• Hypo- or achlorhydria
• Duodenal, jejunal diverticula
  (>50 yrs may bleed,
  perforate rarely)
• Stricture, fistulae, blind loop
• Slow transit time (autonomic
  neuropathy, e.g. DM or
  systemic sclerosis)
• Ig deficiency states
• Bacteria deconjugate bile salts
  (→ steatorrhoea)
  + metabolize B_{12}
  (→ mild deficiency)

Possible clinical signs in malabsorption

	Site of disease	
	Small intestine	*Pancreas/biliary tree*
Weight loss	Marked	Mild
Signs of vitamin deficiency	Frequent	Rare
Anaemia	Common: Hb <8 g/dL	Rare: Hb >10 g/dL
Steatorrhoea	Moderate: 20–35 g/day	Marked: 40–80 g/day
Hypocalcaemia and hypomagnesaemia	Common	Rare
Vitamin B_{12} deficiency	Present (ileal disease)	Absent

Tests in malabsorption

Condition	Test	Measure
Fat malabsorption	Faecal fat analysis	
	Qualitative	Stool microscopy
	Quantitative	3-day faecal fat
Small intestine mucosal problem	Xylose absorption	Blood (xylose)
Hypolactasia	Lactose absorption	H_2 in breath
Bacterial overgrowth	Lactulose absorption	H_2 in breath
	^{14}C-glycocholic test	$^{14}CO_2$ in breath
Pancreatic exocrine failure	Pancreolauryl test	Urine fluoroscein
	^{14}C-triolene breath test	$^{14}CO_2$ in breath

Malabsorption is suggested by the combination of chronic diarrhoea and weight loss despite preservation of appetite (see Chapter 23). Thyrotoxicosis can also cause these symptoms. The causes of malabsorption include:

- **Common**: coeliac disease, pancreatic exocrine insufficiency and Crohn's disease.
- **Uncommon**: hypolactasia, small bowel bacterial overgrowth, giardiasis and HIV.
- **Rare**: tropical sprue, Whipple's disease and amyloidosis.

Clinical features and examination

Most patients describe weight loss despite preservation of appetite (and even hunger), general fatigue and diarrhoea – often steatorrhoea (pale offensive stools that float in the toilet pan and require two or more flushes of the toilet). In malabsorption caused by pancreatic exocrine failure, a history of excess alcohol or previous acute pancreatitis may be found. In malabsorption relating to gastrointestinal (GI) infection, a travel history may be relevant. In the physical examination look specifically for:

- Objective evidence of **weight loss**.
- **Markers of malnutrition**: leukonychia, glossitis, cheilitis, anaemia (folate, vitamin B_{12}, protein).
- **Markers of specific nutritional deficiencies**: scurvy (vitamin C), koilonychia (iron), osteomalacia (vitamin D and calcium), bruising (vitamin K).
- Clinical features of **thyrotoxicosis**: tremor, tachycardia, exophthalmos.

Medicine at a Glance, Fourth Edition. Edited by Patrick Davey. © 2014 John Wiley & Sons, Ltd. Published 2014 by John Wiley & Sons, Ltd. Companion website: www.ataglanceseries.com/medicine

- **Lymphadenopathy**: Virchow's node – representing intra-abdominal malignancy.
- **Abdominal examination**: a mass may be palpable in ileal Crohn's disease. The stool on rectal examination often appears pale and smells offensively. It may also be 'oily'.

Investigations

Investigations should objectively evaluate the effects of malnutrition and seek to identify the underlying disease.

- **Blood tests**:
  - Determine the severity of malnutrition (full blood count, liver function tests, albumin, international normalized ratio, calcium, magnesium, zinc, vitamin B_{12}, folate).
  - Exclude certain conditions (thyroxine, thyroid-stimulating hormone, tissue transglutaminase for coeliac disease).
  - Raise the possibility of certain diseases (erythrocyte sedimentation rate/C-reactive protein in Crohn's disease).
- **Endoscopy and duodenal biopsies** are used to exclude coeliac disease and giardia.
- **Small bowel imaging** is used when non-coeliac small bowel mucosal disease is suspected. The range of investigations include small bowel enema, magnetic resonance or computed tomography (CT) enterography and enteroscopy (either 'push' or 'wireless'/capsule).
- **Testing of stool** for the presence of undigested faecal fat is rarely performed now.
- **Tests of small bowel function**: hydrogen breath tests – H_2 appears in the breath when lactose (hypolactasia) or lactulose (small bowel overgrowth) are given.
- **Pancreatic imaging**: pancreatic ultrasonography, CT and magnetic resonance cholangiopancreatography (MRCP) are indicated when chronic pancreatitis is suspected to underlie pancreatic exocrine failure.
- **Tests of pancreatic function**:
  - **Faecal elastase or chymotrypsin**: low pancreatic elastase activity is found in the stool in moderate–severe pancreatic exocrine failure.
  - **Pancreolauryl test**: fluorescein dilaurate is ingested, and if pancreatic exocrine enzymes are present fluorescein is split off, absorbed and passed into the urine, where it can be detected.

Management

- Treat the underlying cause: see relevant sections.
- Dietary advice and supplementation vitamin and nutrient replacement may be indicated (folate, vitamin B_{12}, iron).
- Think about the bones: osteopenia is a significant long-term problem in malabsorption (see Chapter 216).

Diseases causing malabsorption

Coeliac disease

Coeliac disease (gluten-sensitive enteropathy) is the most common cause of small bowel malabsorption in the West. It is common, especially in northwest Europe. The prevalence in west Ireland is 1:150, in England 1:300. The incidence is increasing, although better diagnostic tests may contribute to this. The peak incidence is 20–40 years, although it can present at any age.

Coeliac disease is the result of an immune reaction to gluten. Initially this causes an increase in the intraepithelial lymphocytes in the small intestinal epithelium. This subsequently progresses to flattening of the intestinal villi (villous atrophy). There are HLA (human leukocyte antigen) associations to HLA DQ2 and DQ8.

Clinical features

- **Iron deficiency**: the diagnosis is often made during investigation of iron deficiency.
- **Malabsorption**: coeliac disease will now rarely present with classic sprue (diarrhoea, weight loss, oedema).
- **Case finding**: although there is no mandate for screening for coeliac disease, the increasing recognition of a strong genetic component has led to a lowered threshold for making the diagnosis in first-degree relatives of affected individuals.
- **Dermatitis herpetiformis**: this rare but characteristic blistering eruption may lead to the diagnosis of coeliac disease.

Investigations

- **Endoscopy and distal duodenal biopsy**: traditionally, this is repeated after a period on a gluten-free diet.
- **Antibodies**: IgA class tissue transglutaminase antibodies are highly sensitive and specific for coeliac disease. However, selective IgA deficiency is present in up to 5% of coeliac patients rendering the serology relatively 'uninformative' in these individuals.
- **Bone densitometry**: even in the absence of significant weight loss, bone density may be significantly reduced at the time of presentation.

Management and prognosis

- **Gluten-free diet**: completely reverses the histological and nutritional changes.
- **Vitamin and iron replacement** with iron, folate and vitamin B_{12} are needed in malabsorption.
- **Osteopenia**: with effective treatments for osteopenia now available, this important feature should be prospectively monitored and treated.
- **Small intestinal cancers** (enteropathy-associated T-cell lymphoma, adenocarcinoma): these are rare complications for which no surveillance has proven to be effective. They are important to consider in refractory disease or individuals who relapse clinically.

Other causes of malabsorption

- **Small bowel bacterial overgrowth** results from either structural or functional disorders that cause relative stasis (e.g. hypo- or achlorhydria, jejunal diverticulosis, post-surgical blind loops, intestinal strictures, autonomic neuropathy, scleroderma). Diagnosis is confirmed with a lactulose breath test or empirical treatment with antibiotics. Small bowel imaging for structural lesions is usually unnecessary. Treatment is with antibiotics (metronidazole and tetracycline), which may need to be repeated.
- **Giardiasis**: persistent infection with *Giardia lamblia* may cause diarrhoea and malabsorption.
- **Hypolactasia**: loss of lactase from the small intestinal brush border may be primary or secondary following a GI infection. This results in milk intolerance, which causes bloating, nausea, wind and diarrhoea. The diagnosis is confirmed by a lactose breath test. Treatment is with a low lactose diet.
- **Other diseases**: including pancreatic exocrine failure and Crohn's disease (see Chapter 128).

American Gastroenterological Association Medical Position Statement. The diagnosis and management of celiac disease. *Gastroenterology* 2006: 131; 1977–80.

130 Pancreatitis and pancreatic cancer

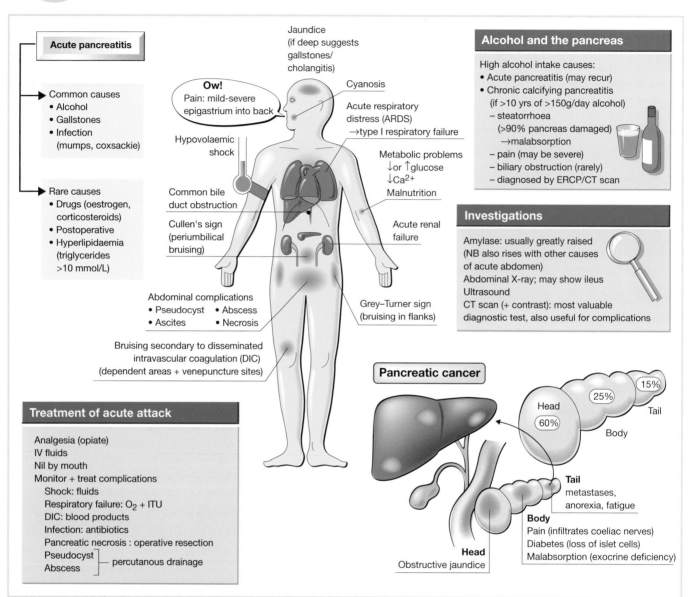

Acute pancreatitis

Common causes
- Alcohol
- Gallstones
- Infection (mumps, coxsackie)

Rare causes
- Drugs (oestrogen, corticosteroids)
- Postoperative
- Hyperlipidaemia (triglycerides >10 mmol/L)

Ow!
Pain: mild-severe epigastrium into back

Jaundice (if deep suggests gallstones/cholangitis)

Cyanosis

Acute respiratory distress (ARDS) →type I respiratory failure

Hypovolaemic shock

Common bile duct obstruction

Cullen's sign (periumbilical bruising)

Metabolic problems
↓or ↑glucose
↓Ca²⁺
Malnutrition

Acute renal failure

Abdominal complications
- Pseudocyst   • Abscess
- Ascites   • Necrosis

Grey–Turner sign (bruising in flanks)

Bruising secondary to disseminated intravascular coagulation (DIC) (dependent areas + venepuncture sites)

Alcohol and the pancreas

High alcohol intake causes:
- Acute pancreatitis (may recur)
- Chronic calcifying pancreatitis (if >10 yrs of >150g/day alcohol)
  – steatorrhoea (>90% pancreas damaged) →malabsorption
  – pain (may be severe)
  – biliary obstruction (rarely)
  – diagnosed by ERCP/CT scan

Investigations

Amylase: usually greatly raised (NB also rises with other causes of acute abdomen)
Abdominal X-ray; may show ileus
Ultrasound
CT scan (+ contrast): most valuable diagnostic test, also useful for complications

Pancreatic cancer

Head 60%
Body 25%
Tail 15%

Tail
metastases, anorexia, fatigue

Body
Pain (infiltrates coeliac nerves)
Diabetes (loss of islet cells)
Malabsorption (exocrine deficiency)

Head
Obstructive jaundice

Treatment of acute attack

Analgesia (opiate)
IV fluids
Nil by mouth
Monitor + treat complications
  Shock: fluids
  Respiratory failure: O₂ + ITU
  DIC: blood products
  Infection: antibiotics
  Pancreatic necrosis : operative resection
  Pseudocyst ⎤
  Abscess   ⎦ — percutanous drainage

Acute pancreatitis

Acute pancreatitis results from a sudden onset of pancreatic inflammation associated with varying degrees of necrosis and 'autodigestion'. The incidence in the UK is currently 20 per 100 000 population with a 43% increase in the last decade, probably as a result of increased alcohol consumption nationally. The common causes of acute pancreatitis are:
- Gallstones: 30–50%, possibly more if one includes 'microlithiasis' – cholesterol crystals within the bile.
- Alcohol: 10–40%.
- Idiopathic: 15%.
- Rarer (but important) other causes include: trauma (endoscopic retrograde cholangiopancreatography (ERCP), postoperative, blunt trauma), drugs (5%, including loop diuretics), ypertriglyceridaemia, viral (mumps, Coxsackie virus).

Once the process has started there is a variable degree of pancreatic necrosis related to proteolytic autodigestion of the gland.

Clinical features
- **Abdominal pain**: characteristically sudden onset (<30 min), epigastric, radiating through to the back.
- **Hypovolaemia/shock**: the degree of circulating volume depletion may be underestimated and contribute significantly to the associated renal failure.
- **Vomiting**: contributes to hypovolaemia.
- **Jaundice**: suggests the presence of an associated cholangitis.

Various scoring systems are used to grade the severity of pancreatitis (Ranson, Glasgow, APACHE II). In general prognosis is determined more by markers of shock (acidaemia, hypoxia, etc.) than by the level of serum amylase recorded on admission. Mortality rate varies from 2% in mild attacks to >50% in severe disease.

Management and prognosis
For investigation see Figure 130.1 and Table 130.1. The key to managing pancreatitis is restoration of euvolaemia and, once stable, determination and treatment of the underlying cause:

Table 130.1 Markers of severe pancreatitis (most reliable when used at 48 h after the onset of pain; >3 = severe disease).

Assessment of severity of pancreatitis	
White cell count	$>15 \times 10^9$/L
Urea	>16 mmol/L
Calcium	<2.0 mmol/L
Albumin	<32 g/L
Glucose	>10 mmol/L
Po_2	<8 kPa
Aspartate transaminase	>200 IU/L
Lactate dehydrogenase	>600 IU/L
C-reactive protein	>150 mg/L

- **Resuscitation**: intravenous fluids, central venous pressure monitoring and oxygen. The routine use of broad-spectrum antibiotics is unproven.
- **Treat underlying cause**: clinical features of cholangitis raise the possibility of a gallstone impacted at the ampulla and are an indication to consider early ERCP. If gallstones are confirmed to be the underlying cause of the pancreatitis, early cholecystectomy is recommended.

Complications

Mild cases of pancreatitis usually resolve without complications; the more severe the acute attack, the more likely are complications:

- **Pancreatic pseudocyst/abscess**: suggested by persistent pain and/or fever, diagnosed by computed tomography (CT), and often drained percutaneously.
- **Adult respiratory distress syndrome**.
- **Portal vein/mesenteric thrombosis**.

Chronic pancreatitis

Chronic pancreatitis may result as a consequence of repeated attacks of acute pancreatitis Some patients present with clinical features of pancreatic insufficiency in the absence of pain. The prevalence is 40–75 per 100 000 and the incidence 8/100 000. Chronic pancreatitis relates to:

- Recurrent acute pancreatitis.
- Alcohol: the most common cause in the UK.
- Idiopathic: accounts for 20% of cases.

Clinical features

The cardinal features of chronic pancreatitis are:

- **Pain**: in 85%; typical pancreatic pain is epigastric radiating through to the back, often precipitated by eating. The severity is very variable.
- **Exocrine pancreatic insufficiency**: produces steatorrhoea and weight loss.
- **Endocrine pancreatic insufficiency** (i.e. diabetes): in 30%.

There are often no abnormal physical signs, despite dramatic symptoms.

Investigations

Pancreatic enzymes raised in attacks of acute pancreatitis are normal in chronic disease.

- **Faecal elastase** (or chymotrypsin) has now largely replaced tests quantifying faecal fat. Tests of exocrine pancreatic function (e.g. pancreolauryl test) are useful in difficult cases, although usually a clinical response to pancreatic enzyme replacement is sufficient.
- **Abdominal CT**: may show pancreatic calcification and small pseudocysts. It might also be used to identify pancreatic masses (i.e. tumour).

- **Magnetic resonance cholaniopancreatography** (MRCP) (or less commonly ERCP): demonstrates pancreatic duct irregularity and pseudocystic change.

Management and prognosis

Pancreatic enzyme replacement with preparations such as Creon and Pancrex often improves both the pain and the malabsorption of chronic pancreatitis. The diabetes associated with chronic pancreatitis frequently requires insulin therapy. Opioid analgesia is frequently needed where pancreatic pain is dominant; a coeliac axis block may be necessary in selected cases.

Pancreatic cancer

Cancer of the pancreas remains a major source of mortality in the developed world. The incidence is increasing, and is now 11/100 000. The disease is more common in men (1.3:1) and African/Caribbean people (50% higher). Smoking and a high fat/meat diet are risk factors. Most primary malignant tumours of the pancreas are adenocarcinomas although neuroendocrine tumours are not uncommon.

Clinical features

Pancreatic cancer is notorious for producing few or non-specific signs in the early stages. Painless jaundice caused by biliary obstruction is the most common presentation as the commonest location for pancreatic tumours is in the pancreatic head. Tumours in the body or tail of the gland will present with weight loss and abdominal pain.

Investigations

- **Abdominal CT**: this is presently the best first-line investigation in patients where pancreatic cancer is suspected clinically. It is useful in establishing a diagnosis and may identify tumours that are potentially resectable (i.e. no invasion into important local structures such as the superior mesenteric vein or distant metastases).
- **MRCP**: this should now become the first-line investigation for painless obstructive jaundice.
- **Endoscopic ultrasound**: this affords accurate assessment of pancreatic masses with particular reference to the local vessels (superior mesenteric vein and artery). It also facilitates targetted biopsy.
- **ERCP**: should be reserved until endoscopic therapy is expected/planned.

Management and prognosis

Too often carcinoma of the pancreas is advanced at the time of presentation and there is no possibility of cure. Overall 90% of individuals presenting with carcinoma of the pancreas will have succumbed to their disease within a year. Five-year survival is only 2%.

- **Surgery**: in some patients pancreatico-duodenectomy (Whipple's procedure) offers the possibility of a surgical cure. Surgery may also be beneficial in patients with advanced disease in providing combined biliary and gastroduodenal bypass.
- **Chemotherapy**: gemcitabine chemotherapy is recommended for use in unresectable pancreatic adenocarcinoma but its role is at present palliative, aiming to slow the progression of the disease. Other chemotherapy regimens undergoing clinical trials may yet bring better clinical outcomes.
- **Palliative measures**: stenting of biliary obstruction by either ERCP or percutaneous transhepatic cholangiography may relieve jaundice. Pancreatic pain may require opioid analgesia. Anorexia and weight loss remain major problems.

UK Working Party on Acute Pancreatitis. UK guidelines for the management of acute pancreatitis. *Gut* 2005: 54 (Suppl. III); 1–9.

131 Gallstone disease

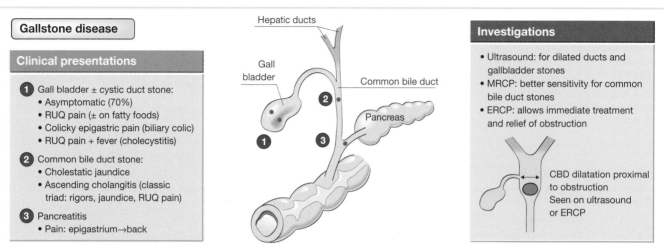

Gallstone disease

Clinical presentations

1 Gall bladder ± cystic duct stone:
- Asymptomatic (70%)
- RUQ pain (± on fatty foods)
- Colicky epigastric pain (biliary colic)
- RUQ pain + fever (cholecystitis)

2 Common bile duct stone:
- Cholestatic jaundice
- Ascending cholangitis (classic triad: rigors, jaundice, RUQ pain)

3 Pancreatitis
- Pain: epigastrium→back

Hepatic ducts

Gall bladder

Common bile duct

Pancreas

Investigations
- Ultrasound: for dilated ducts and gallbladder stones
- MRCP: better sensitivity for common bile duct stones
- ERCP: allows immediate treatment and relief of obstruction

CBD dilatation proximal to obstruction
Seen on ultrasound or ERCP

The prevalence of gallstones is underestimated because around 90% remain asymptomatic. Stones occur in 7% of men and 15% of women aged 18–65 years. There is a 3:1 female predominance in those aged <40 years, which disappears in elderly people.

Pathophysiology
Gallstone formation results from precipitation of cholesterol crystals in supersaturated bile. Stones ultimately contain a combination of calcium salts; they increase in size at a rate of 2.5 mm/year. Less commonly, pigment stones occur from chronic haemolysis (see Chapter 177).

Clinical features
- **Asymptomatic**: gallstones may be an incidental finding.
- **Biliary colic**: recurrent right upper quadrant (RUQ) pain, often precipitated by fatty food.
- **Cholecystitis** typically presents with acute right hypochondral pain and fever. If the neck of the gall bladder becomes obstructed, an empyema of the gall bladder (with a 20–30% mortality rate) may occur.
- **Cholestatic jaundice**: jaundice with pale stools and dark urine indicates biliary obstruction as a result of the migration of a stone into the common bile duct (CBD) (choledocolithiasis). With clinical evidence of superadded infection (fever, rigors) this is known as cholangitis.
- **Pancreatitis**: gallstones are a major cause of pancreatitis in the developed world, usually caused by the migration of stones down the CBD and through the ampulla of Vater.
- **Carcinoma of the gall bladder**: this is rare and in 90% occurs in association with gallstones. Extensive gall bladder calcification ('porcelain gall bladder') is a particularly powerful risk factor.
- **Rare presentations** and complications include biliary peritonitis, resulting from perforation (30% mortality), and small bowel

obstruction (gallstone ileus) caused by a large gallstone being held up at the ileocaecal valve.

Investigations
Only 20% of gallstones are visible on plain X-rays.
- **Transabdominal ultrasonography**: most commonly used to identify gallstones. Bile duct dilatation (intra- or extrahepatic) raises the possibility of CBD stones although transabdominal ultrasonography can rarely prove or exclude this (30–40% of patients with stones in the CBD have 'normal' ultrasound scans). Endoscopic ultrasonography has greater sensitivity and is now more widely available.
- **Liver transaminases**: should be checked in any patient considered for cholecystectomy. If these are abnormal, magnetic resonance cholangiopancreatography (MRCP) and/or endoscopic retrograde cholangiopancreatography (ERCP) should be considered before surgery, because they may reflect stones in the CBD.
- **ERCP**: provides simultaneous imaging of the biliary tree and the opportunity to relieve biliary obstruction by endoscopic sphincterotomy and removal of CBD stones.

Management and prognosis
- **Watchful waiting**: the incidental finding of gallstones requires no treatment.
- **Cholecystectomy**: in patients with symptomatic gallstones or after a significant complication, the definitive treatment is cholecystectomy.
- **ERCP**: this is both an investigation and treatment in patients with cholestatic jaundice in the presence of gallstones. For elderly or otherwise unwell patients, ERCP sphincterotomy may be sufficient because the risk of further problems is probably low.

Medicine at a Glance, Fourth Edition. Edited by Patrick Davey. © 2014 John Wiley & Sons, Ltd. Published 2014 by John Wiley & Sons, Ltd. Companion website: www.ataglanceseries.com/medicine

132 Inflammatory liver disease: viral and immune

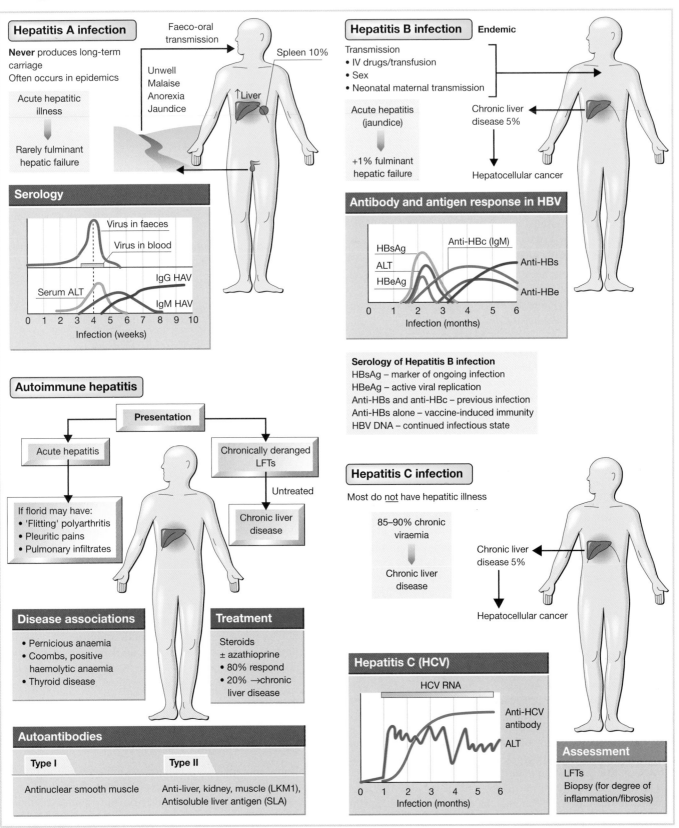

Hepatitis A infection

Never produces long-term carriage

Often occurs in epidemics

Acute hepatitic illness

↓

Rarely fulminant hepatic failure

Faeco-oral transmission

Spleen 10%

↑Liver

Unwell
Malaise
Anorexia
Jaundice

Serology

Virus in faeces

Virus in blood

IgG HAV

Serum ALT

IgM HAV

0 1 2 3 4 5 6 7 8 9 10

Infection (weeks)

Autoimmune hepatitis

Presentation

Acute hepatitis

Chronically deranged LFTs

Untreated

Chronic liver disease

If florid may have:
• 'Flitting' polyarthritis
• Pleuritic pains
• Pulmonary infiltrates

Disease associations

• Pernicious anaemia
• Coombs, positive haemolytic anaemia
• Thyroid disease

Treatment

Steroids
± azathioprine
• 80% respond
• 20% →chronic liver disease

Autoantibodies

Type I	Type II
Antinuclear smooth muscle	Anti-liver, kidney, muscle (LKM1), Antisoluble liver antigen (SLA)

Hepatitis B infection   Endemic

Transmission
• IV drugs/transfusion
• Sex
• Neonatal maternal transmission

Acute hepatitis (jaundice)

↓

+1% fulminant hepatic failure

Chronic liver disease 5%

↓

Hepatocellular cancer

Antibody and antigen response in HBV

HBsAg

ALT

HBeAg

Anti-HBc (IgM)

Anti-HBs

Anti-HBe

0 1 2 3 4 5 6

Infection (months)

Serology of Hepatitis B infection
HBsAg – marker of ongoing infection
HBeAg – active viral replication
Anti-HBs and anti-HBc – previous infection
Anti-HBs alone – vaccine-induced immunity
HBV DNA – continued infectious state

Hepatitis C infection

Most do <u>not</u> have hepatitic illness

85–90% chronic viraemia

↓

Chronic liver disease

Chronic liver disease 5%

↓

Hepatocellular cancer

Hepatitis C (HCV)

HCV RNA

Anti-HCV antibody

ALT

0 1 2 3 4 5 6

Infection (months)

Assessment

LFTs
Biopsy (for degree of inflammation/fibrosis)

Viral hepatitis

Hepatitis A virus (HAV)

Common cause of transient hepatitis; faecal–oral transmission.

- **Subclinical**: 50% of adults have IgG antibodies to HAV without previous jaundice.
- **Jaundice/acute hepatitis**: the most common presentation is an acute hepatitis, occasionally with a prolonged cholestatic phase. Fatigue, malaise, anorexia and nausea are prominent.
- **Fulminant liver failure**: very rarely.

Investigations

- **Liver blood tests** usually show an acute hepatocellular abnormality (i.e. predominant rise in aspartate transaminase, with less marked rises in bilirubin and alkaline phosphatase).
- **HAV IgM serology** in high titre is diagnostic of acute infection.

Management and prognosis

Clinical hepatitis usually settles with symptomatic management and rarely requires hospital admission. Evidence of liver failure (i.e. encephalopathy, coagulopathy) requires referral to a transplant centre. No risk of chronic liver disease/cirrhosis.

- **Similar pathogens**: hepatitis E gives a similar clinical picture, although the risk of fulminant hepatic failure in pregnancy is particularly high. Cytomegalovirus and Epstein–Barr virus are rare causes of fulminant hepatitis.

Hepatitis B virus (HBV)

Worldwide HBV is the most common cause of chronic liver disease and hepatoma. The incidence of HBV in the UK is increasing, being common among intravenous (IV) drug users, migrant populations and individuals with liberal sexual practices. It is a parenterally transmitted hepatotrophic DNA virus. Genetic factors relating to the host immune response may account for the variability in clinical manifestations.

Clinical features

- **Acute hepatitis**: an acute jaundiced illness occurs in 15% of individuals exposed to HBV.
- **Fulminant liver failure** is rare with HBV but more likely in those coinfected with HCV, human immunodeficiency virus (HIV) or the δ agent.
- **Chronic liver disease**: 5% of adults exposed to HBV develop chronic infection, more so in immunocompromised individuals (50% or more) and those acquiring the virus in early childhood (90%).
- **Hepatocellular carcinoma** (HCC) rates are increased ten-fold in HBV carriers.

Investigations

- **Liver function tests** (LFTs): show a non-specific hepatitic picture.
- **HBV serology**: see Figure 132.1 above.
- **Hepatic elastography and serum markers of liver fibrosis** (procollagen III n-peptide, TIMP-1, hyaluronidase): may be useful in detecting and monitoring significant liver fibrosis.
- **Other tests**: liver ultrasonography is needed to screen for focal liver abnormalities (i.e. hepatoma). Liver biopsy may guide treatment in patients with chronic HBV.

Management and prognosis

- **Prevention**: individuals at risk (e.g. health-care workers) should be immunized. Known virus carriers should know the risks to others of exposure to body fluids and should use barrier contraception.
- **General**: acute HBV infection rarely requires hospital admission. Follow-up is necessary to determine whether or not the virus has been cleared.
- **Antiviral therapy**: there is no helpful antiviral therapy during acute infection. Chronic infection may be clinically stable in many patients. Reactivation of disease activity in chronic carriers may require viral suppression with antiviral drugs (e.g. lamivudine, adefovir, tenofovir).
- **Screening** for HCC: regular surveillance with liver ultrasonography and α-fetoprotein measurement.
- **Liver transplantation**: indicated for decompensated cirrhosis and in selected patients with early hepatoma.

Hepatitis C virus (HCV)

Common; accounts for 25% of the liver disease burden in the UK. One of the major causes of chronic liver disease and transplantation in the developed world. The RNA HCV virus is transmitted parenterally. It relies on a reverse transcriptase for replication, which has an inherently high error rate, resulting in high rates of viral mutation. This, among other features, means that the virus commonly escapes the immune response, and chronicity of viraemia is the consequence.

Clinical features

- **Acute hepatitis**: this occurs in only a small number of patients.
- **Asymptomatic carriage**: in the majority of cases the recipient is oblivious to the fact that they have acquired the virus, yet 85–90% of those exposed will develop chronic viraemia.
- **Chronic liver disease**: 20% of patients with chronic viraemia eventually develop liver fibrosis and clinical chronic liver disease. The rate of progression varies but the clinical course is accelerated by concurrent infection with HBV and excess of alcohol consumption.

Investigations

- **Liver blood tests**: show relatively modest elevation in transaminases. The degree of liver blood test derangement bears little relation to the degree of underlying liver fibrosis (scarring).
- **Serological antibody tests** for HCV: the virus is identified in blood by the polymerase chain reaction and levels of viraemia can be quantified. Virus genotyping may determine the duration of antiviral therapy.
- **Liver biopsy**: remains the only way to grade the disease in terms of necroinflammatory change in the liver, and also to stage the condition by defining the degree of liver fibrosis.
- **Hepatic elastography and serum markers of liver fibrosis** (procollagen III n-peptide, TIMP-1, hyaluronidase): may be useful in detecting and monitoring significant liver fibrosis.

Management and prognosis

- **Prevention**: public health measures and education are important. There is no vaccine available or likely in the immediate future.
- **Antiviral therapy**: this is tailored to viral genotype and (to a lesser extent) viral load. HCV genotype 1 is treated with pegylated (sustained release) interferon-α, ribavirin and a protease inhibitor. Treatment may have to continue for up to 48 weeks depending on measurements of the early reponse to treatment. Other genotypes are presently treated with a combination of pegylated interferon and ribavirin. Treatment courses in these genotypes are generally shorter (usually 24 weeks). Overall, antiviral therapy

Natural history of chronic liver disease

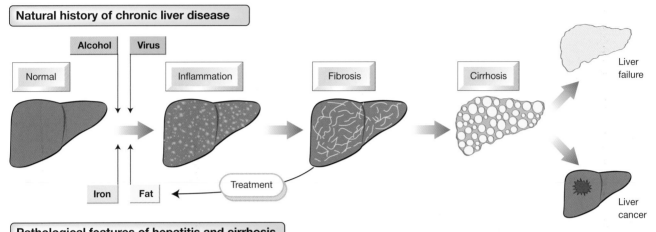

Pathological features of hepatitis and cirrhosis

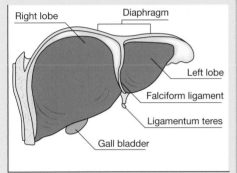

Normal liver: the normal liver is one of the largest organs in the body. It has a key role in producing vital proteins, and detoxifying externally ingested and internally produced toxins

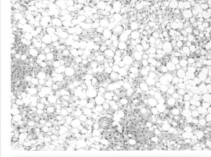

Fatty change of the liver: this slide shows extensive fatty change, now called steatosis (when there is no evidence of inflammation) and steatohepatitis (when there is evidence of inflammation)

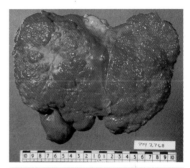

Macronodular cirrhosis; it is reputed that viral infection of the liver results in a macronodular form of cirrhosis (as does Wilson's disease, and α_1-antitrypsin deficiency), whereas alcohol leads to a micronodular form

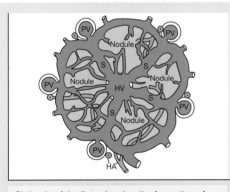

Cirrhosis of the liver showing the formation of portal venous (PV)/hepatic venous (HV) anastomoses or internal Eck fistulae at the site of pre-existing sinusoids (S). Note that the regeneration nodules are supplied by the hepatic artery (HA)

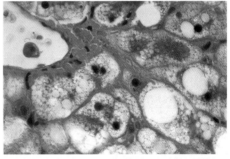

High power appearance of liver in acute alcoholic hepatitis; within this slide can be seen areas of (purplish-red) hyaline within the hepatocytes. These finding, called Mallory's hyaline, are believed to indicate the presence of alcohol abuse

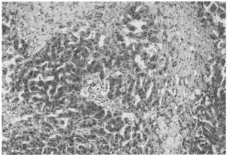

Cardiac cirrhosis: this occurs when the right side of the heart has been failing for a long time. Fibrosis, extending from central vein to central vein isolating nodules of liver cells is seen. Chronic heart failure is the commonest cause of this, and may explain some chronic ill health in heart failure

leads to a 60–75% sustained response (i.e. long-term viral clearance).

- **Liver transplantation**: transplantation remains an important mode of therapy for patients with end-stage chronic liver disease. Viral recurrence in the transplanted organ is common.

Autoimmune hepatitis

Rare. Acute autoimmune inflammation is centred predominantly on the hepatic lobule, causing a range of clinical manifestations,

ranging from fulminant hepatic failure to chronic liver disease and cirrhosis. Presentation is typically with:

- Jaundice.
- Fatigue.
- Arthralgia.
- Associated autoimmune conditions.

Less commonly autoimmune hepatitis presents with a persistent abnormality of liver blood tests:

- **Liver blood tests** usually show a predominant hepatocellular derangement of transaminases. A high titre of antinuclear antibodies often with smooth muscle (anti-actin) antibodies are found. In a few others, classified as having type II autoimmune hepatitis, autoantibodies may be demonstrable (e.g. liver/kidney microsomal antibody, soluble liver antigen). IgG is usually high.
- **Viral serology** must, given the usual acute presentation, be tested.
- **Liver biopsy** shows an acute lobular inflammation with interface hepatitis and may demonstrate features of chronicity (i.e. fibrosis).

Management and prognosis

- **Immunosuppression**: acute autoimmune hepatitis is very sensitive to high-dose steroids. Longer term control often requires azathioprine.
- **Liver transplantation**: for fulminant liver failure and decompensated chronic liver disease.

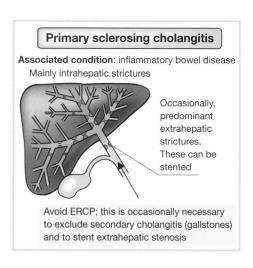

Primary sclerosing cholangitis

Associated condition: inflammatory bowel disease
Mainly intrahepatic strictures

Occasionally, predominant extrahepatic strictures. These can be stented

Avoid ERCP; this is occasionally necessary to exclude secondary cholangitis (gallstones) and to stent extrahepatic stenosis

Primary biliary cirrhosis

Rare (prevalence 90–150 per million) disease of mid-life women (male:female ratio 1:9). The pathology is of a non-suppurative, granulomatous inflammation centred predominantly on the small interlobular bile ducts, resulting in progressive fibrosis and ultimately cirrhosis. The cause is unknown but genetic loci associated with primary biliary cirrhosis (PBC) have recently been identified by genome-wide association studies.

Clinical features

The typical symptomatic presentation is of chronic progressive (intrahepatic) cholestasis with pruritis, lethargy and fatigue, progressing to steatorrhoea, and possibly with fat-soluble vitamin deficiency (A, D and K) syndromes. Some patients present with established chronic liver disease without prior symptomatic cholestasis. Increasingly, asymptomatic individuals are identified by abnormal liver blood tests with a positive mitochondrial antibody. Associated autoimmune conditions include autoimmune thyroid disease, diabetes and rheumatoid disease.

Investigations

- **Liver blood tests**: demonstrate a cholestatic picture (raised alkaline phosphatase with features of chronic liver disease in the advanced stages (i.e. low albumin)). Elevated (sometimes massively) levels of alkaline phosphatase may be the only abnormality on 'simple' blood tests. The antimitochondrial antibody and the M2 antibody directed at the 2-oxoacid dehydrogenase (E2) complex of the inner mitochondrial membrane are specific autoantibodies, and are found in 95% of patients with PBC. IgM is often raised.
- **Liver imaging** (ultrasonography): should be considered if extrahepatic biliary disease needs to be excluded (gallstones, primary sclerosing cholangitis (PSC)).
- **Liver biopsy**: shows features of PBC and fibrosis, the extent of which has prognostic value.

Management and prognosis

PBC progresses slowly, ultimately resulting in cirrhosis. Treatment of pruritis and fatigue is disappointing, although ursodeoxycholic acid may help. Chronic cholestasis increases the risk of osteopenia (see Chapter 216). Liver transplantation is excellent for persistent jaundice and decompensated chronic liver disease.

Primary sclerosing cholangitis

PSC is an uncommon, complex, probably autoimmune disorder, strongly associated with inflammatory bowel disease. The pattern varies considerably. Inflammation may predominantly involve the intralobular bile ducts – intrahepatic (small duct) PSC – or the extrahepatic biliary strictures – extrahepatic (large duct) PSC. Many patients have both small and large duct disease.

Clinical features

- **Abnormal LFTs** are the most common presentation (especially increased alkaline phosphatase). Positive antineutrophil cytoplasmic antibody (ANCA) occurs in 80%; antimitochondrial antibodies are not found.
- **Recurrent bacterial cholangitis** with right upper quadrant (RUQ) pain, fever and jaundice may occur in those with dominant extrahepatic disease.
- **Chronic cholestasis and chronic liver disease** are common.
- **Inflammatory bowel disease** may be diagnosed after PSC.

Investigations

- **LFTs**: often demonstrate a mixed pattern of 'hepatitic' and 'cholestatic' abnormalities.
- **Tumour marker CA19–9** may indicate cholangiocarcinoma.
- **ANCA**.
- **Liver ultrasonography** to exclude focal liver lesions (i.e. cholangiocarcinoma).
- **Magnetic resonance cholangiopancreatography** (MRCP) or **endoscopic retrograde cholangiopancreatography** (ERCP) may demonstrate multiple biliary strictures. Dominant strictures should be brushed and bile aspirated for cytology.
- **Liver biopsy** demonstrates features consistent with PSC – the onion-skin lesion around an obliterated bile duct.

Management and prognosis

The clinical course varies considerably and unpredictably. Symptomatic patients are largely dead in 10–15 years, though some 75% of asymptomatic patients are alive after 15 years. Bacterial cholangitis requires antibiotics. Pruritis may improve with ursodeoxycholic acid. There is no specific therapy. Liver transplantation is used for those with a rapidly progressive clinical course and decompensated chronic liver disease. Cholangiocarcinoma risk is increased and has a very poor prognosis.

NICE. *Adefovir Dpivoxil and Peginterferon Alfa-2a for the Treatment of Chronic Hepatitis B*. NICE Technical Appraisal TA96, 2006.

NICE. *Hepatitis C – Treatment with Peginterferon Alfa and Ribavirin*. NICE Technical Appraisal TA106, 2006.

133 Acute and chronic liver disease

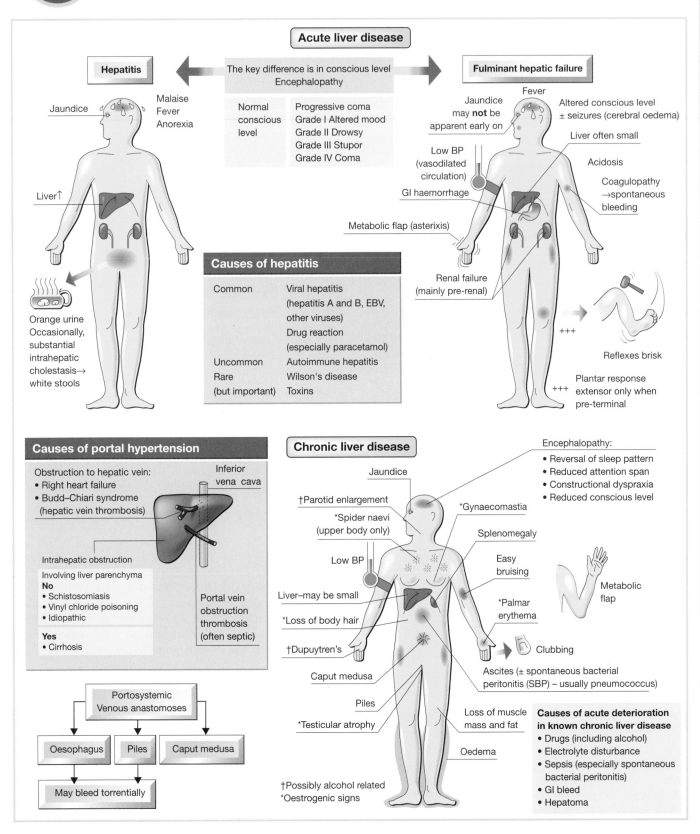

Acute liver disease

Hepatitis

The key difference is in conscious level
Encephalopathy

Normal conscious level	Progressive coma
	Grade I Altered mood
	Grade II Drowsy
	Grade III Stupor
	Grade IV Coma

Jaundice

Malaise
Fever
Anorexia

Liver↑

Orange urine
Occasionally,
substantial
intrahepatic
cholestasis→
white stools

Causes of hepatitis

Common	Viral hepatitis (hepatitis A and B, EBV, other viruses)
	Drug reaction (especially paracetamol)
Uncommon	Autoimmune hepatitis
Rare (but important)	Wilson's disease Toxins

Fulminant hepatic failure

Fever

Jaundice may **not** be apparent early on

Altered conscious level ± seizures (cerebral oedema)

Liver often small

Acidosis

Coagulopathy →spontaneous bleeding

Low BP (vasodilated circulation)

GI haemorrhage

Metabolic flap (asterixis)

Renal failure (mainly pre-renal)

+++

Reflexes brisk

+++ Plantar response extensor only when pre-terminal

Causes of portal hypertension

Obstruction to hepatic vein:
- Right heart failure
- Budd–Chiari syndrome (hepatic vein thrombosis)

Inferior vena cava

Intrahepatic obstruction

Involving liver parenchyma
No
- Schistosomiasis
- Vinyl chloride poisoning
- Idiopathic

Yes
- Cirrhosis

Portal vein obstruction thrombosis (often septic)

Portosystemic Venous anastomoses

→ Oesophagus | Piles | Caput medusa

→ May bleed torrentially

Chronic liver disease

Encephalopathy:
- Reversal of sleep pattern
- Reduced attention span
- Constructional dyspraxia
- Reduced conscious level

Jaundice

†Parotid enlargement

*Spider naevi (upper body only)

*Gynaecomastia

Splenomegaly

Low BP

Easy bruising

Liver–may be small

*Palmar erythema

*Loss of body hair

Metabolic flap

†Dupuytren's

Clubbing

Caput medusa

Ascites (± spontaneous bacterial peritonitis (SBP) – usually pneumococcus)

Piles

Loss of muscle mass and fat

*Testicular atrophy

Oedema

†Possibly alcohol related
*Oestrogenic signs

Causes of acute deterioration in known chronic liver disease
- Drugs (including alcohol)
- Electrolyte disturbance
- Sepsis (especially spontaneous bacterial peritonitis)
- GI bleed
- Hepatoma

Medicine at a Glance, Fourth Edition. Edited by Patrick Davey. © 2014 John Wiley & Sons, Ltd. Published 2014 by John Wiley & Sons, Ltd. Companion website: www.ataglanceseries.com/medicine

Acute hepatitis

This non-specific term refers to a short-term (self-limiting) liver inflammation. There are many causes (see Figure 133.1 above). Jaundice, nausea and anorexia, right upper quadrant discomfort, fever and fatigue occur.

Investigations

- **Liver function tests**: hepatitic enzymes, alanine transaminase; cholestatic enzymes – alkaline phosphatase; synthetic function tests – prothrombin time, albumin.
- **Tests to determine cause**: viral serology, immunoglobulins and autoantibody profile, iron indices, α_1-antitrypsin, copper.
- **Liver ultrasonography**: to exclude structural lesions (e.g. neoplasia, biliary disease, etc.).

Management and prognosis

Stop all potentially harmful drugs. Prognosis is usually good.

Fulminant liver failure

The term fulminant liver failure traditionally describes the progression from normal liver function to liver failure, i.e. hepatic encephalopathy within 8 weeks.

Clinical features

- **Encephalopathy** is the clinical hallmark of liver failure, characterized by a progressive deterioration in cognitive function from a shortened attention span through a reversal of sleep pattern to deep coma. The characteristic clinical sign is the metabolic flap (or asterixis), a coarse and irregular flapping tremor of the hands.
- **Jaundice**: depending on the rate of deterioration, jaundice may not initially be clinically evident.
- **Haemorrhage** may be confined to the gastrointestinal (GI) tract or occur widely as a result of haemostatic failure.
- **Acidosis, hypoglycaemia and renal failure**.

Investigations

- **Prothrombin time** is the single best prognostic marker. Coagulopathy should not necessarily be corrected (with fresh frozen plasma) unless bleeding is otherwise life-threatening.
- **Blood glucose** should be measured frequently. Hypoglycaemia is an ominous sign.
- **Electrolytes**: renal impairment most commonly relates to a degree of acute tubular necrosis on admission, rather than reflecting a true hepatorenal syndrome.
- **Arterial blood gases**: lactic metabolic acidosis is a poor sign.
- **Paracetamol level** should be measured in all cases and is the most common cause of fulminant liver failure in the UK; it is amenable to medical treatment (*N*-acetylcysteine).

Management and prognosis

- **Airway management**: patients can deteriorate quickly. Those with progressive coma should undergo early intubation and ventilation, especially if between-hospital transfer occurs.
- **Optimize circulatory state**: patients have a hyperdynamic circulation with lowered systemic vascular resistance. The degree of volume depletion on admission is often underestimated.
- **N-acetylcysteine** is the antidote to paracetamol poisoning, although increasing evidence suggests that it might benefit patients with fulminant liver failure from all causes.
- **Broad-spectrum antibiotics** and systemic antifungals.
- Indications for liver transplant unit referral and possible transplantation (see Table 133.1).

Table 133.1 Indications for referral to a liver transplant unit in fulminant liver failure.

Paracetamol poisoning
- pH <7.3
- INR >6.5
- Creatinine >300 mmol/L

Other pathologies (viruses, drugs, etc.)
- INR >6.5

And any three of:
- Aetiology being drug or non-A, non-B
- Age <10 years or >40 years
- Jaundice for 7 days before encephalopathy
- Bilirubin >300
- INR >3.5

INR, international normalized ratio.

Chronic liver disease

Much liver pathology follows an indolent course and presents with clinical features of chronic liver disease. Compensated chronic liver disease implies a (relatively) well patient, whereas those with 'decompensated' chronic liver disease have substantial symptoms and/or signs.

Pathophysiology and clinical features

Long-term, low-grade liver damage results in progressive liver fibrosis, which results in a combination of reduced liver cell mass and portal hypertension. These cause the clinical features – the relative dominance of one over the other varies between patients:
- Weakness, anorexia and muscle loss.
- GI bleeding from portosystemic venous anastomoses (i.e. varices).
- Ascites: possibly complicated by spontaneous bacterial peritonitis.
- Jaundice.
- Encephalopathy.

Problems caused by reduced liver cell mass

- **Encephalopathy**: the hallmark of liver cell failure and a common, albeit subtle, feature of most patients with chronic liver disease, causing a reduced attention span and reversed sleep pattern (insomnia and daytime somnolence). A metabolic flap may be found. With more advanced encephalopathy patients demonstrate a constructional dyspraxia and ultimately progress to hepatic coma. Encephalopathy can be worsened by portosystemic shunting (which is sometimes used in treatment).
- **Loss of lean body mass** is usually most evident at the shoulders. The accumulation of body water (oedema and ascites) means that the extent of muscle loss is underestimated.
- **Coagulopathy**.

Problems caused by portal hypertension

- **Varices**: form at sites of portosystemic communication, most commonly in the lower oesophagus. GI bleeding, sometimes torrential, may be the first presentation of chronic liver disease and can provoke decompensation of the chronic liver disease.
- **Ascites**: the result of sodium retention, possibly contributed to by high portal pressure and low albumin. It is important to

exclude spontaneous bacterial peritonitis, as this commonly complicates low protein ascites resulting from cirrhosis.

Investigations

These are directed to identify the cause of the underlying liver disease and to identify the triggers for decompensation (infection, bleeding, drugs, electrolyte disturbance, hepatoma):

- **Haematology**: haemoglobin may be low, as a result of bleeding and hypersplenism. The prothrombin time is prolonged, as a result of synthetic failure ± disseminated intravascular coagulation (DIC).
- **Autoimmune profile**/immunoglobulins.
- **Iron** studies (haemochromatosis) and **copper** studies (Wilson's disease).
- **Viral serology** (hepatitis B and C virus (HBV, HCV)).
- α_1-**Antitrypsin levels**, to exclude α_1-antitrypsin deficiency.

Management

Identify and treat the cause of the clinical decompensation (see Figure 133.1 above).

Treatment of acute complications

- **Variceal bleeding**: blood product support, urgent endoscopy, with band ligation of the varices. Vasoconstrictors (terlipressin) are a short-term but complementary measure. In overwhelming haemorrhage, balloon tamponade (Sengstaken–Blakemore tube) may be tried. Acute percutaneous portosystemic shunting (transjugular intrahepatic portosystemic stent shunt (TIPSS)) can also control bleeding. In the long term, injection/banding of varices and/or β-blockers reduces the risk of haemorrhage.
- **Ascites**: spironolactone and salt restriction are useful.
- **Encephalopathy**: provoking factors are removed/treated. Minimize absorption of dietary nitrogenous substances using lactulose.

Table 133.2 Pugh–Child scoring system (A = 5–6; B = 7–9; C = 10–15).

	1	2	3
Bilirubin (mmol/L)	<35	35–51	>51
Albumin (g/L)	>35	30–35	<30
Ascites	None	Controlled	Poorly controlled
Encephalopathy	None	Minimal	Advanced
Nutrition	Excellent	Good	Poor

Long-term management and prognosis

Prognosis is unpredictable but relates to the Pugh–Child class (see Table 133.2).

- If a clear aetiology is identified, treatment can restore good health even if cirrhosis is present (e.g. haemochromatosis).
- **Hepatoma**: may complicate long-standing cirrhosis from some aetiologies (viral hepatitis, haemochromatosis, alcohol). Frequent liver ultrasonography and α-fetoprotein measurements are indicated for early tumour detection (see Figure 133.2 below).
- Treatment-refractory symptoms may be relieved by **liver transplantation** in selected cases.

British Society of Gastroenterology. Guidelines for the diagnosis and treatment of hepatocellular carcinoma (HCC) in adults. *Gut* 2003: 52 (Suppl. III); iii1–iii8; www.bsg.org.uk (last accessed September 2013).

British Society of Gastroenterology. Guidelines on the management of ascites in cirrhosis. *Gut* 2006: 55; 1–12; www.bsg.org.uk (last accessed September 2013).

Surveillance and recall strategy for hepatocellular carcinoma (HCC)

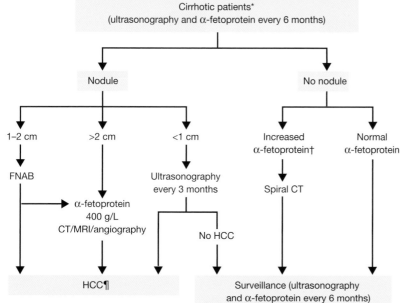

FNAB = fine-needle aspiration biopsy
* Available for curative treatments if diagnosed as having HCC
† α-fetoprotein concentrations to be defined   ¶ Cytohistological or non-invasive criteria

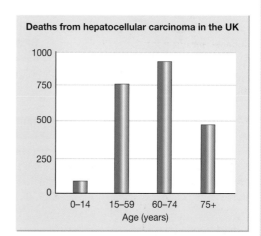

The rate of hepatocellular cancer is greatly increased in liver cirrhosis; annual rates are around 2–6.5%. Worldwide, this leads to around 0.5 million deaths; in the UK 2300 deaths occur from hepatocellular cancer every year. Patients with established cirrhosis (regardless of aetiology) should be regularly screened for this complication, according to the scheme recommended by the European Association for the Study of the Liver. The aim of surveillance is to diagnose cancers at an early stage, when cure is still possible. Advanced hepatocellular carcinoma has a poor prognosis regardless of treatment.

134 Metabolic liver disease (including alcohol)

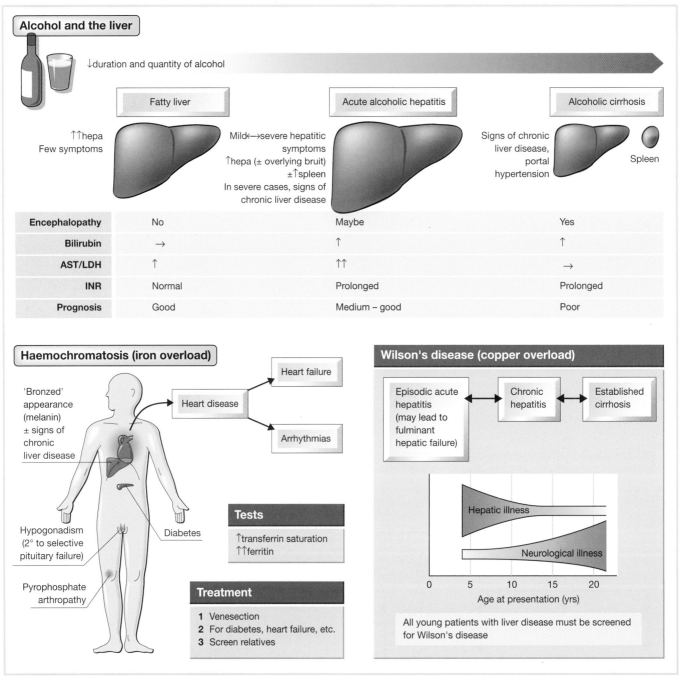

Alcohol and the liver

↓duration and quantity of alcohol

Fatty liver

↑↑hepa
Few symptoms

Acute alcoholic hepatitis

Mild↔severe hepatitic symptoms
↑hepa (± overlying bruit)
±↑spleen
In severe cases, signs of chronic liver disease

Alcoholic cirrhosis

Signs of chronic liver disease, portal hypertension

Spleen

	Fatty liver	Acute alcoholic hepatitis	Alcoholic cirrhosis
Encephalopathy	No	Maybe	Yes
Bilirubin	→	↑	↑
AST/LDH	↑	↑↑	→
INR	Normal	Prolonged	Prolonged
Prognosis	Good	Medium – good	Poor

Haemochromatosis (iron overload)

'Bronzed' appearance (melanin)
± signs of chronic liver disease

Heart disease → Heart failure
Heart disease → Arrhythmias

Hypogonadism (2° to selective pituitary failure)

Diabetes

Pyrophosphate arthropathy

Tests

↑transferrin saturation
↑↑ferritin

Treatment

1 Venesection
2 For diabetes, heart failure, etc.
3 Screen relatives

Wilson's disease (copper overload)

Episodic acute hepatitis (may lead to fulminant hepatic failure) ↔ Chronic hepatitis ↔ Established cirrhosis

Hepatic illness

Neurological illness

| 0 | 5 | 10 | 15 | 20 |

Age at presentation (yrs)

All young patients with liver disease must be screened for Wilson's disease

Alcoholic liver disease

The relationship between alcohol and chronic liver disease is complex. Clearly, excess alcohol consumption is a risk factor for chronic liver disease. However, individual susceptibility varies considerably and typical alcohol-related pathology is increasingly seen in individuals who drink modest amounts of alcohol (non-alcoholic steatohepatitis; see Chapter 127).

Incidence

Common. Alcohol remains the most tolerated substance of abuse in the world. Despite this only a fifth of people with alcohol problems develop features of chronic liver disease.

Pathophysiology

Many theories have been proposed to explain alcohol-related liver injury. Many focus on the acetaldehyde derivatives of alcohol.

Medicine at a Glance, Fourth Edition. Edited by Patrick Davey. © 2014 John Wiley & Sons, Ltd. Published 2014 by John Wiley & Sons, Ltd. Companion website: www.ataglanceseries.com/medicine

There may be important genetic factors. There are three pathological forms of alcoholic liver disease:

- **Fatty liver**: occurs in 50% of heavy drinkers – reversible on alcohol cessation.
- **Acute alcoholic hepatitis**: occurs in 40% of heavy drinkers – most commonly after long periods of heavy drinking.
- **Cirrhosis**: a man consuming 210g ethanol (=2.5 bottles of wine) a day for 22 years has a 50% chance of developing cirrhosis.

Clinical features

Alcohol-related liver injury may present in many different ways:

- Chance finding of abnormal liver blood tests.
- **Decompensated chronic liver disease** (gastrointestinal (GI) bleeding, ascites).
- **Acute alcoholic hepatitis**: this presentation is particularly challenging. Often there is a long history of alcohol use and, then, the apparently sudden onset of jaundice often with anorexia, nausea, malaise, fever and neutrophil leukocytosis.

Investigations

Although clinicians have previously relied on γ-glutamyl transferase and mean cell volume as indicators of alcohol abuse, these are unreliable. A good clinical history (often with corroborative testimonies of relatives) is still the best method for determining alcohol dependence, possibly supported with random ethanol levels.

Management and prognosis

Management of patients with alcohol-related liver injury involves:

- Addressing the difficult challenge of total abstinence from alcohol. In alcoholic cirrhosis 5-year survival is 70% in abstinent patients and only 35% in drinkers.
- Objectively assessing the degree of chronic liver disease (biopsy for fibrosis).
- Hepatocellular carcinoma occurs in 15% of people with alcoholic cirrhosis; surveillance for this may be indicated.

Haemochromatosis

Haemochromatosis is the term used to describe primary iron overload (total body iron of >5g vs normal stores of <3g). In most cases iron overload is the result of increased GI absorption of iron. The excess iron is deposited in many organs, resulting in damage.

Incidence

The mutation in the *HFE* gene responsible for haemochromatosis (*C282Y*) is very common in white people, with a prevalence of up to 1:150 in populations with a strong Celtic ancestry (e.g. the Irish). This makes haemochromatosis the most common single gene disorder to affect northwest European populations. Despite this, symptomatic presentation remains rare. The reason for this disparity is not clear.

Pathophysiology

The *C282Y* mutation in the *HFE* gene prevents cell surface expression of the protein. How this leads to the demonstrable increase in GI iron absorption is still not clear. Once absorbed, excess iron is deposited in the liver and other organs (pancreas, heart, joints). This leads to liver fibrosis and ultimately a risk of hepatoma.

Clinical features

The original 'classic' description of haemochromatosis was of bronzed diabetes with a pigmented cirrhosis and heavy iron deposition in the liver, pancreas (provoking diabetes) and heart (leading to heart failure). Joint involvement, often producing a pyrophosphate arthropathy was in many cases the most disabling symptom. The bronzed discoloration of the skin was due to excess secretion of melanocyte-stimulating hormone from the pituitary. This 'full blown' clinical presentation is rarely seen today and increasingly the diagnosis is made in patients without distinctive clinical symptoms or physical signs.

Investigations

- **Liver blood tests**: non-specific hepatitis usually with a raised alanine transaminase.
- **Iron indices**: transferrin saturation >80%. Ferritin levels are often very high, not infrequently >1000mg/L (normal <300mg/L). Liver biopsy shows a characteristic distribution of iron and provides important information on staging (i.e. the degree of liver fibrosis).
- **Genetic mutation analysis**: 90% of haemochromatosis patients of European descent are homozygous for the *C282Y* mutation in *HFE*.

Management and prognosis

- **Venesection**: 500g of whole blood removed weekly until excess iron stores are removed (which takes up to 12–18 months in heavily iron-loaded individuals). Thereafter, venesection should continue every 3 months indefinitely.
- **Surveillance for hepatoma**: in patients who have developed cirrhosis before the diagnosis has been made there remains a risk of developing hepatoma and in these cases it may be appropriate to regularly test α-fetoprotein and undertake liver ultrasonography.
- **Screening** first-degree relatives: this process has been greatly facilitated by *HFE* mutation analysis.

Wilson's disease

Rare (worldwide incidence 1–30 per million), autosomal recessive disorder of copper metabolism resulting in copper overload. Arises when mutations in the gene coding for a copper transport protein (*ATP7B*, chromosome 13q14.3) lead to failure of biliary excretion of copper and thus progressive copper accumulation. This often results in hepatic and neurological damage. It usually presents in children and young adults; there is an equal sex incidence. Kayser–Fleischer rings may be identified in the eyes by slit-lamp examination. There are various presentations:

- **Hepatic**: acute hepatitis. Fulminant liver failure or chronic liver disease/cirrhosis.
- **Neuropsychiatric**: extrapyramidal disturbance/psychosis.
- **Haematological**: acute intravascular haemolysis.

Investigations

- **Copper studies**: serum copper (low); ceruloplasmin (low in 80%); 24-hour urinary copper (increased).
- **Liver biopsy**: defines degree of fibrosis as well as quantifies copper load.
- **Cerebral computed tomography/magnetic resonance imaging**.

Management and prognosis

- **Liver disease**: penicillamine is used to chelate copper, which is then excreted in the urine. Severe liver disease has been successfully treated with liver transplantation.
- **Neurological disease** is permanent.
- **Screening** of first-degree relatives.

135 Upper gastrointestinal cancer

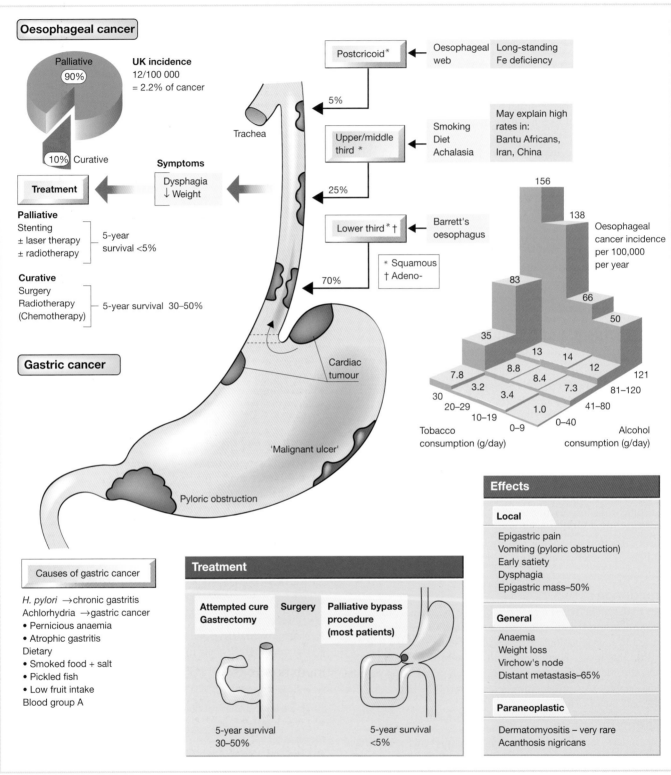

Oesophageal cancer

UK incidence
12/100 000
= 2.2% of cancer

Palliative 90%
10% Curative

Trachea

Postcricoid* ← Oesophageal web | Long-standing Fe deficiency

5%

Upper/middle third * ← Smoking, Diet, Achalasia | May explain high rates in: Bantu Africans, Iran, China

25%

Symptoms
Dysphagia
↓ Weight

Treatment

Lower third* † ← Barrett's oesophagus

* Squamous
† Adeno-

70%

Palliative
Stenting
± laser therapy
± radiotherapy
— 5-year survival <5%

Curative
Surgery
Radiotherapy
(Chemotherapy)
— 5-year survival 30–50%

Oesophageal cancer incidence per 100,000 per year

156
138
83
66
50
35
13 14
7.8 8.8 8.4 12
3.2 3.4 7.3 121
1.0 81–120
30 41–80
20–29 0–40
10–19 0–9

Tobacco consumption (g/day)

Alcohol consumption (g/day)

Gastric cancer

Cardiac tumour

'Malignant ulcer'

Pyloric obstruction

Causes of gastric cancer

H. pylori →chronic gastritis
Achlorhydria →gastric cancer
• Pernicious anaemia
• Atrophic gastritis
Dietary
• Smoked food + salt
• Pickled fish
• Low fruit intake
Blood group A

Treatment

| Attempted cure Gastrectomy | Surgery | Palliative bypass procedure (most patients) |

5-year survival 30–50%

5-year survival <5%

Effects

Local
Epigastric pain
Vomiting (pyloric obstruction)
Early satiety
Dysphagia
Epigastric mass–50%

General
Anaemia
Weight loss
Virchow's node
Distant metastasis–65%

Paraneoplastic
Dermatomyositis – very rare
Acanthosis nigricans

Medicine at a Glance, Fourth Edition. Edited by Patrick Davey. © 2014 John Wiley & Sons, Ltd. Published 2014 by John Wiley & Sons, Ltd. Companion website: www.ataglanceseries.com/medicine

Oesophageal carcinoma

Incidence

Although squamous carcinoma is declining in the western world in keeping with the reduction in cigarette smoking, adenocarcinoma of the distal oesophagus/gastric cardia is increasing throughout the world. The UK incidence is 12 per 100 000, with a 50% increase in incidence over the last 20 years.

Pathophysiology

The two different tumour types behave very differently:

- **Squamous carcinoma** most commonly affects the middle third of the oesophagus. There is a strong association with cigarette smoking.
- **Adenocarcinoma** most commonly affects the lower third of the oesophagus and merges pathologically with carcinoma of the gastric cardia. Most theories relating the cause of the distal oesophageal adenocarcinoma involve chronic gastro-oesophageal reflux of both acid and possibly bile.

Clinical features

The major clinical feature relating to oesophageal malignancy is **dysphagia**. Rapidly progressive dysphagia (i.e. dysphagia to solids progressing to dysphagia to soft food and liquids) and weight loss at the time of presentation are particularly worrying features.

Investigations

Progressive dysphagia always requires urgent investigation (see Chapter 29):

- **Endoscopy** will achieve a histological diagnosis and allows symptoms relief (oesophageal dilatation).
- **Computed tomography** (CT): in patients suitable for consideration of surgery (bearing in mind the high prevalence of significant co-morbidity) a CT of the chest and upper abdomen will exclude gross pulmonary and/or hepatic metastases and may identify local invasion into important other structures such as the pericardium or aorta.
- **Positron emission tomography** scanning is being used increasingly in the preoperative assessment of oesophageal patients being considered for surgery.
- **Endoscopic ultrasonography** is more sensitive than CT for detecting local tumour invasion.
- **Staging laparoscopy**: occasionally undertaken before attempted curative surgery, because malignant spread to lymph nodes may be missed on CT scan.

Management and prognosis

The prognosis is poor, with a 5-year survival of 9%.

- **Surgery**: this offers the best chance of cure, which justifies the efforts put into preoperative staging, although even with 'curative' resection the 5-year survival rate is <20%.
- **Radiotherapy and chemotherapy**: squamous carcinoma of the oesophagus is sensitive to radiotherapy and newer combination regimens are proving beneficial in adenocarcinoma as well.
- **Palliative procedures**: even without the possibility of cure, it is possible to alleviate the distressing symptom of dysphagia.

- **Stenting**: in tumours causing mediastinal encasement, stenting with self-expanding metal stents provides reasonable palliation.

Gastric carcinoma

Incidence

The incidence of gastric carcinoma (other than that of the gastric cardia) is decreasing (17 per 100 000). There is a higher incidence in males than in females.

Pathophysiology

Predisposing factors include atrophic gastritis and previous surgery for peptic ulcer disease. The role of *Helicobacter pylori* in the aetiopathogenesis of upper gastrointestinal (GI) malignancy is controversial. There is an association between *H. pylori* infection and the development of gastric lymphoma (MALToma, where MALT is mucosa-associated lymphoid tissue), but the relationship with adenocarcinoma is less clear.

Clinical features

Gastric cancer often presents late because there are no early clinical symptoms. Although dyspepsia remains a common prompt for diagnostic endoscopy, ironically patients with gastric cancer often have reduced gastric acid output (e.g. gastric atrophy). Many gastric cancers will prove to be at an advanced stage at the time they are identified.

- **Anaemia**: occult GI bleeding and the resulting iron deficiency is probably the most common way in which gastric carcinoma presents (see Chapter 126).
- **Weight loss** is common and suggests advanced or metastatic disease.
- **Vomiting**: indicates impending gastric outflow obstruction.

Investigations

- **Endoscopy**: including biopsies for histological confirmation of the diagnosis.
- **Abdominal CT** for staging, i.e. to detect hepatic and other metastasis.

Management and prognosis

The prognosis is poor, with a 5-year survival of 12%.

- **Surgery** should be considered in most cases because, even in tumours that are advanced at the time of presentation, a surgical bypass (i.e. gastrojejunostomy) can provide good palliation. Increasingly, laparoscopy is being used to stage the tumour before any attempted resection.
- **Chemotherapy and radiotherapy**: these modalities tend to be less useful in gastric carcinoma.

British Society of Gastroenterology. Guidelines for the management of oesophageal and gastric cancer. *Gut* 2002: 50 (Suppl. V); v1–v23, www.bsg.org.uk (last accessed September 2013).

136 Colorectal cancer

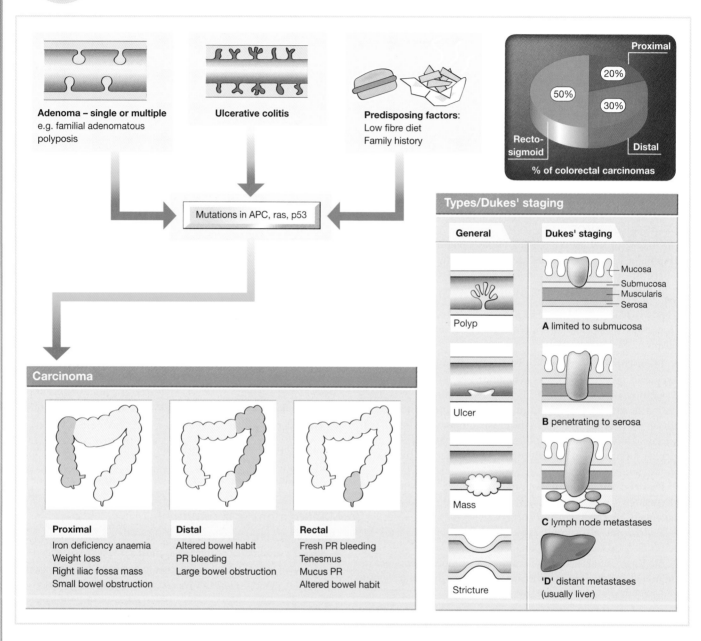

Adenoma – single or multiple
e.g. familial adenomatous polyposis

Ulcerative colitis

Predisposing factors:
Low fibre diet
Family history

Mutations in APC, ras, p53

Proximal
20%
50%
30%
Recto-sigmoid
Distal
% of colorectal carcinomas

Carcinoma

Proximal
Iron deficiency anaemia
Weight loss
Right iliac fossa mass
Small bowel obstruction

Distal
Altered bowel habit
PR bleeding
Large bowel obstruction

Rectal
Fresh PR bleeding
Tenesmus
Mucus PR
Altered bowel habit

Types/Dukes' staging

General	Dukes' staging
Polyp	Mucosa / Submucosa / Muscularis / Serosa — **A** limited to submucosa
Ulcer	**B** penetrating to serosa
Mass	**C** lymph node metastases
Stricture	**'D'** distant metastases (usually liver)

Colorectal cancer is a major public health problem in the developed world and increasingly efforts are being directed to identifying the condition early in individuals considered to be at risk.

Incidence

The incidence of colorectal cancer increases with age and overall this has increased over the last 50 years (currently 55 per 100 000 in men, 40 per 100 000 in women). Colorectal cancer now accounts for 20 000 deaths/year in the UK, with an additional 6000 successful resections. Colorectal cancer accounts for 39% of all cancer deaths in the UK with a 5-year survival of 36% for men and 41% for women. Probably the single greatest determinant of prognosis is early detection, which has led to the principle of screening the population for colorectal cancer.

Pathophysiology

There are several conditions that are recognized to predispose to colorectal cancer.

Adenomatous polyps of the colon

Colorectal cancer usually develops in pre-existing adenomatous polyps in the colon. The risk of finding cancer depends upon the size of the polyp (see Table 136.1).

Ulcerative colitis

Long-standing total ulcerative colitis predisposes to colorectal cancer and patients with a 10-year history of total colitis should be offered colonoscopic surveillance and colonic biopsies taken to detect severe dysplasia.

Medicine at a Glance, Fourth Edition. Edited by Patrick Davey. © 2014 John Wiley & Sons, Ltd. Published 2014 by John Wiley & Sons, Ltd. Companion website: www.ataglanceseries.com/medicine

Table 136.1 Colonic polyp size and risk of cancer.

Polyp size (cm)	Cancer risk (%)
<1	1–10
1–2	7–10
>2	35–55

Table 136.2 Family history and lifetime risk of colorectal cancer.

Family history	Lifetime risk
None	1:40
One first-degree relative >45 years	1:17
One first-degree and one second-degree relative	1:12
One first-degree relative <45 years	1:10
Two first-degree relatives (any age)	1:8
Hereditary non-polyposis colon cancer	1:2

Family history

A greater understanding of the genetic predisposition to colorectal cancer is resulting in an increasing number of individuals referred for colonoscopic screening/surveillance. Surveillance colonoscopy is beneficial at risk ratios of $\geq 1:12$ (see Table 136.2).

Familial cancer syndromes

There are some rare but important hereditary cancer syndromes. The most important of these are familial adenomatous polyposis and hereditary non-polyposis colon cancer (HNPCC). In the former, affected individuals have hundreds of adenomatous polyps throughout the colon evident from an early age. The risk of neoplasia is such that prophylactic colectomy is performed before the age of 20. HNPCC is inherited in an autosomal dominant fashion and is the result of mutations in DNA-mismatch repair genes. Individuals at risk are offered genetic screening in addition to colonoscopic surveillance.

Clinical features

The clinical presentation of sporadic colorectal cancer depends to a degree on the site of the tumour. Proximal colonic cancers may present with features of subacute bowel obstruction or may be identified during the investigation of iron deficiency anaemia. Distal colon cancers will often cause a change in bowel habit (either constipation or diarrhoea) or present with overt rectal bleeding.

Investigations

- **Colonoscopy**: the most sensitive and specific investigation for patients suspected of having colorectal cancer.
- **Computed tomography (CT) colonography**: this examination has now largely replaced barium enema.
- **Full blood count**: iron deficiency anaemia.
- **Search for metastatic disease**: liver function tests and CT of chest, abdomen and pelvis. Although surgery is required in most cases it is useful to identify whether or not the patient has metastatic disease before laparotomy.

Table 136.3 Five-year survival after resection of colorectal cancer.

Dukes' stage		5-year survival rate (%)
A	Limited to bowel wall	95–100
B	Penetrated bowel wall, no metastases	65–75
C	Lymph node metastases	30–40
	Distant metastases	<1

- **Pelvic magnetic resonance imaging** is now considered mandatory in the planning of surgical treatment of rectal cancer.
- **Carcinoembryonic antigen**: this tumour marker is not useful for diagnosis, but is useful in monitoring the patient's response to treatment and for the identification of disease relapse.

Management and prognosis

- **Surgery** is required in most cases of colorectal cancer. The extent of bowel resection depends on the site of the tumour. Attempts are made to resect at least 5 cm of normal bowel either side of the tumour, and regional lymph nodes should also be resected. Prognosis after surgery depends on the histological grade of the tumour and the Dukes' stage (see Table 136.3).
- **Chemotherapy** with 5-fluorouracil improves survival for Dukes' B and C cancers.
- **Radiotherapy**: preoperative chemo-irradiation to 'downstage' rectal tumours is gaining popularity.
- **Follow-up/secondary prevention**: patients with a prior history of either colorectal cancer or tubulovillous adenoma of the colon should undergo surveillance colonoscopy.
- **Palliative approaches**: although surgery has been considered the appropriate treatment of patients with impending colonic obstruction, stenting of tumours with self-expanding metal stents offers an alternative approach for the palliative relief of obstruction.

Screening

Following a successful feasibility study, a national programme for bowel cancer screening has been launched in England. This takes the form of screening the UK population over the age of 60 by faecal occult blood (FOB) testing. Patients identified as FOB positive are invited to attend for colonoscopy. This process identifies patients with early stage (Dukes' A) cancer resulting in improved survival, though up to 30% of colonic cancers are FOB negative. Furthermore the process will identify colonic polyps, which if removed endoscopically will not develop into cancer (i.e. the process might actually *prevent* rather than just detect cancer). In time, flexible sigmoidoscopy or even total colonoscopy might increasingly be seen as the best primary screening tool although there are issues of safety, quality assurance, staffing and patient acceptability that will need to be addressed.

British Society of Gastroenterology. Guidelines for colorectal cancer screening in high risk groups. *Gut* 2002: Suppl. V; v1–2; www.bsg.org.uk (last accessed September 2013).

NICE. *Improving Outcomes in Colorectal Cancer*. NICE Guidance, 2004; www.nice.org.uk (last accessed September 2013).

137 Imaging in gastrointestinal disease

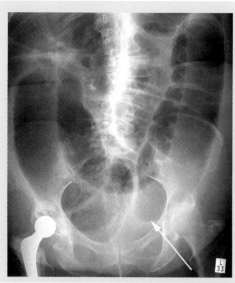

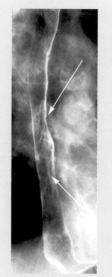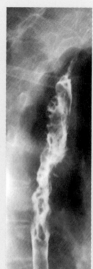

This image shows large bowel obstruction secondary to sigmoid carcinoma. There is gaseous distension of the large bowel down to the left pelvis, at the level of the obstruction (arrow). A plain (erect) abdominal film is a very useful examination in many patients acutely unwell with abdominal pain, especially in the elderly. Although the history usually gives vital clues as to whether or not bowel obstruction is present, many very elderly patients present with very non-specific symptoms, such as vague abdominal pains, without a clear history of absolute constipation. In the presence of abdominal discomfort in the elderly, always consider bowel obstruction, commonly resulting from cancer, ischaemia or sigmoid volvulus (where the 'upside-down' bowel can often be seen)

Although endoscopy with biopsy is the main modality for diagnosing most GI tract malignancies (see other chapters), there remains an important role for barium-based examinations. 1) Left-hand image: this image demonstrates a superficial spreading oesophageal cancer (arrows). 2) Right-hand image: this barium swallow demonstrates a very abnormal oesophagus; there is a large polypoidal mass with structuring, mucosal irregularity and ulceration. The appearances are due to advanced oesophageal cancer

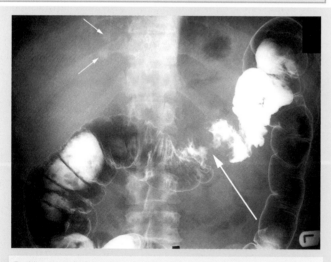

Double contrast barium enema. A cancer of the transverse colon is seen. There is irregular structuring of the bowel, resulting in an 'apple core' lesion. This appearance is highly likely to be due to cancer, and very unlikely to be due to a benign process. This film also shows (arrows) metastasis in the lungs; patients with known GI malignancy usually need a radiological search for secondaries. Plain X-rays can offer much; for example, many GI malignancies spread to the lungs – so the chest X-ray can be useful. Likewise, if any bones hurt, plain X-rays may show secondaries. CT scanning is the usual means to assess occult pulmonary and hepatic metastasis. They do however carry quite a radiation dose (see right), though this is usually not relevant to patients with a known serious malignancy

Typical doses from diagnostic medical exposure

Diagnostic procedure	Typical effective dose (mSv)	Equivalent no. of chest X-rays	Approx. equivalent period of natural background radiation
Radiographical examinations			
Limbs and joints (except hip)	<0.01	<0.5	<1.5 days
Chest (single PA film)	0.02	1	3 days
Skull	0.06	3	9 days
Thoracic spine	0.7	35	4 months
Lumbar spine	1	50	5 months
Hip	0.4	20	2 months
Pelvis	0.7	35	4 months
Abdomen	0.7	35	4 months
IVU	2.4	120	14 months
Barium swallow	1.5	75	8 months
Barium meal	2.6	130	15 months
Barium follow-through	3	150	16 months
Barium enema	7.2	360	3.2 years
CT head	2	100	10 months
CT chest	8	400	3.6 years
CT abdomen or pelvis	10	500	4.5 years
Radionuclide studies			
Lung ventilation (^{133}Xe)	0.3	15	7 weeks
Lung perfusion (^{99m}Tc)	1	50	6 months
Bone (^{99m}Tc)	4	200	1.8 years

UK average background radiation = 2.2mSv/year; regional averages range from 1.5 to 7.5mSv/year

Modified from Royal College of Radiologists handbook, Making the Best Use of the Radiology Department, 4th edn. 2003

138 Functional gastrointestinal disorders

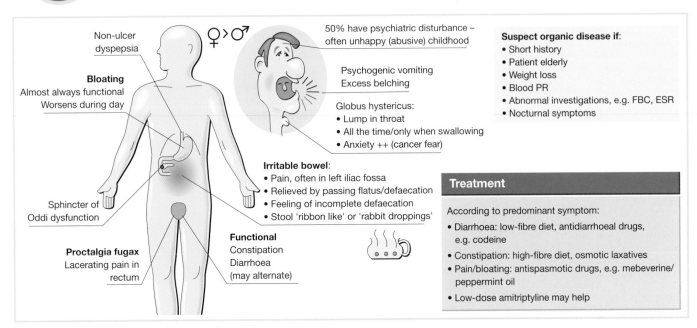

Non-ulcer dyspepsia

♀ > ♂

Bloating
Almost always functional
Worsens during day

Sphincter of Oddi dysfunction

Proctalgia fugax
Lacerating pain in rectum

50% have psychiatric disturbance – often unhappy (abusive) childhood

Psychogenic vomiting
Excess belching

Globus hystericus:
• Lump in throat
• All the time/only when swallowing
• Anxiety ++ (cancer fear)

Irritable bowel:
• Pain, often in left iliac fossa
• Relieved by passing flatus/defaecation
• Feeling of incomplete defaecation
• Stool 'ribbon like' or 'rabbit droppings'

Functional
Constipation
Diarrhoea
(may alternate)

Suspect organic disease if:
• Short history
• Patient elderly
• Weight loss
• Blood PR
• Abnormal investigations, e.g. FBC, ESR
• Nocturnal symptoms

Treatment

According to predominant symptom:

• Diarrhoea: low-fibre diet, antidiarrhoeal drugs, e.g. codeine

• Constipation: high-fibre diet, osmotic laxatives

• Pain/bloating: antispasmotic drugs, e.g. mebeverine/peppermint oil

• Low-dose amitriptyline may help

Irritable bowel syndrome is a widely used term with relatively limited clinical value. It represents one of many functional syndromes of gut sensitivity and/or motility that affect any part of the gastrointestinal (GI) tract. Examples include: globus hystericus, non-ulcer dyspepsia, irritable bowel syndrome, functional diarrhoea, functional constipation, proctalgia fugax and sphincter of Oddi dysfunction.

The common link between these conditions is that they have characteristic symptom complexes without clinical or laboratory features to suggest progressive intestinal pathology.

Incidence and pathophysiology

The prevalence depends on definition. Ten per cent of the population consults doctors with functional GI complaints; 20% who consider themselves normal admit to symptoms consistent with irritable bowel. Other overlapping symptom complexes include chronic fatigue syndrome, fibromyalgia, headache and functional gynaecological symptoms. In some individuals, episodes of gut insult (e.g. severe gastroenteritis) may have triggered the problem (postinfective irritable bowel). Sufferers may have heightened visceral sensory awareness.

Clinical features

Although the symptoms vary enormously there are some patterns that dominate:

• **Bloating**.

• **Marked gastrocolic reflex** (the need to defecate shortly after eating).

• **Identifiable dietary precipitants**: specific foods may cause symptoms, e.g. dairy products, fatty or spicy foods and alcohol.

• **Pain** relieved by defaecation.

• **Chaotic bowel habit**: patients often describe an increased frequency of defecation with clustering in the morning – the 'cork out of the champagne bottle' effect.

• **Stress** may be an overt feature even if this is not recognized by the patient.

Some symptoms should not be put down to a functional cause without further investigation:

• Dysphagia.

• Anorexia and/or weight loss.

• Nocturnal diarrhea.

• Rectal bleeding.

Management and prognosis

The extent of clinical investigation to exclude a progressive intestinal pathology must be individually tailored. A detailed history (including dietary) from the patient is central to the correct diagnosis and management. A full and thorough examination should be undertaken. Thereafter investigations depend largely on the patient's particular symptom complex. As a minimum, a basic blood screen including haematology, biochemistry and inflammatory markers should be performed.

The process of undergoing an in-depth history and physical examination can be therapeutic and often the qualified reassurance of being told that there is no objective evidence of physical disease is sufficient to improve symptoms (or at least the resulting concern).

• **Antispasmodic** drugs: mebeverine or alverine are useful for colicky abdominal pain.

• **Anticholinergics**: low doses of amitriptyline help those with depressive features (low mood, anhedonia, rumination, poor sleep, etc.). Relaxation therapy may also help.

• **Dietary measures**: patients resistant to the above measures or those with clearly identifiable dietary intolerances may benefit from dietary intervention (low lactose diet, exclusion diet). Paradoxically, many patients with an irritable bowel find that their symptoms worsen with a high fibre diet.

British Society of Gastroenterology. Guidelines on the irritable bowel syndrome: mechanisms and practical management. *Gut* 2007: 56; 1770–98; www.bsg.org.uk (last accessed September 2013).

NICE. *Irritable Bowel Syndrome*. NICE Guidance CG61, 2008; www.nice.org.uk (last accessed September 2013).

139 Nutrition

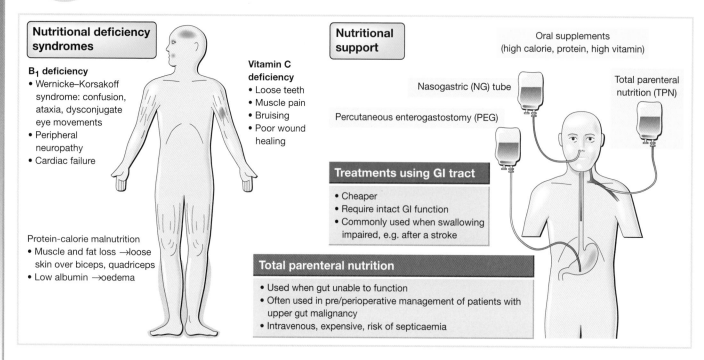

Nutritional deficiency syndromes

B₁ deficiency
- Wernicke–Korsakoff syndrome: confusion, ataxia, dysconjugate eye movements
- Peripheral neuropathy
- Cardiac failure

Vitamin C deficiency
- Loose teeth
- Muscle pain
- Bruising
- Poor wound healing

Protein-calorie malnutrition
- Muscle and fat loss →loose skin over biceps, quadriceps
- Low albumin →oedema

Nutritional support

Oral supplements (high calorie, protein, high vitamin)

Nasogastric (NG) tube

Total parenteral nutrition (TPN)

Percutaneous enterogastostomy (PEG)

Treatments using GI tract
- Cheaper
- Require intact GI function
- Commonly used when swallowing impaired, e.g. after a stroke

Total parenteral nutrition
- Used when gut unable to function
- Often used in pre/perioperative management of patients with upper gut malignancy
- Intravenous, expensive, risk of septicaemia

The extent of malnutrition in hospital inpatients is often underestimated. Many diseases lead to anorexia and a reduction in calorific intake, and this is especially relevant when placed in the context of the increased nutritional requirements resulting from the catabolic state of malignant or inflammatory disease.

Identification of malnutrition in hospital patients

General (protein-calorie malnutrition)

Protein-calorie malnutrition is easy to miss in the hospitalized patient because the primary disease often dominates the clinical picture. Starvation is, however, very common, and can be recognized by weight loss of >10% in <3 months (when the body mass index or BMI is <19 kg/m²), muscle wasting, peripheral oedema (with an albumin <35 g/L) and lymphocytes <1.5 × 10⁹/L.

Specific (vitamin and mineral deficiencies)

Acute vitamin deficiency is much more frequent with the water-soluble vitamins (particularly vitamin B₁ (thiamine) and vitamin C) (see Table 139.1), rather than those that are fat soluble, for which there are substantial body stores.

- **Thiamine deficiency** can develop quickly (within 3 weeks), and leads to Wernicke's encephalopathy. People with alcohol problems are particularly predisposed, but so are patients with prolonged (>3 weeks) vomiting.
- **Folate** stores are relatively small and deficiency can occur quickly, causing a macrocytic anaemia.
- **Vitamin C deficiency** (scurvy) is much commoner than realized, and impairs wound healing. If prolonged, classic scurvy may occur, with the development of unusual 'corkscrew'-shaped hair,

haemorrhages around the hair follicle, swollen spongy gums, leading to loose teeth, spontaneous bruising and bleeding. Anaemia, which is usually hypochromic but can be normochromic, occurs. Vitamin C levels can be measured in the plasma, and also in the leukocyte–platelet layer of centrifuged blood – the 'buffy' layer. Treatment is with ascorbic acid.

- **Iron** (microcytic anaemia, glossitis, cheilosis, koilonychia), **calcium** (proximal myopathy, perioral paraesthesia, tetany) and **magnesium** (myopathy not responding to calcium) deficiency can all occur in hospitalized patients.

Nutritional support

Indications

In patients considered to be malnourished, attention should always be given to nutritional support.

Forms of nutritional support
See Figure 139.1.

Therapeutic diets

Many diets are useful for the treatment of specific gastrointestinal (GI) conditions and for non-specific symptoms (see Table 139.2). Low protein diets tend not to be advised nowadays for either renal failure or hepatic encephalopathy.

British Society of Gastroenterology. Guidelines for enteral feeding in hospital patients. *Gut* 2003: 52 (Suppl. VII); www.bsg.org.uk (last accessed September 2013).

NICE. *Nutrition Support for Adults. Oral nutrition support, enteral tube feeding and parenteral nutrition.* NICE Guidance, 2006; www.nice.org.uk (last accessed September 2013).

Medicine at a Glance, Fourth Edition. Edited by Patrick Davey. © 2014 John Wiley & Sons, Ltd. Published 2014 by John Wiley & Sons, Ltd. Companion website: www.ataglanceseries.com/medicine

Table 139.1 Feature of water-soluble vitamin deficiency (for features of vitamin C deficiency, see text; folate deficiency and B_{12} deficiency, see Chapter 176).

	Vitamin B_1	Vitamin B_2	Niacin	Vitamin B_6
Solubility	Water			
Common name	Thiamine	Riboflavin		Pyridoxine
Occurrence	• Cereals • Beans • Nuts • Pork, duck	• Dairy products • Offal • Leafy vegetables	• Plants • Meat • Fish	Found widely in plant and animal derived foods
Function	Essential cofactor in many enzyme systems, especially involving carbohydrate metabolism		Hydrogen acceptor in many oxidative reactions	Cofactor in metabolism of many amino acids
Cause of deficiency	• Dietary deficiency, e.g. milled rice • Alcoholism (usually due to dietary deficiency) • Prolonged vomiting, e.g. hyperemesis gravidarum, cancer especially with chemotherapy	Low dietary intake	Lost during the milling process of cereals – unless replaced deficiency occurs in those with cereal-only diet • Isoniazid therapy • Malabsorption syndromes (rare) • Carcinoid syndrome	• Dietary deficiency is very rare • Drugs can produce deficiency (e.g. isoniazid, hydralazine penicillamine)
Consequence of deficiency	• 'Dry' beriberi; polyneuropathy, ± cerebral involvement with Wernicke–Korsokoff syndrome (causing dementia, ataxia, external ophthalmoplegia, nystagmus) • 'Wet' beriberi: oedema of the legs * ascites, pleural effusions (largely due to cardiac failure) • Vasodilatation (due to lactic acid) * bounding pulse	Clinical deficiency very rare: • Angular stomatitis • Red inflamed tongue • Seborrhoeic dermatitis • Conjunctivitis	Pellagra (→ the 3 Ds): • **Dermatitis**: in sun-exposed areas of the skin → thickening, dry, hyperpigmentation • **Diarrhoea**: other GI symptoms include a red raw tongue, glossitis, angular stomatitis • **Dementia**: in severe cases; in milder cases, depression, apathy ad thought disorders	• Polyneuropathy • Rarely, some sideroblastic anaemias respond to B_6 • Some premenstrual tension symptoms may respond to B_6 supplementation
Diagnosis	• Clinical response to thiamine • Red cell (transketolase) before and after added thiamine		Clinical features	Clinical features
General treatment	Most vitamin deficiencies are not isolated, and accordingly multiple different vitamin supplements should be given, along with protein and calories			
Treatment	Supplemental thiamine – if due to ethyl alcohol abuse, thiamine must be given prior to carbohydrates	Riboflavin supplementation	Niacin supplementation	Vitamin B_6
Excess	Ataxia	No data		

Table 139.2 Indications for specific diets.

Diet	Indication	Principle
Gluten-free	Coeliac disease	Total gluten withdrawal
Low lactose	Hypolactasia	Low in dairy products
High fibre	Constipation/diverticular change	High content of insoluble fibre (e.g. bran)
Low residue	Subacute small bowel obstruction (e.g. Crohn's disease)	Low in fibre to reduce obstructive symptoms
Exclusion	Intractable irritable bowel	Bland diet for control of irritable bowel symptoms
Low salt	Cirrhosis, heart failure	Useful adjunct to diuretics in control of oedema and/or ascites
Elemental/peptide	Crohn's disease	Liquid diet with nitrogen as either short peptides or amino acids

140 Renal physiology and function tests

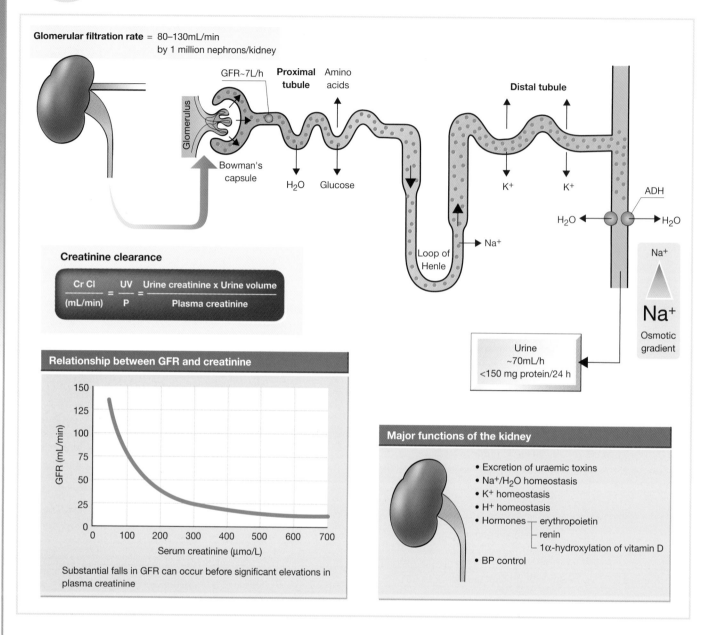

Glomerular filtration rate = 80–130mL/min
by 1 million nephrons/kidney

GFR~7L/h · **Proximal tubule** · Amino acids

Glomerulus

Bowman's capsule

H_2O · Glucose

Distal tubule

Loop of Henle

K^+ · K^+

Na^+

ADH

H_2O · H_2O

Na^+

Na^+

Osmotic gradient

Urine
~70mL/h
<150 mg protein/24 h

Creatinine clearance

$$\text{Cr Cl (mL/min)} = \frac{UV}{P} = \frac{\text{Urine creatinine} \times \text{Urine volume}}{\text{Plasma creatinine}}$$

Relationship between GFR and creatinine

GFR (mL/min) vs Serum creatinine (µmo/L)

Substantial falls in GFR can occur before significant elevations in plasma creatinine

Major functions of the kidney

- Excretion of uraemic toxins
- Na^+/H_2O homeostasis
- K^+ homeostasis
- H^+ homeostasis
- Hormones — erythropoietin
  — renin
  — 1α-hydroxylation of vitamin D
- BP control

Each kidney consists of approximately 1 million nephrons. Each nephron has a glomerulus, which is located mainly in the renal cortex and which filters into a renal tubule. The tubule consists of proximal and distal tubules, and the loop of Henle in which reabsorption of water, electrolytes and other important solutes occurs; this produces urine, which drains into the collecting ducts, undergoes further water absorption and then drains into the renal pyramids. The thick ascending limb of the loop of Henle possesses a specialized plaque of cells that attaches to the extraglomerular mesangium and afferent arteriole to form the juxtaglomerular apparatus; this secretes renin and is involved in the regulation of glomerular blood flow and filtration rate. The kidneys receive 20% of the cardiac output and filter 7 L of fluid per hour to produce 50–100 mL of urine per hour, showing the efficiency with which water and other solutes are reabsorbed by the renal tubules.

The key functions of the kidney are therefore to excrete/secrete the waste products of metabolism, and other substances harmful to the body, while conserving useful constituents of blood. In addition the kidney has major endocrine functions including the secretion of erythropoietin, the α_1-hydroxylation of vitamin D and the production of renin. Although often renal disease leads to failure in all three of these key functions, equally often disease can affect the first two functions independently. It is convenient to consider how the different functions of the kidney can be assessed according to anatomical location.

Medicine at a Glance, Fourth Edition. Edited by Patrick Davey. © 2014 John Wiley & Sons, Ltd. Published 2014 by John Wiley & Sons, Ltd. Companion website: www.ataglanceseries.com/medicine

Glomerular function

Toxin/metabolic waste product elimination

The key variable reflecting the efficiency of the kidney in waste product disposal is the glomerular filtration rate (GFR). The most commonly used measure of GFR is serum creatinine, an end product of skeletal muscle metabolism (higher in those with large muscle bulk). The relationship between GFR and serum creatinine is not linear (see Figure 140.1), and it is important to emphasize that highly significant falls in GFR can occur before serum creatinine rises. If impairment of GFR is suspected, it is insufficient to rely on plasma creatinine; a more accurate measure of GFR should be used instead, such as the creatinine clearance. The principle underlying this measure is that creatinine is an inert molecule, passively filtered by the kidney. A knowledge of urine creatinine quantity ($Urine_{Cr}$) and plasma creatinine concentration (P_{Cr}) (over 24 h) allows calculation of the GFR, from:

$$GFR = (Urine_{Cr} \times urine\ volume)/P_{Cr}$$

Increasingly, laboratories are quoting estimated GFR (eGFR) using calculations that require serum creatinine. Creatinine clearance measurements are usually sufficiently accurate for day-to-day clinical practice, although the GFR measured this way may overestimate the true GFR by up to 100% in severe renal disease, as a result of renal tubule secretion of creatinine (thus overestimating the amount of urine creatinine derived from glomerular filtration). More precise measurement of GFR can be undertaken with radioisotope scans (diethylene triamine penta-acetic acid (DTPA)).

Conservation of normal blood constituents

Glomerular function can be disturbed such that plasma protein is no longer conserved. This leak of protein can range from mild, significant as a marker of renal disease, to devastating, associated with profound hypoalbuminaemia and substantial oedema (the nephrotic syndrome). In addition to defective glomerular function, mild proteinuria also results from defects in tubular function (see Table 140.1) and as an overflow phenomenon (e.g. multiple myeloma, immunoglobulin κ or λ light chains: acute leukaemia, lysozymuria). These three different kinds of mild proteinuria are distinguished on the basis of electrophoretic properties. Urine dipsticks primarily detect albumin, which is found in glomerular disease and not in tubular disease or multiple myeloma. If these conditions are suspected, urine electrophoresis should be performed.

Renal concentrating ability

The loop of Henle, via the countercurrent mechanism, establishes an osmotic gradient that increases from the cortex to the inner medulla. Water excretion is adjusted in the collecting ducts, which pass through the medulla and where permeability of water is controlled by the antidiuretic hormone (ADH). The ability of the kidney to concentrate urine is disturbed in many intrinsic renal diseases, particularly tubulointerstitial ones, as well as in actual or functional deficiency of ADH (diabetes insipidus). The renal concentrating power can be measured by: (i) osmolality of early morning urine, which is the easiest and safest test; and (ii) concentrating ability when faced with 24-hour fluid deprivation, which is uncomfortable (so compliance is an issue) and which may induce hypovolaemic renal failure. It is usual to admit patients to hospital for this.

Amino acid conserving function

Amino acids are filtered at the glomerulus, and reabsorbed in the proximal tubules. Diffuse proximal tubular damage results in generalized aminoaciduria, whereas specific lesions cause specific patterns of amino acid loss. The pattern of aminoaciduria is detected by two-dimensional chromatography.

Renal acid–base control

A major function of the proximal and distal tubules is acid–base balance. Advanced renal failure gives rise to the retention of metabolic acids (exacerbating renal bone disease), which may provoke myocardial depression and death. Specific tubular lesions may, in the absence of filtration failure, produce retention of metabolic acid –so-called renal tubular acidosis.

Electrolyte control

The kidney is central in the control of potassium, as a result of secretion of potassium into the tubular fluid in exchange for sodium or hydrogen ions, and in the regulation of urinary pH. In advanced renal failure, the distal tubule cannot exchange plasma K^+/H^+ for tubule Na^+, leading to hyperkalaemia, which when profound may lead to cardiac arrest.

Hormonal function

The kidney has hormonal functions, notably in the production of renin and erythropoietin, and the α_1-hydroxylation of vitamin D from an inactive to an active form. When renal function is globally disturbed, renal hormone production is usually diminished, provoking anaemia (erythropoietin deficiency) and exacerbating renal bone disease. Other hormones, especially the renin–angiotensin system, are involved in blood pressure (BP) control. Renal diseases such as renal ischaemia (e.g. unilateral renal artery stenosis) or glomerulonephritis are commonly associated with hypertension.

Table 140.1 Proteinuria in renal disease.

	Glomerulonephritis	Tubular disease	Overflow proteinuria
Amount of proteinuria	+ to ++++	+ to ++	+ to ++++
Nephrotic syndrome present	0 to ++++	No	0 to ++ (amyloid in multiple myeloma)
Dipstick positive for protein	Yes	No	No
κ or λ free chains	No	Yes	Monoclonal Ig κ or λ

141 Hypokalaemia and hyperkalaemia

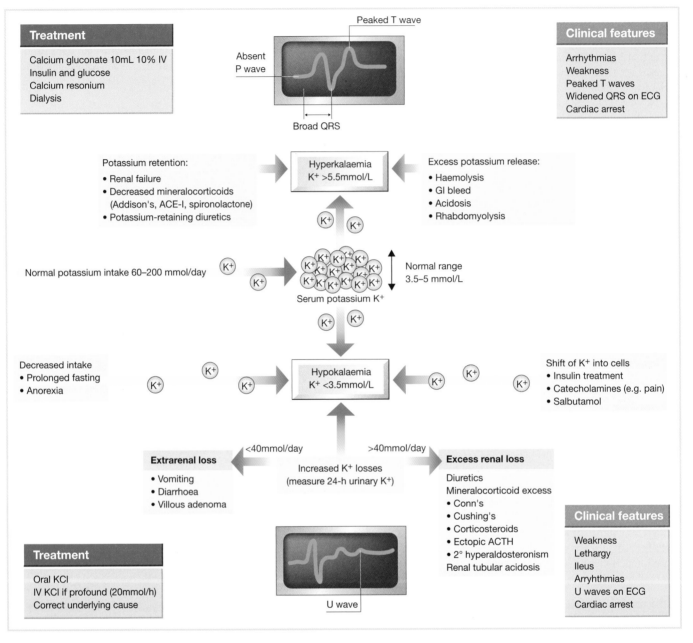

Treatment

Calcium gluconate 10mL 10% IV
Insulin and glucose
Calcium resonium
Dialysis

Peaked T wave

Absent
P wave

Broad QRS

Clinical features

Arrhythmias
Weakness
Peaked T waves
Widened QRS on ECG
Cardiac arrest

Potassium retention:
• Renal failure
• Decreased mineralocorticoids
  (Addison's, ACE-I, spironolactone)
• Potassium-retaining diuretics

Hyperkalaemia
K⁺ >5.5mmol/L

Excess potassium release:
• Haemolysis
• GI bleed
• Acidosis
• Rhabdomyolysis

Normal potassium intake 60–200 mmol/day

Serum potassium K⁺

Normal range
3.5–5 mmol/L

Decreased intake
• Prolonged fasting
• Anorexia

Hypokalaemia
K⁺ <3.5mmol/L

Shift of K⁺ into cells
• Insulin treatment
• Catecholamines (e.g. pain)
• Salbutamol

<40mmol/day   >40mmol/day

Extrarenal loss
• Vomiting
• Diarrhoea
• Villous adenoma

Increased K⁺ losses
(measure 24-h urinary K⁺)

Excess renal loss
Diuretics
Mineralocorticoid excess
• Conn's
• Cushing's
• Corticosteroids
• Ectopic ACTH
• 2° hyperaldosteronism
Renal tubular acidosis

Clinical features

Weakness
Lethargy
Ileus
Arryhthmias
U waves on ECG
Cardiac arrest

Treatment

Oral KCl
IV KCl if profound (20mmol/h)
Correct underlying cause

U wave

Hypokalaemia

Hypokalaemia is a serum potassium of less than 3.5 mmol/L. It is the most common electrolyte disorder in hospitalized patients, mostly attributable to diuretic therapy. It can occur as a result of increased losses from the urinary or gastrointestinal (GI) tract, poor intake (such as in eating disorders) or a shift to the intracellular compartment (insulin treatment or familial periodic paralysis; see Chapter 210). GI losses may occur as a result of diarrhoea, vomiting, laxative abuse or villous adenomas of the colon. Renal losses may occur as the result of diuretic therapy, mineralocorticoid excess (Conn's syndrome, Cushing's syndrome, ectopic adrenocorticotrophic hormone (ACTH), secondary

hyperaldosteronism (renal artery stenosis, hypertension, heart failure)) or renal tubular acidosis. β-Receptor stimulation moves potassium into cells, which explains why hypokalaemia is common in the sick and in those treated with salbutamol.

Common causes

● Diuretic therapy.
● Acute illness.
● Gastrointestinal losses.

Clinical features

Often asymptomatic when mild, hypokalaemia can produce weakness, intestinal ileus, decreased renal-concentrating ability

Medicine at a Glance, Fourth Edition. Edited by Patrick Davey. © 2014 John Wiley & Sons, Ltd. Published 2014 by John Wiley & Sons, Ltd. Companion website: www.ataglanceseries.com/medicine

and electrocardiogram (ECG) changes of T-wave flattening, the appearance of U waves and an increased incidence of tachyarrhythmias. Long-standing hypokalaemia can lead to (poorly reversible) damage to the distal tubule, leading to a failure of renal-concentrating properties, and polyuria, with compensatory polydipsia.

When severe (K^+ <2 mmol/L) skeletal muscle weakness, which may be profound, dominates the clinical picture and flaccid paralysis may be seen. Very rarely, respiratory failure can occur in this situation.

Management

Treat the underlying cause. If potassium is <2.5 (or <3.0 mmol/L in a patient at risk of arrhythmias e.g. post-myocardial infarction), give intravenous (IV) potassium chloride (KCl) as an infusion not exceeding 20 mmol/h at a concentration not exceeding 40 mmol/L because concentrated potassium will damage peripheral veins. If potassium is between 2.5 and 3.5 mmol/L in the general population, give oral replacement therapy (unless the patient is nil by mouth or vomiting) at 80–120 mmol/day in divided doses.

Hyperkalaemia

The main cause of hyperkalaemia is renal failure (because potassium excretion is impaired). Other causes include reduced mineralocorticoids, such as in Addison's disease, spironolactone (aldosterone antagonist) and angiotensin-converting enzyme (ACE) inhibitors angiotensisn receptor blockers (ARBs) or potassium-retaining diuretics such as amiloride. Cell destruction in haemolysis, cytotoxic therapy and rhabdomyolysis can liberate large amounts of potassium and cause hyperkalaemia. The hyperkalaemic effects of ACE inhibitors or potassium-retaining diuretics such as amiloride can be very marked in patients with renal impairment. Hyperkalaemia can be artefactual as a result of the haemolysis of blood during venepuncture, so treat an unsuspected/anomalous finding of hyperkalaemia with suspicion, and repeat the measurement.

Common causes

- Renal failure.
- Drugs in those with borderline or frankly abnormal renal function, e.g. ACE inhibitors and/or spironolactone in elderly people or those with heart failure.

Clinical features

Even very severe hyperkalaemia is usually asymptomatic although it can very rarely be accompanied by muscular weakness. It may be associated with ECG abnormalities of T-wave peaking, QRS widening, prolonged PR interval, loss of P waves and a sine wave appearance (see Figure 141.2 below), leading to cardiac arrest.

Management

In mild hyperkalaemia (potassium <6.0 mmol/L), oral or IV potassium should be restricted. Severe hyperkalaemia (potassium >6.5 mmol/L or hyperkalaemic ECG changes) is a medical emergency, particularly if the rate of rise of potassium has been rapid. The patient should receive IV calcium gluconate (10 mL of 10% over 2 min), which stabilizes the myocardium. Measures to lower potassium should be instituted: the administration of IV glucose with insulin (50 mL of 50% glucose and 10 units of short-acting insulin), the potassium-binding resin, calcium resonium, and dialysis may be required.

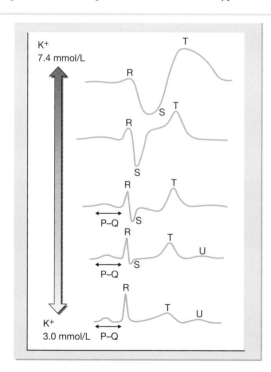

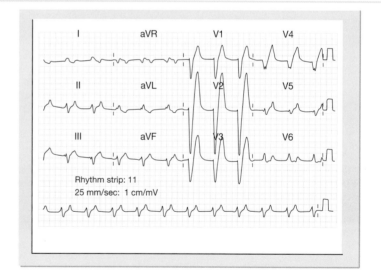

An ECG of a middle aged woman with acute renal failure, and a K^+ of 8.0 mmol/L. This ECG shows absent P waves, very broad QRS complex and tall 'peaked' T waves, especially in leads V1 to V4

142 Hyponatraemia and hypernatraemia

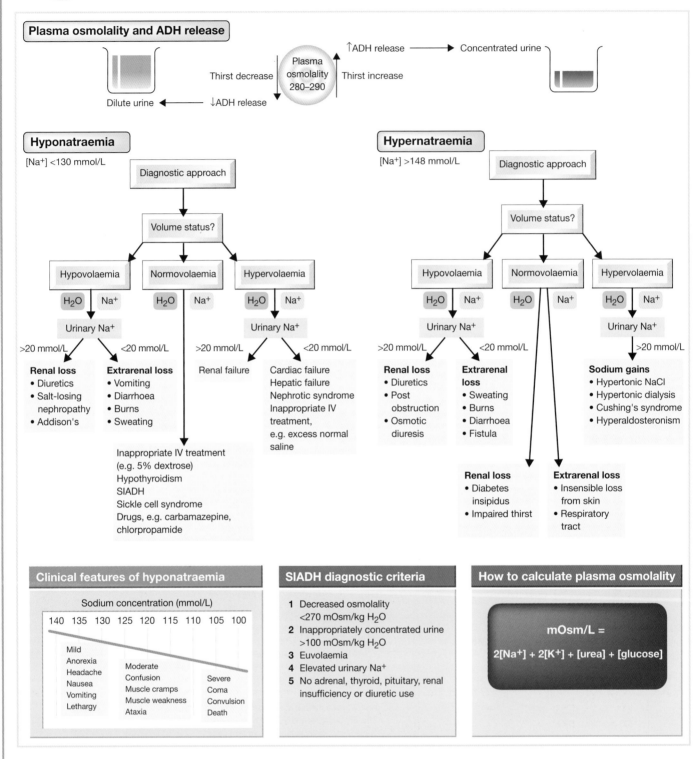

Plasma osmolality and ADH release

Thirst decrease ← Plasma osmolality 280–290 → Thirst increase

↑ADH release → Concentrated urine

↓ADH release → Dilute urine

Hyponatraemia

[Na+] <130 mmol/L

Diagnostic approach → Volume status?

Hypovolaemia (H₂O Na+)
Urinary Na+
- >20 mmol/L → **Renal loss**
  - Diuretics
  - Salt-losing nephropathy
  - Addison's
- <20 mmol/L → **Extrarenal loss**
  - Vomiting
  - Diarrhoea
  - Burns
  - Sweating

Normovolaemia (H₂O Na+)
Inappropriate IV treatment (e.g. 5% dextrose)
Hypothyroidism
SIADH
Sickle cell syndrome
Drugs, e.g. carbamazepine, chlorpropamide

Hypervolaemia (H₂O Na+)
Urinary Na+
- >20 mmol/L → Renal failure
- <20 mmol/L → Cardiac failure
  Hepatic failure
  Nephrotic syndrome
  Inappropriate IV treatment, e.g. excess normal saline

Hypernatraemia

[Na+] >148 mmol/L

Diagnostic approach → Volume status?

Hypovolaemia (H₂O Na+)
Urinary Na+
- >20 mmol/L → **Renal loss**
  - Diuretics
  - Post obstruction
  - Osmotic diuresis
- <20 mmol/L → **Extrarenal loss**
  - Sweating
  - Burns
  - Diarrhoea
  - Fistula

Normovolaemia (H₂O Na+)
Renal loss
- Diabetes insipidus
- Impaired thirst

Extrarenal loss
- Insensible loss from skin
- Respiratory tract

Hypervolaemia (H₂O Na+)
Urinary Na+
- >20 mmol/L → **Sodium gains**
  - Hypertonic NaCl
  - Hypertonic dialysis
  - Cushing's syndrome
  - Hyperaldosteronism

Clinical features of hyponatraemia

Sodium concentration (mmol/L)

140 135 130 125 120 115 110 105 100

Mild
Anorexia
Headache
Nausea
Vomiting
Lethargy

Moderate
Confusion
Muscle cramps
Muscle weakness
Ataxia

Severe
Coma
Convulsion
Death

SIADH diagnostic criteria

1 Decreased osmolality <270 mOsm/kg H₂O
2 Inappropriately concentrated urine >100 mOsm/kg H₂O
3 Euvolaemia
4 Elevated urinary Na+
5 No adrenal, thyroid, pituitary, renal insufficiency or diuretic use

How to calculate plasma osmolality

$$mOsm/L = 2[Na^+] + 2[K^+] + [urea] + [glucose]$$

Medicine at a Glance, Fourth Edition. Edited by Patrick Davey. © 2014 John Wiley & Sons, Ltd. Published 2014 by John Wiley & Sons, Ltd. Companion website: www.ataglanceseries.com/medicine

Abnormalities of serum sodium are closely linked to water balance. The most common causes of altered serum sodium are the result of excessive losses or administration of water.

Hyponatraemia

Hyponatraemia is defined as a serum sodium <130 mmol/L and is found in 5% of hospital inpatients. Hyponatraemia may be asymptomatic, but can produce confusion, coma and convulsions.

In hyponatraemia there is an excess of extracellular water relative to the sodium content of the extracellular compartment. This can occur in three different circumstances:[nl]

1 **Hypovolaemia** (body Na$^+$ and water deficit).
2 **Normovolaemia** (no change in body Na$^+$ but a modest increase in water).
3 **Hypervolaemia** (increase in body Na$^+$ and water).

Common causes

● Syndrome of inappropriate antidiuretic hormone secretion (SIADH).
● Heart failure (severity of hyponatraemia relates to severity of heart failure and prognosis).
● Inappropriate overvigorous intravenous dextrose in postoperative patients.
● Iatrogenic Addison's disease (over-rapid corticosteroid withdrawal in elderly patients on large doses of steroids or with failure to increase corticosteroids when ill).

Management

The underlying aetiology should be sought and corrected where possible. The volume status of the patient should be determined. If signs of hypovolaemia are present (thirst, tachycardia, hypotension, postural fall in blood pressure, reduced skin turgor, etc.) then sodium chloride (NaCl) should be administered intravenously. In mild hyponatraemia, treatment may not be necessary, but if symptoms are present and there is no evidence of hypovolaemia the patient's fluid intake should be restricted. If there is evidence of hypervolaemia (oedema, elevated jugular venous pressure, hypertension), diuretics and water restriction may be necessary. Cautious correction of Na$^+$ is essential to avoid central pontine myelinolysis, a syndrome of encephalopathy, cranial nerve palsies and quadriplegia, which occurs after rapid correction of Na$^+$. In chronic hyponatraemia, the Na$^+$ should be corrected at less than 0.5 mmol/L/h, although in acute hyponatraemia, if neurological symptoms are present, more rapid correction may be appropriate.

Syndrome of inappropriate ADH secretion

This is a relatively common cause of hyponatraemia in hospital patients. However, the diagnosis requires the exclusion of adrenal, thyroid, pituitary or renal insufficiency, no diuretic usage and euvolaemia. For the plasma tonicity, there is inappropriate elevation of ADH (vasopressin) levels which leads to an inappropriate urinary concentration. There are a large number of possible causes (see Table 142.1) which can be broadly grouped into carcinomas (particularly of the lung), pulmonary disorders including pneumonia, central nervous system disorders such as meningitis and head trauma, and drugs.

Treatment of SIADH involves removing the precipitating cause wherever possible. Fluid restriction, of increasing degree with increasingly lower sodium, is usually effective and tolerable.

Table 142.1 Some of the commonest causes of the syndrome of inappropriate antidiuretic hormone release.

Idiopathic	
Postoperative	Pain Lung infection + COPD Drugs (see below)
CNS causes	Infection Stroke Neoplasia
Lung causes	Infection Tumour
Oncological causes	Lung cancer – commonest Prostate, GI tract, haematological malignancies
Drugs	↑ H$_2$O permeability of nephron, e.g. vasopressin ↑ ADH release, e.g. carbamazepine ↑ ADH action, e.g. cyclophosphamide ↓ Prostaglandin synthesis, e.g. aspirin

ADH, antidiuretic hormone; CNS, central nervous system; COPD, chronic obstructive pulmonary disease; GI, gastrointestinal.

Demeclocycline (which inhibits the action of ADH on the distal tubule) may be used if these simple manoeuvres are ineffective. ADH antagonists such as tolvaptan are now available though their therapeutic role is unclear.

Hypernatraemia

Hypernatraemia is defined as a serum sodium >145 mmol/L caused by a relative water deficit and the major defence against it is thirst. It therefore occurs more commonly in patients who are unable to increase their water intake. As for hyponatraemia, the causes can be grouped into three categories depending on volume status:[nl]

1 **Hypovolaemia** (low body sodium with loss of water exceeding that of Na$^+$).
2 **Normovolaemia** (normal body Na$^+$ but water loss).
3 **Hypervolaemia** (increased total body Na$^+$).

As with hyponatraemia, assessment of volume status and determination of urinary sodium are central to the diagnostic approach.

Common causes

● Fluid (water) deprivation, particularly in elderly people.
● Hyperosmolar diabetic coma.

Management

The underlying cause requires identification and correction. In patients with hypovolaemia, the volume deficit should be corrected with physiological saline until haemodynamics are normalized; water may then be required. In hypervolaemic hypernatraemia, the excess sodium requires removal, often with diuretics. In euvolaemic hypernatraemia, water is given intravenously as 5% dextrose. In all cases, careful monitoring of volume status and serum sodium concentration is necessary and correction of Na$^+$ should be made at a rate of less than 0.5 mmol/L/h.

Diabetes insipidus is characterized by polyuria and polydipsia and is the result of defects in ADH action. It can produce hypernatraemia and is discussed in greater detail in Chapter 164.

143 Disorders of acid–base balance

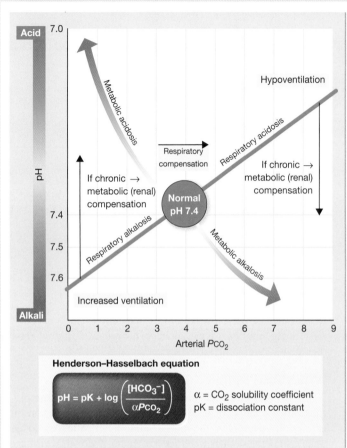

Henderson–Hasselbach equation

$$pH = pK + \log\left(\frac{[HCO_3^-]}{\alpha P_{CO_2}}\right)$$

α = CO$_2$ solubility coefficient
pK = dissociation constant

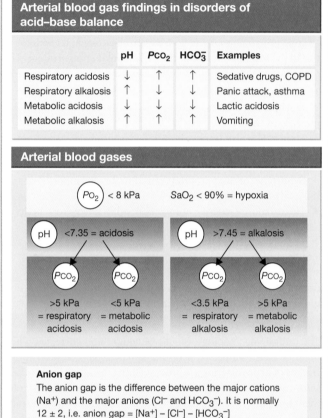

Arterial blood gas findings in disorders of acid–base balance

	pH	P_{CO_2}	HCO$_3^-$	Examples
Respiratory acidosis	↓	↑	↑	Sedative drugs, COPD
Respiratory alkalosis	↑	↓	↓	Panic attack, asthma
Metabolic acidosis	↓	↓	↓	Lactic acidosis
Metabolic alkalosis	↑	↑	↑	Vomiting

Arterial blood gases

P_{O_2} < 8 kPa SaO_2 < 90% = hypoxia

pH <7.35 = acidosis

P_{CO_2} >5 kPa = respiratory acidosis

P_{CO_2} <5 kPa = metabolic acidosis

pH >7.45 = alkalosis

P_{CO_2} <3.5 kPa = respiratory alkalosis

P_{CO_2} >5 kPa = metabolic alkalosis

Anion gap
The anion gap is the difference between the major cations (Na$^+$) and the major anions (Cl$^-$ and HCO$_3^-$). It is normally 12 ± 2, i.e. anion gap = [Na$^+$] – [Cl$^-$] – [HCO$_3^-$]

In many ill patients important acid–base disturbances occur. They may lack specific symptoms, and in any seriously ill patient arterial blood gases should be determined. The type of acid–base disturbance can be determined from the pH and P_{CO_2} (see Figure 143.1).

Metabolic acidosis

Metabolic acidosis is seen most commonly in diabetic ketoacidosis (DKA), lactic acidosis and renal failure. The presence of a significant metabolic acidosis is important and requires urgent diagnosis and treatment. It can be grouped into four major categories by aetiology:

1 Ingestion of acid, such as salicylate, methanol or ethylene glycol poisoning.
2 Accumulation of endogenous acids, such as lactic acid in tissue hypoperfusion or ketones in DKA.
3 Loss of alkali in severe diarrhoea, with biliary or enteric fistulae or renal loss in proximal renal tubular acidosis.
4 Failure of elimination of acid in renal failure and distal tubular acidosis.

Severe acidosis results in cardiac depression and death.

The anion gap can be useful in the diagnosis of metabolic acidoses. The anion gap is the difference between the major cation (sodium) and the major measured anions (chloride and bicarbonate). It is normally 12 ± 2. An elevated anion gap suggests the presence of additional anions such as lactate (in lactic acidosis) or ketones (in DKA), whereas a normal or reduced anion gap (or hyperchloraemic acidosis) suggests bicarbonate loss or renal tubular acidosis (see Tables 143.1 and 143.2).

The body will usually respond to the acidaemia with respiratory compensation, an increase in respiratory rate causing a fall in carbon dioxide, which in turn increases the blood pH. Metabolic acidosis may be associated with the signs or symptoms of the precipitating cause – the increased rate and depth of respiration, sometimes described as Kussmaul's respiration – or if severe it may itself be associated with the signs of shock.

The treatment should be directed towards reversing the underlying cause. In exceptional circumstances sodium bicarbonate may be administered and haemodialysis or haemofiltration used.

Metabolic alkalosis

Metabolic alkalosis rarely gives rise to symptoms from the alkalosis alone. The aetiologies of metabolic alkalosis include:

● Loss of acid such as in vomiting, particularly with pyloric stenosis.

Medicine at a Glance, Fourth Edition. Edited by Patrick Davey. © 2014 John Wiley & Sons, Ltd. Published 2014 by John Wiley & Sons, Ltd. Companion website: www.ataglanceseries.com/medicine

Table 143.1 Anion gap and metabolic acidosis.

Anion gap	Disease
Normal (=hyperchloraemic acidosis)	Renal tubular acidosis Extrarenal HCO_3^- loss Hyperparathyroidism Hypoaldosteronism ± Diabetic ketoacidosis
Increased (>20 mmol/L)	Renal parenchymal disease Ingestion of acid Acid metabolized from endogenous substances Lactic acidosis ± Diabetic ketoacidosis

Diabetic ketoacidosis may give rise to either normal or high anion gap acidosis

Table 143.2 Causes of lactic acidosis.

Mechanism	Disease
Increased rate of lactate production	Any cause of decreased tissue perfusion Hypoxia Increased skeletal muscle activity (e.g. status epilepticus or marathon runners) Destruction of large tumour masses (e.g. lymphoma or leukaemia) Poisoning (e.g. CO or cyanide)
Decreased lactate transport	Decreased cardiac output due to any cause
Decreased lactate metabolism	Liver failure (any cause) Intoxication (phenformin or alcohol) Diabetes mellitus Liver hypoxia
Miscellaneous	Haemofiltration with lactate buffer Pregnancy

Traditionally lactic acidosis is divided into type A (clinical evidence of poor tissue perfusion/oxygenation) and type B (no clinical evidence of poor tissue perfusion/oxygenation). B1 is associated with underlying diseases; B2 is due to drugs and toxins; B3 is due to inborn errors of metabolism

- Increased renal reabsorption of bicarbonate which can occur with hyperaldosteronism or severe hypokalaemia.
- Excess intake of alkali (e.g. the milk–alkali syndrome, where large quantities of alkaline antacids are ingested, often with milk).

There may be respiratory compensation with a reduction in respiratory rate, a rise in carbon dioxide and a fall in pH.

Treatment involves the identification and treatment of the underlying cause.

Respiratory acidosis

The primary control of ventilation is achieved by monitoring of blood pH by the respiratory centre, and appropriate changes in ventilatory rate to alter the blood partial pressure of carbon dioxide, which in turn leads to changes in blood pH. The development of respiratory acidosis is a concern and may indicate the need for ventilatory support (see Chapter 100).

A reduction in ventilation leads to an accumulation of carbon dioxide and the development of acidosis. This may be the result of a wide variety of causes of ventilatory impairment and commonly includes:

- Sedation, particularly with opiates.
- Respiratory muscle weakness, e.g. Guillain–Barré syndrome, poliomyelitis or myasthenia gravis.
- Severe chronic obstructive pulmonary disease (COPD).

The accumulation of carbon dioxide can sometimes be associated with clinical signs, which include a bounding pulse, papilloedema or a metabolic flap. If the carbon dioxide retention has been chronic there may be metabolic renal compensation with an elevated blood bicarbonate concentration.

Treatment usually involves attempts to improve the underlying ventilatory defect. Rarely respiratory stimulants may be used, whereas in particular patients with acute ventilatory failure artificial ventilation may be appropriate.

Respiratory alkalosis

This arises as a consequence of increased ventilation causing the partial pressure of carbon dioxide in the blood to fall, with a resultant rise in blood pH. The causes include:

- A response to hypoxaemia or tissue hypoxia.
- Increased ventilation, e.g. in panic attacks.
- Excessive artificial ventilation.
- Stimulation of respiration by drugs, central nervous system stimulation or pulmonary disease in which there is stimulation of chest receptors.

The fall in carbon dioxide and rise in pH can be associated with a fall in ionized calcium which can produce symptoms of peripheral and circumoral paraesthesia, light-headedness and carpopedal spasm. Chvostek's sign may be present (tapping of the facial nerve elicits a brief facial muscle contraction, reflecting latent hypocalcaemic tetany).

Treatment is directed towards ensuring that there is correction of any concomitant hypoxaemia and reversal of the underlying cause.

Mixed acid–base disorders

The ability of the body to compensate for pH disturbances with respiratory or metabolic compensations and the presence of more than one cause of acid–base disturbance in a particular patient can produce complex disturbances. In such cases a detailed history, complete examination, consideration of the blood gases and determination of the anion gap are critical in establishing the correct diagnosis.

144 Urinary calculi

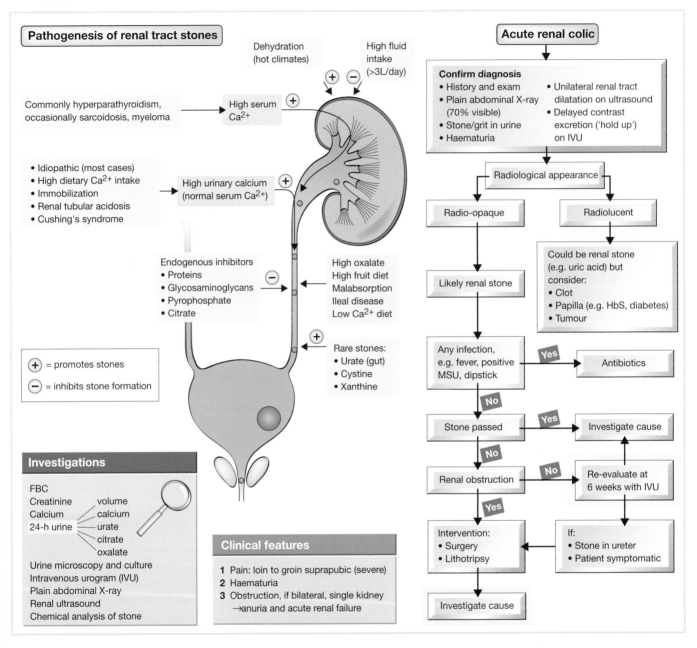

Pathogenesis of renal tract stones

Commonly hyperparathyroidism, occasionally sarcoidosis, myeloma → High serum Ca^{2+}

Dehydration (hot climates) (+)

High fluid intake (>3L/day) (−)

- Idiopathic (most cases)
- High dietary Ca^{2+} intake
- Immobilization
- Renal tubular acidosis
- Cushing's syndrome

→ High urinary calcium (normal serum Ca^{2+}) (+)

Endogenous inhibitors
- Proteins
- Glycosaminoglycans
- Pyrophosphate
- Citrate
(−)

High oxalate
High fruit diet
Malabsorption
Ileal disease
Low Ca^{2+} diet

Rare stones:
- Urate (gut)
- Cystine
- Xanthine
(+)

(+) = promotes stones
(−) = inhibits stone formation

Investigations

FBC
Creatinine
Calcium
24-h urine — volume
— calcium
— urate
— citrate
— oxalate
Urine microscopy and culture
Intravenous urogram (IVU)
Plain abdominal X-ray
Renal ultrasound
Chemical analysis of stone

Clinical features

1 Pain: loin to groin suprapubic (severe)
2 Haematuria
3 Obstruction, if bilateral, single kidney →anuria and acute renal failure

Acute renal colic

Confirm diagnosis
- History and exam
- Plain abdominal X-ray (70% visible)
- Stone/grit in urine
- Haematuria
- Unilateral renal tract dilatation on ultrasound
- Delayed contrast excretion ('hold up') on IVU

Radiological appearance

Radio-opaque — Likely renal stone

Radiolucent — Could be renal stone (e.g. uric acid) but consider:
- Clot
- Papilla (e.g. HbS, diabetes)
- Tumour

Any infection, e.g. fever, positive MSU, dipstick — **Yes** → Antibiotics

No

Stone passed — **Yes** → Investigate cause

No

Renal obstruction — **No** → Re-evaluate at 6 weeks with IVU

Yes

Intervention:
- Surgery
- Lithotripsy

If:
- Stone in ureter
- Patient symptomatic

Investigate cause

Urinary calculi are very common, with a prevalence of 5%. There is a peak prevalence at age 30–40 years and a 3 : 1 male predisposition. Most calculi contain calcium oxalate; the remainder consists of mixed calcium and ammonium phosphate (usually caused by infection), urate, cystine and xanthine stones.

Aetiology

Most calculi are idiopathic; the remainder may be associated with hypercalciuria, hypercalcaemia, recurrent urinary tract infection (UTI), hyperuricosuria or cystinuria. Urinary calculi form when urinary solutes exceed their maximum urinary solubility. Conditions producing excretion of a high solute load or reduced urine volume will promote calculus formation (see Table 144.1). Urine is usually supersaturated for some solutes and crystallization inhibitors such as citrate tend to prevent calculus formation.

Presentation

Urinary calculi can cause haematuria (both macroscopic and microscopic), loin pain, renal colic, suprapubic pain, dysuria, UTIs, urinary tract obstruction, and acute or chronic renal failure as a result of obstruction ± infection. The pain of renal colic may be excruciating and commonly localizes to the flank, although radiation to the anterior abdomen, groin or scrotum can occur.

Investigations

- Full blood count to exclude the very rare association with haematological malignancies (urate stones).
- Creatinine, urea, electrolytes, plasma calcium and urate.
- 24-hour urine collection for urine volume, urine pH, calcium, urate, citrate and oxalate.

Table 144.1 Conditions predisposing to renal stones.

- Metabolic syndromes
- Hypercalciuria: present in 70% of patients with renal stones
- Hyperoxaluria: idiopathic, genetic (type I or II) or secondary to gastrointestinal disease
- Hypocitraturia: distal renal tubular acidosis, K^+ depletion, renal failure
- Chronic hypercalcaemia: usually hyperparathyroidism
- Rare genetic metabolic diseases (e.g. cystinuria, etc.)
- Repeated infection
- Concentrated urine
- Chronically low fluid intake (<2 L/day)/high insensible losses (e.g. in hot countries)
- High dietary intake of animal protein
- Structural abnormality
- Renal tract obstruction (e.g. sloughed papilla, prostate, neurogenic bladder)
- Nephrocalcinosis: renal tubular acidosis (distal – type 1)

- Urine microscopy and culture because recurrent UTIs may be the cause or consequence of urinary calculi.
- Computed tomography (CT) urogram, renal tract ultrasonography and plain abdominal X-ray (AXR) to exclude obstruction and demonstrate the position of calculi.
- Chemical analysis of calculi.

Imaging of calculi

- **Ultrasonography**: 20% sensitivity, 97% specificity. Accessible, good for diagnosing hydronephrosis and renal stones, and requires no ionizing radiation. Poor at visualizing ureteral stones.
- **Plain radiography**: 50% sensitive, 75% specific. Accessible and inexpensive. Problems: stones in the middle section of the ureter, phleboliths, radiolucent calculi, extraurinary calcifications and non-genitourinary conditions.
- **Intravenous pyelography**: 65% sensitive, 90% specific. Accessible; provides information on anatomy and functioning of both kidneys. Problems: variable quality imaging, requires bowel preparation and use of contrast media, poor visualization of non-genitourinary conditions, delayed images required in high-grade obstruction.

- **Non-contrast helical CT**: 95% sensitive, 95% specific. Most sensitive and specific radiological test (i.e. facilitates fast, definitive diagnosis). Provides information on non-genitourinary conditions. Problems: indirect signs of degree of obstruction, less accessible and relatively expensive, no direct measure of renal function.

Management

Renal colic can be particularly painful, so adequate analgesia is important, often requiring non-steroidal anti-inflammatory drugs and/or opiate analgesia. Fluid intake should be increased to >3 L/day. Surgical treatment (required in 20%) of calculi or extracorporeal shock wave lithotripsy – where ultrasonic energy sufficient to fragment the calculus is transmitted from a probe placed on the skin over the renal tract – may prove necessary if the calculus is causing renal obstruction, particularly if infection is present. Renal failure (anuria) can occur if ureteric obstruction to a sole remaining kidney occurs. This is a medical emergency and requires immediate diagnosis and treatment. Several treatments facilitate the passage of stones (particularly <10 mm in diameter), notably α-blockers (e.g. tamsulosin) and calcium channel blockers (e.g. nifedipine).

Prevention

General measures include increasing endogenous inhibitors of stone formation, by giving oral potassium citrate, lemon juice and avoiding low potassium diets. Specific preventive treatments include:

- **Infection** associated with stones: prophylactic antibiotics.
- **Hypercalciuria**: the amount of calcium in the urine can be lessened with thiazide diuretics, and by reducing the amount of sodium in the diet. The relationship between a high protein diet and an excess incidence of upper renal tract stones may be explained by dietary protein increasing renal calcium excretion.
- **Urate calculi**: both gouty and calcium oxalate renal stones can be prevented with allopurinol.
- **Phosphate stones**: the urine should be acidified with ammonium chloride to decrease progression.
- **Oxalate stones**: in oxalate stones, the amount of oxalate in the diet (e.g. rhubarb or spinach) should be reduced, while maintaining normal dietary calcium intake to bind oxalate in the gut. Increasing dietary vitamin B_6 intake decreases urinary oxalate.
- **Cystinuria**: treated with urinary alkalinization or dissolution with penicillamine (although side effects limit its use) or captopril.

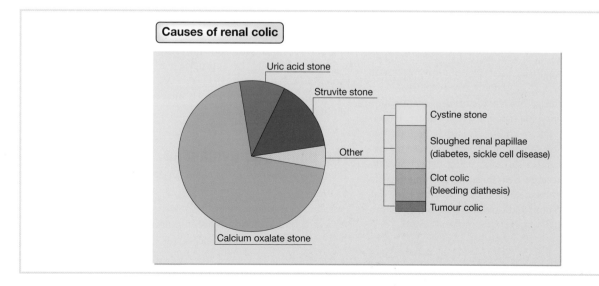

Causes of renal colic

- Uric acid stone
- Struvite stone
- Other
  - Cystine stone
  - Sloughed renal papillae (diabetes, sickle cell disease)
  - Clot colic (bleeding diathesis)
  - Tumour colic
- Calcium oxalate stone

Nephrotic and nephritic syndromes

Normal urinary protein

<150 mg/day

Microalbuminuria

30–300 mg/day
Early sign of diabetic nephropathy

Proteinuria

300 mg–4.5g/day

If >2g/day, + microscopic haematuria or + renal impairment consider renal biopsy

Nephrotic syndrome

>4.5g/ day
Oedema
Hypoalbuminaemia
Renal biopsy usually indicated

Common causes
- Glomerulonephritis
- Diabetes
- Amyloid

Histology in glomerulonephritis associated with the nephrotic syndrome

Normal kidney
Normal electron micrograph of the foot processes of the glomerular endothelial cells; beautiful discrete foot processes are seen on the podocytes

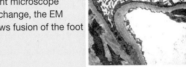

Minimal change disease
Whereas in minimal changes GN, the light microscope shows no change, the EM image shows fusion of the foot processes

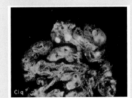

Lupus nephritis
A large number of different histological appearances occur in lupus nephritis – this image shows staining for the C1q component of complement.

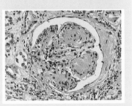

Diabetic glomerular damage
This image shows the characteristic sclerotic lesions found in diabetic glomerular damage. Early on, diabetes leads to glomerular hyperfiltration; later proteinuria and decreases in GFR occur, often culminating in renal failure with the nephrotic syndrome

Cause of proteinuria as related to quantity

Daily protein excretion	Cause
0.15 to 2.0 g	Mild glomerulopathies
	Tubular proteinuria
	Overflow proteinuria
2.0 to 4.0 g	Usually glomerular
>4.0 g	Always glomerular

Features of the nephrotic syndrome

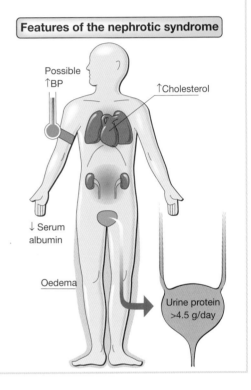

Possible ↑BP

↑Cholesterol

↓ Serum albumin

Oedema

Urine protein >4.5 g/day

Proteinuria and the nephrotic syndrome

The normal amount of protein in urine is <150 mg/day. Most of this is the result of a physiological, rather viscous glycoprotein that is secreted by tubular cells, termed 'Tamm–Horsfall protein'. The presence of higher amounts of protein may indicate significant renal disease, often **glomerulonephritis** (GN). Dipsticks detect mainly albumin and will not detect pathological proteins, such as immunoglobulin light chains (Bence-Jones protein) in myeloma. Microalbuminuria (urinary albumin excretion 30–300 mg/day) is an early sign of **diabetic nephropathy**.

In patients with proteinuria, a careful history and examination should be performed, looking for causes of renal disease. Hypertension, evidence of renal failure and oedema may be found on examination. Renal function should be assessed with serum creatinine and electrolytes, and a 24-hour urine collection performed to determine creatinine clearance and 24-hour protein excretion. A 'spot' urine protein : creatinine ratio correlates well with 24-hour protein excretion, and can be used as a simple estimate of renal protein loss.

If these results confirm significant proteinuria (see Table 145.1) or renal dysfunction, further investigations should include ultrasonography of the renal tract, blood glucose (to exclude diabetes, a common cause of the nephrotic syndrome) and immunological investigations to exclude myeloma and autoimmune conditions such as systemic lupus erythematosus (SLE) or systemic vasculitis (antinuclear factor and antineutrophil cytoplasmic antibody). If significant proteinuria is present (>2g/day) a renal biopsy may be appropriate to define the cause of the proteinuria.

Levels of proteinuria >4.5g in 24 hours may produce the **nephrotic syndrome**.

The nephrotic syndrome

The nephrotic syndrome is characterized by:

- Proteinuria (usually 3–4+ on dipstick testing; 24h urine excretion of protein is often >4g/24h).
- Hypoalbuminaemia (usually albumin <30g/dL).

Medicine at a Glance, Fourth Edition. Edited by Patrick Davey. © 2014 John Wiley & Sons, Ltd. Published 2014 by John Wiley & Sons, Ltd. Companion website: www.ataglanceseries.com/medicine

Table 145.1 Classification of proteinuria.

Type	Pathophysiological features	Cause
Glomerular	Increased glomerular capillary permeability to protein	Primary or secondary glomerulopathy
Tubular	Decreased tubular reabsorption of proteins in glomerular filtrate	Tubular or interstitial disease
Overflow	Increased production of low-molecular-weight proteins	Monoclonal gammopathy, leukaemia

- Peripheral oedema.
- Unlike the nephritic syndrome, haematuria is rare and blood pressure (BP) is normal or only mildly elevated.

Causes

The nephrotic syndrome is usually a consequence of:

- Glomerular disease, commonly GN. The types of GN most commonly found to be responsible for the nephrotic syndrome on renal biopsy are minimal change disease (overwhelmingly the most likely cause for nephrotic syndrome in childhood), membranous nephropathy and focal segmental glomerulosclerosis.
- Diabetes.
- Renal amyloid, which may relate to primary or secondary amyloidosis, or multiple myeloma.
- Drugs (particularly those used in rheumatology, such as non-steroidal anti-inflammatory agents, penicillamine and gold) are occasionally the cause.
- Other causes include SLE.

Complications

Complications of the nephrotic syndrome relate in part to the low albumin, and partly to more complex pathophysiological changes induced by the nephrotic condition:

- **Oedema**: found in dependent sites (i.e. the lower limbs in ambulant patients and the sacral area in bed-bound patients), but can also be found in the face (e.g. periorbitally) and hands.
- **Hypercoagulability**: may lead to renal vein thrombosis and a dramatic worsening of renal function, or may produce deep venous thrombosis. There is no evidence that prophylactic routine anticoagulation in the nephrotic syndrome is indicated.
- **Hypercholesterolaemia**: may play a large role in the accelerated atheroma that may be found in long-standing nephrotic syndrome. The reason why hypercholesterolaemia occurs is not clear; it may relate to hypersynthesis of apolipoproteins, resulting from the general increase in protein synthesis found in many nephrotic patients.

- **Infection**: the nephrotic syndrome is associated with hypogamma-globulinaemia and impairment of the immune system. Infection, which may be overwhelming, can occur, particularly with pneumococci. Immunization against the pneumococcus should be given.

Treatment

Any underlying cause should be fully diagnosed and treated with specific therapy. General management includes the use of diuretics to reduce oedema (although their use must be balanced against the possibility of diuretic-induced hypovolaemia, which itself will worsen renal function) and angiotensin-converting enzyme (ACE) inhibitors may be used to reduce proteinuria and treat hypertension aggressively to slow the progression of renal impairment, particularly in diabetes. Anticoagulation may be instituted for thrombotic episodes and hyperlipidaemia commonly requires treatment. Specific treatment exists for certain types of GN, e.g. minimal change disease commonly responds well to corticosteroids. Unfortunately, some diseases are very resistant to treatment, such as the nephrotic syndrome related to renal amyloid.

The nephritic syndrome

This is an acute renal illness with the following features:

- Haematuria (occasionally macroscopic) and mild proteinuria, i.e. usually only 1–2+ on dipstick testing, which is insufficient to cause a depression in serum albumin, unlike the nephrotic syndrome.
- Inability of the kidney to excrete fluids, leading to fluid retention (oedema), hypertension and occasionally oliguria.
- Decreased glomerular filtration rate (GFR), producing varying degrees of uraemia.

This term was previously more widely used when streptococcal infection was common, because the nephritic syndrome not infrequently followed 2–3 weeks after a throat infection with group A β-haemolytic streptococci. The prognosis of poststreptococcal GN is excellent, the need for dialysis in the acute stage is low, and the likelihood of spontaneous and full recovery of renal function is very high. The differential diagnosis of the nephritic syndrome is wide and includes most of the diseases capable of producing GN (see Chapter 146). Immunological tests and a renal biopsy are usually indicated.

Treatment

It is important to treat any underlying cause with specific therapies. Oedema, hypertension and renal impairment should be treated as for the nephrotic syndrome, although as hypertension is more common and more severe, it should be looked for assiduously and treated aggressively with antihypertensive drugs (often ACE inhibitors). Dialysis is more likely to be needed for uraemia than in the nephrotic syndrome.

146 Glomerulonephritis

Spectrum of presentations of different glomerulonephritides

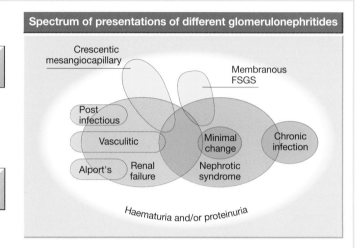

Acute/chronic renal failure

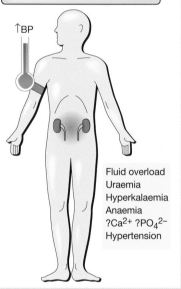

↑BP

Fluid overload
Uraemia
Hyperkalaemia
Anaemia
?Ca^{2+} ?PO$_4$$^{2-}$
Hypertension

Investigations

Creatinine/creatine clearance
FBC
Urine microscopy
Urine dipstick
Urine protein (24-h)
Serum albumin
Anti-GBM
ANCA
ANF
Renal biopsy (provided kidneys not small)
Light microscopy
Electron microscopy
Immunofluorescence
C3 and C4 complement
Antistreptolysin O (ASO) titre
Renal ultrasound
Blood cultures

Classification

Histology

Examples include:

Minimal change
Fusion of glomerular epithelial cell foot process

Membranous
Thickened glomerular basement membrane due to immune complex deposition

Proliferative
Proliferation of cellular elements within Bowman's capsule

Glomerulonephritis (GN) can present in a variety of ways: (i) acute or chronic renal failure; (ii) the nephrotic syndrome (oedema, proteinuria, hypoalbuminaemia); (iii) haematuria; and (iv) proteinuria and hypertension.

It accounts for the cause of renal failure in up to one-third of patients requiring dialysis or transplantation. The cardinal features of glomerular abnormalities are:

- Proteinuria.
- Haematuria.
- Urinary casts.

GN affects both kidneys symmetrically. The disease may affect primarily the kidneys (primary GN) or be associated with systemic illnesses such as Wegener's granulomatosis, systemic lupus erythematosus (SLE) and other vasculitides (secondary GN). The type of GN is usually established by renal biopsy (light microscopy, immunofluorescence, electron microscopy (EM)). The different histological types of GN (see Figure 146.1 above) each have a different spectrum of presentation, and vary in their prognosis and response to treatment.

Acute glomerulonephritis

A confusing aspect of glomerular disease is that many different histological subtypes can produce the same clinical syndrome and, conversely, that each histological form can produce different clinical patterns. It is therefore usual to classify glomerulonephritis in terms of both the clinical syndrome and the pathological diagnosis. The different pathological forms underlying the different clinical syndromes are:

- **Acute renal failure**: GN can underlie acute renal failure, when it is termed 'rapidly progressive GN'. This is usually characterized by the presence of crescents (a crescentic-shaped proliferation of cells in Bowman's capsule) and is most commonly seen with the

Medicine at a Glance, Fourth Edition. Edited by Patrick Davey. © 2014 John Wiley & Sons, Ltd. Published 2014 by John Wiley & Sons, Ltd. Companion website: www.ataglanceseries.com/medicine

GN associated with the vasculitic conditions such as Wegener's granulomatosis, Goodpasture's syndrome (acute renal failure and pulmonary haemorrhage caused by a circulating antiglomerular basement membrane (anti-GBM) antibody) and postinfectious GN after a streptococcal infection. Time is of the essence, because many patients progress from normal renal function to dialysis-dependent renal failure within days, and rapidly progressive GN is therefore a medical emergency. Early aggressive treatment often stabilizes or improves renal function, whereas late (i.e. occurring by the time renal support is needed, or when the patient is oliguric) treatment is usually much less effective.

● **Nephrotic syndrome**: the most common causes of the nephrotic syndrome in adults are shown in Figure 146.2 below.

Renal histology

● **Membranous GN**: the light microscopic appearances are of a thickened basement membrane, which on EM is the result of numerous subepithelial immune complex deposits of IgG and complement C3. Although usually idiopathic, it can be secondary to underlying malignancy in 10% of cases, and can relate to SLE, drugs or infections.

● **Minimal change GN**: light microscope and immunological studies are normal, but podocyte foot processes are fused on EM. Focal segmental glomerulosclerosis (FSGS) is similar, except some glomeruli have segmental sclerotic lesions.

● The renal histology in **incidental haematuria** and/or **proteinuria** varies. The most common finding at renal biopsy is of IgA nephropathy (Berger's disease). Clinically, patients often have marked haematuria after upper respiratory tract infections. Histologically, the condition is characterized by mesangial deposition of IgA with variable segmental mesangial proliferation. Although most patients have a benign prognosis, 20–40% of patients progress to renal failure. IgA nephropathy also occurs in people with long-standing alcohol problems who have liver disease, although rarely is it of clinical importance.

Chronic glomerulonephritis

Patients presenting with chronic renal failure may have small, shrunken kidneys on ultrasonography and chronic fibrotic changes with glomerulosclerosis on biopsy. The disease underlying the renal failure is then presumed to be a GN, particularly if there is a history of previous proteinuria or haematuria. The process is usually burnt out and does not respond to any treatment. Renal biopsy does not usually alter treatment and is contraindicated when small kidneys are found in view of the risks posed by renal biopsy.

Management

Important investigations in a patient with suspected GN include assessment of renal function with serum creatinine and creatinine clearance, urine dipstick and microscopy (examining particularly for red cells and casts), 24-hour urinary protein excretion and renal ultrasonography for renal size. Significant proteinuria (>1 g/day) is strongly suggestive of a GN. Immunological tests are essential in establishing whether the GN is secondary and should include antineutrophil cytoplasmic antibody (ANCA) (Wegener's granulomatosis, microscopic polyangiitis), antinuclear factor (ANF), complement C3 and C4 (SLE), anti-GBM antibodies (Goodpasture's syndrome) and antistreptolysin O (ASO) titre (poststreptococcal GN) (see Chapter 147) and hepatitis B and C serologies. Renal biopsy is necessary to establish an accurate diagnosis; however, this will not usually be undertaken if the kidneys are small.

In GN, aggressive blood pressure treatment can reduce the speed of disease progression, control of lipids is important and nephrotoxic drugs should be avoided.

The **treatment** of GN depends on the precise type:

● **Minimal change GN**: corticosteroid treatment can often produce remission. Half of adult patients relapse once after initial remission; a second course of steroids is then indicated. Further relapses or failure to induce remission are indications for more aggressive immunosuppression.

● **Membranous GN**: the prognosis is variable. At 10 years, 25% have remitted spontaneously, 25% have persistent non-nephrotic proteinuria, 25% have nephrotic proteinuria and 25% have renal failure. In those with deteriorating renal function, regimens including steroids and cyclophosphamide, ciclosporin or rituximab may be beneficial. Drug-induced membranous GN may remit after drug cessation.

● **Rapidly progressive GN**: more aggressive immunosuppressive regimens are commonly advocated and include corticosteroids, cyclophosphamide and plasmapheresis.

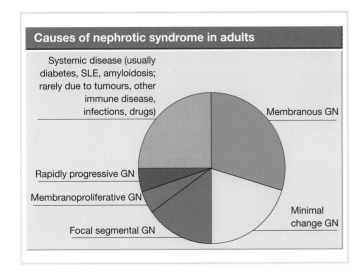

Causes of nephrotic syndrome in adults

Systemic disease (usually diabetes, SLE, amyloidosis; rarely due to tumours, other immune disease, infections, drugs)

Membranous GN

Rapidly progressive GN

Membranoproliferative GN

Focal segmental GN

Minimal change GN

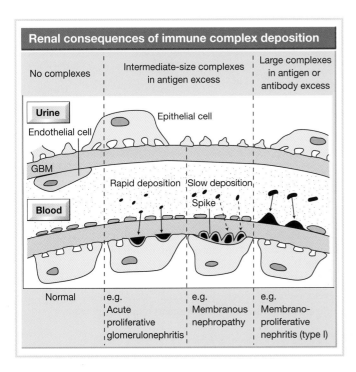

Renal consequences of immune complex deposition

| No complexes | Intermediate-size complexes in antigen excess | Large complexes in antigen or antibody excess |

Urine — Epithelial cell

Endothelial cell

GBM

Rapid deposition | Slow deposition

Spike

Blood

Normal | e.g. Acute proliferative glomerulonephritis | e.g. Membranous nephropathy | e.g. Membranoproliferative nephritis (type I)

147 Renal involvement in systemic disease

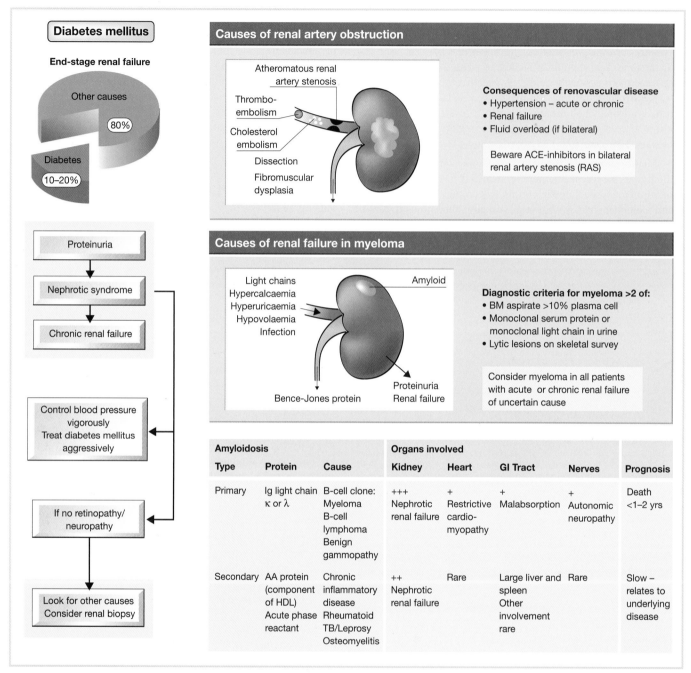

Diabetes mellitus

End-stage renal failure

Other causes 80%

Diabetes 10–20%

Proteinuria → Nephrotic syndrome → Chronic renal failure

Control blood pressure vigorously
Treat diabetes mellitus aggressively

If no retinopathy/ neuropathy

Look for other causes
Consider renal biopsy

Causes of renal artery obstruction

Atheromatous renal artery stenosis
Thrombo-embolism
Cholesterol embolism
Dissection
Fibromuscular dysplasia

Consequences of renovascular disease
• Hypertension – acute or chronic
• Renal failure
• Fluid overload (if bilateral)

Beware ACE-inhibitors in bilateral renal artery stenosis (RAS)

Causes of renal failure in myeloma

Light chains
Hypercalcaemia
Hyperuricaemia
Hypovolaemia
Infection

Amyloid

Bence-Jones protein

Proteinuria
Renal failure

Diagnostic criteria for myeloma >2 of:
• BM aspirate >10% plasma cell
• Monoclonal serum protein or monoclonal light chain in urine
• Lytic lesions on skeletal survey

Consider myeloma in all patients with acute or chronic renal failure of uncertain cause

Amyloidosis

Type	Protein	Cause	Organs involved				Prognosis
			Kidney	Heart	GI Tract	Nerves	
Primary	Ig light chain κ or λ	B-cell clone: Myeloma B-cell lymphoma Benign gammopathy	+++ Nephrotic renal failure	+ Restrictive cardio-myopathy	+ Malabsorption	+ Autonomic neuropathy	Death <1–2 yrs
Secondary	AA protein (component of HDL) Acute phase reactant	Chronic inflammatory disease Rheumatoid TB/Leprosy Osteomyelitis	++ Nephrotic renal failure	Rare	Large liver and spleen Other involvement rare	Rare	Slow – relates to underlying disease

Diabetes mellitus

Diabetes mellitus causes renal disease; the incidence increases with longer duration of disease, with 30% having nephropathy 20 years after diagnosis. It accounts for 20% of patients on renal replacement therapy. The initial diabetic renal lesion is manifest as microalbuminuria, which progresses to increasing levels of proteinuria or even the nephrotic syndrome. There may be a gradual loss of excretory function manifest as rising creatinine and urea. Patients with diabetic nephropathy commonly suffer from diabetic retinopathy or neuropathy. If absent, this should prompt a search for alternative causes of renal impairment or nephrotic syndrome. If doubt remains about whether the renal dysfunction is attributable to diabetes, a renal biopsy should be performed.

In diabetes, very aggressive blood pressure lowering, often with angiotensin-converting enzyme (ACE) inhibitors and/or angiotensin II receptor blockers, can slow the progression of the renal disease. Similarly, excellent glycaemic control may reduce the development and progression of renal disease. Smoking cessation, control of lipids and antiplatelet agents may be important.

Medicine at a Glance, Fourth Edition. Edited by Patrick Davey. © 2014 John Wiley & Sons, Ltd. Published 2014 by John Wiley & Sons, Ltd. Companion website: www.ataglanceseries.com/medicine

Myeloma

Myeloma commonly produces renal impairment. In patients with acute or chronic renal impairment of unknown cause, myeloma should be considered in the differential diagnosis and protein electrophoresis (for paraproteinaemia), urine electrophoresis (for Bence-Jones proteins) and immunoglobulin estimations undertaken. Renal impairment in myeloma has several causes, including the direct toxicity of immunoglobulin light chains to the tubular cells, hypercalcaemia, dehydration, hyperuricaemia, renal amyloid, hyperviscosity and infection. Treatment involves that of the underlying myeloma and rapid correction of hypovolaemia and hypercalcaemia. Plasma exchange has a role in rapidly removing myeloma protein in some patients with renal failure, and treatment of the underlying myeloma with newer agents such as bortezomib and lenalidomide, may improve the chances of renal recovery.

Amyloidosis

Amyloidosis is characterized by the deposition of protein fibrils in many organs, including the kidney. It may be primary in association with myeloma (amyloid AL) or secondary to chronic infections or inflammation or have a hereditary cause (amyloid AA). The most common renal presentation is with proteinuria, often sufficient to produce the nephrotic syndrome. Renal biopsy demonstrates an eosinophilic tissue infiltration that stains positive with Congo red and exhibits green birefringence under polarized light. The prognosis for renal function is usually poor.

Haemolytic uraemic syndrome

Haemolytic uraemic syndrome (HUS) is characterized by haemolysis, platelet consumption and acute renal failure. It may be associated with diarrhoea, particularly in children, when *Escherichia coli* serotype O157 produces verocytotoxin which causes endothelial damage. Atypical HUS may occur in patients with inherited or acquired deficiencies of complement regulatory proteins such as factor H. Investigations reveal haemolysis, thrombocytopenia and renal failure. Renal biopsy shows fibrin thrombi occluding glomerular tufts. In diarrhoea-associated disease, spontaneous remission is common, but in severe forms plasmapheresis is often advocated. There may be benefit from the anti-C5a antibody, ecluzimab.

Renovascular disease

There are two pathologies causing renovascular disease:

1 Atherosclerotic renal artery stenosis: this presents with hypertension, renal impairment or, if bilateral, fluid overload manifesting as pulmonary oedema. A renal bruit may rarely be audible and renal ultrasonography may show small or asymmetrical kidneys. Renal angiography or magnetic resonance angiography can demonstrate the stenosis. Cardiovascular risk factors should be treated. Angioplasty and/or stenting has no definite benefit on subsequent renal function and hypertension; they are usually reserved for patients with resistant hypertension or deteriorating renal function. Obstruction of renal blood flow can also occur with embolism of the renal arteries or renal artery dissection, and classically presents with loin pain and impairment of renal function. Atherosclerosis of intrarenal vessels may occur with or without renal artery stenosis and contributes to renal impairment and hypertension.

2 Fibromuscular dysplasia: produces a beaded appearance of the renal artery on angiography, occurs more commonly in younger females and is an important cause of hypertension.

Renal vasculitis

The UK prevalence of systemic vasculitis affecting the kidney is 10 000 (see Table 147.1). Vasculitis is a difficult disease to diagnose because of its ability to affect many parts of the body. It should be considered in patients with unexplained renal failure, rash, fever, weight loss and upper and lower repiratory symptoms.

Wegener's granulomatosis

This rare condition (600 new cases/year in the UK) is characterized by granulomatous disease of the upper airway (including nose, sinuses, trachea) and lung, and renal impairment resulting from a focal necrotizing glomerulonephritis (GN). It is part of the differential diagnosis in patients with upper airway disease, lung

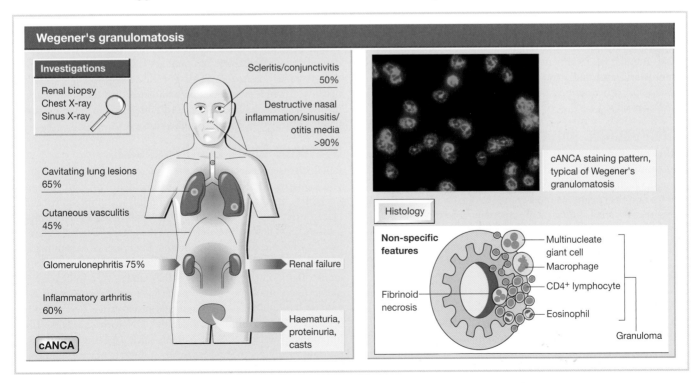

Wegener's granulomatosis

Investigations
- Renal biopsy
- Chest X-ray
- Sinus X-ray

Scleritis/conjunctivitis 50%

Destructive nasal inflammation/sinusitis/otitis media >90%

Cavitating lung lesions 65%

Cutaneous vasculitis 45%

Glomerulonephritis 75% → Renal failure

Inflammatory arthritis 60%

→ Haematuria, proteinuria, casts

cANCA

cANCA staining pattern, typical of Wegener's granulomatosis

Histology

Non-specific features
- Fibrinoid necrosis
- Multinucleate giant cell
- Macrophage
- CD4+ lymphocyte
- Eosinophil
- Granuloma

Table 147.1 Renal vasculitis.

| | Incidence | F:M | Organ involvement | | | | | | Diagnostic test | Treatment |
			Kidney	Lung	Heart	Skin	URT/ sinus	GI tract		
Goodpasture's syndrome	±	1:1	+++	+++	0	0	0	0	GBM antibody	St, CyP, PE
Microscopic polyarteritis	+	1:1	+++	+	0	+	0	+	pANCA (MPO)	St, CyP, PE
Churg–Strauss syndrome	±	1:1	++	+++	++	++	++	0	Eosinophils/ CXR	St
Henoch–Schönlein purpura	+++	1:2	+	0	0	+++	0	++	None	None
Wegener's granulomatosis	+(+)	1:2	+++	++	0	0	+++	0	cANCA (PR3)	St, CyP, PE
SLE	++	9:1	++	+	+	++	+	+	Anti-dsDNA	St, AM, CyP
Scleroderma	++	4:1	+	++	+	+++	0	+++	ANA, Scl-70	ACE inhibitors, none
Cryoglobulinaemia	+	1:1	++	0	0	+++	0	0	See text	St, PE

ACE, angiotensin-converting enzyme; AM, antimalarials (chloroquine); ANA, antinuclear antibodies; ANCA, antineutrophil cytoplasmic antibodies; CyP, cyclophosphamide; CXR, chest X-ray; GI, gastrointestinal; GBM, glomerular basement membrane; MPO, myeloperoxidase; PE, plasma exchange; PR3, proteinase 3; SLE, systemic lupus erythematosus; St, corticosteroids; URT, upper respiratory tract.

masses or rapidly progressive GN. If suspected, an antineutrophil cytoplasmic antibody (ANCA) test should be performed, where the pattern of staining of the cytoplasmic components of neutrophils after applying serum IgG antibodies is studied. Two patterns of staining are found: one where staining is principally cytoplasmic (cANCA – the antigen is principally proteinase-3) and the other where staining is principally perinuclear (pANCA – the antigen is predominantly myeloperoxidase) and can be confirmed with specific enzyme-linked immunosorbent assay (ELISA). pANCA is found in microscopic polyangiitis and cANCA is positive in over 90% of cases of Wegener's granulomatosis, in which its titre can reflect disease activity. A renal biopsy shows a focal necrotizing GN, sometimes with crescent formation and granuloma. Treatment should be prompt because patients can deteriorate rapidly and involves aggressive immunosuppression with corticosteroids, cyclophosphamide (or rituximab) and plasmapheresis.

Microscopic polyangiitis

This rare vasculitis (400 new cases/year in the UK) produces inflammation of the small blood vessels and can present with multisystem or single-organ involvement. The kidneys, skin, brain and nerves are the most common organs affected. Rapidly progressive renal impairment can result. Testing for ANCA usually reveals a positive staining with a perinuclear pattern (pANCA). Treatment is as for Wegener's granulomatosis.

Goodpasture's syndrome

Very rare (50 new cases/year in the UK). This syndrome is characterized by pulmonary haemorrhage (which is more common in people who smoke), haematuria and rapidly progressive renal failure. It is caused by an autoantibody directed against a collagen found only in basement membrane – the antiglomerular basement membrane (anti-GBM) antibody. The antibody can be

detected in blood. Renal biopsies demonstrate a crescentic GN with linear antibody staining along the GBM on immunofluorescence. Lung function tests may reveal an elevated carbon monoxide transfer factor (Kco), consistent with pulmonary haemorrhage because haemoglobin binds CO very avidly. Treatment is with plasmapheresis to remove the antibody, and immunosuppression with corticosteroids ± cyclophosphamide to reduce its production.

Polyarteritis nodosa

This vasculitis (incidence: 150 cases/year in the UK) affects larger blood vessels and presents with non-specific symptoms such as weight loss, fever, malaise and abdominal pain. Arteriography demonstrates microaneurysms and arterial narrowing, and biopsies of affected tissue may be diagnostic. ANCA tests are usually negative. There is an association with hepatitis B infection. Renal involvement causes haematuria and proteinuria or renal impairment. Treatment is immunosuppression.

Systemic lupus erythematosus

Renal disease occurs in half the patients with systemic lupus erythematosus (SLE), with an annual incidence of 3000 patients in the UK. Involvement ranges from mild, with proteinuria and haematuria, to severe, with nephrotic syndrome or rapidly progressive renal failure. In determining the nature of renal involvement, urine microscopy is important. The presence of significant haematuria, proteinuria or red cell casts implies a significant glomerular lesion. Renal biopsy is then undertaken to define the glomerular pathology. Several patterns of renal involvement are seen including a focal and segmental proliferative GN, a membranous GN or a diffuse proliferative GN with crescents. The immunology varies: 90% of patients have a positive ANA test (i.e. IgG staining of the nucleus, often of discrete nuclear or nucleolar elements). Although antibodies to double-stranded DNA

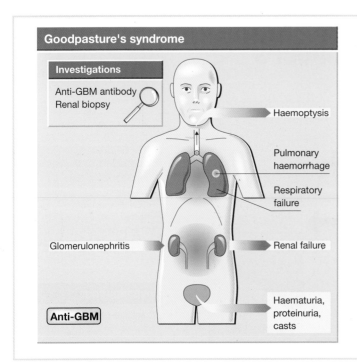

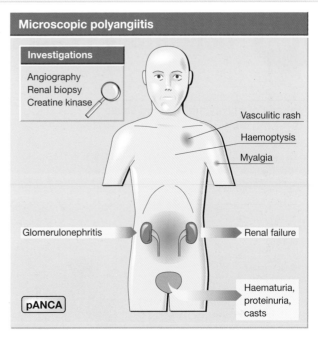

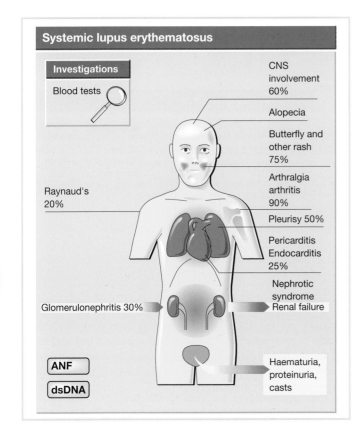

(anti-dsDNA antibodies) are highly specific for SLE, in renal disease their titre may paradoxically be depressed. Some 40% have antibodies to extractable nuclear antigens (such as Smith Sm or Ro–SS-A). Antibodies to platelets, red cells and phospholipid are also common. There is often complement consumption with lowered levels of C3 and C4. The erythrocyte sedimentation rate (but not the C-reactive protein) is elevated. Treatment depends on histology but often involves corticosteroids and immunosuppressive agents such as cyclophosphamide, mycophenolate and azathioprine.

Henoch–Schönlein purpura

Although common in children, Henoch–Schönlein purpura is rare in adults (<300 new cases/year in the UK). The aetiology is not known, but it may reflect an autoimmune response to an infective agent, which in part explains the seasonal variation and that one-third have a preceding upper respiratory tract infection. Malaise, arthralgia, abdominal pain and, most typically, a purpuric rash on the extensor surfaces (elbows, buttocks, knees) characterize the illness. Renal involvement consists of a usually self-limiting focal GN. Occasionally progressive renal failure occurs.

Scleroderma

Renal involvement complicates 25% of scleroderma, occurs early or late on in the course of the disease, and accounts for 40% of deaths. Incidence is about 200 new cases/year. It may present as an active sediment (i.e. haematuria, sometimes severe enough to produce 'red cell casts') or ominously as a 'scleroderma renal crisis', with treatment-resistant hypertension, rapidly progressive uraemia and a characteristic 'onion skin' appearance of blood vessels on renal histology. Immunological tests show antibodies to Scl-70 (the enzyme topoisomerase I) and often to RNA polymerases 1–3. Anticentromere antibodies are associated with mild cutaneous disease. ACE inhibitor therapy may help.

Cryoglobulinaemia

Cryoglobulins are abnormal immunoglobulins that precipitate when cooled. Blood must be transported to the laboratory at 37°C for testing of the presence of a cryoglobulin. If cooling occurs in superficial blood vessels, then obstruction of the vessel and tissue necrosis may occur. Type I cryoglobulins are monoclonal proteins, and found in association with myeloma, Waldenstrom's macroglobulinaemia and lymphoma. Type II cryoglobulins comprise a monoclonal component that has rheumatoid factor activity and binds to normal immunoglobulins. These are found in chronic infections such as hepatitis C and bacterial endocarditis, as well as connective tissue disease and myeloma or lymphoma. Type III cryoglobulins are polyclonal with rheumatoid factor activity and are usually associated with SLE and rheumatoid arthritis.

148 Hereditary renal disorders

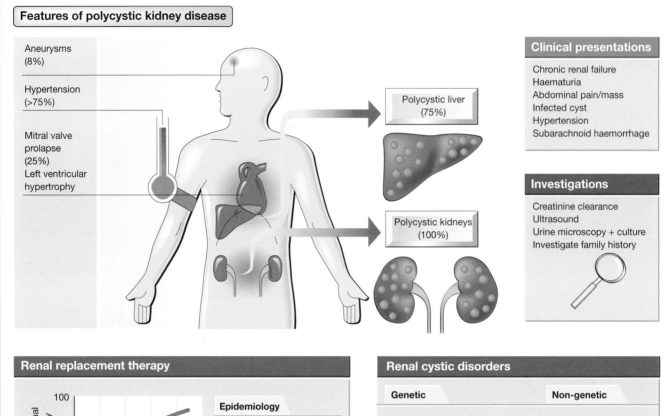

Features of polycystic kidney disease

Aneurysms (8%)

Hypertension (>75%)

Mitral valve prolapse (25%)
Left ventricular hypertrophy

Polycystic liver (75%)

Polycystic kidneys (100%)

Clinical presentations

Chronic renal failure
Haematuria
Abdominal pain/mass
Infected cyst
Hypertension
Subarachnoid haemorrhage

Investigations

Creatinine clearance
Ultrasound
Urine microscopy + culture
Investigate family history

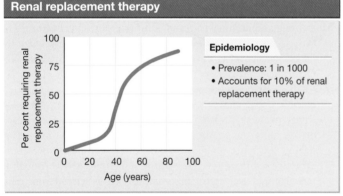

Renal replacement therapy

Epidemiology

- Prevalence: 1 in 1000
- Accounts for 10% of renal replacement therapy

Renal cystic disorders

Genetic	Non-genetic
Autosomal dominant	Medullary sponge kidney
Polycystic kidney disease (ADPKD)	Simple cysts
Von Hippel–Lindau disease	Acquired cystic disease
Tuberous sclerosis	
Autosomal recessive	
Polycystic kidney disease (ARPKD)	

Autosomal dominant polycystic kidney disease

A variety of inherited conditions affect the kidney, but adult polycystic kidney disease (APKD) is by far the most common, affecting one in 1000 individuals and accounting for 8–10% of patients with end-stage renal disease. It usually presents in adult life (the rarer autosomal recessive form presents in infancy). Inheritance is autosomal dominant so children of an affected parent have a 50% chance of inheriting the condition. About 25% of cases are the result of spontaneous mutation. The genetic defect is on chromosome 16 (*PKD1*, which accounts for 95% of cases) or more rarely on chromosome 4 (*PKD2*).

The condition is characterized by a progressive appearance and enlargement of renal cysts. These may bleed, producing haematuria and loin pain, or may become infected. As the cysts gradually enlarge, there is a slowly progressive and inexorable decline in renal function. Patients may also present with abdominal masses, hypertension and chronic renal failure, and subarachnoid haemorrhages occur in some 10% as a result of the associated berry aneurysms that affect intracranial arteries. Polycystic kidneys may be found incidentally on ultrasonography during investigations for other indications. Cysts also occur in the liver, pancreas, spleen and ovaries, although these rarely cause clinical problems.

Investigations

The condition is usually suspected from the clinical features and family history and confirmed with ultrasonography or computed tomography (CT). Renal function should be determined with serum creatinine and creatinine clearance, and urinary infection excluded.

Medicine at a Glance, Fourth Edition. Edited by Patrick Davey. © 2014 John Wiley & Sons, Ltd. Published 2014 by John Wiley & Sons, Ltd. Companion website: www.ataglanceseries.com/medicine

There are no specific treatments to slow the disease progression – as usual it is important to control any hypertension. Infections require appropriate antibiotic treatment and pain caused by haemorrhage may require analgesia. As renal failure progresses, renal replacement therapy with dialysis or transplantation is required, at a mean age in *PKD1* of 55–60 years. Sometimes nephrectomy is required to permit space so that peritoneal dialysis or transplantation can be undertaken. Genetic counselling is important and screening of children of affected individuals should be delayed until cysts are identifiable on ultrasonography – usually >18 years unless there is renal impairment or hypertension.

Simple cysts

These become increasingly common with age and can be detected in >12% of individuals aged over 50 years. They are usually asymptomatic and are detected incidentally. It is important to distinguish them from the multiple cysts of APKD, other cystic diseases and renal cell carcinoma. On ultrasonography simple cysts have smooth walls and no intracystic debris. If doubt exists then CT scanning is necessary.

Other inherited disorders affecting the kidney

Alport's syndrome

This syndrome is characterized by haematuria, sensorineural deafness (overt in 40%) and progressive renal impairment with proteinuria in most and ocular abnormalities in 15%. It is caused by mutations in the basement membrane type IV collagen gene (most commonly) *COL4A5*; 20% are the result of new mutations. It is X-linked in 80% of patients, producing a more severe phenotype in males. The diagnosis is confirmed on renal biopsy, where thickening and splitting of the glomerular basement membrane on electron microscopy is found. End-stage renal failure (i.e. disease requiring dialysis) develops usually between 16 and 35 years of age in virtually all affected males with X-linked Alport's syndrome, and males and females with the autosomally inherited form. Transplantation, although not contraindicated, can rarely result in a Goodpasture's disease-like syndrome caused by the immunological reaction to the previously 'unseen' type IV collagen in the transplanted kidney.

Medullary sponge kidney

This condition, which is often inherited, is characterized by dilated medullary collecting ducts and can affect both, one or part of one kidney. It is often asymptomatic, but small calculi can form which may produce haematuria and predispose to urinary tract infection, or larger calculi may produce obstruction. Renal failure is unusual. The diagnosis is established by an intravenous urogram, which shows a typical blush-like opacity in the medulla corresponding to accumulation of contrast in the dilated collecting ducts.

Tuberous sclerosis

In this rare (1–2/100 000), autosomal dominant condition, tumour-like malformations called hamartomas develop in the central nervous system (often causing learning disorders and epilepsy) and produce skin lesions including facial angiofibromas and hypomelanotic macules. The kidneys can develop angiomyolipomas, cysts and renal malignancies.

Von Hippel–Lindau syndrome

This is a very rare, autosomal dominantly inherited condition characterized by tumours affecting the kidney (renal cell carcinoma), brain (haemangioblastomas) and adrenals (phaeochromocytoma). Occasionally bilateral nephrectomy for tumours leads to the patient requiring dialysis. Mutations in the von Hippel–Lindau gene are also commonly found in cells from patients with sporadic renal cell carcinomas.

Anderson–Fabry disease

This X-linked recessive disorder is the result of mutations in the gene encoding α-galactosidase A. Anderson–Fabry disease results in the intracellular accumulation of glycosphingolipids, which leads to progressive renal failure, autonomic dysfunction and skin lesions called angiokeratomas (dark-red macules or papules). Diagnosis is confirmed by the demonstration of reduced urinary α-galactosidase A. It occurs in two forms: typical Anderson–Fabry disease, where there is no α-galactosidase A activity, and atypical Anderson–Fabry disease, where there is some, albeit greatly reduced, α-galactosidase A activity. Patients with typical Anderson–Fabry disease develop symptoms when very young, in many organs, whereas patients with atypical Anderson–Fabry disease develop symptoms later, typically only affecting the heart.

Typical Anderson–Fabry disease

This affects about 1200 patients in the UK. The first symptoms usually occur around the age of 10 years; unfortunately, they are often ignored or misdiagnosed, and in the typical patient the actual diagnosis of Anderson–Fabry disease is not made until 18 years later. Patients can, however, present at any age: symptoms in children include pain (especially of the hands and feet) and painful crises (often starting in the hands and feet, spreading to other parts of the body, lasting minutes to days), angiokeratomas, peripheral vasospasm and ophthalmological abnormalities. Later on (age 10–30 years) the following can occur: renal dysfunction, fever, reduced sweating, heat sensitivity, exercise intolerance, diarrhoea and abdominal pain, and an increase in angiokeratomas. In later adulthood (age >30 years) the following can occur:

- Heart disease.
- Impaired renal function.
- Stroke or transient ischaemic episodes.
- Epilepsy.

Atypical Anderson–Fabry disease

This affects many thousands in the UK (maybe 6000–10 000). Atypical Anderson–Fabry disease usually presents in adulthood (20–70 years). It is increasingly recognized, and by far the commonest manifestation is left ventricular (LV) hypertrophy. Typically, the heart is the only organ affected. Atypical Anderson–Fabry disease should be considered in all with unexplained LV hypertrophy, especially if LV outflow tract gradient is present. Indeed, atypical Anderson–Fabry disease may account for some 3% of all cases of LV hypertrophy (and a higher percentage in those suspected of having hypertrophic cardiomyopathy). Electrocardiogram evidence of LV hypertrophy (sometimes with pre-excitation) is usually present and is confirmed by cardiac ultrasound. Some (1–30%) α-galactosidase A activity is found.

Treatment

To treat, consider α-galactosidase A enzyme replacement therapy.

149 Tubulointerstitial disease

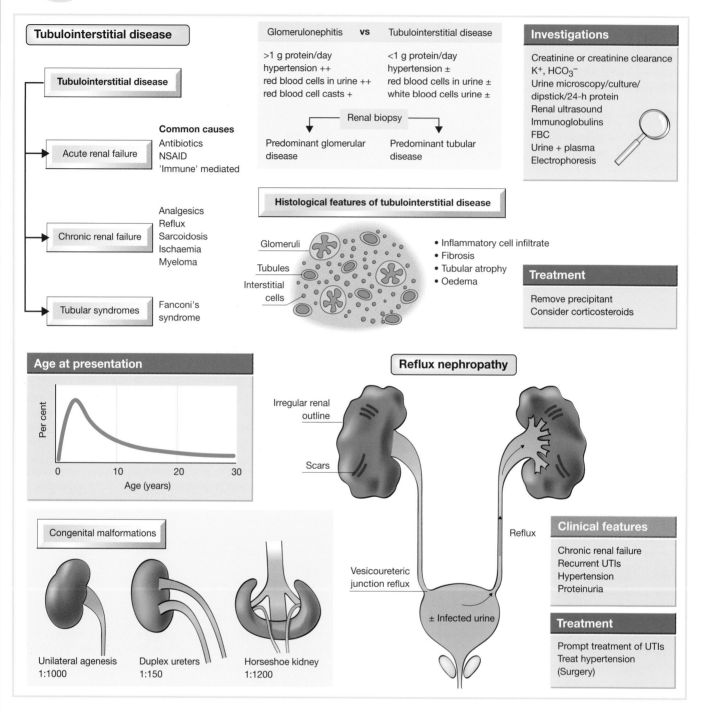

Tubulointerstitial disease

Tubulointerstitial disease

Acute renal failure
- Antibiotics
- NSAID
- 'Immune' mediated

Chronic renal failure
- Analgesics
- Reflux
- Sarcoidosis
- Ischaemia
- Myeloma

Tubular syndromes
- Fanconi's syndrome

Glomerulonephitis	**vs**	Tubulointerstitial disease
>1 g protein/day hypertension ++ red blood cells in urine ++ red blood cell casts +		<1 g protein/day hypertension ± red blood cells in urine ± white blood cells urine ±

Renal biopsy

Predominant glomerular disease → Predominant tubular disease

Histological features of tubulointerstitial disease

- Glomeruli
- Tubules
- Interstitial cells

- Inflammatory cell infiltrate
- Fibrosis
- Tubular atrophy
- Oedema

Investigations

Creatinine or creatinine clearance
K^+, HCO_3^-
Urine microscopy/culture/dipstick/24-h protein
Renal ultrasound
Immunoglobulins
FBC
Urine + plasma
Electrophoresis

Treatment

Remove precipitant
Consider corticosteroids

Age at presentation

Per cent

Age (years)

Congenital malformations

Unilateral agenesis
1:1000

Duplex ureters
1:150

Horseshoe kidney
1:1200

Reflux nephropathy

Irregular renal outline

Scars

Vesicoureteric junction reflux

Reflux

± Infected urine

Clinical features

Chronic renal failure
Recurrent UTIs
Hypertension
Proteinuria

Treatment

Prompt treatment of UTIs
Treat hypertension
(Surgery)

Diseases affecting the renal interstitium and tubules can present with renal impairment, proteinuria, haematuria or tubular syndromes and, in some, prominent abnormalities in electrolyte balance. The most common of these conditions is interstitial nephritis which, in its chronic form, accounts for up to 15% of end-stage renal failure and in its acute form is a common cause of acute renal failure.

Acute interstitial nephritis

Acute inflammation of the renal interstitium is a common consequence of drug hypersensitivity, particularly to antibiotics and non-steroidal anti-inflammatory drugs (NSAIDs). Some 30% of those with drug-induced acute interstitial nephritis have fever, rash and eosinophilia. Acute interstitial nephritis may also relate to infection (leptospirosis, cytomegalovirus, hantavirus). It can also occur in conjunction with other illnesses such as Sjögren's disease or with uveitis (tubulointerstitial nephritis and uveitis or 'TINU syndrome').

Cholesterol emboli

Cholesterol emboli can produce renal failure, and result when an atheromatous plaque in the aorta ruptures, either spontaneously (in elderly people) or after angiography, with systemic emboli resulting in fever, myalgia, skin rash, livedo reticularis, retinal emboli (amaurosis fugax), high white blood cell count and C-reactive protein, and a variable decline in renal function.

Chronic interstitial nephritis and chronic pyelonephritis

Chronic interstitial nephritis may present more insidiously with a progressive decline in renal function, small kidneys on ultrasonography, severe electrolyte disturbance and, in a minority, a salt-losing nephropathy leading to sodium depletion and hypotension. Causes include:

- **Analgesics**: analgesic nephropathy used to be a very common cause of chronic renal failure though its incidence has declined with the withdrawal of phenacetin-containing analgesics. It is four times more common in women than in men. Features include polyuria, mild proteinuria, insidious progressive renal failure, and hypertension (in 60% of cases), often complicated by renal papillary necrosis and renal colic.
- **Reflux nephropathy** and **obstructive uropathy**, either of which may be complicated by infection. When chronic interstitial nephritis results primarily from chronic infection, it is termed 'chronic pyelonephritis'.
- **Primary glomerular disease**.
- **Other causes** (in 15%) include sarcoidosis, ischaemia, hyperuricaemia, myeloma and chronic hypokalaemia. Long-standing hypercalcaemia produces chronic interstitial inflammation, possibly related to calcium salt deposition. Medullary sponge kidney and hyperoxaluria (genetic, high ascorbic acid consumption, long-standing gastrointestinal disease) also occur.
- **Chronic poisoning with heavy metals** (lead, cadmium, mercury): common in industrial workers, especially in certain developing countries, and in Chinese herbs (aristolochic acid), which are often found in over-the-counter herbal preparations.

Features that can help distinguish glomerulonephritis from tubulointerstitial disease are that, in glomerulonephritis, there is usually >1 g of proteinuria/day, hypertension is more common, red blood cells and casts are found in the urine and, in the renal biopsy (which is the diagnostic test), the glomeruli are primarily affected.

Isolated/specific tubular defects

Other rare disorders exist in which there are specific tubular defects, including distal tubular syndromes such as nephrogenic diabetes insipidus and proximal tubular syndromes (Fanconi's defects) which are often congenital, such as renal tubular acidoses. There may be other tubular defects associated with Fanconi's syndrome resulting in aminoaciduria, glycosuria, phosphaturia and bicarbonaturia.

Investigations and treatment

In investigating the patient in whom interstitial nephritis is suspected, important investigations include examining for peripheral blood eosinophilia (which when present may suggest a drug allergy), immunoglobulins, urine and plasma electrophoresis to exclude myeloma, urine microscopy and culture, renal ultrasonography and renal biopsy.

Treatment consists of removing the precipitating cause. There is no effective treatment for many forms of interstitial nephritis but in others corticosteroids can produce important responses. Spontaneous improvement of interstitial nephritis does occur.

Reflux nephropathy

The vesicoureteric junction normally prevents reflux of urine up the ureter; congenital incompetence at this junction can lead to renal damage. 'Reflux nephropathy' is the term given to the scarred and shrunken kidney with chronic tubulointerstitial nephritis that results. This can present during childhood with urinary tract infection (UTI), hypertension, proteinuria or renal failure. For unknown reasons, it is more common in females. UTI is important in the genesis of damage by the refluxing urine.

Investigations

Renal function should be assessed, proteinuria quantified and urine culture performed to exclude active infection. Intravenous urograms (IVUs) characteristically show an irregular renal outline with clubbed calyces, and kidney size is often reduced. A micturating cystogram can demonstrate vesicoureteric reflux whereas DMSA ([^{99m}Tc] mercaptosuccinic acid) scanning can reveal scars. A renal biopsy is not usually appropriate but would show chronic tubulointerstitial nephritis.

Treatment

Any acute UTI should be treated promptly, although in some individuals there may be a role for prophylactic antibiotics. Any associated hypertension should be treated aggressively, asymptomatic infection should be looked for and renal function carefully monitored. The role of surgical ureteric reimplantation to prevent reflux is controversial. There is a strong familial predisposition to reflux and it may be sought in family members.

If there has been substantial scarring, progressive renal failure may develop. However, if renal function is normal during adolescence, the development of renal failure in adulthood is unusual.

Other congenital malformations of the urinary tract

Congenital malformations may affect the kidney, ureter or bladder:

- **Kidney**: unilateral renal agenesis occurs in 1:1000 of the population and is not normally associated with renal impairment. Horseshoe kidneys are fused at their lower pole and are found in 1:1200 individuals and sometimes present with reflux or obstruction.
- **Ureters**: duplex ureters are the most common congenital malformation of the renal tract, occurring in 1:150 individuals, but they rarely cause clinical problems. Pelviureteric junction obstruction is a common cause of urinary tract obstruction in children and young adults. There may be hyperplasia of the smooth muscle of the renal pelvis. It may present with loin pain after high fluid intake or even with hydronephrosis. An IVU may suggest the diagnosis and surgical treatment may be necessary.
- **Bladder**: congenital disorders of the bladder include a neuropathic bladder, prune-belly syndrome (abdominal muscle agenesis, undescended testes and urinary tract malformations, including renal dysplasia and bladder dilatation) and posterior urethral valves.

150 Acute renal failure

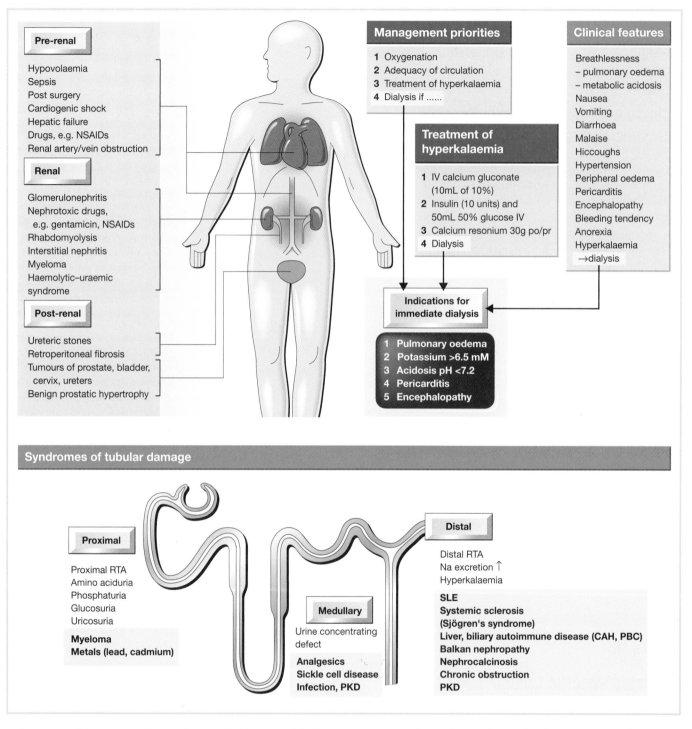

Pre-renal

Hypovolaemia
Sepsis
Post surgery
Cardiogenic shock
Hepatic failure
Drugs, e.g. NSAIDs
Renal artery/vein obstruction

Renal

Glomerulonephritis
Nephrotoxic drugs,
  e.g. gentamicin, NSAIDs
Rhabdomyolysis
Interstitial nephritis
Myeloma
Haemolytic–uraemic
syndrome

Post-renal

Ureteric stones
Retroperitoneal fibrosis
Tumours of prostate, bladder,
  cervix, ureters
Benign prostatic hypertrophy

Management priorities

1 Oxygenation
2 Adequacy of circulation
3 Treatment of hyperkalaemia
4 Dialysis if ......

Treatment of hyperkalaemia

1 IV calcium gluconate
  (10mL of 10%)
2 Insulin (10 units) and
  50mL 50% glucose IV
3 Calcium resonium 30g po/pr
4 Dialysis

Clinical features

Breathlessness
– pulmonary oedema
– metabolic acidosis
Nausea
Vomiting
Diarrhoea
Malaise
Hiccoughs
Hypertension
Peripheral oedema
Pericarditis
Encephalopathy
Bleeding tendency
Anorexia
Hyperkalaemia
→dialysis

Indications for immediate dialysis

1 **Pulmonary oedema**
2 **Potassium >6.5 mM**
3 **Acidosis pH <7.2**
4 **Pericarditis**
5 **Encephalopathy**

Syndromes of tubular damage

Proximal

Proximal RTA
Amino aciduria
Phosphaturia
Glucosuria
Uricosuria

Myeloma
Metals (lead, cadmium)

Medullary

Urine concentrating
defect

Analgesics
Sickle cell disease
Infection, PKD

Distal

Distal RTA
Na excretion ↑
Hyperkalaemia

SLE
Systemic sclerosis
(Sjögren's syndrome)
Liver, biliary autoimmune disease (CAH, PBC)
Balkan nephropathy
Nephrocalcinosis
Chronic obstruction
PKD

Acute renal failure is a syndrome characterized by a rapid decline in glomerular filtration rate over days to weeks with the accumulation of nitrogenous waste and failure to correctly regulate extracellular volume and electrolytes. It is often recognized by a rapidly rising serum urea and creatinine. It may be accompanied by reduced urine output. The symptoms of acute renal failure include those of the precipitating aetiology (e.g. shock or sepsis) and those resulting from renal failure itself, including fluid overload,

nausea, malaise and encephalopathy. The annual incidence of acute renal failure in developed countries is 180 cases/million. The causes of renal failure are conventionally divided into pre-renal, renal and post-renal.

Pre-renal causes

The kidneys need an adequate perfusion pressure for normal function. This depends on the systemic blood pressure (BP) being

Medicine at a Glance, Fourth Edition. Edited by Patrick Davey. © 2014 John Wiley & Sons, Ltd. Published 2014 by John Wiley & Sons, Ltd. Companion website: www.ataglanceseries.com/medicine

high enough, and the post-glomerular arteriole being able to constrict. If either the systemic BP falls too low (the most common cause) or the post-glomerular arteriole dilates inappropriately, glomerular perfusion falls and the kidneys fail. Pre-renal renal failure usually occurs in the context of a seriously ill patient. There are often several systemic insults which produce renal hypoperfusion sufficient to lead to renal failure, including:

- Hypovolaemia from haemorrhage, severe diarrhoea or vomiting.
- Cardiogenic shock.
- Sepsis.
- Drugs such as angiotensin-converting enzyme inhibitors and non-steroidal anti-inflammatory drugs (NSAIDs).
- Severe liver disease leading to renal failure, termed the 'hepatorenal syndrome'.

The common histological pattern seen in the kidney in response to severe injury of this nature is acute tubular necrosis (ATN), increasingly known as acute kidney injury (AKI), which usually recovers over several weeks. In very severe and prolonged hypotensive insults, acute cortical necrosis can also occur, from which recovery is less certain. In established renal failure caused by ATN, the concentrating ability of the kidney is lost and urinary sodium is >40 mmol/L. This contrasts with early pre-renal failure which may be reversible, with attention to haemodynamics and fluid balance when the urine is concentrated (urinary sodium usually <40 mmol/L).

Renal causes

There are many causes of renal failure as a result of disease affecting the kidney itself. These include glomerulonephritis, vasculitis, nephrotoxic drugs (e.g. gentamicin), rhabdomyolysis, interstitial nephritis, haemolytic uraemic syndrome and myeloma.

Post-renal causes

Urinary tract obstruction can occur at any site in the urinary tract and produce renal failure. Common causes include prostatic hypertrophy, carcinoma of the prostate, ureteric stones, tumours of the renal pelvis, ureters or bladder, external compression of the ureters by tumour or retroperitoneal fibrosis. Advanced renal failure will only occur with the obstruction of both kidneys.

Diagnostic approach

The rapid diagnosis of the cause of acute renal failure is important because a reversible cause may be present that will respond to specific treatment. A careful history and examination often point towards the likely cause of acute renal failure. Examination should include palpation and percussion of the bladder, the prostate gland in men and the pelvis for a mass in women. In pre-renal failure, the insults are often apparent, such as significant surgical operation, shock, sepsis or perhaps all three! In any patient with pre-renal failure examination for hypovolaemia is vital, and is suggested by:

- **Decreased skin turgor** (an unreliable sign).
- **Tachycardia**, often >100 bpm.
- **Hypotension**, with systolic blood pressure (BP) <90 mmHg, and a postural systolic BP fall between lying and sitting/standing of >20 mmHg.
- **Low venous pressure**: if the jugular venous pressure is not reliably seen, the central pressure should be measured invasively. The response (urine output) to a small intravenous (IV) bolus of fluid (e.g. 250 mL physiological saline) may clarify if the venous pressure is right for that individual patient.

Any pre-renal precipitants should be rapidly corrected. Renal ultrasonography is important to examine for urinary tract obstruction which will be manifest as urinary tract dilatation, particularly hydronephrosis. It will also provide information about renal size and symmetry (small kidneys indicating chronic renal disease).

If the renal size is normal, the kidneys are not obstructed and the history and examination do not suggest a pre-renal cause, further blood tests including immunology should be undertaken and the urine examined for the presence of red cells, protein and casts, which may suggest a renal cause such as glomerulonephritis. A renal biopsy may be necessary for accurate definition of the cause of the acute renal failure.

Management

As in any seriously ill patient, the priorities in acute renal failure are in ensuring adequate oxygenation and circulation. In acute renal failure, the most dangerous threat to oxygenation is fluid overload resulting in pulmonary oedema. The accurate assessment of the fluid status of the patient is thus crucial. In patients with fluid overload who are in established renal failure, oxygen should be administered and fluid removed. Diuretics will not work, vasodilators such as IV nitrates may provide temporary benefit, but definitive treatment with haemodialysis, haemofiltration or peritoneal dialysis should be performed. Evidence of hypovolaemia should result in treatment with IV fluids.

The other major life-threatening complication of acute renal failure is the presence of hyperkalaemia, which can result in cardiac dysrhythmias (especially ventricular fibrillation and cardiac asystole). The potassium should be measured urgently, electrocardiogram (ECG) changes of hyperkalaemia sought (peaked T waves, widened QRS, absent P waves, sine wave appearance) and, if the potassium is >6 mmol/L or if ECG abnormalities are present, treatment with IV calcium (with ECG monitoring), insulin and glucose, and oral or rectal calcium resonium, and urgent dialysis treatment arranged.

The other serious complications of acute renal failure that may require urgent treatment with dialysis include metabolic acidosis, encephalopathy and pericarditis.

Once these priorities have been addressed, specific treatments for the cause of the renal failure may be necessary. These might include the relief of obstruction, the treatment of sepsis or the administration of immunosuppression for a rapidly progressive glomerulonephritis.

151 Chronic renal failure and the dialysis patient

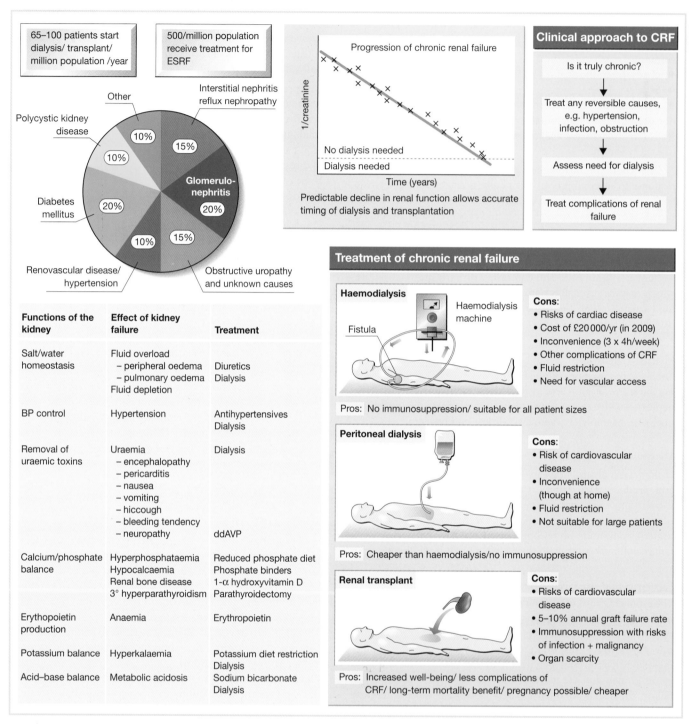

Chronic renal failure (CRF) is defined as an abnormally low glomerular filtration rate (GFR) for >3 months. Numerous disorders produce CRF, including glomerulonephritis (20%), interstitial nephritis and reflux nephropathy (15%), diabetes mellitus (20%), polycystic kidney disease (10%), renovascular disease/hypertension (10%), obstructive uropathy and unknown causes (15%). The incidence of chronic renal failure suitable for renal replacement therapy is 65–100/million population/year, with 500/million patients receiving end-stage renal failure (ESRF)

treatment. In CRF, the normal functions of the kidney are perturbed resulting in:

● Failure of regulation of salt and water excretion which can produce oedema (peripheral and pulmonary) or more rarely fluid depletion. Failure of concentrating power leads to nocturia.

● Hypertension is common and occasionally severe enough to cause encephalopathy. Premature cardiovascular disease (particularly coronary artery disease) accounts for much of the excess mortality of CRF; this may relate to dyslipidaemia (commonly found in CRF), hypertension, chronic anaemia, abnormalities of calcium metabolism and renin–angiotensin system activation.

- Accumulation of nitrogenous waste products in the blood (and of metabolic products with molecular weight of 500–2000: the 'middle molecules') produces symptoms that include encephalopathy, hiccough, pericarditis, nausea, vomiting, pruritus, malaise, impotence, menstrual irregularities and (mixed motor/sensory) neuropathy. Uraemia causes anorexia and complex disturbances in protein metabolism, resulting in malnutrition, so maintenance of lean body mass is difficult. Muscle wasting causes weakness, inactivity and further muscle loss.
- Metabolic acidosis and hyperkalaemia.
- Anaemia, mainly from erythropoietin deficiency, with contributions from a reduced red cell lifespan, occasionally iron deficiency from gastrointestinal bleeding, etc. Anaemia is milder than expected in polycystic kidney disease and can be more severe than expected in diabetics.
- Renal bone disease: this can be profound and disabling. This relates to osteomalacia (failure of renal hydroxylation (1α) of vitamin D), secondary hyperparathyroidism driven by chronic hypocalcaemia (caused by high phosphate and low vitamin D), adynamic bone disease and nutritional osteoporosis. Aluminium bone toxicity may complicate haemodialysis.
- There is an increased bleeding tendency, largely as a result of platelet dysfunction and depressed activity of von Willebrand's factor.
- Infection is common, because immunity is impaired.

The symptoms of CRF may have an insidious onset, or may present as a uraemic emergency with life-threatening complications.

Management (see Table 151.1)

A full history and examination may provide important clues to the aetiology of the renal failure. A history of frequent urinary tract infections in childhood may suggest a diagnosis of reflux nephropathy, whereas a family history may suggest polycystic kidney disease. Haematuria found at previous medical examinations might point towards chronic glomerulonephritis. It is important to establish that the renal failure is truly chronic to ensure that there is no acute and reversible cause of renal failure. Previous estimations of renal function are of the greatest help in determining this; furthermore, the absence of anaemia usually suggests that the renal failure is acute rather than chronic, whilst small kidneys are usually found in chronic (irreversible) disease.

The investigation of patients with CRF includes renal tract ultrasonography to exclude obstruction and document renal size. If the cause is unclear and the kidneys are of normal size, a renal biopsy is undertaken. Tests to exclude myeloma and autoimmune disease (systemic lupus erythematosus, vasculitis) and urinalysis for proteinuria, haematuria and urinary infection are indicated. The severity of the renal failure is determined from creatinine, urea and creatinine clearance.

Once significant renal dysfunction develops, there is usually an inexorable deterioration in renal function over several years (possibly caused by hyperfiltration in the remaining glomeruli). Apart from treatments directed against the specific cause of the renal failure, the main therapy reducing the speed of deterioration is aggressive blood pressure control. ESRF is a term used when patients would not survive without renal replacement therapy (haemodialysis, peritoneal dialysis, renal transplantation). Patients are prepared for renal replacement therapy by creating dialysis access before the renal failure progresses to cause uraemic symptoms. Before dialysis, calcium and phosphate balance are corrected, using 1α-hydroxycholecalciferol and phosphate binders, anaemia is improved by erythropoietin, acidosis is ameliorated with sodium

Table 151.1 Management of chronic renal failure.

GFR	Management
<15 mL/min	Severe renal failure: if new → urgent specialist referral
>15 and <30 mL/min	Significant impairment of renal function → prompt assessment and referral
>30 and <60 mL/min	May reflect age, biological variation or renal disease (suggested by proteinuria, haematuria $\pm \uparrow$ BP). Evaluate, repeat after 1 week in unwell patients and 1 month in the well. Refer all those with renal damage and any with a GFR < 3rd centile for age

The GFR can be estimated from the serum creatinine using the following formulas:

MDRD $\text{GFR (mL/min/1.73 m}^2) = 186 \times (\text{creatinine} (\mu\text{mol/L})/88.4)^{-1.154} \times (\text{age})^{-0.203} \times (0.742 \text{ if female}) \times (1.210 \text{ if African American})$

Cockcroft–Gault $\dfrac{(140 - \text{age}) \times \text{weight} \times 1.23 \times (0.85 \text{ if female})}{\text{Creatinine} (\mu\text{mol/L})}$

Normal GFR in male/female (mL/min):

Centile	40 years	50 years	60 years	70 years
50th	95/85	85/75	70/65	65/55
10th	75/65	65/60	55/50	45/40
3rd	65/55	60/50	45/40	35/35

bicarbonate, hypertension is treated and sodium and water retention are controlled with diuretics.

Indications for dialysis are:

- Uraemic symptoms: the usual indication, often when creatinine is $>500 \mu\text{mol/L}$.
- Life-threatening complications (hyperkalaemia, acidosis, fluid overload, uraemic pericarditis or encephalopathy).

In **haemodialysis** vascular access is achieved forming an arteriovenous fistula (which needs 8 weeks to 'mature' before use) or by using double-lumen jugular, subclavian or femoral lines. The diffusion of solutes and water occurs across a semipermeable membrane, which separates blood and dialysate flow in opposite directions. The major difficulties with haemodialysis are cardiovascular instability (from concurrent cardiovascular disease and drugs used for its treatment, as well as the major fluid shifts that occur during dialysis), difficulties in adhering to the dietary and fluid intake restrictions and difficulties with vascular access. Dialysis membranes can activate the clotting cascade, so heparin is used to prevent this. Most membranes do not allow the removal of β_2-microglobulin, which accumulates causing carpal tunnel syndrome and arthropathy. Over-rapid removal of toxic metabolites causes a profound illness – dialysis 'disequilibrium' – particularly during the first dialysis treatments, and can be prevented by frequent 'small' dialysis schedules.

In **continuous ambulatory peritoneal dialysis** patients instill several litres of isotonic or hypertonic glucose solution four times a day into the peritoneal cavity via a permanent catheter or connect to a machine which does this at night (automated peritoneal dialysis). The peritoneal lining acts as the dialysis membrane. After several hours, the fluid containing solutes and waste products is drained out. Excess body fluid is removed by using hypertonic solutions. Infection of the peritoneal fluid (peritoneal dialysis peritonitis) is the commonest complication requiring treatment with intraperitoneal or intravenous antibiotics.

152 The renal transplant recipient

Management of a rise in creatinine in the renal transplant patient

History and examination

Investigations
- Ultrasound
- Ciclosporin level
- Renal biopsy
- Renal arteriogram

Major causes of graft dysfunction
- Rejection
- Obstruction
- Ciclosporin toxicity
- Renal artery stenosis
- Recurrent disease
- Urinary tract infection

Medical problems

Increased incidence of cardiovascular disease
- Twenty-fold increase in risk of death from MI compared with age-matched control
- Hypertension

Increased incidence of malignancies
- Skin (increased 20-fold)
- Lymphoma (increased 20–50-fold)
- Other, e.g. colon/lung (increased 1.5-fold)

Drug side effects

Corticosteroids –	cushingoid, diabetes
Ciclosporin –	hypertension, renal impairment, diabetes
Azathioprine –	neutropenia

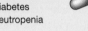

Brainstem death criteria

Patient apnoeic and in deep coma due to irreversible, structural damage to brain

No depressant drugs, neuromuscular blockers, hypothermia, gross metabolic or endocrine disturbance

Lack of brainstem function
No reaction of pupils to light
No corneal reflex
No facial response to pain
No caloric reflex (vestibulocular)
No cough/gag reflex
No respiratory movement after disconnection from ventilator and $PaCO_2$ >6.7kPa whilst oxygenated
Repeat x 2 >1/2 h apart

Post-transplant infections

0–1 month: 'conventional'

Postoperative chest infections/pneumonia
UTIs, wound infections

1–4 months: 'opportunistic'

Viral, e.g. CMV, VZV
Fungal, e.g. *Aspergillus*
Bacterial, e.g. TB, *Listeria*
Parasitic, e.g. *Pneumocystis, Toxoplasma*

3–4 months: 'late-opportunistic'

Cryptococus, zoster, CMV retinitis
Viral-associated malignancy,
e.g. lymphoma (EBV), Kaposi's (HHV-8)

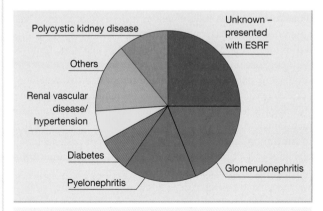

Indications for renal transplantation

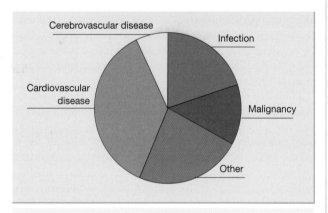

Causes of mortality following renal transplantation

Medicine at a Glance, Fourth Edition. Edited by Patrick Davey. © 2014 John Wiley & Sons, Ltd. Published 2014 by John Wiley & Sons, Ltd. Companion website: www.ataglanceseries.com/medicine

Stages of renal dysfunction

Stage	Description	Creatinine clearance (~GFR) (mL/min/1.73 m^2)	Metabolic consequences
1	Normal or increased GFR – people at increased risk or with early renal damage	>90	
2	Early renal insufficiency	60–89*	Concentration of parathyroid hormone starts to rise (GFR ~ 60–80)
3	Moderate renal failure (chronic renal failure)	30–59*	Decrease in calcium absorption (GFR <50) Lipoprotein activity falls Malnutrition Onset of left ventricular hypertrophy Onset of anaemia (erythropoietin deficiency)
4	Severe renal failure (pre-end-stage renal disease)	15–29	Triglyceride concentrations start to rise Hyperphosphataemia Metabolic acidosis Tendency to hyperkalaemia
5	End-stage renal disease (uraemia)	<15	Azotaemia develops

* May be normal for age (see Chapter 151)

Adapted from National Kidney Foundation—K/DOQI

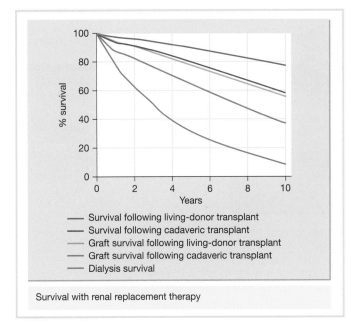

Survival with renal replacement therapy

— Survival following living-donor transplant
— Survival following cadaveric transplant
— Graft survival following living-donor transplant
— Graft survival following cadaveric transplant
— Dialysis survival

Table 152.1 Relative contraindications to transplantation.

- Age >70 years
- HIV positive
- Bacterial infection
- Recent/current malignancy
- Severe cardiac disease
- Renal disease with high risk of recurrence

In the UK, 2000 patients receive renal transplants every year, compared with the 3500 who are taken on for renal replacement treatment. Not all patients with end-stage renal failure (ESRF) are suitable for renal transplantation (see Table 152.1). Transplantation is limited by the availability of donor organs. Organs are most commonly obtained from donors in whom brainstem death has been diagnosed. Increasingly, kidneys are being transplanted from living related (or spouse) donors. In type 1 diabetic patients dual kidney–pancreas transplants may be undertaken.

In the immediate postoperative period, the patient faces the risks of the operation and of infection resulting from heavy immunosuppression. Common infections include cytomegalovirus (CMV) disease, herpes zoster and Balkan nephropathy. In the longer term, the renal transplant recipient faces a variety of medical problems, including those related to immunosuppression, the increased incidence of cardiovascular and cerebrovascular disease, hypertension, increased incidence of a variety of malignancies, notably of the skin and lymphoma, the conse-

quences of previous chronic renal failure, the underlying renal disorder and the problems of graft failure.

Recipients of renal transplants are commonly immunosuppressed with a combination of drugs, including prednisolone, azathioprine, mycophenolate, ciclosporin, tacrolimus, sirolimus and specific therapeutic antibodies (e.g. anti-IL2 receptor). These agents share the general side effects of an increased incidence of infections resulting from immunosuppression, but each has important unique side effects. Examples of these include the cushingoid features that occur with corticosteroid administration; the hypertension, tremor, increased incidence of diabetes mellitus and renal impairment that can occur with ciclosporin and tacrolimus; and the neutropenia that can occur with azathioprine and mycophenolate.

The survival of renal transplants at 1, 5 and 10 years is 90%, 70% and 55%, respectively. Graft survival is enhanced by careful human leukocyte antigen matching of donor and recipient.

The success of renal transplantation is largely the result of the ability to follow renal function precisely and frequently with measurements of serum creatinine. Any significant rise in creatinine should prompt investigation for rejection, ciclosporine/tacrolimus toxicity, problems with the renal vasculature or the obstruction of urine flow. Rejection is usually diagnosed with renal biopsy and is treated with high-dose methylprednisolone or anti-T-cell antibodies. Obstruction can usually be diagnosed with ultrasonography; ciclosporin/tacrolimus levels determined to exclude toxicity and angiography may be required to demonstrate normal renal blood supply.

153 Drugs and renal failure

The following categories contain examples only and are not exhaustive

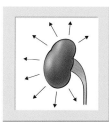

Drugs usually excreted by the kidney which can accumulate in renal failure

- Digoxin
- Lithium
- Morphine (+ metabolites), pethidine (+ metabolites)
- Penicillins, gentamicin, vancomycin, erythromycin, aciclovir

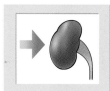

Drugs which require higher dosage in renal failure

- Furosemide (frusemide)

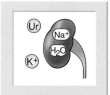

Drugs which can exacerbate metabolic effects in pre-existing renal failure

- K⁺ sparing diuretics →hyperkalaemia
- Corticosteroids →↑uraemia
- NaCl, NaHCO₃ →Na⁺/ H₂O retention

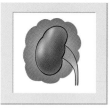

Drugs which can produce idiosyncratic renal toxicity

- NSAIDs
- Penicillins
- Gold, penicillamine

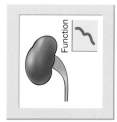

Drugs which can reduce renal function and should be used with caution in renal failure

- NSAIDs
- Angiotensin-converting enzyme inhibitors
- Ciclosporin, aciclovir
- Contrast media

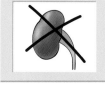
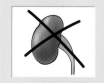

Drugs which can produce renal failure in overdose

- Gentamicin
- Paracetamol
- Ethylene glycol

Drugs often prescribed for patients with chronic renal failure

	Intended effect
Erythropoietin	↓anaemia
1α vitamin D	↑Ca2⁺
Phosphate binders	↓PO₄⁻
Antihypertensives	↓BP
Diuretics (loop)	↓Na⁺ / H₂O
Iron	↓anaemia

When prescribing a drug for a patient with renal failure several issues need to be addressed:

- What is the effect of the renal impairment on renal excretion of the drug?
- What is the effect of the renal impairment on drug action?
- What is the effect of the drug on the kidneys?
- How should the prescription be altered in view of the renal impairment?

The golden rule when prescribing in all patients with renal failure is to 'use drugs very sparingly', and 'always check the dose in a pharmacopoeia such as the *BNF*'.

Effect of renal impairment on excretion

Nearly all drugs are excreted to some extent by the kidneys. Furthermore, in patients with renal impairment there may be differing bioavailability, and alterations in volume of distribution and in plasma protein binding. If there is significant renal impairment, appropriate dosing should be prescribed based on recommended guidelines. For some drugs, such as morphine and pethidine, active drug metabolites may be excreted by the kidney and produce toxicity in renal impairment. The monitoring of blood levels (for drugs such as digoxin or gentamicin) may be essential to achieve appropriate dosing.

Effect of renal impairment on drug action

Uraemia may produce increased or decreased end-organ sensitivity, e.g. loop diuretics such as furosemide (frusemide) must be prescribed in much larger doses in renal impairment to achieve the same therapeutic effect.

Effect of drug on the kidneys

Drugs may produce an idiosyncratic renal toxicity such as the interstitial nephritis produced by antibiotics and non-steroidal anti-inflammatory drugs (NSAIDs) or have a predictable adverse effect such as the exacerbation of renal hypoperfusion by angiotensin-converting enzyme inhibitors and NSAIDs.

In patients undergoing dialysis treatment, it is also necessary to know whether the drug is removed by dialysis. In transplant recipients, there are many important and potentially dangerous interactions with the immunosuppressive agents.

Medicine at a Glance, Fourth Edition. Edited by Patrick Davey. © 2014 John Wiley & Sons, Ltd. Published 2014 by John Wiley & Sons, Ltd. Companion website: www.ataglanceseries.com/medicine

154 Benign prostatic hypertrophy

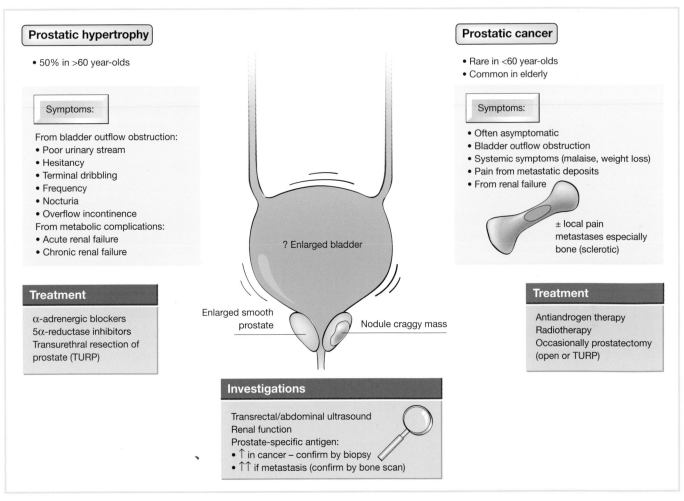

Prostatic hypertrophy

- 50% in >60 year-olds

Symptoms:

From bladder outflow obstruction:
- Poor urinary stream
- Hesitancy
- Terminal dribbling
- Frequency
- Nocturia
- Overflow incontinence
From metabolic complications:
- Acute renal failure
- Chronic renal failure

Treatment

α-adrenergic blockers
5α-reductase inhibitors
Transurethral resection of
prostate (TURP)

? Enlarged bladder

Enlarged smooth prostate

Nodule craggy mass

Prostatic cancer

- Rare in <60 year-olds
- Common in elderly

Symptoms:

- Often asymptomatic
- Bladder outflow obstruction
- Systemic symptoms (malaise, weight loss)
- Pain from metastatic deposits
- From renal failure

± local pain
metastases especially
bone (sclerotic)

Treatment

Antiandrogen therapy
Radiotherapy
Occasionally prostatectomy
(open or TURP)

Investigations

Transrectal/abdominal ultrasound
Renal function
Prostate-specific antigen:
- ↑ in cancer – confirm by biopsy
- ↑↑ if metastasis (confirm by bone scan)

Benign prostatic hypertrophy is characterized by enlargement of the prostate gland and is very common, being present in over 50% of men aged over 60 years, and 80% over the age of 80. It most commonly presents with features of bladder outflow obstruction/ poor urinary stream, hesitancy, terminal dribbling and frequency. Other symptoms can include dysuria and overflow incontinence. Alternatively, patients may present with symptoms of chronic renal failure or acute urinary retention. Cancer of the prostate is common, affecting one in six men, though only 3% of men die from prostate cancer.

Examination
On examination a bladder may be palpable or detected by percussion. An enlarged smooth prostate is found on digital rectal examination.

Investigations
These may include measurement of serum creatinine, ultrasonography of the renal tract, urodynamics and determination of

prostate-specific antigen (PSA) levels because these are raised in prostate malignancy (see Chapter 195). PSA can also be elevated with prostatitis, rises with age and only has a limited specificity (c. 70%) and sensitivity (c. 70%) for the diagnosis of prostate cancer.

Management
The medical management includes the use of α-adrenergic blockers such as prazosin, α_1-adrenoceptor antagonists such as tamsulosin (which relax the smooth muscle of the prostate and bladder neck) or finasteride (a 5α-reductase inhibitor that inhibits the conversion of testosterone to its active metabolite dihydrotestosterone, thus reducing prostatic hypertrophy). Surgery is often necessary to improve urine flow and transurethral resection of the prostate (TURP) is undertaken endoscopically.

Medicine at a Glance, Fourth Edition. Edited by Patrick Davey. © 2014 John Wiley & Sons, Ltd. Published 2014 by John Wiley & Sons, Ltd. Companion website: www.ataglanceseries.com/medicine

155 Urinary tract infection

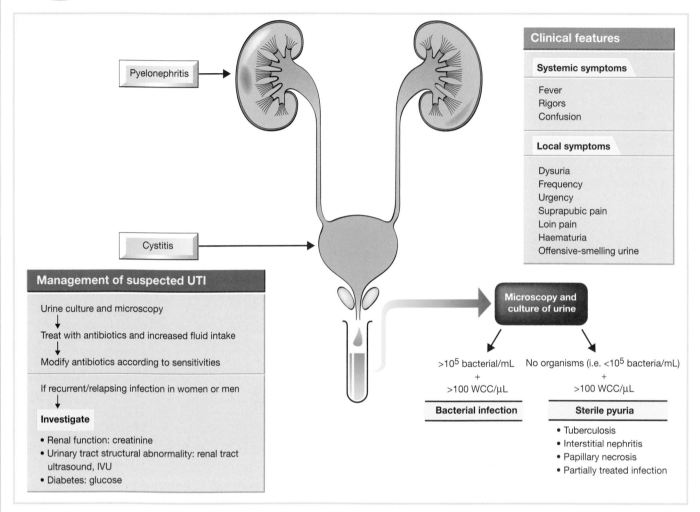

Clinical features

Systemic symptoms

Fever
Rigors
Confusion

Local symptoms

Dysuria
Frequency
Urgency
Suprapubic pain
Loin pain
Haematuria
Offensive-smelling urine

Pyelonephritis

Cystitis

Microscopy and culture of urine

>10^5 bacterial/mL
+
>100 WCC/μL

Bacterial infection

No organisms (i.e. <10^5 bacteria/mL)
+
>100 WCC/μL

Sterile pyuria

- Tuberculosis
- Interstitial nephritis
- Papillary necrosis
- Partially treated infection

Management of suspected UTI

Urine culture and microscopy
↓
Treat with antibiotics and increased fluid intake
↓
Modify antibiotics according to sensitivities
↓
If recurrent/relapsing infection in women or men

Investigate

- Renal function: creatinine
- Urinary tract structural abnormality: renal tract ultrasound, IVU
- Diabetes: glucose

Urinary tract infections (UTIs) are very common, accounting for 1–2% of general practice consultations. They occur much more commonly in females and in young, sexually active women, in whom the annual incidence may be as high as 0.5/woman/year. Most infections arise from the introduction of bowel flora via the urethra into the bladder. The increased frequency of UTIs in women is attributed to short urethral length, and a UTI can commonly follow sexual intercourse. Other host factors associated with an increased risk of UTI include: (i) pregnancy; (ii) incomplete bladder emptying (e.g. neurogenic bladder in multiple sclerosis, spinal cord injury); (iii) urinary calculi; (iv) diabetes mellitus (all suspected UTIs should have urine dipstick tested for glucose); (v) structural abnormality of the urinary tract (e.g. reflux); and (vi) instrumentation of the urinary tract (e.g. urethral catheterization).

The causative organisms are usually coliforms (70%) but other bacterial pathogens include *Proteus mirabilis*, *Staphylococcus epidermidis* and *Streptococcus faecalis*. Certain cell surface antigens may enhance pathogenicity by aiding the adhesion of bacteria to uroepithelial surfaces. The typical symptoms of a UTI are dysuria, urinary frequency and urgency, suprapubic discomfort, loin pain,

fever, haematuria and offensive smelling urine. Sometimes, particularly in the elderly, local symptoms may be absent but the patient may present with confusion or general deterioration. If the infection primarily causes symptoms in the bladder it can be termed 'cystitis', whereas infection affecting the kidney is termed 'pyelonephritis'.

Investigations

A number of investigations are helpful:

- **Urine dipsticks**: most Gram-negative bacteria, the most common organisms implicated in UTIs, convert nitrate, a normal constituent of urine, to nitrite, which is detected by dipstick. The presence of nitrite is therefore a useful guide to the presence of pathogenic Gram-negative organisms. Finding leukocytes in the urine suggests an inflammatory process in the renal/urinary tract. The most common cause of this is infection by conventional bacteria; if these cannot be found (so-called sterile pyuria), other causes should be considered, such as tuberculosis of the renal tract, cancer and renal or bladder stones.

- **Microscopy and culture of a midstream specimen of urine**: if a UTI is suspected, a sample of urine (preferably obtained as a

Medicine at a Glance, Fourth Edition. Edited by Patrick Davey. © 2014 John Wiley & Sons, Ltd. Published 2014 by John Wiley & Sons, Ltd. Companion website: www.ataglanceseries.com/medicine

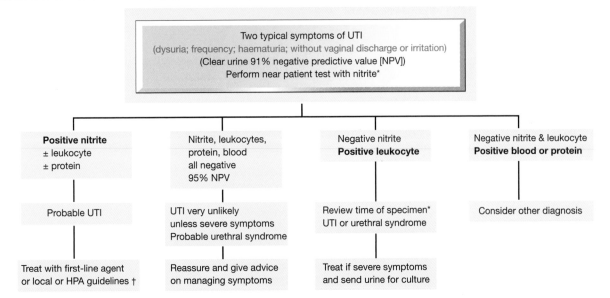

Using urine dipstick to diagnose urinary tract infection (UTI)

Two typical symptoms of UTI
(dysuria; frequency; haematuria; without vaginal discharge or irritation)
(Clear urine 91% negative predictive value [NPV])
Perform near patient test with nitrite*

Positive nitrite
± leukocyte
± protein

Nitrite, leukocytes,
protein, blood
all negative
95% NPV

Negative nitrite
Positive leukocyte

Negative nitrite & leukocyte
Positive blood or protein

Probable UTI

UTI very unlikely
unless severe symptoms
Probable urethral syndrome

Review time of specimen*
UTI or urethral syndrome

Consider other diagnosis

Treat with first-line agent
or local or HPA guidelines †

Reassure and give advice
on managing symptoms

Treat if severe symptoms
and send urine for culture

*Nitrite is produced by the action of bacterial nitrate reductase in urine. As contact time between bacteria and urine is needed, morning specimens are most reliable. Leukocyte esterase detects intact and lysed leukocytes produced in inflammation. Haematuria and proteinuria occur in UTI but are also present in other conditions. When reading test **WAIT** for the time recommended by manufacturer.

HPA, Health Protection Agency guidelines † = www.hpa.org.uk/infections/topics_az/antimicrobial_resistance/guidance.htm

Urethral syndrome: a syndrome characterized by symptoms identical to urinary tract infection (e.g. frequency, suprapubic pain, dysuria) but in which no microbes are found to clonize the urinary tract. Other conditions affecting the uro-gynaecological tract need to be ruled out; in many the cause remains unclear

From Health Protection Agency www.hpa.org.uk

Microorganisms causing hospital-acquired UTIs

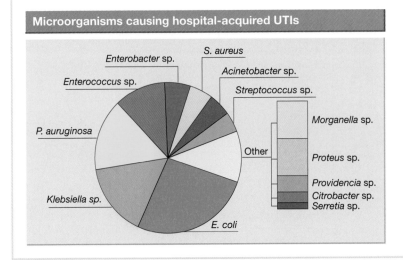

Causes of community-acquired UTIs

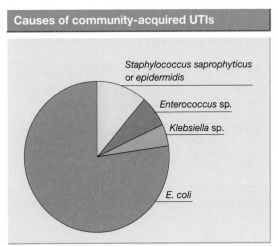

'clean catch' from midstream urine) should be microscoped and cultured. A finding of more than 10^5 organisms/mL urine is significant. Culture enables the causative organism to be identified and its antibiotic susceptibilities defined. Organisms may be cultured from urine without being of pathogenic significance, e.g. because of perineal contamination; but the presence of >100 leukocytes/mm^3 of urine usually characterizes significant bacterial infections.

- **Renal tract imaging**: investigations for a predisposing cause should be undertaken if there are multiple infections in a woman, or a first UTI in a child or man, and these may include tests of renal function (any structural abnormality of the kidneys or renal tract can predispose to infection), glucose, intravenous urogram (IVU) or ultrasonography (to detect renal calculi, abnormalities

of the urinary tract and incomplete bladder emptying) and micturating cystogram (particularly in children to exclude reflux).

Management

Urine should be sent for microscopy and culture before starting antibiotic treatment. In uncomplicated UTIs short-duration (5-day or even single-dose) antibiotic therapy is usually adequate. Trimethoprim, nitrofurantoin or amoxicillin are commonly prescribed, but the prescription may need to be altered in the light of the antibiotic sensitivities of the causative organism. Acute pyelonephritis or prominent systemic symptoms of infection may require intravenous antibiotics. A high fluid intake (>3 L/day) is recommended to prevent urinary stasis in the bladder and to decrease bacterial replication.

156 Diabetes mellitus

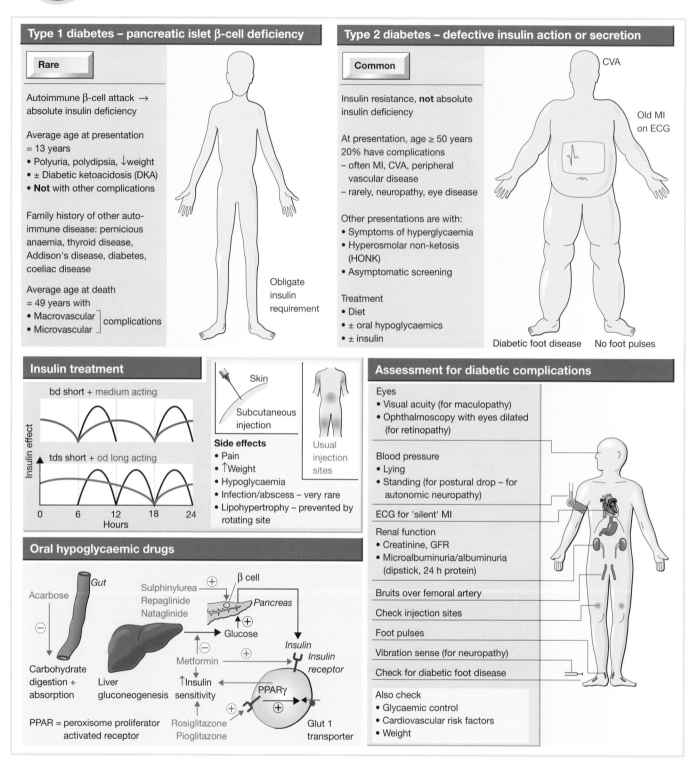

Type 1 diabetes – pancreatic islet β-cell deficiency

Rare

Autoimmune β-cell attack → absolute insulin deficiency

Average age at presentation = 13 years
- Polyuria, polydipsia, ↓weight
- ± Diabetic ketoacidosis (DKA)
- **Not** with other complications

Family history of other auto-immune disease: pernicious anaemia, thyroid disease, Addison's disease, diabetes, coeliac disease

Average age at death = 49 years with
- Macrovascular ⎤ complications
- Microvascular ⎦

Obligate insulin requirement

Type 2 diabetes – defective insulin action or secretion

Common

Insulin resistance, **not** absolute insulin deficiency

At presentation, age ≥ 50 years
20% have complications
– often MI, CVA, peripheral vascular disease
– rarely, neuropathy, eye disease

Other presentations are with:
- Symptoms of hyperglycaemia
- Hyperosmolar non-ketosis (HONK)
- Asymptomatic screening

Treatment
- Diet
- ± oral hypoglycaemics
- ± insulin

CVA

Old MI on ECG

Diabetic foot disease   No foot pulses

Insulin treatment

bd short + medium acting

tds short + od long acting

Insulin effect

0 6 12 18 24
Hours

Skin

Subcutaneous injection

Side effects
- Pain
- ↑Weight
- Hypoglycaemia
- Infection/abscess – very rare
- Lipohypertrophy – prevented by rotating site

Usual injection sites

Oral hypoglycaemic drugs

Acarbose   *Gut*

Carbohydrate digestion + absorption

Liver gluconeogenesis

Sulphinylurea
Repaglinide
Nataglinide

⊕ β cell

Pancreas

⊕

→ Glucose

Metformin ⊖ ⊕

↑Insulin sensitivity

PPARγ

Rosiglitazone
Pioglitazone

⊕ ⊕

Insulin

Insulin receptor

Glut 1 transporter

PPAR = peroxisome proliferator activated receptor

Assessment for diabetic complications

Eyes
- Visual acuity (for maculopathy)
- Ophthalmoscopy with eyes dilated (for retinopathy)

Blood pressure
- Lying
- Standing (for postural drop – for autonomic neuropathy)

ECG for 'silent' MI

Renal function
- Creatinine, GFR
- Microalbuminuria/albuminuria (dipstick, 24 h protein)

Bruits over femoral artery

Check injection sites

Foot pulses

Vibration sense (for neuropathy)

Check for diabetic foot disease

Also check
- Glycaemic control
- Cardiovascular risk factors
- Weight

Definition

Diabetes mellitus is characterized by chronically elevated glucose. Fasting plasma glucose levels are (in mmol/L): diabetes ≥7.0, impaired glucose tolerance 6–7, normal <6; 2 hours post 75 g glucose plasma glucose levels are: diabetes ≥11.1, impaired glucose tolerance 7.8–11.1, normal <7.8. A diagnosis of diabetes mellitus is usually made in a symptomatic person in the absence of intercurrent illness, with a random glucose >11.1 mmol/L or fasting level >7 mmol/L, without requiring a formal oral glucose tolerance test. HbA1c >6.5% may also be used in diagnosis of type 2 diabetes in a symptomatic patient with no intercurrent illness, but HbA1c <6.5% does not exclude the diagnosis.

Classification and pathophysiology

Type 1 diabetes mellitus (pancreatic islet β-cell deficiency)

This is a rare disease, essentially of white northern Europeans (25/10 000 population), presenting when aged <30 years, where absolute insulin deficiency occurs after autoimmune β-cell destruction in the genetically predisposed. Various antibodies are found up to 10 years before clinical disease and disappear several years later. Associated autoimmune conditions may be found in the family (see Figure 156.1).

Clinical features: at presentation patients are often thin and have symptoms of polyuria, polydipsia, weight loss, fatigue and infections (abscesses, fungal infections, e.g. candidiasis). Ketoacidosis may occur, with nausea, vomiting, drowsiness and tachypnoea. Patients have an obligate need for insulin.

Type 2 diabetes mellitus (defective insulin action or secretion)

This is a very common illness (prevalence in 2009 of 2% in the UK and 6.6% in the USA, increasing rapidly as a result of dietary/lifestyle factors) of middle-aged and elderly people, caused principally by resistance to the peripheral action of insulin. Although inadequate secretion of insulin may occur late on, absolute insulin deficiency is not found. There is a substantial genetic contribution. The identical twins concordance rate is 90%, but there is no strong human leukocyte antigen (HLA) association.

Clinical features: 80% are overweight; 20% present with complications (ischaemic heart disease, cerebrovascular disease, renal failure, foot ulcers, visual impairment). May present with insidious polyuria and polydipsia. Many patients can be managed with diet and hypoglycaemic drugs, although some require insulin.

Other types of diabetes
- **Exocrine pancreas failure**: pancreatitis, pancreatectomy and destruction (carcinoma, cystic fibrosis, haemochromatosis).
- **Endocrine disease**: Cushing's syndrome, acromegaly, glucagonoma and phaeochromocytoma.
- **Gestational diabetes**: usually occurs in the last trimester of pregnancy and has a similar pathophysiology to type 2 diabetes. Not surprisingly, some 30–50% of patients develop overt type 2 diabetes within 10 years.
- **Malnutrition-related diabetes mellitus**: found in developing countries.
- **Genetic causes**: all very rare. Maturity-onset diabetes in the young (MODY) accounts for 1% of type 1 and 4% of type 2 diabetes, and relates to defects of β-cell function, most commonly abnormal hepatocyte nuclear factor 1α (HNF-1α) and glucokinase defects, and less frequently HNF-4α and HNF-1β mutations or insulin gene mutations. Other genetic defects are of insulin action (e.g. leprechaunism type A insulin resistance).

Management
- **Patient education**: use of nurse practitioners, self-education, etc. is vital.
- **Clinical assessment**: after diagnosing diabetes mellitus, treating any acute metabolic complications (see Chapter 157) and initiating life-long hypoglycaemic therapy, assessment of end-organ damage should occur every 6–12 months – eyesight (retinopathy and cataracts), cardiovascular system (peripheral pulses, signs of cardiac failure, hypertension), nervous system (peripheral sensory and/or autonomic neuropathy) and feet (ulceration, gangrene, infections). Renal function (creatinine, albuminuria) must be measured.
- **Treatment** should minimize symptoms and avoid complications, while allowing a normal life – this requires patient education and support. Maximizing prognosis depends on optimal blood glucose control and eliminating coexisting cardiovascular risk factors such as smoking, hypertension (aim for a blood pressure of <130/80 mmHg) and hyperlipidaemia. Optimal glycaemic control by itself improves cholesterol levels but, if the cholesterol remains high despite this, aggressive lipid-lowering therapy with statins may be justified. Indeed nearly all people with diabetes who have vascular disease should be on statins.

Specific treatment
- **Dietary advice**: aim for ideal body weight (obesity increases insulin resistance, and weight reduction lessens it in type 2 diabetes). Restrict refined carbohydrate and increase complex carbohydrate intake. Reduce saturated fat; avoid excessive alcohol.
- **Oral hypoglycaemic agents**: indicated in type 2 diabetes if there is inadequate metabolic control by diet alone.
- **Biguanides**: metformin. Reduces hepatic gluconeogenesis and increases muscle glucose metabolism. Mild anorexic action and thus indicated in obese individuals. Reduces insulin resistance and hepatic gluconeogenesis. Side effects: gastrointestinal (GI) upset and rarely lactic acidosis (increased risk with radiological contrast media). Contraindicated in renal failure and hepatic impairment.
- **Sulphonylureas**: gliclazide, glibenclamide, glimepride, tolbutamide. Increases insulin release from β cells (closes K^+ channels → cell depolarization). May cause weight gain or hypoglycaemia particularly in the elderly (avoid glibenclamide as long-acting).
- **Prandial glucose regulators**: repaglinide and nateglinide stimulate insulin release from β cells. Short duration of action makes hypoglycaemia less common than with sulphonylureas. Side effect: hepatic dysfunction.
- **Thiazolidinediones**: pioglitazone, troglitazone (withdrawn), rosiglitazone (withdrawn),. Insulin-sensitizing agents which activate the peroxisome proliferator-activated receptor γ, stimulating transcription of the glucose transporter molecules glut-1 and glut-4. Side effects: hepatotoxicity, increased risk of myocardial infarction (MI) and heart failure.
- **α-Glucosidase inhibitors**: acarbose inhibits carbohydrate digestion, reducing intestinal glucose absorption. Side effects: bloating and diarrhoea.
- **GLP-1 receptor analogues**: exenatide, liraglutide. GI incretin hormones are released on nutrient ingestion, stimulating insulin and inhibiting glucagon release. Side effects are gastrointestinal. Low risk of hypoglycaemia.
- **Insulin**: given subcutaneously and used for all those with type 1 diabetes and some people with type 2 diabetes. There are several kinds; recombinant human insulin is most commonly used, although some patients prefer porcine or bovine insulin. Different preparations have different onset and duration of actions (short, medium, long). Preparations with different combinations of short- and medium/long-acting duration are often used. Insulin analogues are chemically modified forms of insulin (e.g. lispro, aspart, glulisine) which have a rapid onset of action and shorter duration of action, allowing administration immediately before eating. Glargine and detemir are analogues with a 22–24-hour duration. Oral hypoglycaemic agents (e.g. metformin) may be added to insulin in type 2 diabetes to improve insulin sensitivity. Adverse effects of insulin are hypoglycaemia, weight gain and lipohypertrophy at injection sites.
- **Transplantation**: islet cell transplantation may be used in patients with type 1 diabetes. Pancreatic and renal transplantation may be performed in patients with type 1 diabetes with renal failure.

Monitoring glycaemic control in diabetes
Tight glycaemic control improves outcome and is monitored from blood glucose levels. Those on oral agents should monitor fasting blood glucose, whereas those on insulin should check glucose more frequently, e.g. before meals. Monitoring should be more frequent if the patient is unwell. Some patients find blood monitoring difficult, and urine glucose levels are used instead, although this is less reliable than blood because the renal threshold for glucose appearing in the urine varies between 7 and 12 mmol/L. Glycated haemoglobin (HbA1c) is a good measure of glycaemic control over several weeks.

157 Complications of diabetes

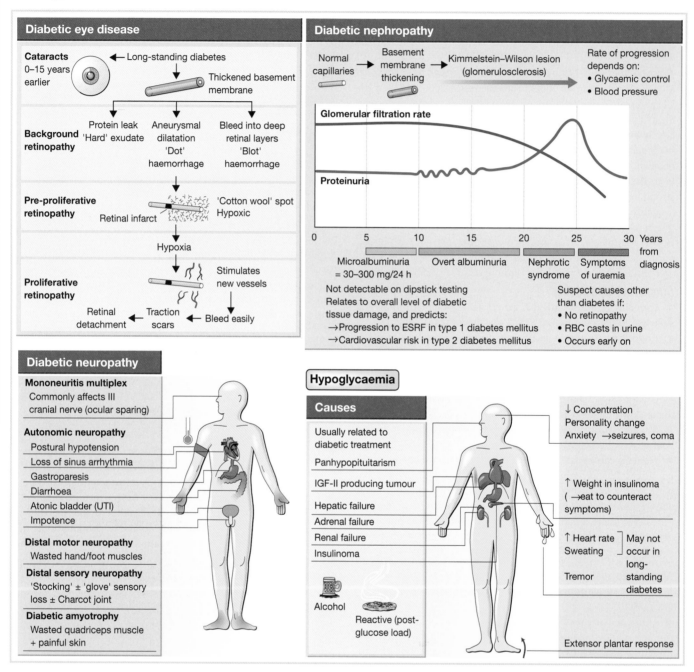

Diabetic eye disease

Cataracts
0–15 years earlier

Long-standing diabetes → Thickened basement membrane

Background retinopathy
Protein leak 'Hard' exudate | Aneurysmal dilatation 'Dot' haemorrhage | Bleed into deep retinal layers 'Blot' haemorrhage

Pre-proliferative retinopathy
Retinal infarct — 'Cotton wool' spot Hypoxic

Hypoxia

Proliferative retinopathy
Stimulates new vessels

Retinal detachment ← Traction scars ← Bleed easily

Diabetic nephropathy

Normal capillaries → Basement membrane thickening → Kimmelstein–Wilson lesion (glomerulosclerosis) →

Rate of progression depends on:
• Glycaemic control
• Blood pressure

Glomerular filtration rate

Proteinuria

0   5   10   15   20   25   30   Years from diagnosis

Microalbuminuria = 30–300 mg/24 h | Overt albuminuria | Nephrotic syndrome | Symptoms of uraemia

Not detectable on dipstick testing
Relates to overall level of diabetic tissue damage, and predicts:
→Progression to ESRF in type 1 diabetes mellitus
→Cardiovascular risk in type 2 diabetes mellitus

Suspect causes other than diabetes if:
• No retinopathy
• RBC casts in urine
• Occurs early on

Diabetic neuropathy

Mononeuritis multiplex
Commonly affects III cranial nerve (ocular sparing)

Autonomic neuropathy
Postural hypotension
Loss of sinus arrhythmia
Gastroparesis
Diarrhoea
Atonic bladder (UTI)
Impotence

Distal motor neuropathy
Wasted hand/foot muscles

Distal sensory neuropathy
'Stocking' ± 'glove' sensory loss ± Charcot joint

Diabetic amyotrophy
Wasted quadriceps muscle + painful skin

Hypoglycaemia

Causes
Usually related to diabetic treatment
Panhypopituitarism
IGF-II producing tumour
Hepatic failure
Adrenal failure
Renal failure
Insulinoma

Alcohol

Reactive (post-glucose load)

↓ Concentration
Personality change
Anxiety →seizures, coma

↑ Weight in insulinoma (→eat to counteract symptoms)

↑ Heart rate
Sweating
Tremor | May not occur in long-standing diabetes

Extensor plantar response

Diabetic complications arise from acute metabolic derangement (hypo- or hyperglycaemia) or, late on, from micro- or macrovascular damage, the risk of which relates to the tightness of glycaemic and conventional vascular risk factor control.

Microvascular complications
Small vessel disease is the hallmark of diabetes and takes 10 years or more to develop.

Eye disease (retinopathy)
One in three people with diabetes develop eye disease and 5% are blind at 30 years. Retinopathy results from capillary basement membrane thickening, leading to leaky vessels (haemorrhage, hard exudates), occluded vessels (retinal ischaemia, new vessels) and macular oedema.

• **Background retinopathy**: blot haemorrhage, 'dot' microaneurysms, hard exudates not involving the macula. No effect on sight.

Medicine at a Glance, Fourth Edition. Edited by Patrick Davey. © 2014 John Wiley & Sons, Ltd. Published 2014 by John Wiley & Sons, Ltd. Companion website: www.ataglanceseries.com/medicine

- **Maculopathy**: macular oedema, haemorrhages, hard exudates. Very difficult to diagnose ophthalmoscopically and suspected from a decrease in visual acuity, which should therefore be checked routinely in all people with diabetes.
- **Pre-proliferative retinopathy**: cotton-wool spots (retinal ischaemia interrupts axoplasmic transport). Venous beading and intraretinal microvascular abnormalities caused by dilated capillaries. Not sight-threatening.
- **Proliferative retinopathy**: retinal ischaemia induces new vessels, which are fragile and bleed easily. Retinal detachment from traction scars occurs, leading to further bleeding. The closer to the disc, the greater the risk to sight.
- **Cataract**: occurs 10–15 years earlier in people with diabetes.

Management: annual eye checks and good glycaemic and blood pressure (BP) control. Laser retinal photocoagulation can be used in pre-proliferative and proliferative retinopathy as well as in maculopathy.

Nephropathy

This occurs 15–25 years after diagnosis in 35–45% of patients with type 1 diabetes and <20% of patients with type 2 diabetes. The initial lesion is glomerular hyperfiltration (increased glomerular filtration rate (GFR)), which leads on to diffuse thickening of the glomerular basement membrane, manifest as microalbuminuria (urinary albumin 30–300 mg/day) – a highly accurate marker of overall vascular damage and thus a predictor of impending cardiovascular death. Persistent albuminuria (urinary albumin >300 mg/day) is initially associated with a normal GFR but, as overt proteinuria (urinary protein >0.5 g/24 h) develops, GFR progressively falls and overt renal failure develops.

Clinical features: asymptomatic early on; later hypertension, oedema and uraemia occur.

Management: antihypertensive treatment with angiotensin-converting enzyme (ACE) inhibitor as first-line therapy. ACE inhibitors are also beneficial if there is any proteinuria, regardless of BP. Good glycaemic control; lipid-lowering agents and aspirin. Chronic renal failure requires renal replacement therapy with dialysis or transplantation.

Neuropathy

This occurs through multiple mechanisms, including damage to the small blood vessels nourishing the peripheral nerves and abnormal sugar metabolism. There are several manifestations:

- **Peripheral sensory neuropathy**: progresses from a 'loss of vibration sense' early on to a 'glove and stocking' sensory loss 'as if walking on cotton wool'.
- **Mononeuropathies**: can affect any nerve, but have a predilection for those controlling eye movements, especially the oculomotor nerve, where the pupillary reactions are spared.
- **Amyotrophy**: painful wasting of the thigh muscles.
- **Autonomic neuropathy**: postural hypotension, absent cardiac vagal tone (no sinus arrhythmia), gustatory sweating, gastroparesis, nocturnal diarrhoea, bladder dysfunction (increased infections, incontinence) and erectile impotence.

Management: treatment is unsatisfactory and mainly supportive.

Macrovascular complications

Diabetes is a major risk factor for the development of atherosclerosis. Cerebrovascular risk is increased two-fold, coronary artery disease three- to five-fold and peripheral vascular disease 40-fold. Diabetes synergizes strongly with other macrovascular risk factors. People with asymptomatic type 2 diabetes have the same cardiovascular mortality as those who do not have diabetes but do have symptomatic vascular disease. These facts justify highly aggressive anti-atherogenic treatments in all people with diabetes.

Foot disease

This occurs as a result of peripheral vascular disease (cold painful foot), peripheral neuropathy (warm foot, often without much pain) and increased susceptibility to infection. It results in ulceration, infection (cellulites, osteomyelitis), gangrene and Charcot's foot (warm/hot foot with destruction of joint).

Management: prevention is by patient education, good footwear and podiatry, with antibiotic treatment of infection, debridement of ulcers and reconstructive arterial surgery for peripheral vascular disease. Amputation is occasionally required for gangrene and ischaemia. Immobilization of Charcot's foot ± bisphosphonates are also used.

Prevention of complications

Good glycaemic control delays the onset of progression of all microvascular disease. Macrovascular disease is less likely in patients with good BP control (<130/80 mmHg), and when all other risk factors are under optimal control. This means that highly aggressive cholesterol and BP-lowering therapy is indicated. Smoking in diabetes leads to a very premature death.

Hypoglycaemia

This is a common complication in people with diabetes who are treated with insulin and occasionally occurs in those on sulphonylureas. Symptoms occur when the blood glucose is ≤2.2 mmol/L, although many people with diabetes, who are used to higher blood glucose, have symptoms at higher blood glucose levels. Causes other than diabetic treatment are rare:

- Alcohol.
- Renal or hepatic failure.
- Very rare causes include reactive hypoglycaemia: rebound hypoglycaemia after a glucose load, insulinoma (pancreatic tumour producing insulin inappropriately), endocrine disease (adrenocortical failure, hypopituitarism) and insulin-like growth factor II (IGF-II)-producing tumours (pleural fibroma, sarcoma).

Clinical features and treatment

The cardinal features of hypoglycaemia are initially anxiety and poor concentration with impaired cognition, proceeding to a decrease in conscious level, which may progress to coma and seizures. The signs are of sweating, tremor and tachycardia, and there may be an extensor plantar response. Immediate treatment with glucose should be given – oral if possible, otherwise intravenously (50 mL of 50% glucose into a large vein). If veins cannot be cannulated, intramuscular glucagon is helpful. The underlying cause also clearly needs to be addressed.

Investigations

The cause is readily apparent in people with diabetes who are treated with insulin and those on sulphonylureas, and extensive investigations are not needed. In those who are not on such treatment, glucose, insulin and C-peptide levels are taken before giving glucose. A raised insulin and C-peptide suggests an insulinoma, whereas raised insulin and low C-peptide suggests exogenous insulin administration. If there is no obvious precipitant it is also important to exclude Addison's disease, and if this is negative to search for IGF-II-producing tumours, including using pancreatic magnetic resonance imaging and chest computed tomography. Urine assay for sulphonylureas may be diagnostic.

158 Diabetic emergencies

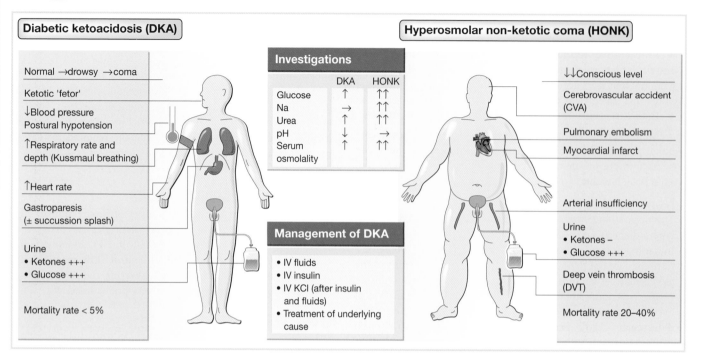

Diabetic ketoacidosis (DKA)

Normal →drowsy →coma

Ketotic 'fetor'

↓Blood pressure
Postural hypotension

↑Respiratory rate and
depth (Kussmaul breathing)

↑Heart rate

Gastroparesis
(± succussion splash)

Urine
• Ketones +++
• Glucose +++

Mortality rate < 5%

Investigations

	DKA	HONK
Glucose	↑	↑↑
Na	→	↑↑
Urea	↑	↑↑
pH	↓	→
Serum osmolality	↑	↑↑

Management of DKA

• IV fluids
• IV insulin
• IV KCl (after insulin and fluids)
• Treatment of underlying cause

Hyperosmolar non-ketotic coma (HONK)

↓↓Conscious level

Cerebrovascular accident (CVA)

Pulmonary embolism

Myocardial infarct

Arterial insufficiency

Urine
• Ketones –
• Glucose +++

Deep vein thrombosis (DVT)

Mortality rate 20–40%

Diabetic ketoacidosis

Diabetic ketoacidosis (DKA) relates to absolute insulin deficiency and therefore occurs in type 1, but not in type 2, diabetes. Lack of insulin causes hyperglycaemia (osmotic diuresis and dehydration) and raises ketone bodies levels, so inducing a metabolic acidosis.

- **Precipitants**: these are common and should always be sought – infections, omitting insulin (sometimes for psychological reasons), myocardial infarction (MI), surgery/trauma, undiagnosed type 1 diabetes.
- **Features**: thirst, polyuria and dehydration (even hypovolaemic shock), vomiting and abdominal pain, tachypnoea (from acidosis – Kussmaul's respiration), decreased consciousness.
- **Investigations**: blood glucose typically >20 mmol/L. Urine – large amount of ketones and high potassium as a result of acidosis, although total body potassium is depleted. Arterial acidosis (pH usually less than 7.3), decrease in bicarbonate as a result of metabolic acidosis and decrease in $P\text{CO}_2$ (carbon dioxide tension) as a result of hyperventilation.
- **Investigation of precipitant**: microbiology, chest X-ray, electrocardiogram (ECG). Full blood count – neutrophilia is common and does not necessarily indicate infection.
- **Management**: fluid replacement, often 3–5 L in <6 hours. Intravenous (IV) insulin, e.g. 6 units soluble insulin, followed by infusion. Potassium replacement (10–20 mmol/h) after initial insulin and fluid replacement (danger of hypokalaemia because insulin drives potassium into cells). Close monitoring of electrolytes. Occasionally need bicarbonate. Nasogastric tube for gastroparesis. Treatment of the underlying cause.
- **Prognosis**: always need insulin long term. Overall mortality during DKA is low (<5%).

Hyperosmolar non-ketotic coma

Found in type 2, but not in type 1, diabetes because insulin levels are insufficient to prevent hyperglycaemia, but are sufficient to prevent ketosis.

- **Precipitant**: infection, MI, excessive sugary drinks.
- **Features**: thirst, polyuria, impaired concentration level. Hyperviscosity leads to thrombotic complications (deep venous thrombosis, pulmonary embolism, stroke).
- **Investigations**: glucose is often very high (>50 mmol/L); sodium often >160 mmol/L; plasma osmolality is increased; acidosis is absent or mild.
- **Investigation of precipitant**: ECG, cardiac enzymes, microbiology.
- **Management**: often need central venous monitoring if patients are elderly or have cardiac disease. IV fluids ± K$^+$ replacement; IV insulin 3 units/h; anticoagulation.
- **Prognosis**: mortality from hyperosmolar non-ketotic coma (HONK) is very high at 20–40%. After the acute episode has resolved, the diabetes can often be managed with diet or oral hypoglycaemic agents.

Lactic acidosis

This is a very rare complication of metformin treatment. Patients present with symptoms of acidaemia (malaise, anorexia, vomiting) and signs of hyperventilation (Kussmaul's breathing). Glucose levels are usually normal. There are no ketones in the urine and blood gases show a (profound) acidosis, with high base excess. The anion gap is increased (see Chapter 143). Treatment is supportive and through the withdrawal of metformin.

Medicine at a Glance, Fourth Edition. Edited by Patrick Davey. © 2014 John Wiley & Sons, Ltd. Published 2014 by John Wiley & Sons, Ltd. Companion website: www.ataglanceseries.com/medicine

159 Hyperprolactinaemia and acromegaly

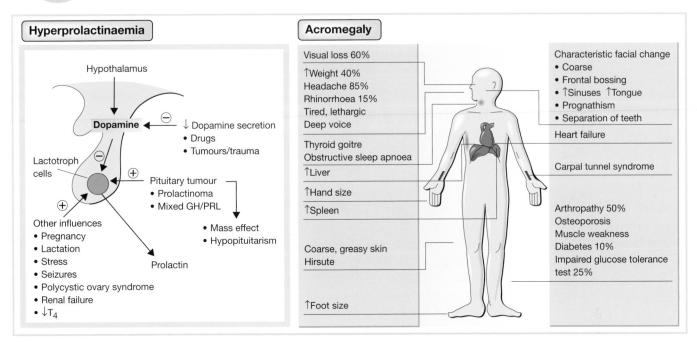

Hyperprolactinaemia

This is more obvious in women, because of presentation with menstrual disturbance or infertility.

- **Females**: milk production (galactorrhoea) in 30–80%, menstrual irregularity (oligo-/amenorrhoea), infertility.
- **Males**: galactorrhoea (<30%), erectile impotence, infertility ± features of a macroadenoma (mass effect, see Chapter 164).

Investigations

Prolactin levels can be very high. If the pathology is a macroadenoma, a full assessment of anterior pituitary function is needed. Women, probably because of the earlier presentation, are more likely to have a microprolactinoma. Stress, renal failure, hypothyroidism and polycystic ovary syndrome are all potent causes of hyperprolactinaemia and should be excluded. Other tests include: magnetic resonance imaging (MRI) of the pituitary and visual field measurement.

Management of prolactinomas

- **Drug treatment**: dopamine agonists (bromocriptine or cabergoline) inhibit prolactin (PRL) secretion and cause tumour shrinkage. Side effects include nausea, vomiting and postural hypotension.
- **Surgery**: trans-sphenoidal removal if there is drug intolerance or if the tumour fails to shrink on dopamine agonist therapy.
- **Radiotherapy**: to prevent tumour regrowth after drug treatment or surgery for macroadenoma.

Acromegaly

This is the clinical condition resulting from prolonged excessive growth hormone (GH) secretion in adults (excessive GH in children results in gigantism). Extremely rare: $5/10^6$ population; males = females; usually diagnosed at age 40–60 years. The underlying pathology is: (i) benign pituitary tumour (macroadenomas more common than microadenomas); (ii) pituitary carcinoma (very rare); and (iii) GH-releasing hormone-secreting carcinoid tumours (very rare).

The clinical syndrome results from insulin-like growth factor I (IGF-I) which mediates the effects of GH: increased sweating, headache (independent of tumour size), tiredness and lethargy; joint pains; effects of a mass in the pituitary fossa (visual field defects, hypopituitarism).

Examination: characteristic facial appearance (see Figure 159.1), deep voice, carpal tunnel syndrome, hand and foot enlargement and organomegaly (goitre, hepatosplenomegaly).

Complications: acromegaly increases cardiovascular morbidity and mortality, from hypertension, impaired glucose tolerance and diabetes mellitus. Cardiac failure (heart muscle disease), ischaemic heart and cerebrovascular disease are all increased. Obstructive sleep apnoea occurs. There may be an increased risk of colonic polyps and carcinoma.

Investigations and management

- **Laboratory tests**: IGF-I is high and GH levels are not suppressed by oral glucose.
- **Other investigations**: MRI scan of the pituitary and visual field assessment.

The aim of treatment is to normalize GH and reduce the associated high mortality:
- **Surgery**: trans-sphenoidal adenomectomy or craniotomy for very large tumours.
- **Pituitary radiotherapy**: useful if the tumour is not fully removed and reduces GH progressively over years.
- **Drugs**: somatostatin analogues (octreotide, lanreotide) suppress GH in 60%. Dopamine agonists (bromocriptine, cabergoline) lower but rarely normalize GH. GH receptor antagonist (pegvisomant) normalizes IGF-I in >90% of patients.

Medicine at a Glance, Fourth Edition. Edited by Patrick Davey. © 2014 John Wiley & Sons, Ltd. Published 2014 by John Wiley & Sons, Ltd. Companion website: www.ataglanceseries.com/medicine

160 Hypothyroidism

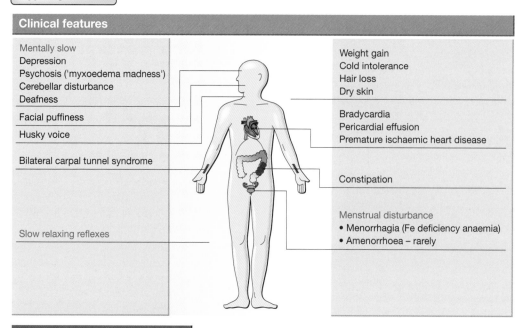

Hypothyroidism

Clinical features

Mentally slow
Depression
Psychosis ('myxoedema madness')
Cerebellar disturbance
Deafness

Facial puffiness

Husky voice

Bilateral carpal tunnel syndrome

Slow relaxing reflexes

Weight gain
Cold intolerance
Hair loss
Dry skin

Bradycardia
Pericardial effusion
Premature ischaemic heart disease

Constipation

Menstrual disturbance
• Menorrhagia (Fe deficiency anaemia)
• Amenorrhoea – rarely

Causes of hypothyroidism

Hypothalamo–pituitary disease (rare)

Thyroid synthetic failure
• Iodine excess, e.g. amiodarone
• Iodine deficiency →epidemic goitrous hypothyroidism
• Drugs, e.g. lithium

Iatrogenic
• Post surgery
• Post radio-iodine

Thyroid destruction (chronic inflammation)
• Hashimoto's (autoimmune) thyroiditis: very common, familial, with other autoimmune illnesses. Autoantibody to thyroglobulin and thyroid, peroxidase Goitre found
• Atrophic (autoimmune) hypothyroidism: elderly people, inhibitory autoantibody to TSH receptor. No goitre. Common
• Riedel's thyroiditis: woody sclerosis of thyroid, related to other sclerosing retroperitoneal fibrosis. Very rare

Hypothyroidism is the clinical state arising from decreased production of and/or the effect of thyroid hormones.

Epidemiology

The female:male ratio is 6:1 in primary hypothyroidism. The prevalence is 1–5%, and the incidence 2/1000. It is most common from middle age onwards and is often associated with a family history of autoimmune disease.

Causes

Thyroid failure can be caused by disease of the thyroid (primary hypothyroidism), the pituitary gland (secondary) or the hypothalamus (tertiary). Primary hypothyroidism is common and in Europe/North America is usually the result of autoimmune disease or previous radioiodine treatment for hyperthyroidism (50% hypothyroid at 10 years). Worldwide, the most common cause is iodine deficiency.

Although hypothyroidism can be congenital, the important causes in adult life are:

• **Autoimmune**: there are two forms of autoimmune thyroiditis, which are easily distinguished by the presence (Hashimoto's thyroiditis/lymphocytic) or absence (atrophic) of a goitre. In both, autoantibodies are found (see Investigations). Family members may have Addison's disease, pernicious anaemia or diabetes. Occasionally Hashimoto's thyroiditis gives rise to pain during the acute phase and, rarely, to transient hyperthyroidism.

• **Post-thyrotoxicosis treatment**: radioiodine, surgery, antithyroid drugs.

• **Iodine deficiency**: endemic goitre (e.g. Derbyshire neck) is the most common worldwide cause of hypothyroidism.

Medicine at a Glance, Fourth Edition. Edited by Patrick Davey. © 2014 John Wiley & Sons, Ltd. Published 2014 by John Wiley & Sons, Ltd. Companion website: www.ataglanceseries.com/medicine

- **Iodine excess**: chronic excess (e.g. amiodarone) may cause hypothyroidism.

Clinical features

See Figure 160.1.

Investigations

- **Haematology**: a full blood count shows a mild macrocytic anaemia (mean cell volume (MCV) = 95–110 fL). If haemoglobin is <10 g/dL, suspect an additional cause; if MCV is >115 fL, this may be pernicious anaemia (see Chapter 176), and if MCV is <85 fL it may be iron deficiency anaemia (menorrhagia).
- **Thyroid function tests**: low thyroxine (T_4) and elevated thyroid-stimulating hormone (TSH) – primary hypothyroidism; low or normal TSH – secondary/tertiary hypothyroidism.
- **Cortisol**: to exclude coexistent hypoadrenalism (Addison's disease or reduced adrenocorticotrophic hormone reserve in secondary hypothyroidism).
- **Thyroid antibodies**: positive peroxidase and thyroglobulin antibodies in Hashimoto's thyroiditis, and blocking TSH in atrophic thyroiditis.
- **Other biochemistry**: cholesterol levels are raised, as may be muscle enzyme levels (e.g. aspartate transaminase and creatine kinase).
- **Electrocardiogram**: bradycardia, low voltage complexes.

Management

This is with T_4, starting at 50 μg/day and increasing to 125–150 μg/day, with the dose titrated against clinical and biochemical (normal TSH) response. Lower starting doses, or triiodothyronine (T_3), which has a short half-life, may be used in elderly patients and patients with ischaemic heart disease because higher doses may provoke angina or myocardial infarction.

Myxoedema coma

This is a rare complication with a mortality rate >50%. It should be suspected in any patient with hypothermia and coma. It is difficult to distinguish from other causes of hypothermia, because the same risk factors (sedatives, age, etc.) are present. It is vital to start treatment immediately (before diagnostic biochemistry is available) with intravenous T_3 (20 μg bolus, repeated 6-hourly). As thyroid failure may relate to pituitary disease (suspect when the Na^+ is low), hydrocortisone should also be given (100 mg bolus, repeated 6-hourly) until an accurate diagnosis is made. Supportive therapy, including space blankets, antibiotics, fluids and correction of acidosis, may also be needed.

Congenital hypothyroidism

Though essentially beyond this textbook, it is none the less important to mention congenital hypothyroidism. The incidence varies from one per 1300 (Middle East) to one per 4000 births. Worldwide, this results most commonly from low environmental iodine levels ('endemic cretinism'). In the developed world, where iodine supplementation of the drinking water is common, endemic cretinism does not occur; sporadic cretinism does, however, and is commonly due to thyroid gland agenesis (50%), ectopia (25%), errors of metabolism (10%), and rarely (15%) from disorders in the hypothalamic–pituitary axis.

While *in utero*, the fetus receives thyroid hormone through the placenta from the mother, and so develops normally. However, after birth, this exogenous supply disappears – the infant is then deprived of thyroid hormone. This results in failure of the brain to develop, leading to profound developmental retardation and a syndrome previously called 'cretinism'. Treatment must be given early or permanent damage occurs. Many (though not all) of the deleterious effects of thyroid hormone deficiency can be prevented by early diagnosis and treatment (i.e. diagnosis by day 13 with normalization of thyroid hormone status by week 3). Since the clinical features can be far from obvious in infants, the best means of diagnosis is by biochemical assay. All children in the UK and developed countries are screened at birth for congenital hypothyroidism by assaying TSH levels.

161 Hyperthyroidism

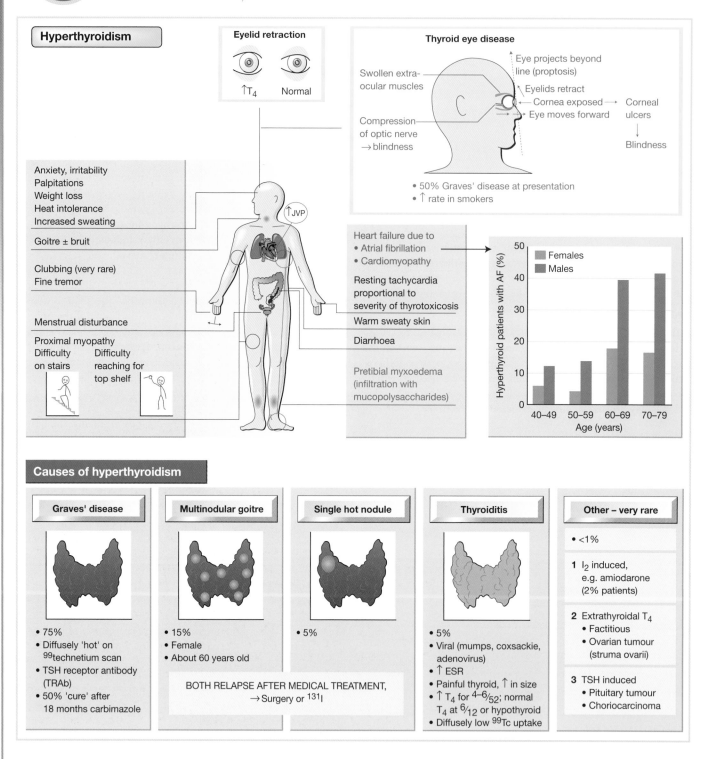

Hyperthyroidism

Eyelid retraction

↑T₄   Normal

Thyroid eye disease

Swollen extra-ocular muscles

Compression of optic nerve → blindness

Eye projects beyond line (proptosis)
Eyelids retract
Cornea exposed →
Eye moves forward

Corneal ulcers
↓
Blindness

- 50% Graves' disease at presentation
- ↑ rate in smokers

Anxiety, irritability
Palpitations
Weight loss
Heat intolerance
Increased sweating

Goitre ± bruit

Clubbing (very rare)
Fine tremor

Menstrual disturbance

Proximal myopathy
Difficulty on stairs   Difficulty reaching for top shelf

↑JVP

Heart failure due to
- Atrial fibrillation
- Cardiomyopathy

Resting tachycardia proportional to severity of thyrotoxicosis

Warm sweaty skin

Diarrhoea

Pretibial myxoedema (infiltration with mucopolysaccharides)

Graph: Hyperthyroid patients with AF (%) vs Age (years)
Females / Males
40–49, 50–59, 60–69, 70–79

Causes of hyperthyroidism

Graves' disease	Multinodular goitre	Single hot nodule	Thyroiditis	Other – very rare
• 75% • Diffusely 'hot' on ⁹⁹technetium scan • TSH receptor antibody (TRAb) • 50% 'cure' after 18 months carbimazole	• 15% • Female • About 60 years old	• 5%	• 5% • Viral (mumps, coxsackie, adenovirus) • ↑ ESR • Painful thyroid, ↑ in size • ↑ T₄ for $^{4-6}/_{52}$; normal T₄ at $^{6}/_{12}$ or hypothyroid • Diffusely low ⁹⁹Tc uptake	• <1% 1 I₂ induced, e.g. amiodarone (2% patients) 2 Extrathyroidal T₄ • Factitious • Ovarian tumour (struma ovarii) 3 TSH induced • Pituitary tumour • Choriocarcinoma

BOTH RELAPSE AFTER MEDICAL TREATMENT, → Surgery or ¹³¹I

Definition and epidemiology

The clinical condition is caused by increased circulating free levels of thyroid hormones. The prevalence is 2%. The male:female ratio is 1:5. It is most common in middle age.

Causes

The most common causes of hyperthyroidism are autoimmune thyroid disease (usually Graves' disease), a toxic nodular goitre and a toxic adenoma:

Medicine at a Glance, Fourth Edition. Edited by Patrick Davey. © 2014 John Wiley & Sons, Ltd. Published 2014 by John Wiley & Sons, Ltd. Companion website: www.ataglanceseries.com/medicine

- **Graves' disease**: 75% of cases. An autoimmune disorder in a genetically susceptible person (associated with CTLA4), resulting from the interaction of antibodies to immunoglobulin IgG thyroid-stimulating hormone (TSH) receptors with the thyroid gland TSH receptor, leading to thyroid gland stimulation, increased thyroxine (T_4) secretion and thyroid growth. Associated with Graves' disease is eye disease (ophthalmopathy) and organ-specific autoimmune disease.
- **Toxic multinodular goitre**: 15% of cases. Hyperthyroidism may develop in a long-standing goitre. Relapses after antithyroid drug therapy, so definitive surgery/radiotherapy is required.
- **Toxic adenoma** (single nodular goitre): 5% of cases. An autonomous hyperfunctioning nodule that produces excess thyroid hormones and suppresses TSH secretion.
- **Hashimoto's thyroiditis**: autoimmune (thyroid peroxidase antibody related), smooth thyroid enlargement; may produce hyper- and then hypothyroidism.
- **Postpartum thyroiditis**: usually self-limiting.
- **Rare causes** include: viral (de Quervain's) thyroiditis, drugs such as amiodarone, excessive T_4 replacement, iodine excess (Jod–Basedow effect), hypothalamic–pituitary disease (TSH-secreting tumour or pituitary resistance to thyroid hormones) or hyperemesis gravidarum (human chorionic gonadotrophin-mediated stimulation of the thyroid).

Clinical features

- Heat intolerance, increased sweating.
- Palpitations ± dyspnoea.
- Weight loss.
- Hyperactivity, insomnia.
- Increased stool frequency.
- Oligo-/amenorrhoea, reduced libido.

  In Graves' disease, the following also occur:

- Opthalmopathy, gritty eyes and lid lag.
- Periorbital oedema, chemosis.
- Diplopia due to extraocular muscle dysfunction.
- Poor vision due to optic neuropathy.
- Pretibial myxoedema (rare, <0.5%) and raised indurated lesions on shins, occasionally elsewhere.
- Thyroid acropachy (very rare), appearance of finger clubbing.

Investigations

- **Thyroid function tests**: increased T_4 and triiodothyronine (T_3), decreased TSH (primary hyperthyroidism).
- **Thyroid autoantibodies**: thyroid peroxidase and antithyroglobulin antibodies suggest an autoimmune aetiology.
- **Imaging**: thyroid uptake scan differentiates Graves' disease (diffusely increased uptake) from toxic adenoma (single hot spot) and multinodular goitre (multiple hot spots).

Management

- **Drug treatment**: first-line therapy in all patients regardless of diagnosis. Carbimazole decreases thyroid hormone synthesis; initial dose 20–60 mg/day, later reduced to a maintenance dose. The dose is titrated according to thyroid function and continued for 18 months, after which 50% patients with Graves' disease are cured. An alternative approach is to give a large dose of carbimazole with T_4 to avoid hypothyroidism ('block and replace' technique). Carbimazole causes agranulocytosis in 0.1%; it should be immediately stopped if sore throat or fever occurs. Propylthiouracil is an alternative antithyroid drug that is often preferred in pregnancy.
- **Surgery**: thyroidectomy for multinodular goitre, toxic adenoma or relapses of Graves' disease after antithyroid drug therapy. The risks are small but include vocal cord palsy (recurrent laryngeal nerve damage), hypothyroidism and hypoparathyroidism.
- **Radioiodine** is concentrated in the thyroid gland, so destroying thyroid tissue. Antithyroid drugs are stopped 7–10 days before administration to allow uptake of radioiodine. Occasionally repeated doses are required. Side effects: worsening of thyroid eye disease (may be the result of the aggravating effect of hypothyroidism), transient/permanent hypothyroidism (50% at 10 years), thyrotoxic crisis (if hyperthyroidism is poorly controlled before administration), pain.

Treatment of thyroid-associated ophthalmopathy

- Supportive: elevation of head of bed, artificial tears and prismatic glasses for diplopia.
- Definitive: medical with high-dose steroids ± other immunosuppressants (to decompress orbit), surgical orbital decompression or orbital radiotherapy.

Thyroid storm

This is a rare life-threatening emergency (mortality rate of 10% or more). Fever, anxiety, agitation, confusion and tachycardia, and occasionally heart failure, can also occur.

- Affects <2% of patients with hyperthyroidism.
- Treatment *must* be started before biochemical diagnosis (which takes too long).
- Mortality 10–20%.
- 50% of patients have lost >15 kg.
- Storm often provoked by minor physical stress.
- Severe symptoms of hyperthyroidism in most, though not always in the elderly (apathetic hyperthyroidism).
- Examination shows tachycardia, often very marked, sweating and sometimes confusion.
- Intensive care unit admission may be required, and should be anticipated.
- β-Blockers, often in high dose, are the mainstay of therapy.
- Give carbimazole or propylthiouracil immediately, by nasogastric tube if necessary.
- 1 hour later give iodide.
- Intravenous glucocorticoids are given in large doses to inhibit the synthesis of new circulating thyroid hormone.
- Fluid and electrolyte replacement as appropriate.

162 Calcium metabolism

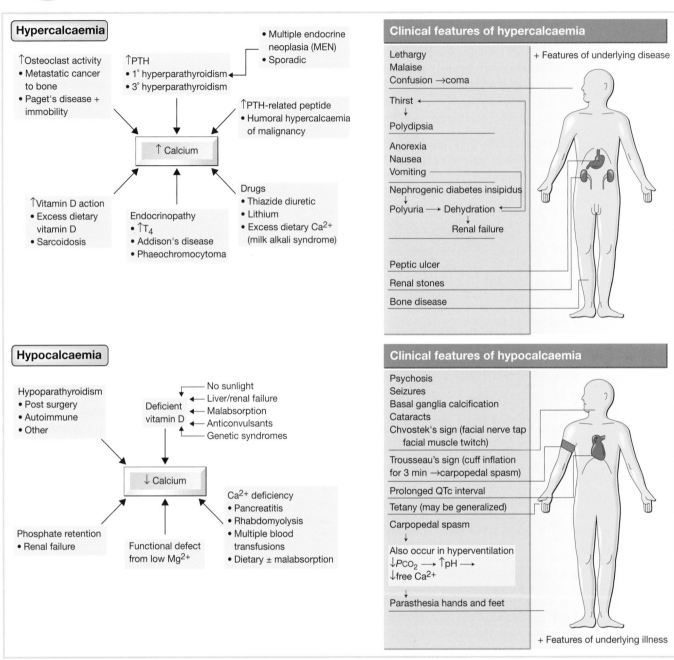

Hypercalcaemia

↑Osteoclast activity
- Metastatic cancer to bone
- Paget's disease + immobility

↑PTH
- 1° hyperparathyroidism
- 3° hyperparathyroidism

- Multiple endocrine neoplasia (MEN)
- Sporadic

↑PTH-related peptide
- Humoral hypercalcaemia of malignancy

↑ Calcium

↑Vitamin D action
- Excess dietary vitamin D
- Sarcoidosis

Endocrinopathy
- ↑T_4
- Addison's disease
- Phaeochromocytoma

Drugs
- Thiazide diuretic
- Lithium
- Excess dietary Ca^{2+} (milk alkali syndrome)

Clinical features of hypercalcaemia

+ Features of underlying disease

Lethargy
Malaise
Confusion →coma

Thirst
↓
Polydipsia

Anorexia
Nausea
Vomiting

Nephrogenic diabetes insipidus
↓
Polyuria → Dehydration
Renal failure

Peptic ulcer

Renal stones

Bone disease

Hypocalcaemia

Hypoparathyroidism
- Post surgery
- Autoimmune
- Other

Deficient vitamin D
- No sunlight
- Liver/renal failure
- Malabsorption
- Anticonvulsants
- Genetic syndromes

↓ Calcium

Ca^{2+} deficiency
- Pancreatitis
- Rhabdomyolysis
- Multiple blood transfusions
- Dietary ± malabsorption

Phosphate retention
- Renal failure

Functional defect from low Mg^{2+}

Clinical features of hypocalcaemia

Psychosis
Seizures
Basal ganglia calcification
Cataracts
Chvostek's sign (facial nerve tap facial muscle twitch)

Trousseau's sign (cuff inflation for 3 min →carpopedal spasm)

Prolonged QTc interval

Tetany (may be generalized)

Carpopedal spasm
↓
Also occur in hyperventilation
↓PCO_2 → ↑pH →
↓free Ca^{2+}

Parasthesia hands and feet

+ Features of underlying illness

Acute hypercalcaemia

The more rapid the rise and the higher the calcium level, the more likely are patients to present with an acute brain syndrome, comprising confusion, drowsiness and coma (rarely muscle weakness or psychosis). In less marked hypercalcaemia, there can be thirst and polyuria, from calcium-induced nephrogenic diabetes insipidus and abdominal symptoms such as anorexia, nausea and vomiting, abdominal pain and constipation. Chronic hypercalcaemia also produces renal stones and bone disease.

Aetiology

Hypercalcaemia occurs in 5–50 per 10 000. The diagnosis is achieved from the clinical situation and from biochemical tests. Key points are:

- Is malignancy present or likely clinically or on routine investigations?
- Is the parathyroid hormone (PTH) level high or suppressed? Normal (inappropriate in normally functioning parathyroid) or elevated PTH levels suggest primary hyperparathyroidism (far

Medicine at a Glance, Fourth Edition. Edited by Patrick Davey. © 2014 John Wiley & Sons, Ltd. Published 2014 by John Wiley & Sons, Ltd. Companion website: www.ataglanceseries.com/medicine

and away the most common cause), tertiary hyperparathyroidism (autonomous parathyroid glands in long-standing chronic renal failure) and rarely familial hypocalciuric or lithium-induced hypercalcaemia. Low PTH levels mean that the parathyroid gland is not responsible. Causes include malignancy, sarcoidosis, thyrotoxicosis and thiazide diuretic induced.

- Presence of associated biochemical and investigative abnormalities: elevated alkaline phosphatase, with deranged liver function tests, suggests malignancy. Paget's disease (mild hypercalcaemia on bed rest) usually has an isolated but large rise in alkaline phosphatase. Immunoglobulin electrophoresis may show a paraprotein band in myeloma. The chest X-ray may show sarcoidosis (bilateral hilar adenopathy) or cancer.
- A full dietary and drug history for excess vitamin D or calcium-containing antacids (milk–alkali syndrome), thiazides and lithium.

Causes

Primary hyperparathyroidism

This is the most common cause of hypercalcaemia; the female : male ratio is 2:1 and 90% of patients are >50 years (when female incidence is 3/1000). Symptoms of hypercalcaemia may occur, although 50% are asymptomatic patients undergoing biochemical assessment for other reasons. In 80%, the pathology is a single parathyroid adenoma; occasionally diffuse hyperplasia of all four glands occurs. Very rarely multiple endocrine neoplasia (MEN) 1 or 2 is present (see Chaper 164). In asymptomatic elderly patients with mild hypercalcaemia, an expectant course may be followed. In all others, definitive treatment is surgical resection, with the parathyroid adenoma being located by the surgeon at the time of operation. Imaging studies (nuclear or ultrasound scans) are required if the adenoma is not found at initial operation. Postoperative hypocalcaemia is usually transient and is treated with calcium supplements and 1α-hydroxy vitamin D.

Hypercalcaemia of malignancy

This is the second most common cause of hypercalcaemia. There are two underlying mechanisms:

1 **Tumour deposits in bone**: most (>95%) hypercalcaemia in malignancy relates to widespread metastatic disease. The most common neoplasms are lung, breast and myeloma. Patients are usually highly symptomatic both from the cancer and, as calcium levels are high and have risen quickly, from hypercalcaemia.
2 **Humoral hypercalcaemia of malignancy** relates to PTH-related peptide, a peptide made up of 144 amino acids, which bears a structural relationship to PTH and mimics its action. The responsible neoplasm is most likely to be squamous carcinoma of the lung, although it can be a genitourinary or gynaecological malignancy. Although humoral hypercalcaemia of malignancy is rare, its clinical importance is that *not all patients with malignancy and hypercalcaemia necessarily have metastatic disease*. This point is vital in deciding whether or not the primary should be resected.

Sarcoidosis and other granulomatous diseases

These are associated with hypercalcaemia, which responds readily to steroids.

Other causes of hypercalcaemia

Thyrotoxicosis and thiazide diuretics can induce hypercalcaemia. Familial hypocalciuric hypercalcaemia is an autosomal dominant inherited condition in which hypercalcaemia is associated with low renal excretion of calcium. Paget's disease can also induce hypercalcaemia.

Management

Acute/symptomatic hypercalcaemia is a medical emergency and requires urgent treatment, principally aggressive rehydration with physiological or 0.9% **saline**, which alone readily lowers calcium. **Loop diuretics** can be added to fluid therapy once adequate hydration has occurred. **Bisphosphonates** are also effective regardless of the underlying pathology. **Steroids** may be added in hypercalcaemia of malignancy and vitamin D-related hypercalcaemia. **Calcitonin** helps in Paget's disease. Definitive therapy varies according to the underlying disease.

Hypocalcaemia

Acute hypocalcaemia results in circumoral tingling, tetany, especially in the muscles supplied by long nerves, and seizures. Chvostek's sign (a tap to the facial nerve just anterior to the ear causing a brief facial muscle contraction) and Trousseau's sign (inflation of a blood pressure cuff resulting in carpopedal spasm) occur. Chronic hypocalcaemia in addition results in basal ganglia calcification and cataracts.

Aetiology

Hypocalcaemia is rare, and usually relates to one of four diseases:

- **Secondary hyperparathyroidism**: the most common cause of hypocalcaemia, occurring in acute or chronic renal failure. Failure of renal vitamin D hydroxylation – together with phosphate retention (through the calcium phosphate double product) – depresses serum Ca^{2+}, stimulating PTH release in an attempt to normalize serum Ca^{2+}. This leads to osteoclast activation, cyst formation and bone marrow fibrosis (osteitis fibrosa cystica), which together with aluminium toxicity contribute to renal bone disease. Characteristic X-ray findings are found in the hand, skull ('pepper pot') and spine ('rugger jersey'). The diagnosis is usually obvious from creatinine and phosphate levels and the characteristic radiology. Treatment is with vitamin D and phosphate binders. If secondary hyperparathyroidism is left untreated, parathyroid gland hyperplasia leads to autonomous production of PTH – resulting in tertiary hyperparathyroidism with frank hypercalcaemia.
- **Post-thyroid/parathyroid surgery**: transient hypocalcaemia may occur.
- **Idiopathic autoimmune parathyroid failure**: very rare. Parathyroid autoantibodies are found. Other autoimmune conditions (vitiligo, etc.) may occur.
- **Osteomalacia**: resulting from inadequate active vitamin D. It is associated with low calcium levels, although these are usually not so low as to cause symptoms. Osteomalacia may be compounded by dietary calcium deficiency or relate to malabsorption.

Treatment

- **Acute symptoms** ($Ca^{2+} < 1.9$ mmol/L): intravenous (IV) bolus of 10% calcium gluconate 10–20 mL with electrocardiogram monitoring followed by IV infusion if necessary. Oral calcium and vitamin D as soon as possible. IV magnesium sulphate may be required.
- **Chronic disease**: vitamin D metabolites (calcitriol or alphacalcidol) and oral calcium.

163 Adrenal disease

Adrenal disease

Addison's disease (hypoadrenalism)

Pigmentation
- Buccal
- Scars
- Palmar creases
- Generalized

Fatigue
Anorexia
Weight loss
Dizzy on standing
(postural hypotension)

Abdominal pain
Diarrhoea

May present with acute crisis
(see text)

± Associated diseases
- Hypothyroid
- Diabetes type I
- Pernicious anaemia
- Vitiligo
- Others

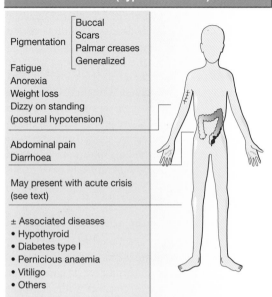

Phaeochromocytoma

Catecholamine-secreting tumour

1/2–1/3 sustained ↑BP
Weight loss
Anxiety
Occasionally myocardial damage
→heart failure

Very rarely, if mainly dopamine
secreted →hypotensive attacks

Classically produces paroxysmal
symptoms:
- Sweating
- Headache
- Palpitations
- Anxiety
- ↑BP

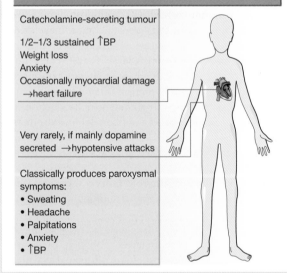

Cushing's syndrome

♀:♂ = 4:1
Depression
Psychosis
Thinned hair
'Moon face'
Acne
Hirsutism

Supraclavicular fat pad

Hypertension
Premature ischaemic heart
disease
Obesity – centripetal
('lemon on a stick')
Peptic ulcer
Purple striae (from weight gain)
Dysmenorrhoea
Impotence

Proximal myopathy
Thin skin
Easy bruising

Causes

Adrenocorticotropic hormone (ACTH) dependent
- Pituitary adenoma (Cushing's disease) (70%) F>M
- Ectopic ACTH (14%)
  Bronchial carcinoma
  Carcinoid – lung, gastrointestinal tract, thymus

ACTH independent
- Adrenal adenoma (10%)
- Adrenal carcinoma (5%)
- Adrenal hyperplasia (1%)

Differential diagnosis
- Pseudo-Cushing's due to alcoholism or depression

Adrenal failure

This is failure of adrenal steroid hormone production:
- Atrophy/destruction of the adrenal gland (primary adrenal failure).
- Inadequate adrenocorticotrophin hormone (ACTH) production (secondary adrenal failure): the most common cause, resulting from acute steroid withdrawal.

Cortisol is needed for the stress response to infection, surgery and trauma. In primary adrenal failure, cortisol deficiency increases ACTH and melanocyte-stimulating hormone production, causing hyperpigmentation – seen in the buccal mucosa, on the palms of hands and in scars. Hyperpigmentation does not occur in secondary adrenal failure (depressed ACTH).

- **Primary adrenal failure**: rare, occurring in $50/10^6$. Autoimmune (Addison's) adrenal destruction, associated with vitiligo, premature ovarian failure and hypothyroidism. Females > males; gradual onset of symptoms; worldwide; tuberculosis destruction of the adrenal glands is more common. Other causes are very rare:
  - Infection (HIV, fungi).
  - Invasion with cancer cells (lymphoma, breast, lung).
  - Haemorrhage: anticoagulants, Waterhouse–Friedrichsen syndrome from meningococcal septicaemia-induced disseminated intravascular coagulation – adrenal failure occurs days/weeks after the initial haemorrhage-induced cortisol release.
  - Infiltration (amyloid, sarcoid, haemochromatosis).
  - Congenital adrenal hyperplasia and drugs (ketoconazole).
- **Secondary adrenal failure**: common; chronic steroid therapy suppresses ACTH levels, producing adrenal cortex atrophy.

Medicine at a Glance, Fourth Edition. Edited by Patrick Davey. © 2014 John Wiley & Sons, Ltd. Published 2014 by John Wiley & Sons, Ltd. Companion website:
www.ataglanceseries.com/medicine

Physical stress or over-quick steroid withdrawal can then provoke acute adrenal failure. Pituitary failure (rare) can occur.

Clinical features of Addison's disease

- Chronic adrenal failure presents with a myriad of vague symptoms, including fatigue, weight loss, anorexia, abdominal pain, diarrhoea and postural hypotension.
- Acute adrenal failure presents with hypovolaemic shock precipitated by intercurrent stress. Untreated, this leads to refractory shock, profound hypoglycaemia and death.

Investigations

Acute adrenal failure should always be suspected in shock with hyponatraemia ($\pm$ hyperkalaemia and hypoglycaemia). Hyponatraemia occurs late in the disease, but only in primary adrenal failure (mineralocorticoid deficiency) not in secondary adrenal failure where the rennin–angiotensin system remains intact. Cortisol is low or normal; ACTH is high in primary failure and low in secondary failure.

- **Short synacthen test**: adrenal stimulation using synthetic ACTH fails to produce cortisol when given only once in adrenal failure from any cause.
- **Long synacthen test**: if ACTH is given repetitively over 3 days, and if it has not been destroyed, the adrenal will produce cortisol.

Adrenal autoantibodies are found in autoimmune Addison's disease. Imaging (computed tomography (CT)) or biopsy is used when rare diseases are suspected.

Management

- **Chronic adrenal failure**: glucocorticoid replacement with hydrocortisone 20 mg/day in divided doses, doubled with treatment of infection or intercurrent illness, or surgery. Mineralocorticoid replacement (fludrocortisone) only in primary adrenal failure.
- **Acute adrenal failure**: a medical emergency. Large volumes of intravenous fluid (physiological saline) and hydrocortisone are given at high doses. The precipitant (infection, etc.) may also need treating. Monitor electrolytes and glucose.

Hyperaldosteronism

This causes treatment-resistant hypertension (2% of hypertension) with hypokalaemia. Occasionally K^+ is normal if salt intake is low. The causes are:

- Benign adenoma (Conn's syndrome) (66%).
- Bilateral adrenal hyperplasia (30%).
- Rarely glucocorticoid remedial aldosteronism or adrenal carcinoma.

Laboratory tests demonstrate hypokalaemia, increased urinary K^+ excretion, suppressed renin and elevated aldosterone. A CT scan of the adrenal glands helps define the pathology. A radiolabelled cholesterol scan and adrenal vein sampling are occasionally useful. Treatment is with surgery (laparoscopic adrenalectomy) for Conn's adenoma and aldosterone antagonists (spironolactone or eplerenone) and potassium-sparing diuretics (amiloride) for other causes.

Phaeochromocytoma

This is a catecholamine-producing tumour of the adrenal medulla. It accounts for <0.5% of hypertension and has an equal sex incidence. It is most common at age 30–50 years. The 10% rule applies: 10% malignant, 10% multiple, 10% bilateral, 10% extra-adrenal and 10% familial (von Hippel–Lindau syndrome, neurofibromatosis, multiple endocrine neoplasia 2). Characteristically, it produces paroxysmal symptoms: labile hypertension (crises precipitated by exercise, abdominal examination, surgery, general anaesthesia, β-blockade), palpitations, sweating, headache, pallor or flushing, anxiety and glucose intolerance.

Investigations, management and prognosis

Catecholamine metabolites are detected in the urine. Adrenal imaging with magnetic resonance imaging (MRI) or meta-iodobenzylguanidine scan (avidly taken up by chromaffin cells) may demonstrate multiple tumours or metastases.

- **Initial management**: at diagnosis α-adrenoreceptor blockade (phenoxybenzamine) before β-blockade (propranolol).
- **Definitive management**: adrenalectomy for tumour removal. Preoperative α- and β-blockade are vital because tumour handling may precipitate a crisis. Surgery is curative in >90% in benign disease; recurrence occurs in <10%. The 5-year survival rate is ≥95% for treated benign tumours but <50% for malignant tumours.

Cushing's syndrome

This is the clinical condition resulting from prolonged exposure to excessive glucocorticoids from:

- Exogenous glucocorticoid administration.
- Endogenous hypersecretion of glucocorticoids: very rare ($1-4/10^6$).

Investigations

- **Confirm Cushing's syndrome**: diagnosed when the 24-hour urinary free cortisol is increased, midnight cortisol is detectable and 9 a.m. cortisol is detectable after 48 hours of low-dose dexamethasone.
- **Determine the cause**: ACTH levels are normal/increased in ACTH-dependent cases or low in ACTH-independent cases. Serum K^+ <3.2 mmol/L suggests ectopic ACTH secretion. In pituitary-dependent cases (termed Cushing's disease), there is a 50% suppression of serum cortisol with high-dose dexamethasone and no suppression in ectopic disease. Adrenal imaging can be helpful.
- **Corticotrophin-releasing hormone (CRH) test**: administer CRH and measure cortisol. Pituitary disease – excessive rise; ectopic disease – flat response.
- **Venous sampling**: inferior petrosal sinus sampling to confirm pituitary-dependent disease. Body sampling to locate ectopic source of ACTH.
- **Imaging**: Cushing's disease is usually the result of a microadenoma, which may not be visible on MRI. CT of chest or elsewhere used to locate ectopic sources of ACTH.

Management and prognosis

- **Drug treatment**: metyrapone (blocks cortisol synthesis) or ketoconazole (inhibits cytochrome P450 enzyme) lower cortisol levels short term before surgery or long term when surgery is inappropriate.
- **Pituitary adenoma**: trans-sphenoidal adenomectomy produces remission in >70% cases; radiotherapy is used for uncured relapse. Bilateral adrenalectomy produces aggressive pituitary tumour enlargement and hyperpigmentation as a result of excessive ACTH secretion (Nelson's syndrome) unless pituitary radiotherapy is also given.
- **Adrenal adenoma**: adrenalectomy is curative.
- **Adrenal carcinoma**: surgery is not curative. Drug treatment with mitotane, an adrenolytic agent, can be helpful.
- **Ectopic secretion**: surgical removal of tumour if possible, otherwise medical treatment or adrenalectomy.

Untreated, Cushing's syndrome has a survival of <5 years as a result of cardiovascular disease or infection.

164 Miscellaneous endocrine disorders

Pituitary tumours

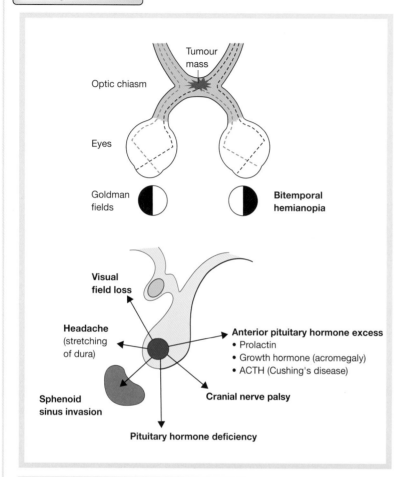

Diabetes insipidus

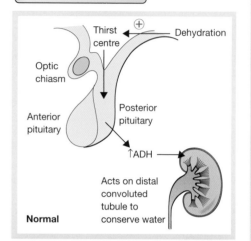

Causes of diabetes insipidus

Cranial
- Familial
- Idiopathic
- Trauma to hypothalamo–pituitary region
- Surgical treatment of pituitary tumours
- Infiltration of posterior pituitary/hypothalamus (secondary deposits, sarcoid)
- Infections (meningitis, TB)

Nephrogenic
- Familial
- Post-obstructive uropathy
- Hypokalaemia/hypercalcaemia
- Sickle cell anaemia
- Amyloid

Pituitary hormone deficiency

Characteristic sequence of loss in pituitary macroadenomas

Earliest → Latest

Hormone	GH	FSH/LH	ACTH	TSH	Prolactin	ADH
Clinical features	Loss of well-being	• No 2° sexual hair • Infertile • Impotent	• Pale • Hypoadrenal	• Hypothyroid	• Lactatory failure	• Diabetes insipidus
Deficiency diagnosed by	• GH after stimulation (insulin, arginine, glucagon) • Insulin-like growth factor-I (IGF-I)	♂ • [Testosterone] ♀ • Pre-menopause: periods • Post-menopause: [LH] [FSH]	• Short synacthen test • Insulin tolerance test	• TSH • T₄	Prolactin	• Serum Na⁺ • Osmolality • Water deprivation test

Medicine at a Glance, Fourth Edition. Edited by Patrick Davey. © 2014 John Wiley & Sons, Ltd. Published 2014 by John Wiley & Sons, Ltd. Companion website: www.ataglanceseries.com/medicine

Table 164.1 Pathophysiology of diabetes insipidus (DI).

	[Na⁺]	Osmolality of plasma	Urine	Urine osmolality on water deprivation	Response to synthetic ADH
Cranial DI	↑	↑	↓	Fails to concentrate	Normal
Nephrogenic DI	↑	↑	↓	Fails to concentrate	Fails to concentrate
Primary polydipsia	↓	↓	↓	Concentrates	Normal

Diseases of the pituitary gland

Pituitary gland diseases are rare, and may be characterized by selective or total (pan-hypopituitary) pituitary failure, visual failure, selective excess in pituitary-dependent hormones (tumours) and hyperprolactinaemia (from mass lesions). Pituitary diseases include:

- Intrinsic neoplastic processes: may result in pituitary failure, mass effects (headaches, visual failure), and a selective increase in a pituitary-dependent hormone or hyperprolactinaemia.
- Inflammation (tuberculosis, sarcoidosis) and invasion by extrinsic tumours result in pituitary failure and, occasionally, in hyperprolactinaemia, by disruption of the tonic dopamine-mediated inhibition to prolactin release.
- Pituitary apoplexy: infarction not related to hypotension.
- Pituitary atrophy: infarction related to hypotension, often postpartum (Sheehan's syndrome). Pituitary failure occurs early or up to 2 years after the hypotensive event.

Pituitary tumours

Pituitary tumours are the most common pituitary disorder and account for 10% of intracranial neoplasms. Tumours are classified according to size:

- **Microadenoma**: <1 cm in diameter; do not cause mass effects or hypopituitarism.
- **Macroadenoma**: >1 cm; can produce mass effects and hypopituitarism. Usually non-functioning, but can cause excessive hormonal secretion. Non-functioning macroadenomas are the most common form.

The clinical features of pituitary tumours are predictable based on which hormones have been lost or gained.

Investigations aim to determine:

- Pituitary function: hormones (and their targets) are measured: growth hormone (GH) (insulin-like growth factor I (IGF-I)); follicle-stimulating hormone (FSH) and luteinizing hormone (LH) (testosterone/oestradiol); adrenocorticotrophic hormone (ACTH) (cortisol ± dynamic tests); thyroid-stimulating hormone (TSH) (thyroxine (T_4)) and prolactin. Antidiuretic hormone (ADH) is assessed from serum Na⁺ and dynamic tests.
- Underlying disease process: assessed by magnetic resonance imaging ± biopsy.
- Mass effect of the tumour: visual field loss (bitemporal hemianopia from compression of the optic chiasma), headache (dural stretching), cranial nerve palsies (lateral extension) or cerebrospinal fluid rhinorrhoea/secondary meningitis (downward erosion into sphenoid sinus).

Management

- **Replacement of anterior pituitary hormones**: hydrocortisone and T_4 to replace ACTH and TSH deficiency; sex hormone and GH therapy.

- **Treatment of underlying cause**: non-functioning tumours are treated surgically (trans-sphenoidally or by craniotomy) and may need postoperative radiotherapy. Functioning tumours are treated by a combination of drugs, surgery and radiotherapy.
- **Functioning tumours**: prolactin (hyperprolactinaemia, see Chapter 159), GH (acromegaly, see Chapter 159) and ACTH (Cushing's disease, see Chapter 163).

Diabetes insipidus

This is the passage of large volumes of inappropriately dilute urine in the presence of concentrated plasma. It is uncommon, and has to be differentiated from other causes of polyuria (urine volume >2.5 L/day) and polydipsia, which include:

- Diabetes mellitus.
- Renal failure.
- Primary polydipsia, usually psychogenic in origin.
- Diabetes insipidus: cranial (relative/absolute vasopressin ADH deficiency) or nephrogenic (renal resistance to vasopressin, e.g. as a result of lithium toxicity) diabetes insipidus.

Pathophysiology and causes are shown in Figure 164.1 and investigations are shown in Table 164.1.

Treatment

This is by unrestricted access to fluid and desmopressin (long-acting ADH analogue).

Syndrome of inappropriate ADH secretion

The syndrome of inappropriate ADH secretion (SIADH) is a common cause of hyponatraemia. For a full discussion see Chapter 142.

Multiple endocrine neoplasia

Multiple endocrine neoplasia (MEN) syndromes are very rare conditions in which a single gene defect causes multiple endocrine tumours within a patient. MEN syndromes most commonly present with disorders of calcium metabolism (see Chapter 162). Probands and their families need to be regularly screened for new malignancies.

- **MEN 1**: parathyroid hyperplasia 95%, pituitary adenoma 70%, pancreatic islet tumour 40%; adrenal and thyroid adenomas; mutation in a recessive oncogene on chromosome 11q13 – encoding menin.
- **MEN 2a**: medullary thyroid cancer; parathyroid hyperplasia; phaeochromocytoma 70% bilateral.
- **MEN 2b**: also has marfanoid habitus and mucosal neuromas. Dominant oncogene on chromosome 10 (ret proto-oncogene).

165 Hypogonadism

Male hypogonadism

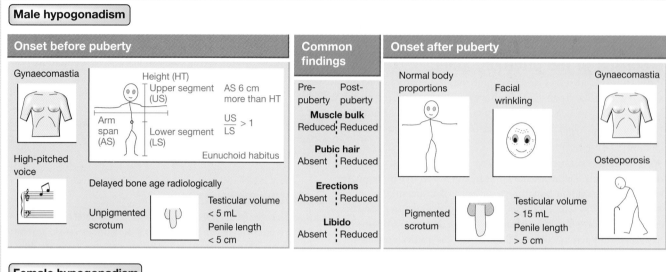

Onset before puberty

Gynaecomastia

High-pitched voice

Height (HT)
Upper segment (US)
AS 6 cm more than HT
Arm span (AS)
Lower segment (LS)
$\frac{US}{LS} > 1$
Eunuchoid habitus

Delayed bone age radiologically

Unpigmented scrotum

Testicular volume < 5 mL
Penile length < 5 cm

Common findings

	Pre-puberty	Post-puberty
Muscle bulk	Reduced	Reduced
Pubic hair	Absent	Reduced
Erections	Absent	Reduced
Libido	Absent	Reduced

Onset after puberty

Normal body proportions

Facial wrinkling

Gynaecomastia

Osteoporosis

Pigmented scrotum

Testicular volume > 15 mL
Penile length > 5 cm

Female hypogonadism

Clinical evaluation in suspected hypogonadal women

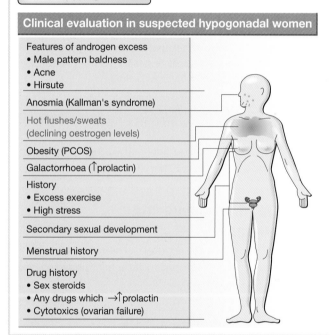

Features of androgen excess
• Male pattern baldness
• Acne
• Hirsute

Anosmia (Kallman's syndrome)

Hot flushes/sweats (declining oestrogen levels)

Obesity (PCOS)

Galactorrhoea (↑prolactin)

History
• Excess exercise
• High stress

Secondary sexual development

Menstrual history

Drug history
• Sex steroids
• Any drugs which →↑prolactin
• Cytotoxics (ovarian failure)

Turner's phenotype (45 X0)

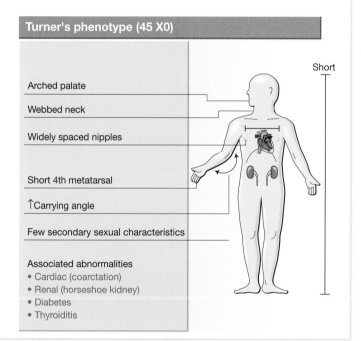

Short

Arched palate

Webbed neck

Widely spaced nipples

Short 4th metatarsal

↑Carrying angle

Few secondary sexual characteristics

Associated abnormalities
• Cardiac (coarctation)
• Renal (horseshoe kidney)
• Diabetes
• Thyroiditis

Hypogonadism is the failure of the ovaries or testis to produce sex steroids (oestrogen or testosterone) from either gonadal failure (primary hypogonadism) or hypothalamic–pituitary failure (secondary hypogonadism). The key difference between primary and secondary hypogonadism is whether luteinizing hormone (LH)/follicle-stimulating hormone (FSH) levels are high (intact hypothalamic–pituitary axis) or low (damaged hypothalamic–pituitary axis) (see Table 165.1).

Male hypogonadism

The clinical features of pre- and postpubescent male hypogonadism are shown in Figure 165.1. Acquired hypogonadism affects 20% of all men.

Primary male hypogonadism

Primary hypogonadism (testicular failure) arises from systemic disease; renal failure and cirrhosis (especially alcohol abuse) are important causes. Of adult men with mumps, 25% develop orchitis and half of these progress to late gonadal failure (primary hypogonadism). Other viral causes of orchitis are also important. Cryptorchidism is a not uncommon cause, as is testicular trauma or torsion. Gonadal radiotherapy or systemic anticancer cytotoxic drugs are more rare but still very powerful stimuli for gonadal failure. Rare diseases causing testicular failure include Klinefelter's syndrome (XXY karyotype, one in 1000 births, causing small testis and gynaecomastia, and eunuch-like appearance from testosterone deficiency); azoospermia contributes to infertility.

Table 165.1 Differences between primary and secondary hypogonadism.

	LH/FSH	Testosterone or oestrogen	Other tests
Primary hypogonadism	↑	↓	Karyotype
Secondary hypogonadism	↓	↓	Prolactin, MRI of pituitary fossa/hypothalamus

Secondary male hypogonadism

Secondary hypogonadism (hypothalamic–pituitary failure) may be caused by severe illness or malnutrition, pituitary disease (especially a hyperprolactinaemia) and Kallman's syndrome. This is a genetic X-linked syndrome (autosomal dominant or autosomal recessive) with a male:female ratio of 4:1, a male prevalence of one in 10 000, and causing isolated failure of hypothalamic gonadotrophin-releasing hormone (GnRH) release with anosmia; magnetic resonance imaging (MRI) may show absent olfactory bulbs.

Management

Androgen replacement therapy will relieve symptoms and prevent osteoporosis, but will not improve fertility, which is irreversible in primary hypogonadism. Gonadotrophins or GnRH are used to induce fertility in secondary hypogonadism.

Female hypogonadism

The symptoms of female hypogonadism are of fatigue and amenorrhoea with infertility. In primary hypogonadism, oestrogen withdrawal symptoms also occur: hot flushes and sweats, mood changes, vaginal dryness and pain on intercourse. The signs of established female hypogonadism include fine facial wrinkling, breast involution and a general reduction in body hair.

Primary female hypogonadism

Primary hypogonadism (ovarian failure) may relate to genetic or acquired diseases, and occurs in 1% of women aged <40 years and accounts for 10% of secondary amenorrhoea.

● **Genetic causes of ovarian failure**: chromosomal abnormalities underlie 60% of cases. Turner's syndrome (45XO) affects one in 2000 women, causes gonadal dysgenesis and is the most common chromosomal abnormality associated with primary hypogonadism. The usual course is delayed puberty leading to premature gonadal failure. Short stature and a characteristic phenotype are found, and there may be associated cardiac (aortic coarctation), endocrine (hypothyroidism), skeletal and renal abnormalities.
● **Acquired premature ovarian failure**: results from autoimmune disease (the most common cause of premature menopause); it may be idiopathic or relate to cytotoxic chemotherapy.

Secondary female hypogonadism

In secondary hypogonadism (hypothalamic–pituitary failure) hypogonadotrophic hypogonadism results from hypothalamic or pituitary disease, including tumours (see Chapter 164), hyperprolactinaemia (see Chapter 159) or extreme physical or psychological stress, including anorexia nervosa.

Management

In ovarian failure, treatment is with oestrogens, which alleviate deficiency symptoms and prevent long-term complications, such as osteoporosis. Progestogens are added for women with an intact uterus to avoid endometrial hyperplasia and subsequent endometrial carcinoma. Oocyte donation is needed for fertility. In secondary hypogonadism, it is vital to have a full assessment of the hypothalamic–pituitary axis functionally and structurally, to diagnose and treat any underlying disease. Gonadotrophins (FSH/human menopausal gonadotrophin + human chorionic gonadotrophin (hCG), or pulsatile GnRH therapy) are used to induce fertility in hypogonadotrophic hypogonadism.

Menstrual failure (amenorrhoea)

Menstrual failure is associated with infertility, oestrogen deficiency (increased osteoporosis and cardiovascular disease risk) and increased risk of endometrial carcinoma (in polycystic ovary syndrome (PCOS)). The definitions of menstrual failure are: primary amenorrhoea – failure of menarche by 16 years; secondary amenorrhoea – failure of menstruation for >6 months in women who have previously menstruated, affecting 3–9% of women of reproductive age; oligomenorrhoea – fewer than nine menstrual periods/year. Important causes of amenorrhoea are:

● **Pregnancy**: should always be excluded by measuring hCG in the urine.
● **Illness, malnutrition and overexercise**: all are usually readily apparent.
● **Endocrine disease** such as hyperthyroidism or excess of androgens (see Chapter 40).
● **Primary or secondary hypogonadism**, investigated as outlined above.
● **PCOS**: symptoms may be mild or severe (Stein–Leventhal syndrome). In PCOS excess androgen production occurs, mainly from the ovary (where multiple small cysts are found), but also from the adrenal glands, resulting in disruption of the menstrual cycle (mild to profound) and mild androgenization, mainly hirsutism (see Chapter 40) or acne. More profound virilization suggests pathology other than PCOS (particularly virilizing tumours). Insulin resistance and dyslipidaemia are also common features. Examination often shows marked obesity, with hirsutism and acne. Cushing's disease and late-onset congenital adrenal hyperplasia may need to be excluded. Investigations show mildly elevated androgen levels, normal oestrogen and normal/elevated LH. Ovarian ultrasonography may demonstrate multiple small (3–5 mm) cysts. Androgen levels are mildly elevated, oestrogen levels are usually normal and LH levels may or may not be raised. There is no completely satisfactory treatment. Weight reduction, metformin (insulin sensitizer), anti-androgens (cyproterone) with contraception, ovarian suppression with the combined oral contraceptive pill, and ovarian diathermy all have a role.
● **Hyperprolactinaemia**: although it may relate to pituitary disease, drugs, hypothyroidism or PCOS, in practice this commonly relates to substantial physical or psychological stress.
● Rarely, **structural disease** such as an imperforate hymen or absent uterus underlies primary amenorrhoea.

166 Bacteraemia and septic shock

Organs affected by septic shock

	Brain 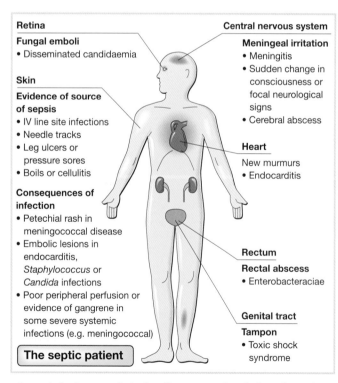	Lungs	Cardiovascular system	Kidneys	Clotting system
Syndrome	Acute confusional state/coma	Adult respiratory distress syndrome (ARDS)	Circulatory failure	Acute renal failure	Haemostatic failure
Examination and investigations	Glasgow Coma Scale Focal neurological defect May need to exclude 1° intracerebral infection: • CT head • Lumbar puncture	Respiratory rate O_2 saturation Arterial blood gases Chest X-ray Occasionally: • CT chest • Bronchoscopy with BAL	Blood pressure Skin warmth/perfusion JVP (central venous pressure) Cardiac output (on ITU) Occasionally, cardiac ultrasound	Urine output Urea/creatinine (2x daily) K^+ Acidosis–blood gases Renal tract ultrasound, to exclude obstruction	Spontaneous bleeding/bruising Prolonged bleeding from venepuncture sites Thrombin time APTT Platelets D-dimers, FDPs
Treatment	Treat underlying condition: • Anticonvulsants for seizures	• High-dose oxygen (unless COPD) • Artificial ventilation	• Fluids (crystalloids/ blood) to keep central pressure high, without pulmonary oedema • If very vasodilated, use vasoconstrictors • If cardiac output low, consider inotropes (prognosis very poor)	• Fluids • Renal vasodilators (dopamine/furosemide) are often tried, to little effect • Haemofiltration	• Platelets • Clotting factors (e.g. FFP) • Control of infection

Retina

Fungal emboli
• Disseminated candidaemia

Skin

Evidence of source of sepsis
• IV line site infections
• Needle tracks
• Leg ulcers or pressure sores
• Boils or cellulitis

Consequences of infection
• Petechial rash in meningococcal disease
• Embolic lesions in endocarditis, *Staphylococcus* or *Candida* infections
• Poor peripheral perfusion or evidence of gangrene in some severe systemic infections (e.g. meningococcal)

The septic patient

Central nervous system

Meningeal irritation
• Meningitis
• Sudden change in consciousness or focal neurological signs
• Cerebral abscess

Heart
New murmurs
• Endocarditis

Rectum

Rectal abscess
• Enterobacteraciae

Genital tract

Tampon
• Toxic shock syndrome

Some infections result in locally contained pathology but others trigger a systemic inflammatory response known as sepsis. This is a clinical syndrome thought to be caused by dysregulation of proinflammatory mediators, which cause tissue damage. The result is a chain of deteriorating clinical conditions:

Infection → sepsis → severe sepsis → septic shock

Definitions

• **Bacteraemia**: presence of viable bacteria in the blood, normally diagnosed by blood culture. Sustained bacteraemia may result in a systemic response, but bacteraemia can also occur transiently with little or no clinical effect, e.g. transient bacteraemia is common after teeth brushing, etc.

Other infections such as fungaemias and localized infections, which result in a significant immune activation, can also trigger sepsis responses.

• **Sepsis**: evidence of infection with a systemic response, including two or more of following:
  • Temperature >38.3 or <36°C.
  • Respiratory rate >20 breaths/min or $P\text{co}_2$ <4.3 kPa.
  • Tachycardia >90 bpm.
  • White blood cell count >12 000/mm^3 or <4000/mm^3.
  • Hyperglycaemia in non-diabetic patients (BM >6.6).

• **Severe sepsis**: sepsis with evidence of organ dysfunction or hypoperfusion:
  • Systolic blood pressure <90.
  • Raised lactate.
  • Central nervous system: acutely altered mental status.
  • Respirator: supplemental oxygen required to maintain saturation over 90%.
  • Renal: urine output <0.5 ml/kg/h.
  • Bone marrow : platelets <100.
  • Coagulopathy: international normalized ratio >1.5.

• **Septic shock**: severe sepsis with hypotension which persists despite adequate fluid resuscitation. This occurs when endotoxins from pathogens or a cytokine-mediated immune response causes vasodilatation and increased vascular permeability ('leaky' capillaries). The result is failure to maintain circulating volume and accumulation of fluid in the extravascular spaces, including peripheral and pulmonary oedema.

Sepsis is the most common cause of death in intensive care units. Mortality rates in patients requiring critical care are 30–40%, and may be much higher if there is septic shock or multiorgan failure. Rates are increasing as there are:

- Increased numbers of unwell patients with diminished resistance to infections. Septic shock most often occurs in patients with underlying conditions, making them susceptible to infection.
- Increased numbers of aggressive surgical procedures.
- Increased numbers of invasive procedures, intravascular lines, etc.

The systemic inflammatory response syndrome is an identical syndrome to sepsis, but it can be triggered by a wide variety of causes, including non-infectious conditions such as pancreatitis, burns or cardiopulmonary bypass.

Epidemiology

Only 50% of patients with septic shock have bacteria found in their bloodstream. The most common organisms are:

- Gram positive: 55–65% (*Staphylococcus* sp., enterococci, pneumococci).
- Gram negative: 35–45% (*Escherichia coli*, *Pseudomonas* sp., *Klebsiella* sp.).
- Fungi: 5–10% (*Candida* sp. in particular).

Clinical manifestations of sepsis

Fever and chills are common, non-specific signs. Patients with severe sepsis can be apyrexial, particularly if elderly – a poor prognostic sign. Symptoms/signs may relate to the source of sepsis.

Clinical assessment

1 Look for signs of sepsis in all patients who are unwell.
2 Aim to identify a source to guide antibiotics.
3 Assess severity using response to fluids and vital organ function, including:
  - The heart and cardiovascular system: skin and core temperature, arterial and venous pressures.
  - Peripheral perfusion: patients may be warm and vasodilated in initial stages, cold and poorly perfused in severe refractory septic shock.
  - Mental state: confusion is common, especially in elderly people.
  - The kidneys: urinary catheterization should be performed to measure hourly urine output as the best minute-to-minute indication of renal function.
  - Lung function, as measured by respiratory rate, oxygenation and alveolar–arterial (A-a) O_2 difference (from arterial blood gases, see Chapter 100). These should be measured frequently, and if deterioration occurs the patient should receive mechanical ventilation.
  - Vital organ perfusion, as reflected by tissue hypoxia and arterial blood gas acidaemia and lactate levels.
  - Haemostatic function: assessed clinically through the presence of bruising. Spontaneous bleeding, such as from venepuncture sites, suggests haemostatic failure, which requires blood product support.

Meningococcal septicaemia

Meningococcaemia is a common cause of community-acquired sepsis, particularly in children or young adults and results in a characteristic illness. Fever, malaise and myalgia are associated with the development of a non-blanching rash, proceeding to hypotension and disseminated intravascular coagulation (DIC; see Chapter 188). Symptoms and signs of meningitis may or may not be present.

Toxic shock syndrome

Toxic shock syndrome is a specific syndrome produced by exotoxins of *Staphylococcus* or *Streptococcus* spp. The syndrome is characterized by fever, vomiting and diarrhoea, desquamation of skin, hypotension and multisystem involvement, leading to a high mortality. Treatment is supportive (fluids and antibiotics to prevent recurrence).

Management

Key components of early management are:

- Oxygenation: ventilatory support, if respiratory failure develops or is imminent.
- Blood cultures and other antimicrobial sampling.
- Early broad-spectrum antibiotics should be started immediately post sampling. Each hour of delay is associated with additional mortality.
- Intravenous fluid resuscitation. Patients with septic shock are functionally hypovolaemic, with substantial ongoing invisible fluid losses (related to fever, etc.). Careful fluid replacement therapy, possibly guided by invasive central pressure monitoring, is important.
- Measurement of lactate, as a marker of severity, is used to prompt intensive care admission.
- High-quality nursing care is crucial.

Using 'sepsis bundles' to remind clinical staff of these initial steps has been demonstrated to improve clinical outcomes in patients.

Other vital measures include:

- Localization of site/origin of sepsis, using clinical pointers, chest X-ray and 'blind' computed tomography (CT) (i.e. in the absence of localizing symptoms) of the abdomen. Infected intravascular lines are a common source of hospital-acquired sepsis and should be removed/exchanged.
- Any abscess present should be diagnosed urgently, using appropriate imaging (ultrasonography/CT), and then drained.
- Haemodynamic support: low blood pressure, despite an increased cardiac output, is commonly found. Provided that vital organs continue to function, this blood pressure should not be supported. However, if renal failure occurs, peripheral vasoconstrictors may be used and inotropes if there is cardiac failure.
- Renal support for acute renal failure.
- Blood product support for anaemia, thrombocytopenia and coagulopathy.

Antimicrobial therapy

High-dose antibiotics should be started immediately. The choice should be guided by cultures (blood, urine and other appropriate fluid/tissue culture) or on the basis of the most likely organism if an obvious source exists. Antibiotic therapy should be reviewed regularly, taking clinical response into account. Empirical therapy is often necessary. Suitable choices in the absence of an obvious focus include:

- **Community**-acquired sepsis: second- or third-generation cephalosporin (e.g. ceftriaxone, cefotaxime) or penicillin with a β-lactamase inhibitor.
- **Hospital-acquired sepsis**: carbenopenem (meropenem, imipenem) or antipseudomonal penicillin and a β-lactamase inhibitor or ceftazidime and an antistaphylococcal drug.

Aminoglycosides may be added for critically ill patients or if resistant organisms are suspected. Vancomycin or teicoplanin should be used for suspected staphylococcal sepsis in a patient at risk of methicillin-resistant *Staphylococcus aureus* (MRSA) (e.g. recent hospitalization).

Prognosis

Gram-negative sepsis has mortality rates of 25–40%; Gram-positive sepsis has slightly lower death rates of 10–20%. Mortality rates are highly dependent on factors such as age and pre-existing medical conditions.

167 Common viral infections in adults

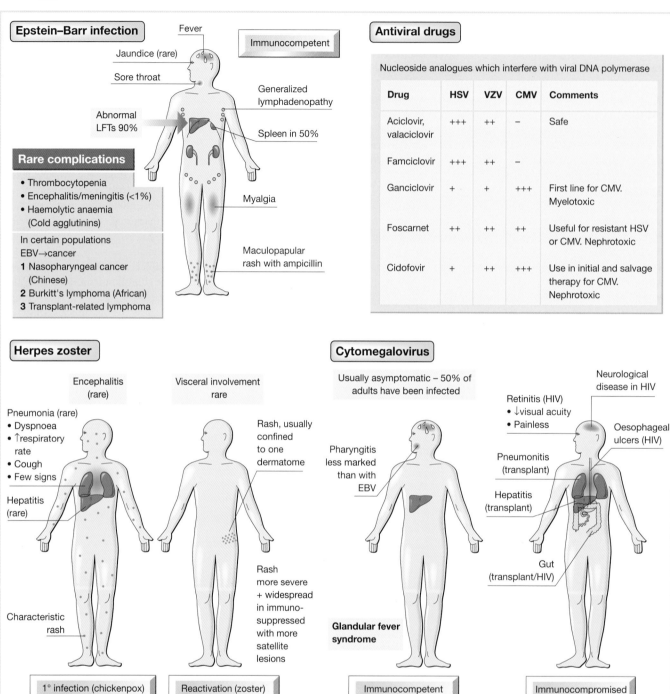

Epstein–Barr infection

Fever

Jaundice (rare)

Sore throat

Abnormal LFTs 90%

Immunocompetent

Generalized lymphadenopathy

Spleen in 50%

Myalgia

Maculopapular rash with ampicillin

Rare complications

- Thrombocytopenia
- Encephalitis/meningitis (<1%)
- Haemolytic anaemia (Cold agglutinins)

In certain populations
EBV→cancer
1 Nasopharyngeal cancer (Chinese)
2 Burkitt's lymphoma (African)
3 Transplant-related lymphoma

Antiviral drugs

Nucleoside analogues which interfere with viral DNA polymerase

Drug	HSV	VZV	CMV	Comments
Aciclovir, valaciclovir	+++	++	–	Safe
Famciclovir	+++	++	–	
Ganciclovir	+	+	+++	First line for CMV. Myelotoxic
Foscarnet	++	++	++	Useful for resistant HSV or CMV. Nephrotoxic
Cidofovir	+	++	+++	Use in initial and salvage therapy for CMV. Nephrotoxic

Herpes zoster

Encephalitis (rare)

Visceral involvement rare

Pneumonia (rare)
- Dyspnoea
- ↑respiratory rate
- Cough
- Few signs

Hepatitis (rare)

Rash, usually confined to one dermatome

Characteristic rash

Rash more severe + widespread in immuno-suppressed with more satellite lesions

1° infection (chickenpox)

Reactivation (zoster)

Cytomegalovirus

Usually asymptomatic – 50% of adults have been infected

Pharyngitis less marked than with EBV

Neurological disease in HIV

Retinitis (HIV)
- ↓visual acuity
- Painless

Oesophageal ulcers (HIV)

Pneumonitis (transplant)

Hepatitis (transplant)

Gut (transplant/HIV)

Glandular fever syndrome

Immunocompetent

Immunocompromised

Epstein–Barr virus

Epstein–Barr virus (EBV) is common – 90% of people are infected by adulthood. Half of infections occur asymptomatically in childhood. Infection in adolescent life is more commonly associated with clinical disease. EBV occurs in oropharyngeal secretions; and many cases result from intimate contact (hence the name 'kissing disease').

Symptoms are of fever, sore throat, headache, myalgia, anorexia and chills, and signs are of lymphadenopathy, prominent pharyngitis and splenomegaly in 50% – the **glandular fever syndrome**. A maculopapular rash often occurs if the patient has been given amoxicillin.

Symptoms usually resolve spontaneously over 2–3 weeks, but prolonged fatigue is not unusual. Complications are: (i) abnormal liver function tests (LFTs) (common) and occasional jaundice; (ii) haemolytic anaemia; (iii) rare neurological: encephalitis or aseptic meningitis; and (iv) lymphoproliferative disorder: EBV-related lymphoproliferative syndromes are common in transplant patients and late-stage human immunodeficiency virus (HIV).

Diagnosis and treatment

- Full blood count: mononucleosis, >10% atypical lymphocytes. Thrombocytopenia is common. Serology: IgM antibodies to EBV

or detection of heterophile antibodies (serum antibodies against red blood cells of other species) – monospot or Paul–Bunnell test.
• Differential diagnosis is from other agents causing a 'glandular fever' type syndrome, principally cytomegalovirus (CMV) or toxoplasmosis. Streptococcal pharyngitis may give similar symptoms.
• No specific antiviral treatment is available. Steroids may be useful in severe pharyngitis, thrombocytopenia and haemolytic anaemia.

Herpes simplex virus

Herpes simplex virus (HSV) infection is common. It has a predilection for mucocutaneous sites, affecting both normal and immunocompromised hosts, and is transmitted by direct oral or genital contact. Two types – HSV1 and HSV2 – have differing epidemiology and clinical patterns, although there is considerable overlap. Most people encounter HSV1 infection in childhood, whereas acquisition of HSV2 depends on sexual contact. Recurrent infections are common as a result of latency of the virus in sensory nerve ganglia. Identified triggers of recurrence include stress, sunlight and local trauma.
• **Oral mucocutaneous HSV**: most primary infections are asymptomatic; fever and pharyngitis or gingivostomatitis may occur. The usual manifestation is of recurrent herpes labialis (cold sores). There is a prodrome of tingling or burning, followed by painful vesicles at the edge of lip. Oral lesions may occur. Vesicles heal with crusting within 10 days.
• **Genital HSV**: the type is HSV2 in 80% of cases. Many infections are asymptomatic. Painful vesicles occur on the glans, penis shaft or vulva, perineum and vagina, 2–7 days after contact. There is dysuria. It is more common in women. Fever, malaise and tender inguinal lymphadenopathy may occur. Vesicles often ulcerate and may persist for several weeks; recurrence is common. Asymptomatic viral shedding can occur and cause transmission to sexual partners.
• **Other clinical syndromes**: (i) primary eye infection (dendritic ulcers); (ii) herpetic whitlow (infection of the finger); (iii) eczema herpeticum: skin infection in atopic dermatitis, which can cause severe illness; and (iv) herpes simplex encephalitis (see Chapter 207).

Treatment

Intravenous (IV) aciclovir (or alternative) is useful for severe systemic illness, e.g. encephalitis. Oral aciclovir used early in oral or genital disease leads to fewer lesions and quicker healing. Topical ointment is useful for dendritic ulcers. Suppressive aciclovir can be helpful for patients who are distressed by frequently recurrent herpes lesions but it does not eliminate viral shedding so sexual partners still need protection.

Immunocompromised hosts

Severe mucocutaneous lesions are common in HIV-infected patients or transplant recipients. Severe proctitis and recurrent perianal disease occur in some HIV-infected gay men. HSV may affect other parts of the gut and, rarely, disseminates to involve organs such as the liver.

Varicella-zoster virus

Varicella-zoster virus (VZV) causes both varicella (chickenpox) and herpes zoster (shingles) – varicella reflects the primary infection and zoster the recurrent infection. Spread of the virus occurs through respiratory droplets, and 90% of primary cases occur in childhood. VZV becomes latent in the dorsal root ganglia after primary infection.

Varicella is usually a disease of children; chickenpox in adults is much more severe, with a 15-fold higher mortality. Fever and malaise precede the development of maculopapular lesions on the face and trunk, which become vesicular and crust over. In adults, particularly pregnant women, complications include:

• Varicella pneumonitis: occurs in one in 400 adults. Tachypnoea, cough and dyspnoea. Chest signs may not be prominent.
• Varicella encephalitis: depressed consciousness and progressive headaches; fatal in up to 15%.
• Varicella hepatitis.

Herpes zoster classically affects elderly people, as a result of reactivation of latent virus. It is also more common in HIV-positive patients including those with high CD4 counts. A prodrome of pain is followed by a unilateral rash in a dermatomal distribution. Vesicles develop over 2–3 days, crust over and then heal.
• The lumbar or thoracic dermatomes are most commonly involved.
• Trigeminal nerve involvement may lead to ocular involvement. Eye assessment is necessary.
• Ramsay Hunt syndrome: the seventh cranial nerve is involved; vesicles may be hidden in the auditory canal. Hearing loss and facial paralysis may occur.

Rare neurological complications include motor weakness and transverse myelitis. Post-herpetic neuralgia is distressing and occurs in up to half of elderly patients.

Immunocompromised hosts

Chickenpox causes significant morbidity and mortality; 30% of bone marrow transplant recipients without prophylaxis have infections in the first year. Dissemination occurs in 50%: lung, central nervous system and liver.

Zoster rash is more severe and lesions may occur outside the dermatome or be disseminated over the skin. Visceral involvement is rare.

Diagnosis and management

The diagnosis is usually clinical. Vesicle fluid can be analysed using polymerase chain reaction to confirm or rule out VZV. Differential diagnoses include impetigo, disseminated herpes simplex (rare) and disseminated Coxsackie viruses. IV aciclovir is used to treat immunocompromised individuals (including those on high-dose steroids) with varicella or zoster. Treatment of chickenpox in adults may reduce complications. Early treatment reduces the number of lesions and subsequent pain in zoster.

Infection during pregnancy

Varicella infection in the first two trimesters of pregnancy is associated with a small but significant increase in the rate of birth defects. Non-immune expectant mothers should avoid contact with chickenpox and shingles patients. If they are exposed, IV immunoglobulin before the onset of symptoms reduces the likelihood of developing the illness.

Cytomegalovirus

Infection with CMV is common but rarely causes clinical disease: 50–95% of adults have been infected. It is, however, a major pathogen in immunocompromised individuals. Disease occurs because of: (i) reactivation; or (ii) transplantation of a CMV-positive organ into a CMV-negative recipient. The clinical features of infection are:
• Disease is rare in healthy people. A glandular fever-like syndrome, with increased monocytes and abnormal liver function tests may occur.
• Transplant recipients: CMV pneumonitis, hepatitis and gastrointestinal disease, such as diarrhoea.
• HIV infected: CMV retinitis, neurological infection and gut disease.

Prophylaxis is often indicated in advanced HIV with evidence of replicating virus and some groups of transplant recipients. Treatment is with CMV antivirals such as valganciclovir. Immunoglobulin is also used for treatment and prophylaxis in some groups of transplant recipients.

168 HIV infection and AIDS

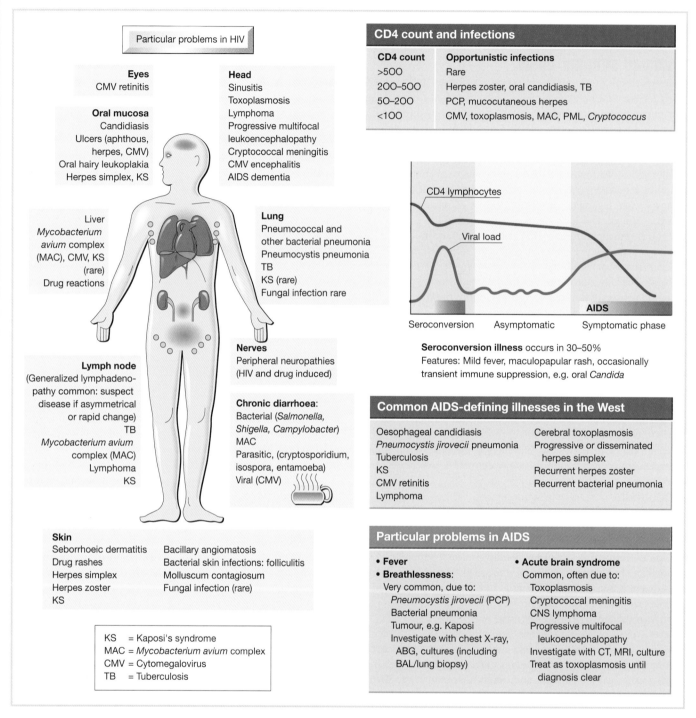

Particular problems in HIV

Eyes
CMV retinitis

Oral mucosa
Candidiasis
Ulcers (aphthous,
  herpes, CMV)
Oral hairy leukoplakia
Herpes simplex, KS

Head
Sinusitis
Toxoplasmosis
Lymphoma
Progressive multifocal
  leukoencephalopathy
Cryptococcal meningitis
CMV encephalitis
AIDS dementia

Liver
*Mycobacterium
avium* complex
(MAC), CMV, KS
(rare)
Drug reactions

Lung
Pneumococcal and
other bacterial pneumonia
Pneumocystis pneumonia
TB
KS (rare)
Fungal infection rare

Lymph node
(Generalized lymphadeno-
pathy common: suspect
disease if asymmetrical
or rapid change)
TB
Mycobacterium avium
  complex (MAC)
Lymphoma
KS

Nerves
Peripheral neuropathies
(HIV and drug induced)

Chronic diarrhoea:
Bacterial (*Salmonella,
Shigella, Campylobacter*)
MAC
Parasitic, (cryptosporidium,
isospora, entamoeba)
Viral (CMV)

Skin
Seborrhoeic dermatitis
Drug rashes
Herpes simplex
Herpes zoster
KS

Bacillary angiomatosis
Bacterial skin infections: folliculitis
Molluscum contagiosum
Fungal infection (rare)

KS = Kaposi's syndrome
MAC = *Mycobacterium avium* complex
CMV = Cytomegalovirus
TB = Tuberculosis

CD4 count and infections

CD4 count	Opportunistic infections
>500	Rare
200–500	Herpes zoster, oral candidiasis, TB
50–200	PCP, mucocutaneous herpes
<100	CMV, toxoplasmosis, MAC, PML, *Cryptococcus*

CD4 lymphocytes

Viral load

AIDS

Seroconversion   Asymptomatic   Symptomatic phase

Seroconversion illness occurs in 30–50%
Features: Mild fever, maculopapular rash, occasionally
transient immune suppression, e.g. oral *Candida*

Common AIDS-defining illnesses in the West

Oesophageal candidiasis
Pneumocystis jirovecii pneumonia
Tuberculosis
KS
CMV retinitis
Lymphoma

Cerebral toxoplasmosis
Progressive or disseminated
  herpes simplex
Recurrent herpes zoster
Recurrent bacterial pneumonia

Particular problems in AIDS

• **Fever**
• **Breathlessness:**
  Very common, due to:
    Pneumocystis jirovecii (PCP)
    Bacterial pneumonia
    Tumour, e.g. Kaposi
    Investigate with chest X-ray,
      ABG, cultures (including
      BAL/lung biopsy)

• **Acute brain syndrome**
  Common, often due to:
    Toxoplasmosis
    Cryptococcal meningitis
    CNS lymphoma
    Progressive multifocal
      leukoencephalopathy
    Investigate with CT, MRI, culture
    Treat as toxoplasmosis until
      diagnosis clear

Human immunodeficiency virus (HIV) infection causes a clinical syndrome characterized by the development of progressive immunodeficiency following a long asymptomatic period. Cellular immunodeficiency eventually leads to severe opportunistic infection and, more rarely, malignancy.

Epidemiology

HIV infection has now reached pandemic proportions, with over 35 million people infected worldwide. The number of new diagnoses of HIV is around 7000 per year.. Transmission of the blood-borne RNA retrovirus occurs predominantly by four mechanisms:

- Homosexual or heterosexual intercourse.
- Intravenous drug abuse.
- Maternal–child transmission.
- Transfusion of blood products (although much less common with improved transfusion screening).

Pathogenesis

After transmission, HIV enters lymphoid tissue where it infects CD4-bearing T lymphocytes and monocyte/macrophages. The virus enters the cell by binding to the CD4 molecule and chemokine receptors, and then replicates and integrates itself into host

DNA. Latent infection or virus production follows. A total of 10^{10}–10^{11} virions are produced each day with considerable turnover of HIV-infected cells. Ultimately, progressive loss of CD4 cells leads to impairment of the immune function.

Clinical patterns

- **Primary HIV infection**: 30–80% patients experience an acute clinical syndrome when viral replication occurs after HIV infection. Symptoms typically occur 2–4 weeks after infection and include fever, malaise, lymphadenopathy and a maculopapular rash. A small proportion have transient immunosuppression with clinical features such as oral *Candida* infection.
- **Asymptomatic HIV**: after seroconversion, most patients have a prolonged asymptomatic period (median 10 years without treatment) before the development of clinical features.
- **Symptomatic HIV** and acquired immune deficiency syndrome (AIDS): as HIV infection progresses, patients become symptomatic. Some symptoms are non-specific, but certain opportunistic diseases are regarded as AIDS defining (see Figure 168.1), along with systemic features such as significant weight loss, persistent fever or persistent diarrhoea.
- **Stage of disease** can be described by: (i) whether the patient is symptomatic; (ii) whether an AIDS-defining illness has occurred; and (iii) the CD4 count. The last reflects the degree of immunosuppression and the likelihood of particular opportunistic infections.

Diagnosis of HIV infection

HIV is diagnosed by the detection of anti-HIV antibodies by ELISA (enzyme-linked immunosorbent assay). Positive samples are confirmed by western blot. Seroconversion (i.e. acquisition of anti-HIV antibodies) occurs between 1 and 3 months after primary infection. Antigen testing can also be performed which reduces the period when early infection may be missed. Plasma HIV RNA is then quantified: a high viral load has a poor prognosis. HIV should be considered in anyone presenting with recurrent infections, especially shingles, unexplained fever or lymphadenopathy.

Treatment of HIV infection

The recent use of a number of drugs in combination (anti-retroviral therapy (ART)) has led to a significant decrease in mortality and reversal of HIV disease progression. The prognosis is now good if HIV is diagnosed early and life expectancy is thought to be reduced by only a few years. Even in advanced disease, anti-retroviral drugs can restore good immune function and improve health in most patients. Five main classes of drugs exist:

1. Nucleoside reverse transcriptase inhibitors.
2. Protease inhibitors.
3. Non-nucleoside reverse transcriptase inhibitors.
4. Integrase inhibitors.
5. CCR5 antagonists.

A combination of three or four drugs is used to reduce the viral load (ideally below the detection limit of the assay). The viral load and CD4 response reflect the efficacy of treatment.

Common problems with ART include:

- Resistance to anti-retroviral drugs: particularly common in patients who have experienced a number of different drugs. Resistance to one drug often limits the use of the whole class. New drugs continue to be developed to treat such patients.
- Side effects (e.g. neuropathy, lipodystrophy) and drug intolerance.
- Adherence problems arising from the complex multidrug regimens.
- Anti-retrovirals commonly interact with other drugs.
- Limited access for patients in many developing countries with a high HIV burden because of the costs of medication and health system limitations.

Common opportunistic infections

Patients with HIV are susceptible to both standard pathogens and unusual opportunistic infections; although ART and routine primary prophylaxis has reduced the incidence of many opportunistic infections, they still present considerable problems. In addition, a third of new patients in the West present late with advanced immunosuppression (particularly older patients and heterosexual men). The major clinical syndromes are shown in Figure 168.1.

- *Pneumocystis carinii* (*jirovecii*) pneumonia (PCP) is a major AIDS-defining illness in the West. Risk increases once the CD4 count drops below 200. Primary prophylaxis with co-trimoxazole (e.g. Septrin) is effective. PCP usually presents with a non-productive cough, fever and dyspnoea; it is usually subacute, with a mean duration of symptoms of 3–4 weeks. Physical examination is often unremarkable. Blood gases often show a moderate hypoxaemia. The chest X-ray (CXR) is abnormal in 90%, classically showing fine interstitial perihilar shadowing, although the spectrum of abnormalities is wide. The demonstration of cysts by immunofluorescence microscopy or polymerase chain reaction (PCR) of induced sputum or bronchoalveolar lavage (BAL) fluid establishes the diagnosis. Treatment is with high-dose co-trimoxazole; the addition of steroids improves the prognosis in severe disease.
- Cytomegalovirus (CMV) occurs in late-stage infection (CD4 <50). The major problem is progressive retinitis (85%), but gut, nervous system and lung infections also occur. It is asymptomatic in early stages; regular ophthalmological screening is useful in advanced HIV. Retinitis is diagnosed clinically; there are white fluffy retinal lesions with perivascular haemorrhages and exudates. Treatment is with specific antiviral agents and treatment of HIV; long-term maintenance therapy is necessary and relapse is common until the CD4 count has significantly improved.
- Toxoplasmosis is a protozoa infection, which most commonly causes encephalitis (80%) in late HIV (CD4 <100). Patients present with fever, headache, confusion, fits and focal neurological signs. Magnetic resonance imaging (MRI) is more sensitive than computed tomography (CT) in demonstrating ring-enhancing lesions, which are often multiple and classically in the basal ganglia or corticomedullary junction. Toxoplasmosis is rare in patients with no serological evidence of previous exposure. Treatment is with pyrimethamine and sulphadiazine; a clinical response confirms diagnosis.
- Kaposi's sarcoma (KS) is caused by herpes virus 8 and occurs in 5–10% of gay men with HIV. Skin lesions are initially macular and progress to reddish-purplish indurated plaques. There is a wide spectrum from isolated skin or oral lesions to dissemination with lymph node, gastrointestinal tract or lung involvement. It is diagnosed clinically or by skin biopsy. Skin disease may completely regress following a good immune response to ART. Localized radiotherapy and injection of lesions may be used for problematic lesions or resistant disease. Chemotherapy is used for disseminated disease and survival has improved dramatically in the last 15 years.
- Non-Hodgkin's lymphoma occurs in up to 10% in late stage disease – 20% are in the central nervous system (CNS). It presents with fever, sweats and organ-related symptoms; extranodal involvement is common. Treatment is with chemotherapy. Prognosis is poor.
- Progressive multifocal leukoencephalopathy (PML) is an uncommon demyelinating disease caused by polyoma JC virus (late-stage HIV). Diagnosis is by imaging (white matter lesion) and PCR of the cerebrospinal fluid for JC virus. The only effective treatment is improving immune function with ART.
- Cryptococcal disease (see Chapter 169).

169 Common fungal infections

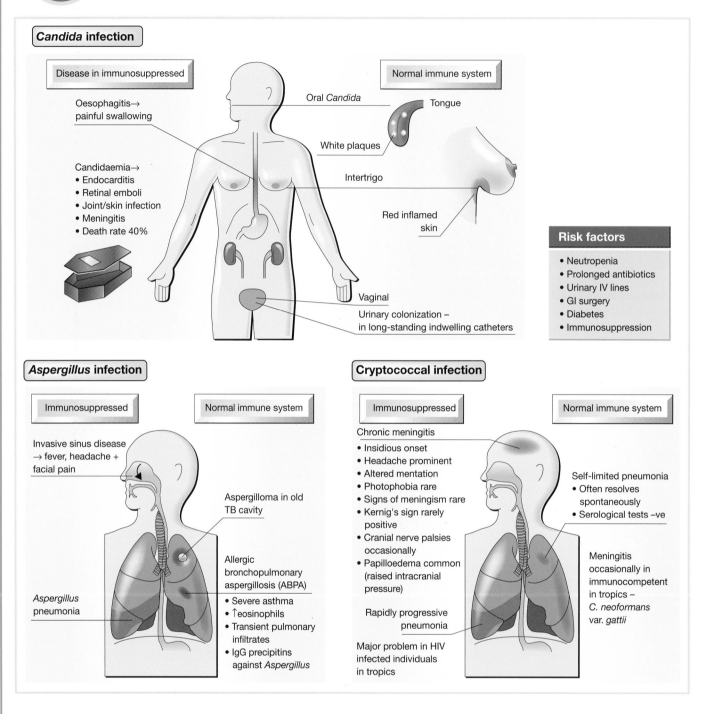

Candida infection

Disease in immunosuppressed

Oesophagitis→
painful swallowing

Candidaemia→
• Endocarditis
• Retinal emboli
• Joint/skin infection
• Meningitis
• Death rate 40%

Normal immune system

Oral *Candida* — Tongue

White plaques

Intertrigo

Red inflamed
skin

Vaginal

Urinary colonization –
in long-standing indwelling catheters

Risk factors

• Neutropenia
• Prolonged antibiotics
• Urinary IV lines
• GI surgery
• Diabetes
• Immunosuppression

Aspergillus infection

Immunosuppressed

Invasive sinus disease
→ fever, headache +
facial pain

Aspergillus
pneumonia

Normal immune system

Aspergilloma in old
TB cavity

Allergic
bronchopulmonary
aspergillosis (ABPA)
• Severe asthma
• ↑eosinophils
• Transient pulmonary
infiltrates
• IgG precipitins
against *Aspergillus*

Cryptococcal infection

Immunosuppressed

Chronic meningitis
• Insidious onset
• Headache prominent
• Altered mentation
• Photophobia rare
• Signs of meningism rare
• Kernig's sign rarely
positive
• Cranial nerve palsies
occasionally
• Papilloedema common
(raised intracranial
pressure)

Rapidly progressive
pneumonia

Major problem in HIV
infected individuals
in tropics

Normal immune system

Self-limited pneumonia
• Often resolves
spontaneously
• Serological tests –ve

Meningitis
occasionally in
immunocompetent
in tropics –
C. neoformans
var. *gattii*

In the UK and in the immunologically competent host, fungi often cause only mild disease, whereas in the immunocompromised individual, severe or life-threatening disease can result. Thus, fungal infections have assumed increasing importance as the number of immunocompromised patients increases. Many different species cause significant disease; only the main endemic fungi in the UK are discussed here.

Candida species

These are the most common invasive fungal species in the UK. The organisms are found readily in the environment and are commensals on mucous membranes in the gastrointestinal (GI), respiratory and genitourinary tracts. *Candida albicans* is the most important species, although non-*albicans* species are becoming

Medicine at a Glance, Fourth Edition. Edited by Patrick Davey. © 2014 John Wiley & Sons, Ltd. Published 2014 by John Wiley & Sons, Ltd. Companion website: www.ataglanceseries.com/medicine

more common. *Candida* spp. can cause both mucocutaneous and invasive disease.

Mucocutaneous candidiasis

This may occur in immunocompetent and immunocompromised individuals; it is particularly common in those with diabetes or with altered cellular immunity such as HIV.

- **Oral *Candida* infection**: the most common clinical manifestation is creamy-white 'curd-like' patches on the mucosa and tongue. The underlying surface is raw if the exudate is scraped off. The diagnosis is usually made clinically, although hyphae can be demonstrated in lesions.
- **Candidal oesophagitis**: usually in advanced HIV or haematological malignancy. May occur without oral lesions, and produces symptoms of dysphagia, odynophagia and retrosternal pain. Diagnosed by appearance on endoscopy and biopsies.
- **Vaginal candidiasis**: see Chapter 49.
- **Intertrigo**: infection in warm damp environments between skinfolds – red macerated skin with satellite lesions.
- **Chronic mucocutaneous candidiasis**: the syndrome is associated with specific T-cell deficiency. There is infection of the skin, mucous membrane and scalp, which may be disfiguring.

Invasive candidiasis

Invasive infections usually arise from endogenous colonization. Entry occurs through damaged skin or mucosa or direct access to the circulation. Both neutrophils and cell-mediated immunity are important in defence against *Candida* spp. The following are risk factors for invasive disease:

- Neutropenia increases the risk of candidaemia.
- Prolonged use of antibiotics.
- Indwelling urinary or intravenous (IV) catheters.
- GI surgery.
- IV drug abuse.

Candidaemia

Candida spp. are commonly isolated from blood cultures. Although this sometimes reflects colonization of indwelling lines rather than disseminated candidal disease, candidaemia also occurs in disseminated candidiasis, especially in immunosuppressed patients. All patients should be carefully evaluated for metastatic infection, including examination of the fundi, the heart for endocarditis, the joints and skin. Candidaemia has a 40% mortality rate.

Disseminated candidiasis

Blood-borne spread can lead to infection in most organs, including the central nervous system, respiratory tract, joints, kidneys and peritoneum. Only 50% of patients with disseminated candidiasis have demonstrated candidaemia. The presence of skin or eye lesions (present in 10%) confirms the diagnosis. *Candida* spp. in the urine occurs in both invasive and disseminated candidiasis.

Treatment

- Oral or vaginal candidiasis: topical therapy or short-term systemic therapy.
- Serious mucocutaneous disease: systemic therapy.
- Candidaemia: usually treated with azoles or echinocandins (e.g. caspofungin). Amphotericin can also be used. IV catheters should be removed.
- Disseminated candidiasis: aggressive antifungal therapy.
- Surgery is usually required for endocarditis.

Antifungal prophylaxis

This is used in HIV patients with recurrent disease, and in high-risk bone marrow and most solid organ transplantations.

Aspergillus species

These mould species are found readily in the environment. Infection is acquired by inhalation of spores. Disease may be caused in three ways:

1 Allergic reactions: allergic bronchopulmonary aspergillosis (see Chapter 117).
2 Colonization of cavities (aspergillomas) (see Chapter 117).
3 Invasive aspergillosis.

Invasive aspergillosis is a disease of immunocompromised patients. Important risk factors include prolonged neutropenia, high-dose steroids or prolonged antibiotic therapy.

Clinical patterns of invasive disease

- Sinus disease: in neutropenic patients, colonizing organisms may become invasive in the nose and sinuses. Patients present with fever, headache and sinus symptoms. Soft tissue and bony invasion may lead to vascular invasion and brain involvement. Diagnosis is suspected when computed tomography shows loss of the normal bony sinus margins, confirmed by tissue biopsy.
- *Aspergillus* pneumonia: acute pneumonia in neutropenic patients:
  - Fever, followed by pulmonary consolidation.
  - Rapidly progressing pneumonia, sometimes with cavitation.

A diagnosis may be made by culture and lung biopsy, which shows histological evidence of invasion, but polymerase chain reaction and serum galactomannan testing is now commonly available. *Aspergillus* is rarely found in blood cultures in pneumonia.

Treatment

Amphotericin has been replaced by voriconzole as the drug of choice for invasive aspergillosis. Caspofungin may be used in refractory disease. Response rates in invasive aspergillosis are very poor and the mortality rate is about 40%.

Cryptococcal disease

Cryptococcus neoformans is a yeast-like fungus that affects both normal and immunocompromised hosts. The organism is acquired through inhalation; there are three main clinical syndromes:

- **Pulmonary disease**: occurs in both normal and immunocompromised hosts.
- **Meningitis**: usually in immunosuppressed individuals, particularly with HIV. There is a long, non-specific history; the most common symptoms are headache and a change in mentation. There may be surprisingly few signs; neck stiffness may not be present. Papilloedema and cranial nerve palsies may occur. Diagnosis is achieved from:
  - Cerebrospinal fluid (CSF): predominant lymphocytes, low glucose, high protein and high pressure; an Indian ink stain demonstrates yeast and capsule in the CSF which can then be confirmed by culture. CSF can be normal in advanced immunosupression.
  - Cryptococcal antigen titres are raised in the serum and CSF.
- **Cryptococcaemia**: may present with fever alone in the immunocompromised or can be associated with meningitis. Skin lesions occur in 10%.

Treatment

- Normal immune system: pulmonary disease may not need treatment and can be observed. Treat meningitis as below.
- Immunocompromised: amphotericin initially, followed by azoles. Prolonged therapy is required and long-term secondary prophylaxis required. The mortality rate in meningitis in HIV is around 25%.

170 Specific bacterial infections

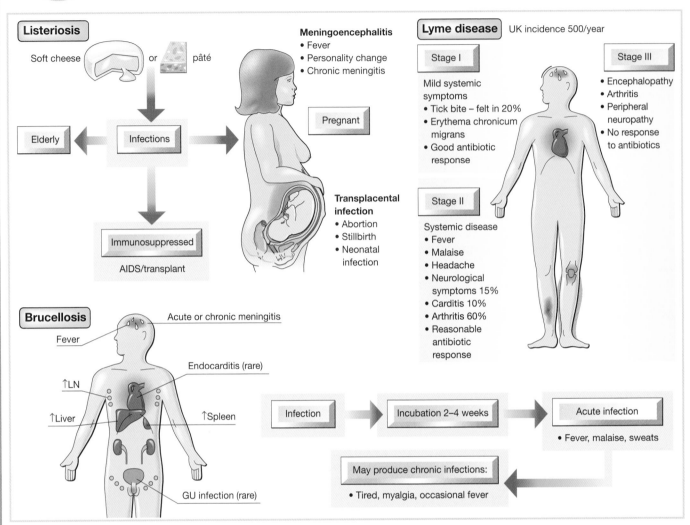

Listeriosis

Listeria monocytogenes is a Gram-positive bacillus causing disease in pregnant women, immunocompromised individuals and neonates. Infection is usually acquired through food, particularly soft cheeses and pâté. Clinical manifestations include:

- Pregnancy associated: bacteraemia producing a flu-like illness, and sometimes transplacental infection or ascending infection leading to abortion, stillbirth or neonatal sepsis. Very rarely maternal meningitis.
- Neonatal infection: high mortality.
- Meningoencephalitis: the most common manifestation, occurring in the late neonatal period, and in immunocompromised and elderly people. There is a wide clinical spectrum from fever with personality change to chronic meningitis.

Diagnosis and treatment

In meningitic syndromes, few organisms are present in the cerebrospinal fluid (CSF), so Gram staining may be difficult. CSF cultures are positive. In systemic disease, blood cultures may be positive. Treatment is with ampicillin and an aminoglycoside.

Brucellosis

This is caused by four species of a Gram-negative coccobacillus: *Brucella abortus*, *B. melitensis*, *B. suis* and *B. canis*. It is acquired from contact with infected animals or milk products or by inhalation of infected aerosols. Most UK infections are imported, but infection can also occur in those with occupational risks (farmers, vets). Systemic spread leads to granuloma formation in different organs. The incubation period is 2–4 weeks. Fever, malaise, sweats and other non-specific symptoms occur; nausea, vomiting and gastrointestinal complaints are frequent; hepatosplenomegaly is common; and lymphadenopathy occurs in 20%. It may cause:

- Bone and joint infection: particularly sacroiliitis and spondylitis.
- Respiratory infection: bronchitis and abscesses.
- Acute or chronic meningitis.
- Rarely endocarditis and genitourinary (GU) infection.

Diagnosis requires a very high clinical suspicion because brucellosis can mimic many other diseases. One should attempt to culture the organism from blood or bone marrow; prolonged

Medicine at a Glance, Fourth Edition. Edited by Patrick Davey. © 2014 John Wiley & Sons, Ltd. Published 2014 by John Wiley & Sons, Ltd. Companion website: www.ataglanceseries.com/medicine

culture is necessary. Laboratory staff need to be warned of the potential diagnosis as *Brucella* is highly contagious. Serology may be diagnostic.

Treatment: doxycycline is the drug of choice in combination with rifampicin or an aminoglycoside or both to prevent relapse. Treatment is for 6 weeks or longer in serious infection.

Tetanus

Tetanus is caused by infection with the anaerobic Gram-positive bacillus, *Clostridium tetani*. Spores from soil infect a wound and germinate under anaerobic conditions, producing the toxin tetanospasmin, which is transported via neurons to the central nervous system (CNS), where it inhibits presynaptic transmitter release from inhibitory neurons, leading to muscular rigidity.

Clinical features

The incubation period is usually 1–21 days.

● **Neonatal tetanus**: common in the developing world; results from infection of the umbilical stump. Initially poor feeding, trismus and spasms; high mortality.
● **Generalized tetanus**: initially spasm of the masseter muscles causing trismus and 'risus sardonicus', gradually spreading to spasms involving the whole of the trunk and body, which can lead to arching of the back – opisthotonos. Spasms may be precipitated by noise or tactile stimuli and may be severe enough to tear muscle or break bones. Autonomic instability – arrhythmias or blood pressure changes may occur.

Diagnosis and management

Tetanus is diagnosed clinically. Human tetanus immunoglobulin is administered intramuscularly to neutralize circulating toxin. The wound should be debrided thoroughly and metronidazole or penicillin given to eradicate the organism. Supportive care consists of benzodiazepines to reduce rigidity and spasms; ventilation may be required. Autonomic disturbances are difficult to treat and may require inotropic support or α- and β-blockade. Mortality in 20% occurs from respiratory problems or autonomic instability. Tetanus can be prevented by primary immunization and boosting with tetanus toxoid. Dirty wounds should be debrided and a booster dose given if five or more doses of toxoid have not been given previously.

Lyme disease

This is an infection with the spirochaete *Borrelia burgdorferi*, transmitted by the tick *Ixodes* sp., found on infected deer or mice. Foci of disease occur in the USA and Europe and cases are also reported in areas of Russia, China, Japan and Australia. The number of new cases has increased over the last 30 years as diagnostic methods and awareness have improved. The clinical features are:

● **Localized early disease** (stage 1): an annular lesion (erythema chronicum migrans) with central clearing usually develops at the site of the bite; present in 60–85% of all cases. Mild systemic symptoms.
● **Disseminated disease** (stage 2): some patients may develop disseminated disease. Blood spread may lead to a fluctuating flu-like illness. Secondary skin lesions may occur. Subsequent development of arthritis occurs in 60% (monoarticular, affecting large joints), neurological symptoms in 15% (meningitis, cranial neuropathy, myelitis, painful radiculopathy) and carditis in 10% (atrioventricular block, myopericarditis). Symptoms and signs are often self-limiting.

● **Late persistent infection** (stage 3): if untreated, there are chronic manifestations of recurrent arthritis (autoimmune, relates to HLA-DR2), skin changes and neurological changes (peripheral neuropathy, encephalopathy).

Diagnosis and treatment

A clinical diagnosis of erythema migrans should prompt treatment. Serology (IgG testing) can take several weeks to become positive but is sensitive and specific in late disease and can be detected in the CSF in neuro-borreliosis. The organism is rarely isolated.

Early disease may be treated with oral doxycycline, amoxicillin or ceftriaxone. Cephalosporins are indicated for arthritis or neurological involvement. There is good evidence that 14–21 days of treatment is adequate and that longer courses of intravenous antibiotics do not give benefit. Treatment of late disease has been shown to stop the development of new symptoms but residual tissue damage may persist.

Syphilis

Syphilis is a sexually transmitted disease caused by the spirochaete *Treponema pallidum*. Most disease occurs in developing countries, but there have been recent increases in incidence in the UK amongst homosexual men. Organisms enter the body of a sexual partner through breaches in the skin or epithelium. *T. pallidum* is disseminated via the blood. The clinical features are:

● **Primary syphilis**: median incubation period of 3 weeks. An ulcerated, typically painless papule – the primary chancre – develops at the site of inoculation on the penis or cervix and labia. Inguinal lymphadenopathy occurs. The lesion heals spontaneously after several weeks.
● **Secondary syphilis**: 6–8 weeks later, with a generalized maculopapular rash (involving the palms and soles), generalized lymphadenopathy (50%) and condylomata lata (moist, broad, highly infectious plaques in warm intertriginous areas). Systemic symptoms include fever, headache and sore throat.
● **Latent syphilis**: symptoms and signs disappear. The only manifestation of infection is positive serology. Asymptomatic CNS infection is common.
● **Tertiary syphilis**: gummata (hard granulomatous lesions) occur after 3–10 years in many sites, including the skin, in which ulceration with damage to the underlying cartilage or connective tissue occurs. Aortitis is a rare complication which develops after 10–30 years and causes ascending aortic aneurysms. Neurosyphilis produces a wide spectrum of disease including:
  ● Meningovascular: 4–7 years.
  ● General paresis of the insane: 10–20 years.
  ● Tabes dorsalis: 15–25 years.

Diagnosis

Diagnosis is made through the identification of *T. pallidum* on dark-ground microscopy of primary or secondary syphilis lesions. Serology: combination of non-treponemal tests (e.g. rapid plasma regain test) and specific treponemal antibody tests (e.g. *T. pallidum* haemagglutination test). CSF should be examined in suspected neurosyphilis; elevation of mononuclear cells and protein may occur and the rapid plasma regain test is usually positive on CSF.

Management

Penicillin is the drug of choice; the regimen and dose depend on the stage. Alternative drugs include tetracycline and ceftriaxone. Steroids are needed to prevent the Jarisch–Herxheimer reaction (anaphylaxis to dead/dying spirochaetes) after treatment in late syphilis. Contacts should be traced and treated.

171 Malaria

Malaria life cycle

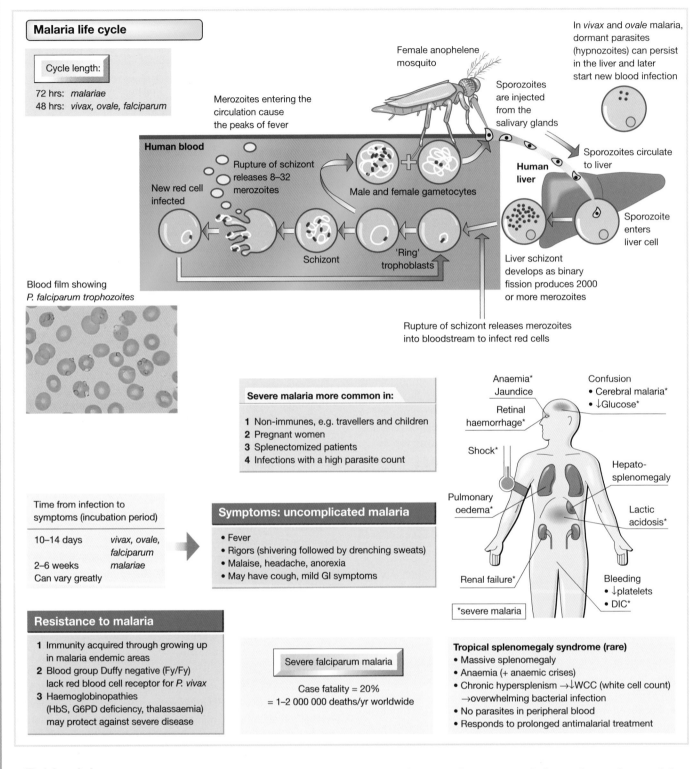

Cycle length:

72 hrs: *malariae*
48 hrs: *vivax, ovale, falciparum*

Merozoites entering the circulation cause the peaks of fever

Female anophelene mosquito

Sporozoites are injected from the salivary glands

In *vivax* and *ovale* malaria, dormant parasites (hypnozoites) can persist in the liver and later start new blood infection

Human blood

Rupture of schizont releases 8–32 merozoites

New red cell infected

Male and female gametocytes

Schizont

'Ring' trophoblasts

Human liver

Sporozoites circulate to liver

Sporozoite enters liver cell

Liver schizont develops as binary fission produces 2000 or more merozoites

Rupture of schizont releases merozoites into bloodstream to infect red cells

Blood film showing *P. falciparum trophozoites*

Severe malaria more common in:

1 Non-immunes, e.g. travellers and children
2 Pregnant women
3 Splenectomized patients
4 Infections with a high parasite count

Anaemia*
Jaundice

Confusion
• Cerebral malaria*
• ↓Glucose*

Retinal haemorrhage*

Shock*

Hepato-splenomegaly

Pulmonary oedema*

Lactic acidosis*

Renal failure*

Bleeding
• ↓platelets
• DIC*

*severe malaria

Time from infection to symptoms (incubation period)

10–14 days	*vivax, ovale, falciparum*
2–6 weeks	*malariae*
Can vary greatly	

Symptoms: uncomplicated malaria

• Fever
• Rigors (shivering followed by drenching sweats)
• Malaise, headache, anorexia
• May have cough, mild GI symptoms

Resistance to malaria

1 Immunity acquired through growing up in malaria endemic areas
2 Blood group Duffy negative (Fy/Fy) lack red blood cell receptor for *P. vivax*
3 Haemoglobinopathies (HbS, G6PD deficiency, thalassaemia) may protect against severe disease

Severe falciparum malaria

Case fatality = 20%
= 1–2 000 000 deaths/yr worldwide

Tropical splenomegaly syndrome (rare)
• Massive splenomegaly
• Anaemia (+ anaemic crises)
• Chronic hypersplenism →↓WCC (white cell count) →overwhelming bacterial infection
• No parasites in peripheral blood
• Responds to prolonged antimalarial treatment

Epidemiology

Malaria is primarily a disease of the tropics and subtropics, but is also the most common imported infection in the UK. It is still estimated to cause over a million deaths per year worldwide, particularly in children in sub-Saharan Africa. In highly endemic areas, malaria mainly causes morbidity and mortality in children, but where transmission is less intense it is a disease of both adults and children. The severity of clinical illness is highly modified by the degree of immunity of an individual. Malaria in an expatriate traveller is far more likely to be

Medicine at a Glance, Fourth Edition. Edited by Patrick Davey. © 2014 John Wiley & Sons, Ltd. Published 2014 by John Wiley & Sons, Ltd. Companion website: www.ataglanceseries.com/medicine

life-threatening than in someone who has grown up in an endemic malarial area.

Pathogenesis

Malaria is a protozoal infection transmitted by the bite of the mosquito *Anopheles* spp. Injected sporozoites initially multiply in the liver and then invade red blood cells. Classically, four species of *Plasmodium* infect humans: *P. falciparum*, *P. vivax*, *P. ovale* and *P. malariae*; recently a primate parasite, *P. knowlesi*, has been shown to cause a significant number of cases in parts of Asia. *P. ovale* and *P. vivax* have forms that remain dormant in the liver for a number of years ('hypnozoites') and cause subsequent relapsing infection. *P. falciparum* is the main cause of severe disease as a result of its ability to infect red blood cells of all ages, and to adhere to vascular endothelium and sequester in vital organs such as the brain, liver, kidneys and muscles.

Clinical features

The incubation period is usually 10–14 days, rarely longer than 6 weeks, but may be several years (unusual in *P. falciparum*). Prophylaxis may delay onset of symptoms. The predominant symptoms are:

- Malaise, headache, fever and rigors.
- Occasionally gastrointestinal (GI) or respiratory symptoms dominate, making the clinical diagnosis difficult.

Irregular fever occurs in the acute stages of malaria; classic periodic fever occurs only if untreated. Examination is often unremarkable apart from mild hepatosplenomegaly. Malaria does not cause rashes; other diagnoses should be considered in this situation (although patients with rashes from other causes, e.g. drugs, may have malaria).

Severe malaria

Only *P. falciparum* causes severe malaria, which is a medical emergency; case fatality rates may be 20% or higher:

- **Cerebral malaria**: coma, often with seizures. Low (<5%) risk of long-term damage in adults, with a greater risk in children (hemiplegia, cortical blindness, mental handicap).
- **Severe anaemia**: due to haemolysis and a depressed marrow response.
- **Respiratory distress**: particularly prominent in children, associated with acidosis and sometimes with severe anaemia.
- **Hypoglycaemia**: as a result of increased glucose consumption, impaired gluconeogenesis and quinine-induced hyperinsulinaemia.
- **Acute renal failure**: multifactorial in origin. Rare in children. Rarely, 'blackwater' fever occurs: intravascular haemolysis, producing haemoglobinuria and deep jaundice. Dialysis is needed in 10% of cases of severe malaria.
- **Jaundice**: caused by haemolysis and hepatic dysfunction, particularly in adults.
- Disseminated intravascular coagulation (DIC; see Chapter 188).
- **Non-cardiogenic pulmonary oedema/ARDS** (adult respiratory distress syndrome), which can be life-threatening.
- **Shock** ('algid malaria'): may be caused by concomitant bacteraemia.

Diagnosis

Consider malaria in every febrile patient who has been in an endemic area. The gold standard of diagnosis is the demonstration of malaria trophozoites on a blood film using stains such as Giemsa or Field's stain.

- Thick blood films are used to screen for the presence of parasites.
- Thin films demonstrate detail of parasites, allowing determination of the species.

Patients may have a low parasite burden, especially if malaria prophylaxis has been used. Repeated thick blood films may be needed to make the diagnosis. Commercial rapid diagnostic 'stick' tests detect parasite antigens or enzymes – these require less expertise to perform and detect *P. falciparum* and *P. vivax* well but are less sensitive for the other species.

Differential diagnosis: uncomplicated malaria needs to be distinguished from the long list of tropical and non-tropical diseases that can cause a fever. The differential diagnosis of cerebral malaria includes bacterial, viral and fungal meningitis, arbovirus and other viral causes of encephalitis, and non-infectious causes of coma.

Treatment and management

Treatment of malaria depends on the malaria species. Antimalarial drug resistance is a significant problem in the treatment of falciparum malaria, particularly in Southeast Asia.

- *P. ovale*, *P. vivax*, *P. malaria* and *P. knowlesi*: treat with chloroquine on three successive days to eliminate red blood cell infection. Primaquine is required in *P. vivax*, *P. ovale* and *P. knowlesi* malaria to eliminate hepatic forms. Glucose-6-phosphate dehydrogenase (G6PD) status should be checked to avoid primaquine-induced haemolysis.
- Uncomplicated *P. falciparum*: chloroquine resistance is present in most areas of the world. First-line treatment should be with artemisinin combination therapy for 3 days or oral quinine and doxycycline for 7 days. Other potential agents include mefloquine and atovaquone-proguanil.
- Severe *P. falciparum* infection: parenteral therapy should be given to those with severe malaria or in high-risk subgroups (parasitaemia >2% and pregnancy). Parenteral artesunate is now the first-line drug of choice in both adults and children, but may be difficult to obtain. If unavailable, intravenous quinine should be used; a loading dose enables rapid attainment of therapeutic concentrations. Supportive care is crucial, including careful fluid balance to prevent renal impairment or pulmonary oedema. Hypoglycaemia is common, (especially if using quinine), and should be anticipated. The role of exchange transfusion in severe malaria is unproven and fiercely disputed. Many advocate its use for patients with manifestations of severe malaria and high parasite counts (>10% red cells infected).

Course and prognosis

Most patients become afebrile and aparasitaemic within 2–3 days. There is a significant case fatality rate from severe malaria, especially in non-immune patients. Antimalarials must be continued for their full course; if inadequate treatment courses are given, or if parasites are partially resistant to the drug, then recrudescence of infection can occur.

Preventing infection

Avoid mosquito bites by physical measures: long-sleeved shirts and trousers, mosquito nets, insect repellents, etc. The choice of a chemoprophylactic regimen depends on local resistance patterns. Chloroquine and proguanil are used in the limited areas where chloroquine resistance is not a problem. Mefloquine, doxycycline and atovaquone-proguanil can all be used for most areas where chloroquine resistance occurs. In parts of Southeast Asia there is extensive resistance to antimalarial drugs and specialist advice is necessary.

172 Tuberculosis

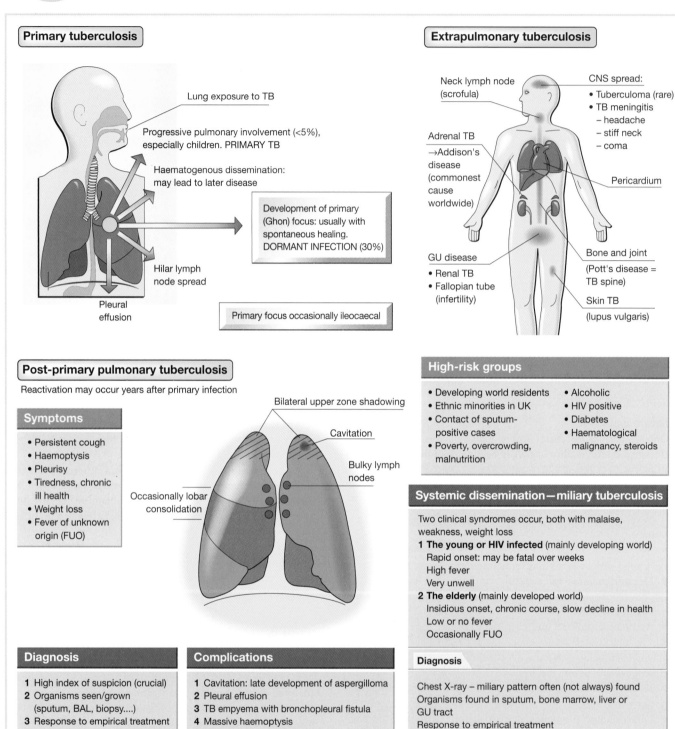

Primary tuberculosis

Lung exposure to TB

Progressive pulmonary involvement (<5%), especially children. PRIMARY TB

Haematogenous dissemination: may lead to later disease

Development of primary (Ghon) focus: usually with spontaneous healing. DORMANT INFECTION (30%)

Hilar lymph node spread

Pleural effusion

Primary focus occasionally ileocaecal

Extrapulmonary tuberculosis

Neck lymph node (scrofula)

CNS spread:
- Tuberculoma (rare)
- TB meningitis
  – headache
  – stiff neck
  – coma

Adrenal TB
→Addison's disease (commonest cause worldwide)

Pericardium

GU disease
- Renal TB
- Fallopian tube (infertility)

Bone and joint (Pott's disease = TB spine)

Skin TB (lupus vulgaris)

Post-primary pulmonary tuberculosis

Reactivation may occur years after primary infection

Symptoms
- Persistent cough
- Haemoptysis
- Pleurisy
- Tiredness, chronic ill health
- Weight loss
- Fever of unknown origin (FUO)

Bilateral upper zone shadowing

Cavitation

Bulky lymph nodes

Occasionally lobar consolidation

High-risk groups
- Developing world residents
- Ethnic minorities in UK
- Contact of sputum-positive cases
- Poverty, overcrowding, malnutrition
- Alcoholic
- HIV positive
- Diabetes
- Haematological malignancy, steroids

Systemic dissemination—miliary tuberculosis

Two clinical syndromes occur, both with malaise, weakness, weight loss
1 **The young or HIV infected** (mainly developing world)
   Rapid onset: may be fatal over weeks
   High fever
   Very unwell
2 **The elderly** (mainly developed world)
   Insidious onset, chronic course, slow decline in health
   Low or no fever
   Occasionally FUO

Diagnosis

Chest X-ray – miliary pattern often (not always) found
Organisms found in sputum, bone marrow, liver or GU tract
Response to empirical treatment

Diagnosis
1 High index of suspicion (crucial)
2 Organisms seen/grown (sputum, BAL, biopsy....)
3 Response to empirical treatment

Complications
1 Cavitation: late development of aspergilloma
2 Pleural effusion
3 TB empyema with bronchopleural fistula
4 Massive haemoptysis

Tuberculosis (TB) remains the cause of over 1.5 million deaths per year despite a reduction over the past two decades. Most infection occurs in tropical regions but there are also a significant number of patients in Europe and the USA, often in poorer, homeless populations and in HIV-infected patients. The HIV pandemic has caused a huge global increase in cases, particularly in sub-Saharan Africa. The emergence of multidrug resistant (MDR) TB and extensively drug resistant TB is a new barrier to improving global control.

Epidemiology

Mycobacterium tuberculosis is spread by respiratory droplets; transmission occurs from close proximity to an infected individual. Household contacts of patients with *M. tuberculosis* in their sputum have a one in four chance of becoming infected. Clinical disease develops in 5–15% of those infected; this risk is higher in HIV.

Pathogenesis

Following inhalation of organisms, multiplication occurs in subpleural and mid-zone terminal airspaces. Bacteria ingested by alveolar macrophages survive and spread to local lymph nodes. Bloodstream spread occurs to the lung apices and other organs, where latent infection may persist for many years. The slow development of a cellular immune response leads to tuberculous granulomata in tissues and cutaneous hypersensitivity to mycobacterial antigens.

Primary infection

Exposure occurs in childhood in endemic areas, but in later life in most western regions. The immune response limits damage to a localized area of the lung with hilar node involvement, termed the primary or Ghon focus; calcification may subsequently be visible on a chest X-ray (CXR). Clinical disease is rare at the time of primary infection in adolescents and adults, although primary pulmonary TB does occur.

Pulmonary TB

Eighty per cent of TB used to be pulmonary, but the proportion of extrapulmonary disease is increasing and is over 50% in HIV patients. The majority of cases are the result of reactivation; reinfection also occurs. The major symptoms are cough, weight loss, malaise, fever and night sweats. Haemoptysis occurs in a third. Examination findings are often unremarkable. The CXR is usually abnormal – classically, apical disease with infiltration and cavitation that heals with fibrotic changes. Complications include severe haemoptysis, bronchopleural fistula and aspergilloma within cavities.

Extrapulmonary disease

- **Pleural TB**: commonly occurs after primary infection. There are systemic symptoms, cough and pleuritic pain. Unilateral effusions are common. Often self-limiting, sometimes with resolution of symptoms. Most develop active disease within 3 years.
- **Lymph node TB**: occurs after primary infection, reactivation and contiguous spread. Cervical in 70%. Systemic symptoms occur in 30–60%. Painless discrete nodes enlarge in size and become matted. Nodes eventually break down with discharging sinuses and chronic skin lesions.
- **Bone/joint TB**: affects any bone or joint. Most common form is spinal (Pott's disease). Vertebral destruction leads to collapse and, sometimes, severe angulation of the spine (gibbus). Paravertebral abscesses may occur. Watch for cord compression; most can be treated medically.
- **TB meningitis**: important; there is a risk of permanent neurological damage or death if not treated promptly. Initial bloodborne spread, followed by rupture of focus into the cerebrospinal fluid (CSF). There are non-specific symptoms for 2–8 weeks, with onset that is often insidious. Fever and headache are prominent. Mild neck stiffness, cranial nerve palsies, papilloedema and long tract signs also occur. Seizures are common in children. Differential diagnosis: fungal or partially treated bacterial meningitis, cerebral abscess.
- **Pericardial TB**: usually caused by spread from the lungs or mediastinal lymph nodes. There are three clinical syndromes: acute pericarditis ± effusion, chronic pericardial effusion and chronic constrictive pericarditis. Systemic symptoms, shortness of breath and signs of effusion or constriction occur; tamponade due to effusion may occur. Pericardial calcification (late) on CXR may be seen in constrictive pericarditis. Echocardiography is helpful.
- **Miliary TB**: disseminated disease from blood spread in those with underlying chronic disease or immunosuppression. Insidious symptoms: weight loss, fever, malaise. Pulmonary, central nervous system (CNS) and liver involvement are most frequent. Choroidal tubercles (15%) are pathognomonic. Classic CXR; multiple 1–2 mm nodules in lung fields.

Diagnosis

Definitive diagnosis depends upon demonstrating or culturing the organism.

- **Pulmonary TB** is normally diagnosed by:
  - Ziehl–Neelsen staining of acid-fast bacilli (AFB) in the sputum.
  - Culture of samples on selective media (takes up to 8 weeks).
- **Open TB** describes the presence of AFB in sputum.
- **Extrapulmonary TB**: sputum culture is occasionally positive, but the diagnosis is usually made from the culture of appropriate samples (needle aspiration of lymph node or marrow and liver biopsy in miliary TB) or by histology (pleural or pericardial biopsy) showing granulomata or AFB. Classic X-ray changes (in Pott's disease) may be diagnostic. The CSF in TB meningitis (lymphocytes, high protein, low sugar) likewise may be highly suggestive. Polymerase chain reaction (PCR) techniques are occasionally used to make a more rapid diagnosis. Automated PCR is beginning to be used for simultaneous identification of species and testing of resistance. Like other diagnostic approaches, it is limited by contamination of specimens and is less accurate in culture-negative TB.
- **Mantoux test**: measures the delayed hypersensitivity reaction to intradermal purified protein derivative. Positive tests indicate previous exposure. Anergy occurs in systemic illness such as miliary TB, but immunosuppression can obtund this response. In the UK, patients may react because of previous BCG (bacille Calmette–Guérin) immunization. A strongly positive reaction can be helpful clinically but results need to be interpreted with care. Interferon γ release assays indicate exposure rather than active disease; they are used in clinical practice to test for latent TB in patients prior to planned immunosuppression.

Treatment

Short-course chemotherapy (6 months) is given for most forms of TB (see Table 172.1); longer courses may be needed for TB meningitis and bone/joint TB. Combinations of four drugs are used to prevent the development of resistance. The clinical response to therapy may be important in confirming the diagnosis; reductions in fever and weight gain are helpful. Steroids are of proven benefit in pericardial disease and are commonly used in TB meningitis and genitourinary (GU) TB.

Resistance to individual TB drugs is a major clinical problem in some countries particularly in eastern Europe, the former Soviet states and some African countries. Some isolates are resistant to multiple drugs. The risk of MDR TB is increased in patients who have had previous treatment, contact with resistant disease or who are from the prison population. Prolonged treatment with second- and third-line agents is necessary, with a poor response in many patients.

Surgery is useful for chronic constrictive pericarditis, Pott's disease if there is severe cord compression or spinal instability, and intractable haemoptysis or bronchopleural fistula.

Infection control issues need to be considered; those with smear-positive TB should be isolated for the first 2 weeks of treatment and if factors suggest the possibility of MDR TB (previous TB treatment or birth in a foreign country), special precautions must be taken.

Table 172.1 Standard short-course therapy for TB.

Drug	Duration	Important side effects or problems
Isoniazid	6 months	Hepatotoxicity, neuropathy (vitamin B_6 prevents)
Rifampicin	6 months	Hepatotoxicity, drug interactions
Pyrazinamide	First 2 months	Hepatotoxicity
Ethambutol	First 2 months	Retrobulbar neuritis (check colour vision) (if resistance is a concern)

173 Tropical infectious diseases

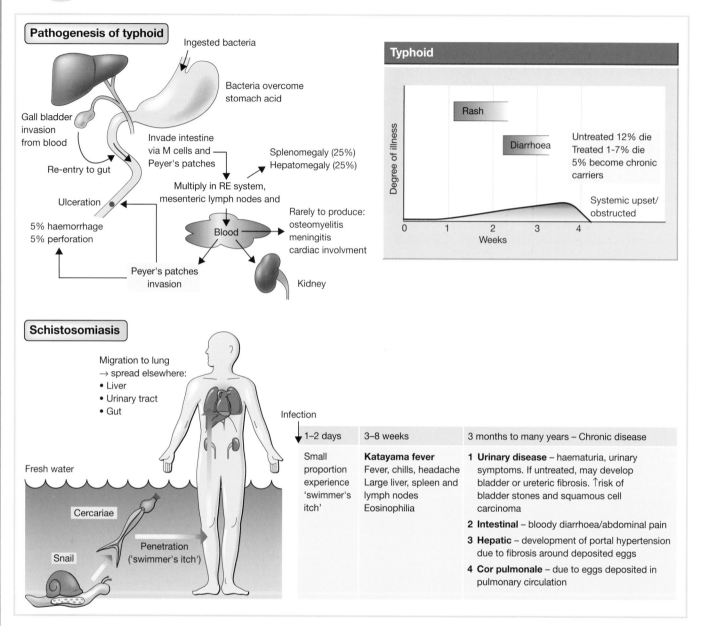

Typhoid

Typhoid occurs from infection with the Gram-negative bacteria *Salmonella typhi* or *S. paratyphi* through the ingestion of contaminated food or water. The *Salmonella* sp. enters through the gut, multiplies within the mesenteric lymph nodes and macrophages and enters the bloodstream to be disseminated to many sites where further replication occurs.

Clinical features

The incubation period is 10–14 days. There is a gradually rising fever, headache, malaise and occasionally cough. Abdominal symptoms (pain, diarrhea, constipation) are prominent during the first week, whereas diarrhoea, mild hepatosplenomegaly and rose spots (in 60%) occur during the second week. Shock, renal impairment and altered mental state, including coma, occur in severe cases. Complications include: (i) perforation or bleeding from the ileum; (ii) osteomyelitis, more common in sickle-cell disease; (iii) cholecystitis; and (iv) myocarditis.

Diagnosis

Leukopenia is common and elevated transaminases may occur. Culture of the organism from stool, blood, urine or bone marrow is diagnostic. Serology (Widal's test) is rarely helpful, even in non-immunized cases.

Treatment

Optimum treatment depends on knowing the geographical origin of the isolate; drug resistance to traditional chloramphenicol, co-trimoxazole or ampicillin is common. Sensitivity testing is

Medicine at a Glance, Fourth Edition. Edited by Patrick Davey. © 2014 John Wiley & Sons, Ltd. Published 2014 by John Wiley & Sons, Ltd. Companion website: www.ataglanceseries.com/medicine

useful. Fluoroquinolones are still considered first-line therapy in most regions although azithromycin is becoming more commonly used as first-line therapy; azithromycin or ceftriaxone should be used for resistant cases Steroids are used in severe disease. Fever may take several days to respond to treatment. Relapse occurs in 10%. Long-term asymptomatic carriage may occur from persistence of the organism in the gall bladder but is rare (<2%).

Dengue

Dengue is caused by an arbovirus transmitted by the mosquito *Aedes* sp.; it is increasingly common as its geographical distribution expands. Two main clinical syndromes occur:

- Dengue fever, seen in most travellers.
- Dengue haemorrhagic fever/dengue shock syndrome (DHF/ DSS), usually seen in children in endemic areas as a result of an immunological response to a second infection.

Clinical features (3–8-day incubation)

These are sudden fever, severe headache, backache, muscle pains and rigors. Fever may be biphasic – it disappears then reappears. Maculopapular rash occurs late on in the illness. In DHF/DSS (rare in the UK) increased vascular permeability results in shock, petechiae and bleeding.

Diagnosis and treatment

Leukopenia and thrombocytopenia are common. In DHF/DSS, severe thrombocytopenia, raised haematocrit and abnormal liver enzymes are found. Diagnosis is clinical because virus isolation is not routinely available. Serology is useful for retrospective diagnosis.

No specific treatment is available. DHF/DSS requires supportive therapy and fluids and has a high case fatality.

Schistosomiasis

Two hundred million people are infected worldwide and it is common in returned travellers, although patients are rarely unwell. Schistosomal cerceriae penetrate the skin after freshwater exposure and migrate via the lungs to the vessels of the bladder or gut (depending on the species), where eggs are produced. Eggs migrate back into the gut lumen or urinary tract, but may cause local inflammation. Worm burdens are low in expatriates; severe disease is rare. The clinical features of disease are:

- Swimmer's itch: transient rash 1–2 days after exposure, often unrecognized.
- Katayama fever: 3–8 weeks after exposure in a small proportion of patients. Acute fever, sweats, malaise – sometimes lymphadenopathy, hepatosplenomegaly or bronchospasm; it is self-limiting.
- Urinary schistosomiasis (*Schistosoma haematobium*): often asymptomatic and diagnosed because of eosinophilia. May have haematuria, urinary symptoms or altered ejaculate. Long-term complications are unusual in travellers.
- Intestinal/hepatic schistosomiasis: vague abdominal symptoms/bloody diarrhoea or asymptomatic. The long-term complication of non-cirrhotic portal hypertension is rare in travellers, but is very common worldwide.

Diagnosis and treatment

- Eosinophilia is common.
- Demonstration of eggs in urine, ejaculate, stool or rectal biopsies.

- Schistosomal serology is useful, but may not be positive until several months after exposure.
- Praziquantel is effective for all species.

Tick typhus

Tick typhus is the major rickettsial disease seen in the UK, particularly in travellers from southern Africa. Tick typhus is caused by the bite of a tick which may be infected by a number of different rickettsial species with a wide geographical distribution. The clinical features are:

- Fever, headache and myalgia.
- Maculopapular rash.
- An eschar (black lesion on skin due to necrosis at the site of a tick bite) helps to confirm the diagnosis.
- Lymphadenopathy may occur.
- Rarely, severe systemic illness occurs.

Diagnosis and treatment

Diagnosis is usually clinical, with serological confirmation retrospectively. Tetracycline is extremely effective as treatment.

Leptospirosis

This occurs after contact with water infected by animal urine containing leptospires. It may be contracted in the UK (sewer workers, water sports) and is common in many parts of the tropics. Leptospires penetrate the skin and mucosa, multiply in the blood and then localize in the liver, central nervous system, muscle and renal cortex.

Clinical features

There is a wide spectrum of illness from fever, headache and muscle pains to severe sepsis with conjunctivitis, pneumonitis, jaundice, renal failure and extensive haemorrhages.

Diagnosis and treatment

Leukocytosis and thrombocytopenia are common. Creatine kinase is elevated in moderate or severe cases. There is abnormal liver function and renal function. Clinical suspicion may be confirmed by identification of leptospires on dark-ground microscopy of the blood. Serology gives retrospective diagnosis. Treatment should be with parenteral penicillin or doxycycline although there is limited evidence that they improve outcomes.

Haemorrhagic fevers

Although uncommon, high mortality and potential for transmission to others mean that such fevers should be considered in sick patients returning from the tropics. They are caused by a number of different RNA viruses, are predominately zoonoses and occur on every continent apart from Australia. Diseases include Ebola, Marburg, Lassa fever, yellow fever and Hanta viruses. Suspect on geographical grounds and history of contact with tick or animal blood/faeces, or ill patients (often doctors/nurses), often in remote areas. Clinically:

- Fevers, severe myalgia and increasing prostration.
- Pharyngitis prominent in Lassa fever. Petechiae and bleeding gums may progress to shock and frank haemorrhage.
- Severe malaria is the major differential diagnosis and must be excluded.

Diagnosis and treatment

Diagnosis is by virus isolation or serology in most cases, with appropriate precautions. Patients are isolated until diagnosis has been excluded – take care to avoid nosocomial transmission. Supportive care is crucial; ribavirin is useful in Lassa fever and some other viruses.

174 Diseases predisposing to infection

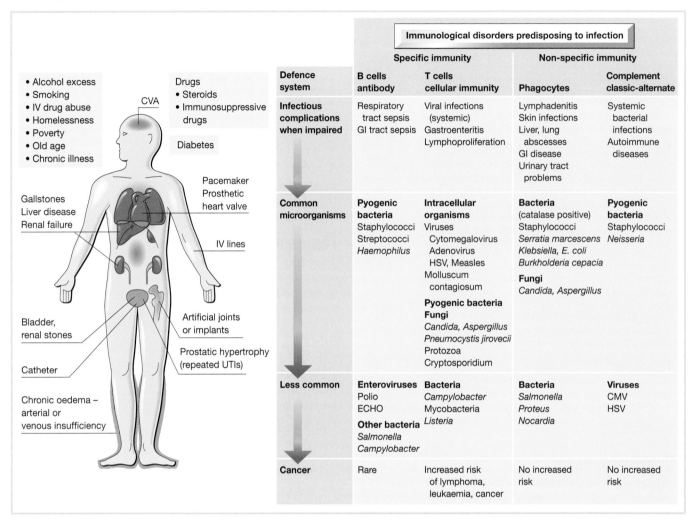

- Alcohol excess
- Smoking
- IV drug abuse
- Homelessness
- Poverty
- Old age
- Chronic illness

CVA

Drugs
- Steroids
- Immunosuppressive drugs

Diabetes

Gallstones
Liver disease
Renal failure

Pacemaker
Prosthetic
heart valve

IV lines

Bladder,
renal stones

Artificial joints
or implants

Prostatic hypertrophy
(repeated UTIs)

Catheter

Chronic oedema –
arterial or
venous insufficiency

Immunological disorders predisposing to infection

	Specific immunity		Non-specific immunity	
Defence system	B cells antibody	T cells cellular immunity	Phagocytes	Complement classic-alternate
Infectious complications when impaired	Respiratory tract sepsis GI tract sepsis	Viral infections (systemic) Gastroenteritis Lymphoproliferation	Lymphadenitis Skin infections Liver, lung abscesses GI disease Urinary tract problems	Systemic bacterial infections Autoimmune diseases
Common microorganisms	**Pyogenic bacteria** Staphylococci Streptococci *Haemophilus*	**Intracellular organisms** Viruses Cytomegalovirus Adenovirus HSV, Measles Molluscum contagiosum **Pyogenic bacteria Fungi** *Candida, Aspergillus Pneumocystis jirovecii* Protozoa Cryptosporidium	**Bacteria** (catalase positive) Staphylococci *Serratia marcescens Klebsiella, E. coli Burkholderia cepacia* **Fungi** *Candida, Aspergillus*	**Pyogenic bacteria** Staphylococci *Neisseria*
Less common	**Enteroviruses** Polio ECHO **Other bacteria** *Salmonella Campylobacter*	**Bacteria** *Campylobacter* Mycobacteria *Listeria*	**Bacteria** *Salmonella Proteus Nocardia*	**Viruses** CMV HSV
Cancer	Rare	Increased risk of lymphoma, leukaemia, cancer	No increased risk	No increased risk

Abnormalities of host immunity predispose to:

- Unusually severe insfection.
- Infection in unusual sites.
- Recurrent infection.
- Infection with unusual pathogens, or organisms not usually regarded as pathogenic.

In a patient with any of the above, a search for diseases that alter immunity is crucial. The type of pathogen, site and extent of infection sometimes helps to identify the underlying disease.

Diseases predisposing to infections with common bacterial pathogens

- Diabetes mellitus predisposes to infection, which may be recurrent or more severe in most tissues, especially the lung, urinary tract and skin (boils, etc.).
- Smoking has a clear role in repeated respiratory tract infections.
- Alcohol excess, even in the absence of chronic liver disease, predisposes to many infections, particularly those involving the

respiratory tract, e.g. pneumococcal pneumonia, Legionnaires' disease and tuberculosis (TB).

- Renal failure is a potent factor predisposing to infection. Not only does uraemia impair immunity, but those with renal failure also have recurrent instrumentation (e.g. intravenous (IV) cannulae, dialysis lines) which introduces infection. Infective endocarditis, often caused by *Staphyloccoccus aureus*, occurs annually in 1% of the dialysis population. The nephrotic syndrome predisposes even more powerfully to infection, possibly as the renal protein losses includes IgG and some complement protiens, although not IgM.
- Chronic liver disease impairs immunity (e.g. bacterial uptake by the reticuloendothelial system), and contributes to infection in those with chronic abuse of alcohol, as well as in those with other forms of chronic hepatitis.
- Steroid therapy, especially in high dose, impairs immunity and, although it may lead to unusual infections, more frequently infection is with common pathogens (e.g. pneumococci, herpes zoster, etc.). The same is true for many other drugs that impair immunity, such as azathioprine, cyclophosphamide, ciclosporin

Medicine at a Glance, Fourth Edition. Edited by Patrick Davey. © 2014 John Wiley & Sons, Ltd. Published 2014 by John Wiley & Sons, Ltd. Companion website: www.ataglanceseries.com/medicine

A, etc. Anticonvulsants impair antibody synthesis and cause secondary hypogammaglobulinaemia.

- Chronic inflammatory illness also impairs immunity, e.g. active rheumatoid arthritis. Crohn's disease, disseminated malignancy, etc. impair nutritional status, producing hypoalbuminaemia and hypogammaglobulinaemia.

Structural factors predisposing to infection with common bacterial pathogens

- IV lines: central and peripheral venous lines are a potent source of bacteraemia, commonly with *Staphylococcus aureus*. This infection may lead to infective endocarditis, even in the absence of underlying valvular disease, or to osteomyelitis. IV drug abuse also predisposes to infective endocarditis, particularly involving the right-sided heart valves and lung abscesses. IV drug abusers may have HIV infection or hepatitis B or C, which can impair immunity and predispose to infection themselves.
- Structural abnormalities should be considered in repeated infections of the same structure, e.g. bladder and renal stones or prostatic hypertrophy may cause recurrent urinary tract infections (UTIs). An obstructing bronchial carcinoma may underlie recurrent/severe pneumonia.
- Prosthetic material: niduses of bacterial infection on prosthetic material (e.g. pacemakers, heart valves and, less commonly, hip replacements) can cause persistent/recurrent bacteraemia or septicaemia. Once colonized, prosthetic material can rarely be sterilized and usually needs to be removed. Usually common bacterial pathogens are involved, although occasionally infection is with fairly indolent bacteria, e.g. *Staphylococcus epidermidis*.
- Immobility predisposes to UTIs because a low fluid intake (deliberate, to avoid unnecessary visits to the toilet) fails to 'flush' the urinary tract free of pathogens.
- Hemiparesis, especially during the acute phase, predisposes to chest infection.
- Gastroenterological pathology such as dysphagia (especially if the result of neurological disease) or gastro-oesophageal reflux can underlie recurrent pneumonia.
- Lack of a spleen (congenital, traumatic, elective removal) or poor splenic function (e.g. in coeliac disease) predisposes to overwhelming sepsis with capsulated organisms (*Pneumococcus*, *Haemophilus*). The presence of Howell–Jolly bodies on a blood film suggests poor/absent spleneic fucntion.

Miscellaneous conditions

- Homelessness is an obvious precipitant for repeated respiratory tract and skin infections.
- Cachexia impairs the ability of the body to fight infection and underlies infections in terminal illness. Milder degrees of malnutrition, such as those relating to undiagnosed inflammatory or neoplastic illness, social deprivation or psychiatric illness, are relatively easy to miss and can underlie some repeated infections. Iron is essential to host defence and iron deficiency increases infection risk.
- Failure of the immune system predisposes to infection with opportunistic pathogens (see following section), as well as with common pathogens – illness in this situation is likely to be more severe and progress more rapidly. Many viral infections depress immunity transiently, predisposing to subsequent bacterial infection, e.g. influenza in elderly people predisposing to bacterial pneumonia, and measles in malnourished individuals leading on to infective diarrhoea. Previous haematological cancer or autologous bone marrow transplantation predisposes, even many years later, to infection with many common pathogens.

Diseases predisposing to infection with unusual pathogens

Defects in immune function should be considered when infection involves unusual organisms (e.g. normally non-pathogenic organisms), or if common pathogens infect patients at unexpected ages (e.g. *Neisseria meningitidis* in adults, TB in well-nourished white adults aged 16–65 years), in unusual sites (e.g. fungal pneumonia) or are particularly severe or recurrent (e.g. extensive pyogenic abscesses). Underlying conditions include diabetes, immunosuppressive drugs and the conditions listed here.

Complement defects

Complement defects predispose to infection with bacteria and, particularly, *Neisseria meningitidis* at an unusual age.

- Acquired complement defects, e.g. as a result of systemic lupus erythematosus.
- Inherited deficiency is very rare. C5, C6, C7 or C8 deficiency predisposes to *N. meningitidis*. C3 deficiency behaves like antibody deficiency, with susceptibility to common pathogenic bacteria.

Neutrophil defects

Neutrophil defects predispose to overwhelming sepsis with *Staphylococcus aureus*, *Serratia marcescens* and fungi, typically *Aspergillus*:

- Neutropenia: inadequate neutrophil numbers (see Chapter 53). The most common causes are drugs and haematological cancer and its treatment. Rare cause include genetic neutropenias, including cyclic neutropenia.
- Defects in neutrophil function: myelodysplasia and haematological cancer depress neutrophil counts and the function of any remaining cells. Other functional defects include the rare inherited ones (see Chapter 175).

Antibody deficiencies

Antibody deficiency predisposes to bacterial infection, especially with staphylococci, streptococci and *Haemophilus influenzae*. Infections, particularly those caused by pneumococci, may be overwhelming:

- Multiple myeloma is a relatively common cause of acquired hypogammaglobulinaemia.
- Chronic lymphocytic leukaemia and other haematological malignancies and their treatment depress B-cell counts, both during and after treatment and cause hypogammaglobulinameia.
- Primary antibody deficiencies are all extraordinarily rare (see Chapter 175).

Defects in cell-mediated immunity

Defects in cell-mediated immunity include:

- HIV infection (see Chapter 168).
- Haematological cancer and its treatment.
- Primary defects (see Chapter 175).

175 Immunological deficiency syndromes

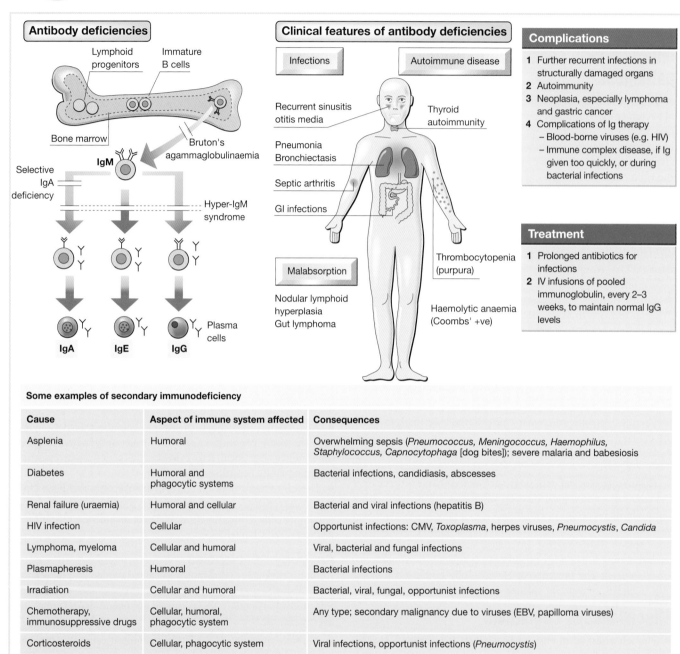

Antibody deficiencies

Lymphoid progenitors
Immature B cells
Bone marrow
Bruton's agammaglobulinaemia
IgM
Selective IgA deficiency
Hyper-IgM syndrome
IgA   IgE   IgG   Plasma cells

Clinical features of antibody deficiencies

Infections
Autoimmune disease

Recurrent sinusitis otitis media
Thyroid autoimmunity
Pneumonia Bronchiectasis
Septic arthritis
GI infections

Malabsorption

Nodular lymphoid hyperplasia
Gut lymphoma

Thrombocytopenia (purpura)
Haemolytic anaemia (Coombs' +ve)

Complications

1 Further recurrent infections in structurally damaged organs
2 Autoimmunity
3 Neoplasia, especially lymphoma and gastric cancer
4 Complications of Ig therapy
   – Blood-borne viruses (e.g. HIV)
   – Immune complex disease, if Ig given too quickly, or during bacterial infections

Treatment

1 Prolonged antibiotics for infections
2 IV infusions of pooled immunoglobulin, every 2–3 weeks, to maintain normal IgG levels

Some examples of secondary immunodeficiency

Cause	Aspect of immune system affected	Consequences
Asplenia	Humoral	Overwhelming sepsis (*Pneumococcus, Meningococcus, Haemophilus, Staphylococcus, Capnocytophaga* [dog bites]); severe malaria and babesiosis
Diabetes	Humoral and phagocytic systems	Bacterial infections, candidiasis, abscesses
Renal failure (uraemia)	Humoral and cellular	Bacterial and viral infections (hepatitis B)
HIV infection	Cellular	Opportunist infections: CMV, *Toxoplasma*, herpes viruses, *Pneumocystis*, *Candida*
Lymphoma, myeloma	Cellular and humoral	Viral, bacterial and fungal infections
Plasmapheresis	Humoral	Bacterial infections
Irradiation	Cellular and humoral	Bacterial, viral, fungal, opportunist infections
Chemotherapy, immunosuppressive drugs	Cellular, humoral, phagocytic system	Any type; secondary malignancy due to viruses (EBV, papilloma viruses)
Corticosteroids	Cellular, phagocytic system	Viral infections, opportunist infections (*Pneumocystis*)

Immunodeficiency should be suspected whenever there is evidence of increased susceptibility to infection. The commonest causes of immunodeficiency are secondary to other medical or surgical problems or their therapy. Symptomatic primary immunodeficiency is rare. There are no hard and fast rules indicating that immunodeficiency is likely to be present, but two or more serious (requiring intravenous antibiotics) infections in a year are highly suspicious. Infections in unusual sites, for example liver or brain abscesses, osteomyelitis, septic arthritis, where there is no obvious structural reason, and infection with unusual or normally non-pathogenic organisms are highly suspicious of immunodeficiency. Primary immunodeficiency may also be accompanied by evidence of immune dysfunction such as autoimmune disease. The immune system is very adaptable and often the severity of the clinical problem is less severe than one might predict because of compensatory mechanisms. The nature of the infection gives a clue to the underlying defect (see Table 175.1). Cases of suspected primary or secondary immunodeficiency should be referred to an immunologist for formal investigation; suspected human immunodeficiency virus (HIV) infection should be referred to a consultant in infectious diseases or genitourinary medicine experienced in the management of the condition.

Medicine at a Glance, Fourth Edition. Edited by Patrick Davey. © 2014 John Wiley & Sons, Ltd. Published 2014 by John Wiley & Sons, Ltd. Companion website: www.ataglanceseries.com/medicine

Table 175.1 Classification of immunological deficiency syndromes.

Type of defect	Typical infections	Type of defect	Typical infections
B-cell defect (reduced antibody)	Bacterial infections: • *Streptococcus pneumoniae* • *Haemophilus influenzae* • *Neisseria meningitidis* • *Staphylococcus aureus* • *Campylobacter* species • *Salmonella* species and other enteric pathogens • *Mycoplasma* species • *Ureaplasma* species Viral infections: • Enteroviruses (polio, echoviruses, Coxsackie viruses) Protozoal infections: • *Giardia lamblia*		Fungal infections: • *Candida* • *Aspergillus* • *Pneumocystis carinii (jirovecii)* Protozoal infections: • *Toxoplasma gondii* • Cryptosporidium • Microsporidium
		Combined T- and B-cell defect	As for B- and T-cell defects Pattern may be variable
T-cell defect	Bacterial infections: • May be some increase in bacterial infections due to poor T-cell help for B-cell responses Viral infections: • All types, often persistent • Enteric viruses (Rotavirus) • Respiratory viruses (respiratory syncytial virus, parainfluenza viruses, adenoviruses) • Herpes viruses (EBV, CMV, HHV6) • Papillomaviruses (warts) • JC and BK viruses (progressive multifocal leukoencephalopathy)	Neutrophil defects	Bacterial infections: • Catalase-positive organisms (*Staphylococcus aureus*) Fungal infections: • Any fungus (typically *Aspergillus*)
		Complement deficiency	Bacterial infections: • *Neisseria* species As for antibody deficiency (C3 deficiency only)

CMV, cytomegalovirus; EBV, Epstein–Barr virus; HHV, human herpes virvs; JC, John Cunningham.

Antibody deficiency syndromes

In antibody deficiencies recurrent bacterial infections occur, usually with common organisms (e.g. *Haemophilus influenzae*, *Streptococcus pneumoniae*), although less usual organisms (e.g. *Mycoplasma*) are also important. Infections most frequently involve the upper and lower respiratory tract, but may involve the gastrointestinal (GI) tract (e.g. *Giardia*) and other sites. Malabsorption may be due to infection, a coeliac-like condition, nodular lymphoid hyperplasia or malignancy. If the underlying disorder is untreated, the frequency and severity of the infections results in structural end-organ damage including bronchiectasis and growth retardation in children. Deficiencies are classified into primary and secondary antibody deficiencies.

Primary antibody deficiency

Primary antibody deficiency is a reduction or absence of one or more immunoglobulin isotypes when no other contributory disorder is present. There are four major forms. All are rare – a prevalence of 12 per million. In primary antibody deficiencies both infections and antibody-mediated autoimmune disease occur:

- **X-linked agammaglobulinaemia** (Bruton's agammaglobulinaemia): mutation in the X chromosome (*Btk* gene) prevents normal B-cell maturation. Presents in patients aged 3–12 months; milder forms present later.
- **Hyper-IgM syndrome**: presents in childhood with recurrent bacterial infections and autoimmune disease (neutropenia, thrombocytopenia). The X-linked form (70% of cases) is a deficiency of the CD40 ligand on T cells (a lymphocyte communication molecule). The IgM antibody response is intact. B cells cannot produce mature IgG or IgA antibody. There is very high IgM, and low/undetectable IgG and IgA, and an increased risk of IgM lymphomas.
- **Common variable immunodeficiency** (CVID): the aetiology is unknown but is partly genetic (50% have a family history of IgA deficiency). There are heterogeneous laboratory findings. Serum IgG levels may be only marginally reduced, but specific antibody production is invariably poor or absent. IgM levels may

be normal. Patients present at any age, particularly in adolescence and early adulthood. Autoimmune disease is common. There is a 40-fold increased risk of lymphoma, and also an increased risk of gastric cancer.

- **Selective IgA deficiency**: this affects one in 400–800. Most are asymptomatic, but there is an increased incidence of allergic disease and connective tissue disease. Recurrent infections are rarely a problem unless additional immune defects are present. The diagnosis is made based upon *absent* serum IgA (not just low levels).
- **Specific antibody deficiency (with normal immunoglobulins)**: this is linked to CVID and selective IgA deficiency and represents a failure of immune responsiveness to a single class of antigens such as bacterial polysaccharides. Serum immunoglobulins and IgG subclasses are normal.

Secondary antibody deficiency

Secondary antibody deficiency syndromes are the commonest cause of antibody deficiency and relate to conditions such as the nephrotic syndrome (protein leak), protein-losing enteropathies/malabsorption (protein leak), immunosuppressive drug therapy, multiple myeloma (negative feedback), lymphoproliferative disease (especially chronic lymphocytic leukaemia) and (probably) malignancy.

Investigations

The initial investigations in suspected primary antibody deficiency are serum immunoglobulins and protein electrophoresis. These measure the ability to produce antibodies, although not their 'usefulness'. The absence of immunoglobulins is always significant, but specific antibody deficiency can occur with normal serum immunoglobulins and functional tests of antibody production may be required. The diagnosis in CVID is complicated, as while serum IgG may be absent or very low, this is not invariable. In such cases it is important to measure specific antibodies to antigens to which the patient has been exposed, e.g. tetanus/diphtheria vaccinations. If specific antibodies are undetectable or very low, the patient may be test immunized with a (killed) vaccine and serology repeated 4–6 weeks later. Failure to mount a response may indicate an antibody deficiency. Secondary antibody deficiencies should be excluded.

Management and prognosis

The mainstay of treatment is long-term replacement therapy with pooled immunoglobulin, which provides passive protection from bacterial infections. Once diagnosed and treated, patients usually lead normal active lives, although recurrent infections can occur despite adequate replacement therapy if there is pre-existing structural damage. If an infection becomes established, early and prolonged treatment with antibiotics is essential, usually for 10 days. Autoimmune diseases usually require corticosteroids. There is an increased incidence of malignancies, particularly lymphoma.

T-cell deficiencies

These are usually secondary to another disease process (haematological malignancy, its treatment or HIV infection) but can be primary. Most are evident in childhood but may present in early adult life.

- **22q11 deletion syndrome** (DiGeorge's syndrome): complex genetic disorder (chromosome 22) with major cardiac, facial and parathyroid gland defects. Intellectual impairment is common. There is a high risk of blood-borne infection from transfusions during cardiac surgery. The degree of immunodeficiency is very

variable: severe cases have a small, atrophic thymus and no T cells and can mimic severe combined immunodeficiency (SCID). Autoimmune diseases often develop later in life. Survival into adult life is common. Bone marrow and thymic transplants have been used.

- **Chronic mucocutaneous candidiasis**: a common, mainly T-cell defect, leading to chronic candidiasis, typically of the mouth and nails. Fifty per cent have an autoimmune endocrinopathy (associated with defects in the autoimmune regulator gene, *AIRE*). Bacterial, viral and mycobacterial infections may also occur.
- **Other syndromes**: other predominantly T-cell syndromes include Wiskott–Aldrich syndrome (eczema, thrombocytopenia with small platelets, immune deficiency), due to mutations in the *WASP* gene on the X chromosome, and ataxia telangiectasia (progressive cerebellar degeneration, immune deficiency), due to mutations in the *ATM* gene. The IPEX syndrome is due to a genetic deficiency of the FOXP3 protein required for regulatory T-cell function; severe autoimmune disease, with bowel involvement, is common.

Severe combined immunodeficiency

This only rarely presents in adult life. Features are those of bacterial, viral, fungal and opportunist infections. Genetic defects include mutations affecting the cytokine common γ chain, Jak-3, adenosine deaminase genes. The bare lymphocyte syndrome often presents slightly later and may be due to defects in genes controlling major histocompatibility complex (MHC) antigen expression.

Investigations

Measurement of T-cell subpopulations (CD4, CD8) and MHC antigens (MHC class I and class II) and functional assays of T cells are required. This can only be undertaken in specialist laboratories and early referral to an immunologist is required.

Management of severe combined and T-cell disorders

Prevention of infection is critical in all T-cell deficiencies:

- Live vaccines (e.g. BCG) should not be given.
- Concomitant antibody deficiency can be treated with immunoglobulin replacement therapy.
- Blood transfused should be cytomegalovirus negative and irradiated to avoid graft vs host disease (mediated by donor lymphocytes).
- Prophylaxis against *Pneumocystis jirovecii* infection should be given.
- Human stem cell transplantation (HSCT) is indicated in severe primary disease, including all patients with SCID and the Wiskott–Aldrich syndrome. This is much more difficult in adults.

Neutrophil disorders

The commonest neutrophil disorders in adults are secondary, but primary neutrophil disorders may also present in adults for the first time. They typically present with recurrent abscesses (liver), unusual granulomatous disease (mimicking sarcoidosis) and atypical Crohn's disease.

- **Chronic granulomatous disease**: occurs due to defects in neutrophil oxidative metabolism, caused by mutations in genes for the components of the multiprotein NADPH (reduced nicotinamide adenine dinucleotide phosphate) oxidase enzyme. X-linked and autosomal recessive forms may occur. Involvement of the bowel with consequent malabsorption and hepatosplenomegaly are common.

- **Other inherited neutrophil defects**: other genetic diseases interfere with chemotaxis (hyper-IgE syndrome, Chediak–Higashi syndrome), phagocytosis (leukocyte adhesion deficiency) or neutrophil numbers (cyclic neutropenia).
- **Acquired defects**: neutrophil abnormalities include deficient numbers (neutropenia, see Chapter 53 – often drug or leukaemia related) or quality (e.g. in myelodysplasia, see Chapter 185).

Investigations

Diagnosis of chronic granulomatous disease is made using the nitroblue tetrazolium test or a flow cytometric assay of neutrophil oxidative metabolism.

Management

Prevention of infection is critical.

- Prophylactic co-trimoxazole (active in neutrophil phagocytic granules).
- Prophylactic itraconazole to prevent fungal infections.
- γ-Interferon may be helpful for treating infection in combination with antibiotics.
- Investigate for bowel involvement.
- HSCT (any age), as long-term outlook without is poor.

Complement deficiency

Complement deficiency is strongly associated with recurrent neisserial infection and atypical connective tissue disease (systemic lupus erythematosus) and glomerulonephritis. Any

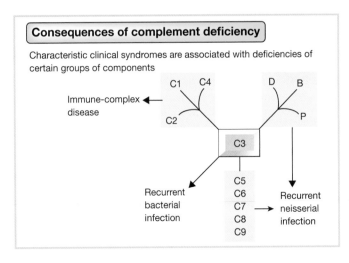

Consequences of complement deficiency

Characteristic clinical syndromes are associated with deficiencies of certain groups of components

component may be deficient. Investigate every patient with more than one episode of bacterial meningitis.

Investigations

Complement deficiency can be proved by demonstration of the absence of haemolytic complement activity in fresh serum (CH100 and alternate pathway CH100).

Management

- Prophylactic penicillin V 500 mg bd for adults.
- Immunize against *Meningococcus* (quadrivalent conjugate vaccine) and *Pneumococcus*.

176 Haematinic deficiency anaemias

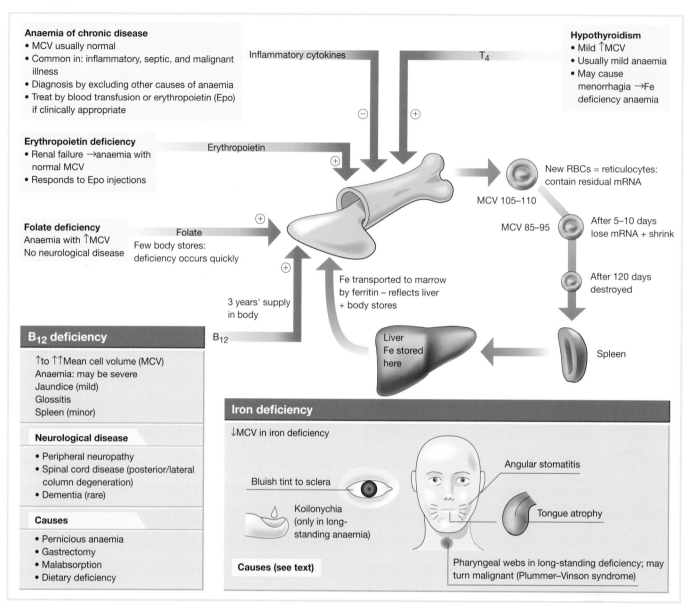

Anaemia of chronic disease
- MCV usually normal
- Common in: inflammatory, septic, and malignant illness
- Diagnosis by excluding other causes of anaemia
- Treat by blood transfusion or erythropoietin (Epo) if clinically appropriate

Erythropoietin deficiency
- Renal failure →anaemia with normal MCV
- Responds to Epo injections

Folate deficiency
Anaemia with ↑MCV
No neurological disease

Inflammatory cytokines

T_4

Hypothyroidism
- Mild ↑MCV
- Usually mild anaemia
- May cause menorrhagia →Fe deficiency anaemia

Erythropoietin

Folate
Few body stores: deficiency occurs quickly

New RBCs = reticulocytes: contain residual mRNA
MCV 105–110

MCV 85–95

After 5–10 days lose mRNA + shrink

After 120 days destroyed

Fe transported to marrow by ferritin – reflects liver + body stores

3 years' supply in body

B_{12}

Liver Fe stored here

Spleen

B_{12} deficiency

↑to ↑↑Mean cell volume (MCV)
Anaemia: may be severe
Jaundice (mild)
Glossitis
Spleen (minor)

Neurological disease
- Peripheral neuropathy
- Spinal cord disease (posterior/lateral column degeneration)
- Dementia (rare)

Causes
- Pernicious anaemia
- Gastrectomy
- Malabsorption
- Dietary deficiency

Iron deficiency

↓MCV in iron deficiency

Bluish tint to sclera

Koilonychia (only in long-standing anaemia)

Angular stomatitis

Tongue atrophy

Causes (see text)

Pharyngeal webs in long-standing deficiency; may turn malignant (Plummer–Vinson syndrome)

Iron deficiency

Iron deficiency causes 500 million cases of anaemia worldwide. Premenopausal women are more commonly affected than men because of menstrual blood loss. Iron is absorbed from the upper small intestine from food. A normal western diet provides around 15 mg/day. Adult men have a daily iron requirement of 1 mg, menstruating females 1.5 mg and an extra 5–6 mg/day are needed in pregnancy. Iron is transported in the blood by transferrin and stored bound to ferritin.

Causes

Blood loss from the gastrointestinal or genitourinary tracts is the most common cause of iron deficiency. The increased demands of pregnancy also lead to maternal iron deficiency. Malabsorption caused by coeliac disease is also an important cause. Iron deficiency solely caused by an inadequate diet is uncommon in the West.

Clinical features

The important clinical features relate to anaemia (fatigue, breathlessness, swollen feet and ankles, pale mucous membranes) and, more rarely, as the result of tissue iron deficiency (angular stomatitis, glossitis and, very rarely, koilonychias – spoon-shaped nails).

Diagnosis

Iron deficiency is suspected by finding microcytic (small red cells) and hypochromic (red cells with reduced haemoglobin) anaemia. Serum iron and ferritin are low and the total iron-binding capacity (transferrin) is high. Ferritin is an acute phase protein and is normal or elevated in patients with inflammatory, malignant or liver disease even in the presence of iron deficiency.

Management

● Diagnose the underlying cause: it is vital to diagnose and manage appropriately the underlying illness. Blood loss is identified from the history, examination and investigation. Occult gastrointestinal malignancy may be found.

● Replace iron: oral iron, to replace and replenish body iron stores, should be given until the haemoglobin and mean cell volume (MCV) are normal, then continued for a further 3 months to build up adequate body iron stores. Side effects include nausea, diarrhoea or constipation. Intravenous iron is rarely needed.

● Blood transfusion is seldom appropriate unless the patient is severely symptomatic with angina or breathlessness.

Vitamin B$_{12}$ deficiency

The most common cause of vitamin B$_{12}$ deficiency in the UK is pernicious anaemia. Other causes include malabsorption of vitamin B$_{12}$ in the terminal ileum (e.g. Crohn's disease), after a total gastrectomy, pancreatic disease, bacterial overgrowth as a result of blind loop syndrome, gut infection with the fish tapeworm and, very occasionally, dietary deficiency, usually in strict vegans.

Pernicious anaemia

There are 25 new cases of pernicious anaemia per 100 000 people every year. It is more common in elderly people. The mean age of onset is 60 years.

Pathophysiology

Vitamin B$_{12}$ is synthesized by microorganisms and humans obtain it from food of animal origin, particularly liver and kidney. Vitamin B$_{12}$ absorption requires intrinsic factor (made by stomach parietal cells) and does not occur in its absence. Vitamin B$_{12}$ binds to intrinsic factor and is absorbed in the terminal ileum. In pernicious anaemia there is an autoimmune gastritis and antibodies occur against:

● Gastric parietal cells, diminishing intrinsic factor secretion.
● Intrinsic factor, preventing vitamin B$_{12}$ binding.

In addition to vitamin B$_{12}$, methyl tetrahydrofolate is needed as a coenzyme in the methylation of homocysteine to methionine – the first step in intracellular folate production. Thus, vitamin B$_{12}$ deficiency results in intracellular folate deficiency. Given this biochemical background, it is not surprising that the haematological disorder is the same in both vitamin B$_{12}$ and folate deficiency.

Clinical features

Common clinical features are symptoms of anaemia, mild jaundice, glossitis and weight loss. Pernicious anaemia is an autoimmune disease and other autoimmune diseases such as vitiligo may occur. Neurological disturbances (peripheral neuropathy or subacute combined degeneration of the cord) are rare now, as a result of earlier diagnosis. Infertility is a rare presenting symptom. Dementia may occasionally be caused by vitamin B$_{12}$ deficiency in the absence of a macrocytic anaemia.

Diagnosis

Most patients have a macrocytic anaemia with a megaloblastic bone marrow (delay in nuclear maturation of red cell precursors). Mild/moderate thrombocytopenia and leukopenia are common. A small increase in the plasma bilirubin is found. The diagnosis is confirmed by finding:

● Low serum vitamin B$_{12}$.
● Antibodies against gastric parietal cells and intrinsic factor: found in 50% of patients with pernicious anaemia. Also check thyroid antibodies and thyroid function in view of the close association between pernicious anaemia and thyroid disease.
● The Schilling test: the absorption of orally administered radiolabelled vitamin B$_{12}$ in the absence (part one of the test) or presence (part two) of intrinsic factor is determined. In pernicious anaemia, only vitamin B$_{12}$ with intrinsic factor is absorbed. In malabsorption (e.g. caused by Crohn's disease), vitamin B$_{12}$ is not absorbed with or without intrinsic factor.

Treatment and prognosis

Intramuscular vitamin B$_{12}$ (daily for 5 days, then every 3 months for life) should be given. Surprisingly, perhaps, B$_{12}$ replacement can also be given by mouth but it remains much commoner to use intramuscular injections. Potassium deficiency can occur within the first few days of starting treatment so potassium supplements are advisable. Iron deficiency can develop because the patient responds to the vitamin B$_{12}$ with a huge increase in red cell production. The prognosis for treated patients is excellent, although there is a slightly higher incidence of gastric cancer.

Folate deficiency

Folate deficiency is a common cause of a macrocytic anaemia. Folate occurs in abundant quantities in green vegetables and is mainly absorbed in the upper part of the small intestine. Folate deficiency may be the result of:

● Dietary deficiency.
● Malabsorption, such as in coeliac disease.
● Excessive requirement, e.g. haemolytic anaemia.
● Increased requirement, i.e. pregnancy.
● Folate antagonist drugs, such as methotrexate.

Diagnosis

A macrocytic anaemia associated with a low serum and red cell folate establishes the diagnosis. The marrow will be megaloblastic.

Treatment

Treatment is with folic acid 5 mg/day. The underlying cause should be investigated and treated.

Hormonal and cytokine causes of anaemia

Erythropoietin deficiency (renal failure), hypothyroidism and chronic disease are all common causes of anaemia (see Figure 176.1).

177 Haemolytic anaemia

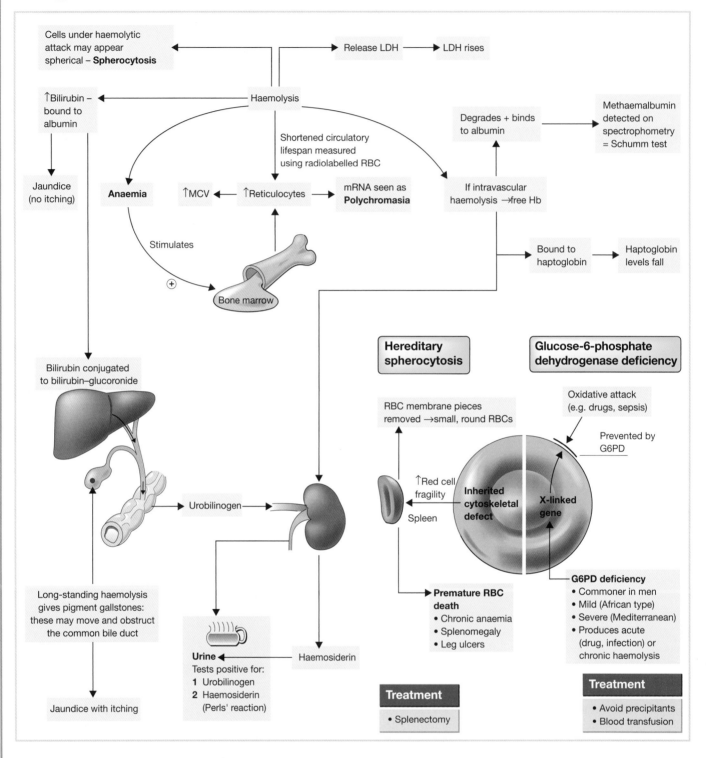

Cells under haemolytic attack may appear spherical – **Spherocytosis**

Release LDH → LDH rises

↑Bilirubin – bound to albumin

Haemolysis

Degrades + binds to albumin → Methaemalbumin detected on spectrophometry = Schumm test

Shortened circulatory lifespan measured using radiolabelled RBC

Jaundice (no itching)

Anaemia ↑MCV ← ↑Reticulocytes → mRNA seen as **Polychromasia**

If intravascular haemolysis →free Hb

Stimulates

Bound to haptoglobin → Haptoglobin levels fall

⊕

Bone marrow

Bilirubin conjugated to bilirubin–glucoronide

Hereditary spherocytosis

Glucose-6-phosphate dehydrogenase deficiency

RBC membrane pieces removed →small, round RBCs

Oxidative attack (e.g. drugs, sepsis)

Prevented by G6PD

Urobilinogen

↑Red cell fragility

Inherited cytoskeletal defect

X-linked gene

Spleen

Long-standing haemolysis gives pigment gallstones: these may move and obstruct the common bile duct

Premature RBC death
• Chronic anaemia
• Splenomegaly
• Leg ulcers

G6PD deficiency
• Commoner in men
• Mild (African type)
• Severe (Mediterranean)
• Produces acute (drug, infection) or chronic haemolysis

Urine
Tests positive for:
1 Urobilinogen
2 Haemosiderin (Perls' reaction)

Haemosiderin

Jaundice with itching

Treatment
• Splenectomy

Treatment
• Avoid precipitants
• Blood transfusion

Medicine at a Glance, Fourth Edition. Edited by Patrick Davey. © 2014 John Wiley & Sons, Ltd. Published 2014 by John Wiley & Sons, Ltd. Companion website: www.ataglanceseries.com/medicine

Table 177.1 Common causes of haemolytic anaemia.

Congenital

- Hereditary spherocytosis
- Glucose-6-phosphate dehydrogenase deficiency
- Pyruvate kinase deficiency
- Sickle cell disease
- Thalassaemia

Acquired

- Infection
- Autoimmune
- Drug induced
- Cardiac (typically across a prosthetic heart valve)
- Haemolytic transfusion reaction
- Microangiopathic (e.g. haemolytic uraemic syndrome, thrombotic thrombocytopenic purpura)
- Paroxysmal nocturnal haemoglobinuria

Haemolytic anaemia is defined as anaemia due to a reduction in the lifespan of red blood cells (normally 120 days). Although the bone marrow can increase red cell production to several times the normal level, this is inadequate and anaemia results. Such an increase in red cell production increases folate requirements, which if unmet can provoke folate deficiency. Haemolysis may be congenital or acquired (see Table 177.1). General clinical features include pallor, jaundice and variably splenomegaly. Pigment gallstones can occur in those who are chronically hyperbilirubinaemic and may lead to obstructive jaundice.

General laboratory abnormalities in haemolysis

Laboratory tests show evidence of increased red cell breakdown:

- Increased unconjugated plasma bilirubin (a breakdown product of haem).
- Raised plasma lactate dehydrogenase (LDH), released from damaged red cells.
- Low or absent plasma haptoglobin (binds avidly to free plasma haemoglobin).
- Radioisotope studies (seldom performed) show a shortened red cell lifespan.

Blood film examination shows polychromasia (resulting from the residual RNA found in young but not old red cells) and a raised reticulocyte count is found, both indicative of increased red cell production. Intravascular haemolysis (e.g. due to cardiac haemolysis) results in free plasma haemoglobin which is filtered by the glomerulus and altered in the tubules to produce haemosiderinuria, a characteristic finding in this condition.

Hereditary haemolytic anaemias

Hereditary spherocytosis

This autosomal dominant inherited illness results in an abnormal red cell membrane and typically presents in childhood with pallor and attacks of jaundice. There is usually, but not always, a family history of hereditary spherocytosis. Splenomegaly is very common. The diagnosis is made from the history, physical findings (splenomegaly) and the general laboratory features of haemolysis and finding spherocytes (small, spherical, darkly staining red cells with no central area of pallor) on the blood film. Many patients do not need treatment but, if anaemia is severe and symptomatic, it can be very successfully treated by splenectomy. As those without a spleen are at increased risk of infection by encapsulated bacteria, immunization against *Pneumococcus* and *Haemophilus influenzae* type B and the meningococcal vaccines should occur beforehand. After surgery life-long prophylactic penicillin should be given and annual influenza vaccination performed.

Red cell enzyme deficiency

The deficiency of almost any enzyme involved in red cell glucose metabolism can result in a haemolytic anaemia. The most important (and common) are glucose-6-phosphate dehydrogenase (G6PD) deficiency and pyruvate kinase deficiency.

G6PD deficiency

NADPH (reduced nicotinamide adenine dinucleotide phosphate), essential to the maintenance of functional haemoglobin, is generated by the catalysis of glucose-6-phosphate by G6PD. A deficiency of G6PD leads to a haemolytic anaemia. G6PD deficiency results from a variety of mutant alleles of its structural gene, and is very common in the subtropics and tropical regions; because of migrations, it is increasingly found in northern Europe and the USA. The gene for G6PD is X-linked, so G6PD deficiency is much more common in males. Most people with G6PD deficiency are asymptomatic until an acute haemolytic episode occurs, triggered by a number of possible factors including infection, some drugs (e.g. sulphonamides, primaquine) and the ingestion of fava beans. An acute haemolytic attack is usually self-limiting and supportive care only is required. A chronic haemolytic anaemia is rare.

Diagnosis and treatment The general features of haemolysis are found. Heinz bodies (caused by denaturation of unstable haemoglobin) are detected in the red blood cells (RBCs). Red cell G6PD activity is low (<20% of normal). Treatment is by transfusion if needed and by avoidance of triggers.

Pyruvate kinase deficiency

Pyruvate kinase deficiency is a rare autosomal recessive disease with a prevalence of 1 : 10 000. The clinical features vary but most present in childhood with anaemia and jaundice. Typically, haemoglobin is 4.5–10.0 g/dL. Splenomegaly is usually only mild. Interestingly, the patient's exercise tolerance is better than expected for the degree of anaemia because pyruvate kinase deficiency increases red cell 2,3-diphosphoglycerate concentrations, thus lowering haemoglobin oxygen affinity and enhancing tissue oxygen delivery. The diagnosis is made by finding a haemolytic anaemia (often with a very marked reticulocytosis), bizarre 'prickle cells' in the blood and a significantly reduced red cell pyruvate kinase activity. Treatment is usually conservative. Folic acid is recommended. Many patients need blood transfusion on occasion, but there is no benefit from regular transfusion. Splenectomy improves the haemoglobin in most anaemic patients.

Acquired haemolytic anaemias

Thrombotic thrombocytopenic purpura

This uncommon acquired disorder is characterized by a pentad of haemolytic anaemia with red cell fragments in the blood film (microangiopathic haemolytic anaemia), thrombocytopenia, neurological abnormalities, renal impairment and fever. The

Anaemia with red cell fragments in the blood

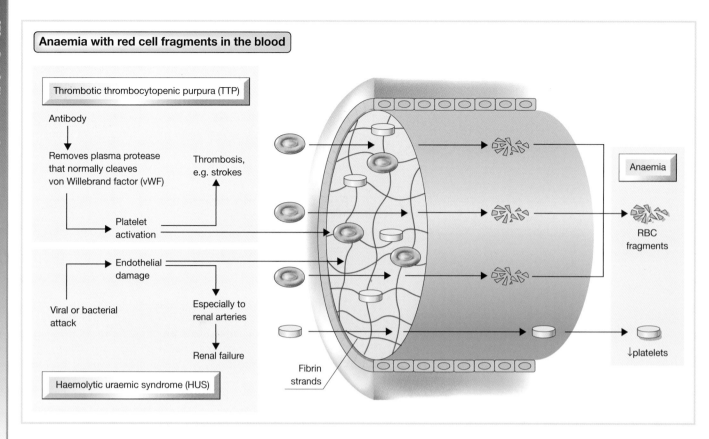

Thrombotic thrombocytopenic purpura (TTP)

Antibody
↓
Removes plasma protease that normally cleaves von Willebrand factor (vWF)

Thrombosis, e.g. strokes

Platelet activation

Endothelial damage

Viral or bacterial attack

Especially to renal arteries

Renal failure

Haemolytic uraemic syndrome (HUS)

Fibrin strands

Anaemia

RBC fragments

↓platelets

---

onset is often abrupt and the disease is usually fatal without treatment. An antibody occurs against a metalloprotease, which cleaves the high-molecular-weight polymers of von Willebrand's factor (vWF), which normally cause platelet aggregation and adhesion to the endothelial cell surface. Endothelial cell injury and platelet aggregation have both been implicated in the pathogenesis of thrombotic thrombocytopenic purpura (TTP). Plasmapheresis, which removes antibody, and infusion of fresh frozen plasma (FFP), which contains the metalloprotease, are the mainstays of treatment. Most patients recover, although there is a 20% mortality rate. Occasional patients have a relapsing/remitting course, caused by an inherited deficiency of the metalloprotease enzyme or by recurrence of the antibody.

Haemolytic uraemic syndrome

This is characterized by a microangiopathic haemolytic anaemia, thrombocytopenia and renal impairment. The aetiology is often obscure but infection with *Escherichia coli* O157 is sometimes responsible and may cause small epidemics. Haemolytic uraemic syndrome (HUS) is associated with a deficiency of complement factor H. Although most clinical and laboratory features of TTP and HUS are similar, neurological injury is unique to TTP, and no antibody against the metalloprotease has been detected in HUS. The treatment involves supportive care. Dialysis may be required. Childhood HUS often does not need specific treatment; plasmapheresis is the mainstay of treatment in adult HUS, although the response is usually less good than for patients with TTP. Most patients recover, although there is a mortality rate of 10–30%. Some patients are left with persistent renal impairment.

Cardiac haemolysis

This usually occurs only after prosthetic heart valve replacement and is caused by a small leak around the valve. The patients are anaemic and found to have red cell fragments in the blood film. The haemolysis is usually mild but re-operation is sometimes needed. Other causes of haemolysis need to be excluded.

Autoimmune haemolytic anaemia

Autoimmune haemolytic anaemia (AIHA) may be warm or cold antibody mediated. The clinical features include fatigue and lethargy and occasionally heart failure. Splenomegaly is common. In addition to the general features of haemolysis, the blood film is characterized by spherocytes (warm antibodies only) and, in some cases, by red cell agglutination.

Warm antibody-mediated haemolysis

This is usually caused by IgG binding to red cells, resulting in splenic phagocytosis, either complete or partial (the latter leads to rounder red cells – spherocytes). Some complement-mediated cell death also occurs. Causes of warm AIHA include:

- Idiopathic disorder.
- Lymphoproliferative diseases (e.g. chronic lymphocytic leukaemia, non-Hodgkin's lymphoma).
- Autoimmune disease (e.g. systemic lupus erythematosus).
- Inflammatory bowel disease.
- Drugs (e.g. methyl-dopa, mefenamic acid, penicillin).

The direct antiglobulin test (Coombs' test), which detects the presence of antibody and complement on the red cell surface, is usually positive. Most patients respond to prednisolone. Blood transfusions are helpful for severe, symptomatic anaemia while waiting for steroids to work. Splenectomy is often effective at relieving haemolysis if steroids fail, and the anti-CD2 antibody rituximab is also being increasingly used.

Cold antibody-mediated haemolysis

The antibody (usually IgM) may be polyclonal and arises as a consequence of infection or monoclonal secondary to a lymphoproliferative disorder or an idiopathic disorder – cold haemagglutinin disease (CHAD).

- **Cold antibody-mediated haemolysis and infection**: polyclonal IgM antibodies causing haemolysis sometimes occur 1–2 weeks after infection, usually with either *Mycoplasma*

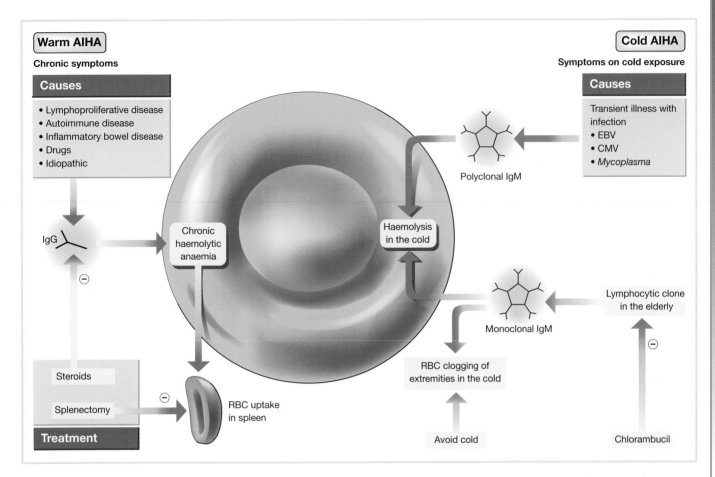

Cold AIHA

Symptoms on cold exposure

Causes

- Lymphoproliferative disease
- Autoimmune disease
- Inflammatory bowel disease
- Drugs
- Idiopathic

Causes

Transient illness with infection
- EBV
- CMV
- *Mycoplasma*

Polyclonal IgM

IgG

⊖

Chronic haemolytic anaemia

Haemolysis in the cold

Lymphocytic clone in the elderly

Monoclonal IgM

⊖

Steroids

Splenectomy

⊖

RBC uptake in spleen

RBC clogging of extremities in the cold

Treatment

Avoid cold

Chlorambucil

---

pneumoniae or infectious mononucleosis. The disorder is usually self-limiting. Avoidance of the cold and, where needed, blood transfusion (given through a blood warmer) are appropriate measures.

- **Cold haemagglutin disease**: here, an often occult clone of lymphocytes produces an IgM antibody, which binds to red blood cells *in the cold*, activates complement and destroys red cells. Typically pallor, mild jaundice and occasionally mild splenomegaly occur. Acrocyanosis of the extremities (purplish discoloration from red cell agglutination in small distal vessels) is common. Diagnosis is by finding a mild-to-moderate anaemia, red cell agglutination in the blood film and a positive Coombs' test for complement, but not for antibody (IgM antibodies elute from the red cell into the serum *in vitro*). The concentration of IgM

antibodies may be too low for detection by serum electrophoresis – they are instead found because of their ability to agglutinate red cells in the cold (cold agglutinins). Avoidance of the cold, folic acid supplements and alkylating agents (e.g. chlorambucil) are the mainstays of treatment. Prednisolone is often ineffective. A very similar illness to CHAD occasionally complicates the clinical course of overt lymphoproliferative disorders; the management is as for CHAD.

Paroxysmal cold haemoglobinuria

This rare disorder, usually self-limiting, is most common in children, and is often preceded by a viral illness. Very rarely it may be associated with syphilis. It is caused by a polyclonal IgG cold antibody (the Donath–Landsteiner antibody).

178 Thalassaemia and sickle cell disease

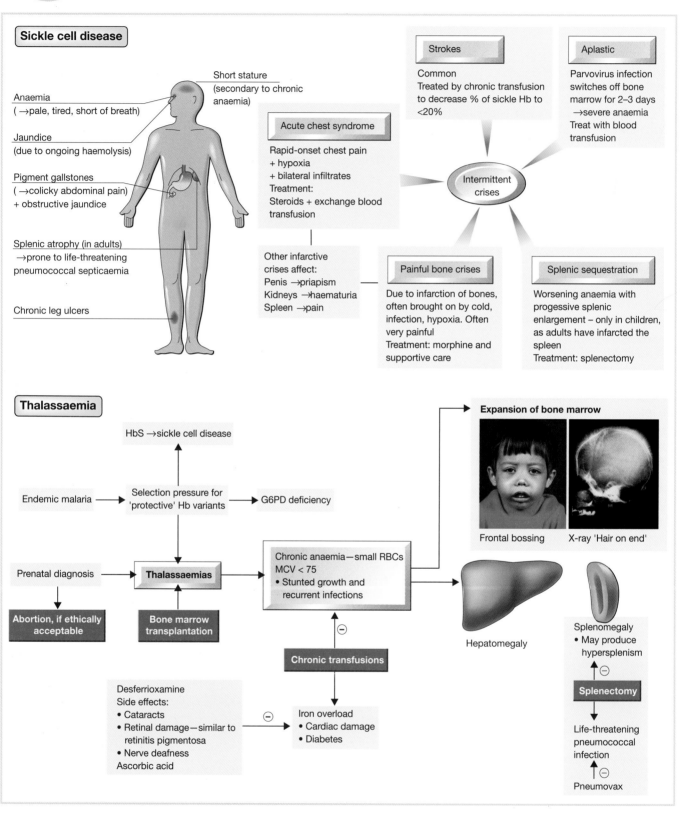

Sickle cell disease

Anaemia
(→pale, tired, short of breath)

Jaundice
(due to ongoing haemolysis)

Pigment gallstones
(→colicky abdominal pain)
+ obstructive jaundice

Splenic atrophy (in adults)
→prone to life-threatening
pneumococcal septicaemia

Chronic leg ulcers

Short stature
(secondary to chronic
anaemia)

Acute chest syndrome

Rapid-onset chest pain
+ hypoxia
+ bilateral infiltrates
Treatment:
Steroids + exchange blood
transfusion

Other infarctive
crises affect:
Penis →priapism
Kidneys →haematuria
Spleen →pain

Strokes

Common
Treated by chronic transfusion
to decrease % of sickle Hb to
<20%

Aplastic

Parvovirus infection
switches off bone
marrow for 2–3 days
→severe anaemia
Treat with blood
transfusion

Intermittent
crises

Painful bone crises

Due to infarction of bones,
often brought on by cold,
infection, hypoxia. Often
very painful
Treatment: morphine and
supportive care

Splenic sequestration

Worsening anaemia with
progessive splenic
enlargement – only in children,
as adults have infarcted the
spleen
Treatment: splenectomy

Thalassaemia

HbS →sickle cell disease

Endemic malaria → Selection pressure for
'protective' Hb variants → G6PD deficiency

Prenatal diagnosis → **Thalassaemias**

**Abortion, if ethically
acceptable**

**Bone marrow
transplantation**

Chronic anaemia—small RBCs
MCV < 75
• Stunted growth and
  recurrent infections

Expansion of bone marrow

Frontal bossing   X-ray 'Hair on end'

Hepatomegaly

Splenomegaly
• May produce
  hypersplenism

⊖

Splenectomy

Life-threatening
pneumococcal
infection

⊖

Pneumovax

Chronic transfusions

⊖

Desferrioxamine
Side effects:
• Cataracts
• Retinal damage—similar to
  retinitis pigmentosa
• Nerve deafness
Ascorbic acid

⊖ → Iron overload
• Cardiac damage
• Diabetes

These genetic disorders of haemoglobin synthesis are classified by whether the α-globin chain (α-thalassaemia) or β-globin chain (β-thalassaemia) production is defective. The carrier state protects against falciparum malaria, explaining the disease's geography. Thalassaemias are subdivided into thalassaemia trait or thalassaemia major based on clinical presentation.

Thalassaemia

Thalassaemia trait

- In β-**thalassaemia trait** one normal and one abnormal β-globin gene occur. Haemoglobin (Hb) electrophoresis is normal but HbA2 (a vestigial haemoglobin with no known function) is increased from 2% to 4–6%.
- In α-**thalassaemia trait** Hb electrophoresis and HbA2 levels are normal. The diagnosis is made by excluding β-thalassaemia trait and iron deficiency (see Chapter 176).

Both traits have mild anaemia (Hb 10.0–12.0 g/dL) and low mean cell volume (MCV 65–70 fL). Partners of those with β-thalassaemia trait should be tested, because trait carriage by both partners can lead to offspring with thalassaemia major. α-Thalassaemia is more complex as there are four α-genes and severe disease only occurs when three or four genes are deleted. Only patients from certain parts of the world (e.g. South and East Asia) need be concerned about seriously affected children and therefore require prenatal counselling.

Thalassaemia major

Thalassaemia major is a life-threatening illness.

- β-**Thalassaemia major**, caused by point mutations (occasionally deletion) in both β-globin genes, results in symptomatic anaemia at 6–12 months, as fetal haemoglobin levels fall. Untreated children are wasted, have skull bossing, splenomegaly and leg ulcers, with the pathognomonic 'hair on end' skull X-ray appearance (see Figure 178.1). Laboratory tests show a severe microcytic anaemia, target and nucleated red cells in the peripheral blood, and no HbA. Blood transfusion, to maintain a normal haemoglobin level and suppress abnormal red cell production, results in normal physical development. Iron overload from frequent transfusions causes serious disability and death by 25 years, unless prevented by chelation with desferrioxamine or other iron chelators. Most well-treated thalassaemic patients survive at least into their thirties or forties. Bone marrow transplantation can be considered if a suitable sibling donor is found.
- α-**Thalassaemia major** (hydrops fetalis) often ends in intrauterine death and is caused by deletion of all four α-globin genes. Rarely, the diagnosis is made early, when intrauterine blood transfusions are life saving. Life-long transfusion is necessary as in β-thalassaemia.

Thalassaemia intermedia

The severity of thalassaemia intermedia lies between thalassaemia trait and thalassaemia major. Several different genetic disorders underlie this condition. The most common is homozygous β-thalassaemia where one or both genes still produce small amounts of HbA. Deletion of three of the four α-globin genes (HbH disease) causes a similar picture, with a moderately severe anaemia of 7–9 g/dL and splenomegaly. *By definition* they are not transfusion dependent. Splenectomy may be used to lessen anaemia.

Sickle cell disease

Sickle cell haemoglobin results from a point mutation (β^S^). It is common in Africa, the Arabian peninsula and southern Europe. Heterozygous carriers have one normal β and one β^S^ globin gene – sickle cell trait (AS).

Sickle cell trait is usually asymptomatic, although haematuria and sudden death may occur more commonly. The blood count and film are normal. The diagnosis is made on finding a positive sickle solubility test and one band of HbA (normal adult haemoglobin) and one of HbS on electrophoresis. General anaesthesia requires no special precautions.

Sickle cell disease occurs in those homozygous for HbS (SS). Sickle cells are more rigid than normal red cells and obstruct blood flow, particularly in small blood vessels. Deoxygenation of sickle haemoglobin causes the characteristic shape change. Blood examination shows sickle-shaped cells, even when not in crisis, features of splenic atrophy (Howell–Jolly bodies in red blood cells) and moderate anaemia (Hb 7–9 g/dL). Electrophoresis shows the HbS band. The sickle solubility test is positive. The natural history of this condition is variable but typically patients are well with occasional crises which can be severe.

- Painful bone crisis is the most common and may be precipitated by cold, infection or hypoxia – often no cause is found. Treatment is with simple or opiate-based analgesia (morphine, because pethidine may cause seizures and is more addictive). Intravenous or oral fluids, oxygen and antibiotics may be given. Most episodes settle within a few days.
- Acute chest syndrome may be fatal and is characterized by the rapid onset and progression of chest pain associated with hypoxia, cough and bilateral lung infiltrates. Exchange blood transfusion is the treatment of choice.
- Splenic sequestration is more common in children than in adults, because splenic atrophy from autoinfarction occurs by the age of 5–6 years. Typical features are a rapidly worsening anaemia and progressive splenomegaly. Blood transfusion is used as necessary. The condition is usually short-lived. If patients have recurrent attacks splenectomy is undertaken.
- Aplastic crises are caused by parvovirus infection, which switches off red cell production for 2–3 days. This does not matter in normal individuals. In haemolytic anaemias, where the red cell lifespan is very short, temporary cessation of red cell production causes an abrupt, life-threatening fall in haemoglobin. Red cell transfusion is life saving. Aplastic crisis is characterized by severe anaemia with a near total absence of reticulocytes.
- Strokes are common in children and adults with sickle cell disease. In fact sickle cell disease is the commonest cause of stroke in children. Blood transfusions to maintain the HbS concentration at <20% should be given for at least 1–2 years after a stroke. Monitoring of the cerebral blood flow is important in children with initiation of an exchange transfusion programme in those at high risk of stroke.
- Although not strictly a crisis, pulmonary hypertension is a contributory factor for early death in sickle cell disease. Echocardiographic monitoring is important and an exchange transfusion programme should be considered for those affected.

Treatment

Most patients with sickle cell disease are treated conservatively with specific treatment for crises. Hyposplenism from splenic infarction is common, so appropriate immunization and prophylaxis against encapsulated bacteria with penicillin are essential. Folic acid is often prescribed. Disease severity is very variable: those with the highest concentration of HbF have the mildest clinical course. Hydroxycarbamide is used in severe disease to increase HbF concentration and decrease painful crises. Bone marrow transplantation may be used in young people with severe disease.

Other haemoglobin variants

Other haemoglobin variants include haemoglobins C, D and E. Heterozygous patients are asymptomatic. In combination with haemoglobin S or β-thalassaemia trait, a far more serious disorder occurs, e.g. the combination of haemoglobins S and C – haemoglobin SC disease. The clinical course is milder than SS, although avascular necrosis of the femoral head is just as common as in SS, and proliferative retinopathy much more common.

179 Bone marrow failure

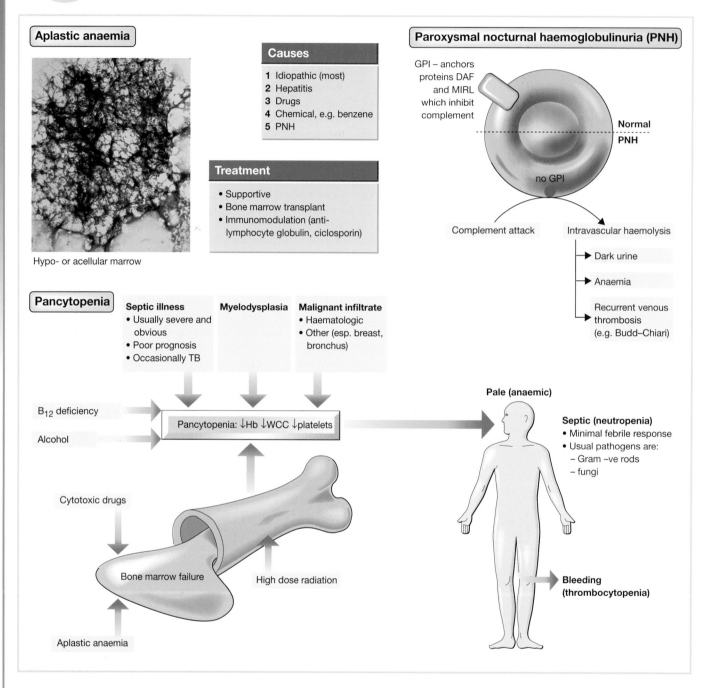

Aplastic anaemia

Hypo- or acellular marrow

Causes

1 Idiopathic (most)
2 Hepatitis
3 Drugs
4 Chemical, e.g. benzene
5 PNH

Treatment

• Supportive
• Bone marrow transplant
• Immunomodulation (anti-lymphocyte globulin, ciclosporin)

Paroxysmal nocturnal haemoglobulinuria (PNH)

GPI – anchors proteins DAF and MIRL which inhibit complement

Normal
PNH

no GPI

Complement attack

Intravascular haemolysis

→ Dark urine

→ Anaemia

→ Recurrent venous thrombosis (e.g. Budd–Chiari)

Pancytopenia

Septic illness
• Usually severe and obvious
• Poor prognosis
• Occasionally TB

Myelodysplasia

Malignant infiltrate
• Haematologic
• Other (esp. breast, bronchus)

B₁₂ deficiency

Alcohol

Pancytopenia: ↓Hb ↓WCC ↓platelets

Cytotoxic drugs

Bone marrow failure

High dose radiation

Aplastic anaemia

Pale (anaemic)

Septic (neutropenia)
• Minimal febrile response
• Usual pathogens are:
  – Gram –ve rods
  – fungi

Bleeding (thrombocytopenia)

Bone marrow failure may be caused intentionally by anticancer chemotherapy or radiotherapy, or may develop unexpectedly from both congenital and acquired causes. The clinical features of bone marrow failure relate to the absence of:

• Haemoglobin (symptoms of anaemia).
• Neutrophils (bacterial or fungal sepsis).
• Platelets (initially a purpuric rash, later on bleeding).

Although one cell line may be more severely affected than another, the peripheral blood film shows variable depression of all three cell lines, i.e. of haemoglobin (Hb), white cell count and platelet cell count – a pancytopenia. It is important to realize that

a peripheral blood pancytopenia does not necessarily mean that there is an underlying marrow failure caused by an aplastic anaemia. Thus, the differential diagnosis of a peripheral blood pancytopenia includes:

• Sepsis: usually clinically obvious and severe.
• Vitamin B₁₂ or folate deficiency (see Chapter 176).
• Myelodysplasia (see Chapter 185) or acute leukaemia (see Chapter 180). Paroxysmal nocturnal haemoglobinuria (PNH) can present as a pancytopenia.
• Bone marrow failure as a result of drug toxicity, deliberate or as an unwelcome side effect, or caused by aplastic anaemia.

Medicine at a Glance, Fourth Edition. Edited by Patrick Davey. © 2014 John Wiley & Sons, Ltd. Published 2014 by John Wiley & Sons, Ltd. Companion website: www.ataglanceseries.com/medicine

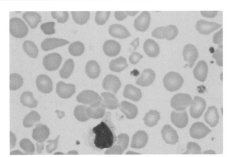

Myelofibrosis: peripheral blood film showing aniso-poikolocytosis, teardrop forms and giant platelets

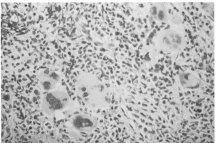

Myelofibrosis: bone marrow biopsy showing increased cellularity and large numbers of megakaryocytes

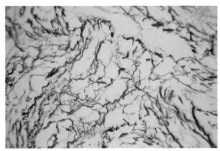

Myelofibrosis: bone marrow biopsy (reticulin stain) showing increased reticulin

- Myelofibrosis often results in bone marrow failure: the clinical examination shows massive splenomegaly.
- Severe malnutrition such as that associated with severe anorexia nervosa.

The key investigation in peripheral blood pancytopenia is the bone marrow examination, which will diagnose aplastic anaemia or an underlying haematological disease process. Bone marrow is usually obtained by aspirating cells from the posterior iliac crest or the sternum, and from a biopsy – termed a 'trephine' – where the architecture of the bone marrow is preserved. In pancytopenia caused by aplastic anaemia, a hypocellular marrow is seen. Aplastic anaemia may be idiopathic (primary) or secondary to another disease process or drugs.

Acquired aplastic anaemia

Epidemiology
This is a rare disorder occurring in three per million people per year, defined as a peripheral blood pancytopenia in conjunction with a hypocellular bone marrow in which there are no malignant cells.

Aetiology
In most patients (70–80%) no cause is found and the condition is thought to be an autoimmune disorder targeting the haematopoietic stem cell. In the rest, causes include:
- Viral infections (hepatitis C is the most common).
- An idiosyncratic reaction to some drugs (e.g. gold, chloramphenicol).
- Chemicals such as benzene.
- PNH: see next section.

Clinical features
Most patients present with bleeding as a result of thrombocytopenia, bacterial and fungal infection because of neutropenia, and symptoms of anaemia. Splenomegaly is not a feature.

Diagnosis
The blood count will show a decrease in haemoglobin, platelet and white cell count (WCC), i.e. a pancytopenia of variable severity. A bone marrow aspirate and trephine biopsy show a hypocellular marrow.

Treatment and prognosis
Patients should be given supportive care with blood products (red cells, platelets) and antibiotics in the first instance, and then withdrawal of any relevant drug, or specific treatment for hepatitis C. In primary aplastic anaemia, immunosuppressive treatment with antilymphocyte globulin and ciclosporin is effective in improving the blood counts in most patients. Bone marrow transplantation is used for younger patients with severe disease who have an appropriate donor. The survival rate of patients with severe aplastic anaemia is 50–80% 5 years after diagnosis, and depends on the initial severity of disease. Unfortunately, about 50% of patients treated with immunosuppressives will develop a clonal haematopoietic illness such as leukaemia or PNH some years after treatment.

Paroxysmal nocturnal haemoglobinuria

This is a rare, acquired, clonal disease of bone marrow, which may arise during the course of aplastic anaemia. The abnormal blood cells lack a series of proteins (glycosyl-phosphatidylinositol (GPI) anchored proteins), which normally anchor complement regulatory proteins on to the cell. The absence of such proteins encourages complement attack on red cells, with the net result being complement-mediated haemolysis.

The clinical features are the result of an intravascular haemolytic anaemia – with characteristic haemoglobinuria. Haemolysis is worse with sepsis, even when minor (e.g. colds and surgical trauma). Patients develop insidious symptoms of anaemia and many (although not all) have intermittently dark urine. Large vessel thrombosis is a feature and abdominal pain as a result of bowel ischaemia or infarction may occur. Occasionally Budd–Chiari syndrome occurs.

The physical signs are pallor (from anaemia), mild jaundice (from intravascular haemolysis), minor splenomegaly and dark red/black urine. Urine testing reveals haemosiderinuria. The blood film shows a pancytopenia, with the red cells having a normal or high mean cell volume (MCV) – a low MCV suggests complicating iron deficiency from urinary iron loss. The diagnosis is made by immunophenotyping of the red and white cells showing a deficiency on GPI-linked proteins.

Treatment is mainly supportive with blood products. Treatment with a monoclonal antibody (eculizumab) against the complement protein C5 has resulted in significant improvement in patients' anaemia and general health and is being more commonly used despite its considerable cost. Bone marrow transplantation is rarely used. The median survival is 8 years, although 10–15% of patients recover spontaneously.

Congenital aplastic anaemia

These disorders are rare and include conditions such as Fanconi's anaemia and dyskeratosis congenita. Fanconi's anaemia is an autosomal recessive disease in which – in addition to aplastic anaemia, which usually develops in the first few years of life – there may be other abnormalities such as small stature, skeletal defects and hyperpigmentation. In dyskeratosis congenita, learning disorders, skin, nail and hair abnormalities, and growth failure may complicate the aplastic anaemia.

180 Acute leukaemia

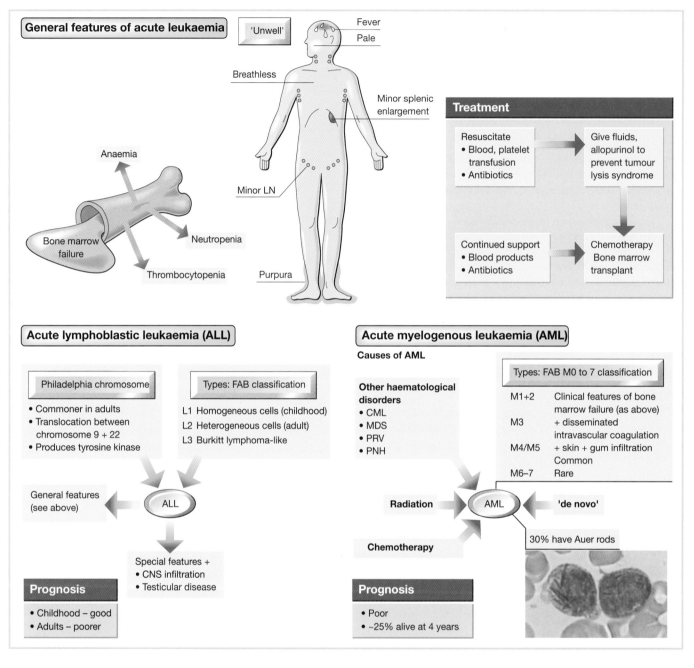

General features of acute leukaemia

'Unwell'

Fever
Pale

Breathless

Minor splenic enlargement

Minor LN

Purpura

Anaemia

Bone marrow failure

Neutropenia

Thrombocytopenia

Treatment

Resuscitate
• Blood, platelet transfusion
• Antibiotics

Give fluids, allopurinol to prevent tumour lysis syndrome

Continued support
• Blood products
• Antibiotics

Chemotherapy Bone marrow transplant

Acute lymphoblastic leukaemia (ALL)

Philadelphia chromosome
• Commoner in adults
• Translocation between chromosome 9 + 22
• Produces tyrosine kinase

Types: FAB classification
L1 Homogeneous cells (childhood)
L2 Heterogeneous cells (adult)
L3 Burkitt lymphoma-like

General features (see above)

ALL

Special features +
• CNS infiltration
• Testicular disease

Prognosis
• Childhood – good
• Adults – poorer

Acute myelogenous leukaemia (AML)

Causes of AML

Other haematological disorders
• CML
• MDS
• PRV
• PNH

Types: FAB M0 to 7 classification

M1+2	Clinical features of bone marrow failure (as above)
M3	+ disseminated intravascular coagulation
M4/M5	+ skin + gum infiltration Common
M6–7	Rare

Radiation

AML

'de novo'

Chemotherapy

30% have Auer rods

Prognosis
• Poor
• ~25% alive at 4 years

Acute leukaemia is defined as a clonal haematopoietic stem cell/progenitor disorder characterized by the rapid accumulation of immature progenitor cells (blasts) and impairing normal marrow function. It is serious, progresses quickly and, in the absence of treatment, results in the death of the patient within a few weeks or months. Acute leukaemia may affect the lymphoid cell line (acute lymphoblastic leukaemia or ALL) or the myeloid cell line (acute myeloid leukaemia or AML).

Epidemiology
ALL is more common in children, with a peak age of onset of 4 years. In contrast, AML occurs more commonly with increasing age, with a peak age of onset of 70 years. For most patients the cause of acute leukaemia cannot be determined, although infection may play a role in childhood ALL. Exposure to cytotoxic drugs, radiation and some chemicals such as benzene increases the likelihood of acute leukaemia developing. Some chronic haematological diseases, such as myelodysplasia, myelofibrosis and paroxysmal nocturnal haemoglobinuria (PNH), have a high likelihood of transforming to AML.

Symptoms and signs
Symptoms of acute leukaemia usually develop over several weeks and can be divided into three types:

Medicine at a Glance, Fourth Edition. Edited by Patrick Davey. © 2014 John Wiley & Sons, Ltd. Published 2014 by John Wiley & Sons, Ltd. Companion website: www.ataglanceseries.com/medicine

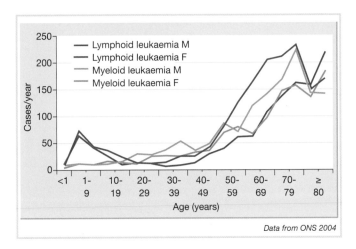

Data from ONS 2004

1 Bone marrow failure symptoms: these are the most common presentation complaints. Leukaemia suppresses normal bone marrow function, causing any combination of anaemia, leukopenia (shortage of white cells) and thrombocytopenia (low platelet count). Typical symptoms are fatigue and breathlessness (from anaemia), bacterial infection (from leukopenia) and bleeding (from thrombocytopenia and sometimes from disseminated intravascular coagulation (DIC)). Examination often reveals pallor, some bruising and bleeding. Fever suggests infection, although in some it may be caused by the leukaemia itself. It is, however, dangerous to assume this (see Management). Lymphadenopathy, when present, is usually small volume and more typical of ALL than AML.

2 Systemic symptoms of malaise, weight loss, sweats and anorexia are common.

3 Local symptoms: occasional patients present with symptoms or signs of leukaemic infiltration of skin, gums or the central nervous system.

Investigations

- Full blood count: usually shows anaemia and thrombocytopenia. Normal white blood cells are usually decreased and the total white blood count may be low, normal or raised. When normal or raised, most of the cells are primitive white cells (blasts).
- Biochemistry: may show renal dysfunction, hypokalaemia and high bilirubin levels.
- Coagulation profile: may show prolonged clotting times and reduced fibrinogen suggestive of DIC.
- Blood cultures because of the risk of infection.
- Chest X-ray (CXR): patients with ALL of T-cell lineage often have a mediastinal mass seen on the CXR.
- Blood group and antibody screen because transfusion of blood and platelets is needed sooner or later.
- Specific diagnostic investigations include a bone marrow aspirate and trephine biopsy, and cell marker and cytogenetic studies for accurate distinction of ALL from AML. Auer rods in the cytoplasm of blast cells are pathognomonic for AML, but are found in only 30%. Cell marker studies (also known as immunophenotyping) can help distinguish B- from T-lineage ALL and the different subtypes of AML (see Figure 180.1 above). This is useful for the haematologist in planning treatment and prognosis.

Chromosome analysis of leukaemic cells is useful in distinguishing ALL from AML, and most importantly gives prognostic information. Molecular diagnostic tests are becoming more frequently used, particularly to assist in the monitoring of minimal residual disease and also are sometimes of help in predicting response to treatment and prognosis.

Management

Resuscitation

A newly diagnosed patient with acute leukaemia is often very ill and certainly vulnerable to severe infection and/or bleeding. The priority is resuscitation using broad-spectrum intravenous antibiotics for infection, platelets and fresh frozen plasma for bleeding, and blood transfusion to correct anaemia. Antibiotic usage in this situation will never be criticized even if the patient's fever turns out to be induced by disease rather than infection. It is easier to stop antibiotics later on than to salvage a septicaemic, shocked patient who has been left without antibiotic treatment.

Chemotherapy

The definitive treatment of acute leukaemia is with cytotoxic chemotherapy using multiple drugs given in combination. The precise protocols differ for ALL and AML. Cytotoxic drugs work in differing ways but all kill leukaemic cells. Unfortunately, some normal cells get damaged or killed as well and this causes the side effects such as hair loss, nausea and vomiting, a sore mouth (from damage to the oral mucosa) and bone marrow failure as a result of killing bone marrow cells. One of the major consequences of chemotherapy-induced neutropenia is severe infection. Patients are treated for months (AML) or for 2–3 years (ALL). A subtype of AML (promyelocytic leukaemia) associated with a t(15:17) responds very well to a combination of a vitamin A analogue (all trans retinoic acid) and low-dose chemotherapy given over 2 years. Arsenic trioxide is also increasingly used in this subtype.

Stem cell transplantation

This is a treatment option after very-high-dose chemotherapy and radiotherapy for some but not all patients with acute leukaemia. The haematopoietic cells may be obtained either from the patient before the high-dose treatment, stored and then reinfused (autologous transplantation) or from an HLA (human leucocyte antigen) matched donor (allogeneic transplantation). The very-high-dose treatment kills off the patient's bone marrow, which will not recover. The infused stem cells will restore bone marrow function. Patients receiving allogeneic transplants have a lower risk of disease recurrence than those receiving autologous transplants. In allogeneic transplantations there is good evidence that the transplanted marrow exerts a powerful antitumour effect (graft vs leukaemia) mediated by transplanted T lymphocytes. Recent work shows that allogeneic transplants using low-dose conditioning are possible with potential cure being produced by an immunological mechanism and also reducing the toxicity of the procedure.

Prognosis

The prognosis gets worse with increasing age and if the leukaemia cells contain certain chromosome abnormalities. For a child with ALL, 70–80% will be cured. For adults less than 50 years old with ALL or AML, around 30–40% will be cured.

181 Chronic leukaemia

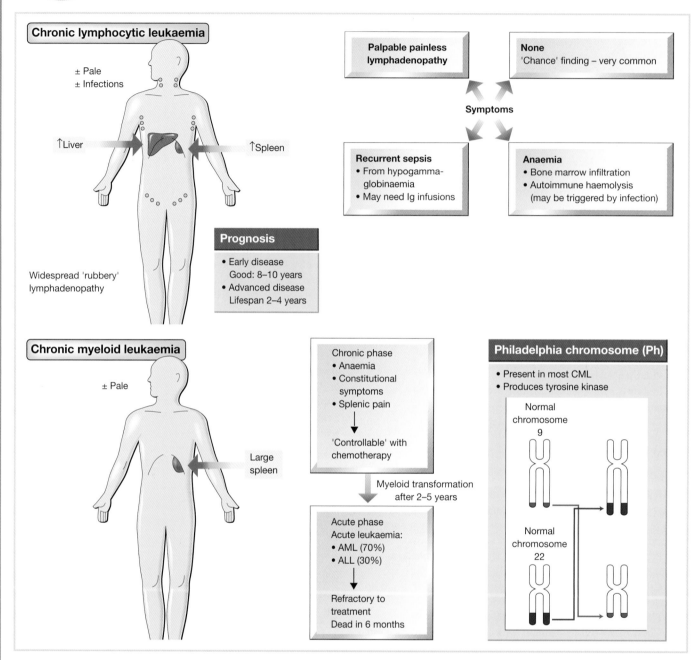

Chronic lymphocytic leukaemia

± Pale
± Infections

↑Liver

↑Spleen

Widespread 'rubbery' lymphadenopathy

Palpable painless lymphadenopathy

None
'Chance' finding – very common

Symptoms

Recurrent sepsis
• From hypogamma-globinaemia
• May need Ig infusions

Anaemia
• Bone marrow infiltration
• Autoimmune haemolysis (may be triggered by infection)

Prognosis
• Early disease
  Good: 8–10 years
• Advanced disease
  Lifespan 2–4 years

Chronic myeloid leukaemia

± Pale

Large spleen

Chronic phase
• Anaemia
• Constitutional symptoms
• Splenic pain

'Controllable' with chemotherapy

Myeloid transformation after 2–5 years

Acute phase
Acute leukaemia:
• AML (70%)
• ALL (30%)

Refractory to treatment
Dead in 6 months

Philadelphia chromosome (Ph)
• Present in most CML
• Produces tyrosine kinase

Normal chromosome 9

Normal chromosome 22

There are two important types of chronic leukaemia: chronic lymphocytic leukaemia (CLL) and chronic myeloid leukaemia (CML).

Chronic lymphocytic leukaemia

The incidence of CLL rises with age. Males are affected twice as often as females and there is a slightly higher incidence of the disease in families where one family member has CLL. The genetic basis is unclear. CLL occurs less commonly in Asian individuals.

Pathophysiology

CLL is a malignant illness of mature B lymphocytes, of unknown cause. The cells look quite mature but functionally are immature.

Symptoms and signs

Half of the patients with CLL are diagnosed by chance when a blood count is performed for another reason. The remainder are symptomatic to some extent, such as with lymphadenopathy and/or systemic symptoms, e.g. fever, weight loss or night sweats. Infection (bacterial or viral) is common and is often the

Medicine at a Glance, Fourth Edition. Edited by Patrick Davey. © 2014 John Wiley & Sons, Ltd. Published 2014 by John Wiley & Sons, Ltd. Companion website: www.ataglanceseries.com/medicine

Table 181.1 Binet staging of chronic lymphocytic leukaemia.

Stage	Lymph node enlargement*	Haemoglobin (g/dL)	Platelets ($\times 10^9$/L)
A	0, 1 or 2 areas		
B	3, 4 or 5 areas		
C		<10.0	<100

* Involved areas include cervical, axillary or inguinal nodes, spleen or liver.

presenting feature. Symptoms of anaemia or, more rarely, thrombocytopenia may be present at diagnosis, but more commonly occur later in the course of the illness. In patients with early stage disease, palpable lymphadenopathy is often absent (see Table 181.1). With more advanced disease, generalized lymph node enlargement occurs and the spleen and liver may become palpable.

Investigations
The full blood count (FBC) is the single most important test. By definition the lymphocyte count is $>5 \times 10^9$/L in the absence of viral infection and is often much higher – levels of $100–300 \times 10^9$/L are common. The haemoglobin and platelet count are usually normal, although mild anaemia and thrombocytopenia may be present. The blood film confirms the characteristic lymphocytosis. It is important to bear in mind that autoimmune haemolysis is a frequent complication and should be considered in new-onset anaemia in a patient with CLL.

Cell marker studies demonstrate clonality and differentiate CLL from other chronic lymphoproliferative diseases such as hairy cell leukaemia and follicular or mantle cell lymphoma.

The biochemistry profile is usually normal although lactate dehydrogenase and alkaline phosphatase may be modestly elevated.

Immunology
B cells mature into immunoglobulin-producing plasma cells. In CLL, this normal maturation process is disrupted and hypogammaglobulinaemia occurs frequently. Abnormalities of T cells are also found that contribute to the high incidence of autoimmune haemolysis and thrombocytopenia.

Prognostic markers
Prognosis depends on tumour stage, the length of time it takes for the lymphocyte count to double, the β_2-microglobulin level and certain chromosome abnormalities. The Binet stage relates to prognosis, and is best with stage A (median survival >10 years) and worst with stage C (median survival <5 years). Patients with a mutation of 17p (P53 gene) have a very poor response to standard chemotherapy and a poor prognosis. Patients with mutated immunoglobulin heavy chain genes have a far better prognosis than patients with unmutated genes.

Treatment
CLL is a chronic, incurable condition in most patients. As a result of its indolent nature many patients die from causes other than CLL. Treatment is only given to patients who are symptomatic. In those who are, the mainstay of treatment is with fludarabine combinations, and the monoclonal antibody rituximab. For less fit patients, chlorambucil or bendamustine are commonly used.

Autologous or allogeneic bone marrow transplantation has been used in young patients.

Chronic myeloid leukaemia
Epidemiology
CML has an incidence of 1/100 000 per year and is most common in middle age. Children are rarely affected. Ionizing radiation and benzene exposure have been cited as causative, although few patients have known exposure to these agents.

Pathophysiology
CML is a clonal disorder arising in a pluripotential stem cell. The cells contain the Philadelphia chromosome.

Clinical features
Systemic symptoms of weight loss, sweating and anorexia are common at presentation. Abdominal pain as a result of splenomegaly is frequent and symptoms from anaemia may occur.

Investigations
The blood count shows a leukocytosis (white cell count often $>100 \times 10^9$/L), the haemoglobin is usually a little low and the platelet count is either normal or high. The blood film shows both mature and immature granulocytes. The bone marrow is hypercellular and the leukaemic cells contain a translocation between chromosome 9 and 22 – the *Philadelphia chromosome*.

Treatment and prognosis
Treatment of CML has changed significantly in the last 10 years.

- Treatment with hydroxurea and interferon has been replaced by imatinib (taken by mouth) which blocks the adenosine triphosphate (ATP) binding site on the tyrosine kinase induced by the *BCR-Abl* gene from the derived chromosome 22. Nearly all patients with chronic phase disease will have a complete haematological response (FBC returns to normal) and three-quarters become Philadelphia chromosome negative after 6–24 months of treatment. Most of these patients still have molecularly detectable disease, however. After 5 years of follow up over 90% of responding patients will be alive and well. The previous median survival of around 5 years for CML patients is likely to at least double with imatinib and could be much longer than this. Resistance to imatinib occurs in a small percentage of patients over the first few years of treatment. This can sometimes be overcome by a dose increase or by switching to newer tyrosine kinase inhibitors such as dasatinib or nilotinib.
- Bone marrow transplantation used to be commonly used for younger patients with CML as it provided the opportunity for cure, albeit at the expense of a substantial morbidity and mortality risk. Far fewer transplants are performed nowadays because of the effectiveness of imatinib but it may still be considered for very young patients or those who do not respond well to imatinib.

Treatment of relapse after bone marrow transplantation
Donor marrow exerts a powerful antileukaemia effect, mediated by T lymphocytes. Patients with CML who relapse after the transplantation are treated by collecting lymphocytes from the original donor and giving them intravenously to the patient. Of these patients, 75% will go back into a sustained remission with such treatment. This is the most powerful example of immunotherapy currently available. Such an approach has been tried in other forms of leukaemia relapsing after transplantation, but it has proved less effective in acute leukaemia than in patients with CML.

182 Lymphoma

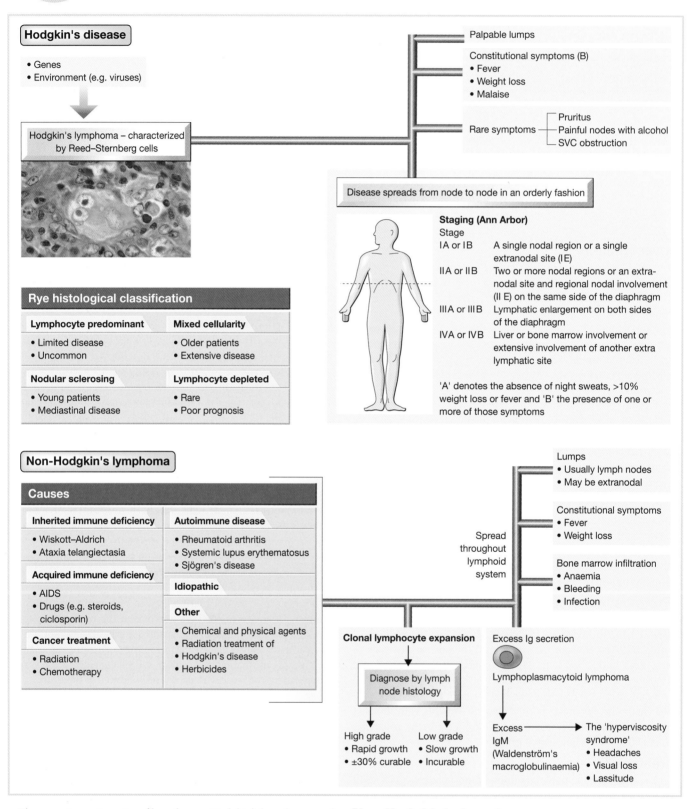

Hodgkin's disease

- Genes
- Environment (e.g. viruses)

Hodgkin's lymphoma – characterized by Reed–Sternberg cells

Palpable lumps

Constitutional symptoms (B)
- Fever
- Weight loss
- Malaise

Rare symptoms
- Pruritus
- Painful nodes with alcohol
- SVC obstruction

Disease spreads from node to node in an orderly fashion

Staging (Ann Arbor)

Stage	
IA or IB	A single nodal region or a single extranodal site (IE)
IIA or IIB	Two or more nodal regions or an extra-nodal site and regional nodal involvement (II E) on the same side of the diaphragm
IIIA or IIIB	Lymphatic enlargement on both sides of the diaphragm
IVA or IVB	Liver or bone marrow involvement or extensive involvement of another extra lymphatic site

'A' denotes the absence of night sweats, >10% weight loss or fever and 'B' the presence of one or more of those symptoms

Rye histological classification

Lymphocyte predominant	Mixed cellularity
• Limited disease • Uncommon	• Older patients • Extensive disease
Nodular sclerosing	**Lymphocyte depleted**
• Young patients • Mediastinal disease	• Rare • Poor prognosis

Non-Hodgkin's lymphoma

Causes

Inherited immune deficiency	Autoimmune disease
• Wiskott–Aldrich • Ataxia telangiectasia	• Rheumatoid arthritis • Systemic lupus erythematosus • Sjögren's disease
Acquired immune deficiency	**Idiopathic**
• AIDS • Drugs (e.g. steroids, ciclosporin)	**Other**
Cancer treatment	• Chemical and physical agents • Radiation treatment of • Hodgkin's disease • Herbicides
• Radiation • Chemotherapy	

Lumps
- Usually lymph nodes
- May be extranodal

Constitutional symptoms
- Fever
- Weight loss

Bone marrow infiltration
- Anaemia
- Bleeding
- Infection

Spread throughout lymphoid system

Clonal lymphocyte expansion

Diagnose by lymph node histology

High grade
- Rapid growth
- ±30% curable

Low grade
- Slow growth
- Incurable

Excess Ig secretion

Lymphoplasmacytoid lymphoma

Excess IgM (Waldenström's macroglobulinaemia) → The 'hyperviscosity syndrome'
- Headaches
- Visual loss
- Lassitude

There are two categories of lymphoma: Hodgkin's lymphoma and non-Hodgkin's lymphoma (NHL).

Non-Hodgkin's lymphoma

The NHLs are a heterogeneous collection of malignancies affecting the lymphoid system; 90% are of B-cell origin with the

Medicine at a Glance, Fourth Edition. Edited by Patrick Davey. © 2014 John Wiley & Sons, Ltd. Published 2014 by John Wiley & Sons, Ltd. Companion website: www.ataglanceseries.com/medicine

remainder derived from T cells. There was a dramatic increase in incidence between 1970 and 2000 which was largely unexplained. Other known causes of NHL are shown in Figure 182.1, though in most cases no cause is found. Cytogenetic abnormalities are frequently found, most involving translocations of antigen receptor genes.

There are more than 20 different classification schemes for NHL. Most recently the World Health Organization classification has been widely adopted. This classification scheme defines distinct entities based on morphological, immunological and genetic features. However, most haemato-oncologists still classify the NHLs into broad groups termed 'low-grade' and 'high-grade' disease.

Low-grade NHL

This includes diseases such as follicular lymphoma and Waldenström's macroglobulinaemia. These are usually indolent disorders, with slow progression, which are usually readily controlled with mild to moderate chemotherapy combined with rituximab. Life expectancy is generally 5–15 years.

Follicular lymphoma

Follicular lymphoma is a low-grade B-cell lymphoma with a median age at presentation of 55–60 years. A translocation between chromosome 14 and 18 – t(14;18) – occurs which over-expresses *bcl-2*, thus inhibiting apoptosis and prolonging survival of lymphoma cells. Most patients present with lymphadenopathy and have stage 3 or 4 disease; one-third have B symptoms at diagnosis. B symptoms are defined as the presence of one or more of: drenching night sweats, fevers (of more than 38°C on more than one occasion) and weight loss (of more than 10% body weight in 6 months). Asymptomatic patients do not require treatment until symptoms or disease progression occurs. Treatment is then with mild to moderate strength combination chemotherapy, e.g. CVP or CHOP in combination with rituximab. Bendamustine with rituximab is increasingly used. Stem cell transplantation (autologous or allogeneic) is occasionally indicated for younger patients with aggressive disease. This is an incurable illness for most, with a median survival of around 12 years.

Waldenström's macroglobulinaemia

This is a low-grade lymphoma, most common in elderly people, in which abnormal lymphocytes have plasma cell features (lymphoplasmacytoid lymphoma) and produce a monoclonal IgM paraprotein. Patients present either with features of lymphoma (lymphadenopathy or B symptoms) or with a hyperviscosity syndrome, caused by high levels of the IgM paraprotein, which comprises lethargy, confusion, headache, light-headedness and visual disturbance.

Plasmapheresis rapidly reduces the concentration of IgM and decreases plasma viscosity. The effect is then maintained with chemotherapy. Oral purine analogues such as fludarabine or gentle intravenous chemotherapy ± rituximab are most frequently used. Median survival is 4–5 years.

High-grade NHL

These are aggressive diseases of rapid onset and progression. Examples include diffuse large B-cell lymphoma and Burkitt's lymphoma. Using intensive chemotherapy, 60–70% of patients <60 years are cured. *Staging* seeks to define the extent of spread of the lymphoma within the body. The Ann Arbor system, which relates to prognosis, is commonly used to define stage (see Figure 182.1).

Diffuse large cell lymphoma

This is the commonest lymphoma subtype and is characterized by rapid onset and, if untreated, rapid progression. Patients present with symptoms of nodal involvement (e.g. palpable lumps or complications of internal nodes causing obstruction of, for example, the ureters or the pelvic veins) or of extranodal involvements (e.g. central nervous system or liver or bone disease). Less commonly they may present with systemic symptoms such as fever or weight loss (B symptoms). Of patients, 60–70% can be cured using multi-agent chemotherapy in combination with rituximab. High-dose treatment with peripheral blood stem cell support cures 30–50% of patients whose disease relapses, although this is only suitable for younger patients without significant co-morbidities. The remaining patients usually die from their disease.

Burkitt's lymphoma

This is considered to be the most rapidly proliferative of all malignancies. Endemic African Burkitt's lymphoma is strongly linked with infection with Epstein–Barr virus (EBV), whereas in non-endemic Burkitt's lymphoma EBV proteins are found in tumour cells in fewer than half of the patients. Children with the endemic tumour present with a tumour involving the jaw and facial bones – those with non-endemic Burkitt's often have extensive extranodal abdominal disease. In both disease types, the tumour cells contain a chromosome translocation t(8;14) which causes increased expression of the c-myc oncogene. Intensive chemotherapy may cure patients with both types of disease. The non-endemic form occurs commonly in patients with HIV infection and other immunocompromised states.

Hodgkin's lymphoma

This lymphoma has a bimodal distribution with a peak in young adults and another peak in elderly people. The hallmark of the disease is the Reed–Sternberg cell. The cause is unknown. Epidemiology/serological studies suggest that EBV is relevant. The EBV viral genome is found in 40% of biopsy specimens. There is a small increased risk in family members of an affected person. Most patients present with lymphadenopathy in the neck or, less commonly, elsewhere. B symptoms may occur. A relatively common presentation is with a large mediastinal mass causing cough and breathlessness. Superior vena cava obstruction is, however, rare. The diagnosis is made by biopsy of an affected lymph node.

Types and staging

Two main types of Hodgkin's lymphoma are recognized. Classic Hodgkin's lymphoma is by far the most common type. Nodular lymphocyte-predominant Hodgkin's lymphoma is a much less common type which behaves in a very different and usually more indolent manner. Patients are staged in the same way as for NHL. The Ann Arbor system is used.

Treatment and prognosis

Most patients with Hodgkin's lymphoma are treated with chemotherapy with or without adjuvant radiotherapy. Early stage disease can be treated with fewer cycles of chemotherapy than late stage. High-dose treatment with peripheral blood stem cell support may be effective in curing some patients who have relapsed after standard chemotherapy. The cure rate varies from 65% for patients with advanced stage disease to 85–90% for patients with early stage disease. Unfortunately, complications of the treatment are noticed more frequently as patients survive for longer periods. Secondary malignancies are a problem occurring in 5–10% of patients by 10–15 years after treatment for their Hodgkin's lymphoma.

183 Myeloproliferative disorders

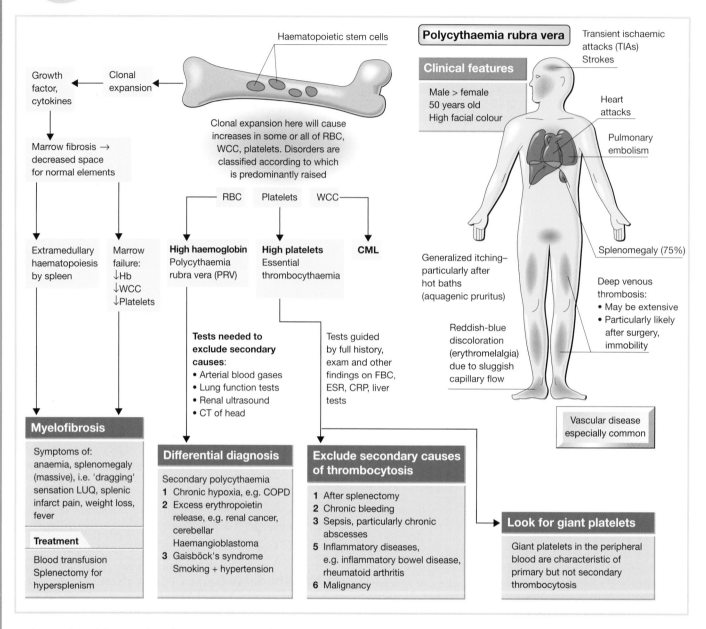

Haematopoietic stem cells

Clonal expansion here will cause increases in some or all of RBC, WCC, platelets. Disorders are classified according to which is predominantly raised

Growth factor, cytokines ← Clonal expansion

Marrow fibrosis → decreased space for normal elements

Extramedullary haematopoiesis by spleen

Marrow failure:
↓Hb
↓WCC
↓Platelets

RBC | Platelets | WCC

High haemoglobin Polycythaemia rubra vera (PRV)

High platelets Essential thrombocythaemia

CML

Tests needed to exclude secondary causes:
• Arterial blood gases
• Lung function tests
• Renal ultrasound
• CT of head

Tests guided by full history, exam and other findings on FBC, ESR, CRP, liver tests

Myelofibrosis

Symptoms of: anaemia, splenomegaly (massive), i.e. 'dragging' sensation LUQ, splenic infarct pain, weight loss, fever

Treatment

Blood transfusion Splenectomy for hypersplenism

Differential diagnosis

Secondary polycythaemia
1 Chronic hypoxia, e.g. COPD
2 Excess erythropoietin release, e.g. renal cancer, cerebellar Haemangioblastoma
3 Gaisböck's syndrome Smoking + hypertension

Exclude secondary causes of thrombocytosis

1 After splenectomy
2 Chronic bleeding
3 Sepsis, particularly chronic abscesses
5 Inflammatory diseases, e.g. inflammatory bowel disease, rheumatoid arthritis
6 Malignancy

Polycythaemia rubra vera

Clinical features

Male > female
50 years old
High facial colour

Transient ischaemic attacks (TIAs) Strokes

Heart attacks

Pulmonary embolism

Splenomegaly (75%)

Generalized itching– particularly after hot baths (aquagenic pruritus)

Reddish-blue discoloration (erythromelalgia) due to sluggish capillary flow

Deep venous thrombosis:
• May be extensive
• Particularly likely after surgery, immobility

Vascular disease especially common

Look for giant platelets

Giant platelets in the peripheral blood are characteristic of primary but not secondary thrombocytosis

The myeloproliferative disorders are a group of four diseases caused by clonal proliferation of haematopoietic stem cells:
- Chronic myeloid leukaemia (see Chapter 181).
- Myelofibrosis.
- Polycythaemia rubra vera (PRV).
- Essential thrombocythaemia.

Myelofibrosis

Myelofibrosis is caused by a clonal proliferation of haematopoietic stem cells – these release growth factors, particularly platelet-derived growth factor and cytokines, resulting in a characteristic polyclonal marrow fibrotic reaction, which gives the disease its name. The mean age of presentation is 60 years. Typical clinical features include anaemia, splenomegaly (often massive and causing pain) and systemic symptoms such as weight loss and fever.

The diagnostic tests are a blood count and film, and examination of the bone marrow. The blood count usually reveals anaemia. The white cell and platelet counts are usually high at diagnosis but can be normal or low. The blood film shows immature white and red blood cells (RBCs) (leukoerythroblastic change) and tear-drop RBCs. The bone marrow is often inaspirable as a result of the fibrosis. The trephine biopsy is hypercellular with increased marrow fibrosis.

Treatment is unsatisfactory. With disease progression anaemia occurs and is corrected by blood transfusion or by alternative approaches (anabolic steroids and erythropoietin), although neither is very effective. Thalidomide and prednisolone works for a while in a small number of patients. Splenectomy is useful in painful splenomegaly or to reduce transfusion requirements. As disseminated intravascular coagulation (DIC) may complicate

Medicine at a Glance, Fourth Edition. Edited by Patrick Davey. © 2014 John Wiley & Sons, Ltd. Published 2014 by John Wiley & Sons, Ltd. Companion website: www.ataglanceseries.com/medicine

myelofibrosis, a coagulation profile should be checked before surgery. Hydroxycarbamide can be used to control a high white cell count (WCC) and to try to reduce spleen size, but it has no impact on the marrow fibrosis. Poor prognostic factors include increasing age, anaemia, leukopenia and an abnormal marrow karyotype. Median survival is 4 years.

Polycythaemia rubra vera

Epidemiology and pathophysiology

This disorder is most common in patients in their fifties. Men are affected slightly more commonly than women. Young adults are occasionally affected. PRV is a clonal stem cell disorder. The red cell mass is high and half of patients have an increased platelet and/or white cell count; 40% have a marrow karyotypic abnormality.

Clinical features

The common complications of PRV are vascular; they occur in 30–50%, and include transient ischaemic attacks (TIAs), strokes, myocardial infarction, deep venous thrombosis and pulmonary emboli. Such events are more common in those with other risk factors for vascular disease. Other common features are facial plethora; itching, particularly after a hot bath or shower (aquagenic pruritus); and a burning discomfort, usually occurring in the fingers or toes associated with a reddish/blue discoloration (erythromelalgia). The latter is caused by sluggish blood flow and platelet aggregation in the small arterioles, which may lead to gangrenous digits. There is a small increased risk of haemorrhage as a result of abnormal platelet function. Bruising is common but more serious gastrointestinal or central nervous system bleeding may occur. Splenomegaly occurs in 75% of patients.

Investigations

The haemoglobin (Hb) and RBC count are high. The WCC and platelets are often raised. Isotopic measurement shows an increased red cell mass. The plasma volume may be high. PRV must be distinguished from other causes of polycythaemia: secondary polycythaemia caused by hypoxaemia (e.g. lung disease, cyanotic heart disease, high altitude); tumours releasing erythropoietin (e.g. renal, cerebellar haemangioblastoma, etc.); or polycythaemia in which the red cell mass is normal but the plasma volume is reduced (e.g. apparent polycythaemia more commonly found in hypertensive men who are heavy smokers – Gaisböck's syndrome). Criteria for the diagnosis of PRV are given in Table 183.1. A mutation in the JAK2 gene has been described in most patients with PRV and is now the single most useful diagnostic test in distinguishing PRV from other types of polycythemia. This single nucleotide mutation results in the stimulation of erythropoiesis independent of erythropoietin.

Treatment and prognosis

Venesection to reduce the haematocrit to <45% is a simple and usually safe treatment. Cytotoxic treatment with hydroxyurea is very effective, where adequate control of the red cell count cannot be achieved by venesection or in those with high platelet counts. Excellent control of the red cell mass and the platelet count will reduce the risk of vascular events. Antiplatelet drugs such as aspirin are also indicated prophylactically.

The prognosis for well-treated patients with PRV is good. The median survival is 10 years. Some patients' PRV transforms into myelofibrosis and a few patients develop acute leukaemia.

Table 183.1 Criteria for the diagnosis of PRV.

Jak2-positive polycythaemia vera

A1 High haematocrit (>0.52 in men, >0.48 in women) OR raised red cell mass (>25% predicted)

A2 Mutation in JAK2

Diagnosis requires both criteria to be present

Jak2-negative polycythaemia vera (JAK2 mutation must by definition be absent)

A1 Raised red cell mass >25% predicted	B1 Thrombocytosis (platelet count >450 × 10^9/L)
A2 Absence of secondary polycythaemia	B2 Neutrophil leukocytosis (>10× 10^9/L)
A3 Palpable splenomegaly	B3 Splenomegaly on ultrasonography
A4 Acquired cytogenetic abnormality	B4 Spontaneous growth of red cell abnormality precursors *in vitro* without added erythropoietin

A1 + A2 + A3 or A4 establishes the diagnosis of PRV.
A1 + A2 + two of B establishes the diagnosis of Jak2-negative PRV

Essential thrombocythaemia

Epidemiology, aetiology and pathogenesis

Most patients will be elderly; the typical age is 50–80 years. The sex distribution is equal. The cause is unknown but must be distinguished from a reactive thrombocytosis (see Figure 183.1). The peripheral blood platelet count will be >600 × 10^9/L and often >1000 × 10^9/L. The differential diagnosis includes:

- Other myeloproliferative disorders.
- Illnesses associated with a reactive thrombocytosis, where the platelet count is usually 400–1000 × 10^9/L, but may be higher, and where cytoreductive treatment is not needed. Prophylaxis against thrombosis with aspirin is appropriate, particularly if the patient is immobile or has other risk factors for thrombosis.

Clinical features

Most patients are diagnosed by chance. In the remainder, the most common presenting symptoms are thrombotic events from the raised platelet count, such as heart attacks, strokes and venous thrombosis. The risk of a thrombotic event is increased by coincidental risk factors such as hypertension, diabetes and cigarette smoking. There is also an increased risk of bleeding in these patients because of impaired platelet function.

Investigations

There is no diagnostic test for essential thrombocythaemia, although about 40% will be found to have a JAK2 mutation. Exclusion of other myeloproliferative diseases, such as polycythaemia, and of a reactive cause is important.

Treatment and prognosis

Elderly patients with a platelet count >1000 × 10^9/L, other risk factors for thrombosis or a previous thrombotic event are at high risk of further vascular occlusive events and require treatment. Young patients with a platelet count <1000 × 10^9/L and no additional risk factors might just be observed or given aspirin. If treatment is needed, hydroxycarbamide is used. Interferon-α is occasionally of value and anagrelide is a useful second-line agent.

If the platelet count is maintained within the normal range the risk of vascular events drops to close to normal. Of patients, 70% survive for more than 10 years. A few (5%) develop acute myeloid leukaemia.

184 Myeloma

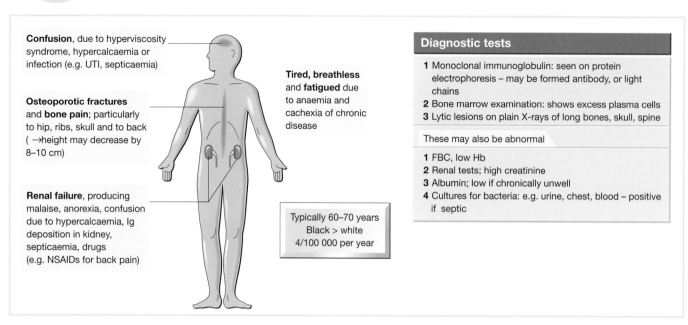

Confusion, due to hyperviscosity syndrome, hypercalcaemia or infection (e.g. UTI, septicaemia)

Osteoporotic fractures and **bone pain**; particularly to hip, ribs, skull and to back (→height may decrease by 8–10 cm)

Renal failure, producing malaise, anorexia, confusion due to hypercalcaemia, Ig deposition in kidney, septicaemia, drugs (e.g. NSAIDs for back pain)

Tired, breathless and **fatigued** due to anaemia and cachexia of chronic disease

Typically 60–70 years
Black > white
4/100 000 per year

Diagnostic tests

1 Monoclonal immunoglobulin: seen on protein electrophoresis – may be formed antibody, or light chains
2 Bone marrow examination: shows excess plasma cells
3 Lytic lesions on plain X-rays of long bones, skull, spine

These may also be abnormal

1 FBC, low Hb
2 Renal tests; high creatinine
3 Albumin; low if chronically unwell
4 Cultures for bacteria: e.g. urine, chest, blood – positive if septic

Myeloma is a malignancy of plasma cells in the bone marrow, with an incidence of 4/100 000. It is more common in elderly people and in American black populations.

Pathophysiology

In myeloma, a clone of cancerous plasma cells forms, filling the bone marrow, and producing just a single (monoclonal) immunoglobulin type, known as M band or a paraprotein. Normal immunoglobulin production is suppressed, i.e. immunoparesis occurs, responsible for the increased risk of infection. Anaemia is common from tumour infiltration, a cytokine-mediated anaemia of chronic disease, and there is often coexistent renal impairment. Kidney failure affects 50% of patients at some time during their illness and is most frequently the result of the renal deposition of Bence-Jones protein (i.e. the light chains of an immunoglobulin molecule), although it can be the result of hypercalcaemia, sepsis or drugs. Usually plasma cells produce a near 1:1 ratio of heavy:light chains (which together make up the normal immunoglobulin molecule), but in myeloma this finely tuned cell regulation is disturbed and it is common for an excess of light chains to be produced (Bence-Jones protein), which are then deposited in the kidney and interfere with its function.

Other factors contributing to renal failure are dehydration, infection, drugs (e.g. non-steroidal anti-inflammatory drugs (NSAIDs)) and hypercalcaemia. The latter is found in 25% of patients at diagnosis, and is caused by myeloma cells releasing cytokines, which stimulate osteoclasts to erode cortical bone. Calcium is then released into the bloodstream, causing hypercalcaemia.

Clinical features and investigations

The mean age of presentation is 65–70 years. Common complications are bacterial infection (from hypogammaglobulinaemia), bone pain and fractures resulting from lysis and resorption of cortical bone, hypercalcaemia (which causes nausea, thirst, polyuria, constipation and confusion), anaemia and renal impairment. Diagnosis depends on demonstrating a monoclonal immunoglobulin band, with depression of the other immunoglobulins

and/or finding Bence-Jones protein in the urine. Free light chains can now be detected in the blood using the 'Freelite' assay. Other findings include either generalized osteoporosis and/or lytic lesions on a radiological skeletal survey. The bone marrow aspirate shows excess plasma cells. Renal function, blood count and plasma calcium should be checked as they may be abnormal.

Treatment and prognosis

The standard treatment is with chemotherapy, usually a combination of melphalan, prednisolone (or dexamethasone), thalidomide or cyclophosphamide. Thalidomide and dexamethasone are commonly used initial treatments, which provide disease control in around two-thirds of patients at least. Disease control usually lasts only a few months, although it can occasionally be much longer. High-dose treatment with autologous peripheral blood stem cell support increases the response rate and duration of remission in younger patients. Newer treatments such as lenalidomide and the proteasome inhibitor bortezomib may help to improve outcomes for all patients. Allogeneic bone marrow transplantation has been used in a few young patients and cures around 25%. Supportive care is very important in patients with myeloma. The regular use of bisphosphonates has been shown to reduce the progression of bone disease.

Life expectancy is slowly improving for patients with myeloma and the median has increased from around 3 years up to 4–5 years over the past decade.

Monoclonal gammopathy of uncertain significance

This condition, increasingly common with rising age, is sometimes referred to as benign paraproteinaemia, although monoclonal gammopathy of uncertain significance (MGUS) is more correct. Patients have a monoclonal paraprotein but no other features of myeloma, e.g. bone lesions, anaemia or renal impairment. Of these patients the risk of developing myeloma or similar disorder is about 1% per year.

185 Myelodysplasia

Myelodysplastic syndrome

Recurrent infections

Pale

Easy bruising, bleeding

Clinical features
- Common
- Usually elderly
- FBC shows ↓Hb (↑MCV) ↓neutrophil and ↓platelets
- Bone marrow exam diagnostic

Treatment
- Mainly supportive (blood, platelets, antibiotics)

Prognosis
- After 2–3 years, many transform to AML (treatment refractory)

Myelodysplasia is a clonal disorder of the bone marrow in which morphologically and functionally abnormal blood cells are produced. It occurs with increasing frequency with rising age. Most patients have a macrocytic anaemia; leukopenia and thrombocytopenia are also very common. In most, no cause can be identified. In some, myelodysplasia develops after exposure to cytotoxic drugs or radiotherapy.

Clinical features
The clinical features can be predicted from the pathological findings. Symptoms of anaemia are common. There is an increased risk of bacterial infection resulting from the leukopenia and because the neutrophils are functionally abnormal. Haemorrhagic complications are common as a result of thrombocytopenia and because platelet function is usually abnormal. The previous French–American–British (FAB) classification defined five types:

1 Refractory anaemia: anaemia with <5% blasts in the marrow.
2 Refractory anaemia with ring sideroblasts: sideroblastic anaemia.
3 Refractory anaemia with excess blasts: marrow containing 5–20% blasts.
4 Refractory anaemia with excess blasts in transformation: marrow containing 21–29% blasts.
5 Chronic myelomonocytic leukaemia: there are dysplastic white cells and the absolute monocyte count exceeds 1.0×10^9/L.

A prognostic score can be developed based on the percentage of marrow blasts, the number of cytopenias and chromosomal abnormalities.

Diagnosis
Most patients have a macrocytic anaemia without vitamin B_{12} or folate deficiency. Abnormal-looking cells (dysplastic) in the blood film are commonly found. The bone marrow is hypercellular and dysplastic.

Treatment and prognosis
There is no satisfactory treatment for myelodysplasia although new agents have increased life expectancy recently:

- **Drug treatment**: azacytidine is a relatively new agent which works by influencing the packaging of genes in the chromosome. In high-risk myelodysplasia it has been shown to increase overall survival by several months. Lenalidomide is an immunomodulatory drug which seems particularly effective in a subtype of myelodysplastic syndrome (MDS) associated with loss of the long arm of chromosome 5 (so-called 5q minus syndrome).
- **Hormone treatment**: in some patients who are nearing transfusin dependence, erythropoeitin injections can suppor their hamoglobin level. This is particularly effective in patients with an inappropriately low baseline serum erythropoietin level.
- **Blood transfusion**: used for anaemia; infections should be promptly treated with antibiotics. Platelet transfusions help in haemorrhage caused by thrombocytopenia, but are not recommended for uncomplicated low platelet counts because platelet antibodies may develop and lessen the effectiveness of future platelet transfusions. Transfused platelets have a lifespan of 24–48 hours.
- **Allogeneic bone marrow transplantation**: this can be curative in young patients when a donor can be found. Patients with an increased blast count may benefit from anti-AML-type chemotherapy regimens, although the remission rate and survival is worse than in *de novo* acute myeloid leukaemia (AML).
- **Myelodysplasia and surgery**: the risks of bleeding and infection make any surgery more hazardous. Platelet transfusions are recommended *pre-* or *peroperatively* for those with even mild thrombocytopenia, because platelet function is abnormal. Postoperative infection should be rigorously sought and treated.

The median survival is 3 years but with a wide range based on the prognostic score. Most patients die from either infection or haemorrhage. One-third of patients will develop AML, which is often chemotherapy resistant. For this reason, most patients with myelodysplasia who progress to AML are managed just with supportive and palliative care.

186 The blood in systemic disease

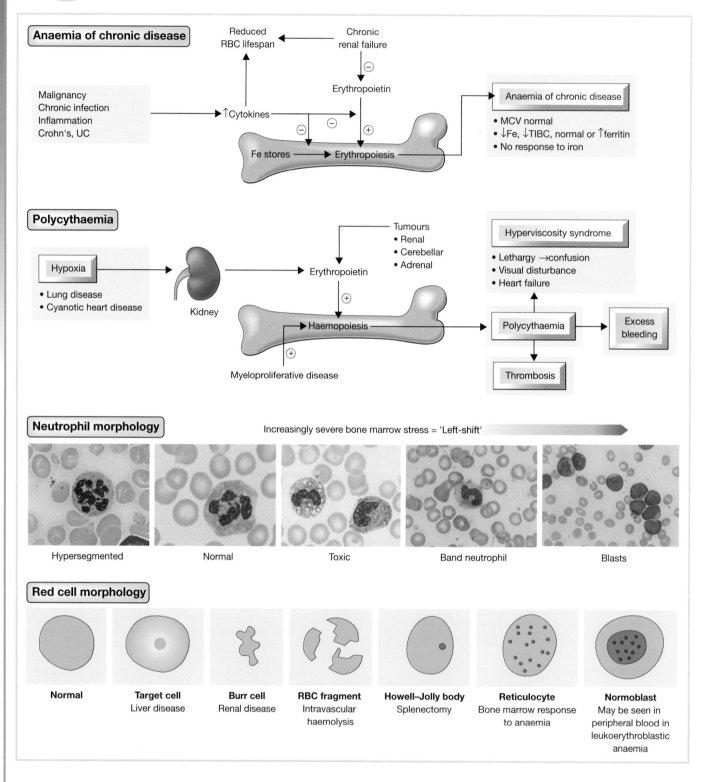

Anaemia of chronic disease

Reduced RBC lifespan

Chronic renal failure

⊖ Erythropoietin

Malignancy
Chronic infection
Inflammation
Crohn's, UC

↑Cytokines

⊖ ⊖ ⊕

Fe stores → Erythropoiesis

Anaemia of chronic disease
• MCV normal
• ↓Fe, ↓TIBC, normal or ↑ferritin
• No response to iron

Polycythaemia

Tumours
• Renal
• Cerebellar
• Adrenal

Hypoxia
• Lung disease
• Cyanotic heart disease

Kidney

Erythropoietin

⊕

Haemopoiesis

⊕

Myeloproliferative disease

Hyperviscosity syndrome
• Lethargy →confusion
• Visual disturbance
• Heart failure

Polycythaemia → Excess bleeding

Thrombosis

Neutrophil morphology

Increasingly severe bone marrow stress = 'Left-shift'

Hypersegmented | Normal | Toxic | Band neutrophil | Blasts

Red cell morphology

Normal

Target cell
Liver disease

Burr cell
Renal disease

RBC fragment
Intravascular haemolysis

Howell–Jolly body
Splenectomy

Reticulocyte
Bone marrow response to anaemia

Normoblast
May be seen in peripheral blood in leukoerythroblastic anaemia

The blood is commonly affected by systemic disease.

Anaemia of chronic disease

Many chronic disease processes produce inflammatory cytokines, which depress haematopoiesis by reducing iron transfer to developing red cells and diminishing the effects of erythropoietin on the bone marrow. Red cell survival is also shortened. Underlying disease processes include:

- Chronic infection, e.g. infective endocarditis, abscesses (particularly in the lung) and osteomyelitis.
- Chronic inflammation, e.g. rheumatoid arthritis, temporal arteritis and other vasculitides (e.g. systemic lupus erythematosus (SLE), polyarteritis nodosa).
- Inflammatory bowel disease, which causes both chronic disease and iron deficiency anaemia.
- Malignancy.
- Chronic renal failure, which causes anaemia principally by impairing the production of erythropoietin, although other mechanisms are also implicated.

The anaemia is usually mild (Hb usually $\geq 8\,g/dL$), and the mean cell volume (MCV) is normal (80–90 fL). Serum iron is low, as are iron transfer proteins (as measured by the total iron-binding capacity (TIBC)). Bone marrow examination, indicated when iron deficiency cannot be excluded non-invasively, shows plentiful supplies of iron. The anaemia does not respond to iron supplementation, but does to treatment of the underlying disease. Erythropoietin helps in renal failure and in some other diseases, e.g. anaemia of malignancy. Blood transfusions may help symptomatic patients.

Anaemia of acute disease

Anaemia can occur within a few days in severe acute illnesses:

- Acute severe infection pneumonia, septicaemia, etc.
- Acute renal failure from any cause although especially from vasculitis.

It is vital to actively exclude acute gastrointestinal haemorrhage, a common cause of anaemia in sick patients. In addition to treating the underlying disease blood transfusion has a role.

Leukoerythroblastic anaemia

Leukoerythroblastic anaemia is anaemia with immature white and red blood cells found in the blood film. Leukoerythroblastic anaemia is a common reaction to severe bone marrow stress in:

- Severe gastrointestinal haemorrhage.
- Severe haemolytic anaemia.
- Overwhelming sepsis.
- Bone marrow malignancy, commonly metastatic, although also intrinsic haematological malignancy, such as myelofibrosis and myeloma.

If the underlying diagnosis is unclear, bone marrow examination is usually diagnostic. The treatment is of the underlying condition and blood transfusion.

Polycythaemia

Polycythaemia is an increase in haemoglobin level by ≥ 2 standard deviations from the mean. Increased haemoglobin occurs in myeloproliferative disease (see Chapter 183), though these are rare. Much more common is polycythaemia secondary to:

- Chronic hypoxaemia from lung disease, usually chronic obstructive pulmonary disease (COPD).

- Heavy cigarette smoking associated with systemic hypertension (Gaisböck's syndrome); this occurs mainly in men. Premature death from coronary or lung disease is common.
- Cyanotic heart disease.
- Rare causes include excess erythropoietin-secreting tumours in the kidney or, rarer still, cerebellar haemangioblastomas, uterine fibroids and other tumours.
- Spurious causes: dehydration is a common cause of a transient polycythaemia.

Polycythaemia may be asymptomatic or produce a hyperviscosity syndrome (tiredness, effort intolerance, headaches, visual disturbance). Thrombosis, usually venous and occasionally arterial, may occur. As most polycythaemia is secondary or relative, investigation should include blood gases and lung function tests. Other tests include estimation of red cell mass using radioactive chromium and occasionally bone marrow biopsy. Renal, abdominal and cerebellar imaging may demonstrate a tumour. Treatment is of the underlying disease.

Leukocytosis

A neutrophil leukocytosis most commonly occurs in patients with bacterial infection and a lymphocytosis in those with a viral infection. A neutrophil leukocytosis also occurs in: (i) tissue necrosis, e.g. myocardial or pulmonary infarction, associated with a mild fever; (ii) malignancy; (iii) non-infectious inflammatory causes, including connective tissue disease; (iv) corticosteroid usage; and (v) diabetic ketoacidosis.

Investigations to exclude infection, vasculitis and malignancy may be needed if the cause is not obvious. Rarely neutrophil or lymphocytic leukocytosis is leukaemic in origin.

An increase in the eosinophil count is defined as $>0.5 \times 10^9$ eosinophils/L. It is uncommon and occurs in:

- Drug allergy: a common cause.
- Skin diseases: atopic eczema, urticaria.
- Asthma: complicating allergic bronchopulmonary aspergillosis should be considered.
- Parasitic infection, often intestinal, although infection elsewhere may be responsible, such as in the skin (cutaneous larva migrans).
- Vasculitis, especially polyarteritis nodosa.
- Malignancy such as Hodgkin's disease.
- More rarely found in the hypereosinophilic syndrome.

Patients usually do not have symptoms from the excess eosinophils, and treatment is of the underlying condition. Occasionally very high eosinophil counts occur, usually with tropical infections (tropical eosinophilia), causing myocardial and endocardial damage (restrictive cardiomyopathy).

Thrombocytosis

Although increases in platelet counts occur in myeloproliferative diseases (see Chapter 183), most increases are secondary to:

- Bleeding, especially chronic blood loss anaemia.
- Infection.
- Post-surgery, especially after splenectomy.
- Malignancy.
- Inflammatory disease, including vasculitis.

Mild increases ($400–700 \times 10^9/L$) are usually asymptomatic, but the higher the platelet count the more likely is thrombosis, both arterial and venous. Treatment is of the underlying cause; if this is not possible, aspirin is used for thrombosis prophylaxis.

Table 186.1 Causes of a macrocytosis (MCV >100 fL).

Cause	Clues from full blood count and film	Other blood results	Causes/comment
Drug-induced	Usually unremarkable	No specific abnormality	Many drugs, e.g. azathioprine, zidovudine
B$_{12}$/folate deficiency	Oval macrocytic red cells, hypersegmented neutrophils, pancytopenia	Low serum B$_{12}$/red cell folate Positive intrinsic factor antibodies in pernicious anaemia	B$_{12}$ deficiency: pernicious anaemia/malabsorption Folate deficiency: inadequate dietary intake/malabsorption
Haemolysis	See Table 186.2. Haemolytic anaemia is usually normocytic but can be macrocytic if there is marked reticulocytosis		
Primary bone marrow disorder	MCV usually >110 fL Other cytopenias Leukocytosis Monocytosis Thrombocytosis Blast cells	No specific abnormality	Myelodysplasia, leukaemia
Alcohol	Alcohol may also cause lymphopenia and thrombocytopenia	Abnormal liver function tests, with raised AST (>ALT) and γ-GT	Macrocytosis due to alcohol usually indicates a chronic intake of 80 units/day or more
Hypothyroidism	Usually unremarkable	Raised TSH, low free T$_4$/free T$_3$	Hypothyroidism may also cause normocytic anaemia
Chronic liver disease	Associated thrombocytopenia may be seen in cirrhosis with portal hypertension and splenomegaly	Abnormal liver function tests/ prothrombin time	Anaemia may also be due to acute or chronic gut bleeding (e.g. from oesophageal varices)

Table 186.2 Causes of a normocytic anaemia (MCV 78–100 fL).

Cause	Clues from full blood count and film	Other blood results	Causes/comment
Bleeding	Polychromasia Anisocytosis	Falling haemoglobin without evidence of haemolysis	Occult bleeding may occur from gut or into retroperitoneal space
Haemolysis	Polychromasia (reflecting increased reticulocyte count) Spherocytes Keratocytes ('bite' cells, due to acute haemolysis induced by oxidant damage, as may occur in G6PD deficiency) Fragmented red cells seen in microangiopathic haemolytic anaemia	Increased unconjugated bilirubin, increased LDH and reduced serum haptoglobin seen in haemolysis of all causes	Haemolysis is due either to intrinsic red cell abnormalities (e.g. G6PD deficiency, sickle cell anaemia) or to extrinsic factors (immune and non-immune causes)
Anaemia of chronic disease	Film usually unremarkable	Low iron Low/normal transferrin Normal/increased ferritin Abnormalities related to underlying cause	Seen in acute and chronic infection, cancer, renal failure, inflammatory disorders (e.g. rheumatoid arthritis, SLE), endocrine disorders and chronic rejection after solid-organ transplantation
Bone marrow disorder	Other cytopenias Leukocytosis Monocytosis Thrombocytosis Blast cells	Paraproteinaemia in myeloma	Myelodysplasia, myeloma, leukaemia

Table 186.3 Causes of a microcytic anaemia (MCV <78 fL).

Cause	Clues from full blood count and film	Other blood results	Causes/comment
Iron deficiency	Increased red cell distribution width Anisocytosis Increased platelet count	Low iron Increased transferrin Low ferritin	Commonest cause of microcytic anaemia; caused by inadequate dietary intake, malabsorption (e.g. coeliac disease) or blood loss
Anaemia of chronic disease (ACD)	Film usually unremarkable	Low iron Low/normal transferrin Normal/increased ferritin Abnormalities related to underlying cause	c. 20% of ACDs are microcytic: causes include Hodgkin's disease and renal cell carcinoma (see Table 186.2)
Thalassaemia	Polychromasia Target cells	Normal ferritin Haemoglobin electrophoresis normal in α-thalassaemia trait and abnormal in β-thalassaemia trait and other thalassaemia syndromes	Haematocrit usually >30% and MCV <75 fL in β-thalassaemia trait
Sideroblastic anaemia	Siderocytes may be seen: hypochromic red cells with basophilic stippling that stains positive for iron (Pappenheimer's bodies)	Increased ferritin	Rare Hereditary and acquired forms

Table 186.4 White blood cell abnormalities.

Finding	Possible causes	Finding	Possible causes
Neutrophilia	Sepsis Metastatic cancer Acidosis Corticosteroid therapy Trauma, surgery, burn Myeloproliferative disorders	Lymphopenia	Infections (e.g. viral, HIV, severe bacterial) Immunosuppressive therapy Systemic lupus erythematosus Alcohol excess Chronic renal failure
Neutropenia	Drugs (e.g. carbimazole) Infections (e.g. viral, severe bacterial, HIV) B_{12} and folate deficiency Systemic lupus erythematosus Felty's syndrome Haematological disorders (e.g. leukaemia)	Monocytosis	Infections Myeloproliferative disorders (e.g. chronic myelomonocytic leukaemia) Metastatic cancer
Lymphocytosis	Infections (e.g. infectious mononucleosis) Chronic lymphocytic leukaemia	Eosinophilia	Drug allergy Parasitic infestation Haematological disorders (e.g. lymphoma, leukaemia) Churg–Strauss vasculitis Disorders with eosinophilic involvement of specific organs Adrenal insufficiency Atheroembolism

Table 186.5 Common causes of thrombocytosis (platelet count $>350 \times 10^9$/L).

Setting	Common causes
Acute admission	Acute blood loss/iron deficiency Acute infection Cancer
Inpatient	After surgery or trauma Acute infection Acute pancreatitis Cancer Chronic inflammatory disorders
Outpatient	Chronic infection Post-splenectomy Cancer Chronic inflammatory disorders Chronic myeloproliferative or myelodysplastic disorder

Table 186.6 Causes of pancytopenia (red cell, white cell and platelet counts all low).

- Aplastic anaemia
- Idiopathic
- Cytotoxic drugs and radiation
- Idiosyncratic drug reaction
- Viral infections
- Acute leukaemia
- Marrow replacement
- Cancer
- Myelofibrosis
- Miliary tuberculosis
- B_{12}/folate deficiency
- Paroxysmal nocturnal haemoglobinuria
- Myelodysplasia
- Human immunodeficiency virus infection

187 Platelet disorders

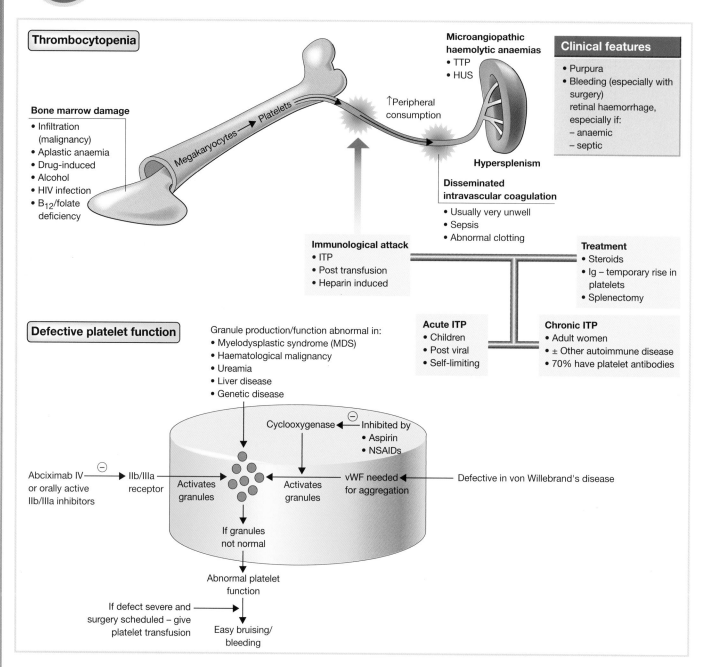

Thrombocytopenia

Bone marrow damage
- Infiltration (malignancy)
- Aplastic anaemia
- Drug-induced
- Alcohol
- HIV infection
- B_{12}/folate deficiency

Megakaryocytes → Platelets

↑Peripheral consumption

Microangiopathic haemolytic anaemias
- TTP
- HUS

Hypersplenism

Disseminated intravascular coagulation
- Usually very unwell
- Sepsis
- Abnormal clotting

Clinical features
- Purpura
- Bleeding (especially with surgery) retinal haemorrhage, especially if:
  – anaemic
  – septic

Immunological attack
- ITP
- Post transfusion
- Heparin induced

Treatment
- Steroids
- Ig – temporary rise in platelets
- Splenectomy

Acute ITP
- Children
- Post viral
- Self-limiting

Chronic ITP
- Adult women
- ± Other autoimmune disease
- 70% have platelet antibodies

Defective platelet function

Granule production/function abnormal in:
- Myelodysplastic syndrome (MDS)
- Haematological malignancy
- Ureamia
- Liver disease
- Genetic disease

Cyclooxygenase ← ⊖ Inhibited by
- Aspirin
- NSAIDs

Abciximab IV ⊖ → IIb/IIIa receptor
or orally active
IIb/IIIa inhibitors

Activates granules

Activates granules

vWF needed for aggregation ← Defective in von Willebrand's disease

If granules not normal

Abnormal platelet function

If defect severe and surgery scheduled – give platelet transfusion → Easy bruising/bleeding

Physiology of haemostasis

When there is injury to a blood vessel, a series of five events are initiated to control haemostasis. The first three processes are: (1) local vasoconstriction, (2) adhesion and aggregation of platelets, and (3) activation of the clotting cascade to create a fibrin clot. Coagulation inhibitors are then activated (4) to restrict coagulation to the site of injury and (5) fibrinolysis occurs later to restore vessel patency. Step 2 (platelet adhesion/aggregation) requires that platelets adhere to the exposed collagen in damaged blood vessels via von Willebrand's factor (vWF), a large polymeric molecule, individual subunits of which possess collagen- and platelet-binding sites (for platelet glycoprotein Ib). The platelets aggregate to each other by cross-linking with fibrinogen, which binds to specific fibrinogen-binding sites on the platelet surface (glycoprotein IIb/IIIa). Upon activation, platelets release agents (including adenosine diphosphate (ADP)) from their dense granules to recruit other platelets to the site and thromboxane, a potent platelet agonist, which provides positive feedback.

Platelet disorders

Platelet disorders are quantitative or qualitative. They present clinically with purpura, petechiae, mucosal bleeding, epistaxis and menorrhagia.

Medicine at a Glance, Fourth Edition. Edited by Patrick Davey. © 2014 John Wiley & Sons, Ltd. Published 2014 by John Wiley & Sons, Ltd. Companion website: www.ataglanceseries.com/medicine

Thrombocytopenia

The causes of thrombocytopenia are summarized in Table 187.1.

Immune thrombocytopenic purpura

Immune thrombocytopenic purpura (ITP) is an autoimmune disorder where antibodies are directed against antigens on the platelet surface, causing platelet removal from the circulation by reticuloendothelial cells, largely in the spleen. An acute self-limiting form occurs in children, typically after a viral infection and often not needing treatment. In adults ITP is a chronic disorder that is most common in middle-aged women. The diagnosis is largely one of exclusion, the bone marrow being normal or having an increased number of normal megakaryocytes. Treatment with steroids is only given to maintain the platelet count at safe levels and there is no need for therapy if the platelet count is above $30 \times 10^9/L$. Splenectomy is used if steroids fail or if too high a dose is needed. Intravenous IgG gives a good, rapid, albeit temporary, response and is useful for emergencies and before splenectomy or other operations.

Thrombotic thrombocytopenic purpura

Thrombotic thrombocytopenic purpura (TTP) has a classic pentad of thrombocytopenia, microangiopathic haemolytic anaemia, neurological disturbance, fever and renal failure. The defect is the absence of a vWF-cleaving protease (ADAMTS-13) normally present in plasma. This results in abnormally large vWF polymers in the circulation, which induce platelet microthrombi, resulting in end-organ ischaemia. The common sporadic form is the result of cleaving protease-directed autoantibodies. The rare autosomal recessive familial form of TTP is caused by an inherited deficiency. Treatment is with plasma exchange which replaces the enzyme and removes antibody and ultra-large vWF multimers. The patient is simultaneously started on steroids.

Disseminated intravascular coagulation

See Chapter 188.

Bone marrow infiltration

Bone marrow infiltration (by tumour) or aplasia (particularly chemotherapy induced) may cause thrombocytopenia.

Table 187.1 Causes of thrombocytopenia.

Decreased production
- Marrow aplasia or infiltration
- Megaloblastic anaemia
- Acute alcohol toxicity

Increased consumption
- Immune:
  immune thrombocytopenic purpura
  thrombotic thrombocytopenic purpura
  post-transfusion purpura
  heparin-induced thrombocytopenia
  drug induced thrombocytopenia
  antiphospholipid antibody syndrome
- Non-immune:
  disseminated intravascular coagulation
  haemolytic uraemic syndrome
  hypersplenism

Post-transfusion purpura

Post-transfusion purpura is suspected if thrombocytopenia occurs about 10 days after a blood transfusion. The patient's own platelets lack the HPA-1a antigen, which is present on the platelets in 98% of the population. When transfused with HPA-1a-positive platelets the recipient makes antibodies against HPA-1a and these, bizarrely, cross-react with the recipient's own HPA-1a-negative platelets, resulting in thrombocytopenia. Treatment is with intravenous immunoglobulin and the avoidance of HPA-1a-positive platelets.

Heparin-induced thrombocytopenia

Heparin-induced thrombocytopenia is a rare but serious adverse reaction to heparin. The patient makes IgG antibodies to heparin–platelet factor 4 complexes. This antibody then interacts with the platelet $Fc\gamma$ receptor, resulting in platelet activation, thrombocytopenia and arterial and venous thrombosis. Heparin must be stopped and an alternative such as argatroban, danaparoid or fondaparinux substituted.

Haemolytic uraemic syndrome

Haemolytic uraemic syndrome (HUS) presents with thrombocytopenia, renal failure and microangiopathic haemolytic anaemia. Although clinically similar to TTP, the pathology is different and is the result of endothelial damage with subsequent platelet activation. It is often seen in children after infection with verotoxin-producing strains of *Escherichia coli*. Treatment is supportive.

Qualitative platelet defects

Disorders of platelet function (see Table 187.2) are rare other than those caused by drugs:
- **Aspirin** irreversibly and **non-steroidal anti-inflammatory drugs** (NSAIDs) reversibly inhibit the cyclo-oxygenase 1 enzyme in platelets, preventing thromboxane synthesis and so ameliorating platelet aggregation.
- **Myelodysplastic platelets** have major functional defects, as do those from uraemic patients.
- **Bernard–Soulier disease** and **Glanzmann's thrombasthenia** are rare, inherited, autosomal recessive disorders caused by the absence of platelet glycoproteins (Gp Ib and Gp IIb/IIIa, respectively). Bleeding can be severe and treatment is with platelet transfusions as required.
- **Storage pool disease** is generally a mild disorder resulting from an inherited defect in the platelets' storage granules. The inability to release ADP and other agents from the granules reduces platelets' activation and recruitment.

Table 187.2 Disorders of platelet function.

Inherited
- Storage pool disease
- Glycoprotein (Gp) Ib deficiency: Bernard–Soulier disease
- Gp IIb/IIIa deficiency: Glanzmann's thrombasthenia

Acquired
- Drugs: aspirin and NSAIDs
- Hypergammaglobulinaemia
- Myeloproliferative disorders
- Uraemia

188 Disorders of coagulation

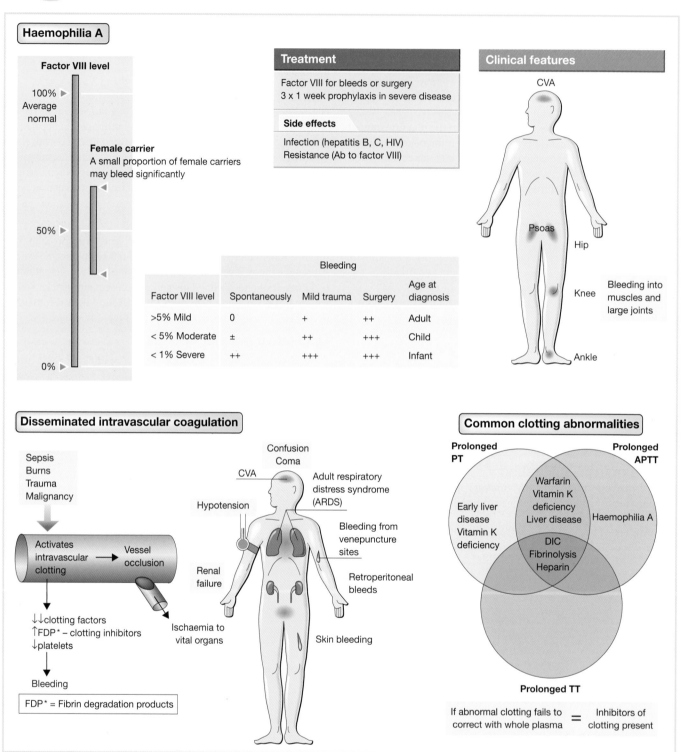

Haemophilia A

Factor VIII level

100%
Average normal

Female carrier
A small proportion of female carriers may bleed significantly

50%

0%

	Bleeding			
Factor VIII level	Spontaneously	Mild trauma	Surgery	Age at diagnosis
>5% Mild	0	+	++	Adult
< 5% Moderate	±	++	+++	Child
< 1% Severe	++	+++	+++	Infant

Treatment

Factor VIII for bleeds or surgery
3 × 1 week prophylaxis in severe disease

Side effects

Infection (hepatitis B, C, HIV)
Resistance (Ab to factor VIII)

Clinical features

CVA

Psoas

Hip

Knee

Bleeding into muscles and large joints

Ankle

Disseminated intravascular coagulation

Sepsis
Burns
Trauma
Malignancy

Activates intravascular clotting → Vessel occlusion

↓↓clotting factors
↑FDP* – clotting inhibitors
↓platelets

Bleeding

FDP* = Fibrin degradation products

Confusion
Coma

CVA

Hypotension

Adult respiratory distress syndrome (ARDS)

Bleeding from venepuncture sites

Renal failure

Retroperitoneal bleeds

Ischaemia to vital organs

Skin bleeding

Common clotting abnormalities

Prolonged PT

Prolonged APTT

Early liver disease
Vitamin K deficiency

Warfarin
Vitamin K deficiency
Liver disease

Haemophilia A

DIC
Fibrinolysis
Heparin

Prolonged TT

If abnormal clotting fails to correct with whole plasma = Inhibitors of clotting present

Medicine at a Glance, Fourth Edition. Edited by Patrick Davey. © 2014 John Wiley & Sons, Ltd. Published 2014 by John Wiley & Sons, Ltd. Companion website: www.ataglanceseries.com/medicine

In vitro tests of clotting

The coagulation cascade has classically been divided into the intrinsic pathway, which was thought to be initiated by contact between denuded endothelium and coagulation factors (contact activation), and the extrinsic pathway initiated by the tissue factor/factor VIIa complex. Both pathways activate factor X, which then cleaves prothrombin (II) to release thrombin (IIa). This simplified version is still the most useful for interpreting routine coagulation tests, which comprise the activated partial thromboplastin time (APTT), the prothrombin time (PT) and occasionally the thrombin time (TT) (exogenous bovine thrombin is added to the patient's plasma – the time taken to clot is the TT). Characteristic abnormalities in PT, APTT and TT occur in different diseases:

- PT prolonged, APTT normal: factor VII deficiency (early liver disease or vitamin K deficiency).
- PT normal, APTT prolonged: factor VIII, IX, XI or contact factor deficiency. Lupus anticoagulant; heparin and direct thrombin inhibitors (PT may also be prolonged).
- PT prolonged, APTT prolonged: interpretation depends on whether or not the TT is abnormal:
  - Normal TT: factor II, V or X deficiency; frank vitamin K deficiency or warfarin therapy; liver disease, anti-Xa inhibitors (though effect is variable).
  - Prolonged TT: deficiency of fibrinogen and disseminated intravascular coagulation (DIC), especially as a result of fibrin degradation products (FDPs) interfering with fibrin polymerization; fibrinolysis; heparin and direct thrombin inhibitors (PT may not be significantly prolonged).

In vivo coagulation

In vivo it is the tissue factor/factor VIIa pathway that initiates coagulation – largely by activation of factor IX (see Figure 188.1). Factor IXa in conjunction with its cofactor, factor VIII, then activates factor X. The centrality of factors VIII and IX to clotting explains why haemophilia A (deficient factor VIII) and haemophilia B (deficient factor IX) are such severe coagulation disorders. This clotting cascade also explains why patients deficient in contact factors do not bleed abnormally. Factor XI is activated by thrombin, which then activates more factor IX in a positive feedback loop. Patients with factor XI deficiency exhibit a variable bleeding disorder.

Inherited disorders of coagulation

Deficiency of coagulation factors presents with haemarthroses and muscle haematomas (in contrast with platelet disorders which present principally with skin bleeds), although gastrointestinal, genitourinary and intracranial bleeds can occur. The most common inherited deficiencies are of factors VIII and IX and von Willebrand's factor (vWF); other inherited coagulation disorders are rare.

Haemophilia A

Haemophilia A is caused by a deficiency of factor VIII. It is an X-linked recessive disorder affecting 1 in 5000 males. In severe disease (<1% factor VIII), spontaneous bleeding into large joints and muscles (e.g. psoas) occurs, unless regular prophylactic treatment with factor VIII concentrate is given. Moderate (1–5% factor VIII) and mild (5–40% factor VIII) disease is associated with bleeding on mild or moderate trauma. Factor VIII is given here only in response to trauma or in anticipation of surgery.

Previously, plasma-derived concentrates resulted in infection with hepatitis C and HIV. Recombinant factor VIII, uncontaminated with viruses, is now widely used.

Haemophilia B

Haemophilia B is caused by a deficiency of factor IX. Factor IX acts with factor VIII to activate factor X, and like factor VIII is encoded on the X chromosome. Haemophilia A and haemophilia B (which is only one-fifth as common) are clinically indistinguishable.

von Willebrand's disease

Von Willebrand's disease (vWD) is the most common inherited bleeding disorder – mild autosomal dominant forms may affect up to 1% of the population. The vWF is either deficient (partial: type 1 vWD; complete: type 3 vWD) or defective (type 2 vWD). The vWF circulates as large polymers and serves two functions. Its principal function is to form the bridge that allows platelets to adhere to damaged endothelial surfaces. Thus, in vWD clinical presentation is with the same pattern of bleeding as in patients with platelet disorders, e.g. skin bruising, epistaxis and menorrhagia. A secondary function of vWF is to stabilize circulating factor VIII. Plasma factor VIII levels therefore parallel those of vWF – although severe factor VIII deficiency occurs only in the rare type 3 disease. Treatment is with desmopressin (which raises vWF) in mild disease, and a factor VIII/VWF concentrate in more severe disease.

Acquired disorders of coagulation

The most common acquired coagulation disorders are DIC, liver disease and vitamin K deficiency. Rarely men or women can develop autoantibodies to factor VIII and so develop an acquired haemophilia.

Disseminated intravascular coagulation

This describes pathological activation of coagulation resulting in widespread microvascular thrombosis. Although consumption of coagulation factors often results in bleeding, it is the end-organ damage from thrombosis, rather than the bleeding itself, that leads to the very high mortality. Many insults can trigger DIC, e.g. septicaemia, malignancy and obstetric emergencies. The key to management is to treat the underlying disease. Blood product support, with fresh frozen plasma and platelets, is given simply to buy time.

Liver disease

Coagulation factors are synthesized in the liver and deficiency occurs as liver disease progresses. The situation is often compounded by thrombocytopenia – caused by splenic uptake in the large spleen occurring in portal hypertension. As a result of the short half-life of factor VII, the PT is a sensitive marker of liver damage.

Vitamin K deficiency

Vitamin K is required as a coenzyme for the γ-carboxylation of the coagulation factors II, VII, IX and X. This post-translational modification is necessary for efficient secretion from the liver and is necessary in order for these factors to bind Ca^{2+}, which then enables them to bind to phospholipid surfaces. Vitamin K deficiency may present with easy bruising and occurs in malnutrition, and especially in the malabsorption resulting from obstructive jaundice. All patients with obstructive jaundice should receive vitamin K before any surgical procedure, including endoscopic retrograde cholangiopancreatography.

189 Anticoagulation and antiplatelet drugs

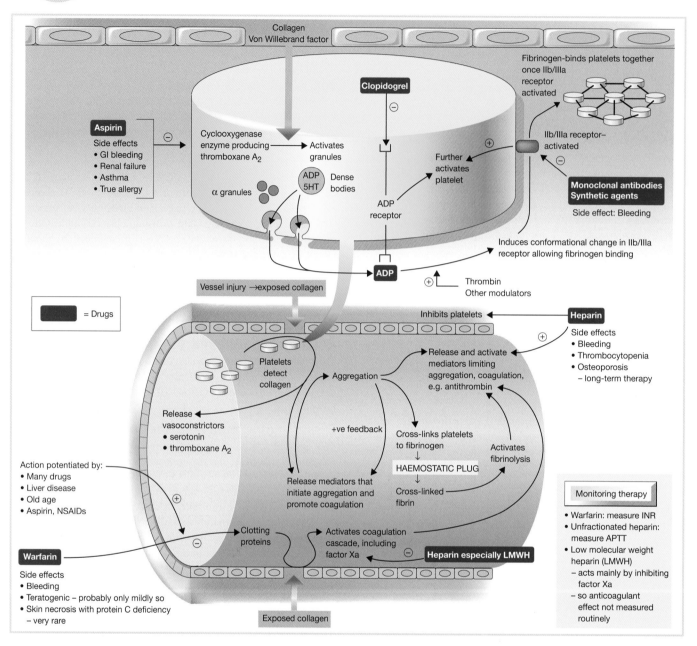

Anticoagulant and antiplatelet drugs are frequently used to prevent/treat abnormal clotting. Which is chosen depends on whether the mechanism underlying the clotting process is platelet or clotting protein dependent.

Antiplatelet agents

Diseases primarily involving platelet activation include most *in situ* arterial thrombosis, i.e. acute coronary syndromes (unstable angina, acute myocardial infarction (MI)), transient ischaemic attacks (TIAs) and most thrombotic strokes. Drugs with antiplatelet action include the following.

Aspirin

Aspirin is powerful and cheap, and inhibits platelet function by irreversibly acetylating platelet cyclo-oxygenase. The duration of action is several days, until new platelets are produced. It is effective in stable angina (reduces MI rates), unstable angina (reduces MI and death rates), MI (reduces death rate by 15%), TIAs (reduces stroke rate) and thrombotic strokes (reduces early and late recurrence rates). If immediate action is required (e.g. MI or stroke), 300 mg should be chewed (absorbed from the mouth). Otherwise, it is given orally in a daily dose of 75 mg. Side effects include upper gastrointestinal (GI) ulceration and bleeding and renal dysfunction (especially if there is pre-existing renal impairment). True

Medicine at a Glance, Fourth Edition. Edited by Patrick Davey. © 2014 John Wiley & Sons, Ltd. Published 2014 by John Wiley & Sons, Ltd. Companion website: www.ataglanceseries.com/medicine

allergy (rash or frank anaphylaxis) is very rare and is found more frequently in those with recurrent nasal polyps.

Dipyridamole

Dipyridamole inhibits the uptake of adenosine into platelets and inhibits phosphodiesterase in various tissues. Aspirin plus sustained release dipyridaomole is more effective than aspirin alone in secondary stroke prevention.

Clopidogrel and other ADP receptor antagonists

Clopidogrel irreversibly inhibits the platelet adenosine diphosphate (ADP) receptor. It has a role in acute coronary syndromes, and after implantation of intracoronary non-drug eluting stents (until stent endothelialization occurs after 1 month) and drug eluting stents as add-on therapy to aspirin. It is used as monotherapy in aspirin allergy/intolerance and has an expanding role in primary prevention of acute MI in high-risk patients. Prasugrel and ticagrelor are alternative ADP receptor antagonists (the latter binds reversibly).

Platelet IIb/IIIa receptor inhibitors

The platelet glycoprotein Gp IIb/IIIa fibrinogen receptor acts as a final common pathway when fibrinogen links platelets, resulting in platelet activation. Inhibition of this receptor powerfully inhibits platelet activation. There are two classes of inhibitors:

- Abciximab is a monoclonal antibody to the IIb/IIIa receptor, given intravenously, and useful in percutaneous coronary intervention (percutaneous coronary angioplasty, intracoronary stenting), reducing MI rate and increasing procedural success rates. It is very expensive. Side effects are of bleeding around the groin (entry site for the catheter to the arterial circulation) and retroperitoneally. Abciximab binds very strongly to the IIb/IIIa receptor and prevents fibrinogen binding; in severe haemorrhage, fresh platelet transfusion is given to stem the bleeding.
- Intravenous, synthetic, small molecule IIb/IIIa receptor inhibitors (eptifibatide, tirofiban) improve the outcome in high-risk unstable angina (i.e. ongoing angina despite drug therapy, pulmonary oedema during angina, persisting major abnormalities on the resting electrocardiogram, or elevation in troponin ≥ 10 the detect limit). Side effect: excess bleeding (e.g. intracranial or retroperitoneal haemorrhage).

Anticoagulants

Most venous clotting involves clotting cascade activation, e.g. deep vein thrombosis, pulmonary embolus, paradoxical right-to-left embolus, left atrial thrombosis (predisposition through atrial fibrillation) and any resulting emboli.. Clotting on artificial heart valves also involves the clotting cascade. For sagittal venous sinus thrombosis see Chapter 203. Warfarin and heparin have been used to treat and prevent venous thrombosis for decades.

Warfarin

Warfarin is a vitamin K antagonist and so inhibits the γ-carboxylation of clotting factors II, VII, IX and X. Its effect is measured by the international normalized ratio (INR), which is the patient's prothrombin time (PT; see Chapter 188), divided by the mean normal PT, raised to the power of the international sensitivity index of the reagent used:

- INR = 2.0–3.0 is usually therapeutic; some heart valves (e.g. Starr–Edwards) require an INR of 3.0–4.0.
- INR ≤ 2.0 provides inadequate therapeutic action and excess thrombosis.

- INR >3.0 is associated with an increased risk of bleeding.

Although warfarin rapidly inhibits vitamin K epoxide reductase, the clotting proteins whose production is inhibited have various half-lives. This 'buffer' delays the onset of therapeutic action (and the prolongation of the INR) by several days. Thus, if an anticoagulant is required to have immediate effect, heparin rather than (or as well as) warfarin should be used. Side effects of warfarin therapy include:

- **Bleeding**, often from over-anticoagulation, i.e. an INR ≥ 3.0. Bleeding can occur anywhere (intracranially, into the GI tract, etc.). Bleeding into the urinary tract, unless the INR is very prolonged (i.e. ≥ 6.0), often indicates intrinsic urinary tract pathology, e.g. urinary epithelial tumour.
- **Drug interactions** are very important and can increase or decrease warfarin metabolism leading to over- or under-anticoagulation. Antibiotics can decrease gut vitamin K production, so increasing the action of warfarin. Concomitant antiplatelet drugs may lead to bleeding. As there are so many drugs that interact with warfarin it is recommended that before prescribing additional drugs, possible interactions are identified from the *British National Formulary*.
- **Skin necrosis** is an exceptionally rare side effect, and often a manifestation of protein C deficiency.

Heparin

Heparin is a powerful, naturally occurring anticoagulant, which potentiates the action of antithrombin. It has an immediate onset of action, unlike warfarin.

- **Unfractionated heparins** (UFHs) are a mixture of different molecular weights (5000–35 000, average 13 000), which inhibit activated serine protease coagulation factors by promoting their irreversible union with antithrombin. They are usually given by continual intravenous infusion, with the dose titrated against the activated partial thomboplastin time (APTT; see Chapter 188). It is difficult to obtain ideal anticoagulation. Side effects: bleeding, thrombocytopenia and osteoporosis in long-term therapy.
- **Low-molecular-weight heparins** (LMWHs) are unfractionated heparins chemically or physically reduced in size to a molecular weight of 2000–8000. Their principal action is also via antithrombin, although they have a higher anti-Xa:IIa ratio. LMWHs have a much more predictable anticoagulant effect in an individual and are given subcutaneously as a body weight-adjusted dose once/twice a day. The APTT does not satisfactorily measure factor Xa inhibition, but fortunately anticoagulant action does not need to be monitored routinely. Side effects: bleeding and thrombocytopenia, both rarer than with UFHs.

Direct thrombin inhibitors

Bivalirudin and argatroban are parenteral direct thrombin inhibitors. Dabigatran etexilate is orally avaialble and is metabolized rapidly by non-specific esterases in the blood to dabigatran. Dabigatran has been licensed as an alternative to warfarin for stroke prevention in atrial fibrillation. It can be given in fixed dose with no monitoring.

Direct Xa inhibitors

Rivaroxaban and apixaban are orally available and act by directly inhibiting factor Xa; both can be given in fixed dose with no monitoring. Rivaroxaban has been licensed as an alternative to warfarin for stroke prevention in atrial fibrillation, for treatment of acute deep vein thrombosis and for secondary prevention of venous thromboembolism.

190 Thrombophilia

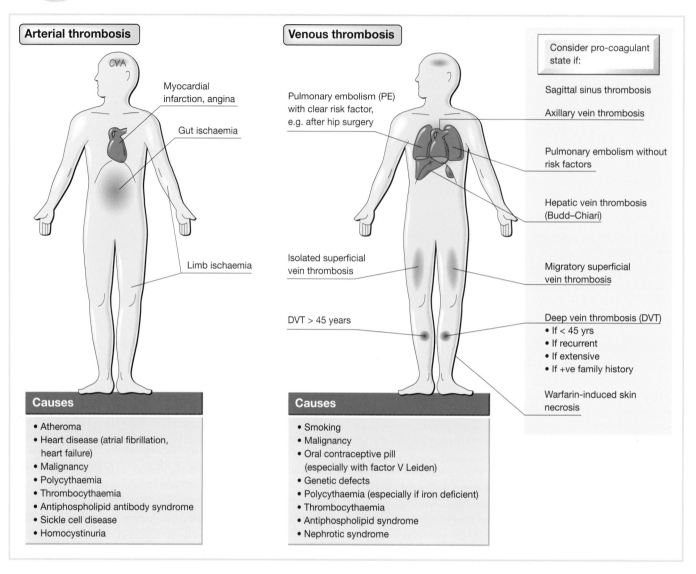

Arterial thrombosis

CVA

Myocardial infarction, angina

Gut ischaemia

Limb ischaemia

Causes

- Atheroma
- Heart disease (atrial fibrillation, heart failure)
- Malignancy
- Polycythaemia
- Thrombocythaemia
- Antiphospholipid antibody syndrome
- Sickle cell disease
- Homocystinuria

Venous thrombosis

Pulmonary embolism (PE) with clear risk factor, e.g. after hip surgery

Isolated superficial vein thrombosis

DVT > 45 years

Consider pro-coagulant state if:

Sagittal sinus thrombosis

Axillary vein thrombosis

Pulmonary embolism without risk factors

Hepatic vein thrombosis (Budd–Chiari)

Migratory superficial vein thrombosis

Deep vein thrombosis (DVT)
- If < 45 yrs
- If recurrent
- If extensive
- If +ve family history

Warfarin-induced skin necrosis

Causes

- Smoking
- Malignancy
- Oral contraceptive pill (especially with factor V Leiden)
- Genetic defects
- Polycythaemia (especially if iron deficient)
- Thrombocythaemia
- Antiphospholipid syndrome
- Nephrotic syndrome

Two natural anticoagulant pathways prevent excess thrombus forming *in vivo*:

- **Antithrombin** is a serine protease inhibitor or serpin. Many coagulation proteins are serine proteases and antithrombin, through the formation of a 1:1 stoichiometric complex, has substantial inhibitory activity against such proteases. Antithrombin's main effect is to neutralize thrombin, although it does also have inhibitory activity against factor Xa.
- **Protein C pathway**: the zymogen protein C is activated by thrombin in the presence of an endothelial cell cofactor, thrombomodulin. Activated protein C (APC) is a serine protease that acts as a natural anticoagulant by cleaving the two cofactors in the coagulation pathway, factors V and VIII, for which it needs its own cofactor, protein S. Both protein C and protein S are vitamin K-dependent proteins.

Inherited thrombophilia

Inherited mutations increasing the risk of thrombosis are common, affecting 5–7% of the population (see Table 190.1). The inherited forms of thrombophilia are associated only with venous thrombosis not (in adults) with arterial disease.

Deficiencies of antithrombin, protein C or protein S predispose to thrombosis. Heterozygotes for these deficiencies with approximately 50% of normal levels are at risk, so the thrombotic tendency is inherited in an autosomal dominant fashion. Homozygous antithrombin deficiency is not seen and is presumably fatal *in utero*, whereas homozygosity for protein C or protein S deficiency leads to the very rare condition of neonatal purpura fulminans. Until 1993, these three deficiencies were the only well-characterized forms of inherited thrombophilia.

Medicine at a Glance, Fourth Edition. Edited by Patrick Davey. © 2014 John Wiley & Sons, Ltd. Published 2014 by John Wiley & Sons, Ltd. Companion website: www.ataglanceseries.com/medicine

Antiphospholipid syndrome

Key features

Female:male ratio 2:1
- Venous (50-70%) and arterial thrombosis (40-60%) are the dominant clinical feature
- Recurrent fetal loss (30%)
- Thrombotic events usually isolated but recurrent
- Very rarely 'catastrophic APS', due to acute thrombotic microangiopathy, leading to renal failure (HUS), respiratory failure (ARDS), CNS and cardiac involvement, coagulopathy (and often death)

Antiphospholipid antibodies vs:
- Mitochondrial phospholipid (anti-cardiolipin); often due to infection; rarely leads to thrombosis
- Phospholipid binding protein; β_2 glycoprotein I
- Phospholipid coagulation pathway proteins → prolonged APTT (called lupus anticoagulant)

Causes

- 1° APS   No other autoimmune disease
- 2° APS   Associated autoimmune illness (usually SLE)
- Other   Drugs, infection, malignancy

Diagnosis

Requires appropriate clinical features + moderate ↑antibodies (twice ≥ 6 weeks apart)

CNS
- Accounts for 50% of arterial thrombotic events in APS
- APS may account for 20% of CVA in those <45 years
- Seizures
- Retinal infarcts

Heart
- Valvar involvement; regurgitation common 4% have sterile vegetations (may →CVA)
- MI; rare

Hepatic vein thrombosis (Budd–Chiari syndrome)

Renal
- May cause hypertension
- Haemolytic uraemic syndrome

Recurrent fetal loss

Haematological
- ↓Platelets
- Haemolytic anaemia
- TTP

Venous thrombosis
- (Recurrent) DVT – common (55%)
- PE (20%)

Table 190.1 Prevalence of inherited thrombophilia.

Deficiency/abnormality	Population prevalence
Factor V Leiden	1 in 20
Prothrombin G20210A	1 in 50–100
Protein C	1 in 300
Protein S	1 in 300
Antithrombin	1 in 3000

Factor V Leiden

In 1993 the phenomenon of resistance to APC was described and one year later the defect identified as a point mutation in factor V (G to A substitution at nucleotide position 1691), resulting in the arginine at position 506 being replaced by a glutamine. The abnormal factor is referred to as factor V Leiden after the Dutch town where it was identified. This substitution occurs at the site where protein C inactivates factor V. Normally factor V is inactivated by an initial cleavage of the peptide bond on the carboxyl side of arginine 506. Thus, the mutation here renders factor V resistant to APC. Factor V Leiden is present in 5% of the population – in heterozygotes it increases the risk of venous thrombosis seven-fold, whereas in homozygotes (one in 1600 of the population) there is a 50–100-fold increase in risk.

The prothrombin G20210A mutation

A polymorphism in the 3′-untranslated region of the prothrombin gene was identified in 1996; it is present in 1–2% of the population and is associated with a four-fold increased risk of venous thromboembolism. The mechanism seems to be higher prothrombin levels in individuals with the mutation.

Investigation of inherited thrombophilia

Not all cases of venous thromboembolism are investigated for genetic thrombophilia – studies are confined to those in whom testing will affect management or usefully inform relatives. Consider testing:

- Patients with unprovoked venous thromboembolism who have a positive family history or are young with children/siblings (especially daughters/sisters).
- Relatives (especially females of child-bearing age) of a patient with proven venous thromboembolism and an identified heritable thrombophilia.

In addition to testing for the five causes of inherited thrombophilia in Table 190.1, patients should also be tested for antiphospholipid antibodies, which are acquired risk factors for both venous and arterial disease (see Figure 190.2 above).

Acquired thrombophilia

See Figure 190.1 at the beginning of this chapter.

191 Aetiology of cancer

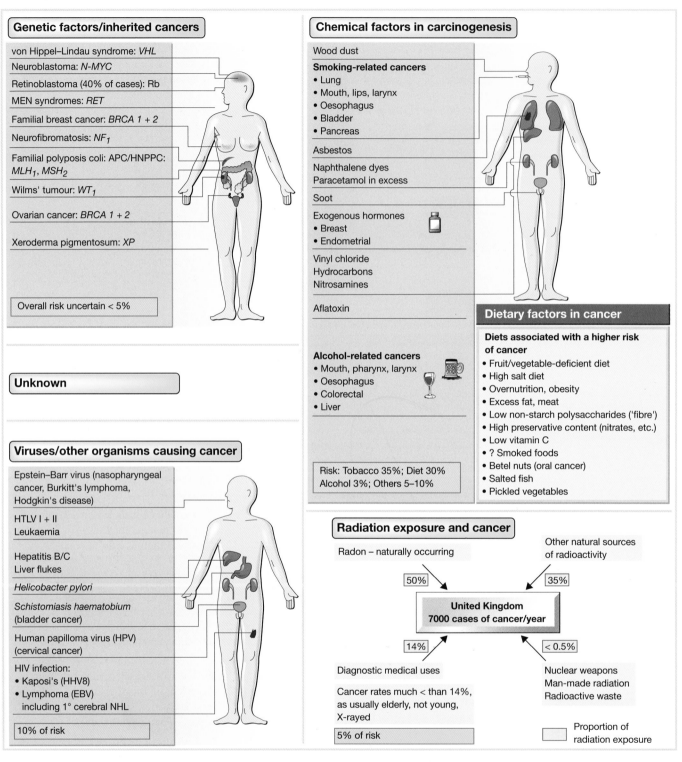

Genetic factors/inherited cancers

von Hippel–Lindau syndrome: *VHL*

Neuroblastoma: *N-MYC*

Retinoblastoma (40% of cases): Rb

MEN syndromes: *RET*

Familial breast cancer: *BRCA 1 + 2*

Neurofibromatosis: *NF₁*

Familial polyposis coli: APC/HNPPC: *MLH₁, MSH₂*

Wilms' tumour: *WT₁*

Ovarian cancer: *BRCA 1 + 2*

Xeroderma pigmentosum: *XP*

Overall risk uncertain < 5%

Unknown

Viruses/other organisms causing cancer

Epstein–Barr virus (nasopharyngeal cancer, Burkitt's lymphoma, Hodgkin's disease)

HTLV I + II
Leukaemia

Hepatitis B/C
Liver flukes

Helicobacter pylori

Schistomiasis haematobium (bladder cancer)

Human papilloma virus (HPV) (cervical cancer)

HIV infection:
• Kaposi's (HHV8)
• Lymphoma (EBV) including 1° cerebral NHL

10% of risk

Chemical factors in carcinogenesis

Wood dust

Smoking-related cancers
• Lung
• Mouth, lips, larynx
• Oesophagus
• Bladder
• Pancreas

Asbestos

Naphthalene dyes
Paracetamol in excess

Soot

Exogenous hormones
• Breast
• Endometrial

Vinyl chloride
Hydrocarbons
Nitrosamines

Aflatoxin

Alcohol-related cancers
• Mouth, pharynx, larynx
• Oesophagus
• Colorectal
• Liver

Risk: Tobacco 35%; Diet 30%
Alcohol 3%; Others 5–10%

Dietary factors in cancer

Diets associated with a higher risk of cancer
• Fruit/vegetable-deficient diet
• High salt diet
• Overnutrition, obesity
• Excess fat, meat
• Low non-starch polysaccharides ('fibre')
• High preservative content (nitrates, etc.)
• Low vitamin C
• ? Smoked foods
• Betel nuts (oral cancer)
• Salted fish
• Pickled vegetables

Radiation exposure and cancer

Radon – naturally occurring

Other natural sources of radioactivity

50%   35%

**United Kingdom
7000 cases of cancer/year**

14%   < 0.5%

Diagnostic medical uses

Cancer rates much < than 14%, as usually elderly, not young, X-rayed

5% of risk

Nuclear weapons
Man-made radiation
Radioactive waste

Proportion of radiation exposure

Cancer causes 20–25% of deaths. The development of cancer is a multistep process of genetic alterations. Many cancers are age related, reflecting this accumulation of genetic damage. Cancer cells can grow in defiance of the normal restraints on cell growth and they can invade and colonize areas normally reserved for other cells. Carcinogenesis is term for the genetic events producing malignant transformation and metastasis.

Environmental causes of carcinogenesis

• **Chemical carcinogenesis**: there are two stages to chemical carcinogenesis – tumour initiation and tumour promotion. Initiation means permanent, potentially inheritable (passed in the germline, i.e. gonadal) DNA damage from carcinogens (direct) or metabolites (indirect). Promotion can produce malignancy only in previously initiated cells and reflects increased cellular proliferation rather than direct effects on DNA (mitogenic as opposed to mutagenic). Common carcinogens include aromatic hydrocarbons and amines and nitrosamines. Aflatoxin B$_1$ induces a point mutation in *p53* (G to T transversion in codon 249) and causes hepatocellular carcinoma. Although the mechanisms are less clear, carcinogens in tobacco smoke are overwhelmingly the most important, probably causing 30% of cancers.

- **Radiation carcinogenesis**: ultraviolet irradiation, mainly UVB, produces pyrimidine dimers in DNA, normally repaired by the nucleotide excision–repair system. Excess UVB exposure overwhelms this pathway, resulting in DNA damage. Mutations in this repair pathway in xeroderma pigmentosa result in high rates of skin malignancy. UVB also causes mutations in oncogenes or tumour suppressor genes, e.g. *p53*. Ionizing radiation damages DNA by direct ionization or through the production of highly reactive free radicals from the ionization of adjacent water.

- **Viral carcinogenesis**: viruses may cause cancer by integrating genetic material into the host cell genome, which then activates oncogenes or inactivates tumour suppressor genes. RNA viruses may cause malignancy by the insertion of proviral DNA near a proto-oncogene, inducing a structural change, and so conversion to a cellular oncogene (*c-onc*). This is termed 'insertional mutagenesis'. Epidemiologically the most important viruses are human papillomavirus (HPV) (cervical cancer) and hepatitis B (liver cancer).

Inherited factors contributing to the development of cancer

An inherited predisposition occurs in 5–10% of cancers. Inheritance of a single mutant gene in germ cells (e.g. disrupting a tumour suppressor gene) increases the risk of tumour development (e.g. retinoblastoma). Subsequent mutation of the remaining tumour suppressor gene in somatic cells causes transformation. There are several well-characterized familial cancer syndromes linked to a specific inherited mutant gene, e.g. familial breast and ovarian cancer (*BRCA* genes) and familial adenomatous polyposis (*APC* gene). Although these are autosomal dominantly inherited, there are autosomal recessive syndromes (e.g. xeroderma pigmentosa). Subtle inherited variations in enzyme activity (genetic polymorphisms) and differences in gene expression profiles (epigenetics) affect the development and growth of cancers.

Genetic mechanisms underlying carcinogenesis

The genetic mechanisms underlying carcinogenesis are crucial to tumour development and growth. Most human tumours so far studied show activation of several oncogenes and the loss of two or more tumour suppressor genes. The important gene groups are:

- **Oncogenes** (cancer-causing genes) are derived from proto-oncogenes, normal cellular genes that promote and control normal growth and differentiation. They are classified as viral or cellular oncogenes (*v-onc* and *c-onc*). Each *v-onc* is named after the virus from which it was isolated, e.g. *v-fes* from the *fe*line *s*arcoma virus. The *c-onc* oncogenes are similarly named, e.g. *c-ras* from the *ra*t *s*arcoma virus or *c-myc* from murine (mouse) *my*elo*c*ytoma virus. Viral oncogenes (unique sequences within the genome of tumour-forming retroviruses) are almost identical to sequences found in normal cellular DNA. They may have become integrated into the genome during evolution by chance recombination with the DNA of the infected host cell. Cellular oncogenes are normal cellular genes that have become oncogenic through structural changes inducing altered *in situ* behaviour. Typically changes in the gene sequence produce an abnormal gene product with an aberrant function. Alternatively, changes in gene expression (protein production) by gene amplification (multiple copies) or overexpression cause high levels of normal growth-promoting proteins (often receptors). Oncoproteins (proteins encoded by oncogenes) include

growth factors and their receptors, signal transduction proteins, nuclear transcription factors (regulating gene expression), cyclins and cyclin-dependent kinases (regulating cell cycle progression from synthesis of new DNA to mitosis).

- **Tumour suppressor gene products** regulate cell growth by inhibition of cellular proliferation. Their loss is the key event in most, if not all, human cancers. Mutated tumour suppressor genes are mostly recessive – that is, carcinogenesis requires inactivation of both normal alleles, e.g. the protein product of the retinoblastoma gene (*pRb*), which controls cell cycle progression, and *p53*, which monitors for genetic damage, halting cell cycle progression and triggering apoptosis if damage is not repaired.

- **Caretaker genes** are a class of tumour suppressor genes but their inactivation is not directly responsible for cancer development. For example, genes regulating DNA repair are not themselves oncogenic when defective, but allow mutations in other genes to develop during replication, thereby increasing the likelihood of tumour development, e.g. the defective mismatch repair genes in hereditary non-polyposis colon cancer (HNPCC), the breast and ovarian cancer predisposition genes, *BRCA-1* and *-2*, and the defective DNA repair mechanism in xeroderma pigmentosum.

- **Genes regulating apoptosis**: apoptosis or programmed cell death is the orchestrated involution of redundant cells. Many genes regulate apoptosis. If these genes are damaged, there is a steady inappropriate accumulation of cells, e.g. overexpression of *bcl-2* in lymphoma or mutations in *bax* associated with failure of apoptosis in several solid tumours.

- **Ageing telomerase**: it is increasingly clear that cancer is a correlate of ageing, and the regulation of cellular longevity through telomere length has an important anti-cancer role.

Factors underlying growth and the spread of tumours

The key processes in cancer are growth and metastasis:

- **Growth**: clonal expansion of a transformed cell. Cancer cells are no longer dependent on normal mitogeic growth signals, they exhibit insensitivity to anti-growth signals and have developed mutations to evade apoptosis. Speed of growth is determined by the balance between cycle time and cell apoptosis, and by the proportion of tumour cells progressing through the cell cycle (growth fraction).

- **Invasion**: malignant cells invade locally (using collagenases and metalloproteases) or metastasize, by invading lymphatic channels and blood vessels, from where they embolize to distant sites. Adhesion molecules, vascular supply, vessel calibre, tumour cell size and target tissue characteristics determine the distribution of metastases. Initial metastatic growth relates to tumour angiogenesis, which in turn depends on the production of various cytokines, including vascular endothelium growth factor (VEGF).

- **Cellular immortality**: malignant cells have (express) the enzyme telomerase, which allows the ends of the chromosomes (telomeres – the cellular clock) to be elongated and so avoid the senescence (crisis death) of typical cellular ageing.

- **Angiogenesis**: tumours need to develop a blood supply to grow beyond 1–2 mm. Angiogenesis is an important part of embryology and healing, is disordered in malignancy and is driven by VEGF, inhibition of which by the monoclonal antibody bevacizumab confers a significant survival advantage in a number of tumours.

- **Host factors**: the interaction between the cells of the immune system and tumour is complex with evidence to suggest that tumour cells evade immune surveillance. Increasingly there is evidence to suggest that the host environment in which the tumour grows contributes to the growth and spread of cancers.

192 Diagnostic strategies and basic principles of cancer management

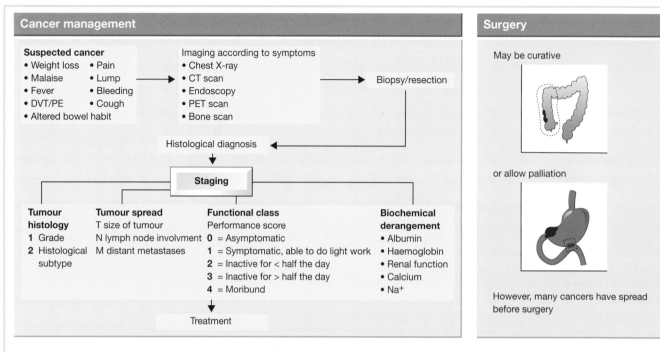

Cancer management

Suspected cancer
- Weight loss
- Malaise
- Fever
- DVT/PE
- Altered bowel habit
- Pain
- Lump
- Bleeding
- Cough

Imaging according to symptoms
- Chest X-ray
- CT scan
- Endoscopy
- PET scan
- Bone scan

Biopsy/resection

Histological diagnosis

Staging

Tumour histology
1 Grade
2 Histological subtype

Tumour spread
T size of tumour
N lymph node involvment
M distant metastases

Functional class
Performance score
0 = Asymptomatic
1 = Symptomatic, able to do light work
2 = Inactive for < half the day
3 = Inactive for > half the day
4 = Moribund

Biochemical derangement
- Albumin
- Haemoglobin
- Renal function
- Calcium
- Na+

Treatment

Surgery

May be curative

or allow palliation

However, many cancers have spread before surgery

Radiotherapy

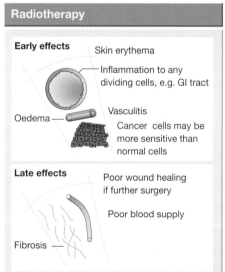

Early effects
Skin erythema
Inflammation to any dividing cells, e.g. GI tract
Oedema
Vasculitis
Cancer cells may be more sensitive than normal cells

Late effects
Poor wound healing if further surgery
Poor blood supply
Fibrosis

Chemotherapy

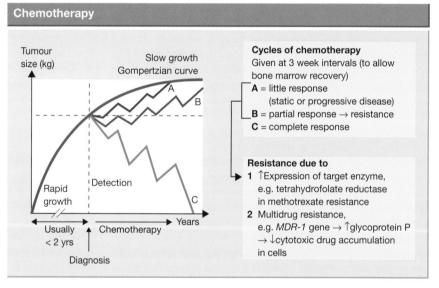

Tumour size (kg)

Slow growth
Gompertzian curve

A
B

Detection

Rapid growth

C

Years

Usually < 2 yrs

Chemotherapy

Diagnosis

Cycles of chemotherapy
Given at 3 week intervals (to allow bone marrow recovery)
A = little response (static or progressive disease)
B = partial response → resistance
C = complete response

Resistance due to
1 ↑Expression of target enzyme, e.g. tetrahydrofolate reductase in methotrexate resistance
2 Multidrug resistance, e.g. *MDR-1* gene → ↑glycoprotein P → ↓cytotoxic drug accumulation in cells

Important diagnostic strategies

Cancer needs to be diagnosed, staged and then the effects of treatment monitored:

- **Diagnosis** is made by histological (tissue) or cytological (cells) examination. Cells (fine needle aspiration) or small tissue samples (needle biopsy) are usually sufficient, although in lymphomas the architectural pattern (lymph node) should be examined.
- **Staging** reflects the mechanisms of spread of the tumour (local invasion, lymph or blood spread), determines treatment and, along with histological subtype and grade, is the most powerful determinant of outcome. Tumour staging is occasionally done surgically, but more often radiologically and by bone marrow examination/scan. Histological characteristics define the

'aggressiveness' of the tumour, based on mitotic rate, nuclear pleomorphism, tubule formation, etc. and on growth factor receptors, e.g. oestrogen and HER-2/neu receptors.

- Increasingly **tumour markers**, particularly in ovarian cancer (CA-125), germ cell tumours (α-fetoprotein, β-human chorionic gonadotrophin) and lymphoma (lactate dehydrogenase) are used in evaluating treatment and surveillance, and relate to tumour burden. The polymerase chain reaction (PCR) amplifies specific molecular markers of malignant cells and detects residual disease in chronic myeloid leukaemia (CML) and follicular lymphoma.
- **Measures** of age, performance score, activity and physiological function are important determinants of the response to treatment, as are laboratory measures (e.g. albumin).

Principles of surgical oncology

Surgery is used for both diagnosis and staging of the tumour. Historically, radical surgery gave optimal chance of cure. It still remains an important modality and can be the primary treatment in ovarian cancer, some sarcomas, melanomas, head and neck tumours, lung cancer, colon cancer and, when appropriate, resection of oligo- (one or few) metastasis. Surgical resection should, for local control, extend to a clear (cancer-free) margin of 1 cm in most cancers. With modern adjuvant therapies (radiation or chemotherapy) to complement surgery, more conservative surgical operations with their reduced morbidities are possible.

Surgery can have an important role in palliation and local control of tumours when complete excision is not possible. For example, surgical fixation of a pathological fracture or, in obstructing bowel tumours, surgery may be used to bypass the lesion to relieve symptoms.

Basic principles of radiotherapy

Radiotherapy plays an essential role in the treatment of many cancers. Radiotherapy may be used for curative or adjuvant treatment (e.g. radiotherapy to the breast and lymph nodes following surgery for breast cancer). It is also used for palliative treatment where the aim is for local control and symptom management, e.g. pain control in bone metastasis and control of haemoptysis in lung cancer. Ionizing radiation induces DNA damage, which triggers apoptosis (programmed cell death). Radiation doses are divided (fractionated) to allow for recovery of normal tissue and thus reduce side effects. Certain tissues (e.g. the lens, nervous and cardiac tissue) are particularly radiosensitive and mandate careful radiation planning. The concurrent use of chemotherapy is increasingly improving the outcome of radiation, as in cervical carcinoma.

Computed tomography (CT) planning, conformal (shaped beam) radiotherapy and intensity modulated radiotherapy enable tailored radiotherapy with minimal irradiation of adjacent tissues. Brachytherapy (the use of seeds, wires or implants, applied close to the malignancy), monoclonal radioimmunotherapy and stereotactic radiotherapy are techniques that exploit this principle further.

Basic principles of chemotherapy

Chemotherapy works by:
- Damaging the DNA of rapidly dividing cells, which is detected by the *p53/Rb* pathway, thus triggering apoptosis.
- Damaging the cellular spindle apparatus, preventing cell division.
- Inhibiting DNA synthesis.

Chemotherapy can lead to cure, either when given alone (choriocarcinoma, childhood acute lymphoblastic leukaemia, some lymphomas and leukaemias, germ cell tumours) or in combination with surgery (osteosarcoma, adenocarcinoma of the breast and ovary, colorectal cancer, squamous cell carcinoma of the upper gastrointestinal (GI) tract). It may prolong life without producing cure, as in acute myeloid leukaemia, small cell carcinoma of the lung and ovarian cancer. Increased understanding of cancer cell biology has improved current treatments. The different classes of chemotherapy are:

- **Folate antagonists, purine and pyrimidine analogues**: these drugs (methotrexate, 5-fluorouracil, hydroxyurea) inhibit DNA synthesis.
- **Alkylating agents**: these damage DNA. They include cyclophosphamide (breast cancer, lymphoma), melphalan (myeloma) and platinum (testicular cancer, lymphoma, squamous cell carcinoma, ovarian and bladder cancer). Drug resistance can occur.
- **Topoisomerase I and II interacting drugs** intercalate double-stranded DNA (dsDNA) and form a cleavable complex with topoisomerase II, an essential nuclear enzyme that causes dsDNA breaks. Examples include the anthracyclines (breast cancer, lymphoma) and etoposide (teratoma, lung cancer). Related drugs, including topotecan and irinotecan, associate with topoisomerase I to cause reversible single-stranded DNA breaks.
- **Alkaloids and taxanes**: inhibit microtubule function and disrupt mitosis. Examples include the vinca alkaloids (leukaemia, lymphoma, bladder cancer) and the taxanes (ovarian cancer, breast cancer).

Side effects of chemotherapy

Chemotherapy causes myelosuppression and so risks infection (neutropenia) and bleeding (thrombocytopenia). Damage to mucous membranes causes a sore mouth and diarrhoea and stimulation of the chemotactic trigger zone produces nausea and vomiting. Any rapidly dividing tissues, such as the hair follicles (alopecia) and germinal epithelium (infertility), are vulnerable to the effects of chemotherapy and late effects such as secondary malignancies are increasingly recognized. All are teratogenic. Some drugs cause specific organ toxicity, such as to the kidney (cisplatin) and nerves (vincristine). Supportive care with the 5-hydroxytryptamine (serotonin) 5-HT$_3$ antagonists, neurokinin-1 receptor antagonists and steroids has improved the control of nausea. Several recombinant human proteins are in routine use to support the effects of myelosuppression; e.g. granulocyte colony-stimulating factor reduces the depth and duration of neutropenia.

Other therapies

- **Immunotherapy**: interleukin-2 induces a small (<5%) complete remission rate in young patients with advanced renal cell carcinoma or melanoma.
- **Monoclonal antibodies**: several monoclonal antibodies are used successfully, including trastuzumab (breast cancer: anti-HER-2), rituximab (lymphoma: anti-CD20) and cetuximab (epidermal growth factor receptor (EGFR) inhibitor: colorectal cancer). Bevacizumab is a monoclonal antibody against vascular endothelial growth factor receptor that inhibits angiogenesis. It has a role in breast and colorectal cancer.
- **Tyrosine kinase inhibitors**: e.g. Imatinib (Glivec®), an oral tyrosine kinase (bcr/Abl gene product) inhibitor, has revolutionized the treatment of CML. Erlotinib (Tarceva®), used in non-small cell lung cancer, targets the EGFR.
- **Others**: multiple different treatments are being developed that exploit known mutations within the cancer cell. For example, inhibitors of poly (adenosine diphosphate ribose) polymerase (PARP) target cancer cells with defects within the homologous recombination DNA repair pathway and have been particularly investigated in *BRCA*-mutated cancers.
- Gene therapy and tumour vaccines are all investigational.

Basic principles of hormonal therapy

Some tumours (e.g. breast, prostate) are hormone responsive. The removal of endogenous hormones in some cases improves prognosis, e.g. one-third of premenopausal women with advanced breast cancer have a remission with oophorectomy. Drugs interfere with hormone action within cancer cells – e.g. tamoxifen, a competitive inhibitor of the oestrogen receptor, with some oestrogenic activity, and aromatase inhibitors (block oestrogen synthesis) are used in breast cancer. Androgens are important for the growth and malignant transformation of prostatic tissue. Androgen deprivation therapy is the primary treatment for metastatic prostate cancer and can be produced by castration or by medical means with gonadotrophin-releasing hormone (GnRH) analogues.

193 Cancer screening and early detection

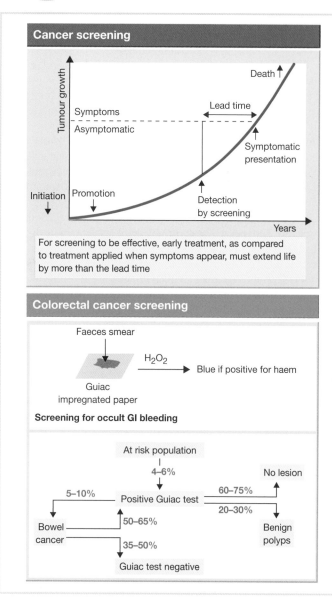

Cancer screening

For screening to be effective, early treatment, as compared to treatment applied when symptoms appear, must extend life by more than the lead time

Colorectal cancer screening

H₂O₂ → Blue if positive for haem

Guiac impregnated paper

Screening for occult GI bleeding

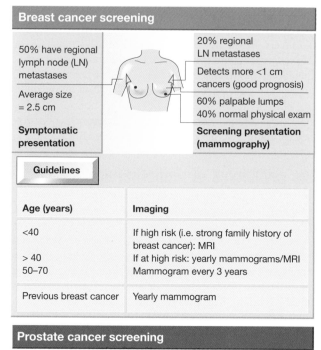

Breast cancer screening

50% have regional lymph node (LN) metastases

Average size = 2.5 cm

Symptomatic presentation

20% regional LN metastases

Detects more <1 cm cancers (good prognosis)

60% palpable lumps 40% normal physical exam

Screening presentation (mammography)

Guidelines

Age (years)	Imaging
<40	If high risk (i.e. strong family history of breast cancer): MRI
> 40 50–70	If at high risk: yearly mammograms/MRI Mammogram every 3 years
Previous breast cancer	Yearly mammogram

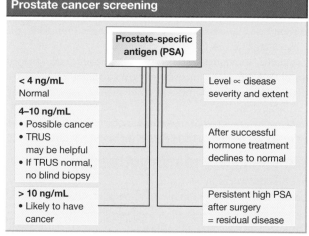

Prostate cancer screening

Prostate-specific antigen (PSA)

< 4 ng/mL Normal

4–10 ng/mL
- Possible cancer
- TRUS may be helpful
- If TRUS normal, no blind biopsy

> 10 ng/mL
- Likely to have cancer

Level ∝ disease severity and extent

After successful hormone treatment declines to normal

Persistent high PSA after surgery = residual disease

Principles of screening

Early disease detection offers the best hope for cure with the least intervention. Treatment success is often dependent on the spread (stage) and biology (grade and behaviour) of disease, both of which worsen with time. Successful screening strategies should:

- Address a common and dangerous disease.
- Use a simple, safe, inexpensive and valid screening test.
- Be acceptable to all social groups.
- Enable curative treatment, which when instituted earlier has a significant impact on survival.

Although observational, cohort and randomized controlled trials have shown the advantage of some screening programmes, there are problems:

- Screening can provoke anxiety.
- Screening may only increase lead time (time before development of symptoms but does not impact on survival).

- Screening may only increase the detection of more indolent cancers, which may never become clinically apparent. When added to the clinically relevant cancers, these apparently increase the percentage of early cases and overall survival. In screening, one of the earliest indicators of a future decrease in mortality is a decrease in the absolute rate (not percentage) of cases of advanced disease.

The impact of screening has been limited by the huge size of target populations, the difficulty of follow-up, poor compliance and poor test sensitivity with high false-positive rates.

Breast cancer

In 1963, the first randomized cancer screening trial investigating mammography in breast cancer was undertaken, using mortality as an end point. Subsequently, several studies have supported this approach and suggest that screening 50–69-year-old women with mammography decreases the breast cancer mortality. There is controversy about women aged 40–49 because:

● Although breast cancer is the leading cause of death in such women, breast cancer incidence and mortality rates are lower in this age group.
● To date the randomized controlled trials have been too small to be statistically unambiguous.
● The sensitivity of mammography is lower in denser breast tissue.
● There is a higher relative rate of ductal carcinoma *in situ*.

Two-view mammography diagnoses twice as many patients with benign breast disease as with cancer. Wire localization of the breast cancer and conservative surgery detect more node-negative breast cancers with a good prognosis that are <1 cm in size (5-year survival rate of 80–90%).

The current guidelines in the UK recommend:

● A two-view mammography for women aged 50–70 every 3 years.
● Yearly mammograms for those who have had a previous breast cancer.
● Screening should start yearly at the age of 40 for those with a strong family history of breast cancer.
● Magnetic resonance imaging (MRI) may be offered to women aged 29–40 if at high risk (e.g. known *BRCA-1* or *BRCA-2* carriers).
● Women should be breast aware.

The UK National Health Service is currently extending breast screening to women aged 47–50 and 70–73 and plans to increase the use of digital mammography in the future. MRI is also increasingly being used.

The finding that some breast cancer is genetically inherited has opened the question of genetic screening. At present assays of *BRCA-1* and *-2* may be offered to young women with a strong family history of breast and ovarian cancer occurring early in life. The best management of those found to carry these genes is unclear although prophylactic surgery (mastectomy and oophorectomy) and tamoxifen may be options.

Colorectal cancer

Colorectal cancer is the second leading cause of cancer death. For localized disease the 5-year survival rate is 90%, for node-positive (Dukes' stage C) disease it is 60%, and for patients presenting with metastatic disease it is 10%. Many screening studies show an increase in the proportion of early cases detected by colonoscopy, sigmoidoscopy or digital rectal examination and faecal blood examination. Of asymptomatic patients aged >50 years, 1–5% have positive faecal occult bloods, of whom 10% have cancer and 20–30% have adenomas. Annual faecal occult blood and flexible sigmoidoscopy every 5 years thus have the potential to reduce mortality significantly, although this has not yet been unequivocally shown. The current guidelines for colorectal screening suggest that:

● Those with a very high incidence of colon and/or rectal cancer (e.g. familial polyposis coli, hereditary non-polyposis coli, cancer family syndrome or ulcerative pan-colitis) should have yearly faecal occult bloods ± colonoscopy.
● Rectal examination should be included in routine check-ups.
● Screening using faecal occult blood test kits is now implemented throughout the UK. This programme is aimed initially at men and women aged 60–69 years, every 2 years.

Some cancer societies recommend sigmoidoscopy or colonoscopy at age 50 years, regardless of symptom status or whether occult blood is positive or not. This is not routine practice in the UK.

Prostate cancer

In the last 10 years the incidence of prostate cancer has increased in the USA. The average age of presentation with prostate cancer is 70 years, close to life expectancy, and competing causes of death influence the epidemiology and management of the disease. Furthermore, the negative impact of treatment (impotence/incontinence) limits their utility. Finally, no study has yet shown conclusively that the benefit from screening outweighs the harm from the possible over investigation and overtreatment. Studies are, however, ongoing, investigating the role of transrectal ultrasonography (TRUS), prostate-specific antigen (PSA) and digital rectal examination in screening. It may be appropriate to screen high-risk patients (black men and men with a family history of prostate cancer).

Cervical cancer

The mortality rate for cervical cancer has decreased in several countries, following the introduction of screening programmes based on Papanicolaou's (Pap) smears. Although there are no randomized controlled trials, the introduction of Pap smear screening in Finland and Iceland was associated with a 50% and 80%, respectively, reduced mortality rate over a 20-year period. The current UK guidelines recommend that:

● The newer technique of liquid-based cytology is now the preferred technique for cervical screening.
● Screening should be offered to all women between the ages of 25 and 64 every 3–5 years.

Central to the pathogenesis of cervical cancer is the presence of high-risk strains of human papillomavirus (HPV) in the cervical epithelium. The HPV vaccine has been introduced for girls aged 12–13 across the UK. Screening should still continue in those receiving the vaccine. The role of HPV testing as a screening modality is under evaluation, although HPV testing is currently used for women with cervical samples showing borderline nuclear changes or mild dyskaryosis and in those following a diagnosis for cervical intraepithelial neoplasia to determine whether they should proceed to colposcopy.

The future for screening

There is increasing evidence to support a lung cancer screening programme, and work is currently underway in the UK investigating the feasibility of a trial of computed tomography screening for lung cancer. The UK Collaborative Trial of Ovarian Cancer Screening is currently an ongoing trial assessing the effectiveness of two possible methods of ovarian cancer screening, an annual CA125 test and an annual transvaginal ultrasound.

Education and awareness

There are two tumours where the principal screener should be the patient:

● **Testicular tumours**: typically detected by accident or self-examination, and although rare are the most common tumour in young men. Education and increased awareness reduces delays in diagnosis.
● **Skin tumours**: education about the dangers of excess sun (ultraviolet) exposure, especially for fair-skinned individuals and those with a personal/family history of melanoma or dysplastic naevi syndrome, has decreased the incidence of sun-related cancers and improved early diagnosis, e.g. a high-profile public education programme in Scotland decreased the proportion of thick, poor prognosis lesions from 34% to 15%.

194 Breast cancer

Incidence

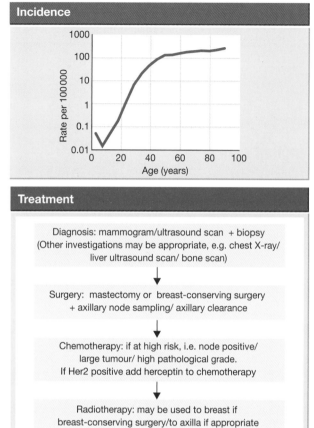

Presentation

Loco-regional disease
- Breast lump
- Discharge
- Peau d'orange
- Axilla lump

Systemic disease
Symptoms which occur:
- Bone pain
- Malaise
- Weight loss
- Confusion
- Breathlessness

Symptoms arise from:
- Hypercalcaemia
- Pleural effusion
- Lymphangitis carcinomatosis
- SVC obstruction
- Brain, spinal cord secondaries
- Organomegaly

Treatment

Diagnosis: mammogram/ultrasound scan + biopsy
(Other investigations may be appropriate, e.g. chest X-ray/
liver ultrasound scan/ bone scan)

↓

Surgery: mastectomy or breast-conserving surgery
+ axillary node sampling/ axillary clearance

↓

Chemotherapy: if at high risk, i.e. node positive/
large tumour/ high pathological grade.
If Her2 positive add herceptin to chemotherapy

↓

Radiotherapy: may be used to breast if
breast-conserving surgery/to axilla if appropriate

↓

Oestrogen receptor positive:
tamoxifen or aromatase inhibitors

Prognosis

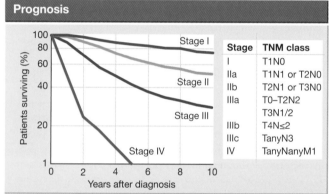

Stage	TNM class
I	T1N0
IIa	T1N1 or T2N0
IIb	T2N1 or T3N0
IIIa	T0–T2N2
	T3N1/2
IIIb	T4N≤2
IIIc	TanyN3
IV	TanyNanyM1

Staging – modified TNM classification

Tumour
Tis – DCIS or LCIS
T1 – Tumour ≤ 2cm in maximum diameter
T2 – Tumour > 2cm but ≤ 5cm
T3 – Tumour > 5cm
T4 – Tumour involving skin or chest wall

Nodes
N0 – No nodes
N1 – Ipsilateral mobile axillary nodes
N2 – Fixed axillary nodes
N3 – Ipsilateral internal mammary/
infraclavicular/supraclavicular nodes

Metastases
M0 – No evidence of distant metastasis
M1 – Distant metastasis (including cervical
or contralateral internal mammary
lymph nodes)

Epidemiology and aetiology

Breast cancer is the most common tumour in women, with more than 48 000 women diagnosed in the UK each year and 11 500 dying of the disease. The lifetime risk to a woman of developing breast cancer is one in eight. Most breast cancer occurs without an obvious cause, although several predisposing factors are recognized, including:

- Oestrogen exposure: particularly unopposed by progestogens, explaining the association with early menarche, late menopause and nulliparity.
- Family and personal history: 10% of breast cancer is genetically determined with links to the highly penetrant genes *BRCA-1*, *BRCA-2* and *p53*. A previous history of breast, endometrial or ovarian cancer indicates a genetically determined increased risk. Chest irradiation and specific types of previous benign breast disease are also risk factors.

- High socioeconomic status is associated with increased risk.

Molecular genetics

The autosomal dominant *BRCA-1* or *-2* genes occur in 2–5% of all breast cancer patients, but in 50–80% of young patients aged <40 years with a strong family history (i.e. more than one affected first-degree relative) of breast and ovarian cancer. Mutations in the p53 tumour suppressor gene (or accummulation of p53 protein) are seen in 20–50% of patients with breast cancer and are more common in those with the familial Li–Fraumeni syndrome.

Pathology

Adenocarcinoma is most commonly infiltrating ductal carcinoma, accounting for >70% of all breast cancers. Lobular, medullary, mucinous, papillary or tubular carcinomas are rarer.

- **Ductal carcinoma *in situ*** is a malignant cell proliferation within the ducts without stromal invasion, usually unilateral, and occasionally multifocal. It is often detectable on mammography due to the presence of calcification. Without treatment, 14–53% of patients develop invasive breast cancer.

- **Lobular carcinoma *in situ*** is a proliferation of malignant cells within the breast lobules. It is rarely palpable or visible on mammography, and usually multicentric and often bilateral. It may be a premalignant lesion, and is an indicator of increased breast cancer risk.
- Breast cancer can also present as Paget's disease of the nipple (tumour of main excretory ducts involving overlying nipple and skin) and rarely as lymphoma, sarcoma, squamous or clear cell carcinomas.

Histological grading

Breast adenocarcinomas are graded histologically using the 'modified Bloom and Richardson' scoring scheme to categorize aggressiveness and probable behaviour, on the basis of tubule formation, nuclear pleomorphism and mitotic rate. Other important histological findings are:

- Receptor status: breast cancer cells may express oestrogen and/or progestogen receptors. Their presence or absence affects treatment.
- 25% of breast cancers overexpress HER-2/neu and these have a worse prognosis.

Investigations

Initial diagnosis of a breast mass or breast abnormality detected by breast screening should involve a 'triple assessment' approach:

1 Clinical examination.
2 Imaging:
   - Two-view mammography (oblique/craniocaudal): rarely useful in women <40 years old (breasts are radiodense).
   - Breast ultrasonography: useful if there is a palpable mass and can distinguish cystic from solid lesions. Malignant lesions have indistinct edges. Not useful for screening.
   - Magnetic resonance imaging is being increasingly used.
3 Biopsy: core biopsy with or without fine needle aspiration:: manual or stereotactic (if indicated).

Staging (see Figure 194.1)

- Routine haematological and biochemical screening (including liver function tests and serum calcium).
- Other tests including: (i) chest radiograph; (ii) ultrasonography of liver; (iii) computed tomography (CT) scan of the chest, abdomen and pelvis; and (iv) isotope bone scan, which may be indicated for high-risk patients.

Treatment

- **Surgery**: for most patients the primary surgical treatment aims to remove the tumour and to obtain staging and prognostic information from the tumour and axillary nodes. Surgery may be modified radical mastectomy or breast conserving (lumpectomy with postoperative radiotherapy). Local excision of the tumour (with a histologically confirmed margin of normal tissue), combined with postoperative radical radiotherapy, achieves as good local control as total mastectomy, though the latter is indicated for large (>4 cm), multicentric tumours, or if there is extensive ductal carcinoma *in situ*. Axillary management depends on whether there is known lymph node involvement or not; if there is, then axillary node clearance/dissection is performed. Otherwise sentinel lymph node biopsy/axillary node sampling is performed. This more limited procedure limits postoperative morbidity. If, however, subsequent histology confirms the presence of nodal involvement patients either need to undergo completion clearance or radiotherapy.
- **Radiotherapy**: adjuvant radiotherapy to the breast remnant reduces the risk of local tumour recurrence following breast-conserving surgery. Radiotherapy to the axilla is given if axillary

node sampling has revealed positive nodes, although not if full axillary dissection has been performed, because it adds little to local control and has an unacceptably high incidence of lymphoedema.

- **Adjuvant systemic therapy**: 30–50% of patients with apparently resectable breast cancer subsequently die of their disease, suggesting that micrometastases were present at diagnosis. Systemic adjuvant therapy reduces the risk of disease relapse and improves overall survival.
- **Endocrine therapy**: tamoxifen, an anti-oestrogen, reduces the risk of disease relapse in all women. It is given for 5 years and is the treatment of choice for premenopausal women. Increasingly for postmenopausal women the aromatase inhibitors (e.g. anastrozole, letrozole) are being used as first-line treatment.
- **Chemotherapy**: most patients (not small (<1 cm), low-grade, node-negative disease) with moderate- to high-risk disease benefit from adjuvant chemotherapy. Equivalent relative benefit is seen in post- and premenopausal women. Combination chemotherapy is used (typically an anthracycline-containing regimen, e.g. epirubicin in combination with or followed by a taxane (docetaxel and paclitaxel)).
- **Targeted therapy**, e.g. herceptin. This is a humanized monoclonal antibody to the HER2 receptor used in the adjuvant treatment of HER2-positive breast cancer. It has been shown to improve both relapse-free and overall survival. Other HER2-blocking agents (e.g. lapatinib, pertuzumab) and other targeted therapies (e.g. bevacuzimab) are currently being tested in the adjuvant and neoadjuvant setting.

Follow-up

Follow-up is used to detect disease recurrence, manage treatment-related toxicity, and screen for a new primary lesion and for psychological support, but it does not improve survival. The cancer risk to the second breast is increased four-fold. Mammography should be performed yearly, bilaterally if the patient had breast-conserving treatment.

Locally advanced breast cancer

This is defined as tumours >5 cm in size or showing evidence of skin or chest wall invasion (i.e. 'fixed') or inflammatory breast cancer (erythematous with lymphatic permeation). A response to primary treatment with chemotherapy may facilitate surgery and in some instances may allow breast-conserving surgery.

Metastatic breast cancer

The treatment depends upon a number of factors including endocrine and HER2 status, the age of the patient and the extent of disease. For example, chemotherapy should be considered in young, healthy patients with rapidly progressive, visceral disease, particularly if relapse has occurred early after surgery or in oestrogen receptor (ER) negative disease that is unlikely to respond to hormonal therapy. The same regimens used in the adjuvant setting are given. Therefore the first line of treatment includes anthracyclines (but not if already used adjuvantly), with taxanes being used as second line. Third- and fourth-line agents include capecitabine and vinorelbine. Herceptin for HER2-positive women is given together with chemotherapy (but should not be used with anthracycline chemotherapy because of the increased risk of cardiotoxicity). Lapatinib, a dual action (HER1 and HER2) oral tyrosine kinase inhibitor, is a newer agent recently introduced for the treatment of HER2-positive metastatic disease. Other targeted treatments, e.g. the anti-angiogenic agent, bevazicumab, have been investigated in the treatment of metastatic disease. For limited disease (e.g. bone only) in ER-positive disease then endocrine treatment would be appropriate first-line treatment. Bisphosphonates are now routinely used in the management of bony metastases.

195 Prostate cancer

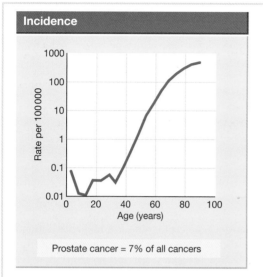

Incidence

Prostate cancer = 7% of all cancers

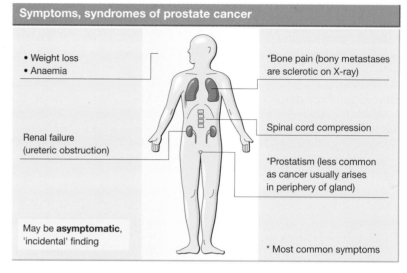

Symptoms, syndromes of prostate cancer

- Weight loss
- Anaemia

Renal failure
(ureteric obstruction)

May be **asymptomatic**,
'incidental' finding

*Bone pain (bony metastases
are sclerotic on X-ray)

Spinal cord compression

*Prostatism (less common
as cancer usually arises
in periphery of gland)

* Most common symptoms

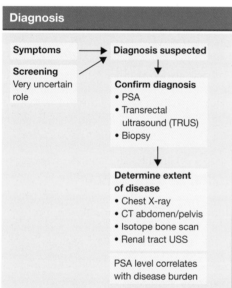

Diagnosis

Symptoms → **Diagnosis suspected**

Screening
Very uncertain
role

↓

Confirm diagnosis
- PSA
- Transrectal
  ultrasound (TRUS)
- Biopsy

↓

**Determine extent
of disease**
- Chest X-ray
- CT abdomen/pelvis
- Isotope bone scan
- Renal tract USS

PSA level correlates
with disease burden

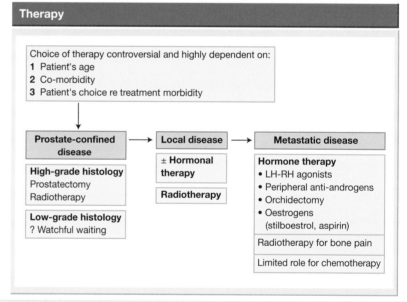

Therapy

Choice of therapy controversial and highly dependent on:
1 Patient's age
2 Co-morbidity
3 Patient's choice re treatment morbidity

**Prostate-confined
disease** → **Local disease** → **Metastatic disease**

High-grade histology
Prostatectomy
Radiotherapy

Low-grade histology
? Watchful waiting

± **Hormonal
therapy**

Radiotherapy

Hormone therapy
- LH-RH agonists
- Peripheral anti-androgens
- Orchidectomy
- Oestrogens
  (stilboestrol, aspirin)

Radiotherapy for bone pain

Limited role for chemotherapy

Prostate cancer is the most common malignancy in men and it may soon exceed lung cancer as the most frequent cause of cancer death. Many patients have small, indolent cancers that will never be clinically significant, so the older age of patients, co-morbidities and the adverse impact of surgery on quality of life make screening with prostate-specific antigen (PSA) and treatment decisions about early stage disease particularly controversial. Prostate cancer is highly sensitive to androgen ablation.

Aetiology

Malignant transformation is a common complication of the ageing prostate. Age, ethnicity, family history, radiation exposure, diet and environmental pollutants contribute to the risk.

Pathology

Almost all tumors are adenocarcinomas:

- Adenocarcinoma is the most common. It arises in the acinar epithelium in the peripheral region of the gland. Cells stain for acid phosphatase and PSA. Various grading systems predict the biological behaviour of the tumour. The most commonly used of these is the Gleason system, where the tumour is graded (both predominant and highest grade) histologically between grade I (well-differentiated, uniform gland formation) and grade V (very poorly differentiated, minimal gland formation) for a total score out of 10.
- Rarer tumours (<2%) include transitional cell carcinoma arising in the ductal epithelium, stromal sarcomas, lymphomas and small cell carcinomas.

Clinical presentation

Early prostatic cancer is typically asymptomatic and may be detectable clinically only by the presence of a rectally palpable

Medicine at a Glance, Fourth Edition. Edited by Patrick Davey. © 2014 John Wiley & Sons, Ltd. Published 2014 by John Wiley & Sons, Ltd. Companion website:
www.ataglanceseries.com/medicine

Table 195.1 TNM staging of prostate cancer.

T1	Tumour neither palpable nor imageable, identified only in resected specimens or by needle biopsy
T2	Tumour confined to the prostate
T3	Tumour extending through the prostate capsule including seminal vesicle invasion
T4	Tumour is fixed or invading adjacent structures other than the seminal vesicles (bladder, rectum or pelvic side wall, etc.)
N1	Single metastatic lymph node measuring <2 cm
N2	Single node 2–5 cm or multiple notes <5 cm
N3	Nodes >5 cm
M0	No evidence of distant metastases
M1	Distant metastases present

mass or induration of the gland. The tumour usually arises peripherally in the gland, so obstructive symptoms ('prostatism') happen late unless secondary to associated benign prostatic hypertrophy. Haematuria and perineal pain sometime occur. Many patients have metastatic disease at diagnosis, and present with symptoms related to these, such as the constitutional symptoms of weight loss, anaemia, bone pain, lymphadenopathy or neurological complications.

Staging (see Table 195.1)

Prostate cancer most typically metastasizes to bone. It may, however, spread through the lymphatics to regional pelvic nodes and then to abdominal nodes. Visceral metastases may also occur.

Clinical approach

Investigations in suspected prostate cancer aim to confirm the diagnosis histologically and determine whether metastases are present (typically inferred by a PSA >10 ng/mL). If disease is confined to the prostate, local therapy with radiotherapy or radical prostatectomy may be appropriate. These treatments may have similar outcomes (>30% incontinence and >80% impotence), although this has not been tested in an adequately powered clinical trial. Early disease is often overtreated with devastating complications, and watchful waiting may be a better option.

Investigations

Examination under anaesthesia with clinical staging (see Table 195.1) and needle biopsy:
- **Transrectal ultrasonography** (TRUS): to identify small peripherally sited lesions, with sextant biopsy.
- **Transurethral resection of the prostate** (TURP): if there is prostatism.
- **Biochemistry**: serum PSA levels >10 IU suggest metastatic disease. Alkaline and acid phosphatase.
- **Radiology**: computed tomography (CT) of the abdomen and pelvis may identify pelvic or abdominal nodes. Magnetic resonance imaging of the pelvis defines the tumour and the degree of local extension better if radical (curative) treatment is an option. Chest X-ray and isotope bone scan are needed for metastases.

Screening for prostate cancer remains controversial. The use of serum PSA analysis combined with digital rectal examination is quite effective in terms of early disease detection. It remains unclear whether early detection and treatment saves lives, although the European Randomised Study of Prostate Cancer

reported a 29% reduction in mortality. The challenge is that screening with PSA in men aged 55–69 at best may save one in 100 lives but will result in impotence in 50–80% of those who get surgery.

Treatment

- Localized prostatic carcinoma: the principal treatment approaches are surgery, radiotherapy and watchful waiting. There is no consensus about the benefit of intervention in early prostatic cancer. Patients should be encouraged to make an informed choice.
- Surgery is recommended for poorly differentiated tumours confined to the prostate, although this has never been tested against radiotherapy in a randomized clinical trial. Patients with well- or moderately well-differentiated tumours survive for an equally long period (5-year survival rate is 85%) whether they receive radical radiotherapy or they are simply kept under observation (watchful waiting).
- Radical radiotherapy has similar survival figures; new initiatives are investigating increasing the radiation dose using more targeted (conformal) radiotherapy or combining radiotherapy with hormonal therapy.
- Brachytherapy using radioactive palladium or iodine seeds implanted directly into the prostate gland can be performed on an outpatient basis, and is used for small low-grade tumours with excellent results in selected patients.
- Hormone treatment (androgen ablation): prostate cancer cell growth shows a striking dependence on androgens. Hormonal therapy directed at interfering with this association typically produces disease response in both metastatic and loco-regional disease. Bilateral orchidectomy or gonadotrophin-releasing hormone (GnRH) agonists, such as goserelin or buserelin, can mediate this. They only block pituitary-driven testicular androgen production. Complete androgen blockade requires the concomitant use of a peripheral anti-androgen (flutamide, bicalutamide, cyproterone acetate) and GnRH agonist and has minimal extra efficacy, so these agents are typically used sequentially. Oestrogens such as diethylstilboestrol produce similar effects but are associated with significant cardiovascular morbidity. Hormone therapy before radiotherapy can reduce the size of the prostate gland, hence also reducing the radiation treatment volume and lowering toxicity; there is also improved local control and disease-free survival. Overall survival may not be prolonged, although this is an area of active clinical research. Anti-androgen side effects include hot flushes, weakness, impotence and loss of sexual drive.

Metastatic prostate cancer

Widespread metastatic disease is often initially very responsive to hormone therapy; it is the first line of therapy in most cases, and is associated with a considerable symptomatic improvement and clinical response. The response may be followed closely and accurately by regular assessment of PSA levels. Patients may continue to respond to hormone therapy for several years, but on average the disease escapes hormonal control after about 18 months. Radiotherapy has a role to play in the palliation of symptoms either from the primary tumour or from troublesome sites of metastases. The response rates of chemotherapy in prostate cancer are modest but docetaxel and cabazitaxel can improve survival and quality of life in fitter, younger patients. Osteoclast inhibition using bisphosphates or antibodies against the RANK ligand decrease the skeletal morbidity of androgen deprivation. Bone-seeking radioisotopes such as strontium-89 and radium-223 may have a role in some patients with extensive bony metastases.

196 Cancer with an unknown primary

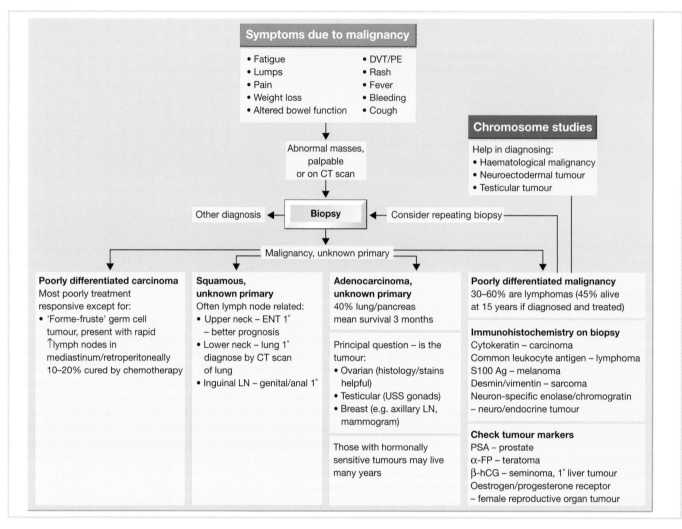

Symptoms due to malignancy

- Fatigue
- Lumps
- Pain
- Weight loss
- Altered bowel function
- DVT/PE
- Rash
- Fever
- Bleeding
- Cough

Chromosome studies

Help in diagnosing:
- Haematological malignancy
- Neuroectodermal tumour
- Testicular tumour

Abnormal masses, palpable or on CT scan

Other diagnosis ← **Biopsy** ← Consider repeating biopsy

Malignancy, unknown primary

Poorly differentiated carcinoma
Most poorly treatment responsive except for:
- 'Forme-fruste' germ cell tumour, present with rapid ↑lymph nodes in mediastinum/retroperitoneally 10–20% cured by chemotherapy

Squamous, unknown primary
Often lymph node related:
- Upper neck – ENT 1° – better prognosis
- Lower neck – lung 1° diagnose by CT scan of lung
- Inguinal LN – genital/anal 1°

Adenocarcinoma, unknown primary
40% lung/pancreas mean survival 3 months

Principal question – is the tumour:
- Ovarian (histology/stains helpful)
- Testicular (USS gonads)
- Breast (e.g. axillary LN, mammogram)

Those with hormonally sensitive tumours may live many years

Poorly differentiated malignancy
30–60% are lymphomas (45% alive at 15 years if diagnosed and treated)

Immunohistochemistry on biopsy
Cytokeratin – carcinoma
Common leukocyte antigen – lymphoma
S100 Ag – melanoma
Desmin/vimentin – sarcoma
Neuron-specific enolase/chromogratin – neuro/endocrine tumour

Check tumour markers
PSA – prostate
α-FP – teratoma
β-hCG – seminoma, 1° liver tumour
Oestrogen/progesterone receptor – female reproductive organ tumour

---

Cancer is present without a clear primary source in 5% of all cases. This is a heterogeneous group of cancers that contains treatable and indeed curable subgroups. In this situation, therapeutic nihilism is inappropriate and a treatable cancer should be actively sought. There are four light microscopic diagnoses that typically describe the spectrum of neoplasms of unknown primary site:

1 Poorly differentiated malignancy.
2 Adenocarcinoma.
3 Squamous carcinoma.
4 Poorly differentiated carcinoma.

Neoplasms of unknown primary site

Poorly differentiated malignancy

These are less commonly seen now that advanced immunohistochemistry techniques are widely used. Of the poorly differentiated neoplasms that are hard to identify histologically, the most important of the non-epithelial cancers are:

- Lymphoma.
- Melanoma.
- Sarcoma.

Between 30% and 60% of totally undifferentiated neoplasms are lymphomas and eminently treatable with chemotherapy, with some 45% of patients alive and disease-free after 15 years.

The most common cause for uncertainty is an inadequate biopsy, particularly with fine needle aspiration of accessible but unrepresentative areas of abnormality. Other than repeat biopsy, the most helpful investigation is immunohistochemistry (see Figure 196.1). Chromosome translocations can be helpful in terms of suggesting a specific diagnosis for a number of haematological diagnoses, but they are also increasingly useful in diagnosing solid tumours such as peripheral neuroectodermal tumours or testicular tumours. Many academic centres and commercial outlets offer molecular profiling of tumours which may provide diagnostic information and therapeutic options.

Adenocarcinoma of unknown primary

Adenocarcinoma of unknown primary is the most common type of cancer presenting with an unknown primary and has the poorest prognosis. Of these cases, 40% are the result of lung or upper gastrointestinal (GI) and pancreatic cancer with a median

Medicine at a Glance, Fourth Edition. Edited by Patrick Davey. © 2014 John Wiley & Sons, Ltd. Published 2014 by John Wiley & Sons, Ltd. Companion website: www.ataglanceseries.com/medicine

survival of approximately 3 months. The diagnosis is achieved by elucidating certain histological features, for example:

- Papillary formation suggests an ovarian or thyroid primary.
- Mucinous signet rings suggest a gastric primary.

The history and examination (including rectal and vaginal examination) should be reviewed. It is appropriate to measure a number of simple tumour-specific antigens and carry out basic imaging:

- Mammography and computed tomography (CT) of the abdomen, which finds a primary in 10–30% of patients.
- Upper or lower GI endoscopy has a very low sensitivity in patients without relevant symptoms.
- In male patients testicular ultrasonography is important.

Adenocarcinomas that are treatable

Certain diagnoses are important to establish because these cancers are treatable:

- **Papillary serous ovarian cancer**: suggested by psammoma body formation in women with malignant ascites and a pelvic mass. Serum CA-125 antigen levels may be raised. Surgical cytoreduction and platinum-based chemotherapy prolongs median survival to >20 months, with some long-term survivors.
- **Occult breast cancer**: serum CA-15.3 antigen levels may be raised. Women with axillary node metastasis usually (40–80% of cases) have a locally advanced breast primary that should be treated surgically. Metastatic disease can be treated by tamoxifen or an aromatase inhibitor (if oestrogen receptor positive) or chemotherapy.
- **Prostate cancer** in men: can present with osteoblastic bone metastases, and hormone therapy may provide excellent palliation. Serum prostate-specific antigen (PSA) levels are usually raised. Other cancers that commonly spread to bone are lung, breast, thyroid and renal cancer. Patients with hormonally sensitive cancers typically have a median survival measured in years.
- **Single site adenocarcinoma of unknown primary**: may warrant an aggressive approach with surgery or radiotherapy.

Squamous carcinoma

Patients with squamous cell histology typically present with lymphadenopathy. It is the site of the lymphadenopathy that suggests the location of the underlying primary:

- Upper cervical lymphadenopathy is commonly the result of an ENT (ear, nose, throat) primary, whereas involvement of lower cervical nodes more commonly represents metastases from lung cancer. In young patients with lymphadenopathy and poorly differentiated squamous cell carcinoma (SCC), it is important to determine whether tissue polymerase chain reaction reveals Epstein–Barr virus, because this suggests a nasopharyngeal carcinoma that has a much better prognosis with chemoradiation treatment than other subtypes.
- Inguinal nodes containing SCC typically arise from a genital or an anal primary.
- Skin SCC is rarely metastatic except in immunocompromised patients.

Poorly differentiated carcinoma

It is important to determine whether a poorly differentiated tumour is a variant of a germ cell tumour, because these are responsive to chemotherapy. These typically present as rapidly progressing tumours in young adults with lymphadenopathy and involvement of the mediastinum or retroperitoneum. There may be chromosomal abnormalities (i12p), or some staining of histological samples for α-fetoprotein (α-FP). These patients have a 10–20% long-term disease-free survival rate when treated with bleomycin, etoposide and cisplatin chemotherapy.

Neuroendocrine carcinoma

Lastly, there is a continuum between carcinoid, low-grade neuroendocrine carcinoma and small cell carcinoma. The first is typically treated with octreotide (and chemotherapy such as temozolomide) with or without interferon, and can be very indolent. The last is similar to small cell carcinoma of the lung, which initially responds to platinum-based chemotherapy.

The decision to treat relates to both the disease and the patient. Palliative chemotherapy is appropriate for fitter and younger patients. Referral to an oncologist is appropriate for every patient who has cancer. In all patients with cancer, or indeed any terminal illness, compassion and support, both emotional and physical (e.g. planning terminal care in conjunction with the local hospice), are vital and are the measure of the physician (see Chapter 198).

General approach to management

Modern approaches to the management of cancer change rapidly and caring for patients with life-threatening diseases is challenging. Patients with more difficult cancers should be referred to multidisciplinary care in cancer centres as these usually offer not only better care, but more compassionate care.

Paraneoplastic syndromes and hormone-producing cancers

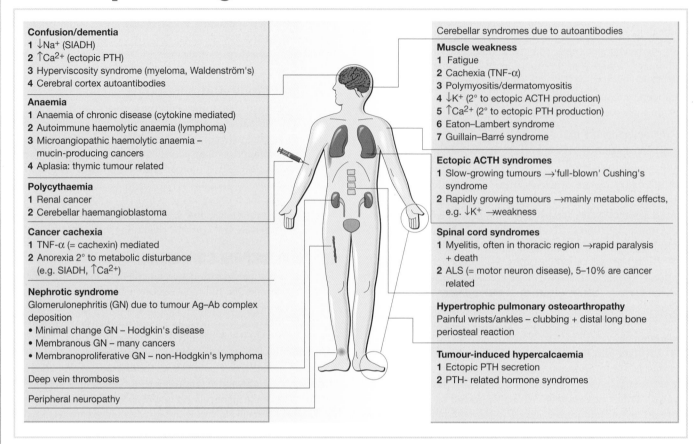

Confusion/dementia
1 ↓Na+ (SIADH)
2 ↑Ca2+ (ectopic PTH)
3 Hyperviscosity syndrome (myeloma, Waldenström's)
4 Cerebral cortex autoantibodies

Anaemia
1 Anaemia of chronic disease (cytokine mediated)
2 Autoimmune haemolytic anaemia (lymphoma)
3 Microangiopathic haemolytic anaemia –
   mucin-producing cancers
4 Aplasia: thymic tumour related

Polycythaemia
1 Renal cancer
2 Cerebellar haemangioblastoma

Cancer cachexia
1 TNF-α (= cachexin) mediated
2 Anorexia 2° to metabolic disturbance
   (e.g. SIADH, ↑Ca2+)

Nephrotic syndrome
Glomerulonephritis (GN) due to tumour Ag–Ab complex
deposition
• Minimal change GN – Hodgkin's disease
• Membranous GN – many cancers
• Membranoproliferative GN – non-Hodgkin's lymphoma

Deep vein thrombosis

Peripheral neuropathy

Cerebellar syndromes due to autoantibodies

Muscle weakness
1 Fatigue
2 Cachexia (TNF-α)
3 Polymyositis/dermatomyositis
4 ↓K+ (2° to ectopic ACTH production)
5 ↑Ca2+ (2° to ectopic PTH production)
6 Eaton–Lambert syndrome
7 Guillain–Barré syndrome

Ectopic ACTH syndromes
1 Slow-growing tumours →'full-blown' Cushing's
   syndrome
2 Rapidly growing tumours →mainly metabolic effects,
   e.g. ↓K+ →weakness

Spinal cord syndromes
1 Myelitis, often in thoracic region →rapid paralysis
   + death
2 ALS (= motor neuron disease), 5–10% are cancer
   related

Hypertrophic pulmonary osteoarthropathy
Painful wrists/ankles – clubbing + distal long bone
periosteal reaction

Tumour-induced hypercalcaemia
1 Ectopic PTH secretion
2 PTH- related hormone syndromes

Cancers produce illness through direct effects (e.g. local invasion) and the release of biologically active substances. Diseases produced by the latter are termed 'paraneoplastic syndromes', the most common of which are: anaemia, cachexia and fatigue, tumour-induced hypercalcaemia, syndrome of inappropriate antidiuretic hormone secretion (SIADH), Cushing's syndrome from ectopic adrenocorticotrophic hormone (ACTH), and hypoglycaemia associated with the production of insulin-like growth factors (IGFs).

Pathogenesis
Paraneoplastic syndromes arise from a variety of mechanisms, many of which are still unknown: (i) through the release of normal cellular proteins, in increased amounts (e.g. ectopic hormone production); (ii) through cytokine production; (iii) via autoantibody production, which typically results in neurological disorders; and (iv) via abnormal metabolism of steroids, the production of enzymes or the expression of fetal proteins.

Anaemia
Anaemia in cancer can relate to many factors, including iron deficiency (especially in gastrointestinal tumours) and folate deficiency (in malnourished patients, and those with very rapidly dividing tumours). However, much anaemia relates to the 'anaemia of chronic disease', whereby the inflammatory response associated with malignancy leads to the production of a number of cytokines that suppress the bone marrow. These include:
• Disturbance of normal iron metabolism by transforming growth factor β, interleukin (IL) 1, IL-6 and interferon γ. These

may act through increasing the levels of hepcidin, which suppresses iron uptake and utilization.
• Tumour necrosis factor α (TNF-α) (whose levels can be greatly increased in patients with cancer) antagonizing the effects of erythropoietin on the bone marrow. Satisfactory haemoglobin levels can be achieved in about 50% of such patients by giving synthetic recombinant erythropoietin.
• In rare patients malignancy induces an autoimmune haemolytic anaemia.
• Rarer still, malignancy can induce red cell aplasia.

Cachexia
The weight loss and malaise associated with cancer relate to the tumour burden, but also, importantly, to the production of cytokines such as TNF or cachexin. Steroids and progesterones may have a useful symptomatic role.

Syndrome of inappropriate ADH secretion
The inappropriate secretion of vasopressin (ADH) results in hyponatraemia, renal sodium loss, hypervolaemia and inappropriately high urine osmolality. Clinically this may only produce biochemical disease, but it may also produce symptoms relating to the hyponatraemia: tiredness, mental clouding, delirium and coma. The mechanism for SIADH in cancer is two-fold: (i) reflex release, by central nervous system tumours, drugs or coexisting lung disease; and (ii) ectopic hormone release by the tumour, as in small cell lung cancer (SCLC), and more rarely tumours of the

Table 197.1 Characteristics of paraneoplastic neurological degeneration-associated tumours.

- Tumours are often difficult to detect
- Tumours are histologically identical to tumours that develop in patients without paraneoplastic neurological degeneration (PND), except that many tumours have evidence of immune infiltration
- Patients often have improved prognosis relative to those with comparable but non-immunogenic tumours (anti-Hu paraneoplastic syndrome, Lambert–Eaton myasthenic syndrome and some paraneoplastic cerebellar degeneration)
- Rare instances of spontaneous regression have been documented (anti-Hu paraneoplastic syndrome and others)
- Prospective analysis of surrogate of anti-tumour immune responses predict cancer patient populations with improved prognosis (Hu syndrome)
- Tumours are associated with circulating PND-antigen-specific killer T cells (paraneoplastic cerebellar degeneration)

duodenum, pancreas, thymus and lymphomas. A precursor molecule is split to produce ADH and neurophysin.

The underlying disease should be aggressively treated; fluid restriction is the mainstay of management. Refractory cases may respond to demeclocycline, which induces nephrogenic diabetes insipidus.

Hypercalcaemia

The most common clinical presentation of an ectopic hormone syndrome is tumour-induced hypercalcaemia (TIH), typically associated with the production of parathyroid hormone-related protein (PTHrP), which has homologues at eight of its 13 amino acids to parathyroid hormone (PTH) and may activate the PTH receptor. The solid tumours causing ectopic PTH-like secretion are those of squamous cell (e.g. lung), genitourinary or gynaecological origin. The differential diagnosis is hypercalcaemia from bony metastases, usually from lung, breast, prostate, thyroid or renal cell primaries, which develop in 10–20% of patients with disseminated malignancy. Bony metastases, which are the most common cause of malignancy-associated hypercalcaemia, cause hypercalcaemia by causing the release of TNF, various prostaglandins and other paracrine agents that activate local osteoclasts. Multiple myeloma and human T-cell leukaemia virus (HTLV) associated lymphoma are the most common haematological malignancies associated with TIH, the latter being, in part, the result of the production of vitamin D within the tumour.

Treatment involves correcting the volume depletion that all hypercalcaemic individuals have (caused by calcium-induced diabetes insipidus). Bisphosphonates have revolutionized management of TIH, but PTHrP-related hypercalcaemia is often refractory. Bisphosphonates inhibit osteoclast function, reduce raised levels of calcium quickly, slow the development of bone metastases, and reduce both the associated symptoms and complications. Steroids are used for steroid-responsive tumours, e.g. multiple myeloma and lymphoma.

Cushing's syndrome

Tumours can produce bizarre syndromes of metabolic upset related to ectopic hormone production. The most common of these is Cushing's syndrome in SCLC, caused by ectopic ACTH production, first reported by Brown in 1928. Overall, 40% of patients with SCLC secrete polypeptides, most of which are not functional, e.g. the precursor molecule to ACTH (proopiomelanocortin) is often present in these tumours but only possesses 4% of the biological activity of ACTH. Overall only 2–3% of patients with SCLC have Cushing's syndrome. When the syndrome is acute and prominent, it is typically associated with hirsutism, acne and hypokalaemia, and warrants medical control (see Chapter 163) both in its own right and because it increases the toxicity of chemotherapeutic regimens.

Hypoglycaemia

Hypoglycaemia in cancer occurs through three mechanisms:

1 Massive size of a slow growing tumour, e.g. mesenchymal sarcomas, lymphomas or mesotheliomas often secrete 'big' IGF factor II.

2 IGF typically from hepatic or adrenal carcinomas.

3 Insulin secretion by insulinomas, with the rare but classic presentation of fasting hypoglycaemia, commonly associated with neuropsychiatric sequelae and relentless weight gain.

Neurological paraneoplastic syndromes

There are a number of paraneoplastic syndromes affecting the nervous system (see Table 197.1):

- **Cerebellar syndrome**: anti-neuronal antibodies (anti-Yo, -Hu, -Ri and -Tr) are associated with this syndrome of cerebellar–cortical degeneration, most commonly seen with carcinoma of the lung, breast or ovary. The cerebellar syndrome has prominent involvement of eye movements, is extremely disabling and precedes the diagnosis of the underlying cancer. The prognosis is poor and is not reversible with successful treatment of the malignancy. Magnetic resonance imaging is typically normal and the diagnosis is often one of exclusion. Toxic, metabolic, degenerative and rare differentials such as Creutzfeldt–Jakob disease and HIV should be considered.
- **Lambert–Eaton myasthenic syndrome**: characterized by symmetrical muscle weakness, hyporeflexia and autonomic dysfunction, with improvement in strength on reinforcement. Eye involvement (unlike in myasthenia gravis) is rare. Nerve-evoked acetylcholine release at the neuromuscular junction is reduced. Serum antibodies against voltage-gated calcium channels occur.
- **Encephalomyelitis**: commonly limbic and associated with dementia or acute behavioural disturbance with hallucination and delusions.
- A **subacute sensory neuropathy** producing a sensory ataxia is associated with lymphoma, SCLC and the presence of anti-Hu antibodies.

Dermatological paraneoplastic syndromes

There are many dermatological paraneoplastic syndromes, all of which are associated with stomach or other intra-abdominal malignancies:

- Trousseau's sign of superficial migratory thrombophlebitis.
- The sign of Leser–Trelat (prominent seborrhoeic keratosis).
- Acanthosis nigricans: hyperpigmented velvety plaques found in the axillae and flexural areas.

After the age of 50, half of dermatomyositis cases are associated with an occult malignancy. Pemphigus is associated with malignancy. Gynaecomastia is associated with the production of human chorionic gonadotrophin by hepatomas or germ cell tumours.

Rare syndromes

These include polymyositis, glomerulonephritis, thrombocytosis, erythrocytosis and pseudo-obstruction.

198 Palliative care

Pain

Causes of pain in cancer patients

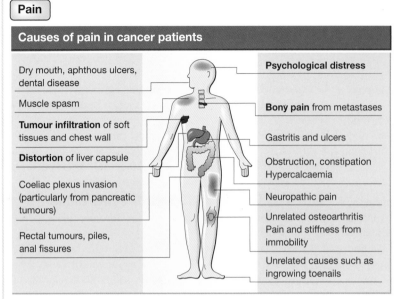

- Dry mouth, aphthous ulcers, dental disease
- Muscle spasm
- **Tumour infiltration** of soft tissues and chest wall
- **Distortion** of liver capsule
- Coeliac plexus invasion (particularly from pancreatic tumours)
- Rectal tumours, piles, anal fissures

- **Psychological distress**
- **Bony pain** from metastases
- Gastritis and ulcers
- Obstruction, constipation Hypercalcaemia
- Neuropathic pain
- Unrelated osteoarthritis Pain and stiffness from immobility
- Unrelated causes such as ingrowing toenails

Analgesic ladder

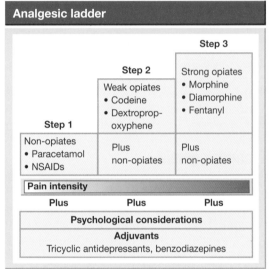

		Step 3
	Step 2	Strong opiates • Morphine • Diamorphine • Fentanyl
Step 1	Weak opiates • Codeine • Dextroprop-oxyphene	
Non-opiates • Paracetamol • NSAIDs	Plus non-opiates	Plus non-opiates

Pain intensity		
Plus	Plus	Plus
Psychological considerations		
Adjuvants Tricyclic antidepressants, benzodiazepines		

> *Palliative care is an approach that improves the quality of life of patients and their families facing the problems associated with life-threatening illness, through the prevention and relief of suffering by means of early identification and impeccable assessment and treatment of pain and other problems, physical, psychosocial and spiritual (World Health Organization definition of palliative care).*

There is a perception that palliation should be reserved for patients who are imminently dying. However this is misjudged. Palliative care is appropriate for any advanced progressive malignant and non-malignant illness. All clinicians need skills in palliative management; however some patients, particularly those with complex needs, need referral to a specialist palliative care service. This chapter will deal with two key symptom control issues: management of pain and of the dying process.

Pain

Assessment

A proper pain assessment is the cornerstone of effective pain control. Pain in progressive illness is complex and focusing exclusively on the physical causes explains why pain relief may be inadequate. When assessing the physical cause consider that pain may relate to the cancer, e.g. local infiltration (visceral, nerve and bone pain), to disabilities relating to chronic illness, e.g. musculoskeletal problems, or to co-morbidities. Consequently, there are often many causes and sites of pain and each of these must be assessed. A careful history should be taken, noting:
- Where the pain is, and radiates to.
- The type and severity of pain.
- The onset of pain.
- Response to analgesics.
- Exacerbating and alleviating factors.

Physical examination often establishes the diagnosis, though it may be necessary to perform investigations such as X-rays,

isotope bone scans, computed tomography scans, etc. A complete assessment includes an appraisal of:
- **Emotional pain**: when faced with advanced illness, patients frequently experience depression, uncertainty, despair, anger and fear.
- **Social pain**: socially isolated patients can feel unsafe, and those who are financially insecure can feel threatened.
- **Spiritual pain**: patients with advanced illness often search for meaning. For some, this meaning may be embedded in a religious framework. Spiritual distress can occur during this search and can significantly affect a patient's perception of pain.

Treatment of pain

A good history will guide management. Specific types of pain may respond to specific treatments (see Table 198.1).

Analgesics

The World Health Organization advocates a three-step ladder for prescribing analgesics (see Figure 198.1). Analgesics should be prescribed regularly. Inadequate pain control at one step requires a move to the next step. Adjuvant co-analgesics can be used at each step for treating that element of the pain that is opioid insensitive.

Opioids

The correct use of opioids has made a major impact on the management of pain in patients with advanced disease. Unfortunately, unfounded fears by professionals and patients about the use of strong opioids, lack of understanding about how opioids should be prescribed and an inability to recognize pain that is opioid resistant can lead to ineffective prescribing.

Prescribing opioids Morphine continues to be the 'gold standard' analgesic. Oral morphine is available in two forms: immediate acting (4-hourly) and slow release (12- and 24-hourly) preparations. When prescribed correctly it is a safe, predictable and reliable drug. Correct prescribing of morphine requires that:
- Morphine should be given orally unless this is not possible or practical.

Table 198.1 Treatment for different types of pain.

Cause of pain	Opioid sensitivity	Primary treatment	Examples of other options
Large infiltrating tumour mass	Partial	Opioids NSAIDs Steroids	Treat tumour bulk, e.g. radiotherapy
Musculoskeletal pain	Insensitive	Peripherally acting analgesics (paracetamol, NSAIDs) Physiotherapy Massage	Benzodiazepines
Colic	Insensitive	Treat underlying cause, e.g. constipation Anticholinergics	In bowel obstruction consider reversal, e.g. with surgery or anti-cancer therapy. Steroids and/or octreotide if reversal is not possible
Bone pain	Partial	NSAIDs Opioids	Radiotherapy Orthopaedic surgery – especially if a metastasis has caused an unstable joint or long bone at risk of fracture Bisphosphonates
Capsular stretching, e.g. liver capsule pain	Partial	NSAIDs Opioids Steroids	Chemotherapy
Nerve pain – symptoms include pain that is described as burning, stabbing or shooting in nature and there may be altered sensation	Partial (?)	Tricyclic antidepressants Antiepileptics (Gabapentin) Opioids	Steroids Nerve blocks Radiotherapy

NSAIDs, non-steroidal anti-inflammatory drugs.

- It must be prescribed regularly to pre-empt pain.
- In acute pain, rapid titration of the dose is best achieved using regular immediate release opioid.
- Extra doses for breakthrough and incident pain must be co-prescribed and used as necessary.
- Side effects, particularly constipation, should be anticipated and prevented.
- Pain should be continuously reassessed.

Failure of opioid therapy may be due to incorrect prescription (wrong dose, interval, route of administration, e.g. unable to absorb), poor compliance or the pain being opioid insensitive.

Side effects of morphine
- Constipation is virtually universal. A laxative should be co-prescribed.
- Nausea and vomiting (less common).
- Drowsiness in 50% of patients. This wears off after a week on a stable dose. Explanation and reassurance are usually all that is necessary.
- Other side effects include confusion, sweating, dry mouth, itch, hallucinations and myoclonus.

Alternative opioids Morphine metabolites can be responsible for side effects and morphine is dependent on the kidney for excretion. Alternative opioids, e.g. fentanyl (transdermal preparation) and oxycodone, may be used when opioid-sensitive pain exists but morphine causes excessive side effects or is contraindicated.

The terminal phase of illness

When a patient has an advanced, progressive illness it is important to assess if a patient has any preferences and wishes about how they want their care to be managed when they deteriorate. This process is known as 'Advance Care Planning'. It is carried out to give confidence to the patient that their professional carers will manage them appropriately in the future if they are not in a position to participate in decision making. Health-care professionals should ensure that the dying patient has a 'good death'. To facilitate this, the professional must be aware of the complex problems occurring round this time. Physical symptoms, including pain, must be controlled and wider issues (e.g. the needs of the family) should be appreciated. Anticipating symptoms and good communication with relatives is fundamental; patient pathways such as the 'Liverpool Care Pathway' enable optimal management. The three commonest symptoms are:

1 **Pain**: where possible ask about pain and check for easily reversible causes. Some patients may need to start opioids, and those on regular opioids, who cannot take oral medication, will need parenteral (often subcutaneous) therapy.

2 **Breathing**: when a patient's condition deteriorates there are likely to be changes in respiration that can be predicted. Often the pattern of breathing alters and it is reassuring to the relatives to be warned of these potential changes. As the patient weakens, the ability to cough up secretions is lost. It can usually be relieved by anticholinergic drugs.

3 **Restlessness and distress**: terminal distress, preterminal agitation, terminal restlessness and terminal anguish are all terms used to describe agitation and distress in patients close to death. Terminal restlessness reflects significant suffering on the part of the patient and causes considerable distress to the relatives who witness it. It is particularly important to assess the patient and rule out easily reversible causes, e.g. catheterization for urinary retention. Sedation should be offered to ease a patient's distress and midazolam is often the drug of choice.

199 Head computed tomography cases

Extradural haemorrhage (EDH): axial CT

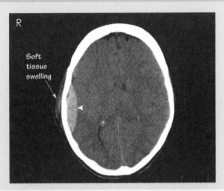

A lens-shaped area of high density is seen within the skull on the right (arrowhead). This is the typical appearance of an extradural haemorrhage which usually arises following injury to the middle meningeal artery. There was an underlying fracture of the temporal bone in this patient seen on bone window settings.

Subdural haematoma (SDH): axial CT

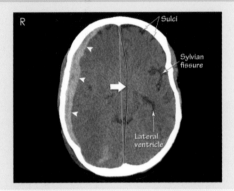

A crescentic rim of high-density material (acute blood) is seen over the surface of the right cerebral hemisphere (arrowheads). There is evidence of mass effect with effacement of the sulci, Sylvian fissure, and lateral ventricle (compare with left), with shift of midline structures (green to red line).

Subarachnoid haemorrhage (SAH): axial CT

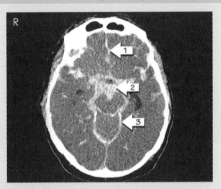

There is widespread high-density material (acute blood) within the subarachnoid space. The blood is seen in the interhemispheric fissure (1), the suprasellar cistern (2), and is layered over the tentorium cerebelli (3). The underlying cause was an aneurysm found on CT angiography.

Intracerebral haemorrhage (ICH): axial CT

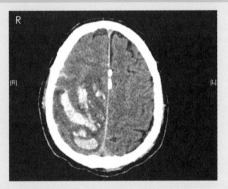

Areas of high density represent acute intracerebral haemorrhage of the right cerebral hemisphere. The high-density areas (blood) are surrounded by low-density areas (oedema). Mass effect is seen with loss of sulci on this side and slight midline shift.

Cerebral infarction: axial CT

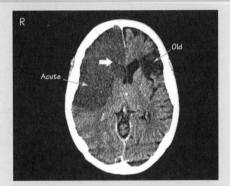

On the right there is a large low-density area indicating an acute infarction of the right middle cerebral artery (MCA) territory. This is causing mass effect with loss of sulci, effacement of the right lateral ventricle anterior horn (arrow) and some midline shift. For comparison an old low-density infarct is seen on the left.

Cerebral tumour: axial CT post-contrast

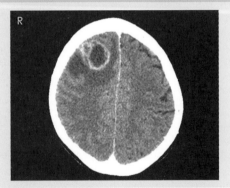

A peripherally enhancing lesion is seen in the right cerebral hemisphere. Note its central low-density area (necrosis) and the surrounding low density (oedema). Mass effect is seen with sulcal effacement on this side and slight deviation of the falx cerebri. Biopsy proved this to be a malignant tumour.

Medicine at a Glance, Fourth Edition. Edited by Patrick Davey. © 2014 John Wiley & Sons, Ltd. Published 2014 by John Wiley & Sons, Ltd. Companion website: www.ataglanceseries.com/medicine

Intracranial haemorrhage

A head computed tomography (CT) scan is performed without an intravenous (IV) contrast agent to detect acute bleeding. This is because blood is dense and therefore difficult to distinguish from the IV contrast agent. The appearance of a haemorrhage on CT imaging changes with time, and so correlation with the onset of clinical symptoms and signs is essential.

Acute blood is bright but becomes darker over the next few days. After 1 month a haematoma becomes the same density as cerebrospinal fluid (CSF).

Extradural haematoma

An extradural haematoma (EDH) is a collection of blood between the skull and dura mater. It is most often due to arterial bleeding following head trauma. The majority are located in the temporoparietal region and are caused by bleeding from the middle meningeal artery secondary to a skull fracture, which is present in up to 90% of cases. CT imaging features of acute EDH include:

- Well-demarcated, 'lentiform' (biconvex), high-density extra-axial (outside the brain) collection.
- Rarely crosses suture lines between cranial bones because the dura mater is firmly attached to the skull at the sutures.
- Air within an EDH suggests an open fracture, or a fracture of the paranasal sinuses or mastoid air cells.

Subdural haematoma

A subdural haematoma (SDH) is a collection of extra-axial blood between the dura mater and arachnoid mater. It is most often due to venous bleeding from bridging veins that traverse the subdural space following head trauma and deceleration injuries. It may also be seen in shaken baby syndrome, patients with coagulopathy and in cerebral atrophy (where minimal trauma can cause significant bleeding due to increased tension on the bridging veins). An SDH may lead to raised intracranial pressure and cause displacement of midline structures to the contralateral side. CT imaging features of acute SDH include:

- 'Crescentic', high-density, extra-axial collection conforming to the cerebral convexity (although it can become lentiform).
- Crosses suture lines as the collection is subdural.
- Moderate and large SDHs can cause midline shift.
- Falx cerebri appears dense, thickened and irregular with interhemispheric SDH (associated with non-accidental injury in children).

Subarachnoid haemorrhage

A subarachnoic haemorrhage (SAH) is bleeding into the subarachnoid space (the space between the arachnoid mater and pia mater, which contains CSF). It most often occurs spontaneously from a ruptured aneurysm in the circle of Willis and patients typically complain of sudden-onset, extremely severe headache. CT imaging typically reveals high-density blood in the CSF spaces (ventricular system, over cerebral hemispheres, Sylvian fissure, basal cisterns). If SAH is confirmed, a CT angiogram or a conventional cerebral angiogram is performed. If CT imaging is negative but the clinical suspicion is high and there are no contraindications, lumbar puncture should be performed for the detection of xanthochromia.

Intracerebral haemorrhage

Intracerebral haemorrhage (ICH) is bleeding into the brain parenchyma (intra-axial). It is also known as haemorrhagic stroke and is the second most common cause of a cerebrovascular event after ischaemic stroke. CT imaging allows differentiation of a haemorrhagic event from an ischaemic event, which dictates subsequent management of these conditions. The greatest risk factors are hypertension and anticoagulation therapy. Other causes include penetrating trauma, deceleration injuries, rupture of an intracerebral aneurysm or bleeding from an arteriovenous malformation or tumour. Patients usually present with neurological deficit.

Cerebral infarction

Cerebral infarction is caused by a sudden perfusion deficit to an area of the brain, resulting in a corresponding loss of neurological function. This is known as ischaemic stroke, which is the commonest cause of a cerebrovascular event. If the neurological deficit lasts less than 24 hours the event is termed a transient ischaemic attack (TIA). Thromboembolic events are by far the commonest cause. Thrombosis most often occurs at cerebral artery branch points and is related to vascular wall damage and hypercoagulable states. Emboli may arise from atherosclerotic plaques of extracranial arteries or thrombus originating from the heart. CT imaging features of cerebral infarction evolve over time. Within the first 3 hours of symptom onset, a faint low-density area may be seen affecting a vascular territory of the brain parenchyma. Between 6 and 12 hours, there is usually sufficient cell swelling (cytotoxic oedema) to produce a CT-identifiable region of low density affecting both the grey and white matter. Subsequent bleeding into the area of infarction may occur from the damaged blood vessels, which causes high density within the low-density infarct. Infarction is often accompanied by oedema, which may cause a mass effect ranging from minor sulcal effacement to shift of midline structures. In the following weeks to months, the infarct is resorbed by macrophages, leaving it appearing as an area of low density (dark) affecting both grey and white matter.

Intracranial tumours

Intracranial tumours may be primary or metastatic. Most are solitary primary tumours arising from the brain parenchyma or other related tissues (vessels, nerves, meninges, pituitary, lymphatics, skull). Metastatic tumours are often multiple and typically from cancers such as lung, breast, melanoma and renal cancers. The clinical presentation of brain tumours varies with their site and size but includes headaches, seizures, focal neurological deficits and signs of raised intracranial pressure (e.g. papilloedema). CT imaging is initially performed without a contrast agent and then with a contrast agent if a space-occupying lesion is suspected radiologically or clinically. Brain tumours usually cause disruption of the blood–brain barrier, resulting in vasogenic oedema from capillary leakage, which spares the grey matter. Most tumours enhance on contrast agent CT imaging and are often surrounded by a halo of low-density subcortical oedema with varying degrees of mass effect.

Classic CT head features

- **Haemorrhage** High density (acute), density drops over few days, CSF density after 1 month (chronic)
- **EDH** 'Lentiform', rarely crosses sutures, usually associated with skull fracture
- **SDH** 'Crescentic', usually crosses sutures
- **SAH** Blood in CSF spaces, e.g. ventricles
- **ICH** Intra-axial/parenchymal blood
- **Infarct** Low density in vascular territory, grey and white matter affected, cytotoxic oedema
- **Tumour** Typically enhancing focal parenchymal lesion, vasogenic oedema

200 # Head magnetic resonance imaging cases

Sagittal brain MRI : T$_1$ (left) and T$_2$ (right)

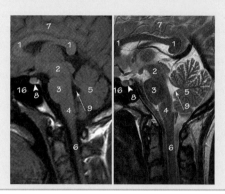

Key

1	Corpus callosum
2	Midbrain
3	Pons
4	Medulla oblongata
5	Cerebellum
6	Spinal cord
7	Cerebrum
8	Pituitary gland
9	Fourth ventricle
10	Caudate nucleus
11	Lentiform nucleus
12	Internal capsule
13	Lateral ventricle
14	Eyes
15	Ethmoid air cells
16	Sphenoid sinus
17	Internal auditory meatus
18	Cochlea
19	Skull

Axial brain MRI: T$_2$ at level of lateral ventricles (left) and T$_2$ at level of cerebellum (right)

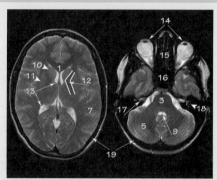

Multiple sclerosis: axial T$_2$ at level above lateral ventricles

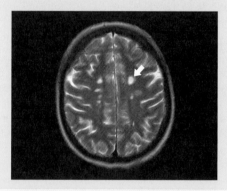

There are multiple bilateral foci of high signal (arrow) present within the white matter (appears dark on T$_2$). These lesions lie immediately above and to the side of the lateral ventricles. The periventricular white matter is a typical location for multiple sclerosis lesions.

Cerebral infarction: DWI (left) and ADC (right)

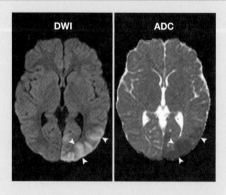

The DWI shows bright signal (arrowheads) in the distribution of the left posterior cerebral artery. The ADC image shows this area as low signal and therefore it is not due to T$_2$ signal (note the bright ventricles). This is evidence of restricted diffusion which is a sign of infarction. DWI is the most sensitive investigation for acute cerebral infarction.

Pituitary tumour: sagittal T$_1$ images pre- and post-gadolinium injection

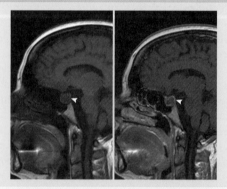

This patient presented with headaches and visual field disturbance (bitemporal hemianopia). The pre-contrast image (left) shows a pituitary adenoma (arrowhead) which demonstrates abnormal enhancement on the post-contrast scan (right). This is classified as a macroadenoma (>1 cm). The bigger a pituitary lesion becomes the more likely it is to cause visual disturbance due to compression of the optic chiasm which lies immediately above the pituitary gland.

Medicine at a Glance, Fourth Edition. Edited by Patrick Davey. © 2014 John Wiley & Sons, Ltd. Published 2014 by John Wiley & Sons, Ltd. Companion website: www.ataglanceseries.com/medicine

The neuroanatomy seen on magnetic resonance imaging (MRI) is similar to that seen on computer tomography (CT) imaging (see Chapter 199). However, MRI allows visualization of structures with greater differentiation and detail even without the use of contrast agent enhancement. The MRI series of the brain are viewed in a similar format to CT images (axial, sagittal and coronal planes). MRI also has the advantage of viewing the brainstem without the significant artefact limitations of CT images. The standard MRI investigation of the brain includes T_1-weighted, T_2-weighted, proton density (PD) weighted and fluid-attenuated inversion recovery sequences (FLAIR). T_1-weighted images with gadolinium enhancement may also be acquired. Each of these acquisition sequences demonstrates different patterns of tissue signal characteristics, which commonly form the basis of interpretation and diagnosis.

- T_1-weighted acquisition sequences: the signal intensity on T_1-weighted acquisitions depends on the fat content of the tissues in question. Subcutaneous fat appears very bright and the myelin sheaths of white matter appear brighter than grey matter. Cerebrospinal fluid (CSF) and pathological fluid appear dark. T_1-weighted images are best at defining anatomy due to their excellent spatial resolution. In the brain, however, they are also useful in conjunction with T_2-weighted images to distinguish blood from other pathology, estimate the age of a haemorrhage and differentiate fatty lesions from other pathology.
- T_2-weighted acquisition sequences: the signal intensity on T_2-weighted acquisitions depends on the water content of the tissues in question. CSF is very bright and can be easily identified within the different components of the ventricular system and subarachnoid space. Fat is darker than on T_1-weighted acquisitions, so white matter appears darker than grey matter. T_2-weighted images are often the best sequence for evaluating pathology. This is because pathological lesions often contain water and are therefore bright and easily seen on T_2. This is true for infective processes, tumours and inflammatory conditions such as multiple sclerosis, which typically reveals bright plaques on T_2-weighted images.
- PD acquisition sequences: this sequence is acquired at the same time as the T_2 sequence. The signal intensity on PD-weighted acquisitions depends on the number of protons per unit tissue. Tissues with a high number of protons are bright (e.g. CSF) and those with a low number of protons are dark. PD sequences are often helpful, but pathological fluid is usually more easily differentiated from other structures on different sequences, such as FLAIR.
- FLAIR acquisition sequences: this is similar to T_2 except the bright signal from CSF is suppressed. This allows clearer evaluation of T_2 bright lesions, especially those near CSF-filled spaces (e.g. white matter plaque adjacent to the ventricular system).

Intracranial haemorrhage

Intracranial haemorrhage may be diagnosed and evaluated by MRI. MRI is superior to CT imaging for detecting haemorrhage in the subacute and chronic phases. However, CT imaging remains the preferred modality in the acute setting because it is much faster. The signal intensity of haemorrhage changes with time on both T_1- and T_2-weighted sequences. This is because the breakdown products of blood clots induce various artefacts. Initially, artefact is due to the presence of oxygenated haemoglobin, which is dark on T_1 and bright on T_2. After several hours, deoxyhaemoglobin is predominant and this is dark on both T_1 and T_2. After approximately 3 days there is an increasing amount of intracellular methaemoglobin, which is bright on T_1 but dark on T_2, and then free methaemoglobin which is bright on both. Eventually, over months, methaemoglobin is exchanged for haemosiderin, which is dark on both sequences. In order to accurately direct management the timing of any haemorrhagic event should be established from the history.

Cerebral infarction and diffusion-weighted MRI

When there is a sudden perfusion deficit to the brain, the glial cells undergo ischaemic change, which causes malfunction of their cell membrane sodium pump. This results in an influx of sodium and water into cells, and restricted diffusion of intracellular water molecules out of the cells by the cell membranes. The net effect is cell swelling, known as cytotoxic oedema. Diffusion-weighted imaging (DWI), a specialized form of MRI, makes use of the Brownian motion of water molecules in the brain to generate a signal. Therefore, a high magnitude of molecular diffusion generates a high intensity signal. While classic Brownian motion refers to free movement of molecules, there is restricted movement in biological tissues due to tissue architecture (e.g. cell membranes) and therefore water diffusion is referred to as apparent diffusion. This phenomenon is represented by an image map of the apparent diffusion coefficient (ADC), whereby restricted diffusion generates a low intensity signal. In the acute ischaemic setting, the restricted diffusion causing cytotoxic oedema results in a low ADC and high DWI signal intensity. This method of diagnostic imaging is very helpful to distinguish acute infarction from old established infarcts.

Intracranial tumours

MRI is more sensitive and specific than CT imaging in detecting and evaluating brain tumours. Intracranial tumours such as meningioma, ependymoma, astrocytoma and metastases are appreciated as being isointense or low signal intensity on T_1-weighted images and high signal intensity on T_2-weighted images, with high signal secondary to the surrounding vasogenic oedema. Imaging after injection of gadolinium is a mainstay of imaging intracranial tumours with MRI as most brain tumours cause disruption of the blood–brain barrier and readily take up the contrast agent.

201 Stroke

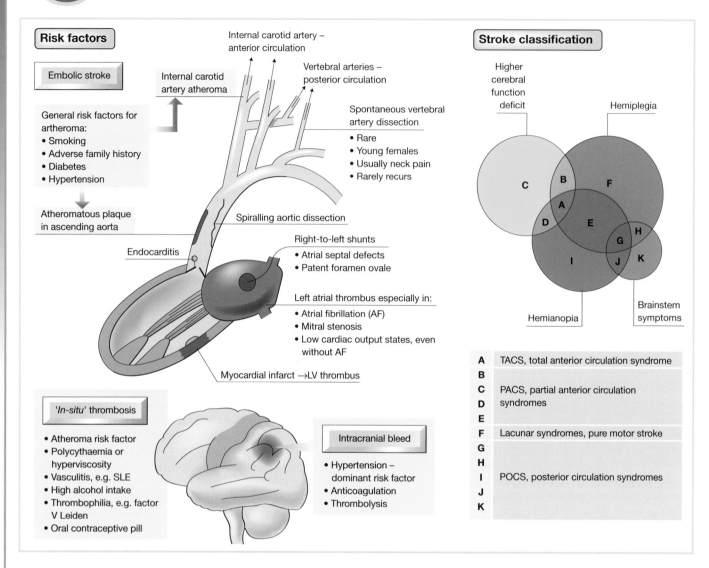

Risk factors

Embolic stroke

Internal carotid artery atheroma

General risk factors for artheroma:
• Smoking
• Adverse family history
• Diabetes
• Hypertension

Atheromatous plaque in ascending aorta

Endocarditis

'*In-situ*' thrombosis

• Atheroma risk factor
• Polycythaemia or hyperviscosity
• Vasculitis, e.g. SLE
• High alcohol intake
• Thrombophilia, e.g. factor V Leiden
• Oral contraceptive pill

Internal carotid artery – anterior circulation

Vertebral arteries – posterior circulation

Spontaneous vertebral artery dissection
• Rare
• Young females
• Usually neck pain
• Rarely recurs

Spiralling aortic dissection

Right-to-left shunts
• Atrial septal defects
• Patent foramen ovale

Left atrial thrombus especially in:
• Atrial fibrillation (AF)
• Mitral stenosis
• Low cardiac output states, even without AF

Myocardial infarct →LV thrombus

Intracranial bleed
• Hypertension – dominant risk factor
• Anticoagulation
• Thrombolysis

Stroke classification

Higher cerebral function deficit

Hemiplegia

Hemianopia

Brainstem symptoms

A	TACS, total anterior circulation syndrome
B	
C	PACS, partial anterior circulation
D	syndromes
E	
F	Lacunar syndromes, pure motor stroke
G	
H	
I	POCS, posterior circulation syndromes
J	
K	

Stroke is the most common condition affecting the brain, with approximately 150 000 new strokes per year in the UK. The burden of mortality and morbidity is high: 30% of people with acute stroke die, 25% are rendered severely disabled.

Key features

Neurological symptoms resulting from cerebrovascular disease are:

• **Of sudden onset**: very occasionally other neurological diseases present suddenly, e.g. brain tumours, demyelination and hypoglycaemia. Evolving neurological signs are not usually the result of vascular pathology, although occasionally major vessel occlusion (e.g. internal carotid artery) presents as a stuttering stroke.

• Focal: referable to a specific anatomical site and associated with loss of function.

• **Usually vaso-occlusive**, either thromboembolic (emboli from the heart in 20% of cases; or from atheromatous plaques in the aorta, extra- or intracranial circulation in the remaining 80%), leading to major vessel occlusion, or *in situ* vascular blockage, usually small vessel and leading to lacunar syndromes.

• **Occasionally caused by haemorrhage** (10% of all strokes), which should be considered in those with marked hypertension, on anticoagulants or presenting with prominent headache.

There are a small number of very common stroke syndromes and a very large number of rare stroke syndromes.

Time course of strokes

• **Transient ischaemic attacks** (TIAs) by definition can last up to 24 hours although usually they last less than a few minutes. TIAs can affect all vascular territories, causing any pattern of neurological dysfunction. The most characteristic is amaurosis fugax, where embolic atherogenic debris from the carotid artery travels to the ophthalmic branch of the internal carotid, causing unilateral blindness, lasting less than a few minutes.

• **Significance**: TIAs imply an active intravascular plaque, i.e. one on which thrombosis is actively occurring and embolizing distally. They are a major risk factor for subsequent disabling stroke; 50% of strokes occurring after a TIA do so within a week, so preventing these strokes is a medical emergency.

• **Investigation**: urgent investigation (carotid ultrasonography and magnetic resonance angiography) to determine whether a high-grade lesion (i.e. >70% stenosis in the internal carotid artery) is present should be undertaken because surgical resection (carotid endarterectomy) significantly reduces the rate of disabling stroke.

- **Minor strokes** have small neurological deficits. Their importance is the same as TIAs – they may be a harbinger of more severe strokes. Sufferers have established vascular disease and need vigorous anti-atherogenic therapy.
- **Completed stroke** implies that the deficit is major, persistent and does not subsequently deteriorate. Unless recovery is good, 'the horse has bolted' and investigations as a prelude to carotid endarterectomy are not indicated.

Anatomy of strokes

An important distinction is between stroke in the anterior (carotid) or the posterior (vertebrobasilar) circulation, because this relates to prognosis (see Table 201.1) and determines the nature of the investigations. Constitutional differences in the cerebral circulation, and the effects of diffuse atheroma on the circle of Willis, mean that it is not always possible to give an accurate clinical determination of the site of occlusion.

Anatomy of stroke 'syndromes'

Carotid territory stroke

Carotid territory stroke presents with a combination of hemiplegia and language dysfunction (dominant hemisphere) or dyspraxia (inability to carry out complex tasks not caused by motor deficits) or denial of the existence (neglect) of the left side (non-dominant hemisphere). Middle cerebral artery (MCA) occlusion has in addition hemianaesthesia and hemianopia (total anterior circulation syndrome (TACS)). An MCA infarct is often large and extensive brain damage may occur, resulting in coma and even death. Recovery is often very poor. Partial anterior circulation presents with a less extensive motor deficit and not all elements of TACS.

Vertebrobasilar (posterior circulation) stroke

There are many eponymous brainstem vascular syndromes of dubious relevance. The combination of any of the following with sudden onset suggests a posterior circulation stroke:
- Diplopia.
- Dysarthria.
- Unsteadiness.
- Dysphagia.
- Unilateral weakness with contralateral facial weakness.

- Bilateral visual loss.
- Amnesia.

Posterior strokes, unlike anterior circulation ones, may have a stuttering evolution. Basilar artery occlusion is frequently catastrophic and fatal. Pontine strokes cause coma, pinpoint pupils, paresis, pyrexia and frequently death.

Lacunar syndromes

Lacunar syndromes are by definition small (<1.5 cm^3). They may cause internal capsule strokes, which are usually either pure motor or pure sensory. Neither of these has an ocular field defect. Recovery is typically more complete than in MCA occlusive syndromes.

Summary of causes of hemiplegia

(see Chapter 59)
- **MCA cortical infarct** (hemiplegia + hemianaesthesia + hemianopia). Haemorrhage into the internal capsule produces a similar triad of signs. Alteration of consciousness is common.
- **Internal capsule lesions**: usually produce rather discrete neurological deficits, such as a 'pure' motor hemiplegia/monoplegia or 'pure' sensory hemianaesthesia.
- **Basis pontis**: dysarthria but not dysphasia may occur, i.e. clumsy hand–dysarthria syndrome.
- **Brainstem lesions**: associated with nystagmus, ocular palsies and cerebellar signs.

Risk factors for stroke

These are as for arterial disease, i.e. increasing age, male sex, family history of vascular disease, hypertension, smoking and diabetes. Structural heart disease predisposes to stroke, especially recent myocardial infarction (MI; ±1% of patients have a stroke during an MI) or atrial fibrillation (especially in those >65 years or with left ventricular (LV) dysfunction). Excess alcohol is a substantial risk factor, particularly in young men. Polycythaemia underlies a few strokes. It has not been established that high cholesterol is a strong primary risk factor for stroke, though lowering cholesterol does appear to reduce the risk of first stroke in trials and it is an important measure in secondary prevention. Neurosyphilis is now very rare, but 45% of cases present as a stroke. For intracerebral haemorrhage, the strongest risk factor is hypertension or vascular abnormality, e.g. arteriovenous malformation or aneurysm, a bleeding diathesis or thrombolytic therapy.

'Young stroke'

Most people aged over 40 years who have had a stroke have the same risk factors as older patients. A few additional conditions should also be considered:
- Infective endocarditis.
- Antiphospholipid syndrome.
- Syphilis.
- Cerebral vasculitis (including systemic lupus erythematosus (SLE)).
- Carotid/vertebral dissection.
- Mitochondrial diseases such as MELAS (mitochondrial encephalopathy, lactic acidosis, stroke-like episodes).
- Inherited thrombophilias, such as protein C and S deficiency, usually produce venous thrombosis in the deep veins of the calf, but occasionally cause stroke, particularly venous sinus thrombosis.
- Structural abnormalities of the extracranial vessels (e.g. moya moya disease, angiographic diagnosis of bilateral distal occlusion/ multiple stenosis of the internal carotid artery, with net-like collaterals around the brain base).
- Drug-induced, e.g. cocaine.

Table 201.1 Stroke prognosis (%).

	TAC	PAC	LAC	POC
30 day				
Dead	40	5	5	5
Dependent	55	40	30	30
Independent	5	55	65	65
1 year				
Dead	60	15	10	20
Dependent	35	30	30	20
Independent	5	55	60	60

LAC, lacunar infarction; PAC, partial anterior circulation; POC, posterior circulation; TAC, total anterior circulation.

202 Management of stroke

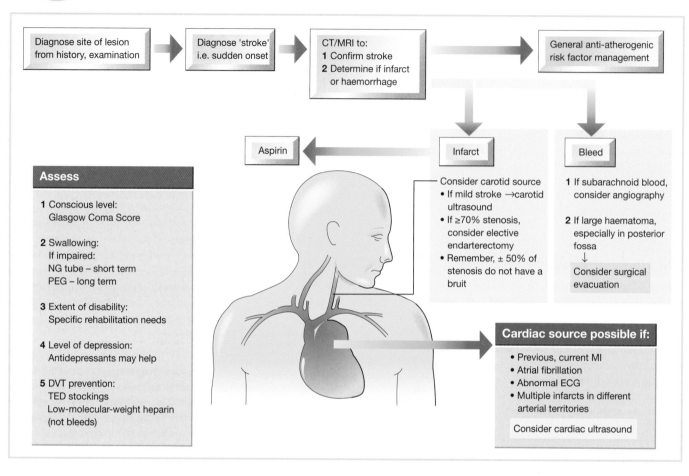

Assess

1 Conscious level:
  Glasgow Coma Score

2 Swallowing:
  If impaired:
  NG tube – short term
  PEG – long term

3 Extent of disability:
  Specific rehabilitation needs

4 Level of depression:
  Antidepressants may help

5 DVT prevention:
  TED stockings
  Low-molecular-weight heparin
  (not bleeds)

Diagnose site of lesion from history, examination

Diagnose 'stroke' i.e. sudden onset

CT/MRI to:
1 Confirm stroke
2 Determine if infarct or haemorrhage

General anti-atherogenic risk factor management

Aspirin

Infarct

Bleed

Consider carotid source
• If mild stroke →carotid ultrasound
• If ≥70% stenosis, consider elective endarterectomy
• Remember, ± 50% of stenosis do not have a bruit

1 If subarachnoid blood, consider angiography

2 If large haematoma, especially in posterior fossa
  ↓
  Consider surgical evacuation

Cardiac source possible if:

• Previous, current MI
• Atrial fibrillation
• Abnormal ECG
• Multiple infarcts in different arterial territories

Consider cardiac ultrasound

The mechanism of stroke (infarct or bleed) must be determined by computed tomography (CT) or magnetic resonance imaging (MRI):

● **Infarct**: the origin of thrombus must be worked out, i.e. from *in situ* thrombosis or emboli originating more proximally, either from the heart or atheromatous plaques in:
  ● The carotid artery, which are diagnosed by ultrasonography.
  ● The aortic arch found by transoesophageal echocardiography; management is unclear.
● **Haemorrhage**: if the clinical condition of the patient is not poor, and especially if there is any suggestion that the bleed is the result of a subarachnoid haemorrhage, it may be appropriate to undertake angiography (conventional or magnetic resonance) to exclude an aneurysm/arteriovenous malformation that might benefit from surgery/intervention.

Acute management

A realistic assessment of prognosis should be sympathetically communicated to relatives. Patients should, if possible, be nursed in dedicated stroke units because these improve outcome.

Cerebral infarcts

● Blood pressure in the long term should be low, but should not be decreased acutely because this may provoke watershed infarcts.
● Aspirin (300 mg, then 75–100 mg per day) and other antiplatelet agents are used to decrease the incidence of further strokes. Current evidence suggests that disability is reduced if thrombolysis (recombinant tissue plasminogen activator) is given <3 hours from symptom onset.

Intracerebral haemorrhage

● Blood pressure should probably be lowered more rapidly in cerebral haemorrhage.
● Posterior fossa bleeds may need neurosurgical evacuation to prevent coning of the brain. Likewise, large intracerebral bleeds with mass effects in young people may benefit from evacuation.

All strokes

● Swallowing dysfunction should be assessed. If the risk of aspiration is not low, feeding should be by nasogastric (NG) tube or, in the longer term, by percutaneous endoscopic gastrostomy (PEG) feeding tube.
● Prevention of deep venous thrombosis (DVT): using thromboembolic (TED) stockings, or possibly low-dose heparin (not cerebral bleeds).
● Good nursing care is the most important factor in outcome.
● Physiotherapy to prevent contractures and help in mobilization.
● Depression occurs in 50–75% of patients. Antidepressants may help.

Long-term management (see Table 202.1)

● **General vascular risk protection**: the annual stroke recurrence rate of 10% is reduced by meticulous control of vascular risk factors (secondary prevention), especially smoking, diabetes and blood pressure (aim for ≤140/85). Cholesterol reduction

Table 202.1 The management of stroke.

Problem	Frequency	Importance	Preventative measures	Interventions for established problem
Fever	Common	Associated with worse outcome	Routine antipyretics	Fanning, antipyretics, treat underlying cause
Low Po_2	Common	↑ Brain ischaemia	Positioning to avoid cardiorespiratory problems	Supplementary O_2
Low BP	Uncommon – may reflect dehydration	May ↑ brain ischaemia	Avoid cause	Treat cause
High BP	Very common	May reflect long-standing ↑ BP, or reaction to CVA; may ↑ brain oedema/bleeding		BP lowering – but these may ↑ brain ischaemia
↑ Blood glucose	20–40%	Associated with ↓ outcome	Avoid dextrose infusions	Insulin
↑ Intracranial pressure (ICP)	↓ Consciousness in most CVAs reflects ↑ ICP	Commonest cause of death ≤1 week	Raising end of bed; avoid overhydration	Anti-oedema drugs, ventilation, decompressive surgery
Sleep disordered breathing	65% of patients	Unknown	Avoid sedatives	CPontinuous positive airway pressure
Dysphagia	50% of patients	Prevents oral feeding; increases risk of chest infection	Routine screening (SALT: speech and language therapy)	Nil by mouth, parenteral or enteral feeding
Epileptic seizures	5% of patients	Leads to neurological deterioration	None	Anticonvulsants
Spasticity and contractures	Depends on preventative measures	Limits function and predisposes to bed sores	Positioning, relief muscle tone (anxiety, pain, overuse)	Physiotherapy, splinting, tone-modifying drugs, botulinum toxin
Emotionalism	20%	Interrupts therapy, social isolation		Antidepressants
Urinary infection	25% in first month	Unwell → ↓ functional level	Maintain hydration, avoid catheters	Antibiotics, fluids
Chest infection	25% in first month	↓ Po_2; → ↓ functional level	Early mobilization, chest physiotherapy, SALT	Antibiotics, chest physiotherapy
Undernutrition	20%	Associated with worse outcome	Nutritional screening; oral supplementation	Oral supplementation, enteral tube feeding
Electrolyte imbalance	Common	May → confusion, seizures	Monitor biochemistry	Supplements, etc.
Deep venous thrombosis (DVT)	50%	May progress to lethal PE; pain, fever	Early mobilization, good hydration, antiplatelet drugs, TED stockings	Anticoagulation
Pulmonary embolism (PE)	5%	May → death	As above	As above
Urinary, faecal incontinence	50%	Demeaning, bed sores	Avoid exacerbating factors, e.g. diuretics	Treat cause if found; bladder retraining, pads, catheters
Pressure sores	<3% with good nursing	Painful, distressing, can → death	Good nursing	Relieve pressure, antibiotics, vitamins
Falls and fractures	Falls common in 35%; fractures rare	Pain, ↓ functional level	Careful supervision; anti-osteoporosis drugs	Standard orthopaedic care for fractures
Painful shoulder	Common	↓ Function and mood	Avoid traction injury	Physiotherapy, analgesics, local steroid injections
Low mood	Very common	Associated with worse outcome	Positive attitude in stroke unit staff	Antidepressants, cognitive behavioural therapy

reduces the rate of further strokes, and statins are indicated for most patients with ischamic stroke for secondary prevention.

● **Carotid endarterectomy**: most patients ≤75 years with small anterior circulation stroke syndromes should have carotid imaging. Those with high-grade lesions (≤70% stenosis) may benefit from carotid endarterectomy.

● **Management and prevention of disability**: 25–50% after a first stroke do not re-achieve independence and require extensive nursing support. Financial and physical aids help.

● **Multidisciplinary management of home environment** can restore independence.

203 Other vascular disorders of the brain

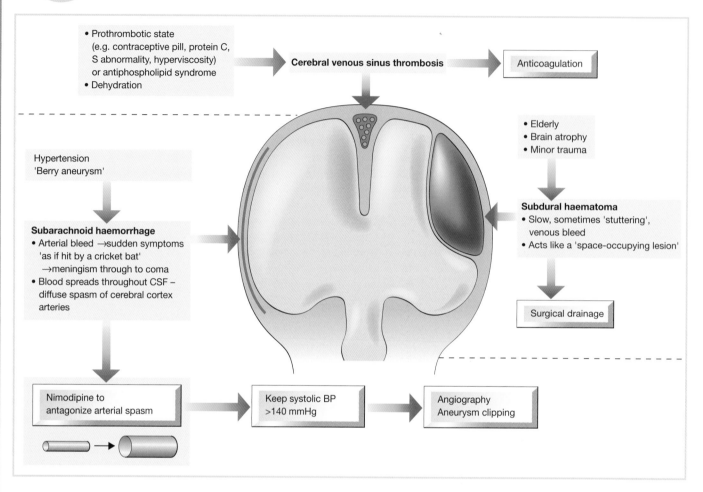

- Prothrombotic state
  (e.g. contraceptive pill, protein C,
  S abnormality, hyperviscosity)
  or antiphospholipid syndrome
- Dehydration

Cerebral venous sinus thrombosis → Anticoagulation

Hypertension
'Berry aneurysm'

- Elderly
- Brain atrophy
- Minor trauma

Subarachnoid haemorrhage
- Arterial bleed →sudden symptoms
  'as if hit by a cricket bat'
  →meningism through to coma
- Blood spreads throughout CSF –
  diffuse spasm of cerebral cortex
  arteries

Subdural haematoma
- Slow, sometimes 'stuttering',
  venous bleed
- Acts like a 'space-occupying lesion'

Surgical drainage

Nimodipine to
antagonize arterial spasm

Keep systolic BP
>140 mmHg

Angiography
Aneurysm clipping

Subarachnoid haemorrhage

Subarachnoid haemorrhage (SAH) is an arterial bleed from a ruptured berry aneurysm (70% of cases) or arteriovenous malformation (10% of cases). There are 3000 cases per year in the UK.

Clinical features and diagnosis

Classic presentation is with a thunderclap headache, often in the occiput. The signs range from none (headache only), through mild meningism to coma. Focal neurological signs are uncommon. Thirty per cent of patients die of the acute bleed: if a re-bleed occurs the mortality rate is ≥60%. A computed tomography (CT) scan should be performed in all suspected cases of SAH. If this is not diagnostic then a delayed (≥12 h after symptom onset) lumbar puncture, looking for xanthochromia (bilirubin on spectrophotometry), should be undertaken.

Treatment

Acutely, blood pressure (BP) should be maintained at 150 mmHg (with intravenous fluids/inotropes if BP is too low), although more chronically BP should be lowered to <140/85. Subarachnoid blood induces damaging cerebral artery spasm, which can be antagonized by nimodipine to improve outcome. The responsible aneurysms can be detected by angiography and treated by endovascular occlusion with platinum coils or by surgical

clipping (open craniotomy) if not accessible by the endovascular route.

Prognosis

Prognosis is poor once coma or a major neurological defect has developed – intervention should therefore occur early on. Overall <40% of cases have a good outcome.

The prevalence of an unruptured intracranial aneurysm on magnetic resonance imaging (MRI) is about 2% and the overall risk of rupture is about 1% per year. The decision whether to treat these asymptomatic lesions is complex and based on size and location.

Subdural haemorrhage

Subdural haemorrhage is a venous bleed, often occurring in the context of brain shrinkage (from age, dementia, chronic alcoholism, etc.). Blood slowly oozes into the subdural space. As this breaks down, osmotically active degradation products are formed, sucking in fluid from the extracellular space. Thus subdural haemorrhages act as space-occupying lesions, expanding slowly over several weeks. Clinically there may be a history of trauma, although this is often absent. Subsequently, there is the slow (a few weeks or more) progression of a focal neurological deficit; equally, elderly patients may present rather non-specifically with

Medicine at a Glance, Fourth Edition. Edited by Patrick Davey. © 2014 John Wiley & Sons, Ltd. Published 2014 by John Wiley & Sons, Ltd. Companion website: www.ataglanceseries.com/medicine

decreased mobility ('off-legs') or decreased mental agility. Focal neurological signs are not invariably present. CT scanning is diagnostic, although a diagnostic trap for the unwary is that 'old' blood (i.e. of the age found in many subdural haemorrhages) may be isodense with the brain. Surgical evacuation should be considered in all affected patients, however elderly.

Venous sinus thrombosis

Cerebral venous sinus thrombosis is a life-threatening condition with an extremely broad range of clinical neurological presentations and a large differential diagnosis.

Demographics

Cerebral vein thrombosis is a rare event, there being estimated to be only some 250–500 cases/year in the UK (60 in peri-/postpartum women). Seventy-five per cent of patients are female and younger ages predominate.

Clinical features

Cerebral vein thrombosis must be considered in acute or subacute headache, seizures and disorders of consciousness or papilloedema. The condition can mimic stroke, abscess, tumour, encephalitis or idiopathic intracranial hypertension. The presenting symptoms depend on which vein is occluded. The pathophysiology can be traced to one of the following two causes:

1 Due to local cerebral vein occlusion leading to local effects – so producing focal signs (e.g. cortical signs (weakness, etc.)) or from deep structures (e.g. dysfunction of the thalamus produces confusion, amnesia, mutism; brainstem dysfunction leads to coma). Occlusion of small cortical veins leads to venous infarction which is highly epileptogenic and may present with seizures.

2 Due to occlusion of cerebral sinuses, leading to intracranial hypertension (so producing headache, found in 90%; the only symptom in 20%; while 80% have focal defects).

Aetiology

There is a wide range of underlying aetiologies including inherited thrombophilias, oral contraception, pregnancy, local intracranial sepsis and systemic inflammatory diseases, such as sarcoidosis and Behçet's disease. It occurs very rarely following lumbar puncture. A predisposing illness is found in 85% of patients.

Diagnosis

The diagnosis can usually be reliably made with MRI with contrast angiography, which shows the thrombus and the venous infarct which, in 40%, can undergo haemorrhagic transformation.

Treatment

Treatment with heparin may improve survival and disability, and patients who continue to deteriorate may be suitable for local thrombolysis. If the intracranial pressure is high, mannitol ± acetazolamide are sometimes used. Surgical removal of the brain infarct has been recommended by some for high intracranial pressures with deteriorating neurological condition.

204 Dementias

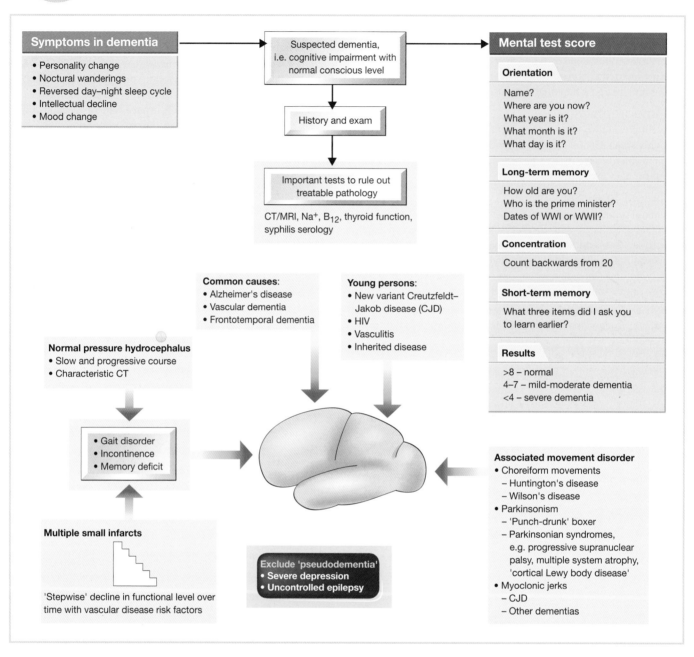

Symptoms in dementia
- Personality change
- Noctural wanderings
- Reversed day–night sleep cycle
- Intellectual decline
- Mood change

Suspected dementia, i.e. cognitive impairment with normal conscious level

History and exam

Important tests to rule out treatable pathology

CT/MRI, Na$^+$, B$_{12}$, thyroid function, syphilis serology

Mental test score

Orientation

Name?
Where are you now?
What year is it?
What month is it?
What day is it?

Long-term memory

How old are you?
Who is the prime minister?
Dates of WWI or WWII?

Concentration

Count backwards from 20

Short-term memory

What three items did I ask you to learn earlier?

Results

>8 – normal
4–7 – mild-moderate dementia
<4 – severe dementia

Common causes:
- Alzheimer's disease
- Vascular dementia
- Frontotemporal dementia

Young persons:
- New variant Creutzfeldt–Jakob disease (CJD)
- HIV
- Vasculitis
- Inherited disease

Normal pressure hydrocephalus
- Slow and progressive course
- Characteristic CT

- Gait disorder
- Incontinence
- Memory deficit

Multiple small infarcts

'Stepwise' decline in functional level over time with vascular disease risk factors

Exclude 'pseudodementia'
- Severe depression
- Uncontrolled epilepsy

Associated movement disorder
- Choreiform movements
  - Huntington's disease
  - Wilson's disease
- Parkinsonism
  - 'Punch-drunk' boxer
  - Parkinsonian syndromes, e.g. progressive supranuclear palsy, multiple system atrophy, 'cortical Lewy body disease'
- Myoclonic jerks
  - CJD
  - Other dementias

Dementia is 'the global impairment of cognition with normal levels of consciousness', in contrast to an acute confusional state, in which conscious level is impaired. The incidence is 5% in those aged ≥65 years and 20% in those aged ≥85 years. With emerging therapies, it is important to attempt a specific diagnosis, although this is not easy because clinical tools are not accurate. Many people labelled as having Alzheimer's disease have a different postmortem diagnosis. Patients who complain of memory disturbance are far more likely to be suffering from anxiety, because those with genuine dementia usually have no insight. Potentially treatable causes of cognitive impairment include:

- Depression: all patients with dementia should have a mental state examination to exclude depressive pseudodementia. However, it should be remembered that depressive symptomatology is a feature of all dementias.

- Normal pressure hydrocephalus may be the result of a diffuse abnormality affecting cerebrospinal fluid uptake; it causes ventricular dilatation, and is suggested by the triad of dementia, incontinence and gait disturbance. Therapeutic lumbar puncture can lead to overt improvement and is used to select patients suitable for shunting.

- Subdural haematoma may present without any antecedent history of trauma as a subacute change in cognitive function with gait disturbance.

- Intracranial tumours are a common cause of subacute cognitive decline. Focal symptoms/signs are usually present.

- Hypothyroidism may produce mild to moderate cognitive impairment.

- Chronic severe hyponatraemia.

- Vitamin B$_{12}$ deficiency.

- Neurosyphilis or general paralysis of the insane.
- Vasculitis.
- Paraneoplastic syndromes (see Chapter 197) rarely cause pure dementia, e.g. tumour-associated limbic encephalitis can present with personality changes.
- Autoimmune encephalopathy due to antivoltage-gated potassium channel antibodies.
- Whipple's disease is associated with cognitive impairment, which may improve with antibiotics.

All patients should therefore have computed tomography (CT) head scans, and vitamin B_{12}, thyroid function and syphilis serology checked, as well as a full blood count, biochemical tests of renal and hepatic function and an erythrocyte sedimentation rate to look for systemic diseases producing cognitive impairment.

Alzheimer's disease

Alzheimer's disease begins most frequently with gradual impairment of episodic memory, but eventually produces global cognitive decline, i.e. early on new memory cannot be laid down, although childhood memories remain accessible. Later on, no memory can be recalled. Although it may be normal early in the disease, volumetric magnetic resonance imaging (MRI) shows specific atrophy of the temporal lobes. Of the cases of Alzheimer's disease, 5% are familial and usually of earlier onset. Mutations have been identified in the *Presenilin 1* and *2* genes and in the amyloid precursor protein gene (*APP*). Certain apolipoprotein E polymorphisms, specifically ε4, predispose to Alzheimer's disease.

- **Pathologically** there is cortical neuron loss, including loss of cholinergic neurons. These form the basis of the usage of acetylcholinesterase inhibitors, which have small but definite beneficial effects.
- **Outlook**: the disease progresses relentlessly, causing death from pneumonia or inanition after 8–10 years. The key to management is to care for the sufferer on a 'symptom-by-symptom' basis and to provide good support and relief for the care giver.

Frontotemporal dementia

Frontotemporal dementia (FTD) is a heterogeneous form of dementia with a spectrum of clinical and pathological features. In behavioural variant FTD, there is prominent personality change and a dysexecutive syndrome develops, i.e. sufferers are reluctant to initiate any actions or they may be frankly disinhibited. Semantic dementia and progressive non-fluent aphasia are forms of FTD associated with specific language disorders and sometimes parkinsonism. Preserved areas of ability such as memory are key diagnostic features that distinguish FTD from Alzheimer's. Onset is usually at age 65 years or older. MRI shows frontal and/or temporal atrophy. The FTDs are pathologically heterogeneous and include forms with tau pathology (FTD-τ) or ubiquitin pathology (FTD-U) and Pick's disease, in which characteristic neuropathology occurs. Some of the FTD-τ cases are the result of mutations in the microtubule-associated tau protein. Of patients with motor neuron disease (MND), 30% develop a mild dysexecutive syndrome and occasionally (3–4%) frank FTD as the predominant clinical finding, with denervation atrophy and fasciculations appearing later. In both FTD-U and MND-associated dementia, ubiquitinated inclusions stain for the nuclear protein TDP-43. A significant number of patients with MND/FTD overlap syndromes characterized by ubiquitin pathology carry a common mutation, a hexanucleotide repeat expansion on chromosome 9.

Vascular dementia

The history is of stepwise evolution of cognitive impairment and focal neurological signs, in someone with the appropriate risk factors. A small stepping gait is characteristic. Memory may be less impaired in relation to defects in visuoperceptual tasking. MRI shows atrophy with diffuse white and grey matter vascular lesions (Binswanger's encephalopathy is CT evidence of white matter infarction, with dementia, in hypertensive patients with a stroke). The diagnostic accuracy is often hampered by finding cerebrovascular disease in Alzheimer's disease patients. Treating vascular disease risk factors and aspirin may slow progression.

Dementia with Lewy bodies

This causes parkinsonism (see Chapter 212). Typical features are fluctuating cognition, nocturnal visual hallucinations and disordered rapid eye movement (REM) sleep. Imaging is normal or shows diffuse atrophy. L-dopa may dramatically exacerbate the psychiatric symptoms, while treatment with antipsychotics can lead to a catastrophic and potentially fatal decline in motor performance.

Prion diseases

In prion disease, mutated forms of the prion protein (PrP) induce a conformational change in other PrP molecules ('permissive templating'), so producing non-functional, non-metabolizable forms which are cytotoxic. Sporadic and inherited forms of Creutzfeldt–Jakob disease (CJD) cause a rapidly progressive dementia with myoclonus, ataxia and cortical blindness progressing over weeks to months. The electroencephalograph (EEG) shows characteristic repetitive complexes. Variant CJD (transmitted from cattle infected with the bovine spongiform encephalopathy agent) seems to occur in younger patients, has a slower evolution and is associated with psychiatric symptoms as the earliest feature, though the initial epidemic in the UK has now come to an end.

Cognitive impairment in younger patients

The distinction between young and old in terms of causation is potentially artificial, and consideration of the conditions listed below should be driven by the presence of specific neurological symptoms and signs, such as dystonia, and the presence of specific risk factors:

- Use of 'recreational' drugs, especially alcohol, and also glue.
- Human immunodeficiency virus (HIV) related dementia occurs as a late feature. Infections and structural lesions must be ruled out (lymphoma, toxoplasmosis, progressive multifocal leukoencephalopathy).
- Cerebral vasculitis.
- End-stage multiple sclerosis.
- Adrenoleukodystrophies resulting from fatty acid dysmetabolism cause a 'multiple sclerosis-type' pattern with prominent dementia.
- CADASIL: a white matter disease associated with mutations in the notch-3 gene – presents as hemiplegic migraine, encephalopathy or a progressive dementia.
- Wilson's disease: the majority of cases present before the age of 30 with neuropsychiatric problems and dystonia of the mouth and tongue associated with a high amplitude limb tremor.
- Uncontrolled epilepsy may produce a 'twilight' state, in which seizures are so frequent as to disallow full recovery in between. Rarely, so-called 'non-convulsive status' – in which patients appear vacant and are seen to perform repetitive movements – may be misinterpreted as a rapidly progressive dementia. The EEG is diagnostic.

205 Epilepsy

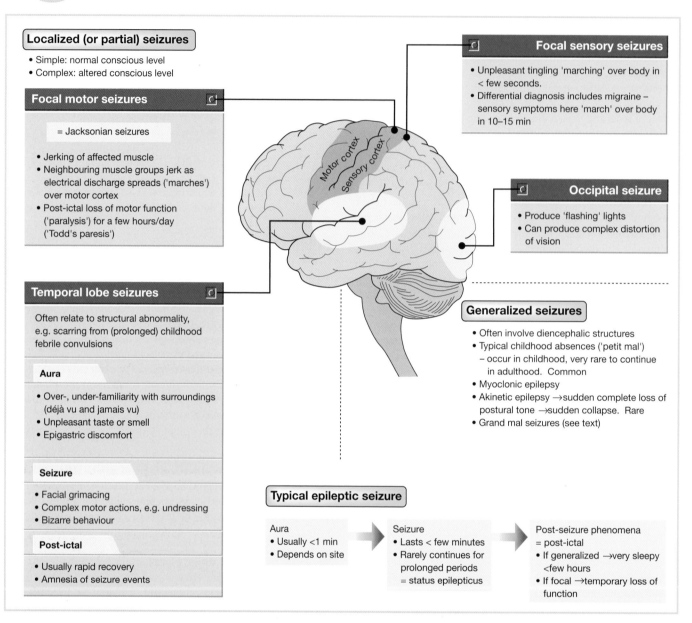

Localized (or partial) seizures
- Simple: normal conscious level
- Complex: altered conscious level

Focal motor seizures

= Jacksonian seizures

- Jerking of affected muscle
- Neighbouring muscle groups jerk as electrical discharge spreads ('marches') over motor cortex
- Post-ictal loss of motor function ('paralysis') for a few hours/day ('Todd's paresis')

Temporal lobe seizures

Often relate to structural abnormality, e.g. scarring from (prolonged) childhood febrile convulsions

Aura
- Over-, under-familiarity with surroundings (déjà vu and jamais vu)
- Unpleasant taste or smell
- Epigastric discomfort

Seizure
- Facial grimacing
- Complex motor actions, e.g. undressing
- Bizarre behaviour

Post-ictal
- Usually rapid recovery
- Amnesia of seizure events

Focal sensory seizures
- Unpleasant tingling 'marching' over body in < few seconds.
- Differential diagnosis includes migraine – sensory symptoms here 'march' over body in 10–15 min

Occipital seizure
- Produce 'flashing' lights
- Can produce complex distortion of vision

Motor cortex   Sensory cortex

Generalized seizures
- Often involve diencephalic structures
- Typical childhood absences ('petit mal') – occur in childhood, very rare to continue in adulthood. Common
- Myoclonic epilepsy
- Akinetic epilepsy →sudden complete loss of postural tone →sudden collapse. Rare
- Grand mal seizures (see text)

Typical epileptic seizure

Aura
- Usually <1 min
- Depends on site

→

Seizure
- Lasts < few minutes
- Rarely continues for prolonged periods = status epilepticus

→

Post-seizure phenomena = post-ictal
- If generalized →very sleepy <few hours
- If focal →temporary loss of function

Epilepsy is 'the recurrent tendency to spontaneous, disordered electrical discharge in the brain manifesting as alteration in motor, sensory or psychological function'. Generalized seizures arise in the brain of anyone subjected to the appropriate stimulus, e.g. hypoxia or electroconvulsive therapy. Therefore a single seizure does not make the diagnosis of epilepsy.

Causes of seizures

- Metabolic, especially ↓ Na$^+$ or ↓ glucose; liver failure, renal failure.
- Drugs, especially alcohol (particularly chronic alcohol excess and alcohol withdrawal), 'street' drugs, penicillins, antipsychotics, antidepressants.
- Cerebrovascular disease.
- Tumours.

- Intracranial infections, especially meningitis, encephalitis, syphilis.
- Cerebral anoxia, especially arrhythmia related.
- Developmental brain abnormalities.
- Degenerative brain disease.
- Hippocampal sclerosis.
- Primary epilepsy syndromes, genetic (e.g. 'channelopathies') or sporadic.

Treatment of the underlying cause, if it can be identified, is the preferred management option; anticonvulsants may also be required.

Epidemiology

The lifetime risk of a generalized convulsion is 3–4%, with peaks at the beginning (neonatal convulsions) and end of life (tumours,

Medicine at a Glance, Fourth Edition. Edited by Patrick Davey. © 2014 John Wiley & Sons, Ltd. Published 2014 by John Wiley & Sons, Ltd. Companion website: www.ataglanceseries.com/medicine

stroke). The incidence is 0.7%. There are 300 000 people in the UK with active seizures; 15–20% attend hospital each year.

Simplified classification

The simplest way to divide seizures is whether on the electroencephalograph (EEG) electrical activity is focal or generalized.

Primary generalized epilepsy

Primary generalized (grand mal) epilepsy refers to electrical seizure activity on the EEG arising in both hemispheres simultaneously. It usually begins in childhood or adolescence; there may be a family history. Brain imaging (computed tomography, magnetic resonance imaging) is normal. It is often photosensitive (triggered by flashing lights). There are three common manifestations:

1 **Typical childhood absences** ('petit mal').
2 **Myoclonic jerks.**
3 **Generalized tonic–clonic seizures**: a brief tonic stiffening of the limbs associated with sudden loss of consciousness followed by a variable period of clonic jerking.

Differential diagnosis of generalized tonic–clonic seizures

- All causes of seizures.
- Loss of cardiac output, e.g. arrhythmias, vasovagal, postural hypotension, etc.
- Psychogenic: seizures usually occur in public places, often hospitals; eyes are held tightly shut; bizarre movements are common. May also occur in those with genuine epilepsy.

Localization-related epilepsy

There is a clear electrical focus on the EEG from which the seizure activity arises. Often an abnormality is identified on imaging (hippocampal sclerosis, benign tumours, arteriovenous malformations, cortical dysplasia). There is usually no family history. The common forms are:

- Simple partial seizures.
- Complex partial seizures (the term 'complex' denotes altered awareness).
- If electrical activity spreads, a secondary generalized seizure occurs.

Diagnosis

The diagnosis of epilepsy is clinical, based on the history from the patient and reliable observers. The EEG supports the clinical diagnosis and differentiates between primary generalized seizures (3 Hz spike and wave discharge triggered by flashing lights) and localization-related seizures (focal spike discharges). Of patients with true seizures, 50% have a normal interictal EEG, emphasizing the importance of the history in making the diagnosis. Similarly, imaging findings must be interpreted in the context of the appropriate history of seizures.

Specific syndromes

Typical childhood absences

This was previously called 'petit mal' epilepsy. Onset is at age 3–6 years. It is associated with brief interruptions of 3–5 seconds in awareness, with minimal or no motor manifestation. Attacks can be provoked by hyperventilation. There is a characteristic EEG pattern of 3 Hz spike and wave activity. It responds to sodium valproate or ethosuximide and is likely to remit fully by adolescence.

Juvenile myoclonic epilepsy

This develops later in childhood, though a history of typical childhood absences is common. It is associated with early morning myoclonic jerks, which may be reported as clumsiness. Generalized tonic–clonic seizures occur in most. The epilepsy responds to sodium valproate. In most, the tendency to seizures is life-long.

Complex partial seizures with secondary generalization

These are common. Seizures arising from the temporal lobes are typically heralded by an aura, which can take the form of abdominal rising sensations, altered taste and, more rarely, visual and auditory hallucinations. Patients appear 'blank' during an attack and may make repetitive movements, e.g. lip smacking. Of cases, 70% are controlled on monotherapy, although a significant number have drug-resistant seizures and are socially and economically handicapped. Approximately 30% of complex partial seizures arise outside of the temporal lobe, usually from the frontal lobe.

Frontal lobe seizures

These present a diagnostic challenge because the EEG is often normal, even during an attack, and the seizure semiology may be bizarre. Patients may appear to remain awake, but to thrash their limbs about uncontrollably and yell. Instantaneous recovery often occurs and patients may be labelled as having non-epileptic attacks.

Jacksonian seizures

These are simple partial seizures arising in the motor cortex. The onset is with rhythmical twitching of the face, which spreads down through the arms and into the legs in a characteristic march-like fashion. There is a high likelihood of finding a structural lesion, so imaging is mandatory.

Treatment

Primary generalized epilepsy responds well to sodium valproate or lamotrigine; it may be worse on carbamazepine. There is little evidence for any other anticonvulsant specificity by seizure type, so drugs are selected on patient characteristics and cost:

- Side effect profile: phenytoin is avoided in young people because it causes gingival hyperplasia and androgenizes the face.
- Potential for teratogenicity: all the older drugs are teratogenic as are the newer agents,, though probably to a lesser degree. Preconception counselling is vital.
- Effect on other drugs: particularly the oral contraceptive pill.

Monotherapy is preferred. Any changes should be made gradually and in the context of an overall seizure pattern, not in response to single seizures.

Status epilepticus (common causes: poor compliance in a known epileptic, sudden anticonvulsant withdrawal, alcohol withdrawal, drug overdose, hypoglycaemia) is defined as continuous seizure activity (arbitrarily for 30 min) or frequent seizures without recovery. This is a medical emergency with a high morbidity. Continuous seizure activity eventually results in cerebral oedema and cardiorespiratory arrest. Management involves:

- **A**irway, **b**reathing and **c**irculation (ABC).
- Urgent glucose (fingerprick testing), electrolytes and toxicology screen.
- 10 mg diazepam intravenously: terminates most seizures and can be repeated once.
- Phenytoin or fosphenytoin intravenous infusion.
- Intubation and transfer to the intensive care unit for thiopental (thiopentone) or propofol infusion.

206 Multiple sclerosis

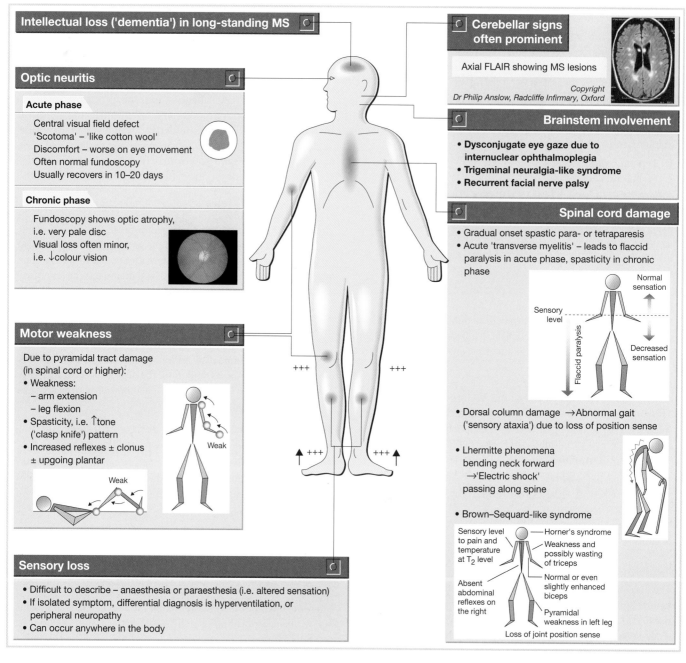

Intellectual loss ('dementia') in long-standing MS

Cerebellar signs often prominent

Axial FLAIR showing MS lesions

Copyright
Dr Philip Anslow, Radcliffe Infirmary, Oxford

Optic neuritis

Acute phase

- Central visual field defect
- 'Scotoma' – 'like cotton wool'
- Discomfort – worse on eye movement
- Often normal fundoscopy
- Usually recovers in 10–20 days

Chronic phase

- Fundoscopy shows optic atrophy, i.e. very pale disc
- Visual loss often minor, i.e. ↓colour vision

Brainstem involvement

- **Dysconjugate eye gaze due to internuclear ophthalmoplegia**
- **Trigeminal neuralgia-like syndrome**
- **Recurrent facial nerve palsy**

Spinal cord damage

- Gradual onset spastic para- or tetraparesis
- Acute 'transverse myelitis' – leads to flaccid paralysis in acute phase, spasticity in chronic phase

Normal sensation
Sensory level
Flaccid paralysis
Decreased sensation

- Dorsal column damage →Abnormal gait ('sensory ataxia') due to loss of position sense
- Lhermitte phenomena bending neck forward →'Electric shock' passing along spine
- Brown–Sequard-like syndrome

Sensory level to pain and temperature at T₂ level — Horner's syndrome
Weakness and possibly wasting of triceps
Absent abdominal reflexes on the right
Normal or even slightly enhanced biceps
Pyramidal weakness in left leg
Loss of joint position sense

Motor weakness

Due to pyramidal tract damage (in spinal cord or higher):
- Weakness:
  – arm extension
  – leg flexion
- Spasticity, i.e. ↑tone ('clasp knife') pattern
- Increased reflexes ± clonus ± upgoing plantar

Weak

Weak

+++ +++

+++ +++

Sensory loss

- Difficult to describe – anaesthesia or paraesthesia (i.e. altered sensation)
- If isolated symptom, differential diagnosis is hyperventilation, or peripheral neuropathy
- Can occur anywhere in the body

Multiple sclerosis (MS) is the most common of a group of inflammatory conditions in which the basic pathological process is one of loss of myelin in the brain and spinal cord. This leads initially to a relapsing and remitting neurological disturbance, but ultimately, in all but a few patients, to permanent and progressive disability as a result of loss of axons. It is a common disease (50 000 sufferers in the UK, lifetime risk in the UK 2–5/1000) affecting young people, for whom currently there is no proven treatment that alters long-term disability. It is presumed to be a disorder of altered immune responsiveness to targets in the central nervous system (CNS), in which there is a genetic susceptibility and a series of environmentally determined triggers, the

nature of which (viral, toxic, etc.) remains obscure, although it also shows some features of a primary degenerative process. The relative risk of developing MS in first-degree relatives is 15, although the absolute risk is still low. There is marked geographical variation (common in people of Scandinavian origin, rare in Japan and Africa).

Clinical spectrum

There are a number of typical patterns of disease:

- **Relapsing and remitting**: initially the patient presents with episodes of monophasic neurological disturbance with return to normal function in between attacks. Thereafter, the patient may not return to normality, so there is a background of progressive dysfunction with superimposed relapses (termed secondary progressive MS). This accounts for most patients with MS.

- **Relapsing progressive**: there is a progressive course with superimposed relapses but no recovery in between episodes.
- **Primary progressive**: there is relentless progression from the outset. This subtype is associated with males, later onset and a paucity of imaging changes, a presentation with progressive spastic paraparesis, and an overall poorer prognosis. There is rarely any response to steroids.

Clinical features

The most common clinical features are:

- Optic neuritis and subsequent optic atrophy: patients experience blurring of vision through to more profound visual loss, with restoration of eyesight over several months. Colour vision may be permanently lost.
- Cerebellar ataxia (see Chapter 62).
- Spastic paraparesis (see Chapter 209).
- Internuclear ophthalmoplegia: the internuclear tracts are nerve fibres linking the nuclei of the nerves controlling the external ocular muscles. MS plaques commonly disrupt them. There is failure of conjugate eye movements, with slow adduction in the ipsilateral eye usually associated with contralateral nystagmus.
- Patchy sensory disturbance.

The clinical signs most commonly associated with MS are shown Figure 206.1.

Diagnosis

- Magnetic resonance imaging (MRI) shows typical changes in most patients (with white matter hyperintensities usually around the ventricles or in the brainstem) although a spinal cord presentation can be associated with normal imaging.
- Visual evoked potentials (VEPs) to document slowing of optic nerve conduction caused by demyelination are a useful adjunct if the MRI cannot distinguish the changes of vascular disease.
- Lumbar puncture to look for oligoclonal bands is much less frequently performed than in the past but is of use when the MRI changes are not diagnostic, particularly early in the disease or if it is confined to the spinal cord. Oligoclonal bands in the cerebrospinal fluid occur in 97% of MS patients, but also in other conditions: paraneoplastic cerebellar degeneration, Behçet's disease, neurosarcoid and CNS infections.

Differential diagnosis

A first attack of demyelination can be caused by parainfectious immune-mediated damage (acute disseminated encephalomyelitis). Strictly speaking, it is not possible to establish the diagnosis of MS after one attack but, if the MRI shows lesions not referable to the site of clinical involvement, there is at least an 80% chance of going on to develop MS. A number of rarer conditions can look like MS:

- Progressive cerebrovascular disease can occasionally be difficult to distinguish on clinical and imaging grounds, but is associated with negative oligoclonal bands and usually normal VEPs.
- Cerebral vasculitis.

- Similar white matter changes to those seen in MS can occur in Sjögren's syndrome, sarcoidosis and Behçet's disease of the nervous system, and occasionally in cerebral lymphoma.

Prognosis

Occasional patients run a relentlessly progressive course from the beginning of the disease and may die within a few years of the first symptoms. In most patients, however, MS does not significantly shorten life. The disease runs a course over decades, during which time there will in most patients be an increasing burden of disability. However, some patients experience a relapsing and remitting course with good functional recovery for many years.

Treatment

- **Overall approach**: this is vital. The patient requires psychological support, with accurate advice about work, home life (and adaptations) and prognosis, and a balanced view on therapy – the last sometimes being particularly difficult. A multidisciplinary approach involving general practitioners, social workers, relatives, physiotherapists, occupational therapists and sometimes psychiatrists is crucial. This approach is true for all diseases but is particularly important in MS.
- **Acute relapses**: corticosteroids (high dose intravenously or orally) have been shown to reduce the severity and duration of acute relapses, although not in every patient. There is no effect on relapse rate or long-term disability. In general, steroids become less effective after repeated attacks.
- **Disease process and progression**: a number of drugs (β-interferon, copaxone, natalizumab) appear to reduce the number of clinical relapses in selected patients and the number of new lesions on MRI. However, there appears to be no effect on long-term disability.

Symptomatic treatment

- Unpleasant sensory phenomena such as shooting pains and paraesthesiae can be treated with anticonvulsants such as carbamazepine and gabapentin.
- Bladder spasticity can be treated with oxybutynin or intermittent self-catheterization – although this risks frequent urinary tract infections. Such infections are common in MS; fever may (temporarily) dramatically worsen weakness.
- Sexual dysfunction in men may respond to sildenafil (Viagra).
- Constipation is common and requires laxatives, and sometimes manual evacuation.
- Muscle spasticity can be treated with baclofen.
- Depression severe enough to require medication occurs in 30% of patients.

Neuromyelitis optica

Neuromyelitis optica (NMO) presents as attacks of optic neuritis with 'longitudinally extensive transverse myelitis'. Each can occur in isolation giving rise to the concept of 'NMO specturm' disorders. In the past, NMO was considered to be a variant of MS but is now recognized to be a specific disease entity characterized by antibodies to aquaporin 4 (AQP), a distinct pathology of complement-mediated destruction and perivascular astrocytosis and a different response from MS to immunotherapy.

207 Infections of the central nervous system

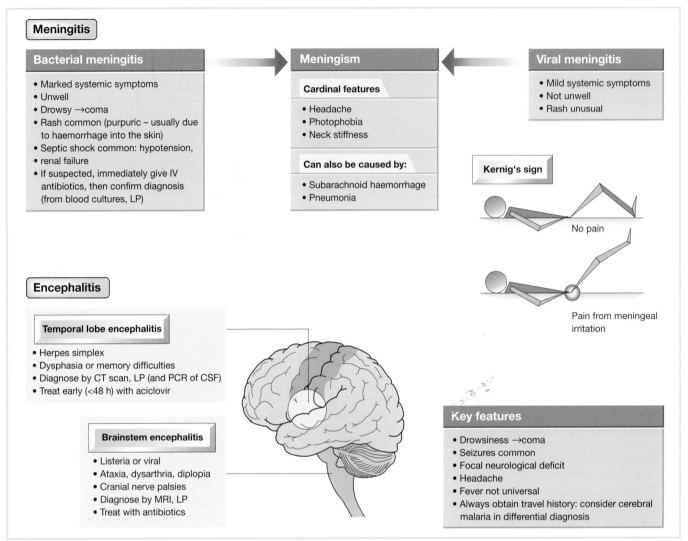

Meningitis

Bacterial meningitis
- Marked systemic symptoms
- Unwell
- Drowsy →coma
- Rash common (purpuric – usually due to haemorrhage into the skin)
- Septic shock common: hypotension,
- renal failure
- If suspected, immediately give IV antibiotics, then confirm diagnosis (from blood cultures, LP)

Meningism

Cardinal features
- Headache
- Photophobia
- Neck stiffness

Can also be caused by:
- Subarachnoid haemorrhage
- Pneumonia

Viral meningitis
- Mild systemic symptoms
- Not unwell
- Rash unusual

Kernig's sign

No pain

Pain from meningeal irritation

Encephalitis

Temporal lobe encephalitis
- Herpes simplex
- Dysphasia or memory difficulties
- Diagnose by CT scan, LP (and PCR of CSF)
- Treat early (<48 h) with aciclovir

Brainstem encephalitis
- Listeria or viral
- Ataxia, dysarthria, diplopia
- Cranial nerve palsies
- Diagnose by MRI, LP
- Treat with antibiotics

Key features
- Drowsiness →coma
- Seizures common
- Focal neurological deficit
- Headache
- Fever not universal
- Always obtain travel history: consider cerebral malaria in differential diagnosis

A number of infectious processes may affect the central nervous system (CNS), including meningitis, encephalitis and cerebral abscess. The range of bacteria, viruses, fungi and parasites that can be responsible is broad, especially in the immunocompromised such as transplant recipients or those with HIV disease.

Meningitis

Acute meningitis presents with fever, headache, stiff neck and photophobia, and can be caused by bacteria or viruses.

- **Bacterial meningitis**: often associated with a septic syndrome (fever, tachycardia, hypotension or shock; see Chapter 166), complicated by septicaemia-induced disseminated intravascular coagulation (see Chapter 188). The two commonest organisms are *Neisseria meningitidis* and *Streptococcus pneumoniae* (more common in elderly people and those who abuse alcohol or with damaged dura (skull fracture, ear sepsis, sinus disease)). Once bacterial meningitis is suspected, broad-spectrum antibiotics (e.g. high-dose ceftriaxone) must be given immediately (i.e. in the community if necessary). The diagnosis is confirmed by

identifying the organism using blood culture, cerebrospinal fluid (CSF) (see Table 207.1), microscopy, culture and polymerase chain reaction (PCR) or blood serology. The prognosis is variable. In meningococcal meningitis, 5–10% die, and a significant proportion have permanent sequelae, including loss of digits (infarction secondary to hypotension), deafness, blindness and intellectual impairment. Immunization against meningococcal serotype A and C is effective (but serotype B, against which there is no vaccine, now accounts for 90% of cases in the UK).

- ***Listeria monocytogenes***: causes meningitis in susceptible individuals (pregnant women, people with alcohol problems, immunocompromised individuals), with a rapidly progressive picture resembling brainstem encephalitis with focal signs and meningism. Treatment is with ampicillin.

- **Viral meningitis**: presents with prominent headache and less obvious signs of meningeal irritation than in bacterial infections. The responsible organism is identified (CSF, PCR or serology) in only 50% of cases, and is often an enterovirus. Many of the common exanthemata of childhood, including measles and

Medicine at a Glance, Fourth Edition. Edited by Patrick Davey. © 2014 John Wiley & Sons, Ltd. Published 2014 by John Wiley & Sons, Ltd. Companion website: www.ataglanceseries.com/medicine

Table 207.1 CSF findings in different infections.

Disease	CSF pressure	Protein	Cell count	Glucose
Bacterial meningitis	Raised	Moderately to severely elevated	>50 polymorphs	Low
Viral meningitis	Normal	Mildly elevated or normal	Lymphocytes	Normal
Tubercular meningitis	Raised Normal	Moderately elevated	Pleocytosis or lymphocytosis	Low
Encephalitis	Raised or normal	Mildly elevated or normal	Lymphocytosis	Normal
Malignant meningitis	Mildly raised or normal	Raised	Raised: either reactive lymphocytes or malignant cells	Low

chickenpox, may be accompanied by a meningitic illness which, although usually mild, can rarely be life-threatening. Management is symptomatic with rehydration and analgesia.

- **Non-infectious causes** of meningism (i.e. headache, photophobia and stiff neck) include subarachnoid haemorrhage and migraine (although this requires exclusion of more serious diagnoses). Malignant meningitis usually presents with sequential cranial nerve palsies, initially painless, later painful, but can cause meningism. Spinal nerve root involvement also occurs.
- **Meningoencephalitis** is meningitis plus some parenchymal involvement.
- **Tubercular meningitis or cryptococcal meningitis**: a chronic presentation may occur; these are more common in the immunocompromised. Tubercular meningitis is increasing in frequency in the West (see Chapter 172).

Encephalitis

Encephalitis implies infection of the brain substance itself. This is rare. The clinical picture is of fever, headache and a diffuse (i.e. confusion, drowsiness up to coma) rather than focal disturbance of cerebral function. The onset may be very dramatic over just a few hours, although more usually the history extends back several days. Other features include: seizures, wandering, behavioural change and frank psychiatric syndromes.

The diagnosis is made from the combination of suggestive clinical features and a lymphocytosis in the CSF. Supportive data come from finding focal inflammation on magnetic resonance imaging (MRI), focal slow wave activity on an electroencephalograph (EEG) and detection of the organism (culture, PCR, serology). There are a large number of viruses responsible, with a marked geographical variation (e.g. Japanese B in the Far East, West Nile in the USA) so a travel history is vital. A cause is only identified in 30% of cases. The prognosis is variable. The principal treatable cause is herpes simplex encephalitis (HSV), which has the following features:

- Rare: causes 20% of viral encephalitis.
- Presents with a viral prodrome followed by behavioural changes with amnesia and sometimes dysphasia.
- Rapid evolution to coma may occur.
- EEG shows repetitive epileptic discharges localized to the temporal lobes. CT/MRI shows necrotizing inflammation in the temporal lobes.
- Treatment: immediate high-dose aciclovir. The prognosis is poor and long-term sequelae are common: 10% die acutely, 10% are so severely impaired as to be rendered institutionalized, 20% are left dependent, and 60% recover but in the majority formal neuropsychological testing reveals residual deficits and most do not function at their premorbid occupational level.

Cerebral abscess

Cerebral abscess is rare and presents with headache, fever and focal neurological signs. Infection arises from direct spread (e.g. infected ears, sinuses) or from infected emboli (endocarditis or cyanotic congenital heart disease). First-line investigation is CT/MRI. Lumbar puncture (LP) must not be performed because the risk of 'coning' (i.e. herniation of the brain through the foramen magnum, precipitating coma and death) is high. Organisms are cultured from the blood or pus aspirated from the abscess. Echocardiography to exclude cardiac infection (see Chapter 93) should be undertaken. Treatment is with prolonged antibiotics and sometimes neurosurgical drainage. The mortality rate is 25%.

Prion diseases

The biologically unique features of these diseases are that they can be simultaneously inherited and infectious. The agent of transmission is thought to be a protein (a 'prion') only, rather than an 'organism' containing DNA or RNA. Prion diseases principally result in dementia (see Chapter 204) and include:

- Sporadic Creutzfeldt–Jakob disease (CJD): rare ($1/10^6$), causes rapid dementia with myoclonus and a characteristic EEG.
- Variant CJD: $\leq$200 cases in total in UK to date, and the incidence appears to be declining. Occurs in younger people with a slower course than sporadic CJD. Characteristic pathological features. A psychiatric presentation (depression, personality changes) is frequently seen.
- Autosomal dominant CJD: familial form of classic CJD.
- Gerstmann–Straussler–Scheinker syndrome: familial spongiform encephalopathy with prominent ataxia.
- Fatal familial insomnia.
- Kuru: endemic in New Guinea highlanders who performed ritual cannibalism. Now very rare.

Parasitic diseases

A number of parasitic diseases may cause neurological problems; ranging from the coma associated with cerebral malaria (see Chapter 171) to fits occurring with cysticercosis.

Neurological consequences of HIV disease

Neurological problems are common in HIV (see Chapter 168) and include the consequences of direct viral infection of the CNS (AIDS dementia, seroconversion meningitis, Guillain–Barré syndrome-like polyneuropathy), opportunistic infections (toxoplasmosis, cryptococcal meningitis, progressive multifocal leukoencephalopathy), primary cerebral lymphoma and drug toxicity (anti-retrovirals: nucleoside analogues and protease inhibitors).

208 Tumours and the nervous system

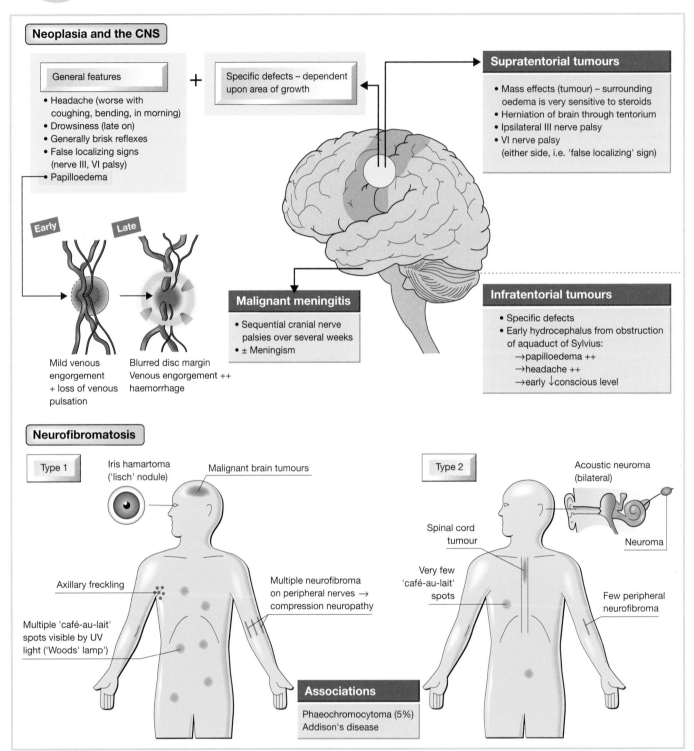

Neoplasia and the CNS

General features

- Headache (worse with coughing, bending, in morning)
- Drowsiness (late on)
- Generally brisk reflexes
- False localizing signs (nerve III, VI palsy)
- Papilloedema

+ Specific defects – dependent upon area of growth

Supratentorial tumours

- Mass effects (tumour) – surrounding oedema is very sensitive to steroids
- Herniation of brain through tentorium
- Ipsilateral III nerve palsy
- VI nerve palsy (either side, i.e. 'false localizing' sign)

Early

Late

Mild venous engorgement + loss of venous pulsation

Blurred disc margin Venous engorgement ++ haemorrhage

Malignant meningitis

- Sequential cranial nerve palsies over several weeks
- ± Meningism

Infratentorial tumours

- Specific defects
- Early hydrocephalus from obstruction of aquaduct of Sylvius:
  →papilloedema ++
  →headache ++
  →early ↓conscious level

Neurofibromatosis

Type 1

Iris hamartoma ('lisch' nodule)

Malignant brain tumours

Axillary freckling

Multiple neurofibroma on peripheral nerves → compression neuropathy

Multiple 'café-au-lait' spots visible by UV light ('Woods' lamp)

Type 2

Acoustic neuroma (bilateral)

Spinal cord tumour

Neuroma

Very few 'café-au-lait' spots

Few peripheral neurofibroma

Associations

Phaeochromocytoma (5%)
Addison's disease

Neoplasia and the CNS

Central nervous system (CNS) neoplasia may present with:

- Epilepsy.
- Symptoms of raised intracranial pressure (headache, intellectual deterioration, vomiting) with papilloedema. Posterior fossa (e.g. cerebellar) metastases produce a rapid rise in intracranial pressure and rapid onset of symptoms.
- Focal deficits, the onset of which is often slow, but occasionally sudden (i.e. stroke-like). The deficit relates to damage caused by the expansion of the tumour (which acts as a space-occupying lesion) and the surrounding oedema. Focal signs usually reflect

Medicine at a Glance, Fourth Edition. Edited by Patrick Davey. © 2014 John Wiley & Sons, Ltd. Published 2014 by John Wiley & Sons, Ltd. Companion website: www.ataglanceseries.com/medicine

the site of the tumour, but occasionally false localizing signs occur from the tumour shifting brain contents and damaging distant nervous structures (e.g. VIth nerve palsy). These false localizing signs are rare but important because they indicate that the tumour is extensive enough to damage distant brain tissue, i.e. death is imminent unless urgent intervention occurs.

Diagnosis is usually straightforward, using computed tomography (CT) or magnetic resonance imaging (MRI) and stereotactic guided biopsy. Occasionally tumours are difficult to see on an unenhanced CT scan – accordingly once a tumour is suspected CT scanning must be contrast enhanced. Electroencephalography, although not indicated, may during the course of epilepsy investigations suggest an underlying neoplasm (focal slow wave activity). Lumbar puncture must not be undertaken because of the risk of 'coning' the brain into the foramen magnum.

Specific tumours

Fifty per cent of CNS tumours are secondary deposits from extracranial malignancies, commonly breast, lung, kidney, thyroid, stomach, prostate and melanoma. Accordingly, many patients with brain tumours should be investigated for an extracranial primary (breast examination, chest X-ray, prostate-specific antigen, abdominal imaging). A quarter of patients with carcinomatosis have brain involvement.

Primary tumours may be malignant or benign. However, the clinical effects of histologically non-malignant tumours may not be benign because pressure effects from expansion within the cranial cavity may lead to disability and death.

- **Astrocytoma**: the most common primary brain tumour, prevalent in the 50–60-year age range. They are divided into four types (I–IV) depending on the degree of malignancy. Glioblastoma multiforme is so undifferentiated as to make the cell of origin impossible to define. Growth is rapid and attempts at surgical excision result in disability and do not improve survival. Dexamethasone results in rapid reduction in neurological deficit as a result of reduction in oedema. Radiotherapy improves quality of life in selected cases and may extend survival by a few months.
- **Oligodendroglioma**: a slow-growing tumour, which may thus show calcification on CT scanning. Oligodendrogliomas occur in a younger population than astrocytomas.
- **Ependymoma**: occurs anywhere throughout the ventricular system and infiltrates into surrounding tissues.
- **Primary CNS lymphoma**: may be single or multifocal and is more common in immunocompromised patients, such as those with HIV, where the Epstein–Barr virus drives tumour growth. Metastatic spread from systemic lymphoma is uncommon and is usually meningeal rather than parenchymal. Primary CNS lymphoma may be exquisitely sensitive to steroids, which should therefore be avoided before a tissue diagnosis has been achieved.
- **Meningiomas**: these account for 20% of intracranial tumours; they arise from the arachnoid granulations and are usually closely related to the venous sinuses. They exert their clinical effects by direct compression of the brain and, although presentation is usually slow, it may be surprisingly acute, leading to the view that there is an inflammatory component. A reactive hyperostosis may occur in the overlying bone. The aim of treatment is complete surgical excision, but the recurrence rate is 30% at 10 years.
- **Acoustic neuroma/schwannoma**: the most common infratentorial tumour. They arise from the vestibular portion of nerve VIII and lie in the cerebellopontine angle, giving rise to symptoms referable to cranial nerves VIII, VII and VI.

Malignant meningitis

The spread of tumours to the nervous system may be via the bloodstream to the meninges. This can cause a diffuse subacute meningitis with headache, stiff neck and vomiting, or a multifocal neurological syndrome of deafness and other, typically lower, cranial nerve palsies. Examination of the cerebrospinal fluid (CSF) reveals a reactive lymphocytosis, a low glucose and a high protein. CSF cytology may reveal tumour cells. Occasionally severe limb weakness can result from diffuse infiltration of the nerve root with tumour. Treatment is usually unsuccessful, except in the case of lymphoma.

Paraneoplastic disorders

The loss of genetic regulation in malignant tumours may lead to the cell surface expression of proteins normally only found in neurons (onco-neuronal antigens). These may initiate an immune response, provoking damage of the nervous system. Antineuronal antibodies can be detected but these may not be pathogenic. Each of the syndromes has in common:

- An evolution over weeks to months.
- A relentlessly progressive course.
- A failure to respond to treatment of the primary tumour or of the immune response (steroids, intravenous immunoglobulin or plasma exchange). The exceptions are Eaton–Lambert myasthenic syndrome and anti-*N*-methyl-D-aspartic acid receptor antibody-associated limbic encephalitis.
- Oligoclonal bands in the CSF.
- Specific antibodies (anti-Hu, anti-Yo, etc.).
- Relatively normal CNS imaging.

Specific syndromes are described in Chapter 197.

Neurocutaneous syndromes

These are dominantly inherited and are the result of mutations in tumour-suppressor genes. They lead to benign and malignant tumours.

- **Neurofibromatosis** has an incidence of one in 3000, occurs in several patterns and may have an associated phaeochromocytoma (which should be suspected if hypertension occurs).
  - Type 1 (peripheral type) is characterized by multiple neurofibromas, café-au-lait patches, axillary freckling, Lisch nodule in the iris, meningiomas and malignant brain tumours, usually astrocytomas of the optic pathway. It is caused by mutations in the neurofibromin gene and has a very high new mutation rate.
  - Type 2 (central type) is the result of mutations in a gene called *Merlin*. Although the hallmark of this disease is the occurrence of bilateral vestibular schwannomas, most patients develop benign or malignant tumours in the spinal cord and elsewhere in the brain. There are also cutaneous manifestations.
- **Von Hippel–Lindau disease** involves tumours in multiple organ systems. As well as cerebellar and spinal cord haemangioblastomas and ocular angiomas, von Hippel–Lindau disease causes renal angiolipomatosis and renal cell carcinoma, phaeochromocytoma and islet cell tumours.

209 Spinal cord disease

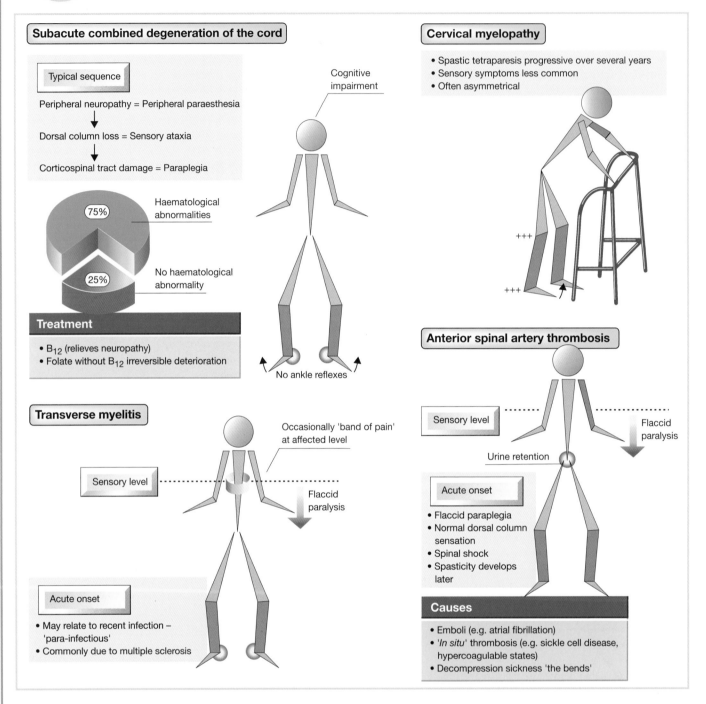

Subacute combined degeneration of the cord

Typical sequence

Peripheral neuropathy = Peripheral paraesthesia

↓

Dorsal column loss = Sensory ataxia

↓

Corticospinal tract damage = Paraplegia

75% — Haematological abnormalities

25% — No haematological abnormality

Treatment

- B_{12} (relieves neuropathy)
- Folate without B_{12} irreversible deterioration

Cognitive impairment

No ankle reflexes

Transverse myelitis

Sensory level

Occasionally 'band of pain' at affected level

Flaccid paralysis

Acute onset

- May relate to recent infection – 'para-infectious'
- Commonly due to multiple sclerosis

Cervical myelopathy

- Spastic tetraparesis progressive over several years
- Sensory symptoms less common
- Often asymmetrical

+++

+++

Anterior spinal artery thrombosis

Sensory level

Flaccid paralysis

Urine retention

Acute onset

- Flaccid paraplegia
- Normal dorsal column sensation
- Spinal shock
- Spasticity develops later

Causes

- Emboli (e.g. atrial fibrillation)
- 'In situ' thrombosis (e.g. sickle cell disease, hypercoagulable states)
- Decompression sickness 'the bends'

Acute spinal cord compression

Spinal cord compression presents with motor dysfunction predominantly affecting the lower limb, *whatever the level of the lesion*. This is associated with a sensory level and upper motor neuron signs below the level of the lesion. Abdominal reflexes are lost when the lesion is above T9. This is a medical emergency whatever the cause – urgent magnetic resonance imaging (MRI) is mandatory, and the results of such imaging dictate management. The spinal cord is most often compressed by:

- Secondary tumours from the breast, prostate and lung.
- Prolapsed intervertebral discs, which usually herniate laterally causing asymmetrical signs, although central disc prolapse can also occur.

Medicine at a Glance, Fourth Edition. Edited by Patrick Davey. © 2014 John Wiley & Sons, Ltd. Published 2014 by John Wiley & Sons, Ltd. Companion website: www.ataglanceseries.com/medicine

Abscess and other inflammatory lesions can also compress the spinal cord. The treatment usually involves surgical decompression or radiotherapy for malignant tumours.

Progressive spastic paraparesis

Bilateral weakness with marked spasticity of the lower limbs and extensor plantar responses can be subacute or chronic. It is always investigated by MRI of the spine, and has a number of important causes:

- **Vitamin B$_{12}$ deficiency**: this causes corticospinal tract damage (spastic paraparesis) associated with a peripheral neuropathy (absent ankle jerks) and dorsal column dysfunction (a high stepping gait, rombergism and pseudoathetosis of the outstretched fingers). This syndrome complex is termed subacute combined degeneration of the cord (SACD). It is important to appreciate that neurological dysfunction in isolation can occur before a rise in mean cell volume (MCV) or anaemia (see Chapter 176). In SACD, folic acid alone may exacerbate the neurological deficit. Accordingly, it is crucial to measure vitamin B$_{12}$, and replace it if deficient, in megaloblastic anaemias with any suggestion of spinal cord involvement. 'Low normal' B$_{12}$ levels with an appropriate clinical picture suggestive of SACD should prompt measurement of methyl malonic acid and homocystine levels, which are a more accurate measure of B$_{12}$ functionality than crude levels of the vitamin.
- **Copper deficiency**: this can cause a clinical picture identical to SACD but with a normal B$_{12}$. Deficiency can occur as part of a generalized malabsorption syndrome or occasionally as a consequence of zinc supplementation.
- **Cervical spondylotic myelopathy**: this is a condition of middle-aged and elderly people, in which degenerative changes in the vertebrae cause slowly progressive constriction of the cervical cord and sometimes the nerve roots at the exit foramina, producing a 'radiculopathy' (wasting, weakness, sensory loss, decreased reflexes). It can present with various combinations of neck pain, tingling of the upper limbs, sphincter dysfunction and gait disturbance. Reflexes in the arms and legs (except those supplied by compressed nerve roots) are very brisk, and often show clonus. Diagnosis is by MRI. The aim of surgery is to prevent worsening because only rarely does it improve symptoms.
- **Hereditary spastic paraparesis**: a genetically heterogeneous disease that can be autosomal dominant or recessive. It selectively affects the long motor tracts and characteristically produces more spasticity than weakness. It is very slowly progressive and typically comes on in early adult life, although cases may present into the fifties.
- **Motor neuron disease**: 1% of cases present with an indolent form called primary lateral sclerosis, in which upper motor neuron signs predominate until late in the illness. Survival may be prolonged (10–15 years as opposed to 2–3 years for amyotrophic lateral sclerosis).
- **Primary progressive multiple sclerosis**.

Transverse myelitis

This is an inflammatory illness localized to the middle of the spinal cord, which presents as acute weakness with an ascending sensory level, i.e. rather similar to acute cord compression (which must be excluded by urgent MRI). A proportion of patients have had a recent flu-like illness and this condition may occur as a parainfectious complication of *Mycoplasma* or *Legionella* spp., Epstein–Barr virus infections, herpes simplex and zoster, and others. Imaging may show a focal lesion in the spinal cord or be normal. In a proportion of patients, transverse myelitis is the first manifestation of multiple sclerosis. A related autoimmune form of cord demyelination ('longitudinally extensive transverse myelitis') is associated with aquaporin-4 antibodies.

Anterior spinal artery thrombosis

The particular anatomical arrangement of the blood supply to the spinal cord makes the mid and upper thoracic regions vulnerable to vascular insufficiency. Two posterior spinal arteries, which provide good collateral circulation, supply the posterior portion of the spinal cord. The anterior part of the cord (spinothalamic tracts, corticospinal tracts), however, is supplied by a solitary anterior spinal artery formed by the anastomosis of a branch from each vertebral artery at the level of the medulla. At a variable level (typically T4) there is a paucity of collateral circulation. If the blood supply here is compromised (e.g. by *in situ* thrombosis or an embolus), this leads to ischaemia in the anterior spinal artery territory which presents as a sudden (maximally over a few hours) flaccid paraparesis and loss of bladder function. Dorsal column function is preserved. Autonomic instability from spinal shock may ensue. Imaging is often normal acutely. There is no treatment and the prognosis for recovery is poor. An embolic source should be looked for (e.g. atrial fibrillation, recent myocardial infarction), vasculitis excluded, and general anti-atherogenic measures undertaken (see Chapters 81 and 82).

Disc prolapse

The prolapse may be central or lateral, so compressing the exit foramina of the nerves, producing radicular pain. The most common example of this is of a L4/5 or L5/S1 disc prolapse, resulting in pain radiating down the buttock and lower limb (sciatica). The signs are of decreased straight leg raising and diminished reflexes. Recovery is usually spontaneous – occasionally laminectomy is required.

Syringomyelia

This is an exceptionally rare illness, in which the central canal in the cervical spinal cord enlarges into a large fluid-filled cavity (the syrinx). This is predisposed to by mild (or more severe) herniation of the cerebellar tonsils into (or beyond) the foramen magnum (the Arnold–Chiari malformation) or previous trauma. The expanding syrinx damages local structures, especially the decussating spinothalamic tracts (producing loss of pain and temperature sensation and, distressingly, severe pain in the same distribution), the corticospinal tracts (spastic weakness) and anterior horn cells (muscle wasting). Cranial nerve signs follow extension of the syrinx into the medulla. Diagnosis is by MRI. Neurosurgical drainage may have a role.

Spinal shock

Sudden transsection of the spinal cord at a cervical or upper thoracic level (often traumatic) can lead to loss of autonomic vasomotor control of blood pressure, which leads to catastrophic hypotension. Substantial fluid replacement is needed.

210 Neuromuscular disease

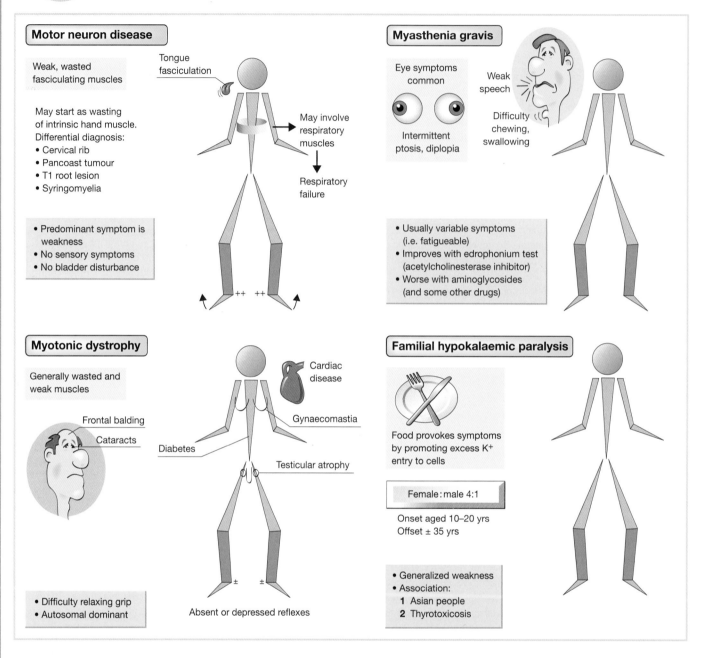

Motor neuron disease

Weak, wasted fasciculating muscles

May start as wasting of intrinsic hand muscle. Differential diagnosis:
• Cervical rib
• Pancoast tumour
• T1 root lesion
• Syringomyelia

• Predominant symptom is weakness
• No sensory symptoms
• No bladder disturbance

Tongue fasciculation

May involve respiratory muscles

Respiratory failure

++   ++

Myasthenia gravis

Eye symptoms common

Weak speech

Difficulty chewing, swallowing

Intermittent ptosis, diplopia

• Usually variable symptoms (i.e. fatigueable)
• Improves with edrophonium test (acetylcholinesterase inhibitor)
• Worse with aminoglycosides (and some other drugs)

Myotonic dystrophy

Generally wasted and weak muscles

Frontal balding

Cataracts

Diabetes

Cardiac disease

Gynaecomastia

Testicular atrophy

±   ±

Absent or depressed reflexes

• Difficulty relaxing grip
• Autosomal dominant

Familial hypokalaemic paralysis

Food provokes symptoms by promoting excess K+ entry to cells

Female: male 4:1

Onset aged 10–20 yrs
Offset ± 35 yrs

• Generalized weakness
• Association:
  1 Asian people
  2 Thyrotoxicosis

The motor unit

There are four possible sites at which pathological processes of the neuromuscular unit may act:

1 The anterior horn cell or lower motor neuron.
2 The peripheral nerve.
3 The neuromuscular junction.
4 The muscle.

Peripheral neuropathies are dealt with in Chapter 211.

Motor neuron disease

Motor neuron disease (MND) is a disorder of complex aetiology, which leads to selective, but not exclusive, degeneration of upper and lower motor neurons. It is characterized by the deposition of ubiquitinated intraneuronal inclusions which stain for the nuclear

protein TDP-43. It is relatively rare (2/100 000 per year) and malignant in behaviour – the average time from diagnosis to death is 2.5 years. Of cases of MND, 5% show familial inheritance (autosomal dominant), but 5% of sporadic cases also have gene mutations (due to low penetrance rare variants). The commonest mutation is a hexanucleotide repeat in a gene of unknown function (*C9orf72*) on chromosome 9, which can also cause fronto-temporal dementia. Other genes in which mutations are associated with MND are *TDP-43*, *FUS* and *SOD1*.

Clinical features

The most common presentation (70%) is with wasting and weakness of one limb. Examination shows mixed upper and lower motor signs in several limbs – a combination of fasciculation, wasting, weakness, extensor plantar responses and brisk reflexes (amyotrophic lateral sclerosis). Tongue fasciculation is a useful sign because it makes a compressive lesion of the spinal cord an unlikely explanation for the observed neurological dysfunction.

Other patients (20%) present with prominent bulbar symptoms before developing signs in the limbs (progressive bulbar palsy) or a pure lower motor neuron picture of symmetrical weakness, wasting and areflexia (progressive muscular atrophy). Similarly, the disease may appear to be restricted to the upper motor neurons and presents a picture of progressive spastic paraparesis. This variant, known as primary lateral sclerosis, is more indolent and survival may be prolonged. Approximately 5% of patients have coexisting frontotemporal dementia and up to 40% have more subtle executive dysfunction.

Diagnosis

Diagnosis is clinical but supported by electromyographic demonstration of denervation in all four limbs. There are no specific treatments and management aims to preserve nutritional status and provide supportive respiratory and terminal care. The glutamate antagonist riluzole prolongs time to ventilation and tracheostomy by 3 months.

Poliomyelitis

Poliomyelitis is rarely seen in countries with effective immunization programmes. It produces asymmetrical motor weakness with bulbar and respiratory compromise in the context of an acute febrile illness. Some patients undergo late deterioration in function decades after the acute illness (post-polio syndrome).

Myasthenia gravis

Myasthenia gravis is an autoimmune disease – antibodies are directed against the acetylcholine receptor in the majority of patients and against the neuromuscular junction protein MUSK in a minority of others. The clinical features are variable, but include:

- Symmetrical proximal muscle weakness, which fatigues on exertion.
- Prominent involvement of the extraocular muscles, producing diplopia and ptosis. Significant limb weakness without eye involvement is rare. In contrast, myasthenia confined to the eyes (ocular myasthenia) is a distinct condition in which many patients do not have acetylcholine receptor antibodies and whose course is more benign.
- Bulbar involvement with dysphagia, dysarthria and a risk of aspiration.
- Myasthenic crises with a rapid evolution of neuromuscular weakness, leading to emergency ventilation.
- An association with thymoma in older patients, and thymic hyperplasia in younger patients.

Treatment is with immunomodulatory therapy (corticosteroids, azathioprine, plasma exchange), thymectomy and drugs that prolong the action of acetylcholine in the neuromuscular junction.

Inflammatory myopathies

Inflammatory myopathies are of presumed autoimmune aetiology, although usually without specific antibodies, where muscle is involved in isolation or in the context of a more diffuse connective tissue disease. They are typically painless. The creatine phosphokinase level is elevated by several thousand. There is a clinical and pathological spectrum from polymyositis to dermatomyositis (see Chapter 222). The latter is associated in elderly people with malignancy and more often involves swallowing dysfunction. Therapy is with steroids, intravenous immunoglobulin and occasionally plasma exchange.

Inclusion body myositis affects middle-aged to elderly people and presents with the insidious onset of slowly progressive, asymmetrical, painless wasting and weakness of muscles, especially the quadriceps. There is no effective treatment.

Muscular dystrophies

Muscular dystrophies are inherited diseases leading to progressive wasting and weakness. The nosology of the dystrophies is being redefined according to specific genetic mutations and associated molecular deficits:

- Dystrophinopathies are caused by mutations in the gene encoding the very large membrane-associated protein dystrophin, thought to have a function in anchoring the muscle cytoskeleton to the extracellular matrix. Duchenne's muscular dystrophy is caused by mutations that lead to complete loss of functional protein and a severe muscle disease, with onset in early childhood, loss of ambulation by adolescence and death in the twenties or thirties from cardiorespiratory failure. Becker's dystrophy is caused by mutations in dystrophin, which produce a truncated and partially functional protein. Onset can be at any time from infancy to late adult life and the prognosis is much more favourable.
- Sarcoglycanopathies are rarer disorders resulting from mutations in genes encoding a variety of other membrane-associated proteins.
- Limb girdle muscular dystrophies.
- Facioscapulohumeral muscular dystrophy.
- Oculopharyngeal muscular dystrophy.

Myotonic dystrophy

Myotonic dystrophy is a multisystem disorder characterized by distal weakness and wasting, male pattern balding, an increased incidence of diabetes mellitus, cardiac conduction defects, cataract and excessive daytime somnolence. It is caused by mutations in the non-coding part of the myotonin protein kinase gene, which contains a triplet repeat (CTG) and undergoes dynamic expansion. Successive generations are progressively more severely affected (genetic anticipation). In one pedigree the phenotype may range from cataract to congenital myotonic dystrophy with death in infancy. Genetic testing usually makes diagnosis by electromyography unnecessary.

Metabolic myopathies

Metabolic myopathies are rare disorders caused by specific enzyme defects in pathways important for muscle function. There is a wide spectrum of clinical presentation, but suggestive features are exertional muscle pain and myoglobinuria:

- Mitochondrial diseases: myopathy is associated with a variable phenotype, including glucose intolerance, pigmentary retinopathy, seizures, stroke-like episodes and deafness. One form is chronic progressive external ophthalmoplegia.
- Disorders of fatty acid metabolism, e.g. carnitine palmitoyl transferase deficiency.
- Disorders of carbohydrate metabolism, e.g. glycogen storage diseases such as acid maltase deficiency.
- Periodic paralysis occurs in a hypokalaemic and a rarer hyperkalaemic form. These are the result of mutations in ion channels (channelopathies). Patients present with attacks of generalized weakness lasting for several hours. Precipitants include large meals, alcohol and cold weather.

211 Peripheral neuropathy

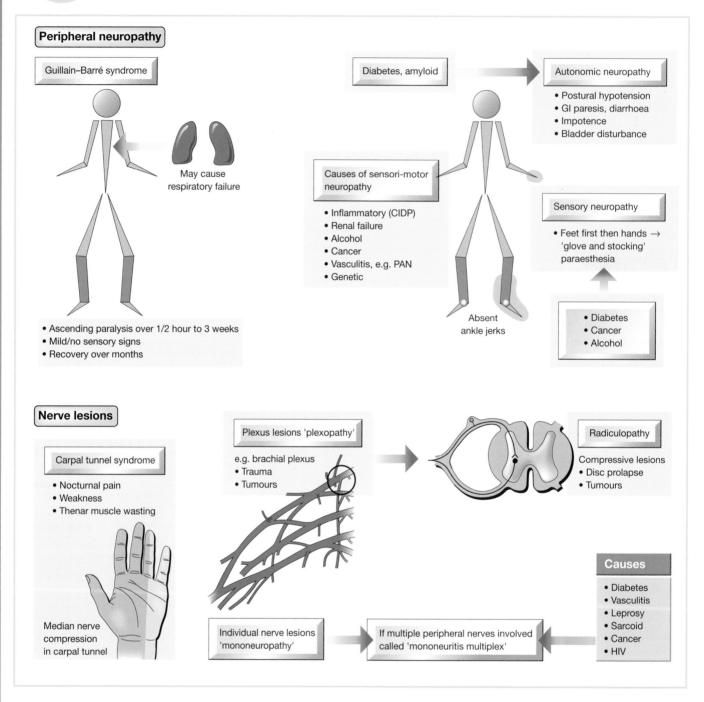

Peripheral neuropathy

Guillain–Barré syndrome

May cause respiratory failure

- Ascending paralysis over 1/2 hour to 3 weeks
- Mild/no sensory signs
- Recovery over months

Diabetes, amyloid

Autonomic neuropathy

- Postural hypotension
- GI paresis, diarrhoea
- Impotence
- Bladder disturbance

Causes of sensori-motor neuropathy

- Inflammatory (CIDP)
- Renal failure
- Alcohol
- Cancer
- Vasculitis, e.g. PAN
- Genetic

Absent ankle jerks

Sensory neuropathy

- Feet first then hands → 'glove and stocking' paraesthesia

- Diabetes
- Cancer
- Alcohol

Nerve lesions

Carpal tunnel syndrome

- Nocturnal pain
- Weakness
- Thenar muscle wasting

Median nerve compression in carpal tunnel

Plexus lesions 'plexopathy'

e.g. brachial plexus
- Trauma
- Tumours

Radiculopathy

Compressive lesions
- Disc prolapse
- Tumours

Individual nerve lesions 'mononeuropathy'

If multiple peripheral nerves involved called 'mononeuritis multiplex'

Causes

- Diabetes
- Vasculitis
- Leprosy
- Sarcoid
- Cancer
- HIV

Clinical approach

Accurate diagnosis of a peripheral neuropathy requires an understanding of neuropathy classification and the speed of onset of symptoms, and a knowledge of which diseases commonly cause neuropathy.

Neuropathy classification

- **Polyneuropathies**: diffuse damage to peripheral nerves. The longest nerves (i.e. supplying the hand and foot) are most vulnerable to damage and are usually affected earliest. Polyneuropathies may be:

- Pure motor or pure sensory.
- Sensorimotor: the most common pattern. Damage is symmetrical. Paraesthesiae and dysaesthesiae are early symptoms. Cramps and spasms commonly occur later. Examination shows diminution of reflexes, weakness, variable wasting and sensory loss. Sensory ataxia is manifest by Rombergism and pseudoathetosis. Trophic changes such as ulcers and joint deformity are found in long-standing neuropathies.
- Autonomic.
- **Radiculopathy**: a disorder of the nerve roots; if present at multiple levels it is termed a polyradiculopathy.

- **Plexopathy**: affecting the nerves of the brachial or lumbosacral plexus.
- **Mononeuropathy**: isolated to a single peripheral nerve, or if a number of anatomically discrete nerves are affected it is called a mononeuritis multiplex.

Consider the evolution of the problem (although there is considerable overlap):

- Acute: vascular, inflammatory, toxic.
- Subacute: inflammatory, toxic, nutritional, systemic illness.
- Chronic: hereditary, metabolic.

Investigation of peripheral nerve disease

Initial screening blood tests should include: full blood count, erythrocyte sedimentation rate, electrolytes and liver function tests to look for any evidence of systemic disease. Specific causes of neuropathy should be excluded with blood glucose, vitamin B_{12}, thyroid function, serum electrophoresis (for a paraprotein) and autoantibodies (especially antineutrophil cytoplasmic antibody and antinuclear antibody). Neuropathy is confirmed and classified (i.e. demyelinating vs axonal) by nerve conduction studies and electromyography (EMG). Parameters measured include: (i) nerve conduction velocity; (ii) the amplitude of nerve and muscle response to stimulation; and (iii) denervation of muscle, i.e. spontaneous electrical activity (fibrillation).

In demyelinating neuropathies (e.g. Guillain–Barré syndrome), there is slowing of conduction velocity and little evidence of denervation. In axonal neuropathy (e.g. caused by drugs such as vincristine), there is normal motor conduction velocity with decreased compound muscle action potential and evidence of denervation on EMG.

Nerve biopsy is not performed frequently. It is most useful to confirm vasculitis before commencing therapy.

Polyneuropathies

Inherited

Peripheral neuropathy occurs as part of many complex neurogenetic disorders. The most common cause of inherited, isolated, peripheral neuropathy is hereditary motor and sensory neuropathy or Charcot–Marie–Tooth disease. The most common genetic subtype is a duplication of part of the short arm of chromosome 17, which causes a very slowly progressive demyelinating neuropathy with wasting below the knees, pes cavus and hand involvement.

Metabolic derangement

- Diabetes mellitus is the most common cause of peripheral neuropathy in the developed world. The usual picture is a progressive, predominantly sensory neuropathy. Loss of vibration sense is the earliest sign. Over time, if diabetes is poorly controlled, autonomic involvement becomes universal. Pain can be difficult to manage.
- Vitamin deficiencies (vitamin B_{12}, thiamine, vitamin E) all cause neuropathy as part of a broader neurological syndrome.
- Chronic renal failure and liver failure can produce peripheral neuropathy.
- Hyperthyroidism is a rare cause.

Toxic and drug induced

Alcohol is a very common cause, as are drugs: amiodarone, metronidazole, cytotoxics, pyridoxine, isoniazid, dapsone, lithium, anti-retrovirals.

Inflammatory/immune polyneuropathy

- Guillain–Barré syndrome: incidence 1–2 per 100 000. It is an autoimmune response occuring typically 1–3 weeks after an infection (cytomegalovirus and *Campylobacter* sp. are commonest). Mild sensory symptoms are often present. Weakness, which is usually a mixture of proximal and distal, ascends proximally over a few days. Respiratory failure requiring ventilation may occur (vital capacity should be frequently measured). Spontaneous recovery – sometimes full, occasionally incomplete – is usual, although 5% die. Autonomic imbalance can produce cardiac arrhythmias. Illness duration is shortened with γ-globulin or plasma exchange, but steroids are ineffective.
- Chronic idiopathic demyelinating polyneuropathy (CIDP) runs a waxing–waning course. Nerve conduction studies are diagnostic. Steroids or γ-globulin help.
- Other neuropathies: vasculitis, critical illness polyneuropathy, infective (leprosy, Lyme disease, HIV, diphtheria), traumatic (entrapment or crush injuries) and paraneoplastic.

Common mononeuropathies

Nerve entrapment is generally the result of local factors, but in some conditions it is much more common and sometimes multiple: (i) hypothyroidism; (ii) acromegaly; (iii) Paget's disease; (iv) rheumatoid disease; and (v) hereditary neuropathy with liability to pressure palsies caused by deletion of the *PMP-22* gene.

In mononeuropathies it is important to consider the possibility that the apparently isolated nerve lesion is part of a mononeuritis multiplex syndrome.

- **Median nerve**: by far the most common mononeuropathy is carpal tunnel syndrome. Lifetime incidence is 6% in women, 0.6% in men (especially manual workers using vibrating machinery). Typical symptoms are of pain, discomfort and tingling in the hand radiating to the forearm and occasionally the shoulder. These commonly wake the patient from sleep and are relieved by shaking the wrist. Symptoms are also precipitated by repetitive flexion at the wrist, e.g. when steering a car. Treatment is by surgical release. Wrist splints are occasionally helpful.
- **Ulnar nerve**: this nerve is vulnerable to compression and injury at the elbow (e.g. arthritis, fracture) where it is superficially located. Patients present with numbness of the little and ring fingers and ulnar border of the hand, wasting and weakness of the first dorsal interosseous, and weakness of the abductor digiti minimi.
- **Lateral popliteal (common peroneal) nerve**: this is very vulnerable to compressive injury at the head of the fibula (e.g. by a plaster cast). Lesions cause painless foot drop as a result of weakness of tibialis anterior. The ankle jerk is retained.

Rarer mononeuropathies

Radial nerve damage is the result of nerve compression in the axilla (e.g. by a chair: 'Saturday night' palsy) or as the nerve winds round the head of the humerus. Patients present with wrist drop.

Femoral nerve damage relate to diabetes, pelvic lesions, particularly inflammation or haematoma (in anticoagulated patients), iliopsoas pathology or, more rarely, lesions in the femoral canal. The quadriceps wastes, extension at the knee is weak, and there is variable sensory loss over the anterior thigh.

Mononeuritis multiplex

This occurs in diabetes, systemic vasculitis, leprosy, sarcoidosis, non-metastatic manifestation of malignancy and HIV. Investigation and treatment are of the underlying disease.

212 Movement disorders

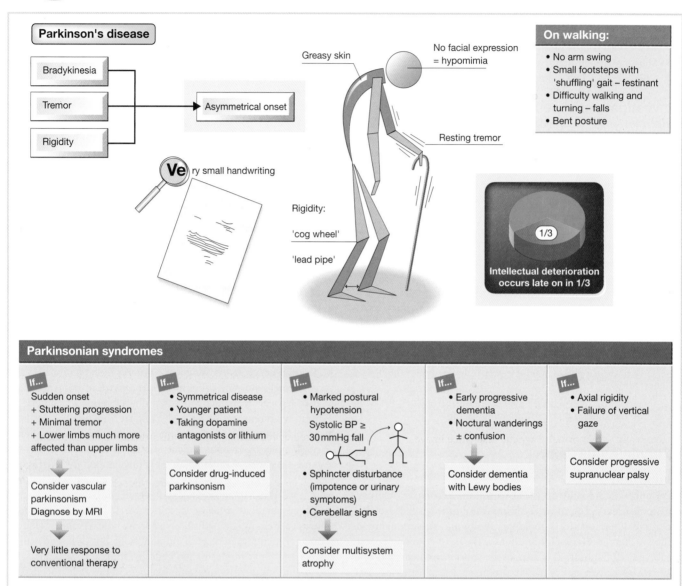

Parkinson's disease

- Bradykinesia
- Tremor
- Rigidity

→ Asymmetrical onset

Very small handwriting

Greasy skin

No facial expression = hypomimia

Resting tremor

Rigidity:
'cog wheel'
'lead pipe'

On walking:
- No arm swing
- Small footsteps with 'shuffling' gait – festinant
- Difficulty walking and turning – falls
- Bent posture

1/3
Intellectual deterioration occurs late on in 1/3

Parkinsonian syndromes

If...
Sudden onset
+ Stuttering progression
+ Minimal tremor
+ Lower limbs much more affected than upper limbs
→
Consider vascular parkinsonism
Diagnose by MRI
→
Very little response to conventional therapy

If...
- Symmetrical disease
- Younger patient
- Taking dopamine antagonists or lithium
→
Consider drug-induced parkinsonism

If...
- Marked postural hypotension
Systolic BP ≥ 30 mmHg fall
- Sphincter disturbance (impotence or urinary symptoms)
- Cerebellar signs
→
Consider multisystem atrophy

If...
- Early progressive dementia
- Noctural wanderings ± confusion
→
Consider dementia with Lewy bodies

If...
- Axial rigidity
- Failure of vertical gaze
→
Consider progressive supranuclear palsy

Parkinsonism

The term 'parkinsonism' describes a syndrome of poverty of movement, resting tremor, rigidity and varying degrees of postural instability.

Parkinson's disease is characterized by asymmetrical onset, slow progression and good response to L-dopa therapy. Only 60% develop tremor. The pathology is loss of dopamine-producing cells of the substantia nigra and Lewy bodies (intraneuronal inclusions). The aetiology, except in genetic cases, is poorly understood. Although predominantly an age-dependent sporadic disease, about 5% of patients have mutations in a range of genes (there are at least 18 separate loci). Onset in young adulthood (<30 years) is associated with a recessive mutation in the *Parkin* gene. Mutations in *LRRK2* cause the disease and the common *Gly2019Ser* mutation is present in 1% of patients with sporadic and 4% of patients with hereditary Parkinson's disease.

Diagnosis

The diagnosis is clinical – structural imaging is normal. Helpful signs are asymmetrical loss of arm swing, micrographia (small handwriting) and facial hypomimia, and the more 'classic' signs of 'cogwheel' stiffness and resting tremor. Bradykinesia is best tested for by checking repetitive finger or foot tapping, which shows degradation in amplitude and interruptions in Parkinson's disease. Other neurodegenerative conditions are included in the differential diagnosis and are suspected if there are:

- Early falls.
- Early cognitive impairment.
- Symmetrical onset.
- Prominent autonomic disturbance including sphincter involvement.
- Pyramidal tract or cerebellar signs.

Medicine at a Glance, Fourth Edition. Edited by Patrick Davey. © 2014 John Wiley & Sons, Ltd. Published 2014 by John Wiley & Sons, Ltd. Companion website: www.ataglanceseries.com/medicine

Treatment and prognosis

Parkinson's disease is progressive and pharmacological manipulation changes as the condition advances. At onset it is usually a problem of poverty of movement. Later on, troublesome dyskinesia, unpredictable freezing and 'on–off' phenomena dominate the picture. Ten per cent of patients develop these problems for each year from diagnosis. Most patients ultimately develop detectable cognitive impairment, with frank dementia in about one-third.

Drug therapy involves increasing dopamine levels in the central nervous system (CNS), by giving either L-dopa with a peripheral decarboxylase inhibitor, or drugs that stimulate CNS dopamine receptors (dopamine agonists, e.g. pramipexole, ropinorole, cabergoline, apomorphine) or inhibit the breakdown of CNS dopamine. Drug side effects are common and include dyskinesias and 'on–off' phenomena. Dopamine agonists should be used with caution and are associated with rare but devastating side effects in susceptible individuals, such as pathological gambling and hypersexuality. In complex disease, dominated by unintended side effects of medication, deep brain stimulation, especially of the subthalamic nucleus, is used.

Drug-induced parkinsonism

Neuroleptics, antiemetics and occasionally calcium channel blockers and lithium can all produce parkinsonism. This is typically an early side effect and is more common with ageing. In contrast to Parkinson's disease, it is symmetrical in onset, tremor is less prominent and improvement occurs on withdrawal of the offending agent. Sometimes drugs unmask idiopathic Parkonson's disease.

Vascular parkinsonism

This rare disorder is characterized by bradykinesia and rigidity of the lower limbs, with marked sparing of the upper limbs. There will usually be a history of stuttering evolution, vascular risk factors and an abnormal magnetic resonance image.

Neurodegenerative akinetic–rigid syndromes mimicking Parkinson's disease

- **Multiple system atrophy** (MSA): formally known as Shy–Drager syndrome, nigrostriatal degeneration or olivopontocerebellar atrophy, depending on the predominant clinical features, until it was realized that all these conditions are linked by the same pathology (specific glial inclusions that stain for α-synuclein) and that they overlap clinically. Current classification divides the condition into MSA-P if parkinsonian features predominate, or MSA-C if cerebellar features dominate. Patients have the insidious onset of parkinsonism with sphincter disturbance, postural hypotension, cerebellar signs and, characteristically, but less commonly, stridor. Cognition is unaffected. The prognosis is poor (death within 2–8 years) and the response to L-dopa is absent or rapidly wanes.
- **Progressive supranuclear palsy**: characterized by prominent axial rigidity, loss of postural reflexes leading to early falls, progressive loss of downgaze and upgaze, dystonia of eyelid opening and facial dystonia imparting a characteristic expression of frowning and surprise. Cognitive impairment occurs later in the condition, which leads to death within 5–7 years.
- **Dementia with Lewy bodies**: parkinsonism with prominent nocturnal wanderings and hallucinations, early and progressive cognitive impairment and myoclonus. Poor response to L-dopa and idiosyncratic but severe reactions to neuroleptics.
- **Corticobasal degeneration**: the picture is of a stuttering evolution of parkinsonism plus parietal lobe abnormalities – including, characteristically, an alien limb abnormality of the arm, dysphasia, extensor plantars, myoclonus and dystonia – and dementia. It is rare. Death occurs in 5–7 years.

Dystonia

Focal dystonias such as writer's cramp and hemifacial spasm (see Chapter 62) can be treated with injections of botulinum toxin. It is a presynaptic blocker of neuromuscular transmission, causing weakness of the injected muscles for up to 3 months, relieving the symptoms over that period.

Huntington's disease

Huntington's disease is caused by an expanded trinucleotide repeat mutation in the *Huntingtin* gene and is inherited as an autosomal dominant. This is a disorder of insidious onset and inexorable progression, in which the first changes are often in personality (poor impulse control, irritability); the subsequent development of chorea, dementia and immobility occurs over 10–15 years.

Drug-induced movement disorders

The neuroleptic class of drugs (e.g. haloperidol), including antiemetics (e.g. prochlorperazine), are dopamine receptor antagonists and, in addition to parkinsonism, can induce acute dystonias, including oculogyric crisis, akathisia (motor restlessness) and tardive dyskinesias. The last are involuntary writhing movements of the face (especially mouth) and limbs, commonly seen in patients treated for schizophrenia.

Movement disorders in young people

The main condition to consider is Wilson's disease because it is treatable. This is an autosomal recessive disease caused by mutations in a gene coding for a copper-transporting protein. It can present as:

- Fulminant hepatic failure in childhood.
- Progressive neuropsychiatric disturbance in adolescence.
- Focal dystonia, dysarthria and drooling.

Diagnosis is by finding a low level of ceruloplasmin and free copper in serum. Patients with neurological Wilson's disease all have Kayser–Fleischer rings visible on slit-lamp examination of the cornea. The condition is treated by copper chelation therapy, usually with penicillamine.

Movement disorders relating to infection

A variety of movement disorders occur as an immune reaction to infections, especially *Streptococcus*. Patients can present with chorea, parkinsonism or some combination including mild psychiatric symptoms such as obsessionality or tics. In a significant proportion of patients it is possible to identify anti-basal ganglia antibodies, though the association is still uncertain.

Gilles de la Tourette's syndrome

Gilles de la Tourette's syndrome presents with a combination of multiple motor and vocal tics (i.e. involuntary vocalizations), both of varying complexity, with onset in childhood usually between 7 and 11 years of age. The prevalence is 1/2000 with a very wide range of severity. Involuntary swearing (coprolalia) is a feature in a minority of cases. Obsessive–compulsive disorder is often also present. The tics can be treated with neuroleptics, e.g. sulpiride, or clomipramine.

Dopa-responsive dystonia

Dopa-responsive dystonia is another rare but treatable genetic disorder caused by mutations in a gene in the pathway of dopa synthesis. It presents with lower limb dystonia, which fluctuates throughout the day. Treatment with L-dopa can result in dramatic improvement.

213 Osteoarthritis

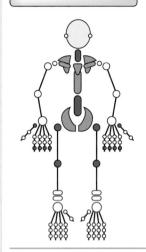

Osteoarthritis

Distribution of joints commonly affected by OA

Distal interphalangeals (DIPs)
1st carpometacarpal (CMCs)
Hips
Knees
Lumbar spine
Cervical spine
PIPs (less frequently)

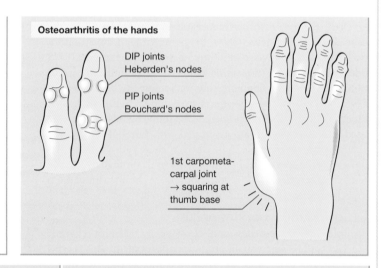

Osteoarthritis of the hands

DIP joints
Heberden's nodes

PIP joints
Bouchard's nodes

1st carpometa-
carpal joint
→ squaring at
thumb base

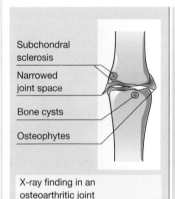

Subchondral sclerosis

Narrowed joint space

Bone cysts

Osteophytes

X-ray finding in an osteoarthritic joint

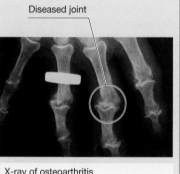

Diseased joint

X-ray of osteoarthritis

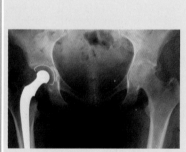

Large joint replacement is very successful in relieving symptoms in advanced osteoarthritis. Complications include:
• Operative: death, MI
• Postoperative: pulmonary embolism, deep vein thrombosis
• Dislocation
• Prosthesis infection
• Loosening

X-ray of joint replacement

Osteoarthritis (OA) is the most common arthropathy of adults. Its aetiology is multifactorial, and it is characterized by progressive cartilage loss and hypertrophic changes in surrounding bone (osteophytosis), resulting in progressive degenerative joint disease. Inflammation is not a marked feature.

Epidemiology

The overall prevalence of OA is 12–15% in at least one joint, and is much higher in the >65 years age group. The prevalence continually increases with advancing age, such that more than 80% of >75-year-olds have radiographic evidence of OA. There is a slight female preponderance overall, particularly in interphalangeal joint disease.

Aetiology and pathogenesis

The cause is unknown but familial aggregation of cases is consistent with an important genetic contribution. Siblings of patients undergoing major lower limb joint replacement for OA are three times more likely than the general population to require similar surgery themselves.

Pathological features are those of progressive cartilage damage and loss. Reactive bony hypertrophy next to cartilage loss results

in characteristic 'osteophyte' development. There is subchondral bone sclerosis and cyst formation which is evident on plain X-rays (see Figure 213.1).

Classification

1 **Primary or idiopathic OA**.
2 **Secondary OA**: this arises from:
   • Trauma, including repetitive use in some occupations associated with heavy loading of the joints. OA may also develop as a late complication of trauma, particularly if osteochondral fracture or meniseal injury has occurred in the knee.
   • Obesity increases the risk of knee OA.
   • Congenital conditions, e.g. hip dislocation or underlying joint dysplasia.
   • Inflammatory arthritis (rheumatoid arthritis, gout).
   • A late complication following bacterial infection of a joint.
   • Acromegaly.
   • Haemophilia.

Clinical features

The following are distinguishing features on the history:

Medicine at a Glance, Fourth Edition. Edited by Patrick Davey. © 2014 John Wiley & Sons, Ltd. Published 2014 by John Wiley & Sons, Ltd. Companion website: www.ataglanceseries.com/medicine

- Joint pain tends to be insidious in onset. Typically there is slow stepwise deterioration in symptoms.
- Pain is aggravated by activity, relieved by rest, is worst at the end of the day and as the condition progresses, and becomes increasingly severe, occurring on minimal movement. Sleep disturbance may exacerbate fatigue and be associated with secondary fibromyalgia.
- Stiffness is minor in the morning but recurs throughout the day with periods of rest, and is described as 'gelling' following inactivity.
- Bony swelling may be noted particularly in the hands (see Figure 213.1) as Heberden's nodes (distal interphalangeal (DIP) joint involvement) and Bouchard's nodes (proximal interphalangeal (PIP) joint involvement). Variable symmetry of large joint involvement occurs that often impairs gait and mobility.

Physical findings

The distribution of joints affected in OA is shown in Figure 213.1. Examination reveals:

- Bony prominence due to a combination of marginal osteophytes and joint deformities (occasionally OA can cause effusions, particularly if it is associated with intra-articular calcium crystal deposition).
- Reduction in range of movement in affected joints with 'end of range' pain and limitation, and palpable 'crepitus'.
- Instability in later stages, particularly where there is associated muscle wasting around the joint and substantial cartilage loss.

Subsets of osteoarthritis

These include:

- **Primary generalized OA**: predominantly in middle-aged women, affecting the first carpometacarpal (CMC) joint, PIP joint, distal DIPs, and joint, knee, hips and spine.
- **Chondromalacia patellae**: limited patellofemoral joint OA, causing pain on climbing stairs, running or squatting.
- **Inflammatory OA**: this affects predominantly postmenopausal women in the distal DIP and/or PIP joints of the hand. Episodes of pain and inflammation may mimic rheumatoid or psoriatic arthritis. X-rays often show erosions as well as the classic hallmarks of OA. It is probably associated with crystal deposition (calcium pyrophosphate, hydroxyapatite).

Investigations

Inflammatory markers (erythrocyte sedimentation rate, C-reactive protein) are normal; serology for antinuclear antibody and rheumatoid factor are unnecessary except in cases with symptoms suggestive of inflammation. Synovial fluid from joint aspiration is clear with normal viscosity and is non-inflammatory (low white cell count) on microscopy; the fluid should be examined for calcium pyrophosphate crystals. Plain X-ray reveals characteristic features of joint space narrowing, bony sclerosis, subchondral cysts and osteophytes (the radiological hallmark) (see Figure 213.1). Consider iron and calcium studies in those with atypical distribution or age of onset (to exclude haemochromatosis or hyperparathyroidism).

The differential diagnosis may include arthropathy of psoriasis, Reiter's syndrome or crystal deposition disease, indicating tests for these conditions where clinically indicated.

Management

The goals of therapy are to relieve pain and maintain function.

Pharmacological management

- Management should rely on simple step-up analgesia such as paracetamol, and topical therapies such as ice, heat or locally applied analgesic creams, including capsaicin cream applied locally.
- Low-dose non-steroidal anti-inflammatory drugs (NSAIDs) should be used in those without contraindication.
- Unresponsive or progressive pain may necessitate full-dose NSAID therapy or other analgesia including opiates. Transdermal sustained release opiates ('patch') may be useful in those with severe pain either awaiting or unsuitable for joint replacement surgery.
- Intra-articular injection of corticosteroid sometimes gives relief of pain, though this may be short-lived. Repeated injections 6 months apart may be beneficial in symptom control. Periarticular injection of painful soft tissues may also be of benefit. In a small number of patients a course of intra-articular injections of hyaluronan (a component of synovial fluid) may be useful.

Physical therapy

- Weight reduction substantially reduces the loading of lower limb load-bearing joints, which may be up to six times body weight during exercise.
- Low-impact aerobic exercise regimens (cycling/swimming) and weight loss programmes are particularly associated with symptomatic improvement and may reduce progression and the requirement for surgery.
- Soft collars and lumbar braces for short periods sometimes help cervical and lumbar OA. Knee braces and foot orthoses are particularly helpful for lower limb problems.

Surgical therapy

Joint replacement dramatically improves pain, function and quality of life in those with advanced disease. Outcome following hip or knee surgery is good or excellent in 95% of patients. The prostheses may be expected to function satisfactorily for 15 years. The main complications are sepsis and aseptic loosening. Revision surgery may subsequently be required and still provides good results in 80% of cases.

214 Gout and pseudogout

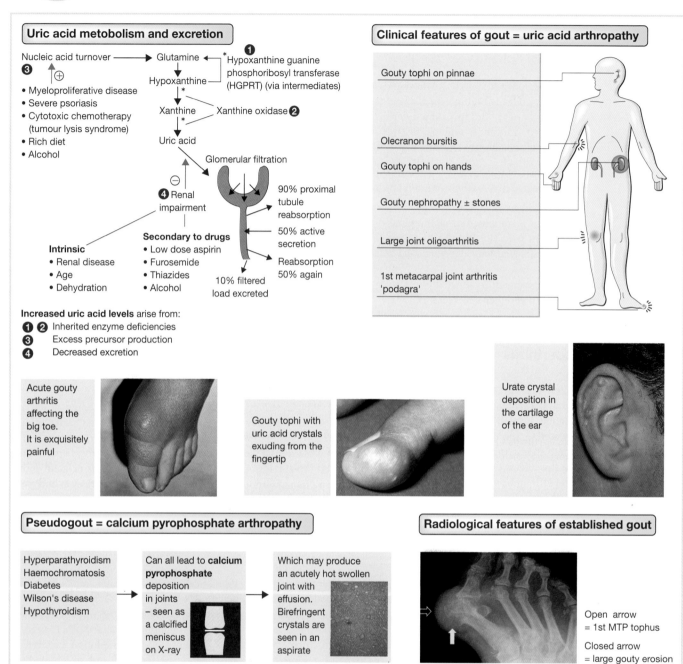

Uric acid metabolism and excretion

Nucleic acid turnover → Glutamine ← * Hypoxanthine guanine phosphoribosyl transferase (HGPRT) (via intermediates) **1**

❸
⊕
• Myeloproliferative disease
• Severe psoriasis
• Cytotoxic chemotherapy (tumour lysis syndrome)
• Rich diet
• Alcohol

Hypoxanthine

Xanthine ← Xanthine oxidase **2**
*
Uric acid

Glomerular filtration

⊖
4 Renal impairment

90% proximal tubule reabsorption

50% active secretion

Reabsorption 50% again

10% filtered load excreted

Intrinsic
• Renal disease
• Age
• Dehydration

Secondary to drugs
• Low dose aspirin
• Furosemide
• Thiazides
• Alcohol

Increased uric acid levels arise from:
1 2 Inherited enzyme deficiencies
3 Excess precursor production
4 Decreased excretion

Clinical features of gout = uric acid arthropathy

Gouty tophi on pinnae

Olecranon bursitis

Gouty tophi on hands

Gouty nephropathy ± stones

Large joint oligoarthritis

1st metacarpal joint arthritis 'podagra'

Acute gouty arthritis affecting the big toe. It is exquisitely painful

Gouty tophi with uric acid crystals exuding from the fingertip

Urate crystal deposition in the cartilage of the ear

Pseudogout = calcium pyrophosphate arthropathy

Hyperparathyroidism
Haemochromatosis
Diabetes
Wilson's disease
Hypothyroidism

→ Can all lead to **calcium pyrophosphate** deposition in joints – seen as a calcified meniscus on X-ray

→ Which may produce an acutely hot swollen joint with effusion. Birefringent crystals are seen in an aspirate

Radiological features of established gout

Open arrow = 1st MTP tophus

Closed arrow = large gouty erosion

Medicine at a Glance, Fourth Edition. Edited by Patrick Davey. © 2014 John Wiley & Sons, Ltd. Published 2014 by John Wiley & Sons, Ltd. Companion website: www.ataglanceseries.com/medicine

Crystal-related arthropathy defines a syndrome of synovitis in response to crystal deposition/formation in the joint. Two types of crystals are commonly implicated: monosodium urate (gout) and calcium pyrophosphate dihydrate (pseudogout). The resulting synovitis may be limited to a single joint (monoarticular) or become more widespread (polyarticular). Gout is the more common entity.

Gout

Epidemiology

Gout almost never occurs in premenopausal females, is of low prevalence (1–6 per 10 000) in women aged <60 years and is 5–6-fold higher than this in males aged 40–50. Environmental factors such as dietary purine intake, alcohol consumption and the use of drugs such as diuretics contribute. Inherited metabolic abnormalities also contribute by causing overproduction or underexcretion of uric acid.

Pathogenesis of hyperuricaemia

Uric acid is produced and excreted as shown (see Figure 214.1). Any factor causing overproduction or underexcretion will raise the serum uric acid (SUA). The risk of developing acute gout increases as SUA increases:

- Levels <420 μmol/L are associated with an incidence of 0.8/1000.
- Levels of >540 μmol/L increase this to 49/1000.

Clinical features

The spectrum of clinical features of hyperuricaemia and gout are shown in Figure 214.1.

- Hyperuricaemia in isolation may not require treatment.
- Classic gout gives rise to a monoarthritis: 50% start in the first metatarsophalangeal (MTP) joint. Ten per cent of first episodes are polyarticular. Crystal arthritis characteristically gives rise to severe pain, swelling and tenderness, often with a peak intensity within 12 hours of onset. Attacks are agonizing and last 7–10 days.
- Acute episodes of gout may be triggered by trauma, exercise, alcohol excess or starvation.
- Crystals may also precipitate in the renal parenchyma, giving rise to gouty nephropathy and renal stones.
- Acute gout may progress to chronic gout, associated with characteristic subcutaneous deposits of urate (tophi) and may become polyarticular in nature.
- Chronic gout usually requires uric acid-lowering therapy.

Differential diagnosis

The differential diagnosis of monoarticular gout includes septic arthritis, trauma and cellulitis, as there is often significant swelling and erythema of the surrounding tissues. The patient may also be febrile. The differential of asymmetrical, large joint, polyarticular gout includes the seronegative arthropathies and osteoarthritis.

Investigations

The clinical picture is often highly suggestive (see Clinical features), however definitive diagnosis requires demonstration of intracellular crystals in synovial fluid neutrophils aspirated from the inflamed joint or from a tophus. As sepsis may coexist with gout, microscopy and culture of synovial fluid should also be undertaken.

- Measurement of SUA is helpful, but not diagnostic. Uric acid levels may be normal in 20% of acute attacks and abnormal in asymptomatic individuals.
- Patients without clear risk factors (e.g. young males with no family history) should have a full blood count to rule out an occult myeloproliferative disorder, as the increased DNA turnover that occurs here can give rise to gout and/or determination of renal excretion of uric acid (mandatory if renal calculi are present). Likewise, patients undergoing cancer chemotherapy should be pretreated with allopurinol (or occasionally recombinant uricase) to prevent gout (particularly with renal deposition of crystals) occurring with tumour cell lysis.
- Plain radiographs in established gout show punched-out cortical erosions (see Figure 214.1), often away from the joint margin, unlike the erosions found in rheumatoid arthritis.
- Plain radiographs in pseudogout sometimes show calcification of the fibrocartilage (e.g. knee menisci, triangular cartilage in wrist) and hyaline cartilage (knee, glenohumeral joint). The structural changes are similar to those of osteroarthritis with cartilage loss, sclerosis, cysts and osteophytes, which may be prominent and exuberant.
- As there is an association between gout and the metabolic syndrome (obesity, hyperglycaemia, hyperlipidaemia, hypertension), these co-morbid conditions should be sought and treated.

Management

European League Against Rheumatism (EULAR) guidelines for gout advise oral colchicine and/or non-steroidal anti-inflammatory drugs (NSAIDs) as first-line agents for treatment of the acute attack. In the absence of contraindications, an NSAID is a convenient option. Where NSAIDs are contraindicated a short course of low-dose oral prednisolone therapy may be preferable and is the treatment of choice for severe polyarticular flares. Intra-articular aspiration and injection of long-acting steroid is both safe and effective in the acute attack.

Therapy to lower uric acid formation by inhibition of xanthine oxidase (allopurinol or febuxostat) or to promote excretion (probenicid) may be given in those with recurrent attacks, high SUA, tophi or erosive arthropathy. The target SUA level is 360 mmol/lL (EULAR guideleines). This treatment should ideally be deferred until the acute attack has settled-otherwise the attack may be prolonged. NSAIDs/colchicine are continued for the first 3 months of hypouricaemic therapy, because the risk of further attacks remains as urate levels flux. Diet and more usually alcohol intake may need to be adjusted.

Pseudogout

Calcium pyrophosphate deposits in joint cartilage are a common age-related phenomenon which may be present in one-quarter of those >60 years old. Rarely it is related to a familial predisposition (activating mutations in Ank, a transmembrane transporter of inorganic pyrophosphate), hyperparathyroidism, haemochromatosis or magnesium. When crystals are released into the joint cavity they produce an acute monoarthritis, diagnosed by finding characteristic rhomboidal crystals in the joint fluid. Treatment is with NSAIDs or intra-articular steroids. Pyrophosphate arthropathy often has a chronic course, which may mimic rheumatoid arthritis or osteoarthritis. Fifty per cent of such cases are punctuated by episodes of acute pseudogout. Pseudogout is the commonest cause of monoarthritis in the elderly.

Arthritis associated with infectious agents

Routes by which infection can reach a joint

1 Haematogenous spread from remote site

2 Local spread from adjacent osteomyelitis

3 Local spread from adjacent skin/soft tissue infection, e.g. cellulitis, bursitis

4 Iatrogenic spread from diagnostic/ therapeutic measure

5 Trauma including puncture, cutting, intravenous drug abuse

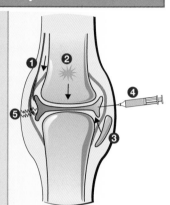

Management of septic arthritis

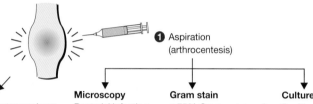

❶ Aspiration (arthrocentesis)

❷ X-ray
Often normal but may show:
- Swelling of joint
- Osteoporosis at 2 weeks
- If suspected, look for bone infection using MRI

Microscopy
Bacterial infection suggested by:
$> 50\,000$ WCC/mm^3
$+ > 85\%$ neutrophils

Gram stain
- 75% Gram +ve cocci
- 25% Gram –ve bacilli

Culture
Positive in nearly 100% of bacterial infection
- Fastidious organisms (myobacteria/fungi) require 8 weeks culture

After fluid drawn off
Initiate treatment

Antibiotic treatment
- Parenteral for 2 weeks, then 6 weeks oral
- Blind cover with benzyl penicillin + flucloxacillin unless unusual organisms are suspected
- Treat according to sensitivities, once they become available

Drain the joint
- Needle aspiration daily
- Repeat M, C & S
- Arthroscopy + washout may be required if fluid very purulent or osteomyelitis present

Immobilize for 1–2 days
- Then passive range of mobile exercises
- Then active/weight bearing as infection resolves

Analgesia
- As required

Medicine at a Glance, Fourth Edition. Edited by Patrick Davey. © 2014 John Wiley & Sons, Ltd. Published 2014 by John Wiley & Sons, Ltd. Companion website: www.ataglanceseries.com/medicine

Definitions

Three distinct clinical patterns are recognized:

1 Septic arthritis from colonization with pathogenic organisms.
2 Arthritis as a significant clinical feature of systemic infection, e.g. rubella, parvovirus B19 infection, Lyme disease.
3 Reactive arthritis: a sterile joint inflammation that develops as an immunologically mediated reaction to infection at a distant site. Triggering infections most commonly arise in the urogenital or gastrointestinal tract. Reactive arthritis is considered in Chapter 219.

Epidemiology of joint infection

Annual incidence varies widely and is related to the prevalence of the underlying predisposing conditions.

Septic arthritis

Pathogenesis and aetiology

Pathogenic organisms may reach a joint by several routes (see Figure 215.1). Predisposing factors include:

- **Impaired host defences**:
  - Inherited impairment of host defences, e.g. complement deficiency, hypogammaglobulinaemia.
  - Immunosuppressive illness or therapy, e.g. HIV, steroids, cytotoxics.
  - Chronic illness, e.g. diabetes mellitus renal failure, cirrhosis, leg ulcers.
  - Elderly or very young.
  - Neoplasia.
- The presence of a **prosthetic or damaged joint** (osteoarthritis/rheumatoid arthritis/gout).

Notably, septic arthritis is usually a disease of the very young, the elderly or those with damaged joints. Young adults with disseminated gonococcal infection may present with septic arthritis.

Clinical features

Septic arthritis affects the knee, hip, shoulder, wrist, ankle and elbow most commonly. Twenty per cent of presentations are polyarticular. Symptoms are usually sudden in onset and progressive, usually with florid systemic features. The joint(s) is red, swollen, tender and hot. It is usually held in flexion, avoiding movement and weight bearing. Disseminated gonococcal infection may feature urogenital symptoms and a pustular rash. Prosthetic joint infection in the early postoperative period is usually self-evident with high fever and a wound discharging pus. Later infection is associated with low-grade fever, recurrent pain, impaired function and less impressive local signs. Infection should always be considered in those with loosening of the prosthesis.

Organisms responsible for septic arthritis

In healthy adults the range of pathogens is narrow:

- *Staphylococcus aureus* is the most frequent joint pathogen in adults.
- About 25% of infections overall are due to Gram-negative bacilli.
- 15% are due to β-haemolytic streptococci.

In the immunocompromised subject, consider less typical organisms:

- Gram-negative bacilli and *Streptococcus pneumoniae* in the debilitated patient (malignancy, alcoholism, diabetes, etc.).
- *Pseudomonas* in intravenous drug abusers.
- Under 2 years of age: high incidence of *Haemophilus influenzae* infection.

Management

A management algorithm of joint sepsis is shown in Figure 215.1. Antibiotic therapy should be selected depending on joint aspirate culture and sensitivity and should continue for at least 2 weeks parenterally and a further 4 weeks orally. Close involvement of infectious disease or clinical microbiology experts is vital. Regular aspiration or open drainage of the joint is essential because of the destructive effects of pus on joint cartilage. Progression to chronic infection has decreased from 10–20% to <2% of acute infections with such early antibiotic therapy and appropriate surgical intervention.

Arthritis as a feature of systemic infection

Viral agents such as parvovirus B19, rubella and other acute viral syndromes (hepatitis, mumps) may have arthritis as a predominant feature. The presentation may be indistinguishable in joint distribution from acute-onset rheumatoid arthritis. Characteristic features of the underlying infection are usually present, and the joint symptoms usually subside without sequelae within 6 weeks of onset. Serology is useful when the result influences management.

216 Metabolic bone disease

Osteoporosis

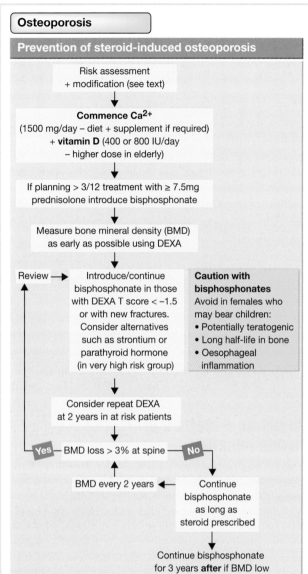

Prevention of steroid-induced osteoporosis

Risk assessment + modification (see text)

↓

Commence Ca²⁺
(1500 mg/day – diet + supplement if required)
+ **vitamin D** (400 or 800 IU/day
– higher dose in elderly)

↓

If planning > 3/12 treatment with ≥ 7.5mg
prednisolone introduce bisphosphonate

↓

Measure bone mineral density (BMD)
as early as possible using DEXA

↓

Review → Introduce/continue
bisphosphonate in those
with DEXA T score < –1.5
or with new fractures.
Consider alternatives
such as strontium or
parathyroid hormone
(in very high risk group)

Caution with bisphosphonates
Avoid in females who
may bear children:
• Potentially teratogenic
• Long half-life in bone
• Oesophageal
inflammation

↓

Consider repeat DEXA
at 2 years in at risk patients

↓

Yes – BMD loss > 3% at spine – **No**

↓   ↓

BMD every 2 years ← Continue
bisphosphonate
as long as
steroid prescribed

↓

Continue bisphosphonate
for 3 years **after** if BMD low

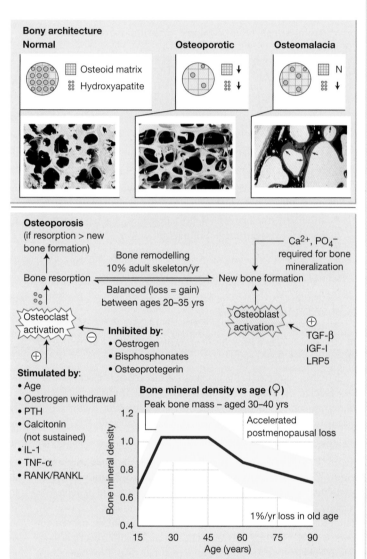

Bony architecture

Normal   **Osteoporotic**   **Osteomalacia**

☐ Osteoid matrix
▦ Hydroxyapatite

Osteoporosis
(if resorption > new bone formation)

Bone resorption ⇄ New bone formation

Bone remodelling
10% adult skeleton/yr

Balanced (loss = gain)
between ages 20–35 yrs

Ca²⁺, PO₄⁻
required for bone
mineralization

Osteoclast activation ⊖

Inhibited by:
• Oestrogen
• Bisphosphonates
• Osteoprotegerin

Osteoblast activation ⊕

⊕ TGF-β
IGF-I
LRP5

Stimulated by:
• Age
• Oestrogen withdrawal
• PTH
• Calcitonin (not sustained)
• IL-1
• TNF-α
• RANK/RANKL

Bone mineral density vs age (♀)
Peak bone mass – aged 30–40 yrs

Accelerated
postmenopausal loss

1%/yr loss in old age

(graph: Bone mineral density (y-axis 0.4–1.2) vs Age (years) (x-axis 15–90))

Osteoporosis

Osteoporosis is very common and predisposes to skeletal fractures from a quantitative decrease in bone matrix components (osteoid and hydroxyapatite) of bone. Fifty per cent of women and 15% of men sustain an osteoporosis-related fracture by age 90. Osteoporosis may be primary or secondary to a specific disease. Osteoporosis is common in elderly women, especially those with a late menarche, early menopause or long history of oligomenorrhoea (e.g. athletes, anorexia nervosa). Other important risk factors include smoking, alcohol, steroid use, sedentary lifestyle (or non-weight-bearing exercise), positive family history (peak bone mass is under strong genetic control) and lean body type. Secondary osteoporosis occurs in:

● Endocrine disease: thyrotoxicosis, Cushing's disease, hypogonadism, hyperparathyroidism, secondary amennorrhoea.
● Rheumatological disease: any inflammatory arthropathy, especially if treated with steroids.
● Gastroenterological disease: malabsorption, cirrhosis.
● Neoplasia.

● Drugs: especially steroids, heparin, warfarin and phenytoin.
● Alcoholism.
● A variety of rare genetic disorders, including osteogenesis imperfecta and hypophosphatasia.

Clinical features

The hallmarks of established osteoporosis are low impact fractures (distal radius (Colles' fracture) or femoral neck) and (wedge) fractures of vertebrae in the thoracic region, causing loss of height, an exaggerated dorsal kyphosis and pain.

Diagnosis

● **Plain radiographs** are useful for demonstrating osteoporosis-related fractures. A low impact or atraumatic fracture enables a clinical diagnosis of osteoporosis to be made.
● **Dual emission X-ray absorptiometry** (DEXA) is used to measure bone density and quantify the degree of osteopenia (mild to moderate bone loss) or osteoporosis (severe bone loss). Bone mineral density (BMD) is commonly reported in relation to two norms: a Z score (compared to the expected BMD for that patient's age and sex) and a T score (compared to young adults of the same

sex). The difference between a patient's score and the norm is expressed as standard deviations above and below the mean. The WHO definitions of osteoporosis and osteopenia relate to these scores: a T score between −1.0 and −2.5 defines osteopenia (low bone mass); a T score of or less than −2.5 defines osteoporosis. Measurement is useful in those at risk (e.g. steroid therapy, premature menopause) and in those aged <70 years with low impact fractures.

Prevention and management

Prevention of osteoporosis and fractures are major public health goals. The WHO recommends that treatment decisions are based on '10-year fracture risk' not measured BMD alone, as fracture risk is related to both BMD and risk of falls in an individual. The WHO Fracture Risk Assessment Tool is available online. Recommendations include:

- **Maximization of peak adult bone mass**: young women should: not smoke, minimize alcohol and caffeine intake, take adequate dietary calcium, perform weight-bearing exercise throughout life.
- **Reducing the rate of bone loss**: peri- and postmenopausal women, those on >7.5 mg/day of prednisolone, and other high-risk individuals should have DEXA scans. If significant osteoporosis is found, therapy is beneficial.
- **Prevention of fractures**: those with established osteoporosis should be assessed for factors that may cause falls (e.g. drugs causing postural hypotension, poor visual acuity) and considered for padded hip protectors (to protect against hip fractures).

In symptomatic osteoporosis, treatment aims to prevent further fractures. DEXA measurements identify those at significant risk and may be useful to monitor treatment in selected cases.

Pharmacological therapy

General measures apply to all patients. Adequate calcium (1000–1200 mg/day) and vitamin D (1000 IU/day or sufficient to ensure measured serum levels are within the normal range) should be assured from diet or supplements.

- **Bisphosphonates**: these agents bind to bone and prevent resorption. They are taken on an empty stomach with plain water and the patient remains upright for 30 minutes to avoid the risk of GI ulceration. There is a very small risk of osteonecrosis of the jaw.
- **Hormone replacement therapy** (HRT): osteoporosis is no longer a primary indication for HRT. The oestrogen agonist/antagonist raloxifene is preferred. Although it carries an equivalent risk of deep venous thrombosis to oestrogen, it confers a reduction in the risk of breast cancer.
- **Anabolic agents** build new bone. The parathyroid analogue teriparatide is injected subcutaneously daily for 24 months. It is contraindicated in skeletal neoplasia and hypercalcaemia.
- **Strontium ranelate** is a daily oral therapy. Its mechanism of action is unclear.
- **Biological therapy**: denosumab is a monoclonal antibody that binds to the RANK ligand. Denosumab thus prevents activation of RANK on the surface of osteoclasts and their precursors, thereby decreasing bone resorption and increasing bone mass and strength. It is licensed for osteoporosis range BMD. Denosumab is associated with a small increase in risk of hypocalcaemia in renal impairment and of infection.

Steroid therapy and osteoporosis

Rapid loss of bone occurs within 3 months of starting steroids, thereafter slowing to a rate 2–3 × normal loss. Osteoporosis risk is related to dose and treatment duration (total cumulative dose). Highly significant bone loss occurs with prednisolone doses >7.5 mg/day for 3 months; however, there is no safe steroid dose for bone loss and any steroid is significant in those with a prevalent or existing fragility fracture, who should all receive prophylaxis. Many conditions requiring steroids are themselves associated with osteoporosis, e.g. rheumatoid arthritis, systemic lupus erythematosus and inflammatory bowel disease. Figure 216.1 shows the methods for preventing bone loss in those taking steroids. Current steroid use doubles the risk of fracture irrespective of bone density.

Osteomalacia/rickets

Osteomalacia results from impaired mineralization of the osteoid matrix. It causes skeletal deformity in the young (rickets) and bone pain, non-specific aches, fractures and proximal muscle weakness in adults (osteomalacia). The causes include:

- **Vitamin D deficiency**: dietary inadequacy, lack of sunshine or malabsorption are the commonest causes in clinical practice, e.g. osteomalacia is relatively common in Asian women who dress traditionally, vegetarians and those (children and the elderly) with poor diets. It also results from coeliac disease.
- **Vitamin D metabolic abnormality**: reduced liver 25-hydroxylation (cirrhosis), reduced renal hydroxylation (renal failure) or increased hepatic metabolism (anticonvulsants).
- **Very rare causes** include vitamin D receptor mutations causing defective vitamin D-mediated calcium absorption, 1α-hydroxylase deficiency and familial (X-linked) hypophosphataemic rickets.

Clinical features and investigations

Delay or deficiency in bone mineralization in childhood (rickets) leads to structural skeletal deformities, including enlargement of the ends of the long bones, widened cranial sutures and frontal bossing in those aged <1 year old, and tibial bowing and genu varum/valgum (knock or bow knees) in older children. Adults experience non-specific pains and aches, predominantly in the proximal limb girdles and lower back. Pressure over the long bones or the rib cage may elicit tenderness. Significant osteomalacia may cause pathological fractures and results in secondary hyperparathyroidism which may complicate the picture biochemically and radiologically. This diagnosis must be considered in at-risk individuals with musculoskeletal symptoms.

- Diagnosis is sometimes evident from plain radiographs showing Looser's zones or pseudofractures (translucent bands occur at sites of stress, e.g. the ribs, axillary borders of the scapulae and pubic rami).
- Histology (usually not necessary) shows a decreased hydroxyapatite component with increased number of unmineralized osteoid lamellae.
- Characteristic biochemistry: low phosphate (early), low calcium (variable) and raised alkaline phosphatase (late due to secondary hyperparathyroidism).
- Low vitamin D and high parathyroid hormone (PTH).

Treatment

- Treat any underlying cause (e.g. coeliac disease).
- Give oral daily vitamin D supplementation according to the degree of depletion and bony abnormality.
- Malabsorption states require high doses.
- Deficiency of vitamin D due to renal or hepatic disease may be overcome by using hydroxylated forms such as alfacalcidol or calcitriol.

Therapy relieves symptoms and corrects bony abnormalities within 3–4 months. Occasionally, hyperparathroidism becomes autonomous in long-standing osteomalacia (tertiary hyperparathyroidism).

Parathyroid and renal bone disease

See Chapters 151 and 162.

217 Other bone disease

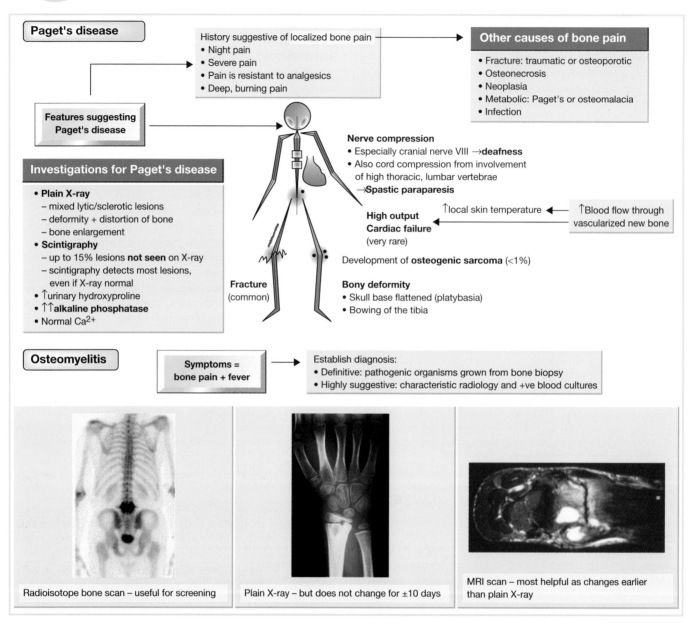

Pagel's disease

History suggestive of localized bone pain
- Night pain
- Severe pain
- Pain is resistant to analgesics
- Deep, burning pain

Other causes of bone pain
- Fracture: traumatic or osteoporotic
- Osteonecrosis
- Neoplasia
- Metabolic: Paget's or osteomalacia
- Infection

Features suggesting Paget's disease

Nerve compression
- Especially cranial nerve VIII →**deafness**
- Also cord compression from involvement of high thoracic, lumbar vertebrae →**Spastic paraparesis**

↑local skin temperature ◄── ↑Blood flow through vascularized new bone

Investigations for Paget's disease
- **Plain X-ray**
  – mixed lytic/sclerotic lesions
  – deformity + distortion of bone
  – bone enlargement
- **Scintigraphy**
  – up to 15% lesions **not seen** on X-ray
  – scintigraphy detects most lesions, even if X-ray normal
- ↑urinary hydroxyproline
- ↑↑**alkaline phosphatase**
- Normal Ca^{2+}

High output Cardiac failure (very rare)

Development of **osteogenic sarcoma** (<1%)

Fracture (common)

Bony deformity
- Skull base flattened (platybasia)
- Bowing of the tibia

Osteomyelitis

Symptoms = bone pain + fever

Establish diagnosis:
- Definitive: pathogenic organisms grown from bone biopsy
- Highly suggestive: characteristic radiology and +ve blood cultures

Radioisotope bone scan – useful for screening

Plain X-ray – but does not change for ±10 days

MRI scan – most helpful as changes earlier than plain X-ray

Paget's disease

This is associated with abnormal remodelling of bone, often in a monostolic pattern, but may be widespread. Up to 40% of cases may have an identifiable affected relative, indicating a significant genetic contribution. It is primarily a disorder of osteoclasts, which become highly activated altering the normal homeostasis of bone remodeling.

- **Early stages**: increased bone resorption occurs, so producing lytic lesions (osteoporosis circumscripta, resorption front).
- **Later stages**: disproportionate stimulation of new bone formation occurs in a disorganized fashion, resulting in areas of bone sclerosis.

Cycles of resorption and formation result in a huge increase in bone turnover and ultimately grossly disorganized bone, which is weak and prone to fracture.

Epidemiology

Paget's disease occurs mainly in the elderly (>70 years). The prevalence is 10% in those aged ≥80 years and <0.3% in those <40 years. It is commonest in western countries and is rare in Africa and Asia. Male preponderance is 3:2, with a marked increased prevalence in relatives. Mutations in the sequestosome gene are well described in a significant proportion of cases and likely cause disease through osteoclast activation via the NF-κB pathway. However, it is far from clear how such germline mutations cause disease with such a patchy and often limited skeletal distribution.

Clinical features

Paget's disease is often asymptomatic with the only abnormality being an isolated raised alkaline phosphatase. Between 5% and 10% develop symptoms bringing them to medical care. Symptomatic presentation depends on the sites and extent of bony involvement (see Figure 217.1). Twenty per cent of patients have a single bone lesion. The pelvis, spine, long bones and skull are most commonly affected. Common symptoms include bone pain, bone deformities and increased warmth over an affected area. Important bony complications are fractures (10%), deformity and osteogenic sarcoma (rare <1%). A sudden increase in pain, deformity or serum alkaline phosphatase should alert the clinician to one of these possibilities. Other complications are very rare, and include:

- Neurological complications: cranial nerve compression, conductive hearing loss (or sensori neural) and spinal stenosis.
- Other: including hypercalcaemia, or hypercalciuria, which in turn may lead to renal stones.

Investigations

- **Raised alkaline phosphatase** (reflects increased osteoblastic activity, which is linked to increased osteoclast activity).
- **Radiology**: X-rays show gross bony distortion and deformity and mixed osteolytic and sclerotic areas, with abnormal trabecular architecture. It is unique in causing enlargement of the affected bones. An area of sharply demarcated osteolysis may be apparent, particualarly in early disease. This may appear as a 'flame-shaped resorbing front' in a long bone or an area of osteoporosis circumscripta. Isotope bone scintigraphy helps define the extent and activity of skeletal involvement (15% of lesions, usually early active areas, are not visible on plain film).
- **Bone biopsy** if imaging cannot exclude tumour.
- **Calcium** in Paget's disease is normal but may rise with a fracture or prolonged inactivity.

Management

Asymptomatic disease does not require treatment. **Indications for treatment** are:

- Active disease at the skull base or in the spine above L2 or any neurological compromise (cranial or spinal nerves).
- Pain.
- Progressive deformity.
- The very rare complications of either immobilization hypercalcaemia or high output cardiac failure.

Treatment of symptomatic patients includes:

- Analgesia.
- Bisphosphonates inhibit bone resorption, and dramatically reduce bone turnover (e.g. alendronate, pamidronate).
- Calcitonin is occasionally useful for severe pain or extensive lytic disease but has been largely replaced by bisphosphonates. Side effects include troublesome flushing, nausea and hypocalcaemia.
- Surgery is used to relieve compression neuropathy.

Osteonecrosis (avascular necrosis)

Avascular necrosis describes the death of cellular elements of bone, occurring in all ages and both sexes, which potentially causes structural collapse.

Aetiology and pathogenesis

Avascular necrosis is associated with pregnancy, corticosteroid therapy, radiotherapy and cytotoxic chemotherapy. It may also occur in sickle cell disease and other haemoglobinopathies and decompression sickness, though many cases are idiopathic. It commonly affects the femoral head and the scaphoid after fracture of these bones.

Clinical features

- The characteristic feature is bone pain.
- Initially pain occurs on weight bearing, subsequently at rest and at night.
- Increasing severity of pain, becoming resistant to escalating analgesia.

Management

Radiographs are frequently normal early on; subsequently patchy osteopenia and osteosclerosis develop, and later still a characteristic 'crescent sign' demarcates viable and dead bone. In advanced disease there is destruction and collapse of the articular surface. Magnetic resonance imaging (MRI) is the imaging technique of choice in early disease and is highly sensitive.

Treatment is:

- Conservative with analgesia and muscle strengthening early in the course, with reduced weight and load bearing until recovery occurs (may be protracted, c. 12 months).
- Surgical 'core decompression'.
- May require joint replacement if severe and associated with structural collapse.

Osteomyelitis

Osteomyelitis is infection of the bone arising either from direct inoculation with the infecting organisms, e.g. an 'open' fracture, or from haematogenous spread. Though common in children, it is relatively rare in adults.

Underlying conditions and responsible organisms

- Diabetes leads to Gram-negative and/or *Staphylococcus aureus* foot infection.
- 90% of adult osteomyelitis is due to *Staphylococcus* infection.
- *S. aureus* septicaemia (e.g. a complication of intravenous cannula in hospitalized patients) is complicated by osteomyelitis in 1% of cases.
- Sickle cell disease (80% of infections are due to *Salmonella* species).
- Immunosuppression predisposes to many different infections.
- Spinal tuberculosis is relatively common in countries with a high prevalence of tuberculosis. In some areas, infection with atypical mycobacteria is common.

Clinical features

Osteomyelitis presents with systemic symptoms (fever, malaise) and local pain. Vertebral osteomyelitis can lead to vertebral collapse and cord compression. Osteomyelitis in patients with diabetes is often painless. Sterile and occasionally septic arthritis can complicate the picture.

Diagnosis and treatment

MRI is the investigation of choice for early disease since X-rays often show no abnormalities. Diagnostic ultrasound also has a potential role. Treatment is with prolonged antibiotics (initially intravenously), debridement of dead bone and stabilization when necessary. Occasionally it proves impossible to eradicate the infection, and lifelong antibiotics are required.

218 Rheumatoid arthritis

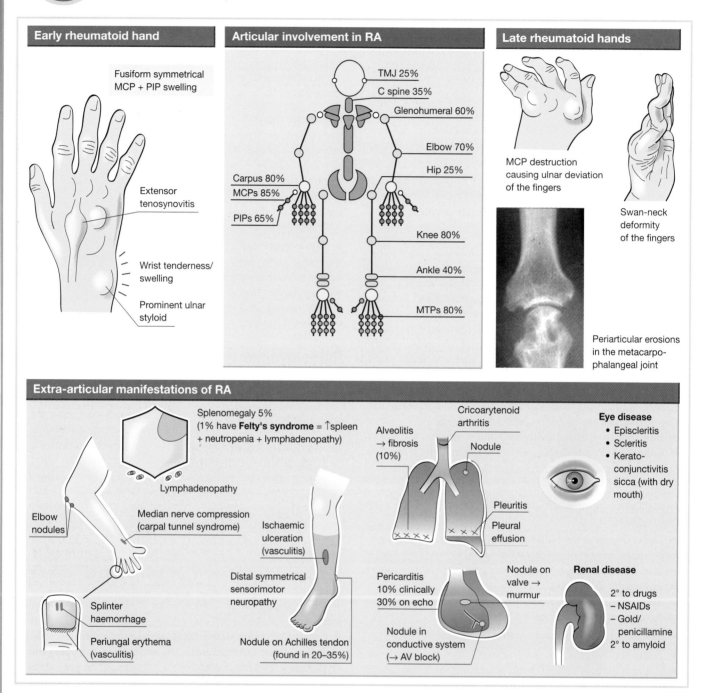

Early rheumatoid hand

Fusiform symmetrical MCP + PIP swelling

Extensor tenosynovitis

Wrist tenderness/ swelling

Prominent ulnar styloid

Articular involvement in RA

TMJ 25%
C spine 35%
Glenohumeral 60%
Elbow 70%
Hip 25%
Carpus 80%
MCPs 85%
PIPs 65%
Knee 80%
Ankle 40%
MTPs 80%

Late rheumatoid hands

MCP destruction causing ulnar deviation of the fingers

Swan-neck deformity of the fingers

Periarticular erosions in the metacarpo-phalangeal joint

Extra-articular manifestations of RA

Splenomegaly 5% (1% have **Felty's syndrome** = ↑spleen + neutropenia + lymphadenopathy)

Lymphadenopathy

Elbow nodules

Median nerve compression (carpal tunnel syndrome)

Ischaemic ulceration (vasculitis)

Distal symmetrical sensorimotor neuropathy

Splinter haemorrhage

Periungal erythema (vasculitis)

Nodule on Achilles tendon (found in 20–35%)

Cricoarytenoid arthritis

Alveolitis → fibrosis (10%)

Nodule

Pleuritis

Pleural effusion

Pericarditis 10% clinically 30% on echo

Nodule in conductive system (→ AV block)

Nodule on valve → murmur

Eye disease
• Episcleritis
• Scleritis
• Kerato-conjunctivitis sicca (with dry mouth)

Renal disease

2° to drugs
– NSAIDs
– Gold/ penicillamine
2° to amyloid

Rheumatoid arthritis (RA) is a systemic autoimmune disorder most obviously characterized by a chronic, symmetrical and erosive arthritis of synovial joints resulting in major disability and handicap. Extra-articular manifestations are common and autoantibodies to immunoglobulin (rheumatoid factors) and cyclic citrullinated peptides (anti-CCP antibodies) occur in most patients. Life expectancy is also reduced, largely due to excess cardiovascular mortality and infection.

Epidemiology

Worldwide prevalence is 1% and the peak age of onset the early forties, although it may present at any stage. Women are 2–3 times more commonly affected than men, but the sex ratio varies with age (at 30 years, F:M ratio is 10:1, at 65 years, 1:1). The genetic contribution to the disease is emphasized by familial aggregation of cases (sibling recurrence risk is 5%) and the association with HLA-DR4 (70% of cases).

Aetiology and pathogenesis

Rheumatoid arthritis represents an immune-mediated response to an undefined antigen, in a genetically predisposed individual. This process triggers inflammation, endothelial cell activation and recruitment of specific inflammatory cells to the joint, facilitated by the upregulation of adhesion molecules on synovial vascular endothelium and on circulating inflammatory cells. Amplification of inflammation occurs in response to the local production of inflammatory cytokines (tumor necrosis factor α (TNF-α) and interleukin-1 (IL-1)).

Synovial tissue proliferates and becomes locally invasive in the joints. Pannus, a thickened inflammatory granulation tissue, is the characteristic pathological lesion in RA. Activated macrophages within the pannus produce destructive collagenases and proteases. These enzymes mediate the erosion of cartilage at the subchondral bone/cartilage junction and inwards until the articular cartilage is destroyed. Cartilage destruction causes instability of joints resulting in the characteristic deformities and radiological destruction of RA.

Clinical features

Initial presentation is usually subacute or insidious:

- Joint swelling, tenderness, pain and stiffness, particularly troublesome in the morning and improving as the day goes on, and recurring in the evening.
- Small joints of the hands, feet and wrists (see Figure 218.1 above) tend to be affected initially asymmetrically, eventually symmetrically, followed by involvement of larger joints such as knees and elbows where effusions occur.
- Onset is often insidious, and asymmetrical with fluctuating joint pain, swelling and stiffness, frequently accompanied by fatigue and lassitude. The clinical examination at onset may be normal, but more usually reveals the characteristic features of synovitis.
- Warmth, swelling and tenderness of the metacarpophalangeals (MCPs) and proximal interphalangeals (PIPs), the wrists and metatarsophalangeal (MTP) joints of the feet in a strikingly symmetrical distribution.
- Tenosynovitis is a prominent early feature, often affecting the extensor tendon sheaths on the dorsum of the hand.

Alternative presentations of RA include:

- **Explosive onset** in 5–10%.
- **Systemic onset** in 5%, usually in middle-aged men with non-articular manifestations (such as weight loss) as the dominant feature. Arthritis may be relatively minor but elevated rheumatoid factor (RF) titres are usually found.
- **Palindromic onset** in 5%, comprising irregular episodes of transient though possibly severe synovitis. Attacks come on suddenly, may be debilitating and abate within 48 hours with no residual deficit. Fifty per cent of these evolve into typical RA (typically RF positive).
- **Polymyalgic onset** in 5%: diffuse proximal limb girdle stiffness without joint inflammation; associated with the presence of RF. Shows a less dramatic response to steroids than classic polymyalgia and progresses to typical RA in time.

Diagnostic criteria for RA are shown in Table 218.1. The differential diagnosis of RA includes:

- Infection-related transient arthritis, e.g. parvovirus B19, hepatitis B, rubella infection; these typically last <6 weeks.
- Reactive arthritis.
- Chronic pyrophosphate arthritis (see Chapter 214).
- Small joint arthritis associated with psoriasis (RF negative).
- Non-erosive arthritis of systemic lupus erythematosus.

Features of established/chronic RA

Established RA pursues an unpredictable clinical course characterized by acute 'flares' of involved joints and variable systemic and extra-articular symptoms. Acute flares give rise to ongoing pain, discomfort and functional impairment as a result of active synovitis (e.g. inability to grip due to MCP and PIP swelling and stiffness). These are partially responsive to anti-inflammatory

Table 218.1 1987 criteria for the diagnosis of rheumatoid arthritis. A patient is said to have RA if he/she has satisfied at least four of these seven criteria. The first four criteria must have been present for at least 6 weeks.

Criterion	Definition
Morning stiffness	In and around the joints lasting at least 1 h
Arthritis of three or more joint areas	Soft-tissue swelling or fluid observed by a physician
	Possible areas are right or left PIP, MCP, wrist, elbow, knee, ankle and MTP joints
Arthritis of hand joints	At least one area swollen in a wrist, MCP or PIP joint
Symmetrical arthritis	Simultaneous involvement of these joint areas bilaterally
Rheumatoid nodules	Subcutaneous nodules over bony prominences/extensor surfaces/in juxta-articular regions
Serum rheumatoid factor	
Radiographic changes	Typical of RA on hand and wrist radiographs (see Figure 218.1)

therapy. This fluctuating clinical picture is usually accompanied by ongoing slowly progressive structural joint damage. This ultimately leads to severe loss of function; historically, only 50% of patients were able to work full time after 10 years of disease. Extra-articular manifestations contribute significantly to the morbidity and mortality of RA. Major vasculitis affects one in nine men, and one in 30 women with RA. Infections are also at least three times more common than in the general population, particularly in those on steroids. Cardiovascular disease risk is significantly increased in RA mainly due to chronic systemic inflammation but also from non-steroidal anti-inflammatory drug (NSAID) induced hypertension. Clinical features of established RA are shown in Figure 218.1. About 1% of patients with RA develop Felty's syndrome, characterized by neutropenia, splenomegaly and other extra-articular features including leg ulcers and vasculitis. It is unusual before 10 years of disease and it very strongly associated with HLA-DR4 (>90%).

Investigations

An acute inflammatory response (raised erythrocyte sedimentation rate (ESR), C-reactive protein (CRP) and diffuse hypergammaglobulinaemia) is found. ESR or CRP are used in the generation of a disease activity score (DAS) which also incorporates counts of swollen and tender joints and a global assessment of disease activity. RF is present in the majority of cases (85–90%) though it may not be positive early in the disease (70% at onset). Anti-CCP antibodies are more specific than RF. X-rays typically reveal only soft tissue swelling at presentation (see Table 218.2). Erosive changes often occur within 2 years of onset, usually first in the feet.

Management

Individual patients with RA have distinct patterns of damage and unique rehabilitation requirements. Treatment must be tailored to these needs within the framework of a multidisciplinary team. The introduction of biological agents, particularly those directed against TNF, have fundamentally changed the treatment of RA in the past decade. See Figure 218.2 below for therapy.

Table 218.2 Assessment in rheumatoid arthritis.

	Indicating active inflammation	Indicating structural damage
Clinical	Symptoms • Prolonged early morning stiffness • Painful and swollen joints • Lassitude, fatigue Signs • Hot swollen tender joints; effusion • Inability to make a fist/ reduction in grip strength	Symptoms • Joint deformity or instability • Functional loss due to tendon rupture or deformity Signs • Joint subluxation • Joint deformity (e.g. swan neck, boutonnière, hallux valgus)
Laboratory tests	↑ ESR, ↑ CRP, ↑ γ-globulins, anaemia High titre RF is associated with more severe disease	
Radiological		Presence of erosion, bony malalignment, secondary osteoarthritis

Principles of therapy: a multidisciplinary approach involving physicians, physiotherapists, surgeons, etc. is desirable. Therapy aims to minimize symptoms and improve prognosis. Disease remission is the primary goal of modern therapy and clinicians now 'treat to target', the target being a DAS score indicative of remission. While this may not be achievable in all, significant improvement in symptoms and function is achievable in most.

1 Symptomatic relief: simple analgesics or NSAIDs. These agents have no effect on long-term outcome (disability and deformity). NSAIDs with relative specificity for the COX-2 isoform of cyclo-oxygenase produce fewer gastrointestinal (GI) complications and may be useful in the elderly and in those with major risk factors for GI ulceration. There are major concerns that NSAIDs may also be associated with an increased cardiovascular risk (*c.* 10%) and they should therefore be used only with caution in those with cardiovascular risk factors. They should also be used with caution in the presence of renal impairment.

2 Modification of underlying disease. Second-line immunomodulatory agents (disease-modifying antirheumatic drugs (DMARDs)) include methotrexate, sulfasalazine, leflunomide, injectable gold salts, ciclosporin and antimalarials. Methotrexate is recommended as the initial agent in patients who have adverse prognostic indicators at onset (high RF/anti-CCP titre, very active disease, early erosions) and is regarded as the 'anchor drug' in RA. Methotrexate is increasingly being used in combination with other DMARDs even in early disease. DMARDs slow the progression of erosions somewhat but have modest impact on morbidity and disability in the long term. They may be used singly or in combination according to the severity of the underlying disease and response.

3 Adjunctive therapy with corticosteroids. For severe systemic illness, intermittent troublesome (mono- or pauciarticular) inflammation and/or vasculitis, steroids may be given as intermittent 'pulses', intramuscular steroids are particularly valuable for the rapid amelioration of symptoms in patients with early disease at the initiation of treatment with DMARDs, which typically require several months for full effect. Low-dose oral prednisolone (7.5 mg/day) may also be useful to control symptoms while other DMARDs are taking effect.

4 Biological agents. The realistic goal of treatment is now drug-induced disease remission. For those patients not responding adequately to DMARD, biological therapies should be considered. These include monoclonal antibodies directed against TNF-α (infliximab, adalimumab, golimumab, certolizumab) and recombinant TNF receptor/IgG fusion protein (etanercept). They are usually prescribed in combination with methotrexate. These drugs are expensive but result in remission of disease in 25% of patients within 3 months and 50% improvement in 40% of patients. They are also highly effective in arresting bone erosion and have a rapid onset of action. Increased risks of infection demand careful monitoring and all patients should be screened for latent tuberculosis (TB) because of the risk of reactivation. For patients who do not respond or for whom anti-TNF therapy is contraindicated (e.g. cancer) a number of alternate or second-line biological theapies are now licensed. B-cell depletion with the anti-CD20 monoclonal antibody rituximab (a B-cell-depleting antibody) gives excellent results. The recombinant CTLA4/IgG fusion protein, abatacept (which inhibits T-cell co-stimulatory pathways), has also proved highly effective as has tocilizumab, an anti-IL-6 antibody therapy.

Prognosis and outcome

The course and outcome of RA in an individual patient is unpredictable. Poor prognostic factors are:

- Generalized polyarthritis (total involved joints >20).
- High ESR and CRP despite therapy.
- Extra-articular features, e.g. nodules/vasculitis.
- Rheumatoid factor and/or anti-CCP antibody positivity.
- Erosions on plain radiographs within 2 years of onset.
- HLA-DR4 status.

The spectrum of severity of RA ranges from mild or subclinical to aggressive and destructive forms, associated with excess mortality (mortality 2–2.5 times that of age- and sex-matched controls). Up to 33% of patients cease work within 5 years of disease onset, and half are able to work full-time within 10 years of disease onset. About 50% of the excess cardiovascular risk can be attributed to traditional risk factors. The remainder reflects chronic systemic inflammation. Tighter control of inflammation with increasing use of biological therapies will probably reduce mortality. Other long-term damage results from:

- Drug side effects, e.g. long-term steroids, methotrexate pneumonitis and deranged liver function from various DMARDs.
- Neurological: cervical myelopathy and peripheral neuropathy.
- Cardiac involvement: ischaemic, nodular valve and pericarditis.
- Amyloidosis (causing renal failure and the nephrotic syndrome).
- Rheumatoid lung disease: fibrosis and pleurisy.
- Vasculitis causing skin ulcers, distal ischaemia, mononeuritis and coronary mesenteric arteritis.

Management of rheumatoid arthritis

Initial assessment

Clinical — Laboratory investigations — Radiology

Initiate treatment

Aims of treatment
1. Induce remission
2. Suppress ongoing inflammation in long term
3. Alleviate pain, maintain (or restore) function, allow patient to live normal productive life

Pharmacological (see tables)

Multidisciplinary approach

Physiotherapy
Local symptomatic treatment
Exercise advice

Nursing
Education
Support

Surgeons
• Joint stabilization (fusion)
• Replacement

Occupational therapy
• Splinting
• Protection
• Aids and adaptations

Psychology
Assessment and support

Follow up and reassess regularly

Progression/failure to respond

Few troublesome joints (≤4)

Initiate or modify DMARD → **Stable** ← Physical treatment ± intra-articular steroid injection

Unstable

Consider and work up for introduction of anti-TNF therapy → **Stable**

Unstable → Consider second generation biological, e.g. rituximab, abatacept

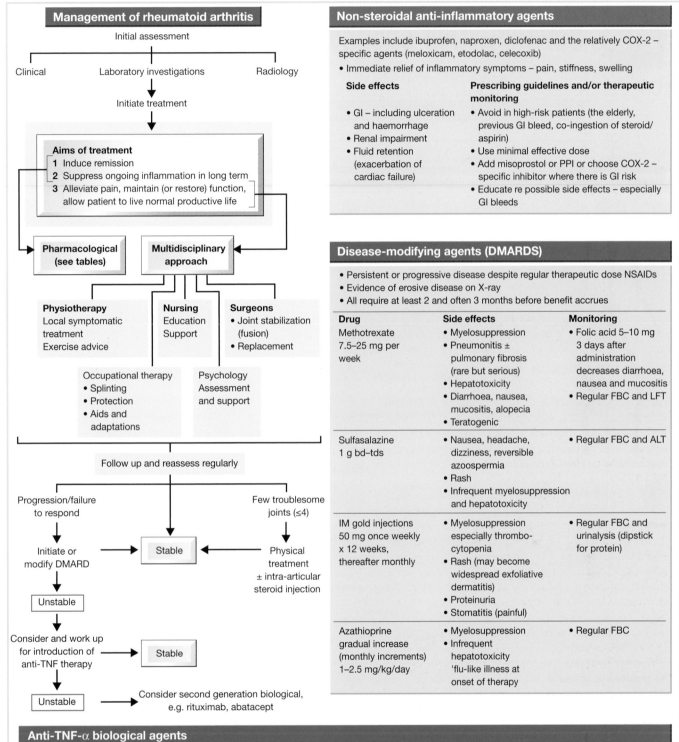

Non-steroidal anti-inflammatory agents

Examples include ibuprofen, naproxen, diclofenac and the relatively COX-2 – specific agents (meloxicam, etodolac, celecoxib)
• Immediate relief of inflammatory symptoms – pain, stiffness, swelling

Side effects	Prescribing guidelines and/or therapeutic monitoring
• GI – including ulceration and haemorrhage • Renal impairment • Fluid retention (exacerbation of cardiac failure)	• Avoid in high-risk patients (the elderly, previous GI bleed, co-ingestion of steroid/aspirin) • Use minimal effective dose • Add misoprostol or PPI or choose COX-2 – specific inhibitor where there is GI risk • Educate re possible side effects – especially GI bleeds

Disease-modifying agents (DMARDS)

• Persistent or progressive disease despite regular therapeutic dose NSAIDs
• Evidence of erosive disease on X-ray
• All require at least 2 and often 3 months before benefit accrues

Drug	Side effects	Monitoring
Methotrexate 7.5–25 mg per week	• Myelosuppression • Pneumonitis ± pulmonary fibrosis (rare but serious) • Hepatotoxicity • Diarrhoea, nausea, mucositis, alopecia • Teratogenic	• Folic acid 5–10 mg 3 days after administration decreases diarrhoea, nausea and mucositis • Regular FBC and LFT
Sulfasalazine 1 g bd–tds	• Nausea, headache, dizziness, reversible azoospermia • Rash • Infrequent myelosuppression and hepatotoxicity	• Regular FBC and ALT
IM gold injections 50 mg once weekly x 12 weeks, thereafter monthly	• Myelosuppression especially thrombocytopenia • Rash (may become widespread exfoliative dermatitis) • Proteinuria • Stomatitis (painful)	• Regular FBC and urinalysis (dipstick for protein)
Azathioprine gradual increase (monthly increments) 1–2.5 mg/kg/day	• Myelosuppression • Infrequent hepatotoxicity 'flu-like illness at onset of therapy	• Regular FBC

Anti-TNF-α biological agents

• Persistently active disease despite treatment with at least 2 DMARDs (including methotrexate)
• Rapid onset of action
• Disease remission within 3–12 months in 1/4 of patients

Drug	Side effects	Monitoring
• Adalimumab • 40 mg per fortnight • Subcutaneous	• Local skin reaction • Reactivation of TB • Lupus-like reaction • Increased infection risk	• Chest X-ray • Latent TB • DNA antibodies
Etanercept 50mg weekly	• Skin reaction • Increased infection risk • Lupus-like reaction	• Chest X-ray • Latent TB • DNA antibodies
Infliximab 3 mg/kg IV Every 2 months	• Increased infections • Reactivation of TB • Lupus-like reaction • Development of neutralizing antibodies and loss of effect	• Chest X-ray • Latent TB • DNA antibodies

219 Seronegative spondyloarthropathies

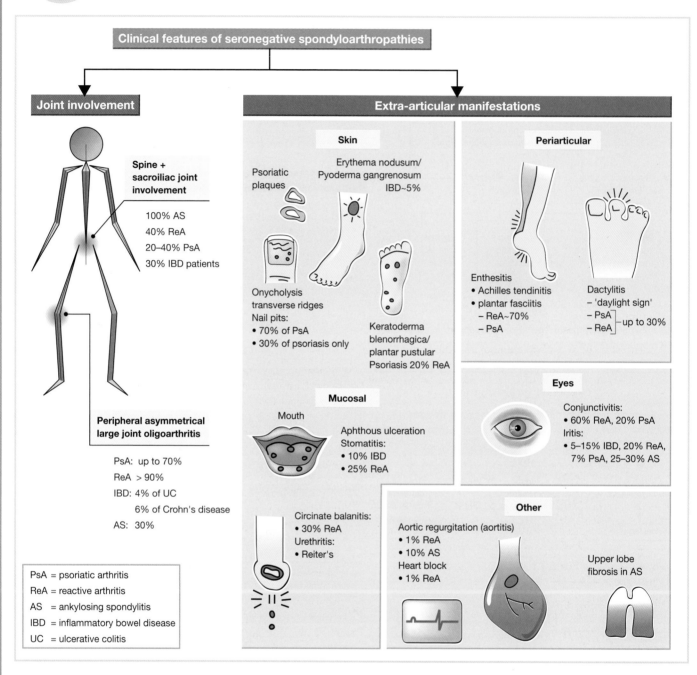

Clinical features of seronegative spondyloarthropathies

Joint involvement

Spine + sacroiliac joint involvement

100% AS
40% ReA
20–40% PsA
30% IBD patients

Peripheral asymmetrical large joint oligoarthritis

PsA: up to 70%
ReA > 90%
IBD: 4% of UC
        6% of Crohn's disease
AS: 30%

PsA = psoriatic arthritis
ReA = reactive arthritis
AS = ankylosing spondylitis
IBD = inflammatory bowel disease
UC = ulcerative colitis

Extra-articular manifestations

Skin

Psoriatic plaques

Erythema nodusum/ Pyoderma gangrenosum IBD~5%

Onycholysis transverse ridges
Nail pits:
• 70% of PsA
• 30% of psoriasis only

Keratoderma blenorrhagica/ plantar pustular Psoriasis 20% ReA

Mucosal

Mouth

Aphthous ulceration Stomatitis:
• 10% IBD
• 25% ReA

Circinate balanitis:
• 30% ReA
Urethritis:
• Reiter's

Periarticular

Enthesitis
• Achilles tendinitis
• plantar fasciitis
    – ReA~70%
    – PsA

Dactylitis
– 'daylight sign'
– PsA
– ReA } up to 30%

Eyes

Conjunctivitis:
• 60% ReA, 20% PsA
Iritis:
• 5–15% IBD, 20% ReA, 7% PsA, 25–30% AS

Other

Aortic regurgitation (aortitis)
• 1% ReA
• 10% AS
Heart block
• 1% ReA

Upper lobe fibrosis in AS

The seronegative spondyloarthropathies are a group of inflammatory arthritides, which share similar clinical features, pathological findings, the absence of rheumatoid factor and a strong association with the histocompatibility antigen HLA-B27. They comprise:

● Ankylosing spondylitis (AS).
● Psoriatic arthropathy.
● Reactive arthritis (sexually acquired reactive arthritis (SARA) follows a sexually acquired infection; enteric reactive arthritis (ERA) follows an enteric infection).
● Enteropathic arthritis (inflammatory bowel disease (IBD)).
● Undifferentiated seronegative arthropathy.

Epidemiology and clinical features

These conditions may present at any age, though they most frequently affect young adults. Males are consistently affected more commonly than females (3:1 for SARA, 2.5:1 for AS), except in the peripheral arthritis of IBD, which is more commonly found in females. The prevalence ranges from 150–500/100 000 for AS to 20/100 000 for SARA/ERA. About 10% of those with psoriasis have an accompanying arthritis, making this perhaps the most common inflammatory arthritis after rheumatoid arthritis. These conditions share many common clinical features (see Figure 219.1 above). Spondyloarthropathies characteristically affect the spine, though peripheral arthritis is common, most frequently asymmetrical, oligoarticular and predominantly in the lower limb.

Table 219.1 Summary of findings in seronegative spondyloarthropathies.

	Ankylosing spondylitis	Reactive arthropathy	Inflammatory bowel disease associated	Psoriatic arthropathy
Sex	M > F	M > F	M = F	F = M
Age	<30 years	<30 years	Any age	Any age
Peripheral joints	c. 40%	>90%	>90%	>90%
Sausage digits (dactylitis)	−	+	−	+
Axial spine	100%	20%	30%	30%
Sacroiliitis				
Enthesitis	++	+++	+	+++
(achilles tendinitis, plantar fasciitis)				
Extra-articular				
Uveitis	+++	++	+	+
Conjunctivitis	0	+++	+	++
Skin	0	++ (keratoderma blenorrhagica)	+ (pyoderma gangrenosum, erythema nodosum)	+++ (psoriasis)
Mucous membranes	0	+ (circinate balanitis)		
Aortic incompetence	+	+	0	0
Urethritis	0	++	0	0
Prostatitis	++	++	0	0

- Periarticular features such as enthesopathy and tendonitis are also very frequent.
- Extra-articular involvement includes the eye, skin, mucous membranes, the genitalia, lungs and proximal aorta.

The particular combination of these extra-articular features and axial/peripheral joint involvement is usually highly characteristic of particular types of seronegative spondyloarthropathy (see Table 219.1).

Ankylosing spondylitis

The onset is usually in late teens or early adulthood. First-degree relatives are affected in 10% of cases. The male:female ratio is 2.5:1. AS usually presents with insidious onset of inflammatory type pain in the lower back/buttock and/or thoracic region. Features of back pain suggesting inflammation include:

- Young age (<40 years).
- Significant early morning stiffness (>20 min).
- Improvement on exercise.
- Localized tenderness over the sacroiliac joints.
- Pain at night.

Any level of the spine may be involved, but characteristically the lumbar spine is involved early on, and the cervical spine relatively late. Chest pain may arise from the thoracic spine itself, the costovertebral joints or the costochondral junctions.

AS may affect the spine at any level but thoracolumbar disease is more common than neck involvement. Chest expansion (<2.5 cm) and thoracic spine rotation are greatly reduced (see Figure 219.2 below). Examination of the lumbar spine shows:

- A decrease in flexibility in all three planes. Reduction in forward flexion is measured by Schober's test (see Figure 219.3 below).
- Advanced disease results in bony ankylosis and the development of deformities characteristic of AS (see Figure 219.2). As the disease progresses and ankylosis develops, the symptoms of active inflammation recede and those of disability predominate.
- Extraskeletal manifestations are shown (see Figure 219.1).

Investigations

- Inflammatory markers (erythrocyte sedimentation rate, C-reactive protein) are raised in under 50% of cases. Rheumatoid factor is negative.
- HLA-B27 is present in >90% compared with 8% of the general population. However, only about one in 20 of HLA-B27-positive individuals will develop AS. HLA typing for B27 should therefore only be carried out where there is a relatively high pre-test probability on clinical grounds.
- Plain radiographs may show juxta-articular sclerosis, erosions and widening of the sacroiliac joints and eventually ankylosis (fusion), but they are insensitive to early disease. Magnetic resonance imaging is the investigation of choice for early disease, because it can detect inflammatory change as well as erosions. Sagittal views of the thoracolumbar spine may show typical 'shiny corners' in the vertebrae, facet joint disease and costovertebritis. Computed tomography is also very sensitive at detecting small erosions.
- AS may be complicated by osteoporosis, and in selected patients a DEXA (dual emission X-ray absorptiometry) scan of the hips may be indicated (lumbar spine measurements are unreliable because of new bone growth).

Management

Management of this condition includes:

- Intense physiotherapy and hydrotherapy.
- Non-steroidal anti-inflammatory drugs (NSAIDs) for persistent symptoms.
- Methotrexate or sulfasalazine are useful for persistent peripheral joint arthritis but not for axial disease.
- Anti-tumour necrosis factor α (anti-TNF-α) biologicals are highly effective for patients with more severe forms of disease refractory to NSAIDs. Nearly 90% of patients show improvement, with c. 50% showing 50% improvement in pain, function and stiffness.
- Topical corticosteroids for uveitis.

Ankylosing spondylitis: Clinical features

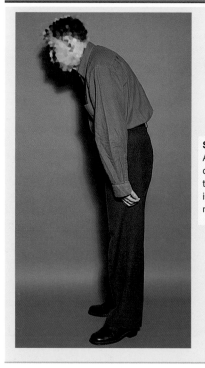

Spine
Ankylosing spondylitis can cause a marked thoracic kyphosis with increased wall-tragus measurement

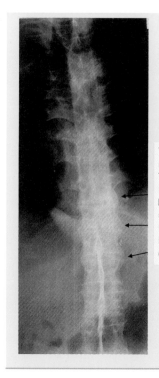

Thoracic and lumbar spine radiograph
There is fusion of the vertical bodies in the thoracic and lumbar spine. Widespread syndesmophyte formation has resulted in the typical bamboo spine appearance (arrowed)

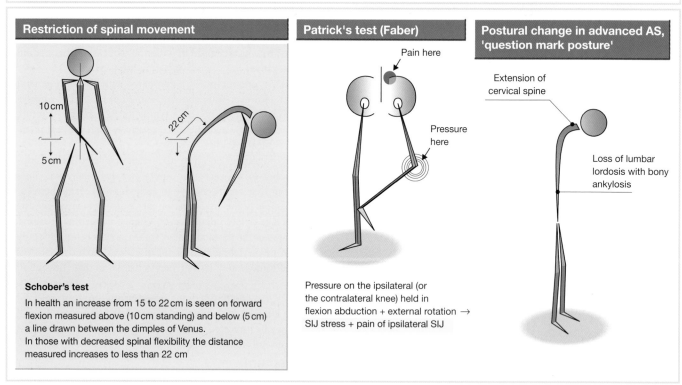

Restriction of spinal movement

10 cm
5 cm
22 cm

Schober's test
In health an increase from 15 to 22 cm is seen on forward flexion measured above (10 cm standing) and below (5 cm) a line drawn between the dimples of Venus.
In those with decreased spinal flexibility the distance measured increases to less than 22 cm

Patrick's test (Faber)

Pain here

Pressure here

Pressure on the ipsilateral (or the contralateral knee) held in flexion abduction + external rotation → SIJ stress + pain of ipsilateral SIJ

Postural change in advanced AS, 'question mark posture'

Extension of cervical spine

Loss of lumbar lordosis with bony ankylosis

- Intra-articular steroids for localized peripheral synovitis and for refractory sacroiliitis; local steroids also for enthesitis (e.g. plantar fasciitis).

Psoriatic arthritis

Ten per cent of those with psoriasis (plaque, guttate, pustular) develop arthritis, which may precede skin lesions or begin simultaneously (33%). It is important to enquire about a family history of psoriasis in anyone presenting with a mono- or oligoarticular arthritis. Psoriatic nail changes (pitting, onycholysis) occur in 70% of those with arthritis. Occult psoriasis may be apparent only in the scalp, natal cleft or umbilicus. Overall morbidity is less than in rheumatoid arthritis but the arthritis tends to be relentlessly progressive.

Clinical patterns of psoriasis-associated arthritis

- Asymmetrical large joint oligoarthritis in 50–70%.
- Axial arthritis/sacroiliitis: asymmetrical and isolated in 5%, or with peripheral joints involvement in 20–40%.

- Peripheral small joint arthritis is indistinguishable from rheumatoid arthritis in 15–25% (negative rheumatoid factor).
- Distal interphalangeal arthritis is associated with dystrophic changes in adjacent nails in 5–10%.
- Arthritis mutilans is a destructive arthritis of the small joints of the hands that rapidly results in joint destruction of such severity as to cause the fingers to collapse and lose length or 'telescope' – so-called 'opera glass hands' – in <5%.
- Dactylitis ('sausage digits') are common and diagnostic.

Clinical management of psoriasis-associated arthritis

Many patients can be managed with NSAIDs alone. Sulfasalazine, gold salts, leflunomide and methotrexate are of modest efficacy. Methotrexate is particularly useful where skin disease is also troublesome. Ciclosporin is more effective for skin disease than the arthritis.

- Anti-TNF biological agents are highly effective for the skin and arthritis in resistant cases. Fifty per cent improvement can be expected within 3 months in 40% of patients.
- Local steroid injections are useful for joint and soft tissue inflammation.
- Systemic steroids may precipitate a skin flare if decreased too rapidly.

Reactive arthritis

Aseptic inflammation of the joints (typically lower limb oligoarticular) may complicate a range of infections at distant sites; typically genital tract and enteric infections are responsible. Seventy per cent of patients are HLA-B27 positive. *Chlamydia*, *Salmonella*, *Shigella*, *Yersinia* and *Campylobacter* species are well-recognized triggers. Although bacterial proteins and DNA can be isolated from the joints, sometimes viable organisms are never cultured.

Extra-articular features are common, including conjunctivitis, aseptic urethritis, mucosal ulceration (circinate balaritis, hard palate) and psoriaform rash on the hands and feet (keratoderma blennorrhagica). The differential diagnosis includes the other seronegative arthritides, septic arthritis/trauma and gout. The diagnosis is clinical but the following investigations may be useful:

- Inflammatory markers are raised and the rheumatoid factor is negative. Synovial fluid is not diagnostic, and a diagnostic tap is indicated primarily to exclude sepsis or crystals, when a sterile leukocytosis is found.
- Urinalysis: pyuria (usually sterile). Culture: urine/stool/synovial fluid/high urethral or vaginal swab, and serology for *Chlamydia* and *Yersinia*. Referral to a genitourinary clinic may be appropriate and contact tracing should be attempted.
- HLA-B27 testing may help to consolidate the diagnosis where there is a strong clinical suspicion.

Management

Establish the diagnosis and rule out sepsis. Initiate bed rest, intra-articular steroids and splinting in the acute attack, followed by passive strengthening exercises at about 10 days. NSAIDs are useful for symptom control but some patients (<5%) may need systemic corticosteroids.

Recurrent or chronic symptoms may require disease-modifying antirheumatic drugs (DMARDs; e.g. sulfasalazine or methotrexate) and, exceptionally, anti-TNF agents are indicated. Remission is usual at 2–6 months, but persistence of symptoms or recurrent flares are common (*c.* 30%). Long-term follow-up of more severe forms of reactive arthritis suggests that up to 20% may develop AS over 20 years. Severe systemic features with weight loss, fevers and deranged liver function tests may mimic deep sepsis or malignancy in some cases. The role of antibiotic therapy in limiting arthritic complications is controversial. However, in sexually acquired forms of the disease contact tracing and eradication of *Chlamydia* is clearly important to prevent long-term damage to the genital tract.

Enteropathic arthritis

Enteropathic arthritis is summarized in Table 219.2:

- Peripheral and/or spinal joint involvement may occur.
- Extra-articular/extraintestinal manifestations occur in the eye (5%), the skin (pyoderma gangrenosum (<5%)) and erythema nodosum (<10%).
- Type I peripheral enteropathic arthritis is oligoarticular, self-limiting and associated with flares of IBD.
- Type II enteropathic peripheral arthritis is polyarticular, protracted and not related to disease activity in the gut. Both types of arthropathy may respond to sulfasalazine or methotrexate. Anti-TNF-α therapy is also highly effective.

Table 219.2 Peripheral arthritis vs sacroiliitis in inflammatory bowel disease (IBD).

	Peripheral arthritis	Sacroiliitis
Frequency of involvement	Crohn's > UC 10% vs 5%	Crohn's > UC 30% vs 10%
Relationship to B27	25% of type I arthritis Type II unrelated	*c.* 100% of B27-positive IBD patients develop sacroiliitis
Relationship to IBD disease extent/activity	Yes (type I), no (type II) Coincident bowel/joint flares in 60–70% in type I	No May even precede bowel symptoms
Responsive to NSAIDs*	Yes	Yes
Responsive to DMARD (sulfasalazine first choice)	Yes	No
Responsive to bowel resection	UC yes, Crohn's no	Neither

*Caution, may flare IBD. UC, ulcerative colitis.

220 Vasculitis

Clinical features of vasculitis

Upper respiratory tract involvement
especially in Wegener's granulomatosis (WG), also Churg–Strauss (CS)
- Epistaxis, sinusitis, deafness
- Otitis media

Cardiac involvement
- PAN
- Angina, MI

Hypertension
- Polyarteritis nodosum (PAN), WG

Lower respiratory tract involvement
- Cough, shortness of breath, haemoptysis (WG)
- Asthma (CS)

Renal involvement
WG, PAN
- Microscopic haematuria, renal failure

Rheumatic involvement
- Myalgia – common in giant cell arteritis, PAN
- Arthritis – common in many vasculitides

Nervous system involvement
- Mononeuritis multiplex
- CNS lesions (cranial nerve palsy, transverse myelitis)
- Stroke

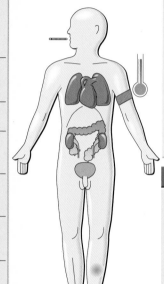

GI tract involvement
PAN, micro PAN, WG, CS
- Colicky abdominal pain, constipation/diarrhoea
- Subacute obstruction (HSP →intussusception)
- GI bleeding

Skin rashes
Rashes are common in vasculitis
Characteristic patterns include:
- Purpura: HSP, limited skin vasculitis
- Diffuse erythema: PAN, WG
- Rashes with ulceration
- Many other rashes also occur

Treatment of vasculitis

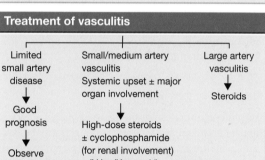

Limited small artery disease → Good prognosis → Observe

Small/medium artery vasculitis
Systemic upset ± major organ involvement → High-dose steroids ± cyclophosphamide (for renal involvement) ± IV I g (Kawasaki)

Large artery vasculitis → Steroids

Management of vasculitis

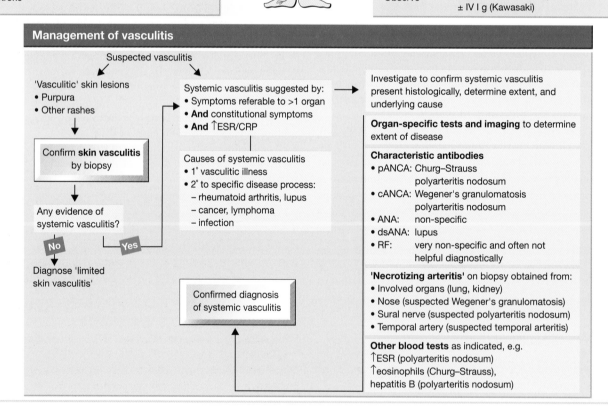

Suspected vasculitis

'Vasculitic' skin lesions
- Purpura
- Other rashes

Confirm **skin vasculitis** by biopsy

Any evidence of systemic vasculitis?

No → Diagnose 'limited skin vasculitis'

Yes →

Confirmed diagnosis of systemic vasculitis

Systemic vasculitis suggested by:
- Symptoms referable to >1 organ
- **And** constitutional symptoms
- **And** ↑ESR/CRP

Causes of systemic vasculitis
- 1° vasculitic illness
- 2° to specific disease process:
  – rheumatoid arthritis, lupus
  – cancer, lymphoma
  – infection

Investigate to confirm systemic vasculitis present histologically, determine extent, and underlying cause

Organ-specific tests and imaging to determine extent of disease

Characteristic antibodies
- pANCA: Churg–Strauss polyarteritis nodosum
- cANCA: Wegener's granulomatosis polyarteritis nodosum
- ANA: non-specific
- dsANA: lupus
- RF: very non-specific and often not helpful diagnostically

'Necrotizing arteritis' on biopsy obtained from:
- Involved organs (lung, kidney)
- Nose (suspected Wegener's granulomatosis)
- Sural nerve (suspected polyarteritis nodosum)
- Temporal artery (suspected temporal arteritis)

Other blood tests as indicated, e.g.
↑ESR (polyarteritis nodosum)
↑eosinophils (Churg–Strauss),
hepatitis B (polyarteritis nodosum)

Medicine at a Glance, Fourth Edition. Edited by Patrick Davey. © 2014 John Wiley & Sons, Ltd. Published 2014 by John Wiley & Sons, Ltd. Companion website: www.ataglanceseries.com/medicine

Table 220.1 Classification of the vasculitides.

Size of vessel affected	Primary	Secondary
Large arteries	Giant cell arteritis	Rheumatoid arthritis (aortitis) Anklyosing spondylitis, Behçet's syndrome
	Takayasu's arteritis	Infection: syphilis
Medium arteries	Kawasaki disease Classic polyarteritis nodosa	Infection: hepatitis B and C
Medium and small arteries	Wegener's granulomatosis* Churg–Strauss syndrome* Microscopic polyangiitis*	Rheumatoid arthritis, SLE, Sjögren's Drugs (see below) Infection, e.g. HIV
Small arteries	Henoch–Schönlein purpura	Drugs, e.g. sulphonamides, penicillins, thiazides
(leukocytoclastic/hypersensitivity)	Essential mixed cryoglobulinaemia	Infection, e.g. tuberculosis, group A streptococci Malignancy, lymphoma Rheumatoid arthritis, SLE, Sjögren's

*Associated with ANCA antibodies, renal impairment and responsive to immunosuppression with cyclophosphamide.

Definition

The vasculitides are a group of conditions characterized by inflammation of the arterial wall and are usefully classified according to the size of the vessel involved (see Table 220.1). They may arise as a primary process or secondary to other conditions such as drug reactions, infection or neoplasia. Diagnosis is based upon clinical features, confirmation of the pathological lesion on tissue biopsy, and the presence of autoantibodies found in association with certain types of vasculitis.

Key points

- Clinical features of systemic vasculitis result from ischaemic damage in the affected organ(s) and the severity of the vasculitis is reflected by the extent or amount of tissue damage. Inflammation is widespread in systemic vasculitis and there may be involvement of several organs.
- Systemic features (fever, weight loss, malaise, anorexia) accompanied by a rise in inflammatory markers indicate widespread inflammation.
- A thorough evaluation of organs potentially involved is necessary to determine the extent and severity of disease. This requires thorough history taking and examination of the patient, followed by laboratory investigations and imaging or biopsy of all target organs.

Epidemiology and pathogenesis

Giant cell arteritis is common with an annual incidence of 18/100 000. Other systemic vasculitides are much less common (3/100 000 in the UK). Vasculitis is particularly prevalent at the extremes of age. For example, Kawasaki disease is almost exclusively paediatric whereas giant cell arteritis generally occurs after the sixth decade. Some vasculitides are clearly associated with viral infections, e.g. hepatitis B and polyarteritis nodosa. There is no exclusive pathology but the following are frequently found:

- 'Leukocytoclastic vasculitis': a characteristic histological appearance resulting from dissolution of leukocytes, seen in small vessels.
- Necrosis of medium and small arterial walls: found in the systemic necrotizing vasculitides (Wegener's granulomatosis (WG), Churg–Strauss (CS) and polyarteritis nodosa (PAN)). Lesions are focal and segmental within vessels; hence tissue diagnosis may be elusive.

History and examination

- Systemic features often predominate: weight loss, fatigue and fever (see Chapter 45).
- Specific symptoms and signs are dependent on the end organs involved (see Figure 220.1 above).
- Involvement of more than one organ in an inflammatory process is a key clue to the presence of an underlying vasculitis.

Investigations

The aims of investigation are to confirm the diagnosis and to determine the extent of disease (which organs are involved?), its current activity and the extent of damage that has already occurred. Laboratory findings in vasculitic syndromes are shown in Figure 220.1.

Immunology

- Antineutrophil cytoplasmic antibodies (ANCAs) are circulating antibodies directed against cytoplasmic components of neutrophils. These are classified according to the pattern of neutrophil staining: (i) cytoplasmic (cANCA) associated with antibodies to proteinase-3 (PR3-ANCA), which are strongly associated with WG; and (ii) perinuclear (pANCA) directed commonly against myeloperoxidase, associated with other primary small vessel arteritides.
- Rheumatoid factors (RFs) are antibodies directed against the Fc component of immunoglobulin (Ig). They occur in many patients with rheumatoid arthritis, and are also found in many other vasculitides (systemic lupus erythematosus (SLE), cryoglobulinaemia, PAN) and chronic infections.
- Antinuclear antibodies (ANAs) are classified according to the pattern of nuclear staining. A diffuse pattern is found with anti-DNA antibodies, characteristic of SLE, though found also in other conditions. Anti-double-stranded DNA antibodies are specific for active SLE. Staining restricted to the centromere suggests systemic sclerosis. A speckled staining pattern is found with antibodies against extractable nuclear antigens. There are several different forms, common in SLE (anti-Ro, Sm) and Sjögren's syndrome (anti-Ro, La).

Radiology

Plain chest radiographs may show pulmonary infiltrates (small and medium vessel vasculitides). Computed tomography and magnetic resonance imaging are useful in investigation of the upper respiratory tract and sinuses (WG). Angiography

Preferred sites of vascular involvement by selected vasculitides

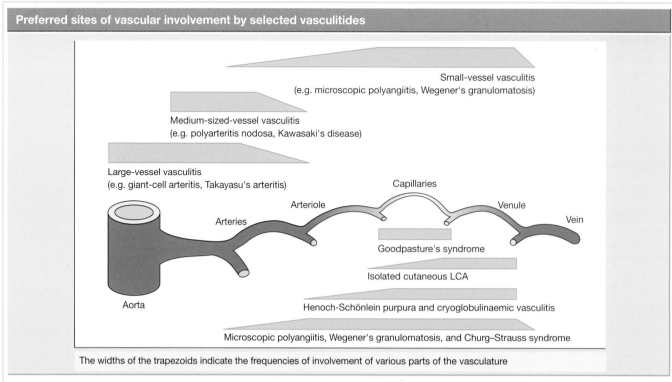

The widths of the trapezoids indicate the frequencies of involvement of various parts of the vasculature

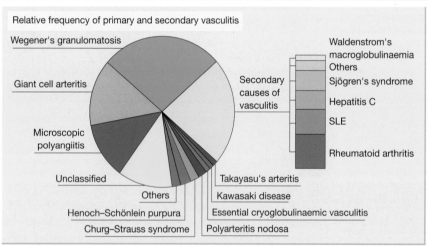

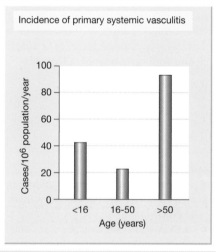

(including magnetic resonance angiography) may be used to delineate the extent of involvement in large vessel vasculitis. Coeliac axis angiography may show clusters of small aneurysms, 'bunches of grapes', in some vasculitides (especially PAN).

Histology

A tissue biopsy shows characteristic vessel wall inflammation, fibrinoid necrosis and 'leukocytoclasis' resulting from dissolution of leukocytes. Suitable sites for biopsy are: blood vessels (e.g. superficial temporal arteries in suspected temporal arteritis), involved skin or other organs such as kidney, muscle, nerve and lung.

Assessing other organ involvement

Screening for involvement of major organs in the small vessel vasculitides is by routine biochemical tests (kidney, liver) or radiology (lung) in the first instance. Characterization of the extent and severity of this involvement requires more invasive investigation (see Figure 220.1).

Prognosis and treatment

These diseases retain a significant morbidity and mortality despite recent therapeutic advances. Immunosuppression is the mainstay of therapy. The large vessel vasculitides are generally responsive to steroids with large doses of oral prednisolone to induce remission (up to 1 mg/kg/day), and smaller 'maintenance' doses often required for prolonged periods. The medium and small vessel vasculitides (WG, CS, microscopic polyangiitis), which are associated with ANCA antibodies, frequently involve the kidney, and respond well to immunosuppression plus oral prednisolone. The choice of agent depends on the severity and extent of disease but in the more aggressive cases (e.g. those with renal involvement or mononeuritis multiplex) intravenous pulsed cyclophosphamide is the current treatment of choice. In refractory cases biological therapies, including rituximab, have been used to good effect. Primary small vessel vasculitis is typically self-limiting in nature (e.g. Henoch–Schönlein purpura (HSP)). In systemic vasculitis, the prognosis is worse for those with renal or other major organ involvement. A comprehensive evaluation of the extent and severity of multiorgan involvement is vital to prevent potentially fatal complications, and to avoid unnecessary use of toxic agents in limited small vessel vasculitis. An algorithm for management and treatment is shown in Figure 220.1.

221 Systemic lupus erythematosus

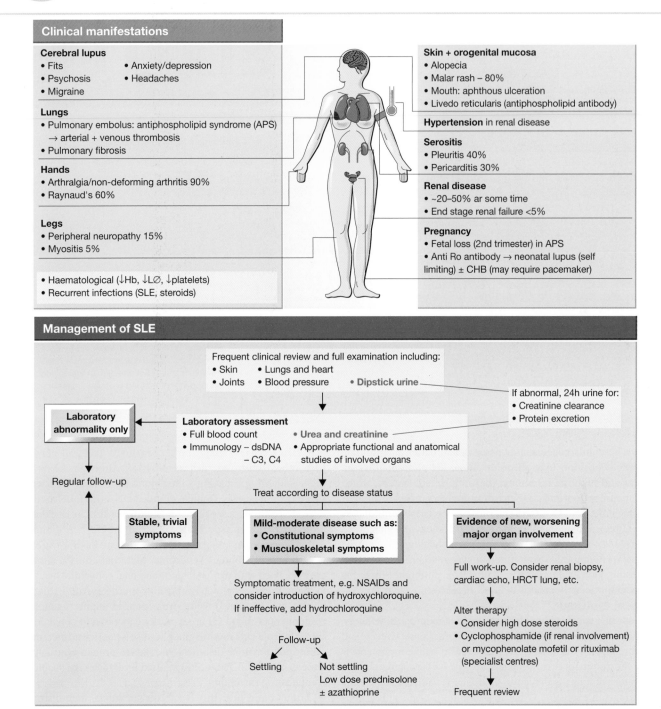

Clinical manifestations

Cerebral lupus
- Fits
- Psychosis
- Migraine
- Anxiety/depression
- Headaches

Lungs
- Pulmonary embolus: antiphospholipid syndrome (APS) → arterial + venous thrombosis
- Pulmonary fibrosis

Hands
- Arthralgia/non-deforming arthritis 90%
- Raynaud's 60%

Legs
- Peripheral neuropathy 15%
- Myositis 5%

- Haematological (↓Hb, ↓LØ, ↓platelets)
- Recurrent infections (SLE, steroids)

Skin + orogenital mucosa
- Alopecia
- Malar rash – 80%
- Mouth: aphthous ulceration
- Livedo reticularis (antiphospholipid antibody)

Hypertension in renal disease

Serositis
- Pleuritis 40%
- Pericarditis 30%

Renal disease
- ~20–50% ar some time
- End stage renal failure <5%

Pregnancy
- Fetal loss (2nd trimester) in APS
- Anti Ro antibody → neonatal lupus (self limiting) ± CHB (may require pacemaker)

Management of SLE

Frequent clinical review and full examination including:
- Skin
- Joints
- Lungs and heart
- Blood pressure
- Dipstick urine

If abnormal, 24h urine for:
- Creatinine clearance
- Protein excretion

Laboratory abnormality only

Laboratory assessment
- Full blood count
- Immunology – dsDNA – C3, C4
- Urea and creatinine
- Appropriate functional and anatomical studies of involved organs

Regular follow-up

Treat according to disease status

Stable, trivial symptoms

Mild-moderate disease such as:
- **Constitutional symptoms**
- **Musculoskeletal symptoms**

Evidence of new, worsening major organ involvement

Symptomatic treatment, e.g. NSAIDs and consider introduction of hydroxychloroquine. If ineffective, add hydrochloroquine

Full work-up. Consider renal biopsy, cardiac echo, HRCT lung, etc.

Alter therapy
- Consider high dose steroids
- Cyclophosphamide (if renal involvement) or mycophenolate mofetil or rituximab (specialist centres)

Follow-up

Settling

Not settling Low dose prednisolone ± azathioprine

Frequent review

Systemic lupus erythematosus (SLE) is a multisystem disease characterized by inflammation involving many systems, and exhibits a relapsing and remitting course. It is strongly associated with autoantibodies to components of the cell nucleus (antinuclear antibodies (ANAs)). Its protean manifestations lead to its inclusion in the differential diagnosis of many 'difficult' cases in clinical practice.

Aetiology and epidemiology

The aetiology of SLE is unknown, but multiple genetic and environmental factors are probably involved. Concordance is 25% in monozygotic twins, but only 2% in non-twin siblings indicating strong genetic influences. The HLA-DR3 association is thought to reflect complement null alleles on these haplotypes. Inherited deficiencies of early complement cascade components (e.g. C1q and C2) are extremely strongly associated with SLE. It is particularly prevalent in the African-American female population of the USA (one in 250), in contrast to the low prevalence in similar ethnic groups in West Africa. In mixed ethnicity UK populations the prevalence is 45–50/100 000 females. Females are ten times more commonly affected than males. Peak onset is 15–40 years. A range of drugs (e.g. minocycline, procainamide, hydralazine) can induce a lupus-like syndrome, particularly in those with certain metabolic polymorphisms of the cytochrome P450 system (e.g. slow acetylators). There is no single immunopathological

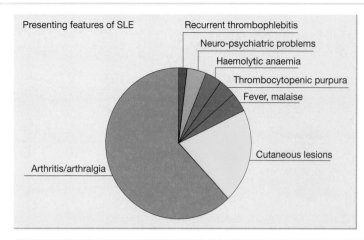

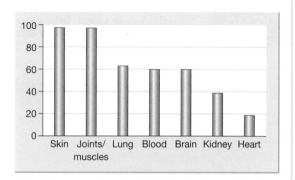

The graph shows the proportion of patients who eventually have involvement of the specified organ

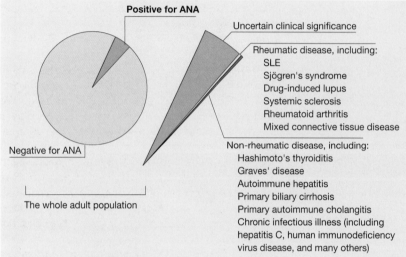

Relevance of ANA in the general population
The diagnosis of SLE rests mainly on the clinical features (Table 221.1); however, the immunological findings are also important. It is however clear that the finding of antinuclear antibodies in the blood is of very uncertain clinical significance in most people without typical clinical stigmata of a specific illness

feature. Vasculitis, coagulapathy, tissue inflammation and immune complex deposition may all occur. There are abnormalities in: cellular and humoral immunity; the complement system, which may underlie abnormal clearance of immune complexes; apoptosis, which may lead to the generation of characteristic antinuclear and antiphospholipid antibodies. Renal pathology is well studied and five histological groups of glomerulonephritis are recognized (in the WHO criteria), from minimal change to proliferative and sclerosing glomerulonephritis. Anti-DNA antibodies may be involved in the pathogenesis of lupus nephritis.

Clinical features

Non-specific constitutional features include joint pains, lethargy, weight loss and lymphadenopathy. Systemic upset (fever and extreme malaise) is usually very marked in active lupus and is often the dominant presenting feature. The best recognized clinical feature of lupus is the 'butterfly'/malar facial rash, commonly following sun exposure. Other rashes, mouth ulcers and a non-deforming arthritis are common. Vital organ involvement, such as renal or central nervous system (CNS), determines prognosis and treatment. Renal involvement may manifest as nephrotic syndrome, or covertly with proteinuria, active renal sediment and progressive loss of renal function. CNS manifestations, such as headaches, seizures, strokes, cognitive decline and altered behaviour are common. Encephalopathy occasionally occurs.

Formal classification criteria for the diagnosis of lupus have been defined by the American College of Rheumatology (see Table 221.1).

Immunology and other investigations in SLE

● **Immunology**: active SLE is always associated with the presence of ANAs so long as the appropriate laboratory test substrate

(e.g. HEP2 cells) is used . Lower sensitivity (c. 90%) may occur with other substrates such as rat liver. Although ANAs occur universally in SLE patients, they alone are neither sufficient nor specific for diagnosis. Double-stranded DNA (dsDNA) antibodies are specific but less sensitive for SLE; titres also correspond only loosely to activity (see Tables 221.2 and 221.3). Antibodies to extractable nuclear antigens, e.g. Ro (SSA) and La (SSB), are found in SLE and in Sjögren's syndrome. Maternal anti-Ro antibodies are associated with neonatal lupus and fetal congenital heart block in a small percentage of Ro-positive mothers. Antihistone antibodies are associated with drug-induced lupus. Complement components C3 and C4 are typically depressed in active SLE but are unreliable as a routine guide to disease activity. In contrast to other inflammatory disorders, C-reactive protein is usually (not always) normal in active SLE; a raised level raises the suspicion of complicating infection.

● **Lupus band test**: this is specific for lupus, demonstrating a characteristic band of IgG and/or IgM deposition at the dermoepidermal junction in involved and uninvolved skin.

● **Haematology**: leukopenia/lymphopenia occur in active SLE. Anaemia is due to chronic disease or Coombs-positive haemolysis. Immune thrombocytopenia can occur, and can predate lupus by many years.

● **Renal function**: renal impairment (decreased glomerular filtration rate) or proteinuria (>3+ dipstick, >0.5 g/24 h) are common in SLE, and of extreme therapeutic importance. An 'active renal sediment' with red cell and/or granular casts may be the *only* indication of serious renal disease. Renal biopsy is the only reliable guide to severity of renal disease and its treatment. It should always be considered in those with renal abnormalities.

Table 221.1 Diagnostic criteria for SLE. Four of out of 11 criteria present at any time is required for a diagnosis of SLE.

Clinical	Laboratory
Malar rash	Haematological abnormalities (see text)
Photosensitive rash	Immunological abnormalities (see text)
Discoid lupus rash	ANA positive
Neurological involvement: seizures or psychosis	
Renal disease: proteinuria or casts	
Serositis: pleuritis or pericarditis	
Mucosal aphthous ulceration	
Arthritis	

Table 221.2 Immunological and other tests for SLE.

Test	% positive
dsDNA binding	70–85
Antinuclear antibodies (high titre, IgG class)	95
Raised serum IgG level	65
Low serum complement (C3/C4 levels)	60
Platelet autoantibodies	60
Cryoglobulinaemia	20
Antibodies to extractable nuclear antigen:	
• Sm	5–30
• RNP	35
• Ro	30
• La	15
Antibodies to phospholipids	30
Rheumatoid factor (low titre)	30
Skin biopsy of normal skin +ve for IgG, C3 and C4 deposits	75–85
Raised ESR	60
Leukopenia	45
Direct Coombs' test +ve	40
Lupus anticoagulant	10–20
C-reactive protein	Normal unless infection present
Proteinuria	30

- **Clotting abnormalities**: venous and arterial thromboses may occur due to autoantibodies that activate *in vivo* clotting. *In vitro* these cause a prolonged activated partial thromboplastin time (APTT). The platelet count is often slightly reduced (*c.* 100×10^9/L). Testing must look for *both* lupus anticoagulant (this can be detected with the dilute Russell viper venom test) and anti-cardiolipin (phospholipid) antibodies (IgG and IgM class). Either test may be abnormal alone, but the significance is the same, and suggests the presence of the antiphospholipid syndrome (APS). SLE underlies many cases of APS; cases can occur without SLE. Clinical features of APS include recurrent fetal loss and arterial and/or venous thromboses. Although clotting times are prolonged *in vitro*, there is a thrombotic tendency *in vivo*. 'False-positive' VDRL (syphilis) serology also identifies one form of the antiphospholipid antibody associated with an increased thrombotic risk. No treatment is required if no clinical features are present.

Management and therapy

Lupus is an unpredictable disease that relapses and remits. Management is aimed at the acute flare but also at preventative strategies such as protection against ultraviolet radiation and prompt evaluation and treatment of infection. Close clinical supervision, with regular assessment of the disease, is vital to determine the

Table 221.3 Interpretation of changes in complement and dsDNA in SLE.

dsDNA	C3	C4	Interpretation dsDNA antibodies
↑	→	→	↑ Activity: watch for change in clinical state
↓/→	↓	↓	Renal involvement should be suspected
↑/→	↑	↑	Look for infection: measure C-reactive protein (not usually increased unless infection present)

need for anti-inflammatory and immunosuppressive therapy, particularly to minimize renal and CNS damage. Pharmacological options are:

- **NSAIDs**: musculoskeletal manifestations.
- **Antimalarials**: hydroxychloroquine is used for musculoskeletal and cutaneous manifestations and improves outcome in epidemiological studies. Side effects include retinal toxicity.
- **Systemic immunosupression** is required for major organ involvement:
  - Corticosteroids: used topically for inflammatory rashes and orally for active disease, such as serositis and constitutional upset. Sometimes used intravenously for acute severe manifestations such as CNS lupus. Azathioprine, methotrexate and mycophenolate mofetil may be used as steroid-sparing agents. Beware osteoporosis risk.
  - Cyclophosphamide suppresses lupus nephritis and reduces the risk of end-stage renal failure. It may also benefit CNS and haematological complications. Mycophenolate mofetl may also be used. Angiotensin-converting enzyme (ACE) inhibitors may help in SLE nephritis by reducing chronic proteinuria and blood pressure.
  - Rituximab is a monoclonal antibody therapy which depletes B cells and is used in severe lupus nephritis unresponsive to standard immunosuppressive regimens. It is frequently used by lupus experts in the management of 'difficult' SLE, though clinical trials were not conclusive.
  - Biological therapies in SLE: a number of SLE-specific biological therapies are currently in development, The first to be licensed is belimumab (anti-BLyS). Therapeutic targets for these drugs are specific to lupus and target B cells and interferon pathways that have been shown to be important in SLE activity and progression.
- **Anticoagulation** is used in the antiphospholipid syndrome: life-long warfarin is used in patients who have experienced thrombosis.
- **Intravenous immunoglobulin** or danazol may be used for immune thrombocytopenia.
- **Symptomatic treatment** as appropriate for depression, epilepsy, Raynaud's phenomenon and mouth ulcers.

Prognosis

Survival is 90% overall at 5 years, but there is an early excess mortality in those with severe disease, probably reducing life expectancy by 15 years overall. There is a highly significant excess of cardiovascular disease, much of which is related to chronic inflammation and steroid use. End-organ involvement differs widely between individuals but renal disease is the most important adverse prognostic indicator. At 15 years only 60% of patients with nephritis are alive compared with 85% of the rest. The main causes of death in SLE are cardiovascular, CNS lupus, infection, lupus nephritis and renal failure.

Scrupulous attention should be paid to correcting traditional adverse cardiovascular risk factors, e.g. hypertension, dyslipidaemia, smoking.

222 Inflammatory muscle disease and selected forms of vasculitis

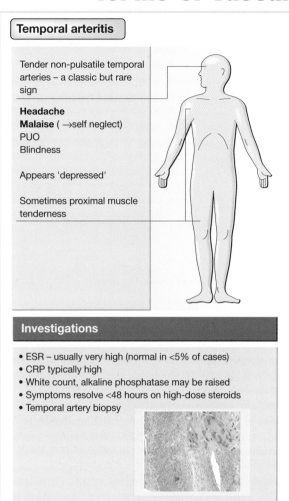

Temporal arteritis

Tender non-pulsatile temporal arteries – a classic but rare sign

Headache
Malaise (→self neglect)
PUO
Blindness

Appears 'depressed'

Sometimes proximal muscle tenderness

Investigations

- ESR – usually very high (normal in <5% of cases)
- CRP typically high
- White count, alkaline phosphatase may be raised
- Symptoms resolve <48 hours on high-dose steroids
- Temporal artery biopsy

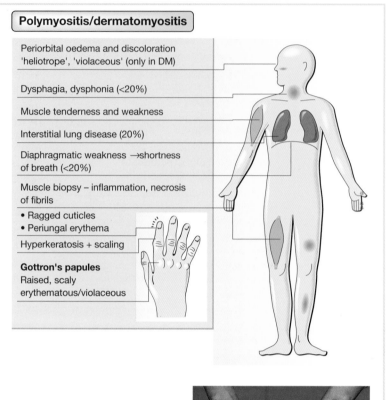

Polymyositis/dermatomyositis

Periorbital oedema and discoloration 'heliotrope', 'violaceous' (only in DM)

Dysphagia, dysphonia (<20%)

Muscle tenderness and weakness

Interstitial lung disease (20%)

Diaphragmatic weakness →shortness of breath (<20%)

Muscle biopsy – inflammation, necrosis of fibrils

- Ragged cuticles
- Periungal erythema

Hyperkeratosis + scaling

Gottron's papules
Raised, scaly erythematous/violaceous

Myositis

Myositis is an inflammation of muscles, and presents with aching, tender, weak muscles sometimes in a characteristic distribution. Muscle enzymes (creatine phosphokinase,(CK or CPK)) are raised and are used to monitor treatment. Where inflammation is suspected, magnetic resonance imaging (MRI) may be diagnostic, or is used to guide biopsy. Electromyography (EMG) findings are also characteristic. Myositis may be a feature of some vasculitides or systemic autoimmune diseases such as systemic lupus erythematosus (SLE) or undifferentiated connective tissue disease. The presence of the anti-ribonucleic protein (RNP) antibody is associated with myositis in these conditions. Myositis is also the key feature in two specific conditions, polymyositis and dermatomyositis.

Polymyositis and dermatomyositis

Polymyositis (PM) and dermatomyositis (DM) are inflammatory myopathies of unknown aetiology. The peak incidence of PM is 40–60 years. DM also occurs in childhood. Overall prevalence is 5–10 per million. Pathological findings are of inflammation in muscles (and skin in DM) and in the vessels that supply them. There is a recognized association of DM conditions with an underlying (usually undiagnosed) malignancy. This is less clear with PM.

Clinical features and classification

Both are characterized by a subacute onset of proximal arm and leg weakness (see Figure 222.1). DM is a distinct clinical entity associated with a rash, most commonly affecting the face and trunk but also on the dorsum of the hands. Rarely skin involvement occurs without myositis. Polymyositis and DM are classified according to age, and whether or not there is an underlying disease process:

- **Childhood-onset DM**: not associated with malignancy; characteristically results in an inflammatory myopathy (with atrophy and contractures), with skin involvement, subcutaneous calcification and vasculitis affecting the skin, muscle and gut.
- **Primary PM**: there is no underlying disease process, with an insidious onset over months of a symmetrical (especially proximal) muscle weakness, which can also involve the oesophageal muscles (resulting in dysphagia) and respiratory muscles (causing respiratory failure).
- **Primary DM**: in addition to the features of primary PM, skin involvement occurs, especially a lilac-coloured rash, and oedema of the upper eyelids, and a scaly violaceous eruption over the extensor surfaces of the joints (knuckles, elbows, knees).
- **PM/DM associated with autoimmune rheumatic diseases** (especially rheumatoid arthritis, systemic sclerosis and SLE).

- **PM/DM associated with malignancy**, of which lung, ovary, breast, gastointestinal tract and myeloproliferative disorders are the commonest.

Investigations

The most helpful tests are markers of muscle damage (biochemical, electrical, histological). Creatine kinase (CK) is raised in >70% cases; EMG is abnormal in almost all polymyositis, with characteristic findings. Muscle biopsy shows inflammatory cellular infiltrate with necrosis of muscle fibres. MRI findings are characteristic, show the extent of mysositis, and are useful in deciding where to biopsy. Autoantibodies (e.g. antinuclear antibody) are positive in 50–75%, with antisynthetase antibodies (e.g. anti Jo-1) characterizing those particularly at risk of interstitial lung disease, arthritis and florid hand rash. It is important to perform a screening history and full physical examination to search for underlying malignancy (present in 20% of DM, less in PM). Further investigations are dictated by these findings.

Management and outcome

Early diagnosis is important to preserve muscle function and avoid major organ involvement:

- High-dose prednisolone initially to achieve disease control. Tapering of steroids occurs according to symptoms and CK level.
- 10–15% may not respond to steroids or relapse on steroid taper. Second-line agents such as methotrexate, azathioprine or mycophenolate are then initiated.
- Intravenous immunoglobulin can be useful, particularly in skin disease.
- In the absence of underlying malignancy, up to 85% of patients have a good or partial response to steroids.

Polymyalgia rheumatica

Polymyalgia rheumatica is an inflammatory disorder of unknown aetiology affecting older adults, resulting in pain and stiffness of the proximal muscle groups. In those >60 years the prevalence is c. 1%, and the female : male ratio is 2 : 1. The disease is uncommon in non-Caucasians. The pathophysiology is unclear and no histological lesion is diagnostic. There may be synovitis.

Clinical and investigative features

- Pronounced early morning stiffness in the limb girdles with ache and weakness, which leads to difficulty rising from squat or raising arms above head.
- Systemic features of weight loss, fatigue and lassitude may occur.
- Up to one-fifth have concurrent giant cell arteritis.

The erythrocyte sedimentation rate (ESR) is usually >60. The C-reactive protein (CRP) is also raised and is a more sensitive indicator of activity. Other laboratory investigations, including muscle enzymes, are usually normal. Normochromic anaemia and/or raised alkaline phosphatase may be found. There is no diagnostic radiology.

Management

- Oral prednisolone therapy gives prompt and dramatic improvement in symptoms, initially 15 mg/day (typically for 2 months), tapering slowly by 1 mg per month as symptoms resolve and inflammatory markers fall. Steroid therapy can usually be stopped after 12–18 months but up to 20% of patients require long-term low-dose maintenance. Immunosuppressive agents, including methotrexate, may then be useful as steroid-sparing drugs.
- Relapses in symptoms are managed by increasing back to the last effective dose of prednisolone.
- Bone protection with calcium/vitamin D preparations or bisphosphonates is usually indicated.

Polymyalgia rheumatic is not life-threatening. Morbidity in the long term may arise due to long-term steroid therapy.

Giant cell arteritis (temporal arteritis)

This is a relatively common vasculitis, mainly affecting those >60 years old (annual incidence 10–25/100 000). The clinical presentation is often a severe, unremitting headache associated with scalp tenderness (lying the head on a pillow is painful, as is combing hair). Transient visual disturbance (amaurosis fugax) or blindness can occur. A minority present with systemic symptoms (malaise, fever, weight loss) and minor scalp tenderness. Masseter muscle claudication may occur. Sometimes patients may sustain strokes. The CRP is often very high. The diagnosis is confirmed by finding characteristic changes (including 'giant cells') on a temporal artery biopsy (70% are biopsy positive). The disease can patchily affect the temporal artery, so a negative temporal artery biopsy does not rule out temporal arteritis.

Treatment is with high-dose oral prednisolone (1 mg/kg/ day), initiated immediately the diagnosis is suspected because of the risk of blindness. These relieve symptoms in <48 hours; if this does not occur the diagnosis should be re-evaluated. Steroids can be tailed cautiously over a few months to a lower maintenance dose, aiming for approximately 10–15 mg/day at 3 months. Low-dose daily aspirin is also recommended to reduce the risk of cerebrovascular events. The disease may 'burn out' over 2 years or so but many patients require life-long low-dose steroid maintenance and some may need additional immunosuppressive drugs for disease control. In these cases azathioprine or methotrexate may be added. Complications include retinal artery inflammation, leading to sudden irreversible blindness. It is to avoid this dreaded complication that treatment is started early and aggressively. Temporal artery biopsy can be deferred for a few days after starting steroids without reducing the diagnostic yield. Other much rarer complications include aortitis, which can lead to aortic dissection or aneurysm formation (in the aorta or the other large head and neck arteries). In these patients biological therapy with infliximab may be considered. Occasional patients present with a stroke (1–2% of all strokes); an ESR or CRP should therefore be performed in all patients with cerebrovascular accident.

Takayasu's arteritis

This is a very rare large vessel vasculitis of the major large arteries (e.g. the aorta, and its major branches) particularly in young Oriental females (commonly 15–35 years), resulting in a systemic illness (fever, malaise) with tenderness over any palpable arteries. Bruits occur and peripheral pulses may disappear (hence its synonym 'pulseless' disease). Renovascular hypertension may occur, as may strokes. Steroids are beneficial in the acute phase but treatment with cyclophosphamide, methotrexate or infliximab may be necessary in steroid-resistant patients or life-threatening disease.

Kawasaki arteritis

This syndrome, essentially only occurring in childhood, is important in adult medicine as it may underlie cases of myocardial infarction/acute coronary syndromes in teenagers and young adults. Predominantly male children (M : F 16 : 1) present with a systemic illness comprising prolonged high fever and a rash with erythema of the hands/feet, progressing to peeling a few days later. The conjunctiva becomes infected, and the lips and oral cavity are typically inflamed with sloughing of the mucosa. Any other organs may be involved; a carditis is particularly common. Coronary dilatation (seen by trans-thoracic cardiac ultrasound) occurs early, and in the absence of treatment 20% develop aneurysms of the coronary arteries. The illness is self-limiting (mortality <0.1% in the acute phase), the main therapeutic issue is to prevent the formation of coronary aneurysms which predispose to later myocardial ischaemia. IV immunoglobulin reduces the risk of coronary aneurysms and should be given promptly in Kawasaki arteritis.

223 Eczema and urticaria

Eczema/dermatitis

Symptoms
Itchy, ill-defined red patches

Acute signs
Erythema, oedema, vesicles, serum exudates

Chronic signs
• Lichenification
• Scaling

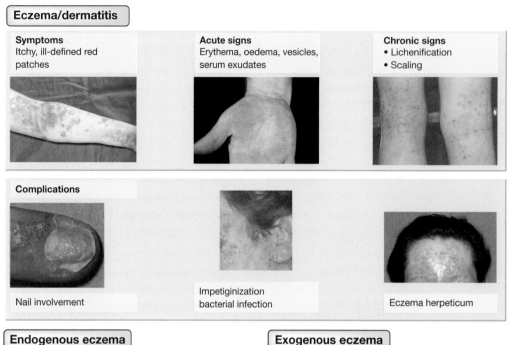

Complications

Nail involvement

Impetiginization bacterial infection

Eczema herpeticum

Treatment

Moisturization
• Soap substitution
• Emollients

Treat infection
• Topical or oral antibiotics
• Oral antivirals

Avoid irritants
• Soap, water
• Solvents, abrasives
• Heat

Decrease inflammation
• Oral antihistamines
• Topical steroids
• Topical tacrolimus pimecrolimus
• Rarely azathioprine, ciclosporin

Phototherapy
• UVB
• PUVA

Endogenous eczema

Atopic eczema

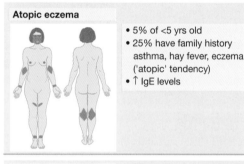

• 5% of <5 yrs old
• 25% have family history asthma, hay fever, eczema ('atopic' tendency)
• ↑ IgE levels

Seborrhoeic eczema

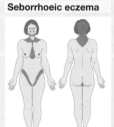

• Itchy, scaly erythematous lesions
• Usually idiopathic
• Common in HIV infection
• Possibly due to abnormal reaction to *Pityrosporum* yeast

Other causes of endogenous eczema
• Pityriasis alba
• Stasis eczema
• Asteatotic eczema
• Pompholyx
• Eczematous drug reactions
• Discoid eczema
• Lichen simplex
• Neurodermatitis
• Nodular prurigo
• Exfoliative dermatitis

Exogenous eczema

Irritant contact dermatitis
• Soaps, detergents
• Hairdressing chemicals
• Cutting oils, coolants

Allergic contact dermatitis

Cosmetic
Nickel ear-rings
Necklace
Deodorants
Jean buttons
Rubber gloves, epoxy resins
Shoe: chrome rubber dyes

Medicament
Otitis externa

Pruritus ani

Medicaments
Gravitational eczema

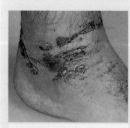

Caustic burns from wet cement

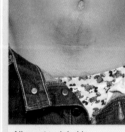

Allergy to nickel in jeans button

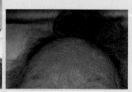

Cosmetic allergy

Phototoxic eruptions
• Drugs (thiazides)
• Plants (parsnip, citrus)

Photoallergic reactions
• Drugs (phenothiazines)
• Perfumes (musk)

Eczema and dermatitis are practically synonymous. They are subdivided aetiologically and clinically. Lesions are very itchy, with ill-defined edges. Histologically, intercellular epidermal oedema (spongiosis) is seen.

Atopic dermatitis

Atopic dermatitis is a relapsing condition beginning in infancy and sometimes continuing into later life. Atopy is an inherited tendency to develop an altered state of immune reactivity (type I

Medicine at a Glance, Fourth Edition. Edited by Patrick Davey. © 2014 John Wiley & Sons, Ltd. Published 2014 by John Wiley & Sons, Ltd. Companion website: www.ataglanceseries.com/medicine

Urticaria and angioedema

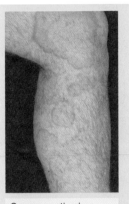

Common urticaria:
giant annular wheals

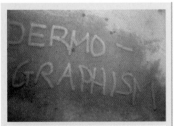

Dermographism: linear wheals
after scratching

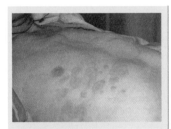

Drug induced urticaria:
penicillin allergy

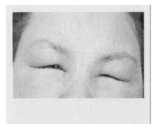

Angioedema of the face:
marked eyelid swelling

and other hypersensitivity reactions). Patients who have a personal or first-degree family history of asthma, hay fever, conjunctivitis or eczema have the atopic diathesis (25% of the population). Atopic patients have elevated serum IgE levels.

Clinical features

Ill-defined erythematous scaly patches occur on the face and in flexural sites. Scratching and rubbing lead to infection, skin thickening and lichenification. Atopic dermatitis is a clinical diagnosis. Infection is common and skin swabs may be indicated. IgE may be elevated.

Management and prognosis

Atopic eczema can be difficult to manage. The principles of therapy are to moisturize the skin with emollients and minimize itching with oral antihistamines. Irritants such as soap, chronic wet work, heat and solvents should be avoided. House-dust mite avoidance may be helpful. Specific treatments include topical therapy with tar, steroids or calcineurin inhibitors and antibiotics for complicating infection. A sunny, dry climate is beneficial. Systemic therapy with oral/intravenous antibiotics and antiviral agents may be indicated. Phototherapy with ultraviolet light or immunosuppression using azathioprine and ciclosporin may be indicated in more severe cases. Secondary infection with herpes simplex virus (eczema herpeticum) constitutes an emergency requiring hospitalization and treatment with systemic aciclovir. The major features of the condition resolve in 40% after 5 years of age and 90% by 15–20 years of age.

Other types of endogenous eczema

- **Lichen simplex**: eczema in response to repeated trauma or scratching.
- **Nodular prurigo**: a widespread manifestation of the above.
- **Stasis eczema** (varicose eczema, lipodermatosclerosis): results from venous hypertension (which may relate to venous valvular damage from deep venous thrombosis, pregnancy, etc.). Leakage of blood from the capillaries into the surrounding tissue deposits fibrin and haemosiderin around the capillaries, so diminishing tissue perfusion and predisposing to skin ulceration. It occurs over the inner shin and medial malleolus, and is itchy, indurated, scaly and purpuric. It is often complicated by contact dermatitis caused by topically applied drugs, and diagnosed by patch testing or by 'autosensitization' (secondary generalization of chronic stasis eczema supposedly resulting from 'sensitization' to epidermal antigens). Autosensitization affects the face, neck and extensor regions of the arms and thighs.

- **Asteatotic eczema**: occurs on the legs of elderly patients where there is dry skin. There is a glazed 'crazy-paving' effect. It responds to emollients and topical steroids.
- **Discoid eczema**: characterized by itchy, symmetrical, coin-shaped lesions on the extensor surfaces of the limbs and feet. The lesions are differentiated from those of ringworm/tinea corporis (which have an active border), psoriasis (often non-itchy with a silvery scale) and mycosis fungoides (asymmetrical and persistent). Discoid eczema is treated with emollients, topical steroids and systemic antihistamines.
- **Pompholyx**: acute vesicular eczema of the palms and soles. It is treated with potassium permanganate soaks, and topical or systemic steroids. Concomitant fungal infection of the foot (tinea pedis) should be sought. Pompholyx often recurs.
- **Seborrhoeic dermatitis**: a common, mildly itchy, scaly, red rash with a predilection for the scalp, face, chest, back, axillae and groins. It is an abnormal cutaneous reaction to commensal *Pityrosporum* yeasts. It may occur in HIV infection and Parkinson's disease. Treatment is with topical steroids plus an anti-yeast agent (e.g. imidazole). When the scalp is affected (dandruff), ketoconazole or selenium sulphide shampoo can be helpful.

Contact dermatitis

Contact dermatitis is a major industrial and occupational category of disease. It may be allergic or an irritant. Almost anything in the environment may be an irritant and many substances are sensitizers, including medicaments. Allergic contact dermatitis is the archetypal type IV cell-mediated immunological reaction. Patch testing is the principal investigation. A battery of common allergens is applied to the non-inflamed back. The patches are removed at 48 hours and the reactions read. The patient is seen again at 72 hours and late responses recorded. Interpretation (false negatives, false positives and significance of positives) is a specialist activity. Treatment: withdrawal of the offending agent is vital, but prophylaxis is important in industry because, once initiated, allergic contact dermatitis may persist despite removal of the responsible allergen(s).

Prevention of hand eczema

Hand eczema may be a diagnostic and management problem. Often atopic, irritant and allergic factors coexist. The use of cotton

Table 223.1 Causes and exacerbating factors of common urticaria (most cases are idiopathic).

Drugs	Aspirin, codeine, morphine, non-steroidal anti-inflammatory drugs
Foods	Fish and shellfish, eggs, nuts, tomatoes
Additives	Tartrazine, benzoates
Inhalants	Pollen, spores, house dust
Infections	Focal sepsis: (e.g. urinary tract infection, upper respiratory tract infection, hepatitis, *Candida* spp., protozoa, helminths)
Systemic	Systemic lupus erythematosus, reticuloses and carcinoma

Table 223.2 Types of urticaria.

Type	Features
Common urticaria	Lesions last for several hours
Angioedema	Deeper dermal and subdermal involvement
Contact urticaria	Immediate response to allergens (e.g. foods)
Physical urticaria	Lesions last several minutes, but <1 h
Dermographism:	In response to scratching or trauma
Cholinergic	In response to heat /exercise
Cold/aquagenic	In response to cold /water
Heat/solar	In response to heat /sun
Urticarial vasculitis	Lesions last several days or longer; purpuric
Hereditary angioedema	C1 esterase inhibitor deficiency
Autoinflammatory syndromes:	
Cryopyrin periodic syndromes	Fever, chills, arthralgia eye pain and redness
Schnitzler syndrome	Fever, bone pain, arthralgia, IgM gammopathy

gloves inside rubber gloves for all wet and dirty tasks is recommended. Consider prophylaxis with barrier preparations where there is industrial/occupational risk.

Urticaria

Urticaria (hives) describes itchy red (erythematous) wheals (i.e. skin swellings resulting from leaky capillaries). Management aims to exclude an underlying cause, identify and remove precipitants or provocatants (see Table 223.1), and provide effective symptomatic treatment.

Epidemiology, aetiology and pathogenesis

Urticaria is very common and results from mast cell degranulation (a type I immunological reaction) in response to an antigen, with the release of histamine and other vasoactive mediators, leading to erythema and oedema. Of patients with this condition, 70% have idiopathic urticaria (where the antigen is not known) and the remainder have other forms (see Table 223.2). The differential diagnosis includes insect bites, prodromal pemphigoid, toxic erythema and erythema multiforme.

Urticaria, when severe, can also affect subcutaneous tissues, so producing angioedema (swelling in the hands, lips and around the eyes, and less commonly but more importantly of the tongue or larynx).
- Angioedema may be idiopathic.
- It may occur in individuals exposed to food antigens to which they have been sensitized, e.g. peanuts.
- Angioedema may occur in those with congenitally deficient C1 esterase levels (hereditary angioedema).

Investigations and management

If something other than acute idiopathic urticaria is suspected (e.g. symptoms for >2 months), a full blood count, eosinophil count and erythrocyte sedimentation rate, thyroid autoantibodies, thyroid function, renal and liver function and complement levels should be examined, and a stool sample taken for ova, cysts and parasites. Counselling and reassurance are the mainstays of treatment. Itching may be exacerbated by psychological factors. High doses of non-sedating anti-H_1-receptor histamines by day are supplemented by sedating antihistamines at night. The patient should be warned about drowsiness, alcohol and driving. Sometimes the addition of high doses of an anti-H_2-receptor agent such as cimetidine is helpful. Systemic steroids are generally eschewed, but have a role in severe cases.

Acute laryngeal angioedema and anaphylaxis can be life-threatening. An intramuscular injection of 0.5 ml of 1 : 1000 adrenaline (epinephrine) (500 µg) is the recommended treatment in adults. Fixed dose (300 µg) 'pen' injections are available for at-risk individuals.

Urticarial vasculitis

Urticarial vasculitis (5% of all urticarias) is a leukocytoclastic vasculitis and is suspected if urticarial lesions last >24 hours and resolve with purpura. It is associated with diseases such as systemic lupus erythematosus and hepatitis B and C. Treatment depends on the cause, but oral corticosteroids or other immunosuppressants are sometimes needed.

Hereditary angioedema

Hereditary angioedema (HAE) caused by congenital (autosomal dominant) deficiency of C1 esterase inhibitor is suspected when there is a family history and angioedema, often spontaneously or in response to infection/ trauma. Urticaria is never present. Patients may present with abdominal pain, mimicking an acute abdomen. Angioedema may affect any part of the body and may affect the larynx, causing respiratory obstruction. The finding of a normal C3 and absent C4 during an attack is highly suspicious of HAE, which can be confirmed by measurement of total and functional C1 esterase inhibitor levels. Modified androgens such as stanozolol and danazol or an antifibrinolytic such as tranexamic acid can be used for prophylaxis. Purified C1 esterase inhibitor may be used as prophylaxis before surgery and when attacks are very frequent. Acute attacks can be treated with purified C1 esterase inhibitor or with icatibant, a bradykinin antagonist. The latter can be self-administered at home as it is given by subcutaneous injection. In emergencies, fresh frozen plasma may be used but may cause a deterioration rather than improvement in symptoms. Respiratory obstruction should be managed by intubation or tracheostomy. Adrenaline and hydrocortisone are relatively ineffective. All patients with HAE should be under the care of an immunologist.

224 Psoriasis

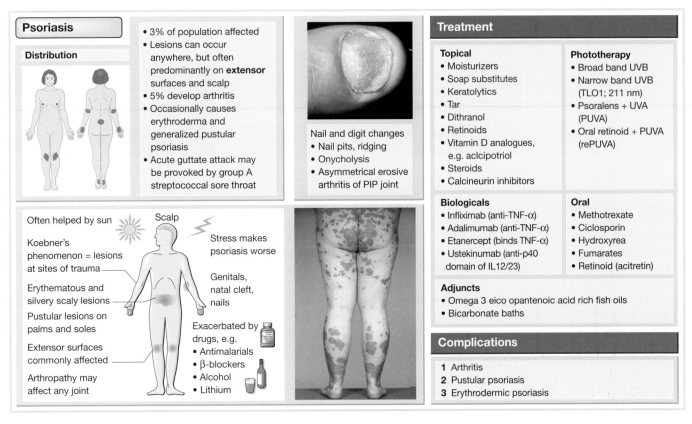

Psoriasis

Distribution

- 3% of population affected
- Lesions can occur anywhere, but often predominantly on **extensor** surfaces and scalp
- 5% develop arthritis
- Occasionally causes erythroderma and generalized pustular psoriasis
- Acute guttate attack may be provoked by group A streptococcal sore throat

Nail and digit changes
- Nail pits, ridging
- Onycholysis
- Asymmetrical erosive arthritis of PIP joint

Often helped by sun

Koebner's phenomenon = lesions at sites of trauma

Erythematous and silvery scaly lesions

Pustular lesions on palms and soles

Extensor surfaces commonly affected

Arthropathy may affect any joint

Scalp

Stress makes psoriasis worse

Genitals, natal cleft, nails

Exacerbated by drugs, e.g.
- Antimalarials
- β-blockers
- Alcohol
- Lithium

Treatment

Topical
- Moisturizers
- Soap substitutes
- Keratolytics
- Tar
- Dithranol
- Retinoids
- Vitamin D analogues, e.g. alcipotriol
- Steroids
- Calcineurin inhibitors

Phototherapy
- Broad band UVB
- Narrow band UVB (TLO1; 211 nm)
- Psoralens + UVA (PUVA)
- Oral retinoid + PUVA (rePUVA)

Biologicals
- Infliximab (anti-TNF-α)
- Adalimumab (anti-TNF-α)
- Etanercept (binds TNF-α)
- Ustekinumab (anti-p40 domain of IL12/23)

Oral
- Methotrexate
- Ciclosporin
- Hydroxyrea
- Fumarates
- Retinoid (acitretin)

Adjuncts
- Omega 3 eico opantenoic acid rich fish oils
- Bicarbonate baths

Complications

1 Arthritis
2 Pustular psoriasis
3 Erythrodermic psoriasis

Aetiology and pathogenesis

A polygenic susceptibility exists. Some human leukocyte antigen (HLA) types (Cw6) are associated with skin disease alone, whereas others (e.g. B27) are associated with additional joint disease. The PSORS1 cluster of genes on chromosome 6 are involved, but other genes implicated are for IL-12 and IL-23R. Infections, stress or drugs may precipitate attacks of psoriasis. A Th2 cytokine profile of activation occurs involving tumour necrosis factor α (TNF-α). Psoriatic plaques are characterized by the dual pathological features of epidermal hyperproliferation and cutaneous inflammation.

Clinical features

Psoriasis manifests as red, silver-scaled lesions, which may be guttate or nummular, or plaques. The scalp is frequently involved, as are the nails. Pustulosis may occur, particularly in the palms and soles, and occasionally psoriasis causes erythroderma. Arthritis, which can be severe, can complicate the disease. The common subtypes of psoriasis are:

- **Chronic plaque psoriasis**: the differential diagnosis includes atopic dermatitis, seborrhoeic dermatitis, mycosis fungoides and tinea.
- **Guttate psoriasis**: this form of psoriasis may be precipitated by a streptococcal sore throat or other infection. Lesions are small (<1 cm), scaly and widespread. Spontaneous resolution usually occurs after a few months. The differential diagnosis includes secondary syphilis and pityriasis rosea.
- **Erythrodermic psoriasis**: widespread erythema occurs, with 'skin failure', which may lead to failure of thermoregulation, infection fluid and protein loss, and a high output form of heart failure. Other causes of erythroderma include eczema, mycosis fugoides (cutaneous T-cell lymphoma) and drug eruption (e.g. toxic epidermal necrolysis).

- **Pustular psoriasis**: this severe form results in a sudden crop of widespread small pustules throughout the skin, with considerable systemic upset.

The chronic inflammation of psoriasis is associated with the metabolic syndrome, a combination of medical disorders that, when occurring together, increase the risk of developing cardiovascular disease and diabetes.

Investigations

A skin biopsy, if necessary, shows irregular epidermal hyperplasia, suprapapillary thinning, clubbing of rete pegs, leukocyte infiltration and epidermal pustulosis.

Management and prognosis

Treatment is hierarchical and depends on severity, site, age, sex and occupation. Systemic drugs have more risks; methotreaxte is hepatotoxic and ciclosporin is nephrotoxic. They are immunosuppressants as are the biologics with a risk of infections (patients should be prescreened for tuberculosis, hepatitis, HIV) and cancers. The facets of the metabolic syndrome require prevention and management.

Reactive arthritis

The reactive arthritis syndrome (arthritis, urethritis, conjunctivitis) occurs in response to urinary or gastrointestinal tract infection in genetically predisposed individuals, and is part of the same disease continuum as psoriasis. Skin lesions in reactive arthritis syndrome are similar to psoriasis. In reactive arthritis, thickened yellow palms and soles with a cobblestone appearance, with or without pustular lesions (keratoderma blennorrhagica) and involvement of the penis (circinate balanitis), are found. Other features of psoriasis may be present.

225 Acne, rosacea and hidradenitis

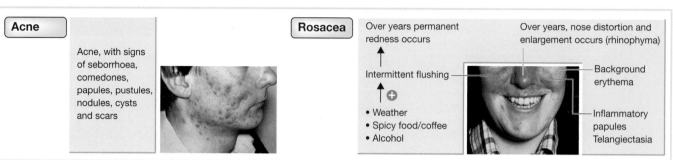

Acne

Acne, with signs of seborrhoea, comedones, papules, pustules, nodules, cysts and scars

Rosacea

Over years permanent redness occurs

Intermittent flushing

- Weather
- Spicy food/coffee
- Alcohol

Over years, nose distortion and enlargement occurs (rhinophyma)

Background erythema

Inflammatory papules
Telangiectasia

Acne vulgaris

Aetiology and pathogenesis

Acne vulgaris is universal in adolescence; 1% of men and 5% of women may require treatment up until the age of 40. Acne vulgaris is a chronic disorder of the pilosebaceous duct with increased sebum production, ductal hypercornification, a deranged symbiotic relationship with commensal microorganisms (*Propionibacterium acnes*) and cutaneous inflammation. Increased sebum production is probably the fundamental abnormality.

The sebaceous glands are driven by androgens. Women with acne manifest a complex form of cutaneous androgenization. Many women with acne have polycystic ovaries on ultrasonography, although most do not have the other features of the polycystic ovary syndrome. There is no evidence for systemic endocrine abnormalities in men. Rarely, endocrine disorders, such as 'full-blown' polycystic ovary syndrome, Cushing's syndrome, virilizing neoplasms or exogenous corticosteroids/androgens, underlie the acne.

Clinical features

The clinical features of acne are seborrhoea, comedones, papules, pustules, nodules, cysts and scars distributed on the face, neck, back and chest. Pyoderma faciale is acute severe facial acne. Acne fulminans is acute severe acne with fever, arthralgia and sterile lytic lesions of bone.

Investigations

Investigations are only indicated if Cushing's syndrome or virilization is suspected. Pelvic ultrasonography can demonstrate polycystic ovaries.

Management and prognosis

Treatment depends on the severity of the condition and an objective record of severity helps follow-up. The principles of therapy are to keep the skin clean, to discourage microorganism growth and the use of keratolytics to relieve comedones.

- Mild acne: topical antibiotics, keratolytics and retinoids.
- Moderate to severe acne: both topical and systemic therapy, with oral antibiotics (which can result in failure of the oral contraceptive pill or teratogenicity) or anti-androgenic hormones (i.e. for women, a suitable contraceptive pill).

- Severe nodulocystic (conglobate) acne or failure to respond to other treatments is an indication for the oral retinoid (vitamin A derivative) isotretinoin (13-*cis*-retinoic acid). This highly effective drug affects all four aetiological factors operating in acne and reduces sebum production by 75–90%. Treatment lasts 4–6 months. Side effects, which are essentially those of hypervitaminosis A, include teratogenesis (women must not get pregnant when on treatment), eczema, cheilitis (sore lips), conjunctivitis, benign intracranial hypertension, mood disturbance and biochemical hepatitis and hyperlipidaemia.

Acne is usually self-limiting. With the exception of isotretinoin, treatment does not alter the natural history, and thus should continue throughout the course of the disorder. Topical therapies are needed long term and antibiotics should be given for at least 6 months. Repeated courses or long-term treatment may be necessary. Maintenance topical treatment is needed after oral therapy is stopped. Combined therapy is rational because there are several pathogenic factors.

Rosacea

Rosacea is a disorder of unknown aetiology, associated with instability of the facial vasculature, facial flushing and the secondary development of inflamed papules and pustules, particularly affecting the cheeks, chin and central forehead. Coffee, spicy foods, alcohol and adverse weather are precipitants to avoid. It responds to oral antibiotics (e.g. tetracycline, erythromycin, metronidazole). Long-term cosmetic damage to the nose (enlargement with discoloration and rhinophyma) and facial telangiectasia can occur if not treated.

Hidradenitis suppurativa

Hidradenitis suppurativa is the apocrine equivalent of acne vulgaris. In mild forms, patients have recurrent boils in apocrine areas (axillae, groins, breasts, behind the ears). Staphylococcal carriage and diabetes mellitus should be excluded. Chronic nodulocystic involvement of the groins with suppuration and fistula formation can occur. Hidradenitis can respond indifferently to oral antibiotics, hormonal manipulation and isotretinoin. Oral steroids may be necessary. Anti-tumour necrosis factor treatment with infliximab shows promise. It may be necessary to resort to surgical excision.

Medicine at a Glance, Fourth Edition. Edited by Patrick Davey. © 2014 John Wiley & Sons, Ltd. Published 2014 by John Wiley & Sons, Ltd. Companion website: www.ataglanceseries.com/medicine

226 Disorders of skin pigmentation

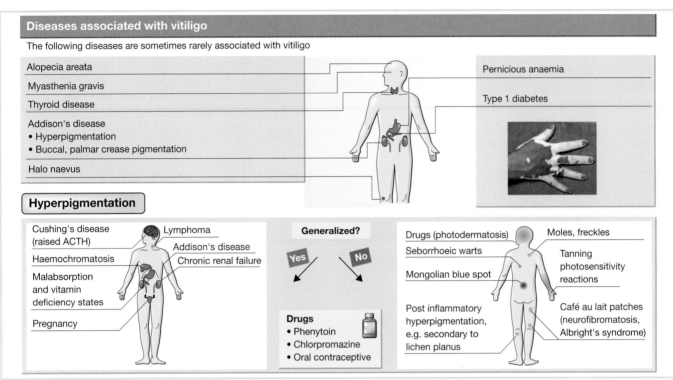

Diseases associated with vitiligo

The following diseases are sometimes rarely associated with vitiligo

Alopecia areata
Myasthenia gravis
Thyroid disease
Addison's disease • Hyperpigmentation • Buccal, palmar crease pigmentation
Halo naevus

Pernicious anaemia

Type 1 diabetes

Hyperpigmentation

Cushing's disease (raised ACTH)
Haemochromatosis
Malabsorption and vitamin deficiency states
Pregnancy

Lymphoma
Addison's disease
Chronic renal failure

Generalized?
Yes   No

Drugs
• Phenytoin
• Chlorpromazine
• Oral contraceptive

Drugs (photodermatosis)
Seborrhoeic warts
Mongolian blue spot
Post inflammatory hyperpigmentation, e.g. secondary to lichen planus

Moles, freckles
Tanning photosensitivity reactions
Café au lait patches (neurofibromatosis, Albright's syndrome)

Excess or diminished pigmentation is usually due to excess or diminished melanocyte activity in the skin, although deposition of other pigments can be involved. Melanocyte activity is influenced by solar ultraviolet light. Both hypo- and hyperpigmentation are common complications of inflammatory dermatoses and are more pronounced in racially pigmented skin.

Hyperpigmentation

Congenital diseases associated with patches of hyperpigmented skin include melanocytic naevi and Fanconi's and Albright's syndromes. Café-au-lait patches are also found in neurofibromatosis.

Acquired diseases can give rise to localized or generalized hyperpigmentation:

● **Localized hyperpigmentation**: many inflammatory skin diseases can leave patches of hyperpigmentation. Chloasma (melasma) is patchy facial hyperpigmentation, due to endogenous or exogenous steroids, sunlight, drugs (e.g. antibiotics) and depilation.
● **Generalized hyperpigmentation**: can result from acquired endocrine or systemic illness (see Figure 226.1) or drugs, particularly photosensitive reactions to drugs, chemicals and plants.

Hypopigmentation

Hypopigmentation may be:

● Congenital and generalized, as in the genetic disease of albinism, where melanization cannot occur as a result of tyrosinase deficiency, or localized, such as the hypopigmented ash leaf patches found in tuberous sclerosis.

● Acquired: post-inflammatory hypopigmentation (common, can occur after any cause of skin inflammation, e.g. contact dermatitis) or with leprosy (depigmented anaesthetic areas). A common cause is vitiligo. A very rare cause is pituitary failure (generalized loss of skin pigment, often with loss of secondary sex characteristics).

Vitiligo

This is a common (1% of the population) autoimmune condition affecting all races, of unknown aetiology and associated with antimelanocytic antibody production and organ-specific autoimmune disease.

Clinical features

Depigmented macules appear on sun-exposed areas, areas previously hyperpigmented (e.g. face, axillae, groins) and areas exposed to trauma or friction (an example of Koebner's phenomenon). Areas of vitiligo are readily demonstrated by an ultraviolet lamp (Wood's light). Hairs within a lesion become amelanotic (white).

Management and prognosis

Treatment is unsatisfactory, but the priorities are:

● Protection from the sun to avoid skin cancer and to minimize the contrast between affected and unaffected skin.
● Cosmetic camouflage.

Of younger patients, 20% may repigment spontaneously, but it is usually unsatisfactorily patchy and perifollicular. Some patients respond to phototherapy.

Medicine at a Glance, Fourth Edition. Edited by Patrick Davey. © 2014 John Wiley & Sons, Ltd. Published 2014 by John Wiley & Sons, Ltd. Companion website: www.ataglanceseries.com/medicine

227 Blistering diseases

Autoimmune blistering diseases

	Bullous pemphigoid	Pemphigus vulgaris	Dermatitis herpetiformis
Incidence	Common	Rare	Very rare
Age	Elderly	40–50 years	Young adults Elderly
Antibody attack target	Basement membrane hemidesmosome	Interepidermal cell desmosomal structure	Not characterized
Diagnosis	Biopsy	Biopsy Serum antibodies	Biopsy (skin and gut) Demonstration of villous atrophy
Treatment	Topical steroid Prednisolone 40–60 mg/day	Topical steroid Prednisolone 80–120 mg/day	Topical steroid Dapsone Gluten-free diet
Underlying malignancy	Possible	Rarely	GI Lymphoma risk
Prognosis	Excellent	Variable	Good

Dermatitis herpetiformis

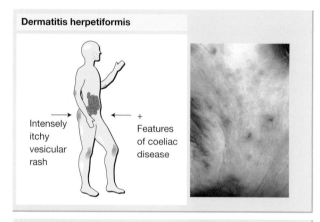

Intensely itchy vesicular rash

+ Features of coeliac disease

Pemphigus vulgaris

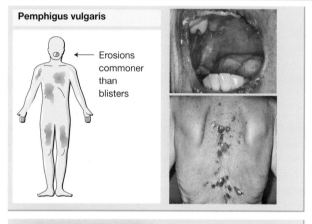

Erosions commoner than blisters

Bullous pemphigoid

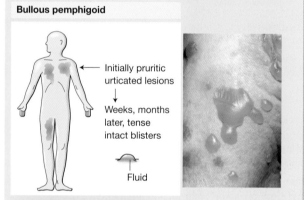

Initially pruritic urticated lesions

Weeks, months later, tense intact blisters

Fluid

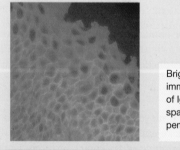

Bright green immunofluorescence of IgG in the intercellular space in a patient with pemphigus vulgaris

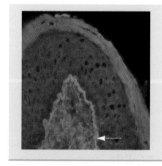

Bright green immunofluorescence of IgG at the BMZ (arrow) in a patient with pemphigoid

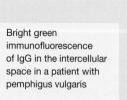

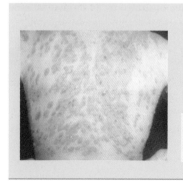

Pemphigus vulgaris: widespread superficial blisters and erosions

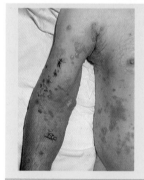

Bullous pemphigoid: tense blisters (bullae) on an erythematosus and urticated base

Medicine at a Glance, Fourth Edition. Edited by Patrick Davey. © 2014 John Wiley & Sons, Ltd. Published 2014 by John Wiley & Sons, Ltd. Companion website: www.ataglanceseries.com/medicine

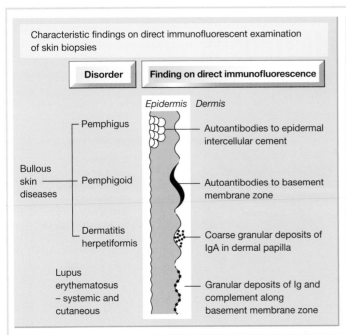

Characteristic findings on direct immunofluorescent examination of skin biopsies

Disorder	Finding on direct immunofluorescence

Bullous skin diseases

- Pemphigus — Autoantibodies to epidermal intercellular cement
- Pemphigoid — Autoantibodies to basement membrane zone
- Dermatitis herpetiformis — Coarse granular deposits of IgA in dermal papilla
- Lupus erythematosus – systemic and cutaneous — Granular deposits of Ig and complement along basement membrane zone

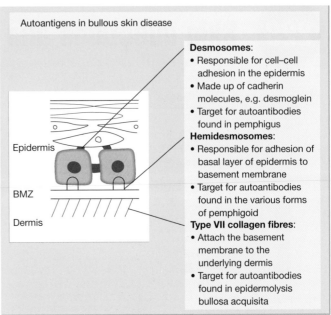

Autoantigens in bullous skin disease

Desmosomes:
- Responsible for cell–cell adhesion in the epidermis
- Made up of cadherin molecules, e.g. desmoglein
- Target for autoantibodies found in pemphigus

Hemidesmosomes:
- Responsible for adhesion of basal layer of epidermis to basement membrane
- Target for autoantibodies found in the various forms of pemphigoid

Type VII collagen fibres:
- Attach the basement membrane to the underlying dermis
- Target for autoantibodies found in epidermolysis bullosa acquisita

Blisters are common, e.g. acute eczema, herpes, impetigo or insect bites. Some drug eruptions are bullous, e.g. toxic epidermal necrolysis, as are some systemic diseases, e.g. porphyria cutanea tarda and amyloid. There are also primary bullous skin diseases.

Congenital blistering diseases

Several very rare, non-infective diseases are associated with blisters from an early age (e.g. epidermolysis bullosa).

Toxic epidermal necrolysis: Lyell's syndrome

This serious, life-threatening idiosyncratic reaction can be the result of a drug reaction or an intercurrent illness. The 'full-blown' disease is rare, but milder cases, usually caused by drug reactions, are much more common. Clinically, there is widespread skin loss, compromising cutaneous homeostasis. There is severe systemic upset. Cardiovascular collapse, infection and failure of thermoregulation contribute to a high mortality. Mucocutaneous involvement is common. Scarring may occur if the patient survives. Intravenous γ-globulins, ciclosporin and granulocyte colony-stimulating factor can be used. The role of systemic steroids is controversial.

Bullous pemphigoid

Bullous pemphigoid is a common disease of elderly people, arising from an autoimmune attack on the hemidesmosome of the basement membrane. Circulating antibodies to the basement membrane zone (BMZ) are often found. There may be an association between seronegative disease, where mucosal lesions are more common, and malignancy. Clinically, the illness can start, not as blisters, but as erythematous, eczematous and urticated areas on the trunk and limbs. Tense blisters appear later in these sites. The diagnosis is confirmed by histology and tissue immunofluorescence. Most patients respond well to prednisolone 40–60 mg daily tapered and replaced by azathioprine longer term.

Pemphigus vulgaris

This is a rare disease, most common in the 45–50-year age group, resulting from antibody-mediated attack on the interepidermal cell desmosomal structure. Clinically, the presenting lesion may be confined to the oral mucosa, scalp, fingernails (paronychia) and genitalia. The blisters are intraepithelial and rupture readily, leaving raw erosions. Skin lesions may not appear for some months. Circulating antibodies are found in the serum. Histology shows an intraepidermal blister with acantholysis (rupture of prickle cells). Direct immunofluorescence demonstrates intercellular IgG and C3. Before the use of systemic corticosteroids, pemphigus vulgaris was fatal. High doses (80–120 mg) of prednisolone are life saving but often produce side effects, which contribute to the mortality. Mycophenolate mofetil and rituximab (anti-CD20 antibody) are promising. Potent topical steroids are used for the mucocutaneous lesions.

Dermatitis herpetiformis

This is a very rare illness of young adults, with a second peak in old age. Patients almost always have a gluten-sensitive enteropathy (coeliac disease). It is strongly associated with certain human leukocyte antigen (HLA) haplotypes. Clinically, intensely itchy groups of small blisters on an urticarial base occur over the elbows, knees, buttocks or face – often only excoriations may be seen. Investigations for coeliac disease may be positive: endomysial antibody, intestinal biopsy or tests for malabsorption (full blood count, serum iron and folate and red cell folate). Skin biopsy shows IgA deposition on the dermal papillae. The eruption responds to dapsone within a few days. A gluten-free diet allows most patients to discontinue dapsone. Follow-up requires awareness of the risk of agranulocytosis and haemolytic anaemia on dapsone and intestinal lymphoma complicating coeliac disease.

228 Skin infections and infestations

Staphylococcal skin disease

Cellulitis
= superficial spreading infection
Occurs on:
- Legs, especially if oedematous
- Around Venflon sites
- Around surgical wounds

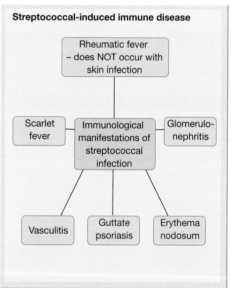

Treatment
- Prolonged antibiotics

Complications
- Staphylococcal bacteraemia

Impetigo
= infection with *Staphylococcus* which elaborates a toxin cleaving upper epidermal layer.
Occurs on the face and armpits

Vesico-pustules with golden crusts

Toxin-mediated staphylococcal syndromes – very rare

Localized staphylococcal infection
↓
Elaborates toxin
↓
Generalized erythema →

Staphylococcal scalded skin syndrome – must be differentiated from toxic epidermal necrolysis (due to drugs, or other infections)

Streptococcal skin disease

Erysipelas and Streptococcal cellulitis

Minor skin trauma
↓
Strep. entry
↓
Pain ++
Burning

Often starts centrally and spreads laterally (often unilateral)

Also occurs on legs/arms, rarely on trunk

Fluid-filled vesicles with well-defined borders

Well defined edge

A linear ascending streak (lymphangitis) suggests streptococcal infection

Necrotizing fasciitis
Strep. and other organisms

Dusky purple
↓ Very rapid progression
Skin, connective tissue, muscle necrosis + severe systemic upset

Treatment
- Antibiotics
- Surgical debridement
- Death rate = 40%

Complications
- Contagious
- Bacteraemia – 5%
- In pre-antibiotic era → 10% death rate

Streptococcal-induced immune disease

Rheumatic fever – does NOT occur with skin infection

Immunological manifestations of streptococcal infection

- Scarlet fever
- Glomerulo-nephritis
- Vasculitis
- Guttate psoriasis
- Erythema nodosum

Staphylococci

Staphylococcal infection of the skin results in spreading superficial infections, deeper infection with abscesses or toxin-mediated damage:

- **Cellulitis**: often on the leg; it is predisposed by trauma, tinea pedis or chronic oedema. Acute episodes require intravenous (IV) antibiotics initially and some patients may need prophylactic low-dose penicillin. Risk factors such as tine pedis, venous eczema and ulceration, and pelvic pathology should be sought and managed.
- **Impetigo**: caused by a toxin cleaving the upper layers of the epidermis; usually on the face and presenting as pustules and golden crusts. Treatment is with topical or oral antibiotics.
- **Abscesses**: may be small and localized to hair follicles (folliculitis) or larger and deeper in the skin, causing boils (furunculosis), which may be extensive (carbuncles). Boils/carbuncles

require incision and drainage. If they recur, nasal carriage of staphylococci and/or diabetes should be considered.

All suspected skin infections should be swabbed for microbiology. Advice from a microbiologist may be needed, e.g. to investigate for Panton–Valentine leucocidin toxin producing strains.

- **MRSA** (methicillin-resistant *Staphylococcus aureus*): this is an increasing problem in dermatology. Treatment should be discussed with a dermatologist and/or microbiologist.
- **Staphylococcal scalded skin syndrome**: this is a reaction to a toxin produced by staphylococci, characterized by generalized erythema and exfoliation in an unwell child or immunocompromised adult. It must be distinguished (a biopsy is informative) from toxic epidermal necrolysis. The organism cannot be cultured from the skin. Systemic antistaphylococcal treatment and IV fluid replacement are given.

Streptococci

Streptococci commonly produce skin and throat infection, and more rarely muscle, joint or heart infection. Damage may result directly, or from toxin elaboration. Organisms may not always be cultured in streptococcal disease and diagnosis is clinical with retrospective rises in the antistreptolysin O and anti-DNAase titres. A portal of entry should be sought.

- **Erysipelas**: a superficial skin infection, of abrupt onset; it is painful and results in systemic upset. There is erythema, peeling and lymphangitis. IV antibiotics are indicated.
- **Scarlet fever**: caused by upper respiratory tract infection with streptococci which elaborate an erythrogenic toxin, resulting in cutaneous vasodilatation.
- **Necrotizing fasciitis**: a serious, often mixed, infection involving streptococci, staphylococci, enterobacteriaceae and obligate anaerobes, or *Streptococcus pyogenes* alone. Often there is no obvious portal of entry in a healthy individual, although the infection may begin in a wound in an unwell patient. The first sign is dusky induration with rapid progressive painful necrosis of the skin, connective tissue and muscle. Prompt diagnosis is essential, IV antibiotics are rarely sufficient and surgical debridement is necessary. There is an appreciable mortality. The infection often occurs on a limb or the scrotum (Fournier's gangrene) or in a postoperative wound (Meleney's progressive synergistic gangrene).
- **Nephritis**, but not rheumatic fever, may follow streptococcal skin infections, so all such skin infections should be treated with systemic antibiotics. Hypersensitivity reactions to streptococci are implicated in erythema nodosum, some vasculitis and guttate psoriasis.

Herpes skin infections

Herpes simplex

Any skin or mucosal site may be infected with, and show recurrence of, herpes simplex virus (HSV) infection. Herpetic lesions are painful vesicles and crusts on an erythematous base. They resolve over 2 weeks. Extragenital disease is usually caused by HSV1 and genital infections are usually caused by HSV2. The diagnosis is clinical, supported by viral culture, electron microscopy and serology. Management: aciclovir orally/intravenously and antibiotics for secondary infection. Long-term prophylaxis should be considered in some cases.

Herpes zoster (varicella) virus

This causes chickenpox or shingles. Shingles results from the reactivation of herpes zoster virus. Physical trauma to the involved dermatome may be the most common trigger. If immune deficiency is present (e.g. lymphoproliferative disorders), zoster may be severe and recurrent. Paraesthesiae and pain precede the eruption. Very rarely, there is pain and no eruption (zoster sine herpete). The rash is variable, but usually asymmetrical. Erythematous oedematous papules and vesicles arise in one crop, become haemorrhagic and necrotic, and then scab and heal with superficial scarring. Outlying lesions are found in most patients. Recurrent zoster is rare and rarely at the same site.

Diagnosis is clinical, but shingles can be confused with HSV, so viral culture, electron microscopy and serology are useful. Mild analgesics control the pain of the prodrome and the illness. A topical antibiotic is often needed for secondary infection and topical steroids suppress the cutaneous inflammation. Postherpetic neuralgia is a consequence of nerve involvement in zoster and is deservedly notorious for its intractability. A short course of oral prednisolone from the beginning of the disease may reduce the risk. Oral aciclovir reduces the time course of the cutaneous eruption, but does not prevent post-herpetic neuralgia.

Zoster affecting the ophthalmic branch of the trigeminal nerve may cause conjunctivitis or rarely optic neuritis, and expert advice should be sought. Zoster of S2 and below may cause acute retention of urine and constipation, and be complicated by haemorrhagic cystitis. Systemic aciclovir is indicated in these and immunosuppressed patients. Varicella zoster immunoglobulin has no impact on established disease but may be given to those who have not had chickenpox but are at significant risk postexposure (e.g. pregnant women).

Warts

Warts are due to human papillomavirus (HPV), of which there are many types: HPV1–4, common warts and verrucas; HPV6 and -11 and genital warts; HPV16 and -18 and penile, vulval and cervical cancer. HPV has a fastidious requirement for human epidermal cells in a particular stage of differentiation. It causes a proliferation of keratinocytes, which partially keratinize and therefore sequester the virus from immunological elimination. Lesions may be sporadic, recurrent or persistent. Treatment is with keratolytics (such as salicylic acid or retinoic acid) or cryotherapy. Cautery and surgical excision may result in lower treatment success rates. Persistent warts can be treated by laser or intralesional bleomycin. Some types, in some sites (e.g. uterine cervix) and in predisposed individuals (e.g. HIV) can cause squamous cancer.

Mollusca

Mollusca are due to a poxvirus. The typical lesion is an umbilicated, dome-shaped papule or nodule. Lesions are common on the trunk in children and usually resolve spontaneously. Cryotherapy is the treatment of choice in adults but is only occasionally tolerated by a child.

Fungal infections

- **Candidosis**: usually an intertriginous infection (i.e. affecting the axillae, submammary folds, crurae and digital clefts). It is a common cause of vulvovaginitis in women. In the immunoincompetent, it may also affect the mucosa and genitalia. It is a common concomitant opportunistic complication of dermatoses (e.g. eczema, psoriasis) at susceptible sites. It is treated with topical nystatin, animidazole or clioquinol, and occasionally with oral imidazole or triazole.
- **Pityriasis versicolor**: a superficial infection of the horny layer by the yeast *Pityrosporum orbiculare*. It is characterized by small, confluent, scaly, depigmented patches, which are often apparent for the first time after tanning. Treatment is with a topical imidazole or with selenium sulphide or occasionally with an oral triazole antifungal (e.g. itraconazole).
- **Dermatophytosis**: the term for ringworm infection (tinea). Lesions are red, scaly and itchy. The groins, feet and axillae are common sites; the lesions are then not necessarily circular and scaly, but are macerated and moist with a scaly edge. The nails may be involved (onychomyosis). Scarring may occur on the scalp due to an infected inflammatory plaque called a kerion. *Microsporum* spp. form spores around hairs (ectothrix) and fluoresce green under Wood's lamp, whereas *Trichophyton* spp. invade the hair shaft (endothrix) and do not fluoresce. Classic treatment is with a topical imidazole or griseofulvin orally. Systemic therapy is necessary for scalp or nail infections. Oral terbinafine or the triazole itraconazole are modern alternatives to griseofulvin.

Parasitosis

- **Scabies** must always enter the differential diagnosis of pruritus. Typically the rash is symmetrical, involving the fingers, backs of hands, axillae, breasts and buttocks. Most lesions may be excoriated papules and nodules, but with care burrows are usually identified. Sites to examine carefully are digital clefts, around the nipples and the genitalia. By taking a skin scraping, burrow contents may be examined under a microscope. The presence of the female mite (*Sarcoptes scabiei*) or her eggs confirms the diagnosis. Only brief apposition of skin surfaces is needed to transmit the infestation; sexual contact is a common means of dissemination. Treatment: topical insecticides applied to cool, dry skin all over the body. Secondary eczema and infection should also be treated. In adult patients with scabies (without HIV) the head can be omitted. It is mandatory to treat partners and co-habitants at the same time. Concomitant sexually transmitted diseases should have been excluded.

● **Head lice** infestation is the result of *Pediculus humanus*, which feeds on perifollicular scalp blood vessels and lays eggs cemented to the hair shaft (nits).

● **Vagabond's disease** (a widespread itchy excoriated dermatosis) is caused by *Pediculus humanus corporis*, which lives in the seams of clothing and lays its eggs there.

● **Crab louse** (*Pthirus pubis*) is named because of its appearance and tenacious adherence to the hairy skin where it is feeding, causing pediculosis pubis.

Mycobacteria and the skin

● **Cutaneous tuberculosis**: common in the developing world but rare in the UK. It may be seen in elderly patients and in immigrants. A chest X-ray, tuberculin and ELISA (enzyme-linked immunosorbent assay) interferon-γ testing and skin biopsy with culture are needed.

● **Atypical mycobacterial infection**: a common cause of skin lesions in people with AIDS or who are immunologically suppressed.

● *Mycobacterium marinum* can result in an indolent granulomatous ulcer. If contracted in a swimming bath it is called swimming pool granuloma; if seen in a pet fish keeper it is called fish-tank granuloma.

● *Mycobacterium ulcerans* is an important cause of leg or arm ulceration in Africa (Buruli ulcer) or Australia (Searle's ulcer).

● *Mycobacterium leprae*: see Figure 228.2 below.

● *Mycobacterium chelonae* is being seen increasingly seen after minor injury or skin surgery in mainly but not always immunocompromised people.

Leprosy	Tuberculoid TT	Borderline			Lepromatous LL	General features of leprosy
		BT	BB	BL		
Immunological responsiveness	High (+ve lepromin test)	Intermediate			Low (–ve lepromin test)	Leprosy (Hansen's disease) results from infection (probably acquired through the respiratory tract) with *Mycobacterium leprae*. Infected patients shed the bacillus from infected nasal secretions; only 1% of contacts develop the disease. Incubation period 2–6 years. The clinical course depends on the host's immunity (see left); skin involvement is a prominent feature, as is peripheral nerve involvement, resulting in hypopigmented patches and anaesthesia. Diagnosis: clinical, finding bacilli in skin smears, culturing bacilli in mice food pad. Lepromin test: intradermal injection of dead bacilli – early reaction (Fernandez) < 48 hours = sensitivity to leprosy protein, late reaction (Mitsuda) 4–5 weeks resistance of host to infection. Treatment is with multiple drugs. Treatment reactions include: • Erythema nodosum leprosum – usually in LL leprosy, painful tender nodules on extensor surfaces • Allergic response to mycobacteria, causing further nerve damage • Iritis Treatment reactions can result in permanent injury – treat promptly with thalidomide
Organisms in lesions	Few – hard to find	Some			Many – easy to find	
Infectivity	Non-infectious	Slightly infectious			Infectious	
Extent of lesions	Localized	Scattered			Generalized	
Involvement	Skin & nerves only				Many tissues	
Skin lesions	1–2 only; commonly on face				Innumerable & widespread	

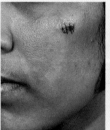

Tuberculoid leprosy: subtle depigmentation with a palpable erythematous rim at the upper edge

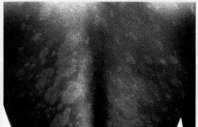

Borderline leprosy (BL). Borderline tuberculoid (BT) downgrading to BL. Showing typical well-defined hypopigmented macules of BT and many small lesions, some of which are papular

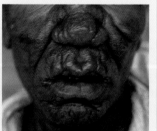

The 'leonine' facies of lepromatous leprosy

Nerve involvement	Thickened nerves in vicinity of skin lesions	Most peripheral nerves thickened
Anaesthesia distribution	Lesions hypoanaesthetic/no sweating	Lesions not hypoanaesthetic – but glove & stocking anaesthesia; trophic ulcers of periphery; muscle nerve paralysis
Clinical course	Disease localized; patients usually not very troubled by the disease – good prognosis, and spontaneous recovery may occur	Patients disabled by the disease with widespread organ involvement

229 The skin and systemic disease

Purpura

Trauma
- Coughing causes petechia in SVC distribution
- Fat embolism after long bone trauma

Sepsis
- Meningococcaemia
- Rickettsia
- SBE

Vasculitis
- Henoch–Schönlein purpura
- Drugs, e.g. bendrofluazide, flucloxacillin
- Autoimmune disease (e.g. SLE, PAN)
- Dysproteinaemias
- Malignancy

Haemostatic failure
- ↓Platelets
- ↓Clotting proteins
- DIC

Others
- Steroids
- Old age
- Scurvy – especially perifollicular
- Amyloidosis – periorbital

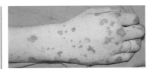

Meningococcal purpura

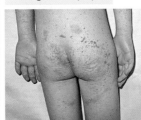

Henoch–Schönlein purpura

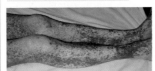

Thrombocytopenic purpura

Cutaneous markers of malignancy

Generalized pruritus

Facial flushing (carcinoid syndrome)

Acute onset multiple seborrhoeic warts (sign of Leser–Trélat)

Clubbing

Acanthosis nigricans

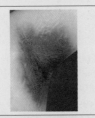

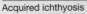

Acquired ichthyosis

Acquired hypertrichosis lanuginosa

Dermatomyositis
- Periorbital oedema
- Heliotrope rash

Superficial thrombophlebitis especially if migratory (carcinoma of the pancreas)

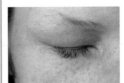

Heliotrope rash of dermatomyositis

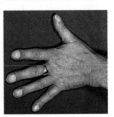

Finger clubbing

Limited cutaneous scleroderma

Associated with anti-centromere antibody distal skin involvement CREST syndrome prominent

Telangiectasia + tightened skin around mouth (microstomia) 'Beaking' of nose

Acid reflux oesophagitis and oesophageal dysmotility ± late stricturing (>10 years)

Late (> 10 years) pulmonary hypertension ± 2° RVF

Distal ulceration + gangrene ± auto-amputation of digits

Distal gangrene → auto-amputation
Calcinosis
Shiny thickened skin
Sclerodactyly (tapered fingers)
Progression

Raynaud's phenomenon
(years – decades)
↓
Limited (arms, face, feet)
skin involvement
↓
Very late (after decades)
internal organ involvement

Raynaud's phenomenon

Diffuse cutaneous systemic sclerosis

Facial symptoms

Oesophageal dysmotility

Heart
- Conduction block
- LV diastolic dysfunction

Pulmonary fibrosis → early pulmonary hypertension

Proximal ± truncal skin involvement

Small bowel dysmotility, wide mouthed diverticular and ± bacterial overgrowth (→malabsorption)

Renal disease
- Oliguric renal failure
- Hypertensive crisis

Hypertension (with rapidly progressive renal disease)

Scl-70 antibody in 30%

Progression

Raynaud's phenomenon
↓
Skin involvement in <1 year
↓
Early internal organ involvement

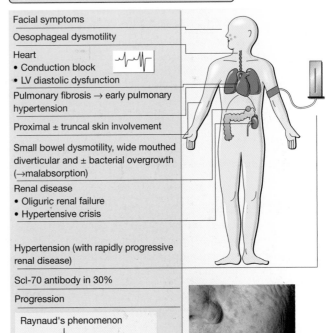

Facial telangiectasia

The skin can be involved in, or react to, many systemic disease processes.

Raynaud's phenomenon

Raynaud's phenomenon is episodic, painful, digital ischaemia in response to cold or emotional stimuli, characterized by classic sequential colour changes of white to blue to red. The disorder may be primary and idiopathic or secondary to underlying disease (see Table 229.1):

- Idiopathic Raynaud's phenomenon is diagnosed in young women who have no features of an underlying disorder on clinical evaluation or investigation.

Table 229.1 Causes of Raynaud's phenomenon.

- Cervical rib
- Vibrating tools
- Vasculitis and connective tissue diseases:
  systemic sclerosis
  Sjögren's syndrome, SLE, dermatomyositis
  rheumatoid arthritis
- Cryoglobulinaemia
- Cold agglutinins
- Hyperviscosity syndromes
- Drugs (β-blockers, ergot alkaloids, cytotoxics)

- Raynaud's phenomenon is more likely to be secondary, usually to systemic sclerosis, if it is especially severe (with digital skin changes) and persistent, or if it begins for the first time in early adulthood, in a male and is unilateral.

Investigations when indicated should include a chest X-ray (cervical rib), autoantibodies (antinuclear antibodies, double-stranded DNA, antineutrophil cytoplasmic antibody), cryoglobulins, cold agglutinins and erythrocyte sedimentation rate. Treatment: heated gloves, oral nifedipine, angiotensin-converting enzyme (ACE) inhibitors and avoidance of cold. If severe, sympathectomy can be considered.

Human immunodeficiency virus

Skin disease is an important corollary of acquired immune deficiency syndrome (AIDS) and human immunodeficiency virus (HIV) infection (see Table 229.2). The incidence of several cutaneous diseases is increased in people who are HIV positive or who have AIDS. The percentage of people with HIV who have skin manifestations, and the number of manifestations, increase as HIV infection progresses. The incidence and severity sometimes correlates with the absolute numbers of T-helper cells, and the prognostic significance of some disorders is well recognized. HIV infection may affect the behaviour of other dermatological conditions such as psoriasis. Generally, HIV-related skin diseases improve with HAART (highly active anti-retroviral therapy) although some patients may experience severe cutaneous immune restoration disease, e.g. due to herpes simplex or cytomegalovirus.

Drug eruptions

Drug reactions are very commonly seen in acute internal medicine and general practice. Regard any drug as capable of causing any cutaneous reaction. Some reactions are predictable (striae with steroids), some likely (photosensitivity with amiodarone, β-blockers exacerbating psoriasis) and some unpredictable or idiosyncratic (erythema multiforme with antibiotics).

Vasculitis

Conditions producing a vasculitic reaction in the skin include:

- **Infection**: meningococcaemia, bacterial endocarditis.
- **Systemic vasculitis** (e.g. systemic lupus erythematosus (SLE), polyarteritis nodosa (PAN)): suspected when internal organs such as the kidneys and/or lungs are involved. Immunology and skin biopsy may be diagnostic, as may renal/lung histology.
- **Erythema nodosum** (EN): painful palpable lesions on the lower legs, arising from a vasculitis of the deep dermis. Although no cause may be found, EN is associated with infection (streptococcal sore throat, mycobacteria, etc.), drugs, sarcoidosis and

Table 229.2 Cutaneous manifestations of HIV infection and AIDS.

Pruritus

Inflammatory dermatoses
- Seroconversion toxic erythema
- Psoriasis
- Seborrhoeic dermatitis
- Severe drug reactions
- Eosinophilic pustular folliculitis
- Papular pruritic eruption
- Vasculitis

Infections
- Folliculitis and cellulitis (including MRSA)
- Tinea and onychomycosis
- Candidosis
- Hairy leucoplakia (EBV)
- Atypical primary, secondary and late syphilis
- Bacillary haemangiomatosis
- Condyloma acuminata (viral warts)
- Molluscum contagiosum
- Cutaneous atypical mycobacterial infection
- Kaposi's sarcoma (HHV8)
- Herpes simplex
- Herpes zoster
- Severe aphthous stomatitis

Other skin manifestations
- Cutaneous and nail hyperpigmentation
- Porphyria cutanea tarda
- Acquired ichthyosis and keratoderma
- Yellow nail syndrome
- Immune reconstitution disease

Neoplasia
- Kaposi's sarcoma (HHV8)
- Cutaneous lymphoma
- Castleman's disease (HHV8)
- Melanoma and non-melanoma skin cancer

EBV, Epstein–Barr virus; HHV, human herpes virus; MRSA, methicillin-resistant *Staphylococcus aureus*.

inflammatory bowel disease. Resolution typically occurs over 5–6 weeks.
- **Other causes**, including drugs, connective tissue disease, paraneoplastic phenomena, clotting abnormalities and cryoglobulinaemia.
- **Skin infarcts**, affecting particularly the extremities, e.g. nail-bed 'splinter haemorrhages' (caused by circulating immune complexes) occur in many acute and chronic infections, including bacterial endocarditis.
- **Purpura** has a wide differential diagnosis (see Figure 229.1). Two common causes are:
  - **Henoch–Schönlein purpura** (anaphylactoid purpura): occurs mainly in children as a result of an abnormal response to a viral infection. A purpuric rash occurs on the extensor aspects of the lower limbs. Nephritis may develop. It normally resolves without sequelae; very occasionally chronic renal damage occurs.
  - **Leukocytoclastic or allergic vasculitis**: may be confined to the skin. The most common clinical pattern is acute, self-limiting, palpable purpura (other lesions may occur), which may be chronic or recurrent and usually affects the limbs with

fever, malaise, arthralgia and gastrointestinal symptoms. The cause is often not discovered but infections, neoplasia and drugs should be excluded.

Skin markers of internal malignancy

There are a number of cutaneous stigmata of internal malignancy:

- **Pruritus**: lymphoma, polycythaemia rubra vera.
- **Ichthyosis**: dry skin with fish-like scales.
- **Acanthosis nigricans**: velvety hyperkeratotic plaques found in flexures and intertriginous areas; also caused by endocrine disorders (acromegaly, Cushing's disease, Addison's disease, hypothyroidism, insulin-resistant diabetes mellitus, polycystic ovary disease), drugs (steroids) or obesity, or rarely it is familial.
- **Dermatomyositis**: skin involvement consists of erythematous plaques over the knuckles, finger joints, elbows and knees. Nail cuticles are ragged. Eyelids are swollen and are discoloured violet (see Chapter 222). Of patients aged >50 years, 30% have an underlying cancer.
- **Migratory superficial thrombosis**: often relates to pancreatic cancer.
- **Secondary deposits in the skin**, e.g. Sister Joseph's nodule (periumbilical deposit from an intra-abdominal malignancy) or Virchow's node (left supraclavicular fossa lymph node deposit from gastric cancer). The scalp is a common site for cutaneous metastasis from internal solid cancers.

Systemic sclerosis

Systemic sclerosis is an autoimmune disease impacting on the skin and internal organs that occurs in two forms: (i) limited cutaneous scleroderma localized to the skin; and (ii) diffuse

cutaneous systemic sclerosis when internal viscera are involved. Scleroderma also occurs in a localized form (morphoea) and in malignancies (e.g. breast cancer), porphyria cutanea tarda, phenylketonuria and in the carcinoid syndrome.

- **Limited cutaneous scleroderma** (morphoea): skin lesions are circumscribed plaques. They can occur anywhere, or may involve the forehead (*en coup de sabre*). Systemic involvement is rare and occurs later.
- **Diffuse cutaneous systemic sclerosis**: female > male. Raynaud's phenomenon precedes cutaneous sclerosis, with puffy swelling of the hands and feet, leading to atrophic thinning of ulcerated digital tips and nail-fold involvement. Muscle weakness occurs (disuse atrophy or muscle involvement). Perioral involvement produces very tight skin around the mouth, restricting opening, and may require lateral release. Dry eyes and mouth (keratoconjunctivitis sicca and xerostomia – Sjögren's syndrome) occur. Oesophageal involvement leads to difficulty swallowing, and small bowel disease produces abdominal pain and diarrhoea (caused by bacterial overgrowth). Pulmonary fibrosis produces shortness of breath (restrictive pattern on lung function testing). An erosive arthritis may cause joint pains. Renal failure occurs and is associated with a worse prognosis. Antinuclear antibodies are found in >90% and anticentromere antibodyies in 70% with CREST (*C*alcinosis, *R*aynaud's, o*E*sophagitis, *S*clerodactyly *T*elangiectasia). No agent reliably arrests disease activity. Treatment is for symptom relief only. Digital vascular insufficiency is treated by cold avoidance, vasodilators (e.g. nifedipine, ACE inhibitors, intravenous prostacyclin, intravenous calcitonin gene-related peptide). In severe cases, digital amputation may be necessary. Oesophageal reflux responds to proton pump inhibitors. The prognosis is generally good, even with some organ involvement, although renal or pulmonary disease can be fatal.

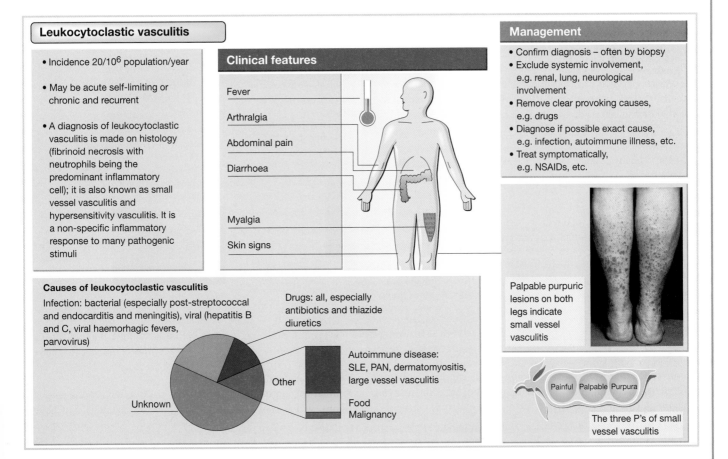

Leukocytoclastic vasculitis

- Incidence 20/10⁶ population/year
- May be acute self-limiting or chronic and recurrent
- A diagnosis of leukocytoclastic vasculitis is made on histology (fibrinoid necrosis with neutrophils being the predominant inflammatory cell); it is also known as small vessel vasculitis and hypersensitivity vasculitis. It is a non-specific inflammatory response to many pathogenic stimuli

Clinical features

Fever
Arthralgia
Abdominal pain
Diarrhoea
Myalgia
Skin signs

Management

- Confirm diagnosis – often by biopsy
- Exclude systemic involvement, e.g. renal, lung, neurological involvement
- Remove clear provoking causes, e.g. drugs
- Diagnose if possible exact cause, e.g. infection, autoimmune illness, etc.
- Treat symptomatically, e.g. NSAIDs, etc.

Palpable purpuric lesions on both legs indicate small vessel vasculitis

Causes of leukocytoclastic vasculitis

Infection: bacterial (especially post-streptococcal and endocarditis and meningitis), viral (hepatitis B and C, viral haemorrhagic fevers, parvovirus)

Drugs: all, especially antibiotics and thiazide diuretics

Other

Unknown

Autoimmune disease: SLE, PAN, dermatomyositis, large vessel vasculitis

Food
Malignancy

Painful Palpable Purpura

The three P's of small vessel vasculitis

230 Skin tumours

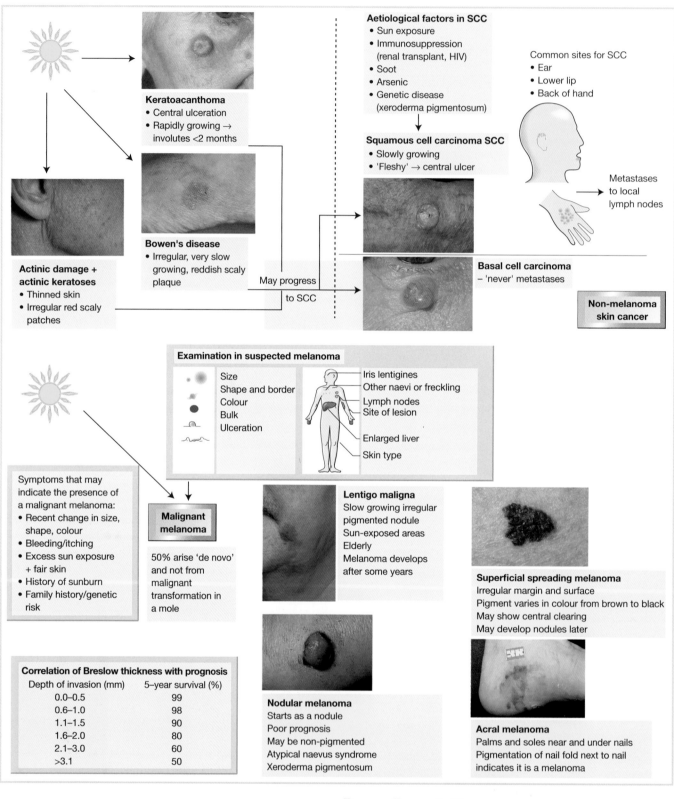

Keratoacanthoma
- Central ulceration
- Rapidly growing → involutes <2 months

Actinic damage + actinic keratoses
- Thinned skin
- Irregular red scaly patches

Bowen's disease
- Irregular, very slow growing, reddish scaly plaque

May progress to SCC

Aetiological factors in SCC
- Sun exposure
- Immunosuppression (renal transplant, HIV)
- Soot
- Arsenic
- Genetic disease (xeroderma pigmentosum)

Common sites for SCC
- Ear
- Lower lip
- Back of hand

Squamous cell carcinoma SCC
- Slowly growing
- 'Fleshy' → central ulcer

Metastases to local lymph nodes

Basal cell carcinoma
– 'never' metastases

Non-melanoma skin cancer

Examination in suspected melanoma

Size
Shape and border
Colour
Bulk
Ulceration

Iris lentigines
Other naevi or freckling
Lymph nodes
Site of lesion
Enlarged liver
Skin type

Symptoms that may indicate the presence of a malignant melanoma:
- Recent change in size, shape, colour
- Bleeding/itching
- Excess sun exposure + fair skin
- History of sunburn
- Family history/genetic risk

Malignant melanoma

50% arise 'de novo' and not from malignant transformation in a mole

Lentigo maligna
Slow growing irregular pigmented nodule
Sun-exposed areas
Elderly
Melanoma develops after some years

Superficial spreading melanoma
Irregular margin and surface
Pigment varies in colour from brown to black
May show central clearing
May develop nodules later

Nodular melanoma
Starts as a nodule
Poor prognosis
May be non-pigmented
Atypical naevus syndrome
Xeroderma pigmentosum

Acral melanoma
Palms and soles near and under nails
Pigmentation of nail fold next to nail indicates it is a melanoma

Correlation of Breslow thickness with prognosis

Depth of invasion (mm)	5–year survival (%)
0.0–0.5	99
0.6–1.0	98
1.1–1.5	90
1.6–2.0	80
2.1–3.0	60
>3.1	50

Skin cancers are the most common of all cancers, with over 100 000 cases per annum in the UK. Sun exposure is the unifying aetiological factor.

Premalignant disease

- **Solar or actinic keratoses**: flat, scaly, often erythematous lesions, which show epidermal dysplasia on histology and have

Medicine at a Glance, Fourth Edition. Edited by Patrick Davey. © 2014 John Wiley & Sons, Ltd. Published 2014 by John Wiley & Sons, Ltd. Companion website: www.ataglanceseries.com/medicine

a low risk of developing into Bowen's disease or squamous cell carcinoma (SCC). They are usually associated with actinic (sun) damage. Treatment is with cryotherapy, curettage, topical 5-fluorouracil, diclofenac or imiquimod or photodynamic therapy.

- **Bowen's disease** (intraepidermal carcinoma *in situ*): a single, red, scaly patch that may be mistaken for eczema or psoriasis, but neither itches nor responds to topical steroids. Sometimes there are multiple lesions. Aetiological factors and treatment are as above, but include surgical curettage or excision. The condition may progress to invasive SCC.

- **Keratoacanthoma**: a rapidly growing nodular lesion on the light-exposed skin of the hand or face. It reaches its maximum size at <1–2 months and appears as a smooth dome-shaped lesion with a central crater filled with keratinaceous material. It can spontaneously involute to leave scarring, but is best excised, as it is probably a form of SCC.

- **Congenital melanocytic naevi**: large pigmented lesions present from birth. They are common anywhere, but a bathing trunk distribution is recognized. There is a significant risk of malignant melanoma developing in lesions larger than 5 cm.

- **Dysplastic naevi**: may be associated with an increased risk of melanoma. The dysplastic naevus syndrome is the presence of many moles (dysplastic naevi), heterogenous in size, shape, colour and surface, often abnormally distributed (scalp, buttocks, feet), usually larger than 0.5 cm, and iris lentigines in the context of a personal or family history of melanoma.

Malignant disease

- **Basal cell carcinoma/epithelioma** (BCC/BCE): an extremely common neoplasm, often on the face, head and neck of older people. BCEs 'never' metastasize, but indolent growth can lead to delayed presentation and deep invasion, leading to high rates of recurrence after conventional treatments. Sun damage is the greatest risk factor for BCE, but sometimes multiple BCEs are associated with previous X-ray treatment for ankylosing spondylitis (spine) and tinea capitis (scalp). Usual treatments are excision, curettage and cautery, or radiotherapy, all with a 5–10% recurrence rate. Tumours around the eye and nasal furrows have a 20% recurrence rate, as a result of infiltration along embryological fusion lines. A very high cure rate can be achieved using micrographic surgery (Mohs' procedure). Late presentation or failed treatment is complicated by fungation, involvement of other structures (such as the eye and lacrimal apparatus), and deep invasion with destruction of cartilage and bone, which may all represent incurable disease.

- **Squamous carcinoma**: occurs in sun-exposed areas in elderly people or as multiple tumours in very young people with xeroderma pigmentosum, a defect in DNA repair mechanisms. Other risk factors include smoking (lip tumours), human papillomavirus and chronic inflammation, e.g. associated with chronic venous ulceration (Marjolin's ulcer of the leg). The best known occupational cancer was cancer of the scrotum in chimney sweeps, which in the nineteenth century was related to exposure to the hydrocarbons in soot. SCC most commonly presents as an irregular ulcer or as a slowly growing nodule. It may be very destructive locally, and can also metastasize to the lymph nodes. Treatment must therefore be ablative (i.e. excision or radiotherapy) and long-term follow-up is necessary.

- **Lentigo maligna** (Hutchinson's melanotic freckle): a slow-growing, pigmented macule on the face in older people. Histologically, it is an intraepidermal melanoma, but it can become invasive

(lentigo maligna melanoma). Biopsy establishes the diagnosis. Treatment is by excision. Plastic repair may be necessary.

- **Malignant melanoma**: in the UK there are 8000 new cases and 2500 deaths per year, with rates doubling every decade. Predisposing factors include (susceptibility to) ultraviolet light exposure: congenital naevi, family history of melanoma, large numbers of acquired naevi, any number of atypical naevi, freckles, previous episodes of sunburn, and significant sun exposure before the age of 20 years.

Melanoma is rare in African Caribbean and Asian individuals, and common in Scots and Australians. Four types of melanoma are recognized clinically: superficial spreading, nodular, acral lentiginous and lentigo maligna melanoma. Superficial spreading and nodular are the most common types and present in early adulthood. In men, the upper back is a common area, but in women it is the lower leg. Some melanomas do not arise from an existing mole. The earliest growth of superficial spreading melanoma is in the horizontal plane, so presentation is usually as a new or changing mole. Melanoma invades locally and metastasizes to lymph nodes early on. On examination, look for actinic damage, freckles, and numbers, types and distribution of moles (and iris lentigines – dark-brown macules), and check the local and distant lymph nodes and the liver. The crucial diagnostic and prognostic investigation is excisional histopathology and this also delivers definitive treatment. Multidisciplinary management is appropriate.

The histological depth of the lesion on first presentation correlates with the prognosis (see Figure 230.1). Melanoma is conventionally excised with wide margins. For extensive disease, surgical or laser debulking, amputation, isolated limb perfusion with chemotherapy, systemic chemotherapy, including with cytokines, and radiotherapy are used. Treatment of metastatic melanoma is not curative and the prognosis is grim.

- **Kaposi's sarcoma**: AIDS-related vascular neoplasm due to human herpes virus 8 (HHV8) infection.

Lymphoma

- **Mycosis fungoides**: a cutaneous T-cell lymphoma where there is slowly evolving infiltration of the skin with T lymphocytes. The cause is not known but human T-cell leukaemia virus 1 (HTLV-1) was first isolated from a patient with Sézary's syndrome (erythroderma, lymphadenopathy and abnormal Sézary cells with cerebriform nuclei in the blood). The differential diagnosis of erythroderma is given in Chapter 69.

The following stages are recognized:

- Fixed itchy scaly patches (like eczema or psoriasis).
- Fixed geographical plaques.
- Nodules, tumours and ulcers.
- Lymph node or systemic organ involvement.

It is possible that at an early stage malignant change has not occurred and the prognosis with gentle treatment (topical steroids, PUVA (psoralens and ultraviolet A), topical nitrogen mustard, electron beam therapy) is good. With more advanced disease, therapy is more radical (radiotherapy, chemotherapy, extracorporeal photochemotherapy) and the outlook is bleak.

- **Adult T-cell lymphoma/leukaemia** (ATLL): may present with a cutaneous prodrome of granulomatous papules and nodules (from which proviral DNA can be recovered), and precedes and accompanies ATLL due to HTLV-1.

- **Hodgkin's disease and non-Hodgkin's lymphoma**: may involve the skin and, it is argued, may originate in the skin.

231 Orogenital disease

Erythema multiforme

Causes

50% unknown
Infections
- Herpes simplex
- Orf
- *Mycoplasma*
- Streptococci

Drugs
- Sulphonamides
- Many others

Rare causes
- Neoplasms
- Autoimmune diseases (e.g. SLE, RA, UC)

If severe (= Stevens–Johnson syndrome)
- Severe mucosal involvement
- Blisters
- High fever
- ± Anterior uveitis
- ± Pneumonia, renal failure
- ± Polyarthritis

Hands/feet often more affected than trunk

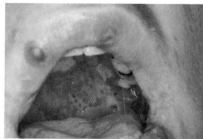
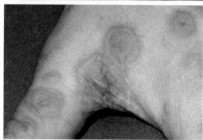
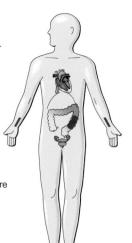

Behçet's syndrome

Diagnosis

Major criteria
- Recurrent aphthous stomatitis
- Pathergy [= sterile pustules at site of skin trauma, e.g. venesection]
- Uveitis
- Genital ulceration

Minor criteria
- Inflammatory large joint arthritis
- Intestinal ulceration
- Meningo-encephalitis
- Epididymitis
- Thrombophlebitis

4 major = Complete Behçet's
3 major = Incomplete Behçet's

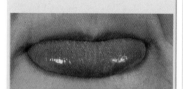

Behçet's disease
This patient demonstrates lingual aphthosis

Clinical features

Neurological disease
- Brainstem dysfunction
- Meningo-encephalitis
- Cranial nerve palsies

Eye disease
- Conjunctivitis
- Scleritis
- Retinal vasculitis

Painful oral ulcers 90%

Pulmonary embolus/infarction

Hepatic vein thrombosis
Budd–Chiari syndrome

Recurrent colitis

Genital ulcers 80%

Large joint (knee/elbow, ankle/wrist)

Erythema nodosum 80%

Deep vein thrombosis

Immunology
- Circulating immune complexes
- Perivascular inflammatory infiltrate
- Anticardiolipin antibody in 20%, recurrent thrombosis (pulmonary embolism, Budd–Chiari)

♂ : ♀ = 2:1

Pathergy

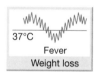
37°C
Fever
Weight loss

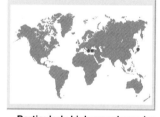

Particularly high prevalence in:
- Greece
- Turkey
- Japan (1 in 100 prevalence)

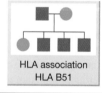
HLA association
HLA B51

Treatment
- Steroids
- Ciclosporin
- Colchicine (skin/mucosal lesions)
- Thalidomide

Oral disorders

- **Oral ulceration**: the most common cause is idiopathic aphthous ulceration. Oral pemphigus is very rare but serious, and is frequently diagnosed late (see Chapter 227). Examination of all patients with oral ulcers should include examination of other mucocutaneous sites and a search for lymphadenopathy. Investigations include microbiology and virology, and a biopsy with immunofluorescence. Treatment of aphthae concentrates on improving oral hygiene, antibiotic and antifungal mouthwashes, and topical steroids.

- **Candida**: an extremely common intraoral commensal, which acts as an opportunistic pathogen in those immunosuppressed from infection (e.g. HIV), disease (e.g. diabetes mellitus) or drugs (e.g. oral antibiotics, cytotoxics). White detachable deposits and plaques are the usual physical signs. Mouthwashes or nystatin lozenges and a systemic imidazole or triazole are effective treatments, but candidosis may recur depending on the context.
- **Leukoplakia**: a non-specific common disturbance of oral mucosal keratinization. Smoking and poor dental hygiene are associated factors. It may result from a syphilitic atrophic glossitis, but small, white mucus patches may occur anywhere in the oral cavity during secondary syphilis; 5% undergo malignant transformation.
- **Erythroplakia**: describes red patches in the mouth. They are more likely to be malignant than leukoplakia and should therefore be biopsied.
- **Lichen planus**: characterized by lilac erythematous patches topped by lacy white striae (Wickham's striae). It is more common on the buccal mucosa than the tongue, although all intraoral sites may be involved. Of patients with the condition, 30% have extraoral lichen planus, and 10–50% of all patients with lichen planus have oral lesions. Erosive or atrophic lichen planus may progress to malignancy.

Vulval disorders

The vulva can be affected by dermatoses such as seborrhoeic dermatitis, psoriasis, lichen sclerosus and lichen planus, or sexually transmitted diseases (STDs). Patients may be severely symptomatic with itch, irritation, dyspareunia and somatopsychic symptoms.

- **Vulval warts**: usually caused by human papillomavirus (HPV) types 6 and 11. All patients and their partners should be screened for STDs. Colposcopy and a cervical smear examination are indicated. Treatment is with liquid nitrogen therapy, topical podophyllin or topical imiquimod.
- **Lichen simplex**: refers to a chronic eczematous process exaggerated and propagated by scratching in response to itch. Treatment is with topical steroids and night-time sedation, possibly with tricyclic antidepressants. Additional causes of vulval itching include urinary incontinence and vaginal discharge, often as a result of candidosis. All women with pruritus vulvae should be screened for diabetes mellitus.
- **Lichen sclerosus**: an idiopathic, chronic, inflammatory dermatosis with subsequent atrophy, which can cause intense itching in the female. Lesions are shiny, white and red-rimmed with central telangiectasia, purpura and erosions. There may be loss of architecture of the labia and burying of the clitoris. Potent topical steroids relieve the itch and reverse the skin changes. Biopsy and continued monitoring are important because intraepithelial neoplasia and frank invasive carcinoma may develop.
- **Vulval intraepithelial neoplasia** (VIN): suspected when hard white plaques or erosions are seen. HPV may be involved. The invasive potential of VIN is small. Cryotherapy and topical imiquimod can be used. Multidisciplinary management (gynaecologists, oncologists, etc.) is desirable; 50% of vulva cancer is associated with HPV and 50% with lichen sclerosis with little overlap.
- **Extrammammary Paget's disease** presents as an irregular psoriasiform patch or plaque. It is adenocarcinoma *in situ*. There may be a subjacent epithelial neoplasm or an underlying gastrointestinal (GI), urological or gynaecological cancer.

Penile disorders

Uncircumcised men have more dermatological problems than those circumcised at birth. The penis is a common site for seborrhoeic dermatitis, psoriasis, lichen sclerosus, lichen planus and viral warts. Balanitis due to *Candida* or other microbials may be a presenting feature of diabetes mellitus.

- **Lichen sclerosus** of the penis may result in male dyspareunia, phimosis (inability to retract the foreskin) and even retention of urine. Chronic disease is associated with penile squamous cell carcinoma (SCC). Potent topical steroids help 50% of patients. Circumcision may be necessary.
- **Zoon's balanitis**: an irritant mucositis of the uncircumcised male. It presents with moist raw patches and is treated by circumcision.
- **Erythroplasia of Queyrat** is the eponym for **Bowen's disease** (SCC *in situ*) of the uncircumcised penis and is suspected if there are fixed red lesions of the penis. Biopsy is diagnostic. Treatment options include topical 5-fluorouracil, topical imiquimod, cryotherapy, radiotherapy or surgery. Oncogenic HPV is usually associated. Follow-up (for malignancy detection) is essential. Like in the vulva, 50% of penis cancer is associated with HPV and 50% with lichen sclerosis with little overlap.
- **Extrammammary Paget's disease** presents as an irregular psoriasiform patch or plaque. It is adenocarcinoma *in situ*. There may be a subjacent epithelial neoplasm or an underlying GI, urological or gynaecological cancer.

Genital ulceration

Aetiology
Genital ulcers can be caused by dermatoses, STDs or other infections, Behçet's disease, pyoderma gangrenosum, artefact or, most importantly, squamous carcinoma.

Investigations
These include microbiology (including mycology) and skin biopsy.

Treatment
Genital hygiene, emollient, and topical antibiotic, antifungal and steroid applications.

Orogenital syndromes

Certain diseases result in simultaneous lesions in the mouth and genitalia. These include:

- **Severe erythema multiforme**: the cause of erythema multiforme is often unknown, but includes herpes simplex infection, other infections such as those caused by *Mycoplasma* spp. and drug reactions. In mild to moderate disease, involvement is limited to the skin. Lesions characteristically start as pleomorphic red eruptions on the arms and legs, which spread centrally to the trunk. Spontaneous remission is usual, although topical steroids may improve itch. In severe disease (Stevens–Johnson syndrome) lesions occur in the mouth, conjunctiva and genitalia as well. Treatment is with systemic steroids and antimicrobials for any infection.
  - **Behçet's syndrome** (see Figure 231.1): characterized by painful oral (90–100%) and genital (60–90%) ulceration and variable involvement of other systems as follows:
    - Ocular manifestations (keratitis, uveitis, optic neuritis) (50–90%).
    - Pustules, pyoderma gangrenosum, erythema nodosum and arthritis (20–50%).
    - Central nervous system involvement (e.g. vasculitis, thrombophlebitis) (10–20%).
    - Pulmonary infarction (10–40%).
    - Renal involvement (10%).
    - Budd–Chiari syndrome (10%).
  There are no diagnostic tests for Behçet's syndrome. Treatment is with systemic steroids; occasionally thalidomide is used. Many patients have mild disease and do well. However, cerebral/renal involvement is associated with severe treatment-resistant disease and a worse prognosis.

232 Endometriosis and adenomyosis

Common sites of endometriosis

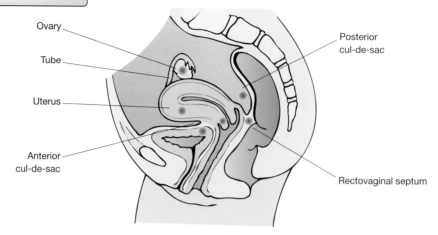

Ovary
Tube
Uterus
Anterior cul-de-sac
Posterior cul-de-sac
Rectovaginal septum

American Fertility Society (AFS) classification of endometriosis

Points assigned for each lesion visualized at surgery

			<1 cm	1–3 cm	>3 cm
Peritoneum	**Endometriosis**		**<1 cm**	**1–3 cm**	**>3 cm**
		Superficial	1	2	4
		Deep	2	4	6
Ovary	R	Superficial	1	2	4
		Deep	4	16	20
	L	Superficial	1	2	4
		Deep	4	16	20
	Posterior cul-de-sac obliteration		Partial 4		Complete 40
	Adhesions		**<1/3 enclosure**	**1/3–2/3 enclosure**	**>2/3 enclosure**
Ovary	R	Filmy	1	2	4
		Dense	4	8	16
	L	Filmy	1	2	4
		Dense	4	8	16
Tube	R	Filmy	1	2	4
		Dense	4	8	16
	L	Filmy	1	2	4
		Dense	4	8	16

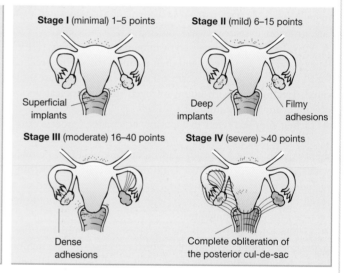

Stage I (minimal) 1–5 points

Superficial implants

Stage II (mild) 6–15 points

Deep implants
Filmy adhesions

Stage III (moderate) 16–40 points

Dense adhesions

Stage IV (severe) >40 points

Complete obliteration of the posterior cul-de-sac

Laparoscopic excision of ovarian endometrioma

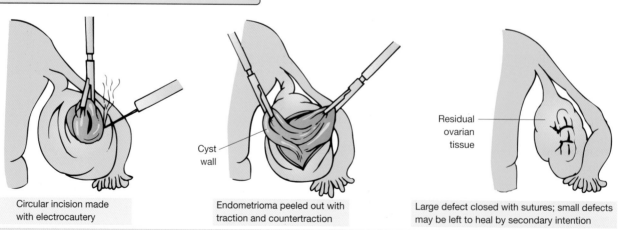

Cyst wall

Residual ovarian tissue

Circular incision made with electrocautery

Endometrioma peeled out with traction and countertraction

Large defect closed with sutures; small defects may be left to heal by secondary intention

Medicine at a Glance, Fourth Edition. Edited by Patrick Davey. © 2014 John Wiley & Sons, Ltd. Published 2014 by John Wiley & Sons, Ltd. Companion website: www.ataglanceseries.com/medicine

Endometriosis

- **Definition**: functional endometrial glands and stroma outside the uterine cavity (see Figure 232.1).
- **Prevalence**: occurs in 5–10% of women of reproductive age; 30–40% of infertile women; and 80% of women with chronic pelvic pain.
- **Age**: typically diagnosed in women during their twenties. Not found before menarche and characteristically regresses after the menopause.
- **Pathogenesis**: theories include (i) *retrograde menstruation* (viable endometrial cells reflux through the tubes during menstruation and implant in the pelvis); (ii) *coelomic metaplasia* (multipotential cells of the coelomic epithelium are stimulated to transform into endometrium-like cells); (iii) *haematogenous dissemination* (endometrial cells are transported to distant sites); and (iv) *autoimmune disease* (a disorder of immune surveillance that allows ectopic endometrial implants to grow).

Symptoms and signs

- The most common symptoms are *pelvic pain* and *infertility*, but many patients are asymptomatic.
- *Cyclic pain* is the hallmark of endometriosis, including secondary dysmenorrhea (begins before or with menstruation and is maximal at the time of maximal flow), deep dyspareunia (pain with intercourse), pain with defecation and sacral backache with menses.
- The severity of symptoms does not necessarily correlate with the degree of pelvic disease. Indeed, many women with minimal endometriosis complain of severe pelvic pain.
- Infertility may result from anatomical distortion of the pelvic architecture due to extensive endometriosis and adhesions, but also occurs in women with minimal disease for unknown reasons.
- Common physical findings include a fixed, retroverted uterus, nodularity of the uterosacral ligaments and enlarged, tender adnexa.

Diagnosis

- History and physical examination may suggest the diagnosis because endometriotic lesions may occur anywhere in the body. The most common site is the ovary.
- Pelvic ultrasonography may demonstrate the presence of one or more *endometriomas* (blood-filled ovarian cysts) which are commonly adherent to the surrounding pelvic structures.
- Laparoscopic surgery with direct visualization of endometriotic lesions and histological examination of biopsy specimens is the standard for making the diagnosis. Early lesions on the peritoneal surface are small and vesicular. Later lesions have a typical 'powder-burn' appearance, which refers to a puckered, black area surrounded by a stellate scar.

Classification

The American Fertility Society classification system (see Figure 232.1) is based on surgical findings with points subjectively assigned to each lesion depending on its size and depth. The presence and extent of adhesions are also scored.

Management

Medical management

The primary goal of medical therapy is suppression of ovulation and induction of amenorrhea. Symptomatic relief of dysmenorrhea, dyspareunia and/or pelvic pain is usually somewhat successful, but often short-lived. Medical therapy does not eradicate the lesions.

- **Non-steroidal anti-inflammatory drugs** (NSAIDs) not only reduce pain but also reduce menstrual flow. They are commonly used together with other therapy. For more severe cases, opiate prescription drugs may be required.
- **Progestins** counteract oestrogen and inhibit growth of the endometrium. Such therapy can reduce or eliminate menstruation in a controlled and reversible fashion.
- **Oral contraceptives** reduce or eliminate menstrual flow and provide oestrogen support. Typically, it is a long-term approach. Newer agents (e.g. Seasonale) were designed to reduce the number of cycles by inducing a menses every 3 months or even less. Alternatively, oral contraceptives can be taken continuously without the use of placebo pills, or, in the case of the use of NuvaRing or the contraceptive patch, without the break week. This eliminates monthly bleeding episodes.
- **Danazol** and **gestrinone** are suppressive steroids with some androgenic activity. Both agents inhibit the growth of endometriosis but their use remains limited because they may cause unsightly hirsutism.
- **Gonadotropin-releasing hormone (GnRH) agonists** induce a profound hypo-oestrogenic 'medical menopause'. Although quite effective, they induce unpleasant menopausal symptoms, and beyond 6 months may lead to osteoporosis. To counteract such side effects or to extend the treatment some oestrogen may have to be given back (add-back therapy).
- 'Empirical' therapy is used when signs and symptoms support the diagnosis of endometriosis, but definitive surgical diagnosis has not been achieved. A trial of oral contraceptives and NSAIDs is often attempted first, but a 3-month course of GnRH agonist (e.g. Lupron) may also be helpful in refractory patients.
- Patients who do not respond to empirical therapy generally warrant diagnostic laparoscopy to confirm the diagnosis before moving on to danazol, long-term GnRH agonist therapy with add-back, or opiates.

Surgical management

- Young women desiring future fertility typically undergo laparoscopic surgery with a primary goal to excise or destroy as much of the endometriosis as possible while restoring normal anatomy and salvaging normal ovarian tissue. Multiple such operations over a period of years may occur in some cases.
- Laparoscopic surgery is generally advised when imaging suggests a larger ovarian endometrioma (>4 cm) or pelvic adhesions are clinically suspected. **Presacral neurectomy** and/or **uterosacral nerve ablation** has been reported to benefit selected patients.
- Pregnancy rates may be improved in women with moderate to severe endometriosis who undergo surgical treatment.
- Older women without concerns about future childbearing are usually the best candidates for more definitive surgery (hysterectomy with bilateral salpingo-oophorectomy).
- Patients should be counselled that pelvic pain may still be unrelieved and hormone replacement therapy with oestrogen is still an option. Alternatively, one or both ovaries may be retained, but the risk of reoperation for persistent pain is about 20%.
- Endometriosis often obliterates natural tissue planes and surgery can be very complex due to adhesions, generalized induration and involvement of the rectum and bladder.

Adenomyosis

- **Definition**: endometrial glands and stroma within the myometrium.
- **Prevalence**: occurs to some degree in about 20% of women.
- **Symptoms and signs**: dysmenorrhoea, menorrhagia, dyspareunia and a smoothly enlarged boggy uterus on pelvic examination.
- **Diagnosis** may be suggested by pelvic ultrasonography and/or magnetic resonance imaging, but adenomyosis is a histopathological diagnosis.
- **Treatment** may be treated with continuous oral contraceptive pills, Depo-Provera or Mirena intrauterine systems but in many there is no effective medical treatment – hysterectomy is curative for symptomatic women.

233 Polycystic ovarian syndrome

Appearance of polycystic ovaries

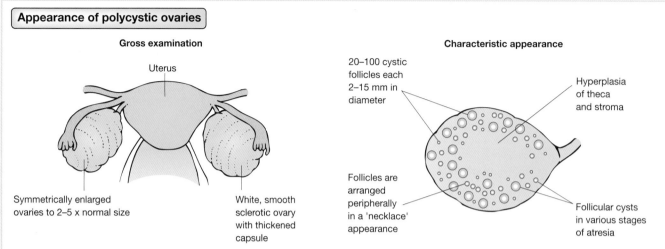

Gross examination

Uterus

Symmetrically enlarged ovaries to 2–5 x normal size

White, smooth sclerotic ovary with thickened capsule

Characteristic appearance

20–100 cystic follicles each 2–15 mm in diameter

Hyperplasia of theca and stroma

Follicles are arranged peripherally in a 'necklace' appearance

Follicular cysts in various stages of atresia

Note: Corpora lutea and corpus albicans are usually absent

Pathophysiology of polycystic ovarian syndrome (PCOS)

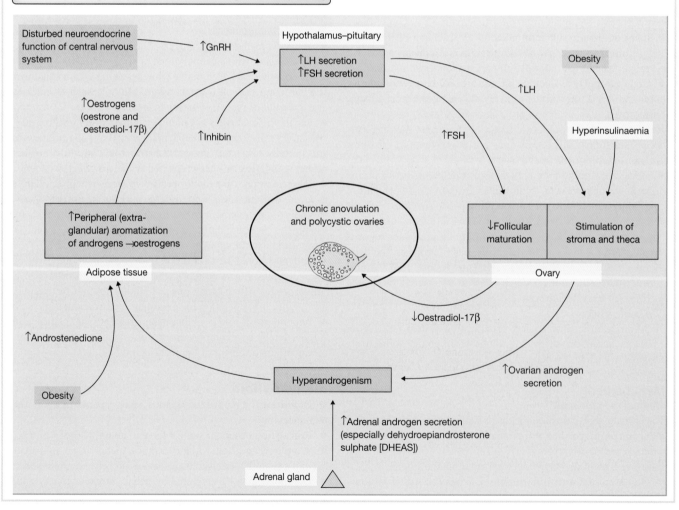

Disturbed neuroendocrine function of central nervous system

↑GnRH

Hypothalamus–pituitary

↑LH secretion
↑FSH secretion

Obesity

↑LH

↑Oestrogens (oestrone and oestradiol-17β)

↑Inhibin

↑FSH

Hyperinsulinaemia

↑Peripheral (extra-glandular) aromatization of androgens →oestrogens

Chronic anovulation and polycystic ovaries

↓Follicular maturation

Stimulation of stroma and theca

Adipose tissue

Ovary

↓Oestradiol-17β

↑Androstenedione

↑Ovarian androgen secretion

Obesity

Hyperandrogenism

↑Adrenal androgen secretion (especially dehydroepiandrosterone sulphate [DHEAS])

Adrenal gland

- **Definition**: a heterogeneous disorder of unexplained hyper-androgenic chronic anovulation in which secondary causes (androgen-secreting neoplasms) have been excluded. Polycystic ovarian syndrome (PCOS) was historically referred to as Stein–Leventhal syndrome.
- **Prevalence**: occurs in 5% of women of reproductive age. It occurs among all races and nationalities, is the most common hormonal disorder of women this age and is a leading cause of infertility.
- Aetiology: unknown; no gene or specific environmental substance has been identified.

Diagnosis

- **History**: this should focus on the menstrual pattern, previous pregnancies (if any), concomitant medications, smoking, alcohol consumption, diet and identification of family members with diabetes and cardiovascular disease.
- **Physical examination** should look for balding, acne, clitoromegaly, body hair distribution and signs of insulin resistance (obesity, centripetal fat distribution, acanthosis nigricans). Bimanual examination may suggest enlarged ovaries (see Figure 233.1).
- **Laboratory tests** such as testosterone or dehydroepiandrosterone (DHEA) sulphate are useful for documenting ovarian hyperandrogenism. Androgen-secreting tumours of the ovary or adrenal gland are also invariably accompanied by elevated circulating androgen levels, but there is no absolute level that is pathognomonic for a tumour or minimum level that excludes a tumour.
- **Imaging studies** such as a pelvic sonogram can exclude a solid ovarian tumour and may demonstrate the characteristic 'polycystic' appearance of the ovaries.
- **Criteria**: in 2003, a consensus workshop in Rotterdam indicated that PCOS should be diagnosed if two out of three criteria are met: (i) oligo-ovulation and/or anovulation; (2) excess androgen activity; and (3) polycystic ovaries by sonogram, other endocrine disorders being excluded.

Pathophysiology

- PCOS represents the end-stage of a 'vicious cycle' of endocrinological events that can be initiated at many different entry points.
- It remains unclear whether the primary pathology resides in the ovary or the hypothalamus, but the fundamental defect appears to be 'inappropriate' signalling to the hypothalamus and pituitary.
- Elevated luteinizing hormone (LH) levels (the hallmark of PCOS) result from increased peripheral oestrogen production (positive feedback) and increased gonadotropin-releasing hormone (GnRH) secretion.
- Suppressed follicle-stimulating hormone (FSH) levels result from increased peripheral oestrogen production (negative feedback) and increased secretion of inhibin.
- PCOS is characterized by a 'steady state' of chronically elevated LH and chronically suppressed FSH levels, instead of their cyclic rise and fall in a normal menstrual cycle.
- Increased LH stimulates ovarian stroma and theca cells to increase the production of androgens. Androgens are converted peripherally by aromatization to oestrogens, which perpetuate chronic anovulation.
- As a result of suppressed FSH, new follicular growth is continuously stimulated but not to the point of full maturation and ovulation (corpus lutea and corpus albicans are rarely detected). Elevated androgens contribute to the prevention of normal follicular development and induction of premature atresia.

- The *ovary* is the major site of androgen overproduction; the adrenal gland has a minor role.
- Increased adipose tissue in obese patients contributes to the extraglandular aromatization of androgens to oestrogens.
- Circulating testosterone is increased (causing hirsutism), because sex hormone-binding globulin (SHBG) levels are decreased in PCOS.

Clinical features

- **Menstrual irregularities** (80%) begin soon after menarche, including secondary amenorrhoea and/or oligomenorrhoea.
- **Hirsutism** (70%) refers to the presence of excessive male pattern (upper lip, chin, chest, back) hair growth in women.
- **Obesity** (50%) contributes substantially to the metabolic abnormalities of PCOS.
- **Infertility** (75%) is due to chronic anovulation.
- **Acanthosis nigricans** is a dermatological marker of insulin resistance and hyperinsulinaemia which is marked by grey-brown, velvety, sometimes verrucous, discoloration of the skin at the neck, groin and axillae.
- **HAIR-AN syndrome** (*h*yperandrogenism, *i*nsulin *r*esistance and *a*canthosis *n*igricans) represents the extreme effects of hyperandrogenic chronic anovulation.

Long-term complications

- Endometrial hyperplasia/adenocarcinoma.
- Insulin resistance/type 2 diabetes.
- High blood pressure, cardiovascular disease, dyslipidaemia.
- Stroke.
- Weight gain.

Management

Medical treatment of PCOS is tailored to the patient's goals in four main categories: (i) lowering of insulin levels; (ii) restoration of fertility; (iii) treatment of hirsutism or acne; and (iv) restoration of regular menstruation with prevention of endometrial hyperplasia and cancer. There is considerable debate as to the optimal treatment. General interventions that help to reduce weight or insulin resistance can be beneficial for all these aims and interrupt the self-perpetuating cycle of hyperandrogenic chronic anovulation.

Medical therapy

- **Oral contraceptives** have been the mainstay of long-term management of PCOS by decreasing LH and FSH secretion and ovarian production of androgens, increasing hepatic production of SHBG, decreasing levels of DHEA and preventing endometrial neoplasia. Cyproterone acetate (e.g. Dianette/Diane), spironolactone or topical eflornithine may be especially helpful in patients with excessive hirsutism.
- **Progestins** have been shown to suppress pituitary LH and FSH and circulating androgens, but breakthrough bleeding is common.
- **Insulin-sensitizing agents** (metformin) decrease circulating androgen levels, improve the ovulation rate and improve glucose tolerance.
- **Clomiphene citrate** has traditionally been the first-line treatment for women wishing to get pregnant.

Surgical therapy

- Ovarian drilling with laser or diathermy has few advantages over medical therapy for infertility and does not appear to have significant long-term benefits in improving metabolic abnormalities.
- Mechanical hair removal (laser vapourization, electrolysis, depilatory creams) is often the front line of treatment for hirsutism.

234 Hypertensive disorders of pregnancy

Risk factors for pre-eclampsia

Nulliparity
African-American/African race
Prior history of pre-eclampsia
Extremes of maternal age (<15 or ≥35 years)
Family history of pre-eclampsia
Multiple gestation
Chronic hypertension
Chronic renal disease
Antiphospholipid antibody syndrome
Collagen vascular disease
Angiotensinogen gene T235 mutation

Diagnosis of pre-eclampsia

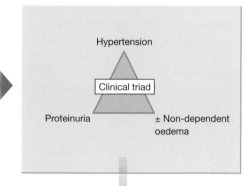

Hypertension

Clinical triad

Proteinuria   ± Non-dependent oedema

Classification of pre-eclampsia

'Mild' pre-eclampsia

- Includes all women with a diagnosis of pre-eclampsia, but without features of 'severe' pre-eclampsia

'Severe' pre-eclampsia

Note: only one of the features listed below is required for diagnosis

Symptoms	Signs	Laboratory findings
• Symptoms of central nervous system dysfunction (severe headache, blurred vision, scotomas) • Symptoms of liver capsule distention (right upper quandrant and/or epigastric pain)	• Severe elevations in BP (defined as BP ≥160/110 on two occasions at least 6 hours apart) • Pulmonary oedema • Eclampsia (generalized seizures or unexplained coma) • Cerebrovascular accident • IUGR	• Proteinuria (>5 g/24 h) • Renal failure or oliguria (<500 mL/24 h) • Hepatocellular injury (serum transaminase levels ≥ 2x normal) • Thrombocytopenia (<100 000 platelets/mm^3) • Coagulopathy • HELLP (haemolysis, elevated liver enzymes, low platelets)

Short-term complications

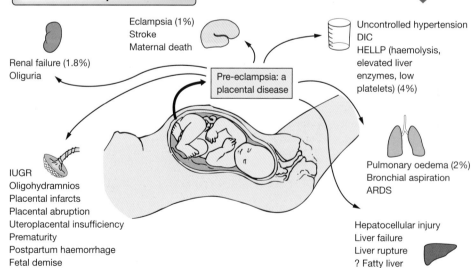

Eclampsia (1%)
Stroke
Maternal death

Renal failure (1.8%)
Oliguria

Uncontrolled hypertension
DIC
HELLP (haemolysis, elevated liver enzymes, low platelets) (4%)

Pre-eclampsia: a placental disease

Pulmonary oedema (2%)
Bronchial aspiration
ARDS

IUGR
Oligohydramnios
Placental infarcts
Placental abruption
Uteroplacental insufficiency
Prematurity
Postpartum haemorrhage
Fetal demise

Hepatocellular injury
Liver failure
Liver rupture
? Fatty liver

Long-term effects

- Complications of pre-eclampsia almost always resolve completely (with the exception of cerebrovascular accident)
- ↑Risk of chronic hypertension
- Does not preclude use of OCPs (if BP returns to normal)
- ↑Risk of pre-eclampsia/eclampsia in a subsequent pregnancy (+ 25%); depends on severity, gestational age, and pressure of underlying medical conditions
- Recurrence rate for eclampsia is 10%
- ↑Risk of other obstetric complications in a subsequent pregnancy (placental abruption, IUGR, preterm labour, ↑perinatal mortality)

Medicine at a Glance, Fourth Edition. Edited by Patrick Davey. © 2014 John Wiley & Sons, Ltd. Published 2014 by John Wiley & Sons, Ltd. Companion website: www.ataglanceseries.com/medicine

Hypertensive disorders of pregnancy are the second most common cause of maternal death in developed countries (after embolism), accounting for 15% of all maternal deaths.

Effects of pregnancy on maternal cardiovascular system

- Blood volume increases 800 mL by 12 weeks (1.5 L in twins).
- Blood pressure (BP) decreases in early pregnancy (due primarily to a decrease in systemic vascular resistance secondary to progesterone), nadirs in mid-pregnancy, and returns to baseline by term.

Classification

Chronic hypertension

- **Definition**: hypertension before pregnancy. The diagnosis should also be entertained in women with BP $\geq$140/90 mmHg before 20 weeks' gestation.
- **Complications**: such pregnancies are at increased risk of superimposed pre-eclampsia, intrauterine fetal growth restriction (IUGR), placental abruption and stillbirth.
- **Management**: continue antihypertensive medications, with the exception of angiotensin-converting enzyme (ACE) inhibitors. These drugs have been associated with progressive and irreversible renal injury and possibly other structural anomalies in the fetus. Diuretic therapy is generally discouraged.
- **Fetal testing** (serial ultrasound examinations for fetal growth with or without fetal non-stress testing) should be initiated after 32 weeks' gestation. Delivery should be achieved by 40 weeks.

Chronic hypertension with superimposed pre-eclampsia

See Pre-eclampsia section.

Gestational hypertension

- Also known as gestational non-proteinuric hypertension.
- **Diagnosis**: persistent elevation of BP $\geq$140/90 mmHg in the third trimester without evidence of pre-eclampsia. It is a diagnosis of exclusion that is best made retrospectively.
- **Aetiology**: it probably represents an exaggerated physiologicsl response of the maternal cardiovascular system to pregnancy.
- Rarely associated with adverse maternal or fetal outcome.

Pre-eclampsia

- Also known as gestational proteinuric hypertension, pre-eclamptic toxaemia.
- **Definition**: a multisystem disorder specific to pregnancy and the puerperium. More precisely, it is a disease of the placenta because it occurs in pregnancies where there is trophoblast but no fetal tissue (complete molar pregnancies).
- **Incidence**: occurs in 6–8% of all pregnancies.
- **Risk factors** (see Figure 234.1).
- **Diagnosis**: the clinical diagnosis has two elements:
  - *New-onset hypertension*: defined as a sustained sitting BP $\geq$140/90 mmHg in a previously normotensive woman (a prior definition included an elevation in systolic BP $\geq$30 or diastolic BP $\geq$15 mmHg over first trimester BP, but these criteria have now been dropped).
  - *New-onset significant proteinuria*: defined as >300 mg/24 h or $\geq$1+ on a clean-catch urine in the absence of urinary tract infection.

Note that a definitive diagnosis of pre-eclampsia should only be made after 20 weeks' gestation. Evidence of gestational proteinuric hypertension before 20 weeks should raise the possibility of an underlying molar pregnancy, drug withdrawal or (rarely) chromosomal abnormality in the fetus.

- **Classification** (see Figure 234.1): pre-eclampsia is classified as 'mild' or 'severe'. There is no category of 'moderate' pre-eclampsia.
- **Aetiology**: the cause of pre-eclampsia is not known. Theories include an abnormal maternal immunological response to the fetal allograft, an underlying genetic abnormality, an imbalance in the prostanoid cascade, and the presence of circulating toxins and/or endogenous vasoconstrictors. What is known is that the blueprint for the development of pre-eclampsia is laid down early in pregnancy. The primary event is a failure of the second wave of trophoblast invasion from 8 to 18 weeks, which is responsible for remodelling of the spiral arterioles in the myometrium adjacent to the developing placenta, and establishment of the definitive uteroplacental circulation. As pregnancy progresses and the metabolic demand of the fetoplacental unit increases, the spiral arterioles are therefore unable to accommodate the necessary increase in blood flow. This then leads to the development of 'placental dysfunction' which manifests clinically as pre-eclampsia. Although attractive, this hypothesis remains to be validated. Whatever the placental abnormality, the end result is widespread vasospasm and endothelial injury.
- **Complications**: eclampsia – defined as one or more generalized convulsions or coma in the setting of pre-eclampsia and in the absence of other neurological conditions – was thought to be the end stage of pre-eclampsia, hence the nomenclature. It is now clear, however, that seizures are but one clinical manifestation of 'severe' pre-eclampsia; 50% of eclampsia occurs preterm. Of those at term, 75% occur either intrapartum or within 48 hours of delivery.
- **Management**: delivery is the only effective treatment for pre-eclampsia, and is recommended:
  - In women with 'mild' pre-eclampsia once a favourable gestational age has been reached (>36–37 weeks).
  - In all women with 'severe' pre-eclampsia regardless of gestational age (with the exception of 'severe' pre-eclampsia due to proteinuria alone or IUGR remote from term with good fetal testing). There has also been a recent trend toward expectant management of 'severe' pre-eclampsia by BP criteria alone at <32 weeks' gestation.
- There is no proven benefit to routine delivery by caesarean section. However, the probability of vaginal delivery in a patient with pre-eclampsia remote from term with an unfavourable cervix is only 15–20%.
- BP control is important to prevent cerebrovascular accident (usually associated with BP $\geq$170/120 mmHg), but does not affect the natural course of pre-eclampsia.
- Intravenous magnesium sulphate should be given intrapartum and for at least 24 hours postpartum to prevent eclampsia.
- **Prevention**: despite promising early studies, low-dose aspirin (acetylsalicylic acid) and/or supplemental calcium does not prevent pre-eclampsia in either high- or low-risk women.
- **Prognosis**: pre-eclampsia and its complications always resolve after delivery (with the exception of cerebrovascular accident). Diuresis (>4 L/day) is the most accurate clinical indicator of resolution. Fetal prognosis is dependent largely on gestational age at delivery and problems related to prematurity.

235 Cardiovascular disease in pregnancy

Management of specific cardiac lesions in pregnancy

Septal defects
- If lesions are small, patients are usually asymptomatic and require no specific treatment
- Large ventricular septal defects (VSD) are associated with aortic insufficiency, congestive cardiac failure, arrhythmias, pulmonary hypertension
- Air filters on all IV lines to prevent paradoxical air embolism

Right-to-left shunts
- Due to pulmonary hypertension with shunting of blood away from lungs
- In pregnancy, decreased systemic vascular resistance worsens shunt with increased hypoxia
- Management: avoid hypotension, maintain preload, oxygen, air filters on IV lines

Mitral/aortic valve stenosis
- Such lesions are particularly dangerous in pregnancy because of the fixed cardiac output and left atrial dilatation (which can result in arrhythmias and/or thrombus formation)
- Management: maintain preload, avoid tachycardia. Consider β-blockers for persistent heart rate ≥ 90–100 bpm. Adequate pain relief in labour to minimize tachycardia
- Autotransfusion immediately postpartum can precipitate pulmonary oedema

Mitral valve prolapse
- Patients are generally asymptomatic
- Treat symptomatic prolapse with β-blocker

Prosthetic valves
- Risks include embolization, valvular dysfunction, and infection (bacterial endocarditis)
- Management: therapeutic anticoagulation for any mechanical valve, antibiotic prophylaxis against endocarditis

Prophylaxis against bacterial endocarditis
- Vaginal delivery is associated with 2–3% risk of bacteraemia
- American Heart Association recommends endocarditis prophylaxis only for: (i) prosthetic heart valve/patch, (ii) prior infectious endocarditis, (iii) heart transplant, or (iv) unrepaired/partially repaired congenital heart disease

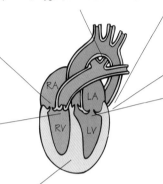

Cardiomyopathy
- Presents with left ventricular dysfunction and global dilatation
- Increased cardiac output in pregnancy may lead to decompensation
- Management: avoid hypotension, careful volume replacement, inotropic support to maximize cardiac output if needed

Regimen for endocarditis prophylaxis during labour and delivery

Low risk regimen	Amoxicillin, 3 g po 1 h before procedure or at onset of labour Repeat 1.5 g po q6 h until after delivery
Standard regime	Ampicillin, 2 g IV plus gentamicin, 1.5 mg/kg IV (do not exceed 80 mg) 30 min before procedure or
Penicillin-allergic	At onset of labour. Repeat above q8 h until after delivery Substitute vancomycin, 1 g IV over 1 h q12 h

Diagnosis of deep vein thrombosis

Pregnancy predisposes to thromboembolism

Virchow's triad describes the underlying principles of clot formation

Venous stasis — Vessel wall damage

Hypercoagulable state

Clinical features of deep vein thrombosis

History: Unilateral swelling and/or pain in the calf or thigh

Examination: May confirm unilateral swelling with or without calf tenderness or a tender 'cord' of thrombus. Homan's sign (ipsilateral calf pain on passive dorsiflexion of the foot) is only 30–40% predictive of DVT

Radiological studies to confirm deep vein thrombosis

Study	Accuracy	Comment
Doppler ultrasound*		
Proximal veins	85–95%	Non-invasive, cheap, but poor for the detection of distal thrombosis
Calf veins	≤50%	
Impedance plethysmography		Non-invasive, cheap, but poor for the detection of distal thrombosis
Proximal veins	90–95%	
Calf veins	<30%	
Venography		Accurate, but invasive with a risk of hemorrhage
Proximal veins	95–99%	
[125I] Fibrinogen		Accurate, contraindicated in pregnancy
Distal to mid-thigh	80–90%	

*also known as lower extremity non-invasive (LENI) test

Diagnosis of pulmonary embolism

Clinical features

History: Tachycardia, shortness of breath, tachypnoea, pleuritic chest pain, cough, and/or haemoptysis

Examination: May show cyanosis, pulmonary rales, and/or a friction rub. The most sensitive sign of PE is unexplained tachycardia

Labs: ECG may show right-heart strain (S_1, Q_3, T_3 with right axis deviation). Although useful to evaluate response to treatment, arterial blood gas (ABG) is not useful in the diagnosis of PE. 70% of women with PE will have evidence of DVT on LENI.

Ventilation-perfusion (V̇/Q̇) scan
- V̇/Q̇ scans are interpreted as normal, intermediate, or abnormal with a low, moderate or high probability of PE
- If the perfusion scan is normal, PE can be reliably excluded
- Data from the 'prospective investigation of pulmonary embolism diagnosis' (PIOPED) study show that overall abnormal studies are sensitive (96%), but not specific (10%)
- A high-probability scan (one showing mismatched perfusion defects) is highly specific (97%)

Pulmonary angiography
- The most accurate test for PE, but is invasive with a number of potentially serious side effects (haemorrhage, acute renal failure, pneumothorax)

Assessing need for pulmonary angiography

V̇/Q̇ scan category	Clinical suspicion		
	High	Intermediate	Low
High	96%	88%	56% *
Intermediate	66% *	28% *	16%
Low	40% *	16%	4%

* pulmonary angiography indicated

Maternal heart disease in pregnancy

Incidence
Occurs in 1% of pregnancies.

Aetiology
- Congenital lesions account for >50% of heart disease in pregnancy.

- Other common causes include coronary artery disease, hypertension and thyroid dysfunction. Rare causes include myocarditis, cor pulmonale, cardiomyopathy, constrictive pericarditis and cardiac dysrhythmias. Historically, rheumatic fever accounted for 90% of heart disease in pregnancy, but is now rare.

Prognosis

Prognosis depends on four factors:

1 *Cardiac function*: a clinical classification was developed by the New York Heart Association (NYHA) in 1928 (see Table 235.1).
2 *Clinical conditions* that may further increase cardiac output (multiple gestation, anaemia, thyroid disease).
3 *Medications*.
4 The specific nature of the *cardiac lesion* (see **Table 235.2**).

Management

- Allow spontaneous labour at term. Scheduled induction is indicated for women requiring invasive cardiac monitoring.
- Adequate pain relief (regional analgesia is preferred).
- Left lateral positioning with supplemental oxygen.
- Maternal pulse oximetry and electrocardiogram (ECG) monitoring.
- Fluid intake and output monitoring.
- Consider invasive haemodynamic monitoring for women with NYHA class III and IV disease.
- Consider elective shortening of the second stage of labour.

Thromboembolic disease in pregnancy

Incidence

- The leading obstetric cause of maternal mortality.
- Deep venous thrombosis (DVT) complicates 0.05–0.3% of all pregnancies (see Figure 235.1). It is 3–5-fold more common in the puerperium, and 3–15-fold more common after caesarean section delivery. If untreated, 15–25% of patients with DVT will have a pulmonary embolus (PE) compared with 4–5% of treated patients (see Figure 235.1).

Aetiology

Pregnancy is a thrombogenic state. Thromboembolic events are five-fold more common in pregnancy than in non-pregnant women. Other predisposing factors include trauma (surgery), infection, obesity, advanced maternal age and underlying thrombophilia (see Table 235.3).

Treatment

- **Unfractionated heparin** is the treatment of choice for acute thromboembolism. It must be given intravenously or subcutaneously to keep the PTT (partial thromboplastin time) at 1.5–2.0 times normal. Heparin does not cross the placenta and, as such, is not teratogenic. Adverse effects include haemorrhage (5–10%), thrombocytopenia (2%) and osteoporosis (dose related). In the setting of acute haemorrhage, protamine sulphate can be given to reverse heparin action.
- **Low-molecular-weight heparin** (LMWH) is replacing unfractionated heparin in non-pregnant women. Although safe, its efficacy in pregnancy is not well validated. As a result of its long half-life and resistance to reversal by protamine sulphate, most authorities recommend converting LMWH to unfractionated heparin at 35–36 weeks.
- Treatment should be continued for the duration of pregnancy and for 6–12 weeks postpartum. After delivery, anticoagulation with oral warfarin (which is teratogenic and should therefore be avoided in pregnancy) can be used. Women on warfarin can breastfeed.
- Alternative therapies (fibrinolytic agents, surgical intervention) are best avoided.

Prophylaxis

- Women with prior unexplained DVT have a 5–10% incidence of recurrence in a subsequent pregnancy. In women with a documented thrombophilic disorder, antepartum *prophylactic* heparin is indicated (5000–10 000 U subcutaneously twice daily). PTT will not increase. Antifactor Xa activity should be 0.1–0.3 U/mL. The management of women with a prior DVT but no thrombophilic disorder is controversial. In the UK, such women are generally given prophylactic anticoagulation in the postpartum period only, for at least 6 weeks. USA practice favours *prophylactic* anticoagulation throughout pregnancy and postpartum.
- In women with a prior PE, *therapeutic* anticoagulation is indicated throughout pregnancy. Maintain PTT at 60–80 seconds (2.0–2.5 times control) or antifactor Xa activity at 0.6–1.0 U/mL. Postpartum anticoagulation is indicated for at least 6 weeks.

Table 235.1 New York Heart Association (NYHA) clinical classification of maternal heart disease.

Class		
I	Uncompromised	No limitation of normal physical activity
II	Slightly compromised	Slight limitation of normal physical activity
III	Markedly compromised	Symptoms with normal activity
IV	Severely compromised	Symptoms at rest

Table 235.2 Maternal mortality associated with specific heart lesions.

Group 1 (mortality rate <%)		Atrial septal defect
		Ventricular septal defect
		Patent ductus arteriosus
		Tetralogy of Fallot (surgically corrected)
		Bioprosthetic valve
		Pulmonary/tricuspid valve disease
		Mitral stenosis (NYHA class I and II)
Group 2 (mortality rate 5–10%)	2A	Aortic stenosis
		Mitral stenosis (NYHA class III and IV)
		Coarctation of aorta (no valvular involvement)
		Tetralogy of Fallot (uncorrected)
		Previous myocardial infarction
		Marfan's syndrome with normal aorta
	2B	Mitral stenosis with atrial fibrillation
		Artificial valve
		Pulmonary hypertension
Group 3 (mortality rate 25–50%)		Coarctation of aorta (with valvular involvement)
		Marfan's syndrome with aortic involvement

Table 235.3 Thrombophilic disorders predisposing to thromboembolism.

Condition	Is test reliable in pregnancy?
Factor V Leiden deficiency	Yes (genetic test)
Prothrombin gene defect	Yes (genetic test)
Protein C deficiency	No (levels may increase in pregnancy)
Protein S deficiency	No (levels decrease in pregnancy)
Antithrombin III deficiency	No (levels may increase in pregnancy)
Lupus anticoagulant	Yes (test for circulating antibodies)
Anticardiolipin antibodies	Yes (test for circulating antibodies)

236 Other medical and surgical conditions in pregnancy

Neurological diseases in pregnancy

Headache

- A common complaint during pregnancy.
- **Causes**: migraine, tension headache, depression. Less common causes include sinusitis, pseudotumour cerebri, cerebrovascular disease, cerebral tumours, temporal arteritis, infection (meningitis, encephalitis), pre-eclampsia, and 'spinal' headache (seen in up to 30% of women within the first week after spinal analgesia, usually mild and self-limiting).
- The majority of headaches represent benign conditions. Headaches that disturb sleep are exertional in nature, or those associated with focal neurological findings are suggestive of an underlying structural lesion.

Seizure disorders

- **Incidence**: occurs in 0.3–0.6% of pregnancies; it is the most frequently encountered major neurological condition in pregnancy.
- **Classification**: primary (idiopathic, epilepsy) or secondary (to trauma, infection, tumours, cerebrovascular disease, drug withdrawal or metabolic disorders). Seizures in pregnancy should be regarded as pre-eclampsia/eclampsia until proven otherwise.
- **Effect of seizure disorder on pregnancy**: obstetric complications include an increased risk of hyperemesis gravidarum, preterm delivery, pre-eclampsia, caesarean section delivery, placental abruption and perinatal mortality. However, most women with seizure disorders will have an uneventful pregnancy.
- **Effect of pregnancy on seizure disorder**: this is variable. Oestrogen lowers the seizure threshold, whereas progesterone raises it. Seizure frequency is increased in 45% of pregnant women, reduced in 5% and unchanged in 50%. If seizures are well controlled before pregnancy, there is little risk of deterioration. However, if poorly controlled, an increase in seizure frequency can be expected. Due to a number of factors (delayed gastric emptying, increase in plasma volume, altered protein binding, accelerated hepatic metabolism), the pharmacokinetics of anticonvulsant drugs change during pregnancy.
- **Effects on fetus and neonates**: women with epilepsy have a 2–3-fold increased incidence of fetal anomalies even off treatment. Moreover, anticonvulsant drugs are teratogenic. The incidence of fetal anomalies increases with the number of anticonvulsant drugs: 3–4% with one, 5–6% with two, 10% with three and 25% with four. Monotherapy is thus recommended. *Valproic acid* is associated with neural tube defects in 1% of cases. Risk is greatest from day 17 to day 30 postconception (days 31–44 from last menstrual period). Folic acid (4 mg daily) may decrease the incidence of neural tube defects. Of women on *phenytoin* 10–30% will have infants with one or more of the following features: craniofacial abnormalities (cleft lip, epicanthic folds, hypertelorism), cardiac anomalies, limb defects (hypoplasia of distal phalanges, nail hypoplasia) or intrauterine growth restriction (IUGR). 'Fetal hydantoin syndrome' is characterized by all of the above features, and is rare. Exposure to other antiepileptic drugs (trimethadione, phenobarbital, carbamazepine) can produce similar anomalies.
- **Management of seizure disorder during pregnancy**: discontinuation of medication before conception should be considered in women who have been seizure-free for ≥2 years, although 25–40% will have recurrence of their seizures in pregnancy.
- Seizures may cause maternal hypoxaemia with resultant fetal injury. The aim of therapy is to control convulsions with a single agent using the lowest possible dose.
- Labour and delivery are usually uneventful. Benzodiazepines should be used with caution in labour because they may cause maternal and neonatal depression.
- All anticonvulsant medications cross into breast milk to some degree. The amount of transmission varies with the drug (2% for valproic acid; 30–45% for phenytoin, phenobarbital and carbamazepine; 90% for ethosuximide). However, the use of such medications is not a contraindication to breastfeeding.

Neurological emergencies in pregnancy

Status epilepticus

- **Definition**: repeated convulsions with no intervals of consciousness.
- It is a medical emergency for both mother and fetus.
- **Management**: as for non-pregnant women. Maintain maternal vital functions, control convulsions and prevent subsequent seizures. Transient fetal bradycardia is common. Resuscitate the fetus *in utero* before making a decision about delivery. Prolonged seizure activity may be associated with placental abruption.

Disorders of consciousness

- Disorders of *content* (confusion) and *level* of consciousness (coma).
- **Differential diagnosis**: similar to that in non-pregnant women, but also includes eclampsia.
- **Management**: treat underlying aetiology. Supportive care.

Psychiatric disorders in pregnancy

Psychiatric medications should be continued in pregnancy. In general, the risk of a clinical relapse poses a greater threat to the pregnancy than continued medication. Guidelines for drug treatment include:

- Use the lowest effective dose.
- Consider delaying treatment until after the first trimester to minimize the risk of teratogenicity.
- Avoid sedating agents immediately before delivery to minimize neonatal sedation.
- Electroconvulsant therapy (ECT) is generally avoided in pregnancy, but is considered safe for the fetus.

Postpartum depression

- **Incidence**: occurs in 8–15% of all postpartum women.
- **Risk factors**: prior depression (30% risk), prior postpartum depression (70–85%).
- Peak onset of symptoms is 2–3 months postpartum, and usually resolves spontaneously within 6–12 months.

Medicine at a Glance, Fourth Edition. Edited by Patrick Davey. © 2014 John Wiley & Sons, Ltd. Published 2014 by John Wiley & Sons, Ltd. Companion website: www.ataglanceseries.com/medicine

- Supportive care and monthly follow-up are necessary. Medications can be started if needed.

Postpartum psychosis
- **Incidence**: occurs in 1–2 per 1000 live births.
- **Risk factors**: primiparity, personal or family history of mental illness, prior postpartum psychosis (25–30% risk).
- Peak onset of symptoms is 10–14 days postpartum.
- **Management**: hospitalization, pharmacological therapy, ECT as needed.

Pulmonary disease in pregnancy
Asthma
- **Incidence**: occurs in 1–4% of all pregnancies.
- Pregnancy has a variable effect on asthma (25% improve, 25% worsen, 50% are unchanged). In general, women with mild, well-controlled asthma tolerate pregnancy well. Women with severe asthma are at risk of symptomatic deterioration.
- **Management**: as for non-pregnant women. Hospitalization, steroids and/or intubation may be required.
- **Complications**: intrauterine fetal growth restriction (IUGR), stillbirth, maternal death.

Amniotic fluid embolism
- An obstetric emergency with an 80–90% maternal mortality rate.
- **Risk factors**: multiparity, prolonged labour, fetal demise, 'excessive' oxytocin augmentation, placental abruption, caesarean section delivery.
- Characterized by acute onset of dyspnoea, hypotension, coagulopathy and hypoxaemia. Therapy is primarily supportive.

Pulmonary oedema
- Classified as cardiogenic or non-cardiogenic.
- **Risk factors**: fluid overload, infection, pre-eclampsia, tocolytic therapy.
- **Management**: as for non-pregnant women. LMNOP: *l*asix (diuresis), *m*orphine, Na^{2+} and water restriction, *o*xygen and *p*osition upright. Consider antibiotics.

Renal disease in pregnancy
Asymptomatic bacteriuria
- **Incidence**: occurs in 4–7% of all pregnancies, which is similar to that in non-pregnant women.
- In pregnancy, asymptomatic bacteriuria is more likely to progress to pyelonephritis (20–30%).
- *Escherichia coli* is the most common causative organism.

Chronic renal failure
- **Complications**: infertility (usually due to chronic anovulation), spontaneous abortion, pre-eclampsia, IUGR, fetal death, preterm birth.
- Pregnancy outcome is dependent on baseline renal function (see Table 236.1) and presence and severity of hypertension. The degree of proteinuria does not correlate with pregnancy outcome.
- In women with end-stage renal disease, renal transplantation offers the best chance of a successful pregnancy (especially if renal function is stable for 1–2 years and there is no hypertension). Triple-agent immunosuppression (ciclosporin, azathioprine, prednisone) should be continued in pregnancy.

Autoimmune diseases in pregnancy
Systemic lupus erythematosus
- Systemic lupus erythematosus does not generally worsen in pregnancy. Pregnancy outcome is related primarily to the severity of underlying renal disease.
- **Complications**: pre-eclampsia, IUGR, preterm birth.

Table 236.1 Pregnancy outcome in women with chronic renal disease

	Category of chronic renal disease		
	Mild	Moderate	Severe
Serum creatinine (mmol/L)	120–150	150–250	>250
Serum creatinine (mg/dL)	<1.4	1.4–2.5	>2.5
Complications (%)	20	40	85
Viable delivery (%)	95	90	50
Long-term sequelae (%)	<5	25	55

Maternal anti-Ro and anti-La antibodies
Associated with complete fetal heart block in 5–10% of cases.

Immune (idiopathic) thrombocytopenic purpura
- Immune thrombocytopenic purpura (ITP) is a maternal disease characterized by the presence of circulating antiplatelet antibodies. It should be distinguished from *alloimmune thrombocytopenia* in which maternal platelet counts are normal, but antiplatelet antibodies (usually anti-PLA1/2) cross the placenta to cause fetal thrombocytopenia and possibly intraventricular haemorrhage. Alloimmune thrombocytopenia is analogous to rhesus (Rh) disease of platelets.
- **Differential diagnosis**: pre-eclampsia, coagulopathy, drugs, gestational thrombocytopenia.
- **Complications**: IgG can cross the placenta and cause fetal thrombocytopenia. However, the correlation between maternal and fetal platelet counts is poor. Fetal intraventricular haemorrhage in the setting of ITP is rare.
- **Management**: corticosteroids may be necessary if maternal thrombocytopenia is severe. Intravenous Ig, plasmapharesis and splenectomy are rarely necessary in pregnancy. Caesarean section delivery has not been shown to improve perinatal outcome.

Rheumatoid arthritis
- Improves in 75% of pregnancies, but >90% of women will relapse within 6 months of delivery.
- Corticosteroids are safe in pregnancy. Gold salts, cytotoxic agents, penicillamine and antimalarials may have adverse fetal effects, but may be used if indicated.

Surgical conditions in pregnancy
- **Incidence**: occurs in 2–3 per 1000 pregnancies.
- **Indications**: appendicitis, biliary disease, ovarian disease.
- **Complications**: haemorrhage, anaesthetic complications, infection, preterm delivery. Complications can be minimized if surgery is performed in the second trimester.
- Technical considerations:
  - Left lateral tilt if ≥20 weeks to improve venous return.
  - Continuous fetal monitoring ≥24 weeks' gestation.
  - Avoidance of teratogenic agents.
  - Specific anaesthetic considerations.

Appendicitis
- **Incidence**: the incidence of appendicitis is not increased (1 in 1500 pregnancies), but an infected appendix is more likely to rupture in pregnancy.
- **Diagnosis**: symptoms and signs are similar to those in non-pregnant women, except that the appendix moves up in pregnancy.
- **Management**: surgical removal through a right paramedian incision is generally recommended (which can be extended if the appendix cannot be located or if caesarean section delivery is indicated).

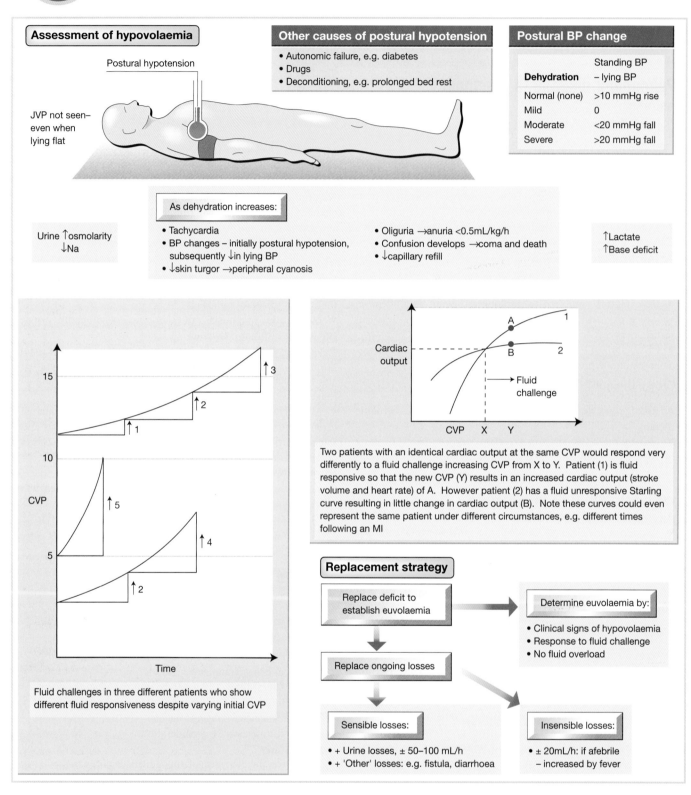

237 Fluid replacement therapy

Assessment of hypovolaemia

Postural hypotension

JVP not seen–
even when
lying flat

Other causes of postural hypotension

- Autonomic failure, e.g. diabetes
- Drugs
- Deconditioning, e.g. prolonged bed rest

Postural BP change

Dehydration	Standing BP – lying BP
Normal (none)	>10 mmHg rise
Mild	0
Moderate	<20 mmHg fall
Severe	>20 mmHg fall

As dehydration increases:

- Tachycardia
- BP changes – initially postural hypotension, subsequently ↓in lying BP
- ↓skin turgor →peripheral cyanosis

- Oliguria →anuria <0.5mL/kg/h
- Confusion develops →coma and death
- ↓capillary refill

Urine ↑osmolarity ↓Na

↑Lactate ↑Base deficit

Fluid challenges in three different patients who show different fluid responsiveness despite varying initial CVP

Two patients with an identical cardiac output at the same CVP would respond very differently to a fluid challenge increasing CVP from X to Y. Patient (1) is fluid responsive so that the new CVP (Y) results in an increased cardiac output (stroke volume and heart rate) of A. However patient (2) has a fluid unresponsive Starling curve resulting in little change in cardiac output (B). Note these curves could even represent the same patient under different circumstances, e.g. different times following an MI

Replacement strategy

Replace deficit to establish euvolaemia

Determine euvolaemia by:
- Clinical signs of hypovolaemia
- Response to fluid challenge
- No fluid overload

Replace ongoing losses

Sensible losses:
- + Urine losses, ± 50–100 mL/h
- + 'Other' losses: e.g. fistula, diarrhoea

Insensible losses:
- ± 20mL/h: if afebrile – increased by fever

Fluid may be required either for the maintenance of euvolaemia or replacement of losses in hypovolaemic patients. The oral route for is optimal for maintenance. Patients unable to eat and drink normally can be fed by either a nasogastric, nasojejunal or a percutaneous endoscopically placed gastric feeding tube. Occasionally, the enteral route is unavailable (recent gastrointestinal (GI) surgery, ileus); intravenous crystalloid may be administered for short periods to provide water and electrolytes, though parenteral nutrition needs to be considered if long-term maintenance is required.

Assessment of hypovolaemia

Profound hypovolaemia will eventually lead to tissue hypoperfusion and multiorgan failure. It may result from absolute losses (haemorrhage, diarrhoea, vomiting, burns, polyuria) or redistribution of fluid, sometimes known as 'third space' loss (sepsis, anaphylaxis, pancreatitis, trauma, spinal cord injury, ascites). The rennin–angiotensin and sympathetic nervous systems are important in regulating the volume of the extracellular space. These compensatory mechanisms may make it difficult to detect mild hypovolaemia. Signs of hypovolaemia are:

- Reduced skin turgor, decreased capillary refill, tachycardia and low jugular venous pressure (JVP).
- Low urine output (<0.5 mL/kg/h) with high osmolality, low urine sodium and a urine urea creatinine ratio of <40, and eventual abnormal urea and creatinine levels in blood. Plasma urea is disproportionably high in dehydration and GI haemorrhage. It may be low in patients with liver disease even in the presence of substantial hypovolaemia.
- Hypotension: reduction in blood pressure (BP) is a late feature. An apparently 'normal' BP may be low if the patient suffers from untreated hypertension. Compensatory mechanisms mask significant hypovolaemia in the supine position, therefore hypotension may only become apparent on sitting or standing (postural hypotension). Such patients often complain of dizziness or syncope when erect. Hypovolaemia in the supine position may also be unmasked by raising the legs for 30 seconds (to increase venous return) and monitoring the effect on heart rate, BP and JVP (or central venous pressure (CVP)). This should not be performed if raising the legs is likely to be painful.
- Reduced weight.
- Lactate and base deficit rise when there is significant tissue hypoperfusion.

As with many critically ill patients, the signs above may be nonspecific and are not by themselves diagnostic, but taken together with the patient's history and diagnosis one may make an assessment of volume status. In some patients this is easy. For example, in a young man with 4 days of diarrhoea who has not been drinking, if examination shows tachycardia, reduced capillary refill, hypotension, reduced JVP and oliguria, there would be little doubt the patient is severely dehydrated. However, if the patient is elderly with pre-existing heart failure and is admitted with acute pancreatitis, the assessment is far more complex. The fluid challenge is extremely useful in the diagnosis and treatment of hypovolaemia.

Fluid challenge

The response to a fluid challenge may be assessed by changes in pulmonary artery occlusion pressure (reflecting left atrial pressure), stroke volume, cardiac output or CVP (reflecting right atrial pressure). The latter is most frequently used outside of the intensive care unit. Traditionally, one is taught 'normal' values of right and left atrial pressures, however absolute values are of little use in guiding fluid therapy because they vary with ventricular compliance and venous tone. An absolute CVP value of 10 mmHg may represent hypovolaemia, euvolaemia or hypervolaemia in three different patients.

A fluid challenge involves giving a relatively small volume of crystalloid or colloid over a short period of time and monitoring the haemodynamic effects. Typically 250 mL of fluid is given over a period of 2–3 minutes. The change in CVP depends on the volume status of the patient. In a hypovolaemic patient there is little increase in CVP following a fluid challenge (<3 mmHg), which may then be repeated. A rise of 3 mmHg in the CVP fol­lowing a challenge implies an adequate circulating volume, whilst a rise >3 mmHg suggests hypervolaemia. The patient should also be monitored for improvements in other haemodynamic variables (↓ heart rate, ↑ BP, ↑ capillary refill) and tissue perfusion (↑ urine output, ↑ Glasgow Coma Score (GCS), reduction in acidosis/lactate), whilst avoiding signs of hypervolaemia.

Management of severely hypovolaemic patients

As with all critically ill patients there needs to be good vascular access (ideally central venous) and appropriate monitoring, which should include electrocardiogram, pulse oximetry, hourly urine output, BP (arterial catheter if severe hypotension or shock), respiratory rate and GCS. A pulmonary artery catheter, oesophageal Doppler or pulse contour analysis may be required in some patients.

Which fluid should be chosen?

Blood is required in acute haemorrhage, but colloid is given to maintain the circulation until this is available. Crystalloids equilibrate within the extracellular space (interstitial, intravascular) and so have less immediate effect on plasma expansion than colloids. Typically, colloid expands plasma volume by three times as much as the same volume of crystalloid, but this effect is not maintained over time, particularly in critically ill patients with increased vascular permeability. This means that in critically ill patients the plasma volume expanding effects of colloids and crystalloids are very similar.

- **Crystalloid-normal saline or lactated Ringer's solution** (Hartmann's solution): cheap compared to colloids. Its use avoids hyperchloraemic acidosis which may occur with large volumes of saline.
- **Colloid-albumin**: 4.5% or 20% salt poor (molecular weight 66.5 kDa). It is the most expensive colloid. There has been some controversy with its use in the past, however a recent multicentre trial shows no difference in safety compared to saline.
- **Colloid-dextrans**: examples include dextran 40 or 70 (molecular weight in kDa). It is the less commonly used of all colloids in Europe, and decreases platelet aggregation.
- **Colloid-gelatins** (Gelofusine, Haemaccel): derived from hydrolysed animal collagen (molecular weight 30–35 kDa). They have a short duration of action, with the highest risk of anaphylactoid reactions.
- **Colloid-hydroxyethyl starches** (HAES-Steril, eloHAES): derived from maize, with various (high) molecular weights. They may affect haemostasis. Colloids containing starch are associated with an increased risk of death and renal failure in septic shock. Long-term storage in tissues can cause pruritus.

Hyperchloraemic acidosis

Colloids contain osmotically active molecules which are usually in normal saline. The administration of large volumes of chloride-rich saline leads to a metabolic acidosis. This phenomenon is not observed with Hartmann's solution, which is a physiologically balanced solution containing much less chloride. Patients with dilutional hyperchloraemic acidosis suffer with nausea, abdominal pain and reduced urine output (hyperchloraemia reduces the glomerular filtration rate). Future developments will undoubtedly see the wider introduction of colloids in physiological solutions.

238 Illness in elderly people

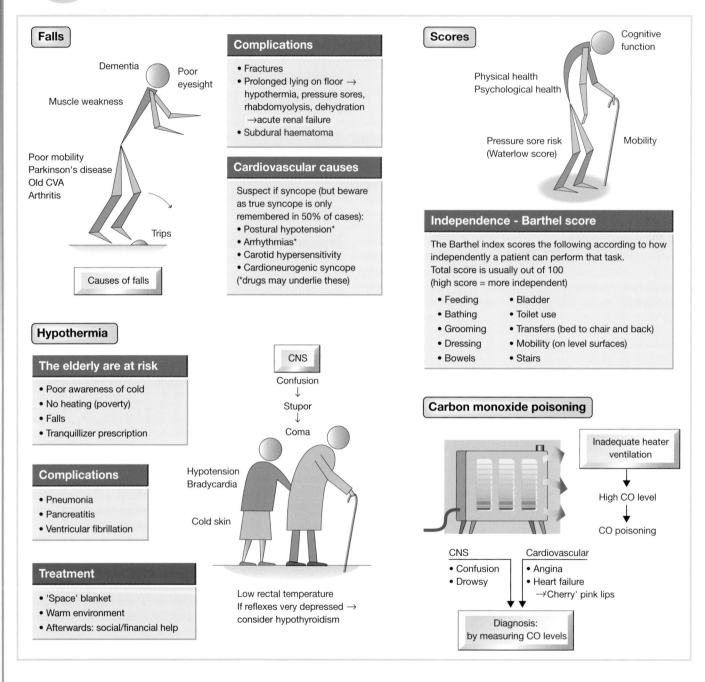

Falls

Dementia
Poor eyesight
Muscle weakness
Poor mobility
Parkinson's disease
Old CVA
Arthritis
Trips

Causes of falls

Complications

- Fractures
- Prolonged lying on floor → hypothermia, pressure sores, rhabdomyolysis, dehydration →acute renal failure
- Subdural haematoma

Cardiovascular causes

Suspect if syncope (but beware as true syncope is only remembered in 50% of cases):
- Postural hypotension*
- Arrhythmias*
- Carotid hypersensitivity
- Cardioneurogenic syncope
(*drugs may underlie these)

Scores

Cognitive function
Physical health
Psychological health
Pressure sore risk (Waterlow score)
Mobility

Independence - Barthel score

The Barthel index scores the following according to how independently a patient can perform that task.
Total score is usually out of 100
(high score = more independent)

- Feeding
- Bathing
- Grooming
- Dressing
- Bowels
- Bladder
- Toilet use
- Transfers (bed to chair and back)
- Mobility (on level surfaces)
- Stairs

Hypothermia

The elderly are at risk

- Poor awareness of cold
- No heating (poverty)
- Falls
- Tranquillizer prescription

Complications

- Pneumonia
- Pancreatitis
- Ventricular fibrillation

Treatment

- 'Space' blanket
- Warm environment
- Afterwards: social/financial help

CNS

Confusion
↓
Stupor
↓
Coma

Hypotension
Bradycardia

Cold skin

Low rectal temperature
If reflexes very depressed → consider hypothyroidism

Carbon monoxide poisoning

Inadequate heater ventilation
↓
High CO level
↓
CO poisoning

CNS
- Confusion
- Drowsy

Cardiovascular
- Angina
- Heart failure →'Cherry' pink lips

Diagnosis: by measuring CO levels

Sick elderly people should in many respects be treated identically to young people, although there are important differences:

- Their premorbid condition is often worse due to multiple ongoing illnesses, multiple medications and varying degrees of dementia, poverty and social isolation. Thus, the rehabilitation potential following the acute illness may be more limited. Additional home support should be planned early on during hospital admission.
- The clinical presentation is often atypical and not classic.
- The differential diagnosis is usually broader.
- The risk to life from any illness is greater.
- Recovery is prolonged and may require substantial support.

Premorbid condition

It is vital to establish the premorbid condition, because this is the target to aim for in subsequent rehabilitation. How independent were they? Several scoring systems (e.g. activities of daily living) can be used to ascertain functional status; the Barthel score is commonly used to measure independence and thus rehabilitation potential and progress (see Figure 238.1).

Medicine at a Glance, Fourth Edition. Edited by Patrick Davey. © 2014 John Wiley & Sons, Ltd. Published 2014 by John Wiley & Sons, Ltd. Companion website: www.ataglanceseries.com/medicine

Polypharmacy

Elderly people are often prescribed multiple drugs for multiple pathologies. This leads to compliance issues (disease progression) and side effects. Always ask whether the current illness can be explained by a side effect of medication.

Differential diagnosis

In young patients, 'Occam's razor' applies: 'the least number of diagnoses needed to explain all the symptoms and signs establishes the correct diagnosis'. In elderly people, multiple pathologies often coexist, e.g. heart failure, leg ulcers, diabetes and its complications, occult cancer, etc. A single unifying diagnosis is often not possible.

Clinical presentations and diseases

Presentations are often atypical, such as 'unwellness' without specific features or a decline in functional or cognitive capacity, rather than with organ-specific symptoms. The differential diagnosis is broader than in many younger patients. For example:

- Acute confusion is a common presentation of many diseases. As the febrile response is diminished, infections often present with minor fever and minor constitutional upset, and major confusion. Abscesses, e.g. subphrenic and pelvic, may present as 'unwellness', without localizing symptoms/signs.
- Many diseases present with decreased function/cognition or apathy and weight loss, rather than more classically. Diseases that may present in this manner include thyrotoxicosis, depression, temporal arteritis and cancer.
- Tuberculosis is not uncommon in elderly people, and may present quite atypically – with non-specific 'unwellness', loss of appetite, etc.
- Diseases may relate to poverty: there are many examples, including accidental carbon monoxide (CO) poisoning resulting from ill-maintained heaters, which are underdiagnosed. CO binds to haemoglobin, decreasing oxygen transport. Presentation is with central nervous system (CNS) (headache, agitation, confusion, occasionally coma) and/or cardiac symptoms (heart failure, unstable angina) – common symptoms in elderly people that are often attributed to other pathology. Diagnosis is by measuring CO levels in the blood. Treatment is with high-dose hyperbaric (i.e. high pressure) oxygen in severe cases (contact Royal Navy diving centres) and, crucially, heater maintenance.
- Hypothermia: see Figure 238.1.

Specific issues

Falls are common. The cause should always be sought, as specific therapy may be effective:

- Musculoskeletal conditions, such as osteoarthritis or age-related decline in muscle strength, are a common cause of falls. Physical rehabilitation, a Zimmer frame or other walking aid, and adjustment of the home environment may prevent falls and consequent fractures.
- Cardiovascular diseases causing recurrent falls include postural hypotension, cardioneurogenic syncope, carotid hypersensitivity syndrome and intermittent arrhythmias (bradyarrhythmias such as complete heart block, occasionally ventricular tachycardia). Carotid sinus massage, tilt-table testing and 24-hour electrocardiogram (ECG) taping may provide important clues to the presence of cardiovascular disease.
- Neurological disease, especially disability from a previous stroke, Parkinson's disease, peripheral neuropathy (e.g. diabetic) or cervical myelopathy. Epilepsy rarely underlies recurrent falls.
- Dementia often underlies or contributes to falls and immobility.

The consequence of falls also should be considered:

- Fractures, which may be lessened by treating osteoporosis, providing hip protectors and adjusting the home environment.
- Assistance may be needed to get up – various alarms are available. Regular visits by friends and neighbours play a vital role.

Diagnostic issues

As clinical symptoms and signs may be less reliable, investigations should be broad. All elderly patients admitted acutely should have:

- Full blood count, electrolytes (K^+, Na^+, Ca^{2+}), renal and liver function, and inflammatory markers (both erythrocyte sedimentation rate and C-reactive protein).
- Chest X-ray and ECG.
- Urine dipstick and, if abnormal, culture.
- Blood cultures unless infection has been ruled by establishing an alternative diagnosis.

Special issues

- Special diagnostic clinics for falls, dementia, syncope, etc. allow for optimal care and treatment.
- The threshold for 'blind' abdomen/pelvis computed tomography is low even without localizing symptoms/signs, because cancer and intra-abdominal/pelvic abscesses are common.
- A therapeutic trial of steroids is diagnostic in temporal arteritis if symptoms resolve ≥ 48 hours after starting steroids.

Consequence and treatment of illness

The risk to life from any illness (e.g. pneumonia, myocardial infarction) is greater with increasing age, justifying aggressive medical therapy. Age alone is not a bar to high technology intervention, such as cardiac surgery (aortic valve replacement is feasible in many aged 85 years or more), abdominal surgery, intensive care, etc. Aggressive treatments, although often having more benefit, equally often have greater risk. This calls for careful clinical judgement in deciding the most appropriate therapy. Cardiac arrest is associated with a poorer outcome in very elderly people (≥ 85 years). Decisions on the appropriateness of cardiopulmonary resuscitation should be made on admission in conjunction with the patient or, if they are incapacitated, their relatives.

Rehabilitation

It is vital that, in order to optimize outcome, specialists in old age medicine, rather than general physicians, undertake rehabilitation, using multidisciplinary teams, including:

- Physiotherapists.
- Occupational therapists.
- Social workers.

The aim should be to return the patient to a stable, long-term environment of his or her choice.

239 Chronic tiredness and other medically unexplained symptoms

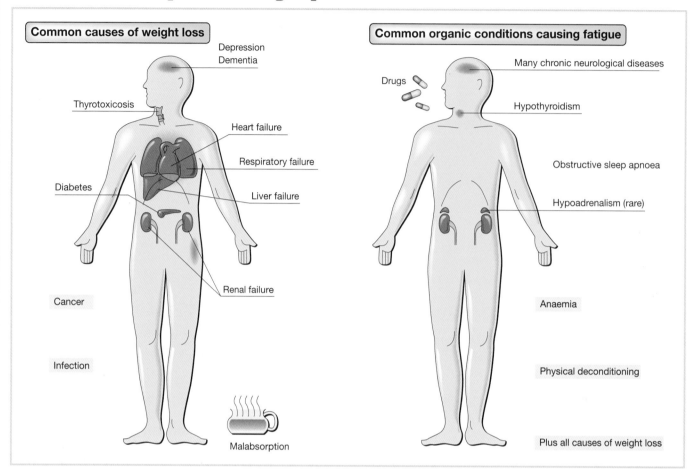

Common causes of weight loss

- Depression
- Dementia
- Thyrotoxicosis
- Heart failure
- Respiratory failure
- Diabetes
- Liver failure
- Renal failure
- Cancer
- Infection
- Malabsorption

Common organic conditions causing fatigue

- Drugs
- Many chronic neurological diseases
- Hypothyroidism
- Obstructive sleep apnoea
- Hypoadrenalism (rare)
- Anaemia
- Physical deconditioning
- Plus all causes of weight loss

Chronic fatigue

Fatigue is a complex and common sensation accounting for 20% of general practitioner consultations. Tiredness results from:

- Many (indeed most) organic diseases (see Figure 239.1).
- Psychological distress.
- Social stresses.
- Psychiatric illness: 20–80% of tired patients have a psychiatric disorder (depression, anxiety or somatization disorder).
- Tiredness may also be a medically unexplained symptom (MUS); the diagnoses applied may vary between this, chronic fatigue syndrome (CFS), post-viral fatigue (especially if there have been symptoms in the past 6 months suggesting a viral infection) and myalgic encephalomyelitis (ME). The variation in the diagnosis made for long-standing fatigue largely follows medical and social styles, rather than reflecting any real change in the epidemiology of the aetiology of this symptom.

From this list, it can be seen that almost any illness or psychic distress can cause tiredness. Accordingly the diagnosis of the cause of any fatigue rests on identifying the associated symptoms, as well as on the demographics (patient's age and sex: male sex and increasing age are associated with serious disease). Features suggestive of an underlying organic illness include:

- Weight loss: unintentional weight loss usually has a serious cause (see Figure 239.1).
- Fevers, night sweats.
- Malaise.
- Persistent pains localized to one area.
- Persistent symptoms of new onset.
- Age ≥35 years.

It is important that serious organic or psychiatric pathology is diagnosed and treated; other causes of tiredness are usually diagnosed by exclusion (see Table 239.1). Accurate diagnosis relies on the history and examination, although investigations are also important. A normal full blood count, renal and liver function and inflammatory markers (C-reactive protein, erythrocyte sedimentation rate) are reassuring, but do not exclude all serious inflammatory/malignant disease (disseminated cancer can present as fatigue with normal blood tests – the diagnostic clue is often weight loss and age ≥50 years). One-third of patients with fatigue have no identifiable organic or psychiatric disorder (including CFS).

Management and prognosis

These depend on the cause. If psychological stresses are significant, counselling may help. Of patients with non-specific fatigue,

Medicine at a Glance, Fourth Edition. Edited by Patrick Davey. © 2014 John Wiley & Sons, Ltd. Published 2014 by John Wiley & Sons, Ltd. Companion website: www.ataglanceseries.com/medicine

Table 239.1 Physical disorders associated with fatigue.

- Vital organ failure (heart, lung, kidney, liver, bone marrow, skin)
- Chronic inflammation or infection
- Viral infections may cause *postviral fatigue* lasting <6 months
- Malignancy
- Endocrine disease (particularly thyroid disease, adrenal disease)
- Anaemia
- Sleep disorders (obstructive sleep apnoea)
- Neurological disease (multiple sclerosis, Parkinson's disease)
- Drugs, e.g. β-blockers

25–50% still complain of fatigue a year later. Chronic fatigue for ≥6 months or associated with multiple associated somatic symptoms has a poorer long-term outlook. Most cases of fatigue are helped by physical reconditioning (a commonly advised exercise prescription is for 20 min sessions of aerobic exercise, sufficiently intense to induce breathlessness, repeated three times a week); this is true whether or not organic illness is present, and so can be applied without prejudice as to the diagnosis.

Medically unexplained symptoms

These are an enormous workload on all doctors:

- Medically unexplained symptoms may account for up to 50% of new patient diagnoses in some specialties, such as gastroenterology or neurology.
- Some symptoms are a marker for physical or sexual abuse; for example, pseudoseizures is a fairly strong marker for childhood sexual abuse.
- Any associated psychological disease should be rapidly diagnosed and treated.
- When a diagnosis of MUS is suspected, it is important to exclude serious illness using the minimum of tests.
- Equally, it is crucial to explain to patients, before the results of the test are known, that it is highly likely that these investigations will be normal, indeed, that they are primarily being done to reassure the patient, and not because the doctor believes they will be abnormal. This will avoid the patient believing that normal results mean that the physician should look harder for an underlying organic illness.
- It is best to acknowledge to the patient that the symptoms are medically unexplained, that these symptoms are frequently seen (thus the individual physician and profession have considerable experience and knowledge of them), and that they have a benign prognosis.
- It is not wise to offer mechanistic explanations that are based on guesswork, as these can often be disproved – leading to the patient losing confidence in their physician. Patients then seek help elsewhere; some patients seek large numbers of opinions (patients with MUSs in neurology clinics have been seen in about six previous specialties), and not surprisingly receive multiple different explanations for their symptoms, leading them to lose faith in doctors generally.
- There is some evidence that labelling these symptoms as functional, rather than medically unexplained, offends fewer patients.
- Dealing with symptoms, rather than seeking an underlying unifying interpretation, may help, e.g. drugs to help constipation or diarrhoea, exercise to help tiredness, anxiolytics to help anxiety, cognitive therapy to help worries about the future, etc., when patients are amenable.

Somatization disorder

The definition of somatization disorder includes:

- ≥2 years of medically unexplained symptoms.
- Persistent refusal to accept advice and reassurance for symptoms.
- Impaired level of functioning.

Various specialties classify clusters of MUSs together: non-cardiac chest pain, fibromyalgia, irritable bowel syndrome, chronic fatigue syndrome and repetitive strain injury. There is evidence that it is best not to give patients' symptoms such a name, as, while it helps to legitimize their symptoms as an illness (which patients find attractive), it may also help perpetuate their symptoms. Cognitive therapy may help, as can treating any of the commonly associated depression and/or anxiety states.

Chronic fatigue syndrome

Many, if not most, patients with isolated tiredness do not have serious organic pathology – some have the chronic fatigue syndrome, defined as 'new onset of persistent/relapsing, debilitating fatigue without previous fatigue, which does not resolve with bed rest and is severe enough to reduce daily activity to 50% of its premorbid level for ≥6 months'. It afflicts twice as many women as men and is very common – the overall incidence of tiredness in the general population is 1.5%. Such patients often have multiple other symptoms, each of which varies greatly from day to day. Patients with CFS are often keen on an 'organic' diagnosis – this is almost a hallmark of the condition, and it is important not to be drawn into endless cycles of negative investigations. This is best done by explaining that the diagnosis is CFS before investigations are ordered, so that negative results come as a reassurance, not as a surprise, or as a sign that the physician should look harder for any underlying pathology. Physical deconditioning often exacerbates symptoms, and regular exercise may have a role. Cognitive therapy and antidepressants likewise may help.

240 Psychiatric disorders

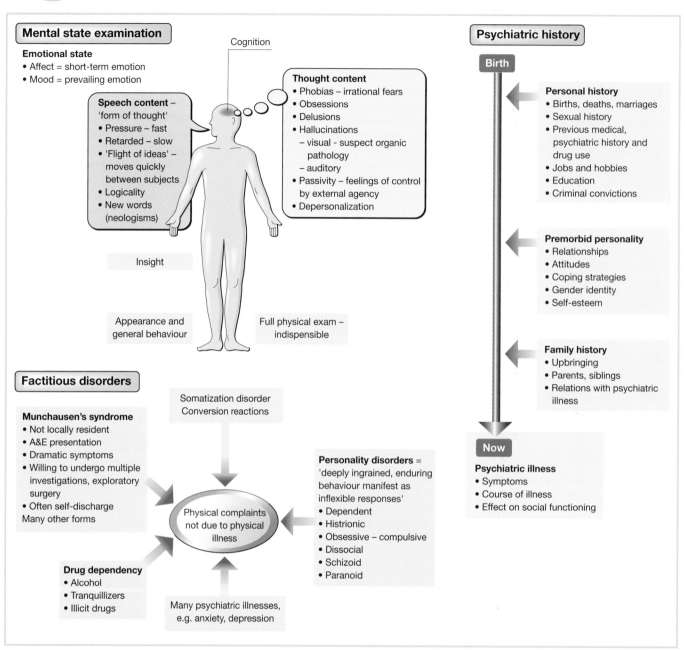

Mental state examination

Emotional state
• Affect = short-term emotion
• Mood = prevailing emotion

Cognition

Speech content – 'form of thought'
• Pressure – fast
• Retarded – slow
• 'Flight of ideas' – moves quickly between subjects
• Logicality
• New words (neologisms)

Thought content
• Phobias – irrational fears
• Obsessions
• Delusions
• Hallucinations
  – visual - suspect organic pathology
  – auditory
• Passivity – feelings of control by external agency
• Depersonalization

Insight

Appearance and general behaviour

Full physical exam – indispensible

Factitious disorders

Somatization disorder
Conversion reactions

Munchausen's syndrome
• Not locally resident
• A&E presentation
• Dramatic symptoms
• Willing to undergo multiple investigations, exploratory surgery
• Often self-discharge
Many other forms

Physical complaints not due to physical illness

Personality disorders = 'deeply ingrained, enduring behaviour manifest as inflexible responses'
• Dependent
• Histrionic
• Obsessive – compulsive
• Dissocial
• Schizoid
• Paranoid

Drug dependency
• Alcohol
• Tranquillizers
• Illicit drugs

Many psychiatric illnesses, e.g. anxiety, depression

Psychiatric history

Birth

Personal history
• Births, deaths, marriages
• Sexual history
• Previous medical, psychiatric history and drug use
• Jobs and hobbies
• Education
• Criminal convictions

Premorbid personality
• Relationships
• Attitudes
• Coping strategies
• Gender identity
• Self-esteem

Family history
• Upbringing
• Parents, siblings
• Relations with psychiatric illness

Now

Psychiatric illness
• Symptoms
• Course of illness
• Effect on social functioning

Psychological illnesses cause symptoms similar to those of organic disease, and may obscure an organic diagnosis or complicate its management. Of acute medical admissions, 5–10% require formal psychiatric review.

Neurotic diseases are an exaggeration of normal emotional responses. Psychotic illnesses have symptoms outside the range of normal human experience.

Common psychological illnesses seen in medical practice

Anxiety disorders
Anxiety disorders cause psychological symptoms (apprehension, fear of impending doom/disaster, irritability, depersonalization) and physical ones (sweating, tremor, palpitations, 'dizziness',

Medicine at a Glance, Fourth Edition. Edited by Patrick Davey. © 2014 John Wiley & Sons, Ltd. Published 2014 by John Wiley & Sons, Ltd. Companion website:
www.ataglanceseries.com/medicine

inability to sleep, poor concentration) which can be confused with certain diseases (e.g. thyrotoxicosis, alcohol intoxication/withdrawal, hypoglycaemia and, extremely rarely, phaeochromocytoma). Symptoms may be situation dependent, e.g. phobic disorders (particular objects or animals trigger attacks) or more commonly free floating, appearing without reason. Symptoms may appear in short overwhelming episodes ('panic attacks') – occasionally triggered by bad news, e.g. an untreatable diagnosis – or as longer, lower intensity anxiety states. Treatment is psychological (explanation, reassurance, relaxation techniques). Short courses of benzodiazepines have a limited role.

Abnormal illness behaviour

Abnormal illness behaviour includes exaggerated anxiety, inappropriate adoption of the 'sick' role and prolonged illness denial. Abnormal psychological reactions need to be identified and treated in order to treat any underlying organic disease effectively.

Somatization disorders

Somatization disorders comprise psychic distress (often depression or anxiety), which manifests as physical symptoms, and are common. Psychic symptoms are often denied or minimized and physical symptoms exaggerated. These disorders cause immense difficulty because the patient is convinced that a physical illness underlies the symptoms. Patients may attend the same department frequently (if the symptom complex remains unchanged) or multiple different departments (if the symptom complex varies) to establish an organic diagnosis. An important diagnostic clue is thick notes without any 'cast-iron' organic diagnosis. Treatment involves excluding physical illness, where possible identifying the underlying psychic symptoms and applying psychological treatments, including reassurance.

Conversion reactions

Conversion reactions (hysterical disorders) comprise psychic distress manifest as physical signs, e.g. paralysis, pseudoseizures, blindness. They are rare. Organic disease should be excluded using a minimum of investigation. The physician should refrain from further investigations otherwise the patient incorrectly perceives that an organic disorder defying diagnosis is present. Treatment (from a psychiatrist specialized in conversion reactions) comprises reassurance that there is no underlying pathology and that symptoms will improve over time. Direct confrontation is unhelpful.

Schizophrenia

This is characterized by a set of beliefs, symptoms and behaviour outside normal experience. Highly suggestive first-rank symptoms are:

- **Auditory hallucinations**, often abusive, repeating the patient's words, or commenting on their behaviour or personality.
- **Thought withdrawal, insertion and broadcasting**: external agencies or people can remove, insert or listen in to their thoughts.
- **Delusional beliefs**, i.e. ideas outside the social norms of that society. For example, a belief in a deity is often not delusional, but the belief that a deity can actually perform miracles can be.
- **External control** of thoughts, emotions or actions.

Symptoms are positive, when delusional beliefs and floridly abnormal behaviour predominate, or negative, when inaction, apathy and social withdrawal predominate. Schizophrenic patients come to the attention of acute medical services through:
- Bizarre behaviour leading to accident and emergency attendance. Organic disease or drug intoxication may need to be excluded.
- Attempted (and successful) suicide is common in psychosis – all self-harm cases should have psychotic illness excluded.

If schizophrenia is suspected, immediate psychiatric review should be requested. The diagnosis is made from the mental state examination (see Figure 240.1). Treatment is with antipsychotic drugs, which inhibit dopamine subtype D1 and D2 receptors and/or central nervous system serotonin traffic. They improve positive symptoms, but have less impact on negative ones. Similar symptoms occasionally arise from organic mental disorders, caused by drugs (e.g. 'street' drugs, steroids, rarely other drugs) or physical illness (e.g. temporal lobe epilepsy, brain tumours). These may need to be actively excluded.

Affective (mood) disorders

Depression

Depression results in a low mood and unhappiness. Conversation is slow, quiet and monotonous, with depressive ideation, low self-esteem, unworthiness and wretchedness. The intellect can be impaired. Physical symptoms can predominate. Somatic features of severe depression are: early morning waking, appetite and weight loss, constipation and loss of libido/sexual prowess. In psychotic depression, symptoms are profound and derogatory or abusive auditory hallucinations can occur. Depression complicates most physical illnesses (especially stroke) and amplifies physical symptoms, resulting in great distress and frequent physician consultations. Treatment is psychological (mild–moderate cases) and with antidepressant drugs, which prolong the action of noradrenaline (norepinephrine) and/or serotonin in neuronal synapses. Electroconvulsive therapy acts quickly and is used for severe depression.

Mania

Mania results in mental restlessness with mood elevation, fast and disinhibited speech, 'flight of ideas' (never dwelling on one topic for long) and overconfident self-belief, with delusions about intellectual, physical, financial or sexual prowess or omnipotence. Sufferers are physically restless and may not eat or sleep. Hypomania, a mild form of mania, comprises mild euphoria, overactivity and disinhibition. Mania can alternate with depression – a bipolar illness. Severe mania is treated with major tranquillizers, and subsequent attacks prevented by the mood stabilizer lithium.

Personality disorders

Personality disorders (see Figure 240.1), manifest as lifelong inflexible responses, cause management difficulties.

Substance misuse

This results in medical, social and economic problems.

- **Cigarettes**: highly addictive. Smokers die some 8 years before non-smokers (of ischaemic heart disease or cancer). Smoking ages skin (facial wrinkling). Counselling, nicotine replacement therapy and antidepressants have a minor role in cessation.
- **Alcohol**: can cause problem drinking (social disruption) or physical dependence (cessation leads to the withdrawal syndrome – tremor, sweating, tachycardia, anxiety, confusion, hallucinations and seizures, which are treated with chlordiazepoxide and vitamins).
- Minor or major **tranquillizers**.
- **Opiates**: common, often injected (HIV or hepatitis infection may result from shared needles). Premature death may result from infection or accidental overdose. Addicts may express opiate-seeking behaviour and commit petty larceny on hospital wards. Withdrawal causes sweating, shivering, tachycardia, hypertension and diarrhoea.
- **Ecstasy**: occasionally causes acute confusion, cardiac arrhythmias, memory loss or 'malignant' hyponatraemia and lethal cerebral oedema.

241 Substance misuse

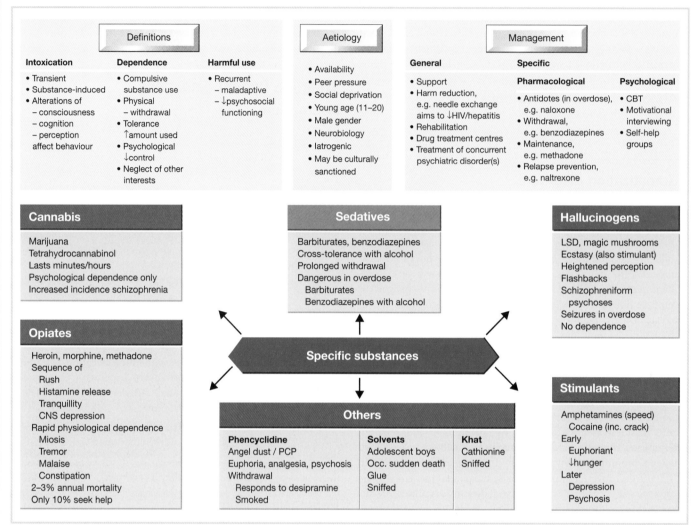

Definitions

Intoxication
- Transient
- Substance-induced
- Alterations of
  - consciousness
  - cognition
  - perception
  affect behaviour

Dependence
- Compulsive substance use
- Physical
  - withdrawal
- Tolerance
  ↑amount used
- Psychological
  ↓control
- Neglect of other interests

Harmful use
- Recurrent
  - maladaptive
  - ↓psychosocial functioning

Aetiology
- Availability
- Peer pressure
- Social deprivation
- Young age (11–20)
- Male gender
- Neurobiology
- Iatrogenic
- May be culturally sanctioned

Management

General
- Support
- Harm reduction, e.g. needle exchange aims to ↓HIV/hepatitis
- Rehabilitation
- Drug treatment centres
- Treatment of concurrent psychiatric disorder(s)

Specific

Pharmacological
- Antidotes (in overdose), e.g. naloxone
- Withdrawal, e.g. benzodiazepines
- Maintenance, e.g. methadone
- Relapse prevention, e.g. naltrexone

Psychological
- CBT
- Motivational interviewing
- Self-help groups

Cannabis

Marijuana
Tetrahydrocannabinol
Lasts minutes/hours
Psychological dependence only
Increased incidence schizophrenia

Opiates

Heroin, morphine, methadone
Sequence of
  Rush
  Histamine release
  Tranquillity
  CNS depression
Rapid physiological dependence
  Miosis
  Tremor
  Malaise
  Constipation
2–3% annual mortality
Only 10% seek help

Sedatives

Barbiturates, benzodiazepines
Cross-tolerance with alcohol
Prolonged withdrawal
Dangerous in overdose
  Barbiturates
  Benzodiazepines with alcohol

Specific substances

Others

Phencyclidine
Angel dust / PCP
Euphoria, analgesia, psychosis
Withdrawal
  Responds to desipramine
  Smoked

Solvents
Adolescent boys
Occ. sudden death
Glue
Sniffed

Khat
Cathionine
Sniffed

Hallucinogens

LSD, magic mushrooms
Ecstasy (also stimulant)
Heightened perception
Flashbacks
Schizophreniform psychoses
Seizures in overdose
No dependence

Stimulants

Amphetamines (speed)
  Cocaine (inc. crack)
Early
  Euphoriant
  ↓hunger
Later
  Depression
  Psychosis

Cannabis is the most common illicit drug used by the British general adult population (11% within the previous year), followed by cocaine (2.4%) and ecstasy (2%). In Britain, an estimated 500 000 people take ecstasy every weekend. Drugs are commonly used in combination. In ICD-10(International Classification of Diseases version 10), substance use disorders are classified according to (i) substance and (ii) type of disorder. The latter include the following:

- **Acute intoxication**: transient disturbances of consciousness, cognition, perception, affect or behaviour following the administration of a psychoactive substance (PS).
- **Harmful use**: damage to the individual's health and adverse effects on family and society.
- **Dependence**: physiological dependence includes a withdrawal state, tolerance (increasing doses of PSs needed for the same effect) and consequently the PS being taken in larger amounts or for longer than intended. Psychological dependence involves a sense of compulsion to take the PS, difficulties in controlling its use, increasing time spent obtaining, ingesting or recovering from the

PS, persistence with PS use despite awareness of harmful consequences, and a persistent but futile wish to cut down its use. There is usually a reduction or neglect of important social, occupational or recreational activities because of the PS use.
- **Withdrawal state**: physical and psychological symptoms occurring on absolute or relative withdrawal of a substance after repeated and usually prolonged and/or high-dose use of that substance. Onset and course of the withdrawal state are time limited and are related to the type of substance and the dose used before abstinence.
- **Psychotic disorder**: psychotic symptoms occurring during or immediately after PS use, characterized by vivid hallucinations, abnormal affect, psychomotor disturbances and persecutory delusions and delusions of reference.
- **Amnesic disorder**: memory and other cognitive impairments caused by substance use, most commonly alcohol.
- **Residual and late onset psychotic disorders**: where effects on behaviour, affect, personality or cognition last beyond the period during which a direct PS effect might be expected (e.g. flashbacks).

Medicine at a Glance, Fourth Edition. Edited by Patrick Davey. © 2014 John Wiley & Sons, Ltd. Published 2014 by John Wiley & Sons, Ltd. Companion website: www.ataglanceseries.com/medicine

Aetiology and management

Availability and peer pressure are key aetiological factors; there is a strong association with younger age (11–24 years) and male gender. Neurobiological mechanisms, iatrogenic factors (e.g. prescribed benzodiazepines (BDZs)), a desire for the pleasurable effects of substances and the pharmacological properties of the PS may all also contribute. Substance misuse and psychiatric illness share several associations, including socioeconomic disadvantage. Substance misuse can exacerbate psychiatric symptoms (commonly depressed mood) or precipitate episodes of illness (e.g. psychosis). Conversely, certain psychiatric symptoms, such as impulsivity or anxiety, may increase drug use, and patients with certain psychiatric diagnoses (e.g. dissocial personality disorder) are much more likely to take illicit drugs.

Management of patients with psychiatric and substance misuse disorders (dual diagnosis) should ideally involve a multidisciplinary team trained to manage both disorders concurrently. As well as being obtained illicitly, some PSs may be acquired legally from chemists (codeine), shops (solvents) or doctors (benzodiazepines, ostensibly therapeutically). In the UK, illicit drugs are controlled under the Misuse of Drugs Act. Drugs are classified as Class A (the most harmful, e.g. opiates, hallucinogens, injected stimulants), Class B (e.g. oral stimulants) and Class C. Cannabis is class C at time of writing, but may be reclassifi d to class B.

Treatment can be in residential rehabilitation, hospital and community settings. Medication has several uses: short-term treatment as antidotes in overdose and alleviation or prevention of withdrawal, or longer term treatment as substance replacement therapy (e.g. methadone) or relapse prevention (e.g. naltrexone, acamprosate). Psychological approaches such as cognitive behavioural therapy (CBT), motivational interviewing and self-help groups (such as Alcoholics Anonymous and Narcotics Anonymous) are effective. Infection (HIV, hepatitis C) is the greatest risk associated with injected drug use; harm reduction strategies aim to minimize infection risk (e.g. needle exchange) and improve safety.

Specific substances

Opiates

Opiates include *heroin, morphine* and *methadone*. They may be smoked ('chasing the dragon'), sniffed ('snorting') or taken orally, intravenously ('mainlining'), intramuscularly or subcutaneously ('skin popping'). After an intensely pleasurable 'buzz' or 'rush' and release of histamine (itching, reddening of eyes), a sense of peace and detachment occurs, succeeded by central nervous system depression. Tolerance and withdrawal develop quickly. Ten per cent of opiate misusers become dependent, but only 10% of these ever seek help; 2–3% die annually. Of the remainder, 25% are abstinent at 5 years and 40% at 10 years. Miosis, tremor, malaise, apathy, constipation, weakness, impotence, neglect, malnutrition and evidence of HIV and other infection (e.g. hepatitis C) are signs of chronic dependence. Early withdrawal symptoms (24–48h) include craving, flu-like symptoms, sweating and yawning. Mydriasis, abdominal cramps, diarrhoea, agitation, restlessness, piloerection ('gooseflesh') and tachycardia occur later (7–10 days). Opiate dependence may be treated by replacement with methadone (opioid agonist) or buprenorphine (opioid partial agonist), which are less euphoriant and have a relatively long half-life. Methadone, lofexidine and buprenorphine are used for detoxification; naltrexone (opioid antagonist) blocks the euphoric effects and so can help prevent relapse. Signs of overdose (often accidental) include miosis and respiratory depression and may require naloxone.

Hallucinogens

Hallucinogens include *LSD* (lysergic acid diethylamide), which produces psychological (e.g. heightened perceptions) and physiological (dilated pupils, peripheral vasoconstriction, increased temperature) effects, but not dependence. Rare adverse effects include 'flashbacks', psychoses and (in overdose) seizures. *Ecstasy* (MDMA (3,4 methylenedioxymetamphetamine)) – a synthetic amphetamine analogue – has mixed stimulant and hallucinogenic effects and can induce hyperactivity and potentially fatal dehydration (or hyponatraemia from the resulting excess water consumption) and hyperpyrexia. *Magic mushrooms* (psylocybin) have effects similar to LSD but are less prolonged.

Stimulants

Amphetamines ('speed'), taken orally or intravenously, cause euphoria, increased concentration and energy, mydriasis, tachycardia and hyperreflexia, followed by depression, fatigue and headache. Acute use may induce a schizophreniform psychosis. Methamphetamine is chemically related but more potent, long-lasting and harmful; it can be ingested, snorted or smoked (as 'crystal meth'). *Cocaine* may be sniffed, chewed or injected intravenously. Its effects (restlessness, increased energy, abolition of fatigue and hunger) resemble hypomania and last about 20 minutes. Visual/tactile hallucinations of insects (formication) and paranoid psychoses occur. Post-cocaine dysphoria ('the crash'), with sleeplessness and intense depression, precedes withdrawal (depression, insomnia and craving). 'Crack' (a purified, very addictive form of cocaine) is smoked. The crack 'high' is extremely short and, on withdrawal, persecutory delusions are common.

Cannabis

The active compound of *marijuana* ('pot', 'grass', hashish, ganja) is tetrahydrocannabinol. The effects are psychological (euphoria, relaxation, well-being, omnipotence, hallucinations) and physiological (increased appetite, lowered body temperature). Substantial psychological dependence occurs. Adverse effects include conjunctival irritation, decreased spermatogenesis, lung disease, flashbacks, transient psychoses and apathy. Cannabis use is associated with increased incidence of depression and schizophrenia.

Sedatives and hypnotics

Overdose may cause respiratory depression. *BDZs* produce dependence, withdrawal (including seizures) and tolerance. BDZ dependence is often iatrogenic, although BDZs are also common street (illicit/recreational) drugs.

Others

Solvents are typically sniffed, principally by groups of boys aged 8–19 years (a red rash around the mouth and nose may be a sign of abuse). Initial euphoria is followed by drowsiness. Psychological dependence is common, but physical dependence is rare. Chronic abuse results in weight loss, nausea, vomiting, polyneuropathy and cognitive impairment. Toxic effects (sometimes fatal) include bronchospasm, arrythmias, aplastic anaemia and hepatorenal or cerebral damage. *Phencyclidine* (PCP, 'angel dust') is usually smoked. Its effects include euphoria and peripheral analgesia and impaired consciousness or psychosis, which may require antipsychotics. *Khat*, used particularly by men from the Somali and Yemeni communities, contains cathinone, an amphetamine-like stimulant causing excitement and euphoria. It is not a controlled substance in the UK. *Nicotine*: around a quarter of British adults smoke. Counselling, nicotine replacement therapy, varenicline (partial nicotinic receptor agonist) and buproprion (noradrenaline and dopamine reuptake inhibitor) may aid smoking cessation.

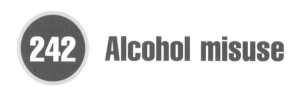

242 Alcohol misuse

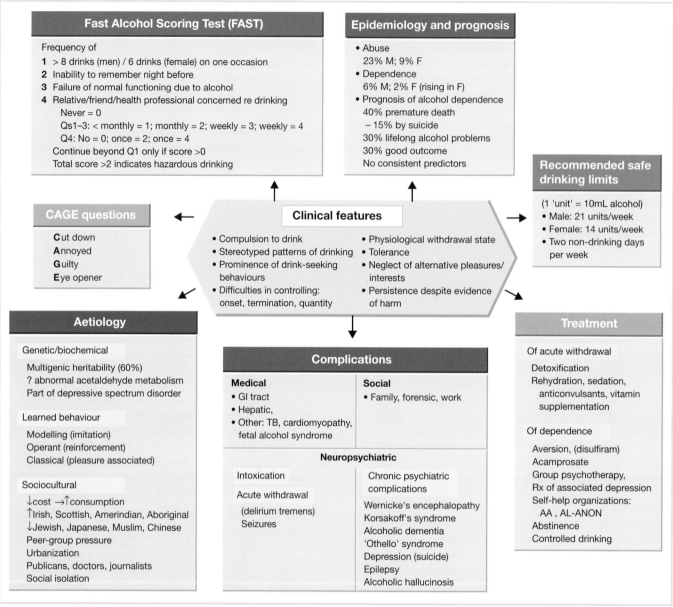

Fast Alcohol Scoring Test (FAST)

Frequency of
1 > 8 drinks (men) / 6 drinks (female) on one occasion
2 Inability to remember night before
3 Failure of normal functioning due to alcohol
4 Relative/friend/health professional concerned re drinking
　　Never = 0
　　Qs1–3: < monthly = 1; monthly = 2; weekly = 3; weekly = 4
　　Q4: No = 0; once = 2; once = 4
　　Continue beyond Q1 only if score >0
　　Total score >2 indicates hazardous drinking

Epidemiology and prognosis

- Abuse
  23% M; 9% F
- Dependence
  6% M; 2% F (rising in F)
- Prognosis of alcohol dependence
  40% premature death
  – 15% by suicide
  30% lifelong alcohol problems
  30% good outcome
  No consistent predictors

Recommended safe drinking limits

(1 'unit' = 10mL alcohol)
- Male: 21 units/week
- Female: 14 units/week
- Two non-drinking days
  per week

CAGE questions

Cut down
Annoyed
Guilty
Eye opener

Clinical features

- Compulsion to drink
- Stereotyped patterns of drinking
- Prominence of drink-seeking behaviours
- Difficulties in controlling: onset, termination, quantity
- Physiological withdrawal state
- Tolerance
- Neglect of alternative pleasures/ interests
- Persistence despite evidence of harm

Aetiology

Genetic/biochemical

Multigenic heritability (60%)
? abnormal acetaldehyde metabolism
Part of depressive spectrum disorder

Learned behaviour

Modelling (imitation)
Operant (reinforcement)
Classical (pleasure associated)

Sociocultural

↓cost →↑consumption
↑Irish, Scottish, Amerindian, Aboriginal
↓Jewish, Japanese, Muslim, Chinese
Peer-group pressure
Urbanization
Publicans, doctors, journalists
Social isolation

Complications

Medical	**Social**
• GI tract	• Family, forensic, work
• Hepatic,	
• Other: TB, cardiomyopathy, fetal alcohol syndrome	

Neuropsychiatric

Intoxication	Chronic psychiatric complications
Acute withdrawal	
(delirium tremens)	Wernicke's encephalopathy
Seizures	Korsakoff's syndrome
	Alcoholic dementia
	'Othello' syndrome
	Depression (suicide)
	Epilepsy
	Alcoholic hallucinosis

Treatment

Of acute withdrawal

Detoxification
Rehydration, sedation, anticonvulsants, vitamin supplementation

Of dependence

Aversion, (disulfiram)
Acamprosate
Group psychotherapy,
Rx of associated depression
Self-help organizations:
　AA , AL-ANON
Abstinence
Controlled drinking

Alcohol abuse is regular or binge consumption of alcohol sufficient to cause physical, neuropsychiatric or social damage.

Safe limits

- A 'unit' of alcohol (10 mL, 8 g) is roughly a small glass of wine, a pub single of spirits or a half pint of beer.
- The conventional safe drinking limits are 21 units per week for men and 14 for women, with at least two drink-free days each week.
- The UK government gives guidelines for maximum daily use (<4 units a day for men, <3 units for women), reflecting concerns about binge drinking.
- Much smaller amounts may be hazardous to a fetus.

Classification

The ICD-10 (International Classification of Diseases version 10) classifies alcohol use disorders using the same system as for other psychoactive substances:
- **Acute intoxication** is characterized by slurred speech, impaired coordination and judgement, labile affect and, in severe cases,

hypoglycaemia, stupor and coma. Differential diagnosis includes other causes of acute confusion, particularly head trauma.
- **Acute withdrawal** reflects the degree of previous dependence and usually occurs within 1 or 2 days of abstinence.
  - It is characterized by malaise, nausea, autonomic hyperactivity, tremulousness, labile mood, insomnia and transient hallucinations or illusions (usually visual).
  - Seizures are a recognized complication.
  - Severe withdrawal, or 'delirium tremens' ('shaking delirium'), occurs in 5% of withdrawals and has a mortality of up to 15%, partly as a result of other medical complications.
- **Alcohol dependence**.
- **Psychotic disorders** related to alcohol use include:
  - Alcoholic hallucinosis (usually threatening, second-person voices in a clear sensorium).
  - Jealousy (paranoid delusions about infidelity).
- **Amnesic syndrome**: for example Korsakoff's psychosis.
- **Residual and late-onset disorders**: these include depression and dementia.

Epidemiology

- Prevalence rates worldwide vary widely and are related to overall consumption levels, availability and price.
- In the UK, heavy drinking (an average of 8 units/day for men and 6 units/day for women) is reported by 23% of men and 9% of women; younger people are more likely to exceed safe limits.
- The prevalence of alcohol dependence is 6% in men and 2% in women. Rates are particularly high in medical inpatients, and are increasing in women and adolescents.
- Alcohol abuse and dependence often begin in the early to mid twenties, at a time when most people begin to moderate their drinking as their responsibilities increase.

Detection and screening

- A fifth of primary care attenders have an alcohol use disorder.
- The detection of disorders can be difficult because they are not usually clinically obvious, but is crucial to:
  - Enable appropriate treatment.
  - Avoid long-term complications.
  - Avoid withdrawal from unplanned abstinence (e.g. after surgery).
- Professionals should have a high index of suspicion in medical inpatients, and those with mental illness or two or more drink-driving offences.
- Many cases can be detected by documenting a typical drinking week.
- Screening questionnaires are also helpful (see Figure 242.1).
- Collateral history can be revealing.
- Physical examination may reveal alcoholic stigmata, particularly signs of liver disease (jaundice, spider naevi, palmar erythema, gynaecomastia) and peripheral neuropathy.
- Macrocytosis without anaemia and raised γ-glutamyl transferase, alanine and aspartate aminotransferase or carbohydrate-deficient transferrin indicate recent harmful use.

Aetiology

This is multifactorial. Factors include the following:
- A strong genetic component (around 60%), which appears to be multigenic. Genetically determined alterations in alcohol metabolism may partially explain this, with those at low risk producing more (hangover causing) acetaldehyde; 50% of Japanese people have an unpleasant 'flush reaction' on drinking alcohol due to a mutation in the acetaldehyde dehydrogenase 2 gene. There is often a positive family history of depression.
- Occupation: high-risk groups include the armed forces, doctors, publicans and journalists.
- Cultural influences: low rates are reported in Jews and Muslims, and high rates in Scottish and Irish people.
- The cost of alcoholic drinks.
- Behavioural models stress:
  - Learning by imitation (modelling).
  - Social reinforcement.
  - The association between drinking and pleasure (classic conditioning).
  - Avoiding withdrawal symptoms (operant conditioning).
- Risk increases in the presence of chronic psychiatric or physical illness, particularly if complicated by chronic pain. There is an association with mood and anxiety disorders.

Complications

- **Neuropsychiatric complications**:
  - Wernicke's encephalopathy.
  - Peripheral neuropathy.
  - Erectile or ejaculatory impotence.
  - Cerebellar degeneration.
  - Dementia.
- **Other physical complications**: drinking damages almost every organ system in the body.

- **Social complications** include unemployment, marital difficulties, criminality, prostitution, homicides, domestic violence, accidental deaths, road accidents and suicides.
- **Psychiatric complications**: repeated heavy drinking is associated with:
  - A 40% risk of temporary depressive episodes.
  - Suicidal ideas and attempts.
  - Severe anxiety.
  - Insomnia.
  These often improve within 2–4 weeks of abstinence.
- **Fetal alcohol syndrome** (from drinking in pregnancy) is characterized by:
  - Decreased muscle tone.
  - Poor coordination.
  - Developmental delay.
  - Heart defects.
  - A range of facial abnormalities.

Management

- Abstinence is the usual goal for treatment of dependence, although sometimes it is controlled drinking.
- Achieving abstinence requires **acute detoxification**:
  - This should be in hospital if there is a risk of delirium tremens or withdrawal seizures, or the person is a child or vulnerable (e.g. cognitively impaired or lacking support).
  - This is initially high and a rapidly tailing sedation (almost always a benzodiazepine, such as chlordiazepoxide or diazepam) is usually needed to control withdrawal symptoms and prevent seizures.
  - Treatment of delirium tremens is usually with lorazepam or antipsychotics (e.g. haloperidol or olanzapine).
  - Treatment also includes rehydration, correction of electrolyte disturbance, and oral or parenteral thiamine.
- **Motivational interviewing** is client-centred counselling that explores ambivalence to seeking treatment, drinking cessation, or both. It may help problem drinkers in denial achieve insight and a desire to change.
- **Psychological therapies** (individually or in groups) may promote maintenance of abstinence or controlled drinking (i.e. within safe limits). They are useful for:
  - Sustaining motivation.
  - Learning relapse prevention strategies.
  - Developing social routines not reliant on alcohol.
  - Treating coexistent depression and anxiety.
- **Self-help groups** (e.g. Alcoholics Anonymous) are effective; they reduce pro-drinking activities and social ties.
- **Medication** may help maintain abstinence after detoxification:
  - Disulfiram blocks alcohol metabolism, inducing acetaldehyde accumulation if alcohol is ingested, with resultant flushing, headache, anxiety and nausea.
  - Acamprosate acts on the γ-aminobutyric acid system to reduce cravings and risk of relapse.
  - Naltrexone, an opioid-receptor antagonist, has similar therapeutic effects (licensed in the USA but not the UK).
- **Prevention measures** include:
  - Increasing taxation on alcohol.
  - Restricting its advertising or sale.
  - School alcohol education: this reduces long-term alcohol use, risky alcohol-related behaviour and binge drinking.

Prognosis

- Continued alcohol problems increase the rate of early death by a factor of three or four. The most common causes are heart disease, stroke, cancers, liver cirrhosis, accidents and suicide.
- Only 15% of those with alcohol use disorder seek treatment; those who do have a better prognosis.

243 Drug toxicity (adverse drug reactions)

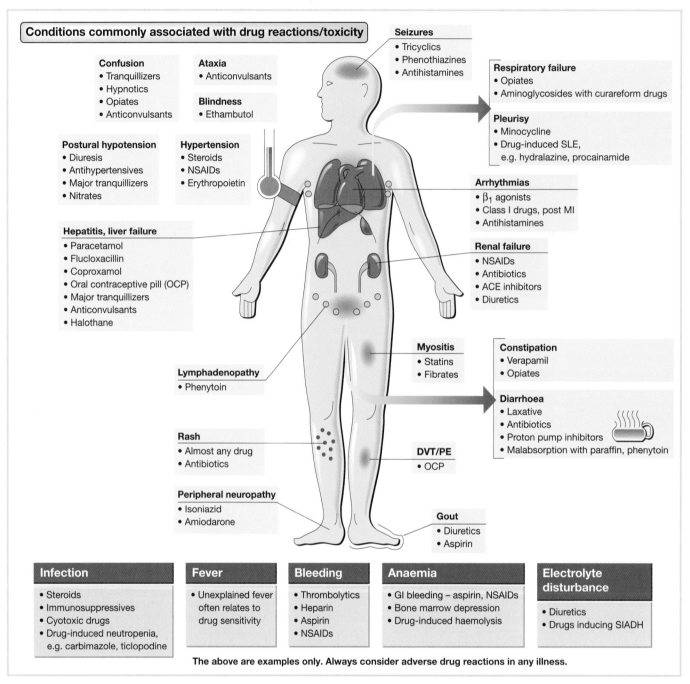

Conditions commonly associated with drug reactions/toxicity

Seizures
- Tricyclics
- Phenothiazines
- Antihistamines

Confusion
- Tranquillizers
- Hypnotics
- Opiates
- Anticonvulsants

Ataxia
- Anticonvulsants

Blindness
- Ethambutol

Respiratory failure
- Opiates
- Aminoglycosides with curareform drugs

Pleurisy
- Minocycline
- Drug-induced SLE, e.g. hydralazine, procainamide

Postural hypotension
- Diuresis
- Antihypertensives
- Major tranquillizers
- Nitrates

Hypertension
- Steroids
- NSAIDs
- Erythropoietin

Arrhythmias
- β_1 agonists
- Class I drugs, post MI
- Antihistamines

Hepatitis, liver failure
- Paracetamol
- Flucloxacillin
- Coproxamol
- Oral contraceptive pill (OCP)
- Major tranquillizers
- Anticonvulsants
- Halothane

Renal failure
- NSAIDs
- Antibiotics
- ACE inhibitors
- Diuretics

Myositis
- Statins
- Fibrates

Constipation
- Verapamil
- Opiates

Lymphadenopathy
- Phenytoin

Diarrhoea
- Laxative
- Antibiotics
- Proton pump inhibitors
- Malabsorption with paraffin, phenytoin

Rash
- Almost any drug
- Antibiotics

DVT/PE
- OCP

Peripheral neuropathy
- Isoniazid
- Amiodarone

Gout
- Diuretics
- Aspirin

Infection
- Steroids
- Immunosuppressives
- Cyotoxic drugs
- Drug-induced neutropenia, e.g. carbimazole, ticlopodine

Fever
- Unexplained fever often relates to drug sensitivity

Bleeding
- Thrombolytics
- Heparin
- Aspirin
- NSAIDs

Anaemia
- GI bleeding – aspirin, NSAIDs
- Bone marrow depression
- Drug-induced haemolysis

Electrolyte disturbance
- Diuretics
- Drugs inducing SIADH

The above are examples only. Always consider adverse drug reactions in any illness.

Adverse reactions to drugs are so common that it is crucial to determine whether any new symptom relates to a drug prescribed for another condition. Adverse reactions are classified as follows.

Predictable side effects

Predictable side effects at normal doses arise from those mechanisms responsible for therapeutic action. The following text is not comprehensive, but does give a number of different examples.

Interference with normal physiological function: drugs used in normal doses

- β-Receptor stimulation dilates peripheral blood vessel and β-blockade leads to vasoconstriction (cold peripheries).
- Bleeding with thrombolytic therapy.
- Immunosuppression from steroid therapy, presenting as severe/unusual infection: oral *Candida* infection with inhaled steroids for asthma; bone marrow suppression, with anaemia, infection and bleeding as a result of antineoplastic agents.

Medicine at a Glance, Fourth Edition. Edited by Patrick Davey. © 2014 John Wiley & Sons, Ltd. Published 2014 by John Wiley & Sons, Ltd. Companion website: www.ataglanceseries.com/medicine

- Daytime sleepiness with nocturnal hypnotics.
- Movement disorders arising from long-term anti-parkinsonian drugs.

Interference with normal physiological function: drugs used in high concentrations (or when excretion is impaired)

- Excess inhaled β-receptor agonists in asthma leads to palpitations: β-receptor stimulation increases the strength and rate of cardiac contraction.
- Diarrhoea with broad-spectrum antibiotics, from altered bowel flora.
- Hypothyroidism from antithyroid drugs or thyrotoxicosis from excess thyroxine.
- Hypoglycaemia from insulin.
- Hypercalcaemia with vitamin D.

Diseases enhancing drug side effects

There are a number of examples of this:

- β-Blockade leading to bronchoconstriction in people with asthma; in phaeochromocytomas β-blockers lead to unopposed α-adrenergic stimulation, which produces intense vasoconstriction and increases peripheral resistance so raising blood pressure, which may result in heart failure or stroke.
- Pre-existing heart failure may be exacerbated in those given verapamil, a negatively inotropic calcium channel blocker. Negative inotropism with calcium channel blockers partly correlates with negative chronotropism, i.e. the less they lower heart rate, the less negative inotropism occurs.
- Class I antiarrhythmics drugs can cause (lethal) ventricular arrhythmias in those with structural heart disease, e.g. previous myocardial infarction (MI).
- In bilateral renal artery stenosis, acute renal failure occurs if angiotensin-converting enzyme (ACE) inhibitors are given; constriction of the post-glomerular arteriole is mediated by angiotensin II. In renal artery stenosis this is critical in maintaining a high glomerular filtration pressure. If this vasoconstriction decreases, glomerular membrane filtration pressure is lost, and renal excretory function falls; if both kidneys have stenosed renal arteries, acute renal failure results.
- Paracetamol is more toxic in those with chronic liver disease, e.g. alcoholism.

Electrolyte abnormalities increasing the likelihood of drug toxicity

- Hypokalaemia increases the action of digoxin (see section Increased tissue action due to renal failure), and increases the likelihood of proarrhythmia occurring as a side effect of antiarrhythmic, antidepressant or antihistamine drugs.
- Chronic hyponatraemia predisposes to saline-induced brain-stem damage (central pontine myelinosis).

Age increasing the side effects of drugs

- Cardiovascular compensatory reflexes are diminished in elderly people, so postural hypotension is more common with antihypertensive therapy; this may present as fractured neck of femur or as recurrent falls.
- Renal tubular function declines in elderly people, so hyponatraemia from diuretics is more common; this may present as confusion.
- Increasing age diminishes brain reserves, so increasing the sensitivity to hypnotics and sedatives.

Sex increasing the possibility of side effects

- Gynaecomastia in men treated with oestrogens.

Increased tissue action of the drug

Side effects arising from increased tissue action of the drug, from increased tissue sensitivity or from overdosage may result from:

- A narrow therapeutic range: small changes in drug metabolism/dosage can easily produce toxic levels. Monitoring drug concentration where possible helps prevent this, e.g. digoxin, anticonvulsants, aminoglycosides.
- Renal or hepatic failure can slow metabolism of a drug or an active metabolite resulting in toxicity. In renal and/or hepatic failure, prescribe sparingly and always determine from the *British National Formulary* (BNF) whether the dose should be adjusted.

Increased tissue action due to renal failure

- **Digoxin** is renally excreted and is commonly given with diuretics to elderly people with heart failure. Old age, renal failure and hypokalaemia all predispose to toxicity, and manifest as (any) cardiac arrhythmia, visual disturbance (objects appear yellow), confusion, nausea and vomiting. The latter produces dehydration and pre-renal renal failure, further increasing digoxin levels and exacerbating toxicity. Treatment: wait for renal elimination and normalize potassium. If symptoms are life-threatening, give dialysis or digoxin antibodies.
- **Lithium** is renally excreted. If toxic levels develop (excess dosage, dehydration, deliberate overdose), ataxia, confusion (which may progress to coma), convulsions and nephrogenic diabetes insipidus occur. Circulating fluid is lost, producing pre-renal renal failure, so lithium levels rise further, exacerbating toxicity. Treatment: intravenous fluids and withholding lithium. Dialysis is occasionally needed.
- **Aminoglycosides** are renally excreted and used in severe infections, which themselves may cause renal failure. Drug levels should be very carefully monitored to avoid toxicity, which is manifest as vestibulocochlear nerve damage (deafness, difficulty with balance) and renal failure. Furosemide (frusemide) if given as a rapid, high-dose, intravenous 'push' can result in a similar ototoxicity.
- **Opiate poisoning** occurs in renal failure (opiates are excreted renally), in cardiac failure (which impairs renal function), in elderly people (increased tissue sensitivity), in type II respiratory failure (CO_2 retention increases the sensitivity of the respiratory centre to respiratory depression induced by opiates and other central nervous system (CNS) depressants), and with excess opiates (inadvertent or deliberate overdose). Opiate overdose impairs conscious level, which may lead to coma and depressed respiratory centre function, producing hypoventilation and leading to apnoea. Patients are often drowsy and hyperventilating with pinpoint pupils. Intravenous naloxone, a specific opiate-receptor antagonist, rapidly improves conscious level and ventilatory function. Beware: as the half-life of naloxone in the circulation (±30 min) is less than that of opiates (up to several hours), naloxone administration may need to be repeated.

Toxicity arising from predictable drug–drug interactions

Often it is the way one drug interacts with another that results in toxicity:

- Altered drug concentration through inhibition/induction of cytochrome P450 (CYP): drugs inhibiting CYP isoforms increase the concentration of other drugs that depend on CYP for elimination. This may lead to toxicity, e.g. macrolide antibiotics inhibit CYP, slowing cisapride (a now withdrawn gut prokinetic agent) elimination, leading to toxic levels and ventricular arrhythmias. CYP induction by anticonvulsants decreases the effect of the oral contraceptive pill (OCP). Racial and familial differences in drug metabolism may be mediated by CYP isoform polymorphisms.

• Altered P-glycoprotein expression: P-glycoprotein decreases gastrointestinal (GI) drug absorption, increases CNS and kidney drug excretion, and extrudes drugs from cells, e.g. antineoplastic agents. Drugs that inhibit P-glycoprotein alter the concentration of other drugs, e.g. verapamil increases the concentration of ciclosporin.

• Altered protein binding: decreased protein binding increases levels of highly protein-bound drugs, e.g. antibiotics compete for the albumin binding of warfarin, increasing warfarin levels and the anticoagulant effect. Antibiotics also kill gut bacteria, decreasing vitamin K production (the natural antagonist to warfarin), so increasing warfarin's effect.

• Administration of drugs with complementary function. Antiplatelet agents promote bleeding in those on warfarin. Drowsiness results from polypharmacy with antipsychotics, nocturnal hypnotics and sedating antihistamines. Excessive bradycardia or asystole results from the combination of verapamil and β-blockers.

• Other interactions, e.g. amiodarone doubles the plasma levels of digoxin, and so may cause toxicity.

Toxicity arising from other predictable mechanisms

• Genetic interactions: factor V Leiden dramatically increases the risk of OCP-induced venous thrombosis. Glucose-6-phosphate dehydrogenase deficiency produces haemolysis with many drugs. Many drugs may precipitate acute porphyric attacks.

• Inhibition of related enzyme systems: non-steroidal anti-inflammatory drugs (NSAIDs) inhibit cyclo-oxygenase enzyme (COX) isoforms 1 and 2. COX-1 produces gastric mucosal protection factors, whereas COX-2 inhibition is responsible for the therapeutic efficacy of the drug. Early NSAIDs inhibited both isoforms, promoting GI bleeding. Recent NSAIDs are more selective and may cause fewer GI bleeds. NSAID-induced renal failure results from an inhibition of prostaglandin production and is more likely in those with pre-existing renal failure. Chronic NSAID consumption can produce chronic renal failure (with prominent tubular damage and a salt-wasting nephropathy), papillary necrosis and uroepithelial cancer.

• Toxicity from other drug constituents: thyroid dysfunction with amiodarone relates to the high levels of contained iodine. Amiodarone commonly induces hypothyroidism in areas with normal environmental iodine levels, and less commonly hyperthyroidism.

• Long-term toxicity is often predictable. Use of chronic high-dose steroids leads to Cushing's syndrome, with osteoporosis, easy bruising and excess cardiovascular morbidity and mortality from hypertension and an adverse lipid profile. Anti-cancer drugs produce a significant late, i.e. 10-year, incidence of secondary tumours, often haematological, from the long-term effects of DNA damage.

Immune reactions

Immune reactions producing drug toxicity are subdivided according to the underlying mechanism (see Figure 243.2 below):

• **Type I hypersensitivity reactions** usually occur after the third or fourth exposure to the drug. The sensitizing drug activates mast cell-bound IgE antibodies, causing degranulation, mild itching, urticaria and angioedema or anaphylaxis. Treatment: antihistamines, bronchodilators and steroids. Anaphylactoid reactions result when drugs cause direct mast cell degranulation, e.g. opiates, contrast medium or aspirin. Reactions are not mediated by immunoglobulin, so previous exposure is not required. Some less severe reactions are sporadic, occur long after the start of treatment, and are difficult clinically to associate with drug therapy, e.g. intermittent angioedema with ACE inhibitors.

• **Type II hypersensitivity reactions** to drugs are rare. The most common example is penicillin-induced haemolytic anaemia, where red cell membrane-bound penicillin comes under IgG or IgM antibody-directed attack, so activating complement and producing cell lysis.

• **Type III hypersensitivity reactions** (serum sickness): offending drugs bind with specific IgG producing antigen–antibody complexes, e.g. penicillin, streptokinase, horse sera and sulphonamides. Immune complex deposition and subsequent inflammation within tissues cause the clinical features of fever, arthralgias, vasculitic skin rashes and renal impairment. Serum complement C3 and C4 are low. Eosinophilia may occur. Skin biopsies show a 'leukocytoclastic' vasculitis. No specific IgE to the antigen can be demonstrated, although specific IgG may be detected.

• **Type IV hypersensitivity reactions** are unusual causes of drug allergy. Frequent exposure sensitizes CD4+ T lymphocytes to a drug, e.g. topically applied penicillin. Lymphocytes migrate to the site of exposure and recruit other cells including neutrophils and macrophages. Contact dermatitis occurs. This responds rapidly to steroids. Exposure to the offending agent via a patch test induces a diagnostic localized dermatitis after 48 hours.

Unpredictable and other mechanisms giving rise to toxicity

Unfortunately much drug toxicity falls into this category. The common ones should be learnt, but the clinician must always be aware of the potential for new and unexpected reactions. Examples include:

• Pneumonitis with high-dose amiodarone is manifest as breathlessness, sometimes with a non-productive cough, and can be misinterpreted as worsening heart failure. Chest X-ray shows diffuse infiltrates. The carbon monoxide transfer factor is decreased. The diagnosis is confirmed by high-resolution computed tomography of the chest. Treatment: steroids (little evidence that they improve outcome) and time, because improvement is contemporaneous with amiodarone leaving the body, which, given its very long *in vivo* half-life of about 30 days, is often several months.

• Drug-induced skin rashes are often immunologically mediated, although other mechanisms also operate, e.g. β-blockers exacerbating psoriasis.

• Anticonvulsant hypersensitivity syndrome from carbamazepine or phenytoin presents as fever, rash, lymphadenopathy, malaise and hepatitis. Re-challenge with either drug is often fatal if the first illness involved hepatitis.

• Malabsorption with phenytoin.

• Myositis on statin therapy.

• The serotonin syndrome (see Figure 243.3 below).

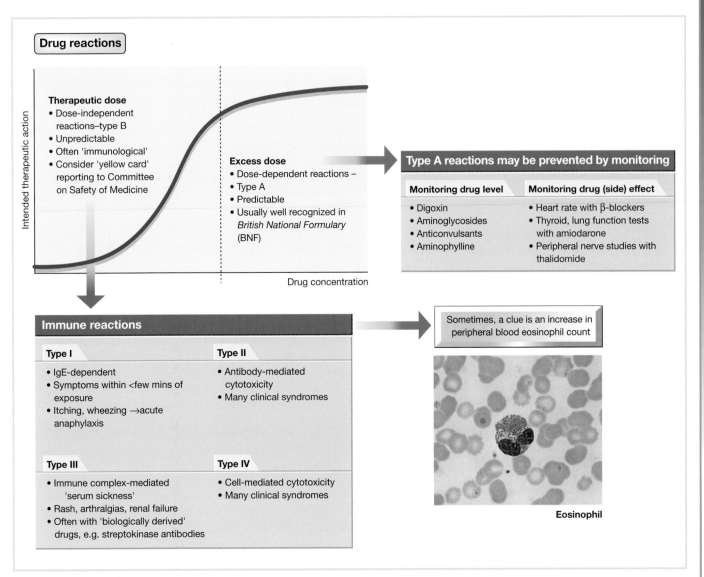

Drug reactions

Intended therapeutic action

Therapeutic dose
- Dose-independent reactions–type B
- Unpredictable
- Often 'immunological'
- Consider 'yellow card' reporting to Committee on Safety of Medicine

Excess dose
- Dose-dependent reactions –
- Type A
- Predictable
- Usually well recognized in *British National Formulary* (BNF)

Drug concentration

Type A reactions may be prevented by monitoring

Monitoring drug level	Monitoring drug (side) effect
• Digoxin	• Heart rate with β-blockers
• Aminoglycosides	• Thyroid, lung function tests with amiodarone
• Anticonvulsants	• Peripheral nerve studies with thalidomide
• Aminophylline	

Immune reactions

Type I
- IgE-dependent
- Symptoms within <few mins of exposure
- Itching, wheezing →acute anaphylaxis

Type II
- Antibody-mediated cytotoxicity
- Many clinical syndromes

Type III
- Immune complex-mediated 'serum sickness'
- Rash, arthralgias, renal failure
- Often with 'biologically derived' drugs, e.g. streptokinase antibodies

Type IV
- Cell-mediated cytotoxicity
- Many clinical syndromes

Sometimes, a clue is an increase in peripheral blood eosinophil count

Eosinophil

Diagnosis

A full clinical history should be taken of the reaction and all drugs administered, including details about previous exposure and time from exposure to symptom onset. Eosinophils may be raised.

Management

- Discontinue the offending drug/agent. Avoid subsequently.
- Advise on any cross-reacting drugs.
- Use a Medic-Alert bracelet for severe drug allergies.
- Inform the Committee on Safety of Medicines (BNF yellow card).
- In immune reactions, initiate drug desensitization (exposure to escalating doses of the drug on multiple occasions) for essential agents, e.g. insulin, but not if alternative treatments are available.

Serotonin syndrome

Causes of serotonin syndrome	Clinical features
Any drug which increases serotonergic neuron activity, either administration or removal of serotonergic drugs; also if drugs which inhibit cytochromes CYP2D6/CYP3A4 are added to those already taking serotonergic drugs	Clinical triad of: • Mental state changes • Autonomic hyperactivity • Neuromuscular abnormalities
• Selective serotonin reuptake inhibitors (SSRIs): all • Antidepressant drugs: all • Monoamine oxidase inhibitors: all • Anticonvulsants: valproate • Antiemetics: ondansetron, metoclopramide • Analgesics: fentanyl, tramadol • Antitussives: dextromethorphan • Antibiotics: linezolide (MAO inhibitor), ritonavir • Some 'street' drugs: LSD, MDMA • Dietary supplements: St Johns Wort, ginseng, tryptophan • Lithium	Incidence; 0.4 cases per 1000 patient-months for many serotonergic drugs Probably about 2–5000 cases/year in the UK, and 20–80 deaths Occurs in 15% of SSRI overdoses
Severe serotonin syndrome is especially likely when combinations of the above drugs are taken	Pathophysiology: relates to ↑serotonergic neuron activity, possibly 5-HT$_{2A}$, and 5-HT$_{1A}$; also ↑CNS noradrenaline (norepinephrine) activity may be relevant

Features of the serotonin syndrome – a spectrum, with subtle symptoms/signs in mild cases, usually occurring ≤ few minutes after new medication or change in dose

		Mild	Moderate	Severe
Mental state		Normal	Mild agitation, hypervigilance, pressured speech	Delirious, great agitation
Autonomic changes	Heart rate	↑	↑↑	↑↑↑
	Sweating	+	++	+++
	Pupil dilatation	+	++	+++
	Blood pressure	Normal – ↑	↑	↑↑ →frank shock
	GI tract		↑bowel sounds Diarrhoea	↑↑ bowel sounds
Temperature		Normal	↑to 40°C	High – up to 41°C
Neuromuscular changes	Muscle findings	Tremor	Inducible clonus	Rigid muscles (especially lower limbs)
	Reflexes	↑	↑↑	↑↑↑
Laboratory tests				Acidosis ↑Muscle enzymes
Therapy	REMOVE PROVOKING DRUG(S)	Supportive Benzodiazepines	Rehydrate, cool; 5-HT$_{2A}$ antagonists	If temp ± 41°C, neuromuscular paralysis and intubation/ventilation

Diagnosis; needs (1) knowledge that a serotonergic agent was given ≤ 5 weeks ago, (2) 1 or more of:
• Tremor with hyperreflexia
• Spontaneous clonus
• Muscle rigidity and T°C ≥ 38; and ocular or inducible clonus
• Ocular clonus and agitation or sweating
• Inducible clonus and agitation or sweating

Differential diagnosis: anticholinergic syndrome, neuroleptic malignant syndrome (see Chapter 43), malignant hyperthermia (see Chapter 43)

Index

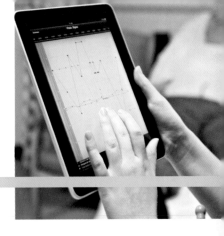

Note: page numbers in *italics* refer to figures, those in **bold** refer to tables

Medicine at a Glance, Fourth Edition. Edited by Patrick Davey. © 2014 John Wiley & Sons, Ltd. Published 2014 by John Wiley & Sons, Ltd. Companion website: www.ataglanceseries.com/medicine